T0382684

The EBCOG Postgraduate Textbook of Obstetrics & Gynaecology

Volume 1: Obstetrics & Maternal-Fetal Medicine

Edited by

Tahir Mahmood
Victoria Hospital, Kirkcaldy, Scotland

Charles Savona-Ventura
University of Malta, Msida, Malta

Ioannis Messinis
University of Thessaly, Greece

Sambit Mukhopadhyay
Norfolk & Norwich University Hospital, Norwich, United Kingdom

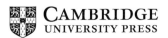
CAMBRIDGE
UNIVERSITY PRESS

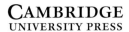

University Printing House, Cambridge CB2 8BS, United Kingdom

One Liberty Plaza, 20th Floor, New York, NY 10006, USA

477 Williamstown Road, Port Melbourne, VIC 3207, Australia

314–321, 3rd Floor, Plot 3, Splendor Forum, Jasola District Centre,
New Delhi – 110025, India

103 Penang Road, #05–06/07, Visioncrest Commercial, Singapore 238467

Cambridge University Press is part of the University of Cambridge.

It furthers the University's mission by disseminating knowledge in the
pursuit of education, learning, and research at the highest international
levels of excellence.

www.cambridge.org
Information on this title: www.cambridge.org/mahmoodvol1
DOI: 10.1017/9781108863049

© Cambridge University Press 2022

First published 2022

Printed in the United Kingdom by TJ Books Limited, Padstow Cornwall

A catalogue record for this publication is available from the British Library.

Library of Congress Cataloging-in-Publication Data
Names: Mahmood, Tahir (Tahir Ahmed), editor. | Savona-Ventura, Charles,
editor. | Messinis, Ioannis, 1947– editor. | Mukhopadhyay, Sambit, editor.
Title: The EBCOG postgraduate textbook of obstetrics & gynaecology /
edited by Tahir Mahmood, Forth Park Hospital, Kirkcaldy, Charles
Savona Ventura, Msida Medical School, Malta, Ioannis Messinis,
Sambit Mukhopadhyay.
Other titles: EBCOG postgraduate textbook of obstetrics and gynaecology
Description: Cambridge, United Kingdom ; New York, NY : Cambridge
University Press, [2021] | Includes bibliographical references and index.
Identifiers: LCCN 2021024740 (print) | LCCN 2021024741 (ebook) |
ISBN 9781108495783 (hardback) | ISBN 9781108863049 (ebook)
Subjects: LCSH: Obstetrics – Examinations – Study guides. | Gynecology –
Examinations – Study guides. | BISAC: MEDICAL / Gynecology &
Obstetrics | MEDICAL / Gynecology & Obstetrics
Classification: LCC RG106 .E23 2021 (print) | LCC RG106 (ebook) | DDC
618.10076–dc23
LC record available at https://lccn.loc.gov/2021024740
LC ebook record available at https://lccn.loc.gov/2021024741

ISBN - 2 Volume Set 9781108955591 Hardback
ISBN - Volume 1 9781108495783 Hardback
ISBN - Volume 2 9781108499392 Hardback

....

To

Aasia, Marylene, Nikoletta and Samita

For their support, tolerance, patience and love during the arduous editing process in bringing together the two volumes of this book.

Tahir, Charles, Ioannis and Sambit

Contents

Section 7 Placenta

Section 8 Public Health Issues in Obstetrics

Section 9 Co-Morbidities during Pregnancy

Colour plates can be found between pages 336 and 337

Contributors

Catherine E. Aiken MB/BChir MA PhD MRCOG MRCP
University Department of Obstetrics & Gynaecology,
The Rosie Hospital, Cambridge, UK

Jennifer Allison BSc MBChB MRCOG
NHS Fife, UK

Frédéric Amant MD PhD
Department of Obstetrics & Gynaecology, University
Hospitals Leuven, Leuven, Belgium

Laura Andreoli MD PhD
Unit of Rheumatology and Clinical Immunology,
ASST Spedali Civili, Brescia, Italy. Department of
Clinical & Experimental Sciences, University of Brescia,
Brescia, Italy

Aris J. Antsaklis MD PhD
First Department of Obstetrics and Gynaecology,
Division of Maternal-Fetal Medicine, Alexandra Hospital,
National and Kapodistrian University of Athens, Athens,
Greece

Panos Antsaklis MD, PhD
First Department of Obstetrics and Gynecology, National and
Kapodistrian University of Athens, Alexandra Maternity
Hospital, Greece

Vrinda Arora MBBS DNB MRCOG
Norfolk and Norwich University Hospital and Foundation
Trust, Norwich, UK

Sabaratnam Arulkumaran MD PhD FRCOG
Academic Department of Obstetrics & Gynaecology,
St George's University of London, London, UK

Parivakkam S. Arunakumari MD FRCOG MFFP
Department of Obstetrics & Gynaecology, Norfolk & Norwich
University Hospital, Norwich, UK

Apostolos P. Athanasiadis MD PhD
First Department of Obstetrics and Gynecology, National and
Kapodistrian University of Athens, Alexandra Maternity
Hospital, Greece

Antonios Athanasiou MD
Department of Surgery & Cancer, Imperial College London,
London, UK

Simon Attard Montalto MBChB MD FRCP FRCPCH DCH
Department of Paediatrics, University of Malta Medical
School, Msida, Malta

Rossella Attini PhD
Department of Obstetrics and Gynecology, Città della Salute
e della Scienza- Sant'Anna Hospital, Torino, Italy

Diogo Ayres-de-Campos MD PhD
Department of Obstetrics & Gynaecology, University of Porto,
Porto, Portugal

Yves Muscat Baron MD FRCOG FRCPI PhD
Department of Obstetrics & Gynaecology, Mater Dei Hospital,
Malta

Christine M. Bates MBBS FRCP DRCOG DipVen DFSRH
Royal Liverpool University Hospital, Liverpool, UK

Giuseppe Benagiano MD PhD FRCOG
Department of Maternal and Child Health and Urology,
Sapienza, University of Rome, Rome, Italy

Chiara Benedetto MD PhD FRCOG
Department of Obstetrics & Gynaecology, University of Turin
S. Anna Hospital, Turin, Italy

Amarnath Bhide MD PhD FRCOG
Fetal Medicine Unit, St George's Hospital Medical School,
London, UK

Charles Bircher MBBS MRCOG
Department of Obstetrics & Gynaecology, Norfolk & Norwich
University Hospital, Norwich, UK

Hans Ulrich Brauer DMD DPhil MA MSc
Dental Academy for Continuing Professional Development,
Karlsruhe, Germany

Jeremy Brockelsby MB/BSc PhD MRCOG
University Department of Obstetrics & Gynaecology, The
Rosie Hospital, Cambridge, UK

Ivo Brosens MD PhD
Faculty of Medicine, Catholic University of Leuven, Leuven, Belgium

Sara Y. Brucker MD
Department of Obstetrics and Gynaecology, Department of Women's Health, University of Tuebingen, Germany

George Gregory Buttigieg KM MD LRCP MRCS Dip.FP MA FRCOG FRCPI FRCPEd
Department of Obstetrics and Gynaecology, University of Malta. Department of Obstetrics and Gynaecology, Plovdiv Medical University and Hospital St George, Bulgaria

Gianfranca Cabiddu
Department of Medical Sciences and Public Health, University of Cagliari, Cagliari, Italy

Jean Calleja-Agius MD MSc FRCOG FRCPI PhD
Department of Anatomy, Faculty of Medicine & Surgery, University of Malta, Malta

Martin Cameron BMSc MD MRCOG
Maternal-Fetal Medicine Unit, Norfolk & Norwich University Hospital, Norwich, UK

Emilie Marion Canuto MD
Department of Obstetrics & Gynaecology, University of Turin S. Anna Hospital, Turin, Italy

Edwin Chandraharan MBBS MS DFSRH DCRM FSLCOG FRCOG
Global Academy of Medical Education & Training, London / Basildon & Thurrock University Hospital, Essex, UK

Panagiotis Cherouveim MD
Department of Obstetrics & Gynaecology, University Hospital of Ioannina, Ioannina, Greece

Anne Chien MSc
Scottish Hydatidiform Mole Follow-Up Service, Ninewells Hospital, Dundee, UK

Patrick Chien MD MbChB FRCOG
Scottish Hydatidiform Mole Follow-Up Service, Ninewells Hospital, Dundee, UK

Rohan Chodankar MBBS MD MRCOG
Department of Obstetrics & Gynaecology, Edinburgh Royal Infirmary, Edinburgh, UK

Bernard Clarke BSc MD FRCP FESC FACC FRCOG(Hon)
Department of Cardiology, Manchester Royal Infirmary, Manchester, UK

Johann Craus MD DFSHRH MRCOG PhD
Department of Obstetrics & Gynaecology, Mater Dei Hospital, Birkirkara, Malta

Alexandros Daponte MD DrMed FCOG
Department of Obstetrics & Gynaecology, University of Thessaly, Larissa, Greece

George J. Daskalakis MD, PhD
First Department of Obstetrics and Gynecology, National and Kapodistrian University of Athens, Alexandra Maternity Hospital, Greece

Ralf Dechend MD
Helios Clinic, Berlin, Germany

Pauline L. M. de Vries MD
Department of Obstetrics & Gynaecology, Leiden University Medical Centre, Leiden, Netherlands

Gilbert G. G. Donders MD PhD
Department of Obstetrics & Gynaecology, University Hospital Antwerp, Antwerp, Belgium

Fidelma P. Dunne MBBCh BAO MD PhD
Galway Diabetes Research Centre, School of Medicine, National University of Ireland Galway, Galway, Ireland

Aoife M. Egan MBBCh BAO PhD
Division of Endocrinology and Metabolism, Mayo Clinic, Rochester, MN, USA

David K. Gatongi MSc MRCOG
Victoria Hospital, Kirkcaldy, Fife, UK

Maria Chiara Gerardi MD
Unit of Rheumatology and Clinical Immunology, ASST Spedali Civili, Brescia, Italy. Department of Clinical & Experimental Sciences, University of Brescia, Brescia, Italy

Ksenija Gersak MD PhD
Department of Obstetrics and Gynecology, Ljubljana University Medical Centre, and Faculty of Medicine, University of Ljubljana, Ljubljana, Slovenia

Eva-Maria Grischke MD
Department of Obstetrics and Gynaecology, Department of Women's Health, University of Tuebingen, Germany

Richard Haines BSc MBBS MRCOG
Department of Obstetrics & Gynaecology, Norfolk & Norwich University Hospital, Norwich, UK

Francoise H. Harlow BSc (Hons) MBBS MRCOG
Department of Obstetrics & Gynaecology, Norfolk & Norwich University Hospital, Norwich, UK

Guttorm Haugen MD PhD
Division of Obstetrics & Gynaecology, Oslo University Hospital, Oslo, Norway

Kahyee Hor MB ChB MRCOG
University of Edinburgh, Edinburgh, UK

Peter Hornnes MD DSc FRCOG
Department of Obstetrics & Gynaecology, North Zealand
University Hospital, Hillerød, Denmark

Irene Hösli MD
Professor of Gynaecology & Obstetrics, University Hospital
Basel, Basel, Switzerland

Ruth Howie MRCOG
Department of Obstetrics & Gynaecology, Edinburgh Royal
Infirmary, Edinburgh, UK

Dr Hasnain M. Jafferbhoy FRCPE
Consultant Physician, Division of Gastero-enterology,
Department of Medicine, Victoria Hospital,Kirkcaldy,
Scotland

Leigh Jenkins
Scottish Hydatidiform Mole Follow-Up Service, Ninewells
Hospital, Dundee, UK

Gauri Karandikar MD DGO FCPS FICOG
Department of Obstetrics & Gynaecology, Karandikar
Hospital & Research Centre, Nasik, India

Omobolanle Kazeem MBChB, MPH, MRCPCH
Norfolk & Norwich University Hospital, Norwich, UK

Jørg Kessler MD PhD
Department of Obstetrics & Gynaecology, Haukeland
University Hospital, Bergen, Norway

Asma Khalil MD MRCOG MSc
Fetal Medicine Unit, St George's Hospital, London, UK

Manjiri Khare FRCOG
Women's & Perinatal Services, University Hospitals of
Leicester NHS Trust, UK

Laura Kitto
Gastroenterology Department, Royal Infirmary, Edinburgh,
UK

Przemyslaw Kosinski MD PhD
First Department of Obstetrics & Gynecology, Medical
University of Warsaw, Warsaw, Poland

Maria Kyrgiou MSc PhD MRCOG
Department of Surgery & Cancer, Imperial College London,
London, UK

Katariina Laine MD PhD
Department of Obstetrics, Oslo University Hospital, Oslo,
Norway

Olav Lapaire
Department of Obstetrics & Antenatal Care, University
Hospital of Basel, Basel, Switzerland

Jeanet Lauenborg MD PhD
Department of Obstetrics, Gynecology & Pediatrics,
Nykoebing Falster Hospital, Region Zealand, Denmark

Emma Leighton MBBS
St. George's University Hospitals NHS Foundation Trust,
London, UK

Elke Leuridan MD PhD
Centre for the Evaluation of Vaccination, Vaccine & Infectious
Diseases Institute, University of Antwerp, Antwerp, Belgium

Chu Chin Lim FRCOG
Victoria Hospital, Kirkcaldy, UK

Christianne A. R. Lok MD PhD
Department of Gynaecological Oncology, Netherlands Cancer
Institute, Amsterdam, Netherlands

Frank Louwen MD
Department of Gynecology & Obstetrics, Goethe University
Hospital, Frankfurt, Germany

Kirsten Maertens PhD
Centre for the Evaluation of Vaccination, Vaccine & Infectious
Diseases Institute, University of Antwerp, Antwerp, Belgium

Charlotte Maggen MD
Department of Obstetrics & Gynaecology, University
Hospitals of Leuven, Leuven, Belgium

**Tahir A. Mahmood CBE MD FRCPI MBA FACOG FRCPE
FEBCOG FRCOG**
Department of Obstetrics & Gynaecology, Victoria Hospital,
Kirkcaldy, Fife, UK

William C. Maina MBChB MRCOG
Royal Bolton Hospital NHS Trust, Bolton, UK

Anastasios Malakasis BSc MBBS MSc
Department of Obstetrics & Gynaecology, Norfolk & Norwich
University Hospital, Norwich, UK

**Pierre Mallia MA MD MPhil PhD MRCP FRCGP CBiol
DipICGP**
Bioethics Research Programme, University of Malta Mater Dei
Hospital, Msida, Malta

Apostolos M. Mamopoulos MD PhD
Third Department of Obstetrics & Gynaecology, School of
Medicine, Faculty of Health Sciences, Aristotle University of
Thessaloniki, Greece

Gwendolin Manegold-Brauer, MD PD
Department of Obstetrics & Gynaecology, Division of
Gynecologic Ultrasound and Prenatal Diagnostics, University
Hospital of Basel, Basel, Switzerland

Lucy Maudlin MRCOG MSc
West Suffolk NHS Trust, UK

Lesley McMahon PhD DipRCPath
Scottish Hydatidiform Mole Follow-Up Service, Ninewells Hospital, Dundee, UK

Sarah McRobbie MRCOG DFSRH PGcert MBChB BSc
Aberdeen Maternity Hospital, Aberdeen, UK

Christina I. Messini MD
Department of Obstetrics & Gynaecology, University of Thessaly, Larissa, Greece

Cécile Monod MD
Department of Gynaecology & Obstetrics, University Hospital Basel, Basel, Switzerland

Neela Mukhopadhaya MRCOG
Department of Obstetrics & Gynaecology, Luton & Dunstable Hospital, Luton, UK

Sambit Mukhopadhyay MD DNB MMedSci FRCOG
Department of Obstetrics & Gynaecology, Norfolk & Norwich University Hospital, Norwich, UK

Britt Ingjerd Nesheim MD PhD
Faculty of Medicine, University of Oslo, Oslo, Norway

Hedvig Nordeng MSc PhD
Department of Pharmacy, University of Oslo, Norway

Vennila Palaniappan
Department of Obstetrics & Gynaecology, Norfolk & Norwich University Hospital, Norwich, UK

Maria Papamichail MD
Alexandra Maternity Hospital, Athens, Greece

Evangelos Paraskevaidis MD PhD
Department of Obstetrics & Gynaecology, University Hospital of Ioannina, Ioannina, Greece

Vasilios Pergialiotis MD MSc PhD
First Department of Obstetrics and Gynaecology, Alexandra Hospital, National and Kapodistrian University of Athens, Athens, Greece

Giorgina Barbara Piccoli MD
Department of Clinical and Biological Science, University of Turin, Turin, Italy

Edward Prosser-Snelling BA(Hons) MBBS MRCOG
Department of Obstetrics & Gynaecology, Norfolk & Norwich University Hospital, Norwich, UK

Patrick Puttemans MD
Unit of Reproductive Medicine, Heilig Hart Hospital, Leuven, Belgium

Rumana Rahman
Luton & Dunstable University Hospital, UK

Sari Räisänen RN MSc PhD
School of Health Care & Social Service, Tampere University of Applied Sciences, Tampere, Finland

Katharine Rankin BMSc MBChB MRCOG PGDipClinEd FHEA
Specialist Registrar in Obstetrics & Gynaecology, South East Scotland Deanery, UK

Anke Reitter MD FRCOG
Department of Obstetrics & Gynaecology, Krankenhaus Sachsenhausen, Frankfurt, Germany

Anna Roberts MRCOG
St Mary's Hospital, Manchester, UK

Rahul Roy MRCPCH, DCH
Consultant Neonatologist Paediatrician with expertise in Cardiology, Norfolk and Norwich University Hospital, Norwich, UK

Shittu Akinola Saheed MRCOG FMCOG DFSRH
Hamand Medical Centre Al Rayyan, Qatar

Francesca Salvagno MD
Department of Obstetrics & Gynaecology, University of Turin S. Anna Hospital, Turin, Italy

Charles Savona-Ventura MD DScMed FRCOG FRCPI FRCPE
Department of Obstetrics & Gynaecology, Faculty of Medicine & Surgery, University of Malta, Msida, Malta

Yvonne Savona-Ventura B.Pharm M.Pharm
Department of Pharmacy, Faculty of Medicine & Surgery, University of Malta, Msida, Malta

Martina Schembri MD EFOG-EBCOG MRCPI
Department of Obstetrics & Gynaecology, Mater Dei Hospital, Malta

Silvia Serrano MD
Department of Obstetrics & Gynaecology, Santa Maria Hospital, Lisbon, Portugal

Katrina Shearer MbChB MRCOG
Aberdeen Maternity Hospital, Aberdeen, UK

Paul Simpson MA (Cantab) BMBS MRCOG MD
Department of Obstetrics & Gynaecology, Norfolk & Norwich University Hospital, Norwich, UK

Vasilis Sitras MD PhD
Division of Obstetrics & Gynaecology, Oslo University Hospital, Oslo, Norway

Anne Cathrine Staff MD PhD
Division of Obstetrics & Gynaecology, Oslo University Hospital, Oslo, Norway

Babill Stray-Pedersen MD PhD
Department of Obstetrics & Gynaecology, University of Oslo National Hospital, Oslo, Norway

Iryna Tepla MD
Department of Obstetrics & Gynaecology, Shupyk National Medical Academy of Postgraduate Education, Kyiv, Ukraine

Kamaleswari Camille Aiyaroo Thyne MBBS MRCOG
Royal Infirmary of Edinburgh, Edinburgh, UK

Angela Tincani MD
Unit of Rheumatology and Clinical Immunology, ASST Spedali Civili, Brescia, Italy. Department of Clinical & Experimental Sciences, University of Brescia, Brescia, Italy

Andrii V. Tkachenko MD PhD
Department of Obstetrics & Gynaecology, Shupyk National Medical Academy of Postgraduate Education, Kyiv, Ukraine

Jone Trovik MD PhD
Department of Obstetrics & Gynecology, Haukeland University Hospital, Bergen, Norway

Ioannis Tsakiridis MD MSc
Third Department of Obstetrics & Gynaecology, School of Medicine, Faculty of Health Sciences, Aristotle University of Thessaloniki, Greece

Sibil Tschudin MD
Department of Obstetrics and Gynaecology, University Hospital Basel, Basel, Switzerland

Austin Ugwumadu PhD FRCOG
Department of Obstetrics & Gynaecology, St. George's Hospital NHS Trust, London, UK

Thomas van den Akker MD PhD
Department of Obstetrics & Gynaecology, Leiden University Medical Centre, Leiden, Netherlands

Sarah Vause MD FRCOG
St Mary's Hospital, Manchester, UK

Ganga Verma
Women's & Perinatal Services, University Hospitals of Leicester NHS Trust, UK

Åse Vikanes MD PhD
Intervention Centre, Oslo University Hospital, Oslo, Norway

Nikolaos Vrachnis
Third Department of Obstetrics & Gynaecology, University of Athens, Athens, Greece

Diethelm Wallwiener MD
Department of Obstetrics and Gynaecology, Department of Women's Health, University of Tuebingen, Germany

Martin Weiss MD
Department of Obstetrics and Gynaecology, Department of Women's Health, University of Tuebingen, Germany

Mirosław Wielgoś MD PhD
First Department of Obstetrics & Gynecology, Medical University of Warsaw, Warsaw, Poland

Juriy W. Wladimiroff MD
Rosie Maternity, Addenbrooke's University Hospital, Cambridge, UK

Branka M. Yli MD PhD
Labour Ward, Oslo University Hospital, Oslo, Norway

Dimitrios Zygouris MD PhD MSc
Third Department of Obstetrics & Gynaecology, University of Athens, Athens, Greece

Preface

The art of practising modern medicine is influenced by its complexity and changing socio-economic factors. Money, power and resources influence health outcomes globally, nationally and locally. Europe with its wide geographic variation has different healthcare, training and education systems. Clinical guidelines are aimed to reduce variation and increase cost-effectiveness of healthcare delivery. However, economic and policy differences amongst various states influence the uptake of guidelines and the standards of care specialists are expected to provide for their patients. The practice of obstetrics and gynaecology within the various European countries also varies extensively from one country to another and sometimes even from one hospital to another within the same country.

The European Board and College of Obstetrics and Gynaecology (EBCOG) has long recognized that, within the wide diversity of healthcare service systems, basic postgraduate training standards in the speciality are necessary to ensure safety and quality of healthcare for women and their babies in the European Region. To help define competencies towards achieving standardization of training and delivering high-quality equitable care, EBCOG has published documents describing 'Standards of Care in Obstetrics, Neonatal and Gynaecology' and a 'European Training Requirement' through the publication of The Project for Achieving Consensus in Training (PACT). In addition, EBCOG publishes state-of-the-art position statements that are based on evidence.

European Training Curriculum of EBCOG defines the core competencies required by all specialist obstetricians-gynaecologists wherever they may be practising, and the elective optional competencies that support the delivery of advanced specialists and subspecialist care. The EBCOG curriculum is supported by the promotion of a standard format training portfolio. On the other hand, the introduction of the EBCOG Fellowship examination (EFOG) has gone a long way towards promoting a wide-based standardization of healthcare provision in the speciality within a wide-ranging spectrum of healthcare service provision and ensuring the training of specialists competent to respond to the ever-changing frontiers of medical services.

The present project provides an up-to-date reference textbook written by authors familiar with a European perspective of care in general obstetrics and gynaecology. It aims to address the competencies defined by EBCOG curriculum and builds the clinical practice related to these competencies upon the basic sciences foundations. It thus is an ideal reference book for postgraduate trainees not only in Europe but also globally who are targeting to sit the EFOG or any other postgraduate examinations. This book will also serve as a postgraduate reference book for specialists currently practising the speciality anywhere in the world and who need to update their knowledge and competencies with the ever-evolving clinical practice of today's modern world.

We are very grateful to all the contributors who studiously prepared and revised the chapters. Without their sterling contributions, the work would not have seen the light of day.

Tahir Mahmood, Charles Savona-Ventura, Ioannis Messinis, Sambit Mukhopadhyay

1 Surgical Anatomy of the Female Pelvis

Jean Calleja-Agius

1.1 Development of the Female Pelvis and Its Contents

The female genitourinary system is mainly derived from the intermediate cell mass, which in turn is derived from the mesoderm following gastrulation. The pelvic girdle, however, is derived from the caudal mesoderm, which, as the name implies, is the mesoderm found caudal to the cloacal membrane. Upon folding, the caudal mesoderm folds ventrally at the point of the cloacal membrane, distal to the paraxial mesoderm and notochord, in such a way that the pelvic girdle wraps around the distal end of the trunk to fuse with the sacral somites and encase the developing female genitourinary system, and leads to the formation of the rump. Blastogenic defects involving the cloaca and caudal folding may also be associated with urogenital and possibly ano-rectal malformations, which can lead to reproductive problems [1].

Soon after gastrulation and folding at the end of the fourth week after fertilization, the gonadal ridge starts appearing as a thickened ridge at the border between the developing mesonephros within the substance of the intermediate cell mass and the intra-coelomic cavity within the lateral plate mesoderm. This gonadal ridge will start developing into an indifferent gonad. The proliferation of the coelomic epithelium over the genital ridge gives rise to primitive sex cords. At the same time, primordial germ cells start arising from the region of the allantois and start migrating towards the developing gonadal ridge. By the sixth week the primordial germ cells invade the primitive sex cords. If the sex chromosomes in the primordial germ cells are XX, this will lead to the formation of the ovary, in contrast to a testis if the sex chromosomes are XY. Failure of migration of these germ cells can occur in certain congenital conditions such as Turner syndrome, leading to ovarian dysgenesis.

By the seventh week, primordial follicles appear from the second generation of cords from the coelomic epithelium, and start proliferating rapidly by mitosis between the second and fourth month. By the end of the 16th week, there are around 4 million oogonia, which then enter the first phase of meiosis. These oogonia remain arrested until puberty, when, periodically, batches of primary oocytes resume the meiotic cycle, forming at least one dominant secondary oocyte which ovulates. There is a degree of oocyte degeneration throughout all of the duration of the meiotic arrest, with only around half of the original amount of oogonia making it until the time of birth. A healthy female

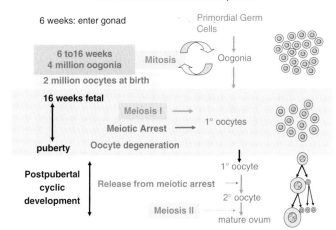

Time frame for ovarian development

Figure 1.1 Time frame for ovarian development

neonate starts off with around 2 million oogonia, which by the time of puberty (average 11.5 years) continue degenerating, with only around 500 oogonia ever managing to be released from meiotic arrest and develop into secondary oocytes, start meiosis II and be ovulated as a mature ovum. Completion of meiosis II happens only physiologically upon fertilization by a sperm (Figure 1.1).

The paramesonephric (or Mullerian) ducts develop as invaginations from the epithelium lining the urogenital ridges, growing laterally to the mesonephric (Wolffian) ducts, but then crossing ventrally towards the caudal end of the mesonephric duct. These paramesonephric ducts fuse caudally in the midline, with the fused caudal tip projecting on the posterior wall of the urogenital sinus. The fallopian tubes and their fimbriae develop from the cranial part of the paramesonephric ducts, while the fused paramesonephric ducts lead to the formation of the uterus and cervix. The medial border of each of the two paramesonephric tubes will atrophy, in order to form one uterine cavity (Figure 1.2). Incomplete atrophy may lead to different degrees of uterine septation, causing bifid, unicornuate and other types of uterine anomalies. These may present with fertility problems and recurrent miscarriages [2]. Treatment of such septa is still debatable, with further trials under way [3]. Due to the close association with the development of the urinary system, such uterine congenital anomalies may have concomitant urinary anomalies.

The female genital duct system derived from
the paramesonephric duct

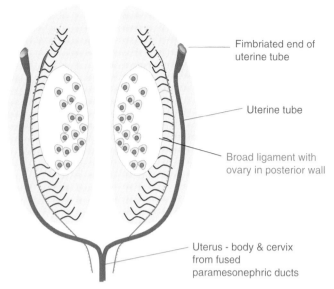

Fimbriated end of
uterine tube

Uterine tube

Broad ligament with
ovary in posterior wall

Uterus - body & cervix
from fused
paramesonephric ducts

Figure 1.2 The female genital duct system derived from the
paramesonephric duct

At the point of contact, a sino-vaginal bulb arises by cell proliferation from the paramesonephric ducts and the urogenital sinus. This leads to the vaginal plate, which canalizes in the fourth month, and the fornices develop. The hymen remains as a thin plate between the vagina and the urogenital sinus. Abnormal development at this point can lead to imperforate hymen or Robert's uterus, among others [4]. In the meantime, the mesonephric ducts will disappear during female urogenital development; however, some remnants may persist as epi-oophoron or para-oophoron in the broad ligament, which are vestigial structures which can lead to Gartner's cysts, which are usually benign.

In the meantime, mesodermal thickenings form around the cloacal membrane, with a genital tubercle forming cranially, leading to the formation of the clitoris and paired cloacal folds laterally. After separation of the urogenital sinus by the urorectal septum, the perineal body forms, and the cloacal folds are transformed into anterior urethral folds, leading to the labia and posterior anal folds.

1.2 The Pelvic Girdle: Bone and Ligaments – Implications in Obstetrics

The pelvis is an anatomically complex set of bones, which function as one, that contributes directly to human obstetrics, as well as locomotion. The unique shape of the human pelvis, superoinferiorly short and mediolaterally wide, is adapted for habitual bipedalism [5].

The pelvis consists of the right and left pelvic bones, the sacrum and the coccyx. Each pelvic bone consists of the ilium, ischium and pubis, which at birth are connected by cartilage at the acetabulum, which fully ossifies at the end of puberty. Superiorly, the sacrum articulates with the fifth lumbar vertebra at the lumbosacral joint. Anteriorly, the pelvic bones articulate

at the pubic symphysis, and posteriorly, they articulate with the sacrum at the sacroiliac joints [6]. The pelvic inlet is circular in shape in women, as opposed to being heart shaped in males, due to the less prominent sacral promontory and broader iliac alae. Also, the subpubic arch is around 20 degrees wider in women, and the ischial spines project less into the pelvic cavity.

The measurements of the pelvis include: the sagittal inlet, between the promontory and the top of the symphysis pubis, 11 cm; the transverse diameter, 11.5 cm; the bispinous outlet, 9 cm; and the sagittal outlet, between the tip of the coccyx and the inferior margin of the pubic symphysis, 10 cm [6]. During labour, these diameters increase in a clinically significant manner with squatting [7]. The ligaments of the pelvic wall are the sacrospinous and the sacrotuberous. They convert the greater and the lesser sciatic notches into foramina, and also help stabilize the sacrum on the pelvic bones.

1.3 Overview of the Blood and Lymphatic Supply

The abdominal aorta bifurcates into two common iliac arteries, which in turn divide at the pelvic inlet in front of the sacroiliac joint into the internal and external iliac arteries. The external iliac becomes the femoral artery, while the internal iliac reaches the upper margin of the greater sciatic foramen, dividing into an anterior and a posterior division. The anterior division gives rise to the umbilical artery, the proximal part of which gives rise to the superior vesical artery; the inferior vesical artery the uterine artery, vaginal artery, internal pudendal artery, inferior gluteal artery, middle rectal artery and obturator artery. The posterior division of the internal iliac artery gives rise to the iliolumbar, lateral sacral and superior gluteal arteries. Apart from the internal iliac artery, the other arteries which enter the pelvic artery are the superior rectal artery, ovarian artery and the median sacral artery. The lymphatic supply is named after the blood vessels that are associated with it, namely, the external iliac nodes, internal iliac nodes and the common iliac nodes.

1.4 Overview of the Innervation in the Female Pelvis

The nerves of the pelvis are derived from the sacral plexus, lumbosacral trunk and autonomic nervous system. The sacral plexus is formed from the anterior rami of the fourth and fifth lumbar nerves and the anterior rami of the first, second, third and fourth sacral nerves. The sacral plexus lies in front of the piriformis muscles on the posterior pelvic wall. The lumbosacral trunk is made up of the fourth and fifth lumbar nerves. Branches to the lower limb leave the pelvis through the greater sciatic foramen, the largest of which is the sciatic nerve. The pudendal nerves, the nerves to the piriformis muscle and the pelvic splanchnic nerves are branches of the sacral plexus, which between them supply the pelvic muscles, pelvic viscera and perineum. The pudendal nerve (S2-4) leaves the pelvis through the greater sciatic foramen and enters the perineum through the lesser sciatic foramen.

The obturator nerve (L2-4), which lies on the lateral wall of the pelvis and supplies the parietal peritoneum, is responsible for referred pain, for example, from an inflamed ovary or appendicitis to be felt on the inner side of the thigh. The autonomic nerves consist of the pelvic part of the sympathetic trunk, the pelvic splanchnic nerves form the parasympathetic part, and the superior and inferior hypogastric plexuses, which both contain sympathetic and parasympathetic nerve fibres and visceral afferent nerve fibres. The superior and inferior hypogastric nerves arise from the superior hypogastric plexus.

1.5 The Pelvic Floor

The pelvic diaphragm, and, in the anterior midline, the perineal membrane and the muscles of the deep perineal pouch, make up the pelvic floor. This separates the pelvic cavity above from the perineum below. The attachment of the pelvic diaphragm to the inside of the cylindrical pelvic walls separates the greater sciatic foramen from the lesser sciatic foramen, in such a way that the latter becomes a route of communication between the pelvic cavity and the gluteal region, while the former allows communication between the gluteal region and the perineum.

The levator ani and the coccygeus muscles from both sides of the pelvis form the pelvic diaphragm, which is shaped like a funnel and, particularly the levator ani, helps to support the pelvic viscera and maintain closure of the vagina and rectum. Each of levator ani muscles is subdivided into at least three parts, based on the site of origin and the relationship to the viscera found in the midline. These are the pubococcygeus, puborectalis and iliococcygeus. The levator ani consists of a medial part containing smooth muscle cells under autonomic nerve influence and a lateral part containing striated muscle cells under somatic nerve control [8]. In fact, the levator ani muscles are innervated directly by branches from the anterior ramus of S4, and by branches of the pudendal nerve (S2-4). The coccygeus muscles overlie the sacrospinous ligaments, spanning from the tips of the ischial spines to the lateral margins of the coccyx and adjacent sacral margins, thus completing the posterior part of the pelvic diaphragm. The coccygeus muscles are innervated by the anterior branches of S4 and S5 [9].

Within the deep perineal pouch, anteriorly there is a group of skeletal muscle fibres forming the external urethral sphincter, the sphincter urethrovaginalis and the compressor urethrae, which together facilitate the closure of the urethra. The deep transverse perineal muscles join in the midline along the posterior edge of the perineal membrane and stabilize the position of the perineal body. The perineal body is a connective tissue structure into which the muscles of the pelvic floor, the perineum, the posterior end of the urogenital hiatus, the deep and superficial transverse perineal muscles, the sphincter urethrovaginalis, the external anal sphincter and the bulbospongiosus muscles attach .The perineal body is the site which may be stretched or torn during childbirth. A posterolateral episiotomy is meant to bypass the perineal body and avoid complications like third- and fourth-degree tears. However, current evidence does not show that routine episiotomy reduces perineal/vaginal trauma. Further

research in women undergoing instrumental delivery may help clarify if routine episiotomy is useful in this particular group [10].

Pelvic organ prolapse is a possible consequence of weakening of the pelvic floor muscles, which can start as early as in adolescence, and is aggravated particularly with childbearing and menopause. It may present with urinary incontinence symptoms, particularly urge urinary incontinence [11]. Women suffering from incontinence tend to have a greater anterior slope of the pelvis, which is directly proportional to the electrical activity of the pelvic floor muscles during rest and in orthostasis [12]. Early education regarding pelvic floor symptoms may lead to prevention using lifestyle modification and Kegel's exercises or empowerment to seek treatment.

A thorough knowledge of the pelvic anatomy is essential during pelvic floor surgery, especially in abdominal laparoscopic sacrocolpopexy, which is the gold standard of pelvic organ prolapse repair. This is because it presents a significant challenge to surgeons because the technique requires meticulous negotiation through abdominopelvic vascular structures and nerves supplying the pelvis and its contents, particularly the rectum, and ureters [13].

1.6 The Perineum

When viewed from below with the thighs abducted, the perineum is diamond shaped, bound anteriorly by the symphysis pubis, laterally by the ischial tuberosities and posteriorly by the tip of the coccyx. The perineum is anatomically divided into an anterior urogenital triangle and a posterior anal triangle, which contains the anal canal and the ischiorectal fossa. The latter is filled with dense fat and has the pudendal nerve and internal pudendal artery and vein passing on its lateral wall through the pudendal canal. The anal canal has an involuntary anal sphincter and a voluntary external sphincter, which in turn is made up of subcutaneous, superficial and deep parts, that then blend in with the puborectalis fibres of the two levatores muscles [14].

Anorectal vaginal fistulas may be obstetric, inflammatory (e.g. Crohn disease and diverticulitis), neoplastic, iatrogenic and/or radiation induced. Surgical management is heavily dependent on the cause and complexity of the fistulizing disease, which are related to the correct identification of location of the fistula in the vagina, the type and extent of fistula branching, the number of fistulas and any concomitant sphincter tears, inflammation and abscesses [15].

The female urogenital triangle contains the vulva, which is the collective term for the external genitalia (the clitoris, mons pubis, labia minora and majora, vestibule of the vagina, the vestibular bulb and the greater vestibular glands) and the urethral and vaginal openings [16].

Branches of the internal and external pudendal arteries supply both sides of the vulva, and the skin is drained into the medial group of the superficial inguinal nodes, with the Cloquet node being considered the sentinel node. The ilioinguinal nerves and the genital branch of the genitofemoral nerves supply the anterior part of the vulva, while the posterior part is supplied by branches of the perineal nerves and the posterior cutaneous nerves of the thigh.

The clitoris is situated at the apex of the vestibule anteriorly, and its root is made up of the bulb of the vestibule, which is attached to the undersurface of the urogenital diaphragm and is covered by the bulbospongiosus muscles and the right and left crura, which become the corpora cavernosa and are covered by an ischiocavernosus muscle. The glans, together with its prepuce, caps the body of the clitoris and has numerous sensory nerve endings, mainly through the dorsal nerves of the clitoris. Appropriate sexual stimulation of the clitoris and the region of the vaginal orifice and labia minora, reinforced by afferent nervous impulses from the breasts and other regions, results in sensory impulses reaching the central nervous system, which then pass down the spinal cord to the sympathetic outflow (T1 to L2), to synapse between the preganglionic and postganglionic first and second lumbar ganglia, which innervate the smooth muscle of the vagina, and via the pudendal nerve to reach the bulbospongiosus and ischiocavernosus muscles.

The greater vestibular glands, also known as Bartholin's glands, lie underneath the posterior parts of the bulb of the vestibule and the labia majora. Each drains its lubricating mucous secretion via a small duct into a groove between the posterior part of the labia minora and the hymen. Blockage of this gland can lead to a Bartholin's cyst or an abscess.

The urethra is just under 4 cm long, extending from the neck of the bladder to the external meatus. It opens into the vestibule at a point about 2.5 cm below the clitoris, immediately in front of the vagina. The relatively short distance between the urethra and the bladder makes it easier for catheterization; however, it does make women more prone to cystitis compared to men. The paraurethral glands open into the vestibule on either side of the urethral orifice.

1.7 The Vagina

The vagina is a muscular tube that is approximately 8 cm long and extends upwards and backwards between the vulva and the uterus. The upper half of the vagina lies above the pelvic floor within the pelvis, posterior to the bladder and in front of the rectum, and with its anterior wall pierced by the cervix. The upper third of the vagina is supported by the levator ani muscles and the transverse cervical, pubocervical and sacrocervical ligaments, while the urogenital diaphragm supports the middle third. The lower half of the vagina lies between the urethra anteriorly and the anal canal posteriorly, within the perineum, and the perineal body supports the lower third of the vagina. The main blood supply is via the vaginal artery, which is a branch of the internal iliac artery and by the vaginal branch of the uterine artery, and then drained by the vaginal veins into the internal iliac veins. The internal and external iliac nodes drain the upper third of the vagina, the internal iliac nodes drain the middle third while the superficial inguinal nodes drain the lower third of the vagina. This difference is due to the embryological development of the vagina, as described in Section 1.1, with the hymen demarcating the point of fusion between the sinovaginal bulb from the

mesoderm and the developing vaginal dimple from the ectoderm. This clearly has implications in cases of the spread of malignancy, especially vaginal and metastatic cervical cancer, and its treatment [17,18].

The paracolpium (paravaginal tissue) is surrounded by the vaginal wall, the pubocervical fascia and the rectovaginal septum (Denonvilliers' fascia). The paracolpium contains the distal part of the pelvic autonomic nerve plexus and its branches: the nerves to the urethra, the cavernous nerve and the nerves to the internal anal sphincter (NIAS). There is evidence that with vaginal delivery and with aging, the pelvic plexus is likely to change from a sheet-like configuration to several bundles [19].

1.8 Overview of the Gross Structures in the Female Pelvis

In the anterior aspect of the female pelvis, there is the bladder and ureters, the uterus, fallopian tubes and broad ligament and the ovaries. The rectum, sigmoid colon and the terminal coils of the ileum occupy the posterior part of the pelvic cavity (Table 1.1).

1.8.1 The Urinary Bladder and Ureters

The apex of the urinary bladder lies immediately posterior to the symphysis pubis, with the neck resting on the upper surface of the urogenital diaphragm. The posterior aspect, or base, of the bladder lies immediately in front of the anterior vaginal wall, which in turn separates it from the rectum. The body of the uterus rests superiorly on the bladder, separated by the uterovesical pouch. The inferolateral surfaces lie in front of the retropubic pad of fat and pubic bones, and posteriorly, rest on the levator ani muscles.

Each of the two ureters crosses over the pelvic inlet in front of the bifurcation of the common iliac artery, running downwards and backwards in front of the internal iliac artery and behind the ovary down till the ischial spine. Here, it turns forward and medially beneath the base of the broad ligament, where it is crossed by the uterine artery. This point is known as 'water under the bridge', because the ureter lies immediately below the uterine artery at 1.5 cm lateral to the cervix. It then runs forward, lateral to the lateral vaginal fornix, to enter the base of the bladder, just above the trigone. There is indeed a risk of iatrogenic ureteric injury during pelvic surgery, both for benign and malignant gynaecological pathologies [20].

1.8.2 The Uterus and Tubes

The uterus is a muscular organ which has the shape of an upside-down pear, measuring about 8 cm in length, 5 cm in width and 2.5 cm in thickness in nulliparous adults of reproductive age. It is divided into a fundus (lying above the uterine tubes), body and a narrow lower part, the cervix.

In most women, the uterus is anteverted and anteflexed, by means of the round ligament; however, in some women, the fundus and the body of the uterus are bent backwards on the vagina, to lie in the rectouterine pouch, making the uterus retroverted and retroflexed. The body of the uterus is related

Table 1.1 Overview of the gross structures in the female pelvis

Pelvic organ	Blood supply	Lymphatic drainage	Nerve supply
Sigmoid colon	Arterial: sigmoid branches of inferior mesenteric artery Venous: tributaries of inferior mesenteric vein, which joins portal system	Along sigmoid arteries to inferior mesenteric nodes	Sympathetic and parasympathetic nerves from inferior hypogastric plexus
Rectum	Arterial: superior rectal artery, middle rectal artery, inferior rectal artery Venous: veins correspond to the arteries	Pararectal nodes to inferior mesenteric nodes; vessels from the lower part of the rectum follow middle rectal artery to internal iliac nodes	Sympathetic and parasympathetic nerves from inferior hypogastric plexus
Urinary bladder	Arterial: superior and inferior vesical arteries, branches of internal iliac artery Venous: form vesical venous plexus, drained into internal iliac vein	Internal and external iliac lymph nodes	Inferior hypogastric plexuses
Uterus	Arterial: uterine artery from the internal iliac, ovarian artery from abdominal aorta Venous: correspond to the arteries	Lymph vessels from the fundus accompany ovarian artery to drain in para-aortic nodes; vessels from body and cervix drain into internal and external iliac lymph nodes; few lymph vessels drain into superficial inguinal lymph nodes	Sympathetic and parasympathetic nerves from inferior hypogastric plexuses
Uterine tubes	Arterial: uterine artery from the internal iliac, ovarian artery from abdominal aorta Venous: correspond to the arteries	Lymph vessels flow corresponding arteries and drain into internal iliac and para-aortic nodes	Sympathetic and parasympathetic nerves from inferior hypogastric plexuses
Ovary	Arterial: ovarian artery – branch of abdominal aorta at the level of first lumbar vertebra Venous: ovarian vein – drains into inferior vena cava on right side, into left renal vein on left side	Lymph vessels follow the ovarian artery and drain into para-aortic nodes at the level of first lumbar vertebra	Sympathetic fibres: from aortic plexus (accompanies ovarian artery); some parasympathetic fibres: from inferior hypogastric plexus (via uterine artery)
Vagina	Arterial: vaginal artery, branch of internal iliac artery and the vaginal branch of uterine artery Venous: form a plexus around vagina that drains into internal iliac vein	Lymph vessels from the upper third of vagina drain to external and internal iliac nodes, from middle third to internal iliac nodes and from lower third to superficial inguinal nodes	Inferior hypogastric plexus

anteriorly to the uterovesical pouch and the superior surface of the bladder, posteriorly is related to the pouch of Douglas, and laterally to the broad ligament and uterine vessels. The uterine artery, which is a branch of the internal iliac artery, supplies the uterus after running medially in the base of the broad ligament, reaching the cervix at the internal os and then ascending along the lateral margin of the uterus within the broad ligament, anastomosing with the ovarian artery, which also supplies the uterus. A small descending branch is given off by the uterine artery to supply the cervix and the vagina. Blood drains into the uterine vein and internal iliac vein.

The lymph from the fundus drains into the para-aortic nodes at the level of the first lumbar vertebra, while the body and the cervix drain into the internal and external iliac lymph nodes. Some lymph vessels pass through the inguinal canal, following the round ligament, and drain into the superficial inguinal nodes. Branches from the inferior hypogastric plexuses provide sympathetic and parasympathetic nerve supply. Knowledge of this lymphatic drainage is important in cases of endometrial cancer [21].

The thick myometrium is made up of smooth muscle supported by connective tissue. Leiomyomata, or fibroids, may occur in this layer, and when treatment is necessary, this can happen through myomectomy, total hysterectomy or uterine artery embolization [22].

The endometrium lines the body of the uterus and is continuous above with the mucous membrane lining the uterine tubes and below with the mucous membrane of the cervix. Deposits of ectopic endometrium can lead to endometriosis [23].

Peritoneum covers all of the uterus except anteriorly below the level of the internal os, where the peritoneum passes forward onto the bladder and laterally between the attachment of the layers of the broad ligament. Apart from the tone of the

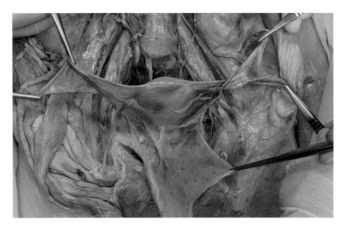

Figure 1.3 Dissection of the female pelvis (carried out on a Thiel embalmed cadaver at the Department of Anatomy, University of Malta). A black and white version of this figure will appear in some formats. For the colour version, please refer to the plate section.

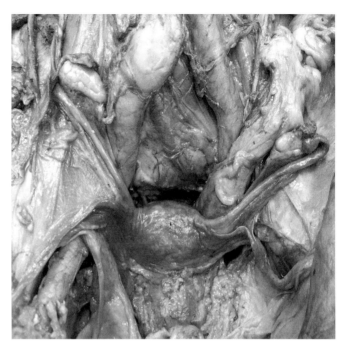

Figure 1.4 Dissection of the uterus, tubes and ovaries (carried out on a Thiel embalmed cadaver at the Department of Anatomy, University of Malta). A black and white version of this figure will appear in some formats. For the colour version, please refer to the plate section.

levator ani muscles, the uterus is supported by three ligaments, namely, the transverse cervical (cardinal), pubocervical and sacrocervical ligaments, which result from the condensations of pelvic fascia (Figures 1.3 and 1.4).

The cervical canal communicates with the cavity of the uterine body through an internal os and with the vagina through the external os. There is a transformation zone, also known as the squamocolumnar junction or the transitional zone, where there is a high affinity for viruses like human papillomavirus due to the increased rate of cell replication at this point. The cervix is related anteriorly to the anterior fornix of the vagina, posteriorly to the rectouterine pouch with coils of ileum and sigmoid colon, and laterally related to the ureters as they pass forward to enter the bladder. Blood is supplied to the cervix by the descending branch of the uterine artery, which in turn drains into the uterine vein.

The anterior and lateral cervix drains to the lymph nodes along the uterine arteries, travelling along the cardinal ligaments at the base of the broad ligament to the external iliac lymph nodes and ultimately the para-aortic lymph nodes. The posterior and lateral cervix drains along the uterine arteries to the internal iliac lymph nodes and ultimately also the para-aortic lymph nodes. The posterior section of the cervix drains to the obturator and presacral lymph nodes. However, there are individual variations of lymphatic drainage from the cervix [24].

In cases of cervical malignancy, advances in magnetic resonance imaging (MRI) and positron emission tomography/computerized tomography (PET/CT) have made it possible to examine many of the prognostic factors noninvasively. In radiology. combining deep learning and anatomic prior information may improve segmentation accuracy for cervical tumours [25, 26].

1.8.3 The Ovary

The ovaries are responsible for the production of ova and the hormones oestrogen and progesterone. They are covered externally by the germinal epithelium, which is a modified area of peritoneum. Both ovaries are often found hanging down in the rectouterine pouch, lying against the lateral wall

of the pelvis. They are each attached to the back of the broad ligament by the mesovarium, while the suspensory ligament (infundibulopelvic ligament) attaches the mesovarium to the lateral wall of the pelvis. The blood and nerve supply, together with the lymph drainage, pass over the pelvic inlet, through the lateral end of the broad ligament via the suspensory ligament and finally enter the hilum of the ovary via the mesovarium. The blood supply is via the ovarian artery, which is a direct branch of the aorta, arising at the level of the first lumbar vertebra. On the right side, blood drains into the inferior vena cava, and into the left renal vein on the left side. Because ovarian cancer might spread via the lymphatics via the suspensory ligament and mesovarium, as well as through the round ligament of the uterus, the sentinel node can be detected in the para-aortic and paracaval regions, obturator fossa and surrounding internal iliac arteries, and inguinal regions. These findings support the strategy of injecting tracers in both ovarian ligaments to identify sentinel nodes [27, 28].

1.9 The Peritoneum

From the anterior abdominal wall, the peritoneum passes down onto the upper surface of the urinary bladder, then onto the anterior surface of the uterus at the level of the internal os, upwards onto the anterior surface of the body and fundus of the uterus, and then downwards over the posterior surface of the uterus, covering the upper part of the posterior surface of the vagina, forming the rectouterine wall (pouch of Douglas). This is the lowest part of the abdominopelvic peritoneal cavity in the erect position. The broad ligaments are two layered folds of peritoneum extending from the lateral margins of the uterus to the lateral pelvic walls. Peritoneal spread of infection or malignancy is particular to the pelvic organs, particularly in the case of ovarian cancer spread [29, 30].

1.10 Conclusion

Accurate knowledge of the anatomy of the female pelvis and its contents is essential for safe management of patients presenting with obstetric and/or gynaecological conditions.

References

1. Vilanova-Sanchez A, McCracken K, Halleran DR, et al. Obstetrical outcomes in adult patients born with complex anorectal malformations and cloacal anomalies: a literature review. *J Pediatr Adolesc Gynecol.* 2019 Feb;**32**(1):7–14.

2. Bailey AP, Jaslow CR, Kutteh WH. Minimally invasive surgical options for congenital and acquired uterine factors associated with recurrent pregnancy loss. *Womens Health (Lond).* 2015 Mar;**11**(2):161–7.

3. Rikken JFW, Kowalik CR, Emanuel MH, et al. The randomised uterine septum transsection trial (TRUST): design and protocol. *BMC Womens Health.* 2018 Oct 5; **18**(1):163.

4. Ludwin A, Ludwin I, Bhagavath B, Lindheim SR. Pre-, intra-, and postoperative management of Robert's uterus. *Fertil Steril.* 2018 Sep;**110**(4):778–9.

5. DeSilva JM, Rosenberg KR. Anatomy, development, and function of the human pelvis. *Anat Rec (Hoboken).* 2017 Apr;**300**(4):628–32.

6. Drake RL, Vogl W, Mitchell AWM. Pelvis and perineum. In *Gray's Anatomy for Students*, 3rd ed. London: Churchill Livingstone Elsevier, 2015, pp. 406–504.

7. Hemmerich A, Bandrowska T, Dumas GA. The effects of squatting while pregnant on pelvic dimensions: a computational simulation to understand childbirth. *J Biomech.* 2019 Apr 18;**87**:64-74. pii: S0021-9290(19)30147-2.

8. NyangohTimoh K, Moszkowicz D, Zaitouna M, et al. Detailed muscular structure and neural control anatomy of the levator ani muscle: a study based on female human fetuses. *Am J Obstet. Gynecol.* 2018 Jan;**218**(1):121.e1-121.e12.

9. Sinnatamby CS. Abdomen. In *Last's Anatomy Regional and Applied*, 12th ed. London: Churchill Livingstone Elsevier, 2011, pp. 301–16, 322–4.

10. Jiang H, Qian X, Carroli G, Garner P. Selective versus routine use of episiotomy for vaginal birth. *Cochrane Database Syst Rev.* 2017 Feb **8**;2: CD000081.

11. Arbuckle JL, Parden AM, Hoover K, Griffin RL, Richter HE. Prevalence and awareness of pelvic floor disorders in adolescent females seeking gynecologic care. *J Pediatr Adolesc Gynecol.* 2019;**32**(3):288–92.

12. Lemos AQ, Brasil CA, Alvares CM, et al. The relation of the pelvis and the perineal function in incontinent women: a neglected subject. *Neurourol Urodyn.* 2018 Nov;**37**(8):2799–2809.

13. Muavha DA, Ras L, Jeffery S. Laparoscopic surgical anatomy for pelvic floor surgery. *Best Pract Res Clin Obstet Gynaecol.* 2019 Jan;**54**:89–102.

14. Snell RS. The perineum. In *Clinical Anatomy by Regions*, 9th ed. Philadelphia: Wolters Kluwer Health, Lippincott Williams and Wilkins, 2012, pp. 302–33.

15. VanBuren WM, Lightner AL, Kim ST, et al. Imaging and surgical management of anorectal vaginal fistulas. *Radiographics.* 2018 Sep-Oct;**38**(5):1385–1401.

16. Wu Y, Dabhoiwala NF, Hagoort J, et al. Architecture of structures in the urogenital triangle of young adult males; comparison with females. *J Anat.* 2018 Oct;**233**(4):447–459.

17. Rajaram S, Maheshwari A, Srivastava A. Staging for vaginal cancer. *Best Pract Res Clin Obstet Gynaecol.* 2015 Aug;**29**(6):822–32.

18. Höckel M, Horn LC, Einenkel J. (Laterally) extended endopelvic resection: surgical treatment of locally advanced and recurrent cancer of the uterine cervix and vagina based on ontogenetic anatomy. *Gynecol Oncol.* 2012 Nov;**127**(2):297–302.

19. Hinata N, Hieda K, Sasaki H, et al. Nerves and fasciae in and around the paracolpium or paravaginal tissue: an immunohistochemical study using elderly donated cadavers. *Anat Cell Biol.* 2014 Mar;**47**(1):44–54.

20. Kaestner L. Management of urological injury at the time of urogynaecology surgery. *Best Pract Res Clin Obstet Gynaecol.* 2019 Jan;**54**:2–11.

21. Bodurtha Smith AJ, Fader AN, Tanner EJ. Sentinel lymph node assessment in endometrial cancer: a systematic review and meta-analysis. *Am J Obstet Gynecol.* 2017 May;**216**(5):459–76.e10.

22. Anton K, Rosenblum NG, Teefey P, Dayaratna S, Gonsalves CF. The enlarged fibroid uterus: aberrant arterial supply via the omental artery. *Cardiovasc Intervent Radiol.* 2019 Apr;**42**(4):615–19.

23. Alimi Y, Iwanaga J, Loukas M, Tubbs RS. The clinical anatomy of endometriosis: a review. *Cureus.* 2018 Sep 25;**10**(9):e3361.

24. Ercoli A, Delmas V, Iannone V, et al. The lymphatic drainage of the uterine cervix in adult fresh cadavers: anatomy and surgical implications. *Eur J Surg Oncol.* 2010 Mar;**36**(3):298–303.

25. Narayan K, Lin MY. Staging for cervix cancer: role of radiology, surgery and clinical assessment. *Best Pract Res Clin Obstet Gynaecol.* 2015 Aug;**29**(6):833–44.

26. Chen L, Shen C, Zhou Z, et al. Automatic PET cervical tumor segmentation by combining deep learning and anatomic prior. *Phys Med Biol.* 2019 Feb 12;**65**(8):085019.

27. Kimmig R, Buderath P, Mach P, Rusch P, Aktas B. Surgical treatment of early ovarian cancer with compartmental resection of regional lymphatic network and indocyanine-green-guided targeted compartmental lymphadenectomy (TCL, paraaortic part). *J Gynecol Oncol.* 2017 May;**28**(3):e41.

28. Kleppe M, Kraima AC, Kruitwagen RF, et al. Understanding lymphatic drainage pathways of the ovaries to predict sites for sentinel nodes in ovarian cancer. *Int J Gynecol Cancer.* 2015 Oct;**25**(8):1405–14.

29. Blackburn SC, Stanton MP. Anatomy and physiology of the peritoneum. *Semin Pediatr Surg.* 2014 Dec;**23**(6):326–30.

30. Le O. Patterns of peritoneal spread of tumor in the abdomen and pelvis. *World J Radiol.* 2013 Mar 28;**5**(3):106–12.

Chapter 2

Maternal Physiology during Pregnancy, Including Immunology of Pregnancy

Ksenija Gersak

Pregnancy is a specific relationship between two or more organisms inside their unique ecosystem. Although they belong to the same species, the relationship can be qualified as a symbiotic and parasitic form of biological interaction [1]. The question might be rooted more in the psychology rather than physiology of pregnancy. On the other hand, however, a fetus does control maternal adaptation to pregnancy, and for its successful development and growth it needs an effective exchange of nutritive and metabolic products with the mother, combined with a reliable life-support system composed of the placenta, umbilical cord and amniotic sac.

This chapter reviews the biochemical, physiological and immunological adaptations of a woman's body to pregnancy.

2.1 Endocrine Changes during Pregnancy

2.1.1 Steroid and Protein Hormones

Hormones associated with pregnancy are steroid hormones, protein hormones and prostaglandins. Their production takes place in the corpus luteum, placenta and fetus. Separately, fetal and placental tissues do not possess the necessary enzymatic capabilities for an adequate synthesis of these hormones. Together, however, they are complementary and form a complete unit that utilizes the maternal compartment as both a source of basic building materials and a resource for the clearance of hormones [2]. Hormone production in the corpus luteum and fetoplacental unit are presented in Table 2.1.

Progesterone is a steroid hormone with a number of physiological effects that are mainly amplified in the presence of oestrogens. It is produced by the corpus luteum until about 7 weeks' gestation. During a transition period of 3 weeks, its production is shared between the corpus luteum and placenta, and after 10 weeks' gestation, placenta becomes the key source of its synthesis [3].

The majority of placental progesterone is derived from maternal cholesterol and is relatively independent of uteroplacental perfusion, fetal well-being or even the presence of a live fetus. Unlike steroidogenesis elsewhere, it is not clear whether the production of placental progesterone requires the control of tropic hormones. Some evidence exists indicating that a small amount of human chorionic gonadotropin (hCG) must be present [4].

The main biological function of progesterone is the prevention of myometrial contractility during pregnancy, manifesting as an increased membrane electrical resting potential

Table 2.1 Hormone production in corpus luteum and fetoplacental unit

Hormone	Production site
Progesterone	Corpus luteum Placenta
Oestradiol	Corpus luteum Placenta
Human chorionic gonadotropin	Decidualized endometrium Placenta
Fetal cortisol, corticosterone, aldosterone	Fetal adrenal gland
Hypothalamic-like releasing hormones	Placenta
Human placental lactogen	Placenta
Human chorionic thyrotropin	Placenta
Human chorionic adrenocorticotropin	Placenta
Placental growth hormone	Placenta
Alpha-fetoprotein	Fetal liver and yolk sac
Relaxin	Corpus luteum
Prolactin	Fetal pituitary Maternal pituitary Decidualized endometrium Myometrium
Insulin-like growth hormones	Placenta
Epidermal growth factor	Placenta
Inhibin A	Placenta
Activin A	Placenta
Follistatin	Decidualized endometrium Placenta
Atrial natriuretic peptide	Placenta Myometrium

Source: Adapted from [2].

8

and prevention of electrical coupling between myometrial cells. Progesterone also decreases the uptake of extracellular calcium, which is needed for myometrial contraction, by downregulating the expression of genes that encode subunits of voltage-dependent calcium channels. Its concentration in the myometrium is about three times higher than maternal plasma levels in early pregnancy. Throughout pregnancy it remains high, and is about equal to the maternal plasma level at term.

During pregnancy, the plasma concentration of two active metabolites of progesterone increases: 5α-dihydroprogesterone and 5β-dihydroprogesterone. The kidneys excrete both of them into the urine. 5α-dihydroprogesterone contributes to the resistance to vasopressor action of angiotensin II during the course of pregnancy.

Progesterone also serves as the substrate for fetal adrenal gland production of glucocorticoids and mineralocorticoids. In the amniotic fluid, progesterone level is highest between 10 and 20 weeks' gestation and then decreases gradually [2].

Oestrogens are steroid hormones produced primarily by the ovaries, and during pregnancy by the placenta. They influence progesterone production, mammary gland development, uterine angiogenesis and fetal adrenal gland function [5]. Together and with progesterone, they induce uterine and systemic artery vasodilation [6].

Like progesterone, initial oestrogen production depends on precursors from outside the placenta: maternal cholesterol and androgen compounds. The major oestrogens during pregnancy are oestradiol, oestrone, oestriol and oestetrol. Oestriol and oestetrol are almost solely produced from fetal steroid precursors.

In maternal circulation, a rise in oestradiol begins during 6 to 8 weeks' gestation, when placental function becomes apparent, followed by a rise of oestriol and oestrone during 7 to 10 weeks' gestation. By the end of 20 weeks' gestation, approximately 90% of oestrogen production can be attributed to synthesis in the fetal adrenal gland from the precursor dehydroepiandrosterone sulphate (DHEAS). At term, an equal amount of oestrogen arises from maternal DHEAS and fetal DHEAS, and their production is increased about 100 times over non-pregnant levels.

Prior to excretion into maternal urine, maternal liver rapidly metabolizes the oestrogens into a variety of more than 20 metabolites.

Human chorionic gonadotropin (hCG) is a glycoprotein with an alpha subunit identical to that of the luteinizing hormone (LH), follicle-stimulating hormone (FSH) and thyroid-stimulating hormone (TSH). While it could be produced in different tissues, only the placenta has the ability to glycosylate the protein, and it is the process of glycosylation that is responsible for the longer circulating half-life of hCG. Since the beta subunit promoter does not contain steroid hormone response elements, it allows hCG secretion to escape feedback regulation mechanisms controlled by sex steroids, in contrast to FSH and LH [2].

The main biological function of hCG is the maintenance of corpus luteum function. It first enters maternal circulation at the time of blastocyst implantation, and its plasma levels increase rapidly, doubling every 2 days during the first trimester. Between 10 and 12 weeks' gestation, plasma levels begin to decline, settling during 16 weeks' gestation and maintaining stable values until the end of pregnancy.

hCG plays an important role in male sexual differentiation by stimulating testosterone secretion from fetal testes, and is also presumed to regulate placental development by influencing differentiation of cytotrophoblast cells.

Production and secretion of hCG are the result of complex interactions between sex steroids, cytokines, placental GnRH, growth factors and other locally produced peptides. About 20–30 isoforms have so far been discovered in maternal blood. A major route of clearance for hCG is maternal renal metabolism, during which a final reduced fragment of the beta subunit is produced, known as the beta-core fragment. hCG fetal plasma levels follow the same pattern as those in maternal circulation, with the peak at the end of the first trimester of gestation.

Human placental lactogen is a non-glycosylated polypeptide with a similar structure to the human growth hormone, and mimics the action of prolactin. It is primarily secreted into maternal circulation and stimulates the secretion of insulin and insulin-like growth factor 1. Placental production appears 5–10 days after conception [7, 8].

Human placental lactogen influences maternal metabolic processes, especially lipolysis. Through its action, maternal blood free fatty acid levels increase, becoming a more prominent source of energy for maternal metabolism, enabling the fetus to utilize relatively more glucose. With its diabetogenic action, it stimulates protein production and, as an angiogenic hormone, plays an important role in the formation of the fetal vascular network. Human placental lactogen also exhibits weak actions similar to those of the growth hormone, thus stimulating the formation of protein tissues.

2.1.2 Thyroid Gland

During a normal pregnancy, changes in maternal thyroid function can be viewed as a balance between hormone requirements and the availability of iodine [9].

Due to the structural analogy with thyroid-stimulating hormone (TSH), hCG causes thyroid stimulation as early as during the first trimester, with a resulting slight decrease in serum TSH levels. At the same time circulating levels of thyroid-binding globulin (TBG) are increased by oestrogen-stimulated hepatic synthesis and by oestrogen-mediated prolongation of TBG half-life.

Thyroid volume and intrathyroidal blood flow increase gradually towards the third trimester and decrease after delivery [10]. The changes in volume are associated with changes in TSH levels and alterations in maternal body mass index.

The apparent increased functional iodine uptake by the thyroid gland is relative rather than absolute, and reflects the decrease in the total systemic iodine pool. A decline in the availability of iodide is induced by the onset of fetal intake and increased renal clearance. Nevertheless, circulating unbound levels of triiodothyronine (T3) and thyroxine (T4) are minimally altered. Free serum T4 level rises slightly during the first trimester, its concentration peaking concurrently with peak hCG levels, and then returning to normal values at 11–13 weeks' gestation.

During normal pregnancy, basal metabolic rate increases by a total of 25% in a progressive manner. Relative to the increased body surface areas of the mother and fetus, however, it remains unchanged.

2.1.3 Pituitary Gland and Prolactin

The **pituitary gland** enlarges during pregnancy. The enlargement is primarily caused by oestrogen-stimulated hypertrophy and hyperplasia of the lactotrophic cells in the anterior pituitary. Production of gonadotropins declines, while synthesis in corticotropic and thyrotropic cells remains constant. Somatotropic cells are generally suppressed due to the negative feedback by placental synthesis of growth hormone.

Prolactin is a single-chain polypeptide. It has a similar structure to growth hormone and human placental lactogen. Maternal serum prolactin levels begin increasing gradually at 8 weeks' gestation with the increasing size of the gland, reaching their peak at term [11]. Only the myometrium, endometrium and the maternal and fetal pituitary are responsible for its secretion. Endometrium requires the presence of progesterone to initiate prolactin production, whereas in the myometrium, progesterone suppresses prolactin production [2].

The major physiological roles of prolactin are priming of the breasts for lactation, maintenance of lactation during the puerperium, modulation of prostaglandin-mediated uterine muscle contractility and contribution to surfactant synthesis in the fetal lung. It also has an impact on maternal metabolism, reducing the permeability of the amnion in the fetus-to-mother direction, and influencing regulation of fetal water and electrolyte balance by acting as an antidiuretic hormone.

2.2 Physiological Adaptation to Pregnancy

2.2.1 Uterus

The **uterus** grows in order to accommodate the growing conceptual mass (the fetus, placenta and amniotic fluid) without increasing intrauterine pressure. The non-pregnant uterus of a nulliparous woman weighs about 40 g and that of a multiparous woman about 70 g. At term, its weight is about 1 200 g.

During the first trimester, the uterus grows more rapidly than the conceptual mass. Mitotic proliferation of myocytes is responsible for a major proportion of total uterine growth due to oestrogen stimulation. The conceptual mass fills the entire uterine cavity approximately at the end of 12 weeks' gestation, when *decidua capsularis* fuses with *decidua parietalis*, which obliterates the uterine cavity.

Production of new myocytes is limited. After the first trimester, further uterine growth is due to hypertrophy of myocytes rather than due to replication. Myocytes increase in size, accompanied by accumulation of fibrous tissue, particularly in

the external muscle layer, and by accumulation of elastic tissue. The increase in uterine size is related predominantly to the pressure exerted on it by the expanding conceptual mass [12].

After 20 weeks' gestation, the uterus begins to elongate and assumes a cylindroid shape. Myofibril density is the highest in the corpus and the lowest in the isthmus. The uterus comes in contact with the anterior abdominal wall, displaces the intestines laterally and superiorly and extends upwards almost to the liver. Also, it usually rotates to the right. By term, the myometrium is only 1 to 2 cm thick, and the architectural arrangement reflects the salient features of uterine behaviour during normal labour.

The uterine wall is arranged in three layers. The outer layer arches over the fundus and extends into various ligaments. Most of the wall is formed by the middle layer, which is composed of a dense network of muscle fibres arranged in the same direction as blood vessels. The inner layer contains sphincter-like fibres around fallopian tube orifices and the internal cervical long axis.

The uterus undergoes irregular **contractions** early in pregnancy. During the second trimester, the contractions can be detected by manual examination, first described by Dr John Braxton Hicks in 1871 [13]. The Braxton Hicks contractions are unpredictable, sporadic and usually non-rhythmic. Their frequency increases during the last two weeks of pregnancy. Similarly, studies of uterine electrical activity have shown low and uncoordinated patterns during early gestation, which become progressively more intense and synchronized by term [14 , 15].

The **isthmic segment** elongates at the end of the first trimester of pregnancy, before the conceptual mass has filled the available place in the uterine corpus. The elongation is accompanied by thickening of the wall of the lower uterine segment and corpus. During the second trimester, the isthmus undergoes incorporation into the lower uterine segment, which is accompanied by thinning of its musculature. This process stops at the border between isthmus and cervix. Later on, the junction is seamless, and no distinct margin can be ascertained [16].

The **cervix** becomes softer during pregnancy due to loosening of the connective tissue by the means of collagen fibril dissociation. Increased vascularity and oedema additionally contribute to its softening and cyanosis, together with hypertrophy and hyperplasia of the cervical glands [12]. Soon after conception, endocervical mucosal cells produce dense mucus that obstructs the cervical canal. All the changes intensify as the pregnancy progresses. At term, cervical glands occupy up to one half of the total cervical mass, and with the onset of labour or slightly before it, the mucus plug is expelled.

Sufficient **uteroplacental blood flow** is essential for a normal pregnancy outcome [17]. Blood is transported to the uterus bidirectionally via a dual arterial anastomotic loop, the ovarian loop originating from the aorta and the uterine loop from the internal iliac arteries.

Perpendicular vessels branch out from the main utero-ovarian arteries and pass into the uterine corpus to form the actuate arteries. They encircle the uterus by coursing within the myometrium just beneath its outer serosal surface. Vessels from each side form anastomoses along the uterine midline. Smaller radial arteries originate from the actuate arteries and penetrate the myometrium centripetally before branching into either straight basal or spiral arteries at the myoendometrial border. Basal vessels spread to form a network along the myoendometrial border, while the spiral arteries penetrate further into the endometrium and terminate close to the uterine lumen in capillaries that are drained by venules into larger veins that enter the inferior vena cava.

The underlying reason responsible for the unique structure of spiral arteries is trophoblast invasion. Fetal trophoblast cells migrate into the arterial lumen, ablate the endothelium and smooth muscle of the arterial wall and reorganize the matrix elements.

Due to endovascular invasion, vessels lose their ability to contract, resulting in decreased vascular resistance, facilitating an increased blood flow. The combined effect of increasing both the length and the diameter of the vessels by a factor of 2 theoretically reduces vascular resistance by a factor of 8. And according to Poiseuille's law, together with additional factors, such as reduced blood viscosity and the growth of new vessels, it contributes to a significant reduction in blood flow resistance.

The flow increases from a baseline value of 20–50 mL/min to 450–800 mL/min in singleton pregnancies, with values in excess of 1 L/min measured in twin pregnancies [17]. Since blood pressure normally decreases during pregnancy, uterine haemodynamic changes can principally be attributed to a profound decrease in uterine vascular resistance. The increase of uteroplacental blood flow is gradual and fairly linear. Absolute blood flow to the myometrium increases proportionally to uterine mass, whereas relative uterine blood flow (millilitre/minute/100 g) may fluctuate or remain fairly constant during the entire pregnancy.

2.2.2 Breast

Breast growth and milk production depend on numerous hormonal factors that occur in two periods: at puberty and during pregnancy.

At puberty, the major influence on breast growth is oestrogen, which potentiates prolactin release stimulation by gonadotropin-releasing hormone (GnRH). The first main response to the increasing level of oestrogen is an increase in size and pigmentation of the areola and the formation of a mass of breast tissue underneath the areola. Breast tissue expresses oestrogen receptors ER-alpha and ER-beta, but only in the presence of prolactin. Besides prolactin, complete differentiation of the gland requires insulin, cortisol, thyroxine, growth hormone and the presence of local growth factors.

The breast enlarges rapidly during the first two months of pregnancy. Later on, progressive enlargement continues at a slower rate. The enlargement is due to an increase in glandular tissue volume.

The key hormone for breast differentiation and growth during this period is progesterone, with oestrogen additionally

being required for the synthesis of progesterone receptors. Similar changes occur during each normal menstrual cycle, especially in the late luteal phase, when mitotic activity, fluid secretion and DNA production in glandular and non-glandular tissue reach their peak [2].

Final differentiation of the alveolar epithelial tissue into mature milk cells is accomplished by gestational increase in oestrogen and progesterone levels, combined with the presence of prolactin after prior exposure to cortisol and insulin. As pregnancy progresses, the nipples become significantly larger and more pigmented. All in all, in most normal pregnancies, pre-pregnancy breast size and post-pregnancy amount of milk production do not correlate [18].

2.2.3 Osmoregulation and Water Metabolism

Pregnant women experience a decrease in tonicity of body fluids. Early in pregnancy, plasma **osmolality** decreases to its lowest level of approximately 10 mOsmol/kg below non-pregnant levels [19]. This puts it below the pre-pregnancy osmotic thirst threshold, and a new steady state needs to be established. Lowering the threshold stimulates increased water intake and dilution of body fluids. The exact mechanism responsible for altered osmoregulation in pregnancy is unclear, chorionic gonatotropin and relaxin possibly being responsible for the changes. As far as we know, relaxin stimulates increased vasopressin secretion, resulting in increased drinking and water retention.

Water content of lean tissue increases from approximately 72% at 10 weeks' gestation to about 75% at the end of pregnancy, with total amount of **extracellular extravascular fluid** reaching about 1.6 to 2.6 litres [20]. Most of this fluid is stored in the connective tissue under the influence of oestrogen. There is also an approximately 1.2 litre increase in water content in the **intravascular compartment**, and about 0.8 litres of fluid in the **amniotic cavity** itself, also contributing to the total body water content increase (Table 2.2). Additional extracellular water can be found also in the cerebrospinal fluid, lymph system, various body secretions and intestinal fluid.

About 30% of pregnant women exhibit physiological leg oedema, due to the effect of gravity and increased venou pressure below the level of the uterus as a consequence of partial vena cava occlusion.

2.2.4 Weight Gain

The physiological average of total weight gain in healthy primigravida eating without restriction is 12.5 kg [20]. Components of weight gain can be divided into two groups: the conceptual mass (fetus, placenta, amniotic fluid) and the maternal part (enlarged uterus, breast tissue, maternal fat deposition, extracellular extravascular and intravascular fluid) (Table 2.2).

On average, the fetus represents approximately 25% of the total gain, the placenta about 5% and the amniotic fluid about 6%. Fetal growth follows a sigmoid curve, with growth slowing in the final week of gestation. The rate of placental growth also declines towards the end of pregnancy.

Table 2.2 Changes in body water, blood and weight gain

Compartment	Increase during pregnancy
Extracellular extravascular fluid	1600 to 2600 mL
Intravascular fluid (plasma and red cell volume)	1200 mL
Water content of uterus and breast	2000 mL
Amniotic fluid, water content of the fetus and placenta	3500 mL
Red cell volume	250 mL
Plasma volume	1000 mL
Total body water gain	8000 to 9000 mL
Fetus, placenta and amniotic fluid	5.0 kg
Uterus	1.0 kg
Breast	0.4 kg
Maternal fat deposition	3.5 kg
Average weight gain	12.5 kg

Source: Adapted from [16, 21].

2.2.5 Serum Electrolytes

Concentrations of most serum electrolytes decrease during pregnancy. The decrease is not substantial, and the mean values are within normal ranges established for non-pregnant women.

The total amount of **sodium** and **potassium** increases during pregnancy, but their serum concentrations decrease slightly because of the expanded plasma volume. In the second and third trimesters, there is a net gain of approximately 1000 mEq of sodium and 300 mEq of potassium. On the other hand, progesterone, being a potent aldosterone antagonist that acts on the mineralocorticoid receptor, prevents sodium retention and protects against hypokalaemia. Despite an increased glomerular filtration of sodium and potassium, urine excretion thus remains unchanged due to enhanced tubular reabsorption.

Serum **calcium** levels, both ionized and non-ionized, decline during pregnancy. The reduction follows a lowered plasma albumin concentration, more specifically a decrease in the amount of circulating protein-bound non-ionized calcium. The fetal skeleton accumulates approximately 30 g of calcium at term, 80% of which is deposited during the third trimester. For this reason, maternal intestinal absorption is doubled during the same period, in part by 1,25-OH vitamin D. Dietary intake is necessary and especially important for pregnant adolescents, in whom bones are still developing [12].

Furthermore, total and ionized serum **magnesium** concentrations are also lower during pregnancy due to extracellular depletion. Serum phosphate concentration, however, remains within non-pregnant ranges due to increased calcitonin levels and elevated renal threshold for non-organic phosphate excretion.

Iodide is produced from dietary iodine in the intestine, from which it is absorbed into the circulation. Together with peripheral catabolism and deiodination of thyroid hormones and iodothyronines, dietary iodine constitutes the extrathyroidal inorganic iodine pool [9]. The pool is in a dynamic equilibrium with two main organs, the thyroid gland and the kidneys. In pregnancy, renal clearance of iodide increases significantly due to increased glomerular filtration rate.

A second mechanism of iodine deprivation occurs later in gestation, by the passage of a proportion of available iodine from the maternal circulation into the fetus and the placenta. In non-pregnant women, adequate iodine intake is estimated to be 100–150 mg/day. Based on several studies, the consensus recommendation of the World Health Organization is that iodine supply should be increased in pregnant and lactating women to at least 200 mg/day.

2.2.6 Haematological Changes and Iron Metabolism

Haematological changes during pregnancy affect plasma volume, red cell volume, haematocrit, haemoglobin and serum iron concentrations, as well as coagulation and fibrinolysis.

Plasma volume increases progressively by 40–50% throughout normal pregnancy, equating to about a 1 200 mL total increase (Table 2.2). Changes in red cell volume are less well defined, rising approximately by 200–400 mL (Figure 2.1).

During the first trimester, plasma volume expands by 15–20% compared to non-pregnant volumes. The most rapid increase can be observed during the second trimester. This increase keeps up with the increased metabolic demands of the enlarged uterus with its hypertrophied vascular system, and provides sufficient nutrients and electrolytes to support the growing fetus and placenta.

Total plasma volume increases from 2 600 mL to 3 800 mL at 34 weeks' gestation [12]. This increase is mediated by a direct action of progesterone and oestrogen on the kidneys, causing the release of renin and subsequent activation of the renin-angiotensin-aldosterone mechanism. This leads to renal sodium retention and an increase in total body water.

During the last few weeks of pregnancy, plasma volume may decline by about 200 mL or remain constant.

Plasma volume changes disproportionately with the increase in **red blood cell mass**, resulting in physiological haemodilution (Figure 2.1). There is a fall in **haemoglobin** concentration and **haematocrit**. Haemodilution has a protective function by decreasing blood viscosity in order to counter the concurrent predisposition to thromboembolic events, and can be beneficial for intervillous perfusion [22].

Red blood cell (RBC) mass starts to increase at 8–10 weeks' gestation aligned with erythropoietin production, and continues to increase until delivery by 15–20% in women who are not taking iron supplements and by 20–30% in women who have been taking iron supplements.

RBC life span is gradually decreased. Reticulocyte count, however, is slightly elevated due to a moderate rise of erythropoiesis in the bone marrow. Maternal erythropoietin does not

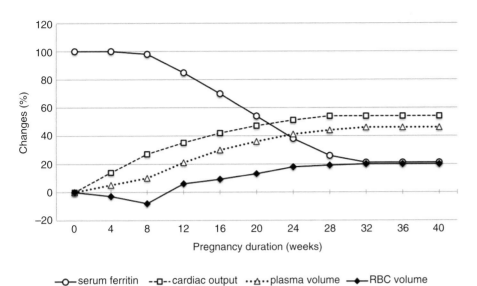

Figure 2.1 Changes in plasma volume, RBC volume, serum ferritin level, cardiac output and heart rate during pregnancy (adapted from [2, 24]).

cross the placenta [23]. Despite haemodilution, mean corpuscular volume (MCV) and mean corpuscular haemoglobin concentration (MCHC) remain on the same level.

Most women begin their pregnancy with a total body **iron** amount of 2.5 g, requiring an additional net intake of at least 1000 mg over the course of 40 weeks [16]. The amount of 400–500 mg is required to compensate for the increased red cell volume, 350 mg for the transfer to the fetus and placenta, and 200 mg for the baseline maternal body iron loss.

Serum **ferritin** level is proportional to body iron stores. During pregnancy, its level gradually decreases, reaching its lowest level in the third trimester (Figure 2.1).

The placenta retains about 90 mg of iron for its own function, and transports 270 mg of iron on average to the fetus. Maternal transferrin production steadily increases during pregnancy, with most of the transfer to the fetus occurring during the last trimester.

After being transported from syncytiotrophoblast by ferroportin, iron is probably oxidized to the ferric form before being loaded onto fetal transferrin.

Pregnancy induces a **hypercoagulable state**. Plasma concentrations of fibrinogen; coagulation factors XII, X, VIII and VII; and von Willebrand factor gradually increase, with an exception being factors XI and XIII, the levels of which decrease. The most pronounced changes can be observed in the third trimester and are currently attributed to hormonal changes, especially increased oestrogen levels, as the pregnancy progresses [25].

Blood levels of **coagulation inhibitors** such as antithrombin are unchanged, those of protein C are slightly increased or unchanged, while protein C inhibitor as well as free and total protein S levels are decreased. Low levels of protein S can be observed until at least 8 weeks postpartum.

Increase in **fibrinolysis** also occurs, and is reflected in increased concentrations of antithrombin III, plasminogen and fibrin degradation products. Inactive pro-enzyme plasminogen levels increase during normal pregnancy due to its reduced utilization and increased production. Furthermore,

markedly increased levels of plasminogen activator inhibitor-1 (PAI-1) produced by endothelial cells can be seen, along with high levels of plasminogen activator inhibitor-2 (PAI-2), which is very seldom found in non-pregnant circulation but is produced in large quantities by the placenta. Thrombin-activated fibrinolysis inhibitor (TAFI) is reported to be unaffected by normal pregnancy [25].

Platelet function remains normal during normal pregnancy. Although there is an increase in their production, the platelet count falls due to haemodilution, as well as due to their increased activity and consumption particularly during the last trimester [26]. Production of thromboxane A progressively increases during the second trimester and can induce aggregation. Increased platelet consumption and their production also lead to a greater proportion of younger and larger platelets.

2.2.7 Cardiovascular System

Multiple factors contribute to the overall alterations in maternal haemodynamic functions during pregnancy.

Pregnancy is associated with **vasodilation** of the systemic circulation as an effect of progesterone, prostaglandins and low-resistance uteroplacental circulation. Systemic vasodilation occurs as early as at 5 weeks' gestation and precedes full placentation and complete development of the uteroplacental circulation. Corpus luteum produces a peptide hormone relaxin, which has an endothelium-dependent vasodilatory role in pregnancy, and influences small arterial resistance vessels.

A substantial decrease in **peripheral vascular resistance** during the first trimester is continued to a nadir in the second trimester, followed by a plateau or slight increase in the last trimester [22].

Due to vasodilation and subsequent decrease in peripheral vascular resistance, **blood pressure**, including systolic, diastolic, mean arterial and central systolic blood pressure, is decreased [27].

Diastolic blood pressure and mean arterial pressure decrease more than systolic blood pressure. Compared with pre-conception baseline values, arterial pressure drops 5–10 mm Hg between 24 to 26 weeks' gestation. Later on, during the third trimester, it begins to increase and during postpartum period returns close to its pre-conception levels.

In the supine position, femoral venous pressure rises steadily: from 8 mm Hg early in pregnancy to 24 mm Hg at term [12]. The elevated venous pressure can return to normal by the woman lying on her left side.

Blood stagnation in the legs during the last trimester results from occlusion of the pelvic veins and inferior vena cava by the enlarged uterus. Vena cava compression can also diminish venous return and decrease stroke volume and cardiac output. Although most women do not become hypotensive, up to 8% of them do demonstrate occurrences of the supine hypotensive syndrome, manifested by a sudden drop in blood pressure, bradycardia and syncope [22].

The growing uterus displaces the **heart** to the left and upwards and rotated on its long axis. Left atrium diameter and left ventricular end-diastolic diameter increase due to the increased preload. Although multiple cardiovascular parameters are altered during pregnancy, myocardial contractility as well as left and right ventricular ejection fractions do not change.

Heart rate increases progressively throughout the course of pregnancy by 10–20 beats per minute (bpm), reaching a maximum in the third trimester. The overall change in heart rate represents a 20–25% increase above baseline.

Cardiac output increases during pregnancy (Figure 2.1). The sharpest rise in cardiac output occurs in the beginning of the first trimester, with further increase in the second trimester. By 24 weeks' gestation, increase in cardiac output can be up by to 45% in a normal, singleton pregnancy [27]. In a twin pregnancy, cardiac output is higher still, with values approximately 15% higher than in singleton pregnancies.

Increase in stroke volume is responsible for the early increase in cardiac output. During pregnancy, stroke volume increases gradually until the end of the second trimester and then remains constant until shortly after delivery, or decreases slightly late in pregnancy. In the late third trimester, cardiac output is primarily maintained by maternal tachycardia.

2.2.8 Respiratory System

Changes in the respiratory system may be categorized as anatomical and physiological.

Anatomical changes include mucosal oedema, hyperaemia and capillary congestion from the upper airway to the pharynx, false cords, glottis and arytenoids. Decreased pharyngeal lumen diameter and fragility of the upper airway commence in the first trimester and persist to the end of pregnancy. Symptoms of rhinitis and nosebleeds commonly occur due to the effect of oestrogen.

Thoracic subcostal angle increases by about 50% and is mediated by relaxin. As a result, chest diameter increases by up to 2 cm and the thoracic circumference by about 6 cm.

Increased progesterone levels mediate many of the **physiological changes** that occur in the respiratory system. Progesterone relaxes bronchial and tracheal smooth muscle, and directly stimulates the respiratory centre of the medulla to increase respiratory drive (Figure 2.2).

Minute ventilation increases by 30–50%, with the increase primarily due to an approximately 40% increase in **tidal volume** (Figure 2.2) [28].

Functional residual capacity decreases on average by 20% (300–500 mL) due to the elevated diaphragm and decreased chest wall compliance, which is not completely balanced by the increase in the chest wall diameter.

At the same time, a number of respiratory parameters do not change during pregnancy. Total lung capacity, vital capacity, lung compliance and diffusion capacity remain unaffected.

As a result of increased minute ventilation, **maternal arterial partial pressure** of carbon dioxide ($PaCO_2$) decreases to

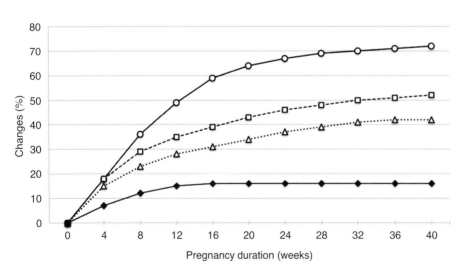

Figure 2.2 Changes in respiratory rate, and alveolar, tidal and minute ventilation during pregnancy (adapted from [28]).

—○— alveolar ventilation --□-- minute ventilation ···△··· tidal ventilation —◆— respiratory rate

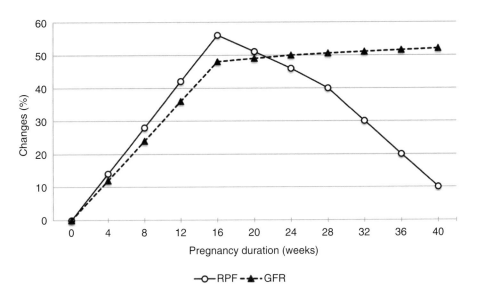

Figure 2.3 Changes in renal plasma flow (RPF) and glomerular filtration rate (GFR) during pregnancy (adapted from [30, 31]).

a level of 26–32 mm Hg. Alveolar oxygen tension increases, with partial pressures of oxygen (PaO_2) in arterial blood rising as high as 106 mm Hg. Oxygen-carrying capacity also increases as total haemoglobin amount increases, while the actual arterial oxygen content gets decreased by the expanded plasma volume. Therefore, oxygen delivery is maintained at normal levels in spite of cardiac output increase, and as such, a pregnant woman is much more dependent on cardiac output for the maintenance of sufficient oxygen delivery than a non-pregnant woman [28].

Hyperventilation facilitates the transfer of carbon dioxide from the fetus to the mother and is partially compensated for by an increased renal secretion of hydrogen ions. A mild chronic respiratory alkalosis is therefore normal in pregnancy, with an **arterial pH** of 7.44, compared to 7.40 in the non-pregnant state [22].

At the same time, bicarbonate excretion by the kidneys increases to compensate for the elevated pH. Thus, the metabolic state of respiratory alkalosis is accompanied with a compensatory metabolic acidosis.

Dyspnoea affects up to 75% of pregnant women. This physiological dyspnoea does not interfere with normal daily activities, and is not associated with exercise, cough, wheezing or other pulmonary symptoms. It typically begins in the first or second trimester and often improves as the pregnancy progresses. Respiratory rate (RR) increases slightly during pregnancy, raising the bar of what is to be considered abnormal tachypnoea to above 20 breaths per minute (Figure 2.2).

2.2.9 Urinary System

Pregnancy affects the anatomy and physiology of the urinary system.

Anatomical changes involve kidneys with their pelvis and calyceal systems, ureters and the bladder. Length of the kidneys increases by 1–1.5 cm during pregnancy, and decreases to its previous value over a period of 6 months postpartum. This growth occurs primarily on account of increased vascular and interstitial space, and secondarily due to mechanical obstruction of the ureters. Hydronephrosis occurs in 43–100% of pregnant women, and is more prevalent during the last trimester [29].

Progesterone can reduce ureteral tone, peristalsis and contraction pressure. The dilated system can hold approximately 200–300 mL of urine, leading to a possible urinary stasis and an asymptomatic bacteriuria. The right ureter is more commonly affected as a result of the angle at which it crosses the iliac and ovarian vessels at its entry into the pelvic space. The elongated ureters often form curves of various radii, with smaller curves possibly sharply angulated.

Maternal hormones cause renal haemodynamic changes in pregnancy [30]. **Renal plasma flow** increases by up to 80% during the first trimester, followed by a plateau, and again decreases later during the last trimester of pregnancy (Figure 2.3) [31]. In the renal circulation itself, relaxin influences endothelin and nitric oxide production. This leads to vasodilation and decreased renal afferent and efferent arteriolar resistance.

Normal pregnancy is marked by an upregulation of the **renin-angiotensin-aldosterone system**. Renin is released from extra-renal sources, specifically the ovaries and decidua. The placenta produces oestrogen, which increases angiotensinogen synthesis by the liver, leading to an increased angiotensin II synthesis. Despite this upregulation, systolic blood pressure decreases during pregnancy due to the presence of progesterone and its influence on vascular muscle relaxation [31].

Glomerular filtration rate (GFR) increases by 50% by the beginning of the second trimester and persists until term, even though renal plasma flow decreases during the last trimester (Figure 2.3). Increased kidney blood flow, decreased oncotic pressure, and changes in glomerular ultrafiltration coefficient (the product of surface area available for filtration and permeability of the filtration membrane) are suggested to be responsible for the increased GFR [29, 32].

Changes in **urinary excretion** of different substances also occur. Urea and creatinine are excreted only by the means of glomerular filtration and as such, their serum levels are significantly reduced during pregnancy. Uric acid clearance can decrease during the last trimester as a result of an increase in tubular reabsorption. A glomerulotubular imbalance leads to mild increases in excretion of vitamins and other nutrients, with proteinuria and aminoaciduria [12].

Glucose excretion increases 10- to 100-fold over its non-pregnant values of about 100 mg/day. Glycosuria is present in about 40% of pregnant women, and occurs in spite of increased plasma insulin and decreased plasma glucose levels. In non-pregnant individuals, approximately 5% of filtered glucose normally escapes reabsorption in proximal convoluted tubules, but is later reabsorbed in the collecting tubules and loops of Henle. In instances of glycosuria, this reabsorption is impaired [22].

2.2.10 Gastrointestinal System

Pregnancy brings anatomical and functional changes to the gastrointestinal system.

Nausea, vomiting and dyspepsia affect the upper gastro-intestinal tract during the first trimester. Later, the enlarging uterus displaces the stomach and may anatomically alter the pressure gradient between the abdomen and thorax. Increased pressure within the stomach promotes reflux of gastric contents into the oesophagus, which lies in the intrathoracic cavity where pressures are negative relative to the abdomen [33]. Additionally, lower oesophageal sphincter tone is decreased due to increased progesterone levels, and symptoms of heartburn may as such increase nearing term.

Both progesterone and increased levels of enzyme histaminase, produced by the placenta, decrease gastric acid output. This lowered acid secretion is coupled with increased protective gastric mucus secretion.

Motility of the stomach, small intestine and colon is decreased. Gastric emptying is slower, and mean small bowel transit time significantly increases each trimester, in relation to elevations in progesterone levels. Together with a concurrent decrease in colon motility, the process contributes to an increased prevalence of symptoms of constipation in late pregnancy [33]. There is also a significant increase in water and sodium absorption secondary to the increased aldosterone levels during pregnancy, leading to reduced stool volume, which contributes to prolonged colonic transit time.

Pregnancy affects biliary motility and cholesterol secretion. Fasting volume and residual volume in the gallbladder are increased, promoting bile stasis. Gallbladder emptying is also impaired due to downregulation of contractile G protein synthesis in gallbladder muscle cells, with stasis progressing during the first 20 weeks of pregnancy.

2.2.11 Skin

Skin changes represent an important part of physiological changes during pregnancy. They are very common and include hyperpigmentation, hair and nail changes, vascular changes and shifts in apocrine and eccrine gland activity [34].

Up to 90% of pregnant women develop increased **pigmentation**, which is typically generalized and mild. This hyperpigmentation is very common in the area of genitals, perineum, neck, axillae, inner thighs, periumbilical skin and areolae. The skin above the midline of the abdomen, the *linea alba*, becomes darkly pigmented to form the *linea nigra*, which extends from the umbilicus to the *symphysis pubis*. *Chloasma gravidarum* is less common and occurs as irregular brownish patches of various sizes on the face and neck.

Although aetiology of hyperpigmentation is not completely known, increased melanogenesis during pregnancy is thought to be the result of increased levels of beta and alpha subunits of melanocyte-stimulating hormone, oestrogen, progesterone and beta-endorphin. The added pigmentation often fades post-partum; however, it is less likely to completely regress to the pre-pregnancy state.

Furthermore, *striae gravidarum* occur in up to 70% of white women, less frequently in black or Asian women, during the second and third trimesters of pregnancy. They are linear atrophic pink-to-violet-coloured bands, most commonly appearing in the areas of maximum skin stretch, such as the thighs, breasts and abdomen. They typically regress to persistent flesh-coloured atrophic bands postpartum. The increase in corticosteroids, oestrogen and relaxin decreases adhesiveness between collagen fibres and promotes formation of ground substance of the extracellular matrix. Collagen and non-sulphated mucopolysaccharide content in the dermis are also increased. From a histological perspective, there is a rupture and retraction of elastic fibres within the reticular dermis [34].

2.3 Immunology of Pregnancy

2.3.1 Allograft Paradigm

First observations of the maternal immune system during pregnancy defined fetus and placenta as semi-allografts (the **allograft paradigm**). Under normal immunological conditions, the fetus should be recognized as foreign to the maternal immune system and as such rejected. Therefore, it was hypothesized that the fetus must somehow escape the maternal immune system altogether [35].

In the 1990s, the allograft paradigm was redefined from maternal-fetal tolerance to **maternal-placental tolerance**, focusing on the interaction between the maternal immune system and the placenta rather than the fetus [36]. Cells from external embryonic trophectoderm directly interact with uterine cells. Placental cells are thus able to avoid rejection by the maternal immune system, and the fetus itself has no direct contact with maternal cells [37].

The maternal immune system interacts, at different stages and under different circumstances, with the invading trophoblast. This active mechanism prevents a maternal response against paternal antigens, and the trophoblast and the maternal immune system can establish a cooperative status. Moreover, interactions between the placenta and maternal immune system create a pregnancy-supportive immunity environment while still being fully capable of defending the mother and fetus against pathogens [38].

2.3.2 Mechanisms of Maternal Immune Response

After redefining the allograft paradigm, maternal immune response to trophoblast was explained through several mechanisms:

- a mechanical barrier effect of the placenta,
- systemic suppression of the maternal immune system during pregnancy,
- a local and systemic cytokine shift from a Th1 to a Th2 profile,
- the absence of 'major histocompatibility complex class I molecules' on trophoblast cells, and
- local immune suppression mediated by the Fas/FasL system [22].

The mechanism of a **barrier effect of the placenta** was challenged by the evidence of bidirectional trafficking across the maternal-fetal interface including migration of maternal cells into the fetus and the presence of fetal cells in maternal circulation.

The idea of **systemic suppression** of maternal immune system during pregnancy was the conventional wisdom for a long time. This mechanism was widely studied, and from an evolutionary point of view, early humans with suppressed immune system would find it very difficult to survive exposed to numerous microorganisms and unsanitary conditions. Analogically, recent studies clearly demonstrate that maternal antiviral immunity is not affected by pregnancy [22].

A local and systemic **cytokine shift** from a Th1 to a Th2 profile is characterized by a unique inflammatory environment.

The first trimester of pregnancy is a pro-inflammatory phase. Implantation, placentation and conceptual mass growth in the first and early second trimester resemble an 'open wound' that requires a strong inflammatory response [37]. The blastocyst has to first break through the epithelial lining in order to implant itself, then damage the endometrial tissue to invade it and finally replace the endothelium and vascular smooth muscle of maternal blood vessels to secure itself an adequate placental-fetal blood supply. All these activities create a 'battleground' of invading, dying and reparatory cells [37].

During the second immunological phase, the placenta, fetus and mother are in a symbiotic relationship, the predominant immunological feature being induction of an anti-inflammatory state.

The last immunological phase of pregnancy prepares the mother for delivery. Parturition is characterized by an influx of immune cells into the myometrium. The pro-inflammatory environment is achieved by renewed inflammation, which also promotes contraction of the uterus [37].

Human leukocyte class I antigens (HLA-A and HLA-B) cannot be detected on the surface of immunologically neutral villous cells, which are in contact with maternal blood at the intervillous interface. Immunologically active extravillous cells, however, which invade the decidua, can express HLA-C, HLA-G and HLA-E class I molecules [22]. HLA-G antigen expression is limited only to cytotrophoblast.

According to the **mechanism of local immune suppression** hypothesis, and the existence of several plausible potential mechanisms for immunological escape of the fetus, immune cells, which specifically recognize paternal alloantigens, are deleted from the maternal immune system. It is presumed that paternal-antigen-recognizing T cells may be deleted by the induction of apoptosis by the Fas/Fas ligand system [22]. Most recently, a subpopulation of T regulatory cells was described, which are able to suppress the actions of alloreactive T cells to promote fetal-paternal immunotolerance.

2.3.3 Immune Cells

Leukocytes act like independent, single-celled organisms and are an important part of the innate immune system. During the first trimester, 70% of decidual leukocytes are natural killer cells, 20–25% are macrophages and 1–2% are dendritic cells. All three cell types infiltrate the decidua and accumulate around the invading trophoblast [22].

Natural killer cells are critical for the development of the placenta by regulating spiral artery formation and controlling the invasion of trophoblast into the endometrium [17]. Despite their close contact with trophoblast, they do not exert cytolytic function against trophoblast cells. They are major regulatory cells, and differ from peripheral blood natural killer cells both in phenotype and in function. They express activating receptors, but fail to produce the full range of cytokines, and do not excrete vascular endothelial and placental growth factors [22].

Macrophages are the predominant population of antigen-presenting cells in the decidua. They are involved in a wide range of activities including implantation, placental development and cervical ripening. At least two major subtypes of macrophages have been characterized: M1 and M2. M1 macrophages are under the influence of pro-inflammatory cytokines. They secrete tumour necrosis factor alpha (TNF-α) and interleukin 12 (IL-12), and participate in the process of inflammation in response to microorganisms. M2 macrophages are involved in tissue repair and inhibition of inflammation. Appropriate removal of dying trophoblast cells prevents the release of paternal antigens that could trigger a maternal immune response against the fetus [22].

At the same time, trophoblastic factors can induce peripheral blood monocyte differentiation into macrophages, which resemble those found in the decidua.

A specific subpopulation of **T regulatory cells** (CD4+/CD25+) is responsible for maintaining a normal immunological self-tolerance by actively suppressing self-reactive lymphocytes. These cells play a critical role also in preventing a maternal immune system response to fetal cells [22].

References

1. McElroy A, Townsend PK. *Medical Anthropology in Ecological Perspective*, 6th ed. Boulder: Westview Press; 2015.

2. Fritz MA, Speroff L. *Clinical Gynecologic Endocrinology and Infertility*, 8th ed. Philadelphia: Wolters Kluwer; 2010.

3. Albrecht ED, Pepe GJ. Placental steroid hormone biosynthesis in primate pregnancy. *Endocr Rev.* 1990;**11**(1):124–50.

4. Bhattacharyya S, Chaudhary J, Das C. Antibodies to hCG inhibit progesterone production from human syncytiotrophoblast cells. *Placenta.* 1992;**13**:135–9.

5. Pepe GJ, Albrecht ED. Actions of placental and fetal adrenal steroid hormones in primate pregnancy. *Endocr Rev.* 1995;**16**(5):608–48.

6. Berkane N, Liere P, Oudinet JP, et al. from pregnancy to preeclampsia: a key role for estrogens. *Endocr Rev.* 2017;**38** (2):123–44.

7. Spellacy WN, Buhi WC, Schram JD, Birk SA, McCreary SA. Control of human chorionic somatomammotropin levels during pregnancy. *Obstet Gynecol.* 1971;**37**:567–73.

8. Handwerger S. Clinical counterpoint: the physiology of placental lactogen in human pregnancy. *Endocr Rev.* 1991;**12** (4):329–36.

9. Glinoer D. The regulation of thyroid function in pregnancy: pathways of endocrine adaptation from physiology to pathology. *Endocr Rev.* 1997;**8**:404–33.

10. Fister P, Gaberscek S, Zaletel K, et al. Thyroid volume changes during pregnancy and after delivery in an iodine-sufficient Republic of Slovenia. *Eur J Obstet Gynecol Reprod Biol.* 2009;**145**(1):45–8.

11. Rigg LA, Lein A, Yen SS. Pattern of increase in circulating prolactin levels during human gestation. *Am J Obstet Gynecol.* 1977;**129**(4):454–6.

12. Cunningham FG, Leveno KJ, Bloom SL, et al. *Williams Obstetrics*, 25th ed. New York: McGraw-Hill Education; 2018.

13. Hicks JB. On the contractions of the uterus throughout pregnancy: their physiological effects and their value in the diagnosis of pregnancy. *Transactions of the Obstetrical Society of London* 1871;**13**:216–31.

14. Garfield RE, Maner WL, Maul H, Saade GR. Use of uterine EMG and cervical LIF in monitoring pregnant patients. *BJOG.* 2005;**112** Suppl 1:103–8.

15. Trojner Bregar A, Lucovnik M, Verdenik I, et al. Uterine electromyography during active phase compared with latent phase of labor at term. *Acta Obstet Gynecol Scand.* 2016;**95**:197–202.

16. Pauerstein CJ, ed. *Clinical Obstetrics.* New York: Churchill Livingstone; 1987.

17. Osol G, Mandala M. Maternal uterine vascular remodeling during pregnancy. *Physiology (Bethesda).* 2009;**24**:58–71.

18. Riordan J, Wmbach K, eds. *Breastfeeding and Human Lactation.* Burlington: Jones & Bartlett Learning; 2010.

19. Lindheimer MD, Davison JM. Osmoregulation, the secretion of arginine vasopressin and its metabolism during pregnancy. *Eur J Endocrinol.* 1995;**132**:133–43.

20. Institute of Medicine, Committee on Nutritional Status During Pregnancy and Lactation. *Nutrition During Pregnancy: Part I: Weight Gain, Part II: Nutrient Supplements.* Washington, DC: The National Academies Press; 1990.

21. Hytten F, Chamberlain G, eds. *Clinical Physiology in Obstetrics.* Oxford: Blackwell Scientific Publications; 1980.

22. Creasy RK, Resnik R, Iams JD, et al. *Creasy and Resnik's Maternal-Fetal Medicine: Principles and Practice.* Philadelphia; Elsevier Saunders: 2014.

23. Fisher AL, Nemeth E. Iron homeostasis during pregnancy. *Am J Clin Nutr.* 2017;**106**(Suppl 6):1567S-74S.

24. Heidemann BH, McClure JH. Changes in maternal physiology during pregnancy. *BJA CEPD Rev.* 2003;**3**:65–8.

25. Hellgren M. Hemostasis during normal pregnancy and puerperium. *Semin Thromb Hemost.* 2003;**29**:125–30.

26. Karlsson O, Jeppsson A, Hellgren M. A longitudinal study of factor XIII activity, fibrinogen concentration, platelet count and clot strength during normal pregnancy. *Thromb Res.* 2014;**134**:750–2.

27. Sanghavi M, Rutherford JD. Cardiovascular physiology of pregnancy. *Circulation.* 2014;**130**:1003–8.

28. Bobrowski RA. Pulmonary physiology in pregnancy. *Clin Obstet Gynecol.* 2010;**53**:285–300.

29. Hussein W, Lafayette RA. Renal function in normal and disordered pregnancy. *Curr Opin Nephrol Hypertens.* 2014;**23**(1):46–53.

30. Odutayo A, Hladunewich M. Obstetric nephrology: renal hemodynamic and metabolic physiology in normal pregnancy. *Clin J Am Soc Nephrol.* 2012;**7**(12):2073–80.

31. Cheung KL, Lafayette RA. Renal physiology of pregnancy. *Adv Chronic Kidney Dis.* 2013;**20**(3):209–14.

32. Roberts M, Lindheimer MD, Davison JM. Altered glomerular permselectivity to neutral dextrans and heteroporous membrane modeling in human pregnancy. *Am J Physiol.* 1996;**270**:F338–43.

33. Vanagunas A, Pandolfino J. Gastrointestinal complications in pregnancy. In Sciarra JJ, ed. *Gynecology and Obstetrics*, CD-ROM ed. Hagerstown: Lippincott Williams & Wilkins; 2004.

34. Tyler KH. Physiological skin changes during pregnancy. *Clin Obstet Gynecol.* 2015;**58**:119–24.

35. Medawar PB. Immunity to homologous grafted skin. iii. the fate of skin homographs transplanted to the brain, to subcutaneous tissue, and to the anterior chamber of the eye. *Br J Exp Pathol.* 1948;**29**(1):58–69.

36. Colbern GT, Main EK. Immunology of the maternal-placental interface in normal pregnancy. *Semin Perinatol.* 1991;**15**(3):196–205.

37. Mor G, Cardenas I. The immune system in pregnancy: a unique complexity. *Am J Reprod Immunol.* 2010;**63**(6):425–33.

38. Racicot K, Kwon JY, Aldo P, Silasi M, Mor G. Understanding the complexity of the immune system during pregnancy. *Am J Reprod Immunol.* 2014;**72**(2):107–16.

Chapter

3

Developmental Abnormalities of the Reproductive System and Their Relevance to Obstetric Practice

Parivakkam S. Arunakumari, Vennila Palaniappan & Richard Haines

3.1 Introduction

3.1.1 Definition

Congenital malformations of the female genital tract are defined as deviations from normal anatomy resulting from embryological maldevelopment of the Mullerian (paramesonephric) ducts [1].

3.1.2 Background

Developmental abnormalities of the reproductive tract span a wide anatomical spectrum, ranging from the almost imperceptible arcuate uterus to the distinctly obvious imperforate hymen. This diversity also extends to the clinical spectrum, ranging from abnormalities which are incidentally diagnosed, as in uterus didelphys, to those associated with classic clinical presentations, as in Mullerian agenesis.

3.1.3 Prevalence

True prevalence is often difficult to ascertain due to differences in diagnostic data acquisition and varied patient populations. Their prevalence in the general female population is thought to be 4–7% and up to 15% in women with recurrent pregnancy loss [1–3].

3.1.4 Causes

Several cellular processes are involved in the development of the normal female reproductive system: cellular division, differentiation, duct elongation, fusion, resorption, canalization and apoptosis [4]. Disruption of any of these complex and intricately linked processes may result in Mullerian duct anomalies.

3.1.5 Genetics

Mullerian duct anomalies may result from genetic mutation – often sporadic, but can be inherited, developmental defects or environmental insults that operate at critical stages of embryonic development. Most Mullerian anomalies are of multifactorial inheritance rather than single gene disorders [5].

3.2 Classification

A classification system serves as a framework for description of anomalies, for categorization of diagnosis, communication between professionals, comparison between treatment modalities and effective standardization of conditions.

Several classification systems have been in use, of which three are popular: American Fertility Society / American Society for Reproductive Medicine (AFS/ASRM), Vagina Cervix Uterus Adnex–associated Malformation (VCUAM) and European Society of Human Reproduction and Embryology / European Society for Gynaecological Endoscopy (ESHRE/ESGE).

3.2.1 AFS/ASRM Classification

The AFS/ASRM classification based on Buttram and Gibbons is still in widespread use [6, 7]. This subdivides uterine malformations into seven major classes. This classification system groups anomalies with similar clinical manifestations, treatment modalities and prognosis for reproductive performance.

3.2.2 VCUAM Classification

The VCUAM classification system is based on the Tumour Node Metastases principle in Oncology [8]. It is intended to focus on the anomalies (e.g. vaginal) not addressed in the ASRM classification.

3.2.3 ESHRE/ESGE Classification

The ESHRE/ESGE classification is a new, updated and more systematic system now known as CONUTA – CONgenital UTerine Anomalies [1, 2]. This system provides a comprehensive description and categorization of almost all of the currently known genital tract anomalies (Figure 3.1).

The general characteristics of this classification system include the following:

- Anatomy is the basis for the systematic categorization of anomalies.
- Deviations of uterine anatomy deriving from the same embryological defect are the basis for the design of the main classes.
- The basis for the main subclasses is the anatomical variations expressing different degrees of uterine deformity and sharing similar clinical significance.
- Cervical and/or vaginal anomalies are classified in independent supplementary subclasses.
- Absolute numbers are not used, in contrast to the ASRM system. For example, uterine deformity is defined as a proportion of the uterine anatomy to allow for the wide interindividual variations in reproductive physiology.

3.3 Uterine Anomalies

As the uterus is the key organ for the design of the ESHRE classes, this will be dealt with first.

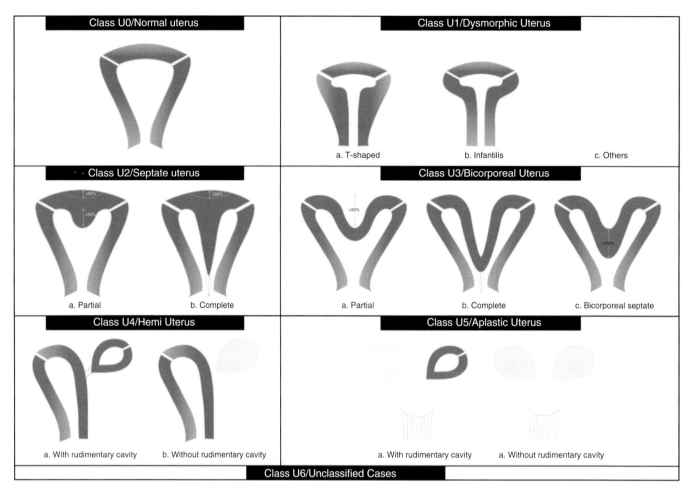

Figure 3.1 ESHRE/ESGE classification of uterine anomalies

	Uterine anomaly		Cervical/vaginal anomaly	
	Main class	*Sub-class*	*Co-existent class*	
U0	Normal uterus		*C0*	*Normal cervix*
U1	Dysmorphic uterus	**a.** T-shaped **b.** Infantilis **c.** Others	*C1*	*Septate cervix*
			C2	*Double 'normal' cervix*
U2	Septate uterus	**a.** Partial **b.** Complete	*C3*	*Unilateral cervical aplasia*
			C4	*Cervical aplasia*
U3	Bicorporeal uterus	**a.** Partial **b.** Complete **c.** Bicorporeal septate	*V0*	*Normal vagina*
U4	Hemi-uterus	**a.** With rudimentary cavity (communicating or not horn) **b.** Without rudimentary cavity (horn without cavity/no horn)	*V1*	*Longitudinal non-obstructing vaginal septum*
			V2	*Longitudinal obstructing vaginal septum*
U5	Aplastic	**a.** With rudimentary cavity (bi- or unilateral horn) **b.** Without rudimentary cavity (bi- or unilateral uterine remnants/aplasia)	*V3*	*Transverse vaginal septum and/or imperforate hymen*
			V4	*Vaginal aplasia*
U6	Unclassified malformations			
U			*C*	*V*

3.3.1 Class U0 – Normal Uterus

Class U0 incorporates all cases with normal uterus. A normal uterus is defined as a uterus with a straight or curved inter-ostial line, but with an internal indentation at the fundal midline not exceeding 50% of the uterine wall thickness. The existence of this normal category gives the opportunity to independently classify cervical and/or vaginal congenital malformations [1].

3.3.2 Class U1 – Dysmorphic Uterus

This class incorporates patients with normal uterine external outline but with an abnormal shape of the uterine cavity excluding septa.

Class U1 is further subdivided in to three categories: these anomalies were included in class VII of the AFS classification – mainly related to diethylstilboestrol (DES) exposure [7].

3.3.3 Class U1a – T-Shaped Uterus

This class is characterized by a narrow uterine cavity due to thickened lateral walls with a correlation of two thirds uterine corpus and one third cervix.

In a T-shaped uterus, the endometrial cavity is T-shaped rather than triangular. It is more common in women exposed in utero to DES and is associated with an increased risk of infertility, recurrent miscarriage and preterm labour and delivery [4].

3.3.3.1 Ultrasound Findings

The exact shape of the endometrial cavity is usually not discernible on a standard two-dimensional (2D) ultrasound. The coronal view of the uterus, usually reconstructed from a three-dimensional (3D) volume ultrasound, is necessary to evaluate this. A normal uterine cavity is triangular or V-shaped, with the three apices being the two cornua and the junction of the lower uterine segment and the cervix (level of internal os). When the uterus is T-shaped, there is a waist in the sides of the triangle such that the corpus of the endometrial cavity is narrowed and takes on the shape of a T rather than a V. The outer myometrial surface of the uterus (the serosal surface) is typically unaffected [9].

3.3.4 Class U1b – Uterus Infantilis

This class is characterized by a narrow uterine cavity without lateral wall thickening and an inverse correlation of one third uterine corpus and two thirds uterine cervix.

By compromising the anatomical integrity of the uterine cavity, this class of congenital anomalies of the uterus is implicated in infertility and pregnancy loss, as they are known to interfere with normal implantation and placentation. Usually dysmorphic uteri are smaller in size [1].

Early data from the Hysteroscopic Outpatient Metroplasty to Expand Dysmorphic Uteri (HOME-DU) technique, wherein incisions are made on the uterine walls with a 5 Fr bipolar electrode, indicate that this a safe and effective technique to expand uterine volume [10].

3.3.5 Class U1c – Arcuate Uterus

This class includes all minor deformities of the uterine cavity including those with an inner indentation at the fundal midline level of <50% of the uterine wall thickness.

ASRM defines arcuate uterus as a uterus where the depth from interostial line to the apex of the indentation is less than 1 cm and the angle of the indentation is >90° [11]. Developmentally, the arcuate uterus can be considered to be at the minor end of the spectrum of failure of Mullerian absorption; it is typically considered a normal variant and therefore functionally not part of the septate spectrum [12].

The arcuate uterus has an external, normal-appearing fundus and a small, smooth indentation at the top of the endometrial cavity.

Arcuate uterus is given a separate category in the AFS classification as, in contrast to other uterine malformations, the arcuate uterus does not cause adverse clinical outcomes. The angle of indentation at the fundal midline to the fundal myometrium is described as obtuse, to differentiate the acute angle of indentation seen with a septate uterus.

The CONUTA classification system does not explicitly mention this, but includes the arcuate uterus as a new subcategory under the general term 'others' in Class 1/ Dysmorphic Uterus, which includes all minor deformities of the endometrial cavity including midline indentations of less than 50% of uterine wall thickness. This is to ensure that septate uterus with a midline indentation of more than 50% of uterine wall thickness remains a separate category.

ASRM also take the view that 'the arcuate uterus should be differentiated from septate uterus for the purposes of prognosis and surgical management'.

Overall, the arcuate uterus represents a variant of a normal rather than a Mullerian anomaly [13]. It is often an incidental finding with no appreciable impact on fertility and pregnancy [14]. Adverse pregnancy outcomes are rare and surgical correction is not warranted.

3.3.6 Septate Uterus: Class U2

3.3.6.1 Definition

Septate uterus is defined as uterus with normal fundal outline and an internal indentation at the fundus in the midline exceeding 50% of the uterine wall thickness [1].

3.3.6.2 Classification

Class U2 is further subdivided in to two subclasses based on the degree of the uterine cavity deformity:

Class U2 a – partial septate uterus is characterized by the existence of a septum dividing the uterine cavity partly above the level of the internal cervical os.

Class U2 b – complete septate uterus is characterized by the existence of a septum fully dividing the uterine cavity up to the level of the internal cervical os.

A complete septate uterus may extend into a duplicated cervix (bicervical septate uterus) or may continue thorough the cervix. The bicervical septate uterus must be distinguished from uterus didelphys, wherein the two uteri are separated externally. Both of these anomalies are typically associated with a longitudinal vaginal septum.

ASRM define a septate uterus as that where the depth from the interostial line to the apex of the internal fundal indentation at the midline exceeds >1.5 cm and the angle of indentation is <90° [11].

3.3.6.3 Prevalence

This is the most common of all the Mullerian anomalies, accounting for over 50% [4]. The true prevalence is difficult to ascertain as many septa are often asymptomatic, but appear to range between 1 to 2 per 1000 to 15 per 1000 females [11].

3.3.6.4 Pathogenesis

A septate uterus results from the normal fusion of the two Mullerian ducts but with abnormal absorption or incomplete resorption of the midline septum, prior to 20th embryogenic week.

The histological structure of the septa ranges from fibrous to fibromuscular tissue. The blood supply to the septum is often markedly reduced compared to that of the normal myometrium. Septal implantation with consequent impaired embryo growth may well explain the pregnancy loss. Distortion of the endometrial cavity and associated cervical and endometrial abnormalities are also thought to contribute to their poor reproductive performance.

3.3.6.5 Clinical Presentation

ASRM summarize the common clinical presentation in their statement: 'Most women with a septate uterus have efficient reproductive function.'

NICE guidance on hysteroscopic metroplasty of a uterine septum for recurrent miscarriage states: 'Uterine septa is more common in women with infertility and in women with repeated miscarriage, and may therefore be one cause of this problem.'

In a meta-analysis of the effect of congenital uterine anomalies on reproductive outcomes, it was evident that septate uterus was the only anomaly that was associated with a significant decrease in the probability of natural conception when compared with controls (Relative Risk 0.86, 95% Confidence Interval 0.77–0.96) [15].

3.3.6.6 Investigation

Hysterosalpingography (HSG) and ultrasound may be suggestive of the diagnosis. Although 2D ultrasound scan can identify the two uterine cavities, it is usually not possible to differentiate between the septate and bicornuate uterus because the outer myometrial contour cannot be visualized in traditional sonographic planes.

In the coronal planes, 3D ultrasound images can be used to measure the intercornual distance, the length of the septum and the depth of the external fundal indentation. ASRM's summary statement on diagnosis with imaging modalities concludes: 'There is fair evidence that 3D ultrasound, sonohysterography and MRI [magnetic resonance imaging] are good diagnostic tests for distinguishing a septate and a bicornuate uterus when compared with laparoscopy and hysteroscopy. (Grade B).'

Hysteroscopic assessment is conclusive in establishing the diagnosis by visualizing a vertical pillar of tissue extending in between the anterior and posterior uterine walls dividing the uterine cavity into two.

ASRM recommend: 'Imaging or Imaging with Hysteroscopy should be used to diagnose uterine septa rather than Laparoscopy with Hysteroscopy because this approach is less invasive.'

Routine evaluation of the renal system is not necessary in patients with uterine septum, as this is an absorption and not a formation defect.

3.3.6.7 Obstetric Significance

It is important to note that many women with uterine septa do not experience any reproductive difficulties.

Septate uterus is generally not thought to increase the rate of preterm labour or caesarean section but is associated with the highest risk of spontaneous miscarriage of all Mullerian anomalies [14]. However, the ASRM guideline on uterine septum summarizes as follows: 'There is fair evidence that a uterine septum contributes to miscarriage and preterm birth (Grade B)' [11, 16].

Early pregnancy loss is significantly more common in septate uterus than a bicornuate uterus. The rate of spontaneous pregnancy loss under 20 weeks is 70% for bicornuate uterus and 88% for septate uterus [6].

Septate uterus can also be associated with intrauterine fetal malformation due to its mechanical effect. ASRM summary statement: 'Some evidence suggests that a uterine septum may increase the risk of other adverse pregnancy outcomes such as malpresentation, intrauterine growth restriction, placental abruption and perinatal mortality (Grade B).'

3.3.6.8 Treatment

ASRM recommend: 'In a patient with infertility, prior pregnancy loss or poor obstetric outcomes it is reasonable to consider uterine septum incision' (Grade C), although 'there is insufficient evidence to recommend a specific method for hysteroscopic septum incision'. 'Commonly used techniques to resect uterine septum include incision or removal of the septum utilizing cold scissors, unipolar or bipolar cautery or laser.'

Abdominal metroplasty (surgical removal of the septum) for septate uterus is now superseded by hysteroscopic resection [17]. Compared to the abdominal approach, hysteroscopic resection reduces the risk of pelvic adhesions, accelerates postoperative convalescence and obviates the mandate for caesarean section.

Hysteroscopic metroplasty is advocated in women with a septate uterus and recurrent second trimester pregnancy loss [18]. The septum is excised until the cavity achieves a normal internal contour. Live birth rates were found to increase from 3% to 80% after surgery whilst the miscarriage rates reduce from 88% to 14% [19]. The operative hysteroscopy can be supplemented with laparoscopic surveillance or ultrasound guidance.

NICE recommends:

1.1 Current evidence on the safety of hysteroscopic metroplasty of a uterine septum for recurrent miscarriage includes some serious but rare complications. Current evidence on efficacy is adequate to support the use of this procedure provided that normal arrangements are in place for clinical governance, consent and audit.

1.2 Patient selection and treatment should be done by a multidisciplinary team including specialists in reproductive medicine, uterine imaging and hysteroscopic surgery.

1.3 Clinicians undertaking hysteroscopic metroplasty of a uterine septum for recurrent miscarriage should be trained in hysteroscopic surgery in accordance with the Royal College of Obstetricians and Gynaecologists training module.

NICE guidance on hysteroscopic metroplasty of uterine septum for primary infertility states: 'Current evidence on efficacy is inadequate in quantity and quality. Therefore, this procedure should only be used with special arrangements for clinical governance, consent and audit or research.'

3.3.7 Bicornuate Uterus – Class U3

3.3.7.1 Definition
A bicorporeal uterus is defined by ESHRE/ESGE as a uterus with an abnormal fundal outline. It is characterized by the presence of an external indentation at the fundal midline exceeding 50% of the uterine wall thickness.

3.3.7.2 Classification
Class U3 is further subdivided into three subclasses based on the degree of uterine corpus deformity:

Class U3a: Partial bicorporeal uterus characterized by an external fundal indentation partly dividing the uterine corpus above the level of the cervix.

Class U3b: Complete bicorporeal uterus characterized by an external fundal indentation completely dividing the uterine corpus up to the level of the cervix.

Class U3c: Bicorporeal septate uterus characterized by the presence of an absorption defect in addition to the main fusion defect. Here the width of the midline fundal indentation exceeds by 150% the uterine wall thickness. As with any other class, these patients could have coexistent cervical and/or vaginal defects.

3.3.7.3 Prevalence
Bicornuate uterus accounts of 10–20% of all Mullerian anomalies [4].

3.3.7.4 Pathogenesis
A bicornuate uterus is caused by the incomplete lateral fusion of the two Mullerian ducts. There is normal fusion at the inferior portion but incomplete fusion at the superior portion of the caudal vertical part of the Mullerian ducts. Typically, there are two separate but communicating endometrial cavities and a single uterine cervix.

Table 3.1 Clinical presentation

Clinical presentation	Bicornuate uterus	Uterus didelphys
Miscarriage rate	36%	32%
Preterm labour	23%	16%
Term deliveries	40%	45%

3.3.7.5 Clinical Presentation
See Table 3.1 for a summation of clinical presentations [20].

3.3.7.6 Investigation
On 3D transvaginal sonography (TVS) and MRI imaging, the fundal contour of the uterus is noted to have a 'cleft' of >1 cm separating the two divergent but typically equal fundal endometrial horns with an endometrial indentation by ASRM criteria of >1.5 cm [21].

Diagnostic differentiation between a septate and a bicornuate uterus cannot be accomplished by hysteroscopy or HSG alone. At laparoscopy, the broad (intercornual distance of wider than 4 cm) and indented fundus with the typical heart-shaped configuration can be observed.

3.3.7.7 Obstetric Significance
The reproductive outcomes of a bicornuate uterus are in general better than that of a unicornuate uterus but worse than uterus didelphys [22]. Uterine dysfunction is thought to occur due to reduced cavity size, impaired ability to distend, abnormal myometrial and cervical functioning, inadequate vascularity and abnormal endometrial development.

Bicornuate uterus has been implicated in miscarriage, preterm labour, malpresentation and low fetal survival rates.

The high rate of preterm labour in bicornuate uteri (20% with partial and 66% with complete bicornuate uterus) [23] has led to bicornuate uterus being proposed as an independent risk factor for cervical os insufficiency. As this has not been validated, however, cervical cerclage can only be recommended in patients with demonstrable evidence of cervical incompetence.

3.3.7.8 Treatment
The bicornuate uterus may require a unification procedure to enhance the size of the uterine cavity if poor reproductive outcomes have been demonstrated [24]. Surgical reconstruction of the bicornuate uterus has been proposed in women with recurrent miscarriage and/or preterm labour. Strassman's technique involves a wedge-shaped incision through the body and the fundus of the uterus to include the myometrium in the midline. The two cavities are then joined to form a single cavity by layered closure of the uterine wall in the vertical plane. Although traditionally undertaken by open laparotomy, this is increasingly being done by the laparoscopic method.

Post-surgery reproductive outcomes have been generally good with a live birth rate of 85%. Delivery is by caesarean section following metroplasty to avoid risk of uterine rupture in labour.

3.3.8 Uterus Didelphys

3.3.8.1 Prevalence

Uterus didelphys accounts for approximately 11% of all the Mullerian anomalies.

3.3.8.2 Pathogenesis

Uterus didelphys results when there is failed fusion of the paired Mullerian ducts. It is characterized by the presence of two non-communicating endometrial cavities, each with a uterine cervix. There is no obstructive element in this Mullerian anomaly.

Seventy-five per cent of these patients also have a longitudinal vaginal septum.

3.3.8.3 Diagnosis

Ultrasonography (USG), 3D and MRI imaging all provide adequate information on the existence of the two endometrial cavities, two cervices and two fundal contours. Hysterosalpingogram may exclude the communication between the two endometrial cavities.

3.3.8.4 Obstetric Significance

The specific miscarriage rate for uterus didelphys is not dissimilar to women with normal uterine cavities. Thus, surgery is rarely indicated. Of all the major uterine malformations, uterus didelphys has the best reproductive prognosis.

3.3.9 OHVIRA

3.3.9.1 Definition

OHVIRA (obstructed hemivagina with ipsilateral renal agenesis) is a combination of uterine anomalies (uterus didelphys or septate uterus) associated with a hemivagina and ipsilateral renal anomalies.

Herlyn–Werner–Wunderlich syndrome is a constellation of uterus didelphys and obstructed hemivagina with ipsilateral renal anomalies.

3.3.9.2 Clinical Features

The classic presentation is progressively worsening severe dysmenorrhoea not responsive to nonsteroidal anti-inflammatory drugs (NSAIDs) against the background of regular, cyclical periods from the non-obstructed tract. On bimanual examination, a mass is felt bulging from the lateral wall of the vagina towards the midline.

3.3.9.3 Diagnosis

Ultrasound is invaluable in providing information on the anatomy of both the genital and urinary tracts. It is important to be aware of the potentially confusing picture on ultrasound of the obstructed haematocolpos which will be found below the non-obstructed cervix. The non-obstructed cervix may not be seen or felt if the vagina is greatly distorted from its contralateral obstruction.

3.3.9.4 Treatment

Where the hemivagina is obstructed by an oblique or transverse vaginal septum, surgical resection of the wall of the obstructed hemivagina is necessary to relieve the obstruction and to allow free drainage of menstrual flow.

3.3.10 Unicornuate Uterus – Class U4

3.3.10.1 Definition

Hemi-uterus is defined as unilateral uterine development. The contralateral part could be either incompletely formed or absent.

3.3.10.2 Classification

Class U4 incorporates all cases of unilaterally formed uterus. This is a different class to that of the aplastic uterus due to the existence of a fully developed functional uterine hemicavity.

Class U4 is further subdivided in to two subclasses depending on the presence or absence of a functional rudimentary cavity:

Class U4a: Hemi-uterus with a rudimentary functional cavity characterized by the presence of a communicating or non-communicating functional contralateral horn.

Class U4b: Hemi-uterus without rudimentary functional cavity characterized either by the presence of non-functional contralateral uterine horn or by aplasia of the contralateral part.

3.3.10.3 Prevalence

There is a prevalence of 0.1% in the general population.

3.3.10.4 Pathogenesis

Arrested or defective development of only one of the Mullerian ducts results in a unicornuate uterus – this is a formation defect.

Sixty-five per cent of unicornuate uteri have an associated uterine horn. Two thirds of rudimentary horns are non-communicating.

Thirty to forty per cent of unicornuate uteri are associated with renal anomalies.

3.3.10.5 Clinical Presentation

Unicornuate uterus is often asymptomatic and discovered during the course of an infertility evaluation.

Women with unicornuate uterus have an increased incidence of infertility, endometriosis and dysmenorrhoea from retrograde menstruation.

Cyclical abdominal pain / pelvic pain can occur when the hemi-uterus has a non-communicating rudimentary horn due to obstruction to the menstrual outflow. However, there is no pelvic mass, as there is no distension of the upper vagina.

Unicornuate uterus should be suspected in women with poor reproductive performance.

On bimanual examination the uterus is often markedly deviated to one side.

3.3.10.6 Investigation

Unicornuate uterus can be suspected on 2D ultrasound with a small uterine volume and presence of a single tubal ostium.

Three-dimensional ultrasound or MRI is invaluable in identifying rudimentary horn and in particular determining the presence / absence of a cavity and/or functional endometrial tissue. HSG typically shows a banana-shaped uterine cavity with a single tube.

Laparoscopy is not necessary to confirm the diagnosis, but is essential to remove the obstructed non-communicating rudimentary uterine horn and diagnosis and management of associated endometriosis.

3.3.10.7 Obstetric Significance

There is a significant impairment of the reproductive performance of the unicornuate uterus with the fetal survival rate of about 29%. Compromised myometrial function and reduced endometrial capacity do not allow adequate gestational growth. Further, congenital alterations in the uterine artery blood flow are also thought to mediate the uterine and placental growth disturbances.

3.3.10.8 Treatment

Pregnancy in the rudimentary horn is not compatible with term gestation. Rupture tends to occur at a later gestation (prior to 20 weeks) than with ectopic pregnancy, and the intraperitoneal haemorrhage tends to be severe. The risk of serious maternal morbidity justifies the need for excision of the cavitary rudimentary horn. This is often logically combined with a salpingectomy on the same side of the rudimentary horn to prevent ectopic pregnancy. However, if the rudimentary horn is non-cavitary, routine laparoscopic excision cannot be justified.

The presence of a functional cavity in the contralateral horn is the factor with the greatest clinical relevance, due to complications such as haematocavity and ectopic pregnancy in the rudimentary horn. In this situation, laparoscopic excision is recommended even if the horn is communicating.

3.3.11 Class U5 – MRKH

3.3.11.1 Introduction

Class U5 or aplastic uterus incorporates all cases of uterine aplasia.

It is a formation defect characterized by the absence of any fully or unilaterally developed uterine cavity.

This group belongs to class I of the AFS classification.

3.3.11.2 Classification

Class U5 is further subdivided into two subclasses depending on the presence or absence of a functional cavity in an existent rudimentary horn:

Class U5a: Aplastic uterus with a rudimentary cavity in a unilateral or bilateral functional horn.

Class U5b: Aplastic uterus without rudimentary cavity characterized either by the presence of uterine remnants or by complete uterine aplasia.

Mayer–Rokitansky–Küster–Hauser (MRKH) syndrome, also known as Mullerian agenesis, is one of the most common disorders of sexual development with an incidence is 1 in 4500 to 5000 female births [5].

3.3.11.3 Types of MRKH Syndrome

The MRKH syndrome exists as three types:

Typical MRKH with no other genital malformation = 55% of cases

Atypical associated with urinary tract malformation = 26%

MURCS (Mullerian aplasia, renal aplasia and cervicothoracic somite dysplasia) associated with urinary and skeletal abnormalities = 13% [5]

3.3.11.4 Pathogenesis

Arrested development of the Mullerian ducts and their failed fusion leads to the MRKH syndrome. The ovaries are spared and develop normally in MRKH syndrome due to their separate embryological non-Mullerian origin.

3.3.11.5 Clinical Presentation

Typical presentation of MRKH syndrome is primary amenorrhoea, defined as absence of menstruation in normally developed 13- to 14-year-old girls. In 2–7% of patients with Mullerian agenesis, cyclical recurrent lower abdominal pain develops due to active endometrium in the rudimentary uterine bulbs.

Physical examination reveals a normal vulva, except that the area where the vaginal introitus should be shows no opening.

A small dimple or a short vagina may be seen. A rectal examination may be helpful to ascertain the presence of midline structures – uterus, cervix and vagina.

3.3.11.6 Clinical Features

The classical clinical features are the following:

1. Absence of functioning uterus. However, 90% of patients have rudimentary uterine bulb without endometrial activity.
2. Short or absent vagina: shallow vaginal pouch only about 2 cm deep.
3. Normal secondary sexual characteristics.
4. Normal appearance of external genitalia except for absent vaginal introitus.
5. Normal ovarian function (normal gonatotropins, normal serum oestrogen and testosterone levels).
6. Normal female karyotype: 46XX.

3.3.11.7 Investigations

A transabdominal or transrectal ultrasound of the abdomen and pelvis will help to confirm the absence of uterus. It should be acknowledged the ultrasound scan may not confidently pick up the rudimentary horn. The difficulty in identifying a small uterus on ultrasound should not be underestimated.

Three-dimensional ultrasound or MRI may be helpful to identify functional endometrium in rudimentary uterine bulbs. Assessment of the renal and urinary tracts should not be overlooked.

Laparoscopy is not necessary for the diagnosis of Mullerian agenesis, but may be indicated for the treatment of associated endometriosis or for the excision of rudimentary uterine horns.

3.3.11.8 Treatment

Management of MRKH involves attention to three aspects: psychological, sexual and reproductive.

Care is best delivered through a multidisciplinary team (MDT) consisting of paediatric and adolescent gynaecologist, nurse specialist, psychologist, fertility specialist and radiologist.

Psychosexual

The diagnosis of MRKH can be devastating to both the patient and her parents. It is important that the healthcare team acknowledges this and offers adequate ongoing support. The prospect of not having a vagina and no reproductive ability can be profoundly distressing. Psychological support is strongly recommended from the time of diagnosis and should precede all other treatments.

Counselling groups of patients rather than individual counselling may help dispel the feeling of 'being like a freak'.

Neovagina Creation

The timing of treatment is determined by the patient in conjunction with her sexual partner, family and the MDT following thorough counselling. Strong motivation and a positive attitude are prerequisites for success. Neovagina creation can be nonsurgical through vaginal dilators or through surgical procedures.

Nonsurgical Method

The ACOG recommends nonsurgical vaginal dilators as first choice as it is simple, safe, effective and patient driven with a success rate of about 85% [25].

The technique (Frank method) involves the use of glass, Perspex, plastic or silicon vaginal dilators to exert continuous pressure against the vaginal dimple towards the sacrum to progressively invaginate the vaginal dimple to create a canal of 'adequate' size of about 6 cm. This is done for about 20–60 minutes per day. It takes between 2 months and 2 years to create a functional vagina, depending on patient motivation and frequency of dilation. The Ingram modification involves the use of a bicycle seat mounted on a stool with the dilator on the saddle of the bicycle seat, on which the patient sits astride.

Surgery

Vaginoplasty can be offered if vaginal dilator therapy fails, but only after the patient consents and commits to regular, frequent and scheduled postoperative dilation, as all the surgical procedures require ongoing vaginal dilators to avoid vaginal stricture.

McIndoe's vaginoplasty uses a split-thickness skin graft taken from the buttock to line the surgically created space.

Williams vulvovaginoplasty involves the creation of a neovagina space between the urethra, bladder and rectum. A modification of Williams technique involves the use of absorbable sutures for both skin layers rather than the chromic catgut used in Williams technique. A further layer of sutures is used to approximate the subcutaneous fat and perineal muscles. This is a simple, quick and effective method for the treatment of vaginal agenesis with a success rate of about 90%.

Techniques involving the use of human amnion, peritoneum, ileum, sigmoid, buccal mucosa and artificial dermis as neovaginal linings have been described, but are not in mainstream use.

The Vecchietti procedure involves a flexiglass olive placed in the vaginal dimple, with two sutures placed through the olive being brought out through the potential neovaginal space, through the pelvic cavity and out through the abdominal wall. The sutures are progressively tightened to rapidly create the neovaginal space over 1 week.

The Davydov method uses the pelvic peritoneum to create a functioning vagina laparoscopically.

Where the presence of rudimentary uterine bulbs become symptomatic, laparoscopic excision of these is often required.

3.3.11.9 Obstetric Significance

Patients with MRKH syndrome have no functioning uterine tissue and therefore traditional conception is impossible. Option for motherhood is restricted to gestational surrogacy (which involves oocyte retrieval, in vitro fertilization (IVF) and blastocyst implantation in a surrogate mother) or adoption.

Uterine transplantation is currently in the research phase but holds potential to become a mainstream operation with five live births being currently reported [26].

3.4 Cervical Anomalies

Cervical anomalies often occur along with uterine and/or vaginal anomalies and very rarely in isolation.

The ESHRE/ESGE subclasses are as below:

Subclass C0: Normal cervix – incorporates all cases of normal cervical development.

Subclass C1: Septate cervix – incorporates all cases of cervical absorption defects, characterized by the presence of a normal externally rounded cervix with the presence of a septum.

Subclass C2: Double cervix – incorporates all cases of cervical fusion defects. It is characterized by the presence of two externally rounded cervices, which could be either fully divided or partially fused.

Subclass C3: Unilateral cervical aplasia – incorporates all cases of unilateral cervical formation. It is characterized by unilateral cervical development: the contralateral part is incompletely formed or absent.

Subclass C4: Cervical aplasia – incorporates all cases of complete cervical aplasia and those with severe cervical formation defects. It is characterized by the absolute absence of any cervical tissue or the presence of severely defective cervical tissue such as cervical cord or cervical fragmentation.

Of these, only cervical aplasia has significant clinical and obstetric significance – hence it is discussed below.

3.4.1 Cervical Agenesis

3.4.1.1 Definition

Cervical aplasia is a very rare condition in which a functional uterus exists without a cervix causing outflow obstruction.

3.4.1.2 Pathogenesis

Typically, the upper vagina is also not developed due to common embryological origin of both the cervix and the upper vagina from the Mullerian duct. There is usually a single midline uterus, although hemi-uterus or septate uterus have also been described.

3.4.1.3 Presentation

Typical presentation is usually with primary amenorrhoea, cyclical abdominal pain or pelvic pain and/or distended uterus – typical of an obstructed anomaly. Endometriosis is common due to retrograde menstruation incumbent on the obstruction.

3.4.1.4 Investigation

Diagnosis is by 2D or 3D ultrasound or MRI, which confirms the presence of a uterine corpus and an absence of the uterine cervix.

3.4.1.5 Treatment

Traditionally, hysterectomy with removal of the obstructed uterus has been recommended, as attempts at surgical reconstruction of the cervix have not been successful. The creation of a uterovaginal fistulous tract has been attempted despite the serious risk of ascending infection with sepsis. Successful pregnancies have been achieved with ZIFT (zygote intrafallopian transfer) following these surgeries. The most important factor determining the management is the amount of cervical tissue present. If the internal os is present, then the prognosis is more optimistic.

Current strategy is to manage the adolescent girl with cervical agenesis with long-term hormonal suppression with either the combined hormonal contraception or gonatotropin-releasing hormone (Gn-RH) analogue with addback hormone replacement therapy (HRT), until she is ready to embark on assisted reproductive techniques (ARTs) and planned caesarean section for delivery.

3.5 Vaginal Anomalies

ESHRE/ESGE classifies vaginal abnormalities as

Subclass V0: Normal vagina – incorporates all cases of normal vaginal development.

Subclass V1: Longitudinal nonobstructing vaginal septum.

Subclass V2: Longitudinal obstructing vaginal septum.

Subclass V3: Transverse vaginal septum and/or imperforate hymen.

Subclass V4: Vaginal aplasia – incorporates all cases of complete or partial vaginal agenesis.

3.5.1 Transverse Vaginal Septum (TVS)

3.5.1.1 Prevalence

TVS is a rare congenital anomaly with an incidence of 1 in 20 000 females.

3.5.1.2 Pathogenesis

TVS is a vertical fusion defect that results from the failure of the sinovaginal bulbs (from the urogenital sinus) and uterovaginal canal (from the Mullerian ducts) to meet or canalize. TVS can be located in three levels – low, middle, high – in the vagina.

Rock et al described 46% of the TVS to be in the upper vagina, 40% in the middle and 14% in the lower third of the vagina. The thickness of the septum is also variable, ranging from 1 cm to 6 cm. In contrast to other Mullerian anomalies, TVS is often not associated with urological anomalies [24].

3.5.1.3 Clinical Presentation

TVS can present as mucocolpos in a neonate or infant.

Adolescent girls can present with gradually worsening cyclical abdominal pain and primary amenorrhoea with slowly expanding central pelvic mass. The higher the septum is, the shorter the time from menarche to presentation due to reduced capacity of the small upper vagina. Endometriosis often develops, causing chronic pelvic pain.

Examination often reveals a normal vulva and external genitalia. The higher the septum is, the more the lower part of the vagina has formed and therefore more likely that the high TVS will be missed. The low TVS can be often be seen beyond the introitus. This differs from an imperforate hymen in that the membrane of the TVS is thicker and does not transilluminate. A rectal examination may be helpful to palpate the midline structures and thereby differentiate from vaginal agenesis.

3.5.1.4 Diagnosis

Ultrasound or MRI will help to define the level and the thickness of the septum. In addition, imaging will provide information on the presence or absence of the cervix, thereby differentiating a high TVS from cervical agenesis with vastly different management strategies.

3.5.1.5 Treatment

Surgical management depends on the distance from the hymen to the obstruction. In general, the higher the septum the more difficult it is to reconstruct a functioning vagina.

TVS in the lower one third can be incised transversely, septum excised, vagina advanced and end-to-end anastomosis undertaken. Garcia's Z plasty technique is useful for a thick TVS to minimize the tension between the opposing ends of the vagina and minimize circumferential scar formation. Ongoing postoperative vaginal dilators are essential to avoid vaginal stenosis. Mid- and upper vagina TVS requires complex surgeries with abdominoperineal approach with creation of neovagina through split skin grafts over vaginal moulds [2]. Interdigitating Y-plasty without the need for excision of the septal tissues has recently been described with good results.

3.5.1.6 Obstetric Significance

Pregnancy outcomes for the lower thin TVS are generally good. High, thick TVS requiring complex reconstructive surgery are often associated with long-term complications and poor pregnancy outcomes. Gynaecological problems also arise from endometriosis from retrograde menstruation and adhesions impairing fertility.

3.5.2 Longitudinal Vaginal Septum (LVS)

3.5.2.1 Pathogenesis

LVS results from the defective lateral fusion and incomplete resorption of paired Mullerian ducts. LVS is often associated with uterus didelphys.

3.5.2.2 Clinical Presentation

Women with LVS often do not encounter any difficulty but may complain of

1. difficulty with tampon insertion
2. failure to contain menstrual efflux despite tampon use
3. difficulty with sexual intercourse
4. difficulty with vaginal delivery and childbirth

3.5.2.3 Treatment

Incidental diagnosis of LVS does not require surgical intervention unless the patient complains of symptoms attributable to HVS.

Excision of LVS can be accompanied by the wedge resection to ensure no ridge remains. Care must be taken to ensure an adequate pedicle and good haemostasis. The septum must be excised in its entirety to the point where both cervices are clearly seen entering the vagina.

3.5.3 Imperforate Hymen

3.5.3.1 Prevalence

Imperforate hymen occurs in approximately 1 in 2000 females [22].

Although usually sporadic, clustering in family members has been reported. It is the most common congenital obstructive genital tract abnormality.

3.5.3.2 Pathogenesis

The hymen is the vestigial remnant of the junction between the sinovaginal bulb and the urogenital sinus. Patency is usually established in fetal life. Imperforate hymen is due to the failure of the inferior end of the vaginal plates to canalize.

3.5.3.3 Clinical Presentation

As in all forms of obstructive outflow disorders, acute urinary retention may be the presenting clinical symptom, caused by the obstruction of the urethra by the haematocolpos. In the neonate this could present as hydro- or mucocolpos. In the adolescent, typical presentation is with cryptomenorrhoea (menstrual symptoms without the efflux of menstrual blood) – cyclical abdominal / pelvic pain, primary amenorrhoea but with normal secondary sexual characteristics.

Examination reveals a bulging, bluish, thin membrane which transilluminates with retained menstrual blood.

3.5.3.4 Diagnosis

Ultrasound is often sufficient to confirm the diagnosis. Routine assessment of the renal tract is not necessary, as the hymen is not of Mullerian origin.

3.5.3.5 Management

Aspiration should be avoided, as this does not provide adequate drainage but only exposes the haematocolpos to associated infection.

The traditional method of a cruciate incision is no longer recommended, as it tends to close up. An elliptical or circumferential incision is made close to the hymenal ring to remove the hymen to allow adequate drainage [27].

3.5.3.6 Obstetric Significance

The fertility potential of patients with imperforate hymen is probably normal, as these patients present early facilitating prompt diagnosis and complete curative treatment.

References

1. Grimbizis GF, Gordts S, Di Spiezio Sardo A, et al. The ESHRE/ESGE consensus on the classification of female genital tract congenital anomalies. *Hum Reprod.* 2013;**28** (8):2032–44.

2. Grimbizis GF, Di Spiezio Sardo A, Saravelos SH, et al. The Thessaloniki ESHRE/ESGE consensus on diagnosis of female genital anomalies. *Hum Reprod.* 2016;**31**(1):2–7.

3. Chan YY, Jayaprakasan K, Zamora J, et al. The prevalence of congenital uterine anomalies in unselected and high-risk populations: a systematic review. *Hum Reprod Update.* 2011;**17** (6):761–71.

4. Kliegman R, Stanton B, St. Geme J, Schor NF, Nelson WE. *Nelson Textbook of Pediatrics*, 20th ed. Philadelphia: Elsevier Health Sciences; 2015.

5. Creighton S, Balen A, Breech L. *Pediatric and Adolescent Gynecology: A Problem-Based Approach*. Cambridge: Cambridge University Press; 2018.

6. Buttram VC, Jr., Gibbons WE. Mullerian anomalies: a proposed classification. (An analysis of 144 cases). *Fertil Steril.* 1979;**32**(1):40–6.

7. The American Fertility Society classifications of adnexal adhesions, distal tubal occlusion, tubal occlusion secondary to tubal ligation, tubal pregnancies, Mullerian anomalies and intrauterine adhesions. *Fertil Steril.* 1988;**49**(6):944–55.

8. Oppelt P, Renner SP, Brucker S, et al. The VCUAM (Vagina Cervix Uterus Adnex-associated Malformation) classification: a new classification for genital malformations. *Fertil Steril.* 2005;**84**(5):1493–7.

9. Benacerraf BR, Goldstein SR, Groszmann YS. T-shaped uterus. In *Gynecologic Ultrasound: A Problem-*

Based Approach. Philadelphia: Elsevier Saunders; 2014. pp. 189–91.

10. Di Spiezio Sardo A, Florio P, Nazzaro G, et al. Hysteroscopic outpatient metroplasty to expand dysmorphic uteri (HOME-DU technique): a pilot study. *Reprod Biomed Online.* 2015;30(2):166–74.

11. Pfeifer S, Butts S, Dumesic D, et al. Uterine septum: a guideline. *Fertil Steril.* 2016;106(3):530–40.

12. Surrey ES, Katz-Jaffe M, Surrey RL, et al. Arcuate uterus: is there an impact on in vitro fertilization outcomes after euploid embryo transfer? *Fertil Steril.* 2018;109(4):638–43.

13. Donnez J. Arcuate uterus: a legitimate pathological entity? *Fertil Steril.* 2018;109(4):610.

14. Tomaževič T, Ban-Frangež H, Virant-Klun I, et al. Septate, subseptate and arcuate uterus decrease pregnancy and live birth rates in IVF/ICSI. *Reprod Biomed Online.* 2010;21(5):700–5.

15. Chan YY, Jayaprakasan K, Tan A, et al. Reproductive outcomes in women with congenital uterine anomalies: a systematic review. *Ultrasound Obstet Gynecol.* 2011;38(4):371–82.

16. Tomaževič T, Ban-Frangež H, Ribič-Pucelj M, Premru-Sršen T, Verdenik I. Small uterine septum is an important risk variable for preterm birth. *Eur J Obstet Gynecol Reprod Biol.* 2007;135(2):154–7.

17. Khalifa E, Toner JP, Jones HW, Jr. The role of abdominal metroplasty in the era of operative hysteroscopy. *Surg Gynecol Obstet.* 1993;176(3):208–12.

18. Pabuçcu R, Gomel V. Reproductive outcome after hysteroscopic metroplasty in women with septate uterus and otherwise unexplained infertility. *Fertil Steril.* 2004;81(6):1675–8.

19. Homer HA, Li TC, Cooke ID, Bontis JN, Devroey P. The septate uterus: a review of management and reproductive outcome. *Fertil Steril.* 2000; 73:1–14.

20. Grimbizis GF, Camus M, Tarlatzis BC, Bontis JN, Devroey P. Clinical implications of uterine malformations and hysteroscopic treatment results. *Hum Reprod Update.* 2001;7(2):161–74.

21. Deutch TD, Bocca S, Oehninger S, Stadtmauer L, Abuhamad AZ. P-465: Magnetic Resonance Imaging versus three dimensional transvaginal ultrasound for the diagnosis of Mullerian anomalies. *Fertil Steril.* 2006;86(3):S308.

22. Venetis CA, Papadopoulos SP, Campo R, et al. Clinical implications of congenital uterine anomalies: a meta-analysis of comparative studies. *Reprod Biomed Online.* 2014;29(6):665–83.

23. Schorge JO, Williams JW. *Williams Gynecology.* New York; London: McGraw-Hill Medical; McGraw-Hill [distributor]; 2008.

24. Rock JA, Thompson JD, Linde RWt. *Te Linde's Operative Gynecology.* Philadelphia: Lippincott Williams & Wilkins; 1997.

25. American College of Obstetricians and Gynecologists. ACOG committee opinion. Nonsurgical diagnosis and management of vaginal agenesis. Number 274, July 2002. Committee on Adolescent Health Care. American College of Obstetrics and Gynecology. *Int J Gynaecol Obstet.* 2002;79(2):167–70.

26. Brannstrom M. Uterus transplantation. *Curr Opin Organ Transplant.* 2015;20(6):621–8.

27. Emans SJH, Laufer MR. *Emans, Laufer, Goldstein's Pediatric & Adolescent Gynecology.* Philadelphia: Lippincott Williams & Wilkins; 2012.

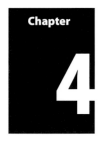

Pharmacology and Pharmacokinetics in Obstetric Practice

Charles Savona-Ventura & Yvonne Savona-Ventura

4.1 Introduction

Pharmaceutical agents have become an essential tool in the medical armamentarium. Pharmaceutical companies over the past century not only have developed more consistently effective agents that are used to manage acute-onset conditions, but also have improved the quality of life of those suffering from chronic progressive disease. The use of any medication must be tempered by its potential side effects. Thus, the clinician must assess the benefit-risk ratio between therapeutic efficacy and safety risks before resorting to any therapeutic intervention in any patient. The benefit-risk assessment (BRA) is made on the weight of randomized evidence obtained from formal clinical trials and observations collected from pharmacovigilance activities after the drug is put on the market [1]. In obstetric practice, the benefit-risk ratio assessment for a pharmaceutical agent must further consider the specific benefit-risk ratio assessment relevant to the developing fetus. The fetal risk assessment presented by a particular agent may not be immediately possible since adverse effects may not be specific and easily linked to the agent, or may present themselves later on in life.

The realization that chemical substances could have an adverse effect on the developing fetus came in the wake of the thalidomide experience in the late 1950s and early 1960s. Thalidomide, administered as an antiemetic to treat morning sickness in pregnant women, was found to be causing severe birth defects giving rise to what has been termed the thalidomide embryopathy or syndrome involving the skeleton and soft tissue organs including heart, kidney and gastrointestinal tract [2]. The administration time-determined effects of thalidomide were demonstrated in the original published observations by E. Nowack in 1965. The word *teratogenesis* originates from the Greek word for monster, *teratos*, thus implying the creation of monsters, notably referring to the birth of infants with structural abnormalities. There has since been increasing realization that the process can result in a whole range of effects including early pregnancy loss, intrauterine deaths, abnormal growth patterns and effects on mental development and adult-onset effects such as late-onset carcinogenesis, infertility [3] and metabolic disease.

During pregnancy, pharmaceutical agents may be used to manage a number of clinical situations. During the antenatal period, medications may be prescribed prophylactically to prevent potential problems from developing with advancing pregnancy (e.g. haematological supplementation to prevent development of anaemia), or to manage pregnancy-related disorders (e.g. managing pregnancy-induced hypertension), or to treat associated acute or chronic medical conditions coincidental to the pregnancy (e.g. managing urinary tract infections, epilepsy or thyroid disease). It is imperative that any woman on medication for any condition should consult her healthcare professional to review the medication profile before she embarks on a pregnancy. Timely pre-conceptional counselling would allow for a careful review of the medication being taken by the woman and provide the opportunity to alter these to safer options. Combined polypharmacy should be avoided. Prescriptions should be targeted specifically to deal with the medical condition being addressed. Multivitamin preparation formulations, especially those directed at general use, may include a significant dose of vitamin A that itself alone can act as a teratotoxic agent on the fetus.

Medications may further be administered to the mother with the aim of directly affecting the developing fetus (e.g. folic acid administration to reduce risk of neural tube defects or the administration of dexamethasone to promote lung surfactant production). Pre-conceptional care is also an opportunity to promote the use of folic acid supplementation at a dose of 0.4–1.0 mg daily which has been proven to decrease or minimize specific birth defects, particularly neural tube defects (NTD). Women known to be at intermediate-high risk for neural tube defects should be prescribed higher folic acid doses of 4.0–5.0 mg daily, provided these women have been shown not to suffer from vitamin B12 deficiency. Women at high risk of neural tube defects include those with a family or personal previous history of an NTD-pregnancy or insulin-dependent diabetes, and those women receiving medication that is a folate antagonist such as anti-epileptic medication, e.g. valproic acid or carbamazepine [4]. Pre-conceptional advice should also include advice about nutrition with an emphasis on partaking of food items with a high antioxidant content to decrease the effect of oxidative stress known to act as a teratotoxic agent [5].

Medications in the first trimester of pregnancy may be partaken to support the pregnancy or to manage a condition or distressing symptomatology that crops up during the pregnancy. The increasing use of reproductive technology has introduced an element of medicalization of pregnancy with attempts to support the early pregnancy state, a process that has extended to the management of recurrent pregnancy loss. These women are very often managed empirically using a combination of anticoagulation, progesterone supplementation and immunomodulatory treatments [6, 7]. Such prescriptions must be tempered with an awareness of the potential teratotoxicity that this polypharmacy may contribute to and the knowledge that teratotoxicity may demonstrate itself in later years. One must bear in mind the past experience of the antenatal use of diethylstilboestrol (DES) in the management of miscarriages and the eventual development of vaginal adenosis-adenocarcinoma and primary infertility in the offspring. The thalidomide experience resulting from an attempt to manage the 'normal' nausea and vomiting of pregnancy must also temper any attempts at managing non-life-threatening symptomatology during early pregnancy. Any medications used during pregnancy should be restricted to those formulations that experience has shown to be non-teratotoxic. These should be used in isolation, for the shortest period of time, and in the lowest dose possible.

Medications may also be administered to the mother during parturition (e.g. oxytocin to augment labour and delivery) and after delivery during lactation (e.g. postoperative antibiotics or postoperative anticoagulation prophylaxis). The administration of any medication to the pregnant or lactating mother will have corresponding pharmacological effects on the developing fetus in utero or on the neonate. The pharmacological effects on the child will replicate those experienced by the mother, but the drug can also have other potentially adverse inadvertent teratogenic effects depending on the stage of fetal development at which the drug exposure takes place.

4.2 Placental Transfer Mechanisms

Fetal development can be broadly viewed into three main phases. The first phase, lasting from conception up to day 16 of development, is that referred to as the *germinal period* when blastogenesis is taking place. Implantation of the blastocyst into the secretory endometrium starts at day 6, the process taking a few days to complete. Implantation initiates the development of the placenta, which starts to function from the fifth week onwards. During the pre-implantation phase, the energy required for cellular reproduction is provided by the secretions from the fallopian tube cells and endometrial glands. Energy metabolism is, at this stage, an aerobic form of metabolism based on oxidizable energy-providing substrates such as non-essential amino acids, pyruvate and glutamine obtained by diffusion following the principles of cell membrane transfer. Once implantation takes place, the nutritional demands of the zygote are met with by substances obtained from the maternal circulation. Energy metabolism now shifts to one primarily based on aerobic glycolysis and oxidative metabolism. Glucose and essential amino acids thus become increasingly more important [8].

In animal studies, alterations in the biochemical *milieu interieur* of the developing zygote during blastogenesis caused by metabolic disturbances such as diabetes mellitus has shown to predispose towards zygote damage and a higher risk of resorption of the developing zygotes. Similarly, exposure to any teratotoxic substances may interfere with cellular development, causing damage to the developing blastocyst. Depending on the degree of damage, cellular death and resorption of the zygote before implantation or expulsion during the subsequent

menstruation after implantation may occur. The proportion of human conceptions that terminate into resorbed or early expulsion zygotes is not known, but animal studies suggest that about 60% of zygotes fail to implant successfully. Furthermore, during the pre-implantation stage, the zygote may react to the biochemical environment, and through the capacity of developmental plasticity and epigenetic mechanisms initiate adaptive processes that can potentially result in long-term health consequences [9].

The second phase of development after implantation is the process of *embryogenesis*, which is characterized by a period of marked structural development and the development of a fetal support system. Any serious error during embryogenesis can result in early embryonic death, leading to a spontaneous first trimester miscarriage. However, if the developmental error is non-lethal, then morphological malformations may result. The developmental process is particularly sensitive at this stage to various physical, biological and chemical exogenous teratogens or to endogenous teratogenic factors. About 15–20% of human pregnancies are estimated to end in a spontaneous miscarriage. While a proportion of these miscarriages may be the result of inherent genetic factors, some will be due to teratotoxic exposure during the embryogenic period. The effects of teratotoxic factors on the developing embryo are dependent on the stage of development the embryo has reached at its time of exposure and on how long the embryo is exposed to the agent. Exposure to teratotoxic agents during embryogenesis will thus tend to affect the organs and systems under development during the period of exposure, resulting in structural and functional abnormalities. The transfer of chemical-based teratotoxic agents is dependent on the physiological mechanisms available for the placental transfer of substrates.

The placenta is a complex organ that controls the passage of substances from the mother to the embryo. It also serves as a metabolic organ altering the chemical structure of toxic substances potentially making these less innocuous or more toxic. The rate of transfer is also dependent on the uterine blood flow, which is increased during pregnancy and accounts for about 15% of cardiac output. The passage of substances through the placenta is mainly dependent on the process of simple diffusion following the principles of cell membrane transfer. However, for some specific substrates, active or facilitated transport mechanisms may also play a role. In conformity to cell membrane transfer mechanisms, transfer of substances is therefore dependent on the water or lipid solubility properties of the substance, the molecular size or whether it is protein- or cell-bound, the degree of polarity or ionization and the pH of the substance. It also is dependent on the overall concentration and the degree of metabolization it undergoes within the syncytiotrophoblast placental cells (Figure 4.1). Other potential mechanisms of placental transfer include pinocytosis (e.g. immunoglobulins), and transfer through breaks between the vascular compartments allowing passage of placental or fetal cells to mother (e.g. rhesus isoimmunization) and maternal cells to the fetus (e.g. melanoma or leukaemic cells).

The principles of placental transfer mechanisms remain in play during the third phase of development referred to as the

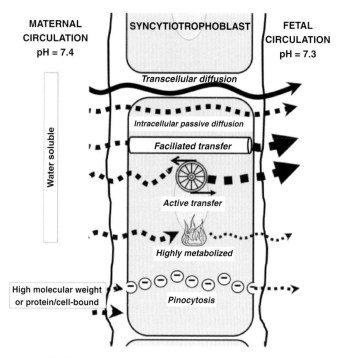

Figure 4.1 Placental transfer variables

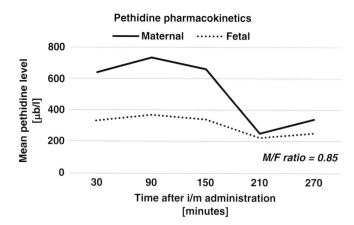

Figure 4.2 Pethidine transplacental pharmacokinetics illustrating quick equilibration between compartments and eventual drug entrapment in fetal compartment (after Savona-Ventura, Sammut, Sammut 1991) [12].

fetal phase. During this last phase of intrauterine life, fetal growth and organ differentiation takes place. After the sixth month of pregnancy, the loss of the cytotrophoblasts – Langerhan's cells – from the placenta will further facilitate the transport of drugs across the placenta. With increasing differentiation of the organs, the sensitivity of the developing fetus to teratotoxic agents diminishes. The agent will, however, continue to exert a pharmacological effect on the fetus similar to that experienced by the mother. The pharmacological effect desired in the mother may be directly or indirectly detrimental to some degree to the fetus. Thus, the inappropriate use of antithyroid medication administered to the mother to manage hyperthyroidism may result in fetal hypothyroidism with adverse effects to growth and neurodevelopment [10]. Prolonged hypotensive treatment or prolonged nicotine exposure of the mother will predispose to reduced placental blood flow, also causing reduced intrauterine fetal growth and neurodevelopment [11]. Intrauterine undernutrition from any cause, including the result of pharmacological agents taken by the mother, has been linked to epigenetic adaptations in the developing fetus predisposing it to adult-onset metabolic disease. Prolonged exposure to drugs of addiction such as narcotics will typically result in a withdrawal syndrome in the neonate after delivery that may necessitate pharmacological intervention.

The mechanisms in play during placental transfer would tend to bring about a maternal-fetal equilibrium depending on the regression coefficient of the particular agent. Elimination of the drug will mainly depend on the efficiency of the maternal detoxification and excretion systems. The fetal contribution towards detoxification is limited since enzyme maturation affecting acetylation and conjugation processes necessary for detoxification may

not yet be fully mature and effective. In spite of the maternal capacity for eliminating the drug, a tendency to drug 'entrapment' in the fetal compartment may occur, especially if the chemical has a high pH (basic properties) and has a high ionizing potential (Figure 4.2), a process that further prolongs fetal exposure time to the drug.

This process of drug entrapment in the fetus becomes even more significant when medications are used late in pregnancy and in the peripartum period. Once delivered and separated from its mother's detoxifying and excretory systems, the fetus is obliged to deal with any residual agent using its own resources that may not yet be fully functional and effective. This effect is exemplified by the association of floppy infant syndrome and the use of benzodiazepines prescribed during the last trimester of pregnancy. Symptoms of floppy infant syndrome resulting from benzodiazepine toxicity develop directly after birth and can persist for hours to days. The mean plasma half-life of benzodiazepine derivatives are two to four times longer for neonates than for adults. Since floppy infant syndrome can cause severe morbidity, prescription of benzodiazepines in the last trimester of pregnancy is thus not recommended [13].

Fetal development can be extended to a fourth phase to include the period after the delivery of the child and during breastfeeding. During the *lactational period*, the neonate can also be exposed to pharmacologically active substances that may have an adverse effect on the child. Nearly all drugs transfer into breast milk to some extent by a process of passive diffusion across the biological membranes. The process is dependent on the maternal serum drug concentration and on the pharmacokinetic properties of the medication such as the protein binding, lipid solubility, molecular weight and ionization properties of the chemical. Transfer is greatest if the drug has low protein binding and high lipid solubility properties, has a small molecular weight composition and is weakly basic. The infant dose exposure (mg/kg/day) to medications can be estimated as a product of the maternal plasma concentration (mg/L), the milk to plasma concentration ratio, and the estimated volume of milk ingested by the infant (commonly estimated as 0.15 L/kg/day).

4.3 Pharmacokinetics of Teratogenesis

Any substance can be toxic if taken in a high enough dose. The safe therapeutic window of a pharmacological agent falls between the defined minimum effective dose (MED) and maximum tolerated dose (MTD) of the substance. The narrower that window, the less safe is the drug for general use. The effective dose (ED_{50}) refers to the dose required to produce a desired therapeutic response in 50% of subjects. Similar pharmacokinetic principles can be applied to toxic agents with the introduction of the 'median lethal dose', or LD_{50} to refer to the dose that is needed to kill 50% of subjects. The LD_{50} value determines the sphere of action of a toxic substance into three zones: a non-lethal zone determined by the maximum tolerated safe dose; a zone of biological probability as determined by the LD_0 and LD_{100} where the effect of the agent on the organism is variable; and the lethal zone, LD_{100}, where all organisms are expected to die. The lower the LD_{50} value, the greater is the toxicity of the agent. The LD_{50} values are different for different agents and furthermore vary according to various factors, including the species and mode of administration. The LD_{50} value for any particular agent can be calculated mathematically using dose-related mortality rates under experimental conditions [14]. Of course, the administration of a toxic substance can have variable adverse outcomes other than death of the organism. Specific organ damage can occur without immediate death and hence the median lethal dose concept has to be tempered with considerations relating to 'median adverse outcome dose', or AOD_{50}, which is necessarily a different value than the LD_{50} for the same agent. The AOD_{50} is considered equivalent to the ratio of the dose necessary to cause a 100% organ damage and that necessary to cause a 100% mortality – AOD/LD_{100}. The adverse outcome principle can be extended

to teratogenic damage of the developing fetus, with teratotoxicity being dependent on the 'median teratogenic dose', or TD_{50}, which is similarly also equivalent to the TD/LD_{100}. In this scenario, the sphere of action of a toxic substance on the developing fetus now extends into four zones: a non-lethal zone; an adverse outcome or teratogenic zone; a zone of biological probability; and the lethal zone (Figure 4.3). This sphere of action must be tempered by also considering the toxic effect the agent has on the pregnant mother which similarly falls within the four zones but with different, generally higher, AOD_{50} and LD_{50} values.

The median teratogenic dose is not a constant variable for all teratotoxic agents but is dependent on a number of variables. There is little correlation between the fetal-TD/LD_{100} values for a particular teratotoxic agent in different animal species so that toxicology studies in animals cannot be transposed to humans. The classical studies on thalidomide demonstrated that there was a wide variation between different animal species in the lowest dose required to produce a teratogenic effect. The teratogenic doses vary from 0.5–1.0 mg/kg/day in humans to as much as 30–50 mg/kg/day in rodents and 350 mg/kg/day in the hamster [15]. The effective dose necessary to cause teratogenic effects for the same teratogen in a specific species also varies throughout gestation, making predictions of teratotoxic effects of particular substances difficult with prolonged use. In the rat model, the lowest effective dose affecting development after exposure to cyclophosphamide ranged from 30 mg/kg on day 4 post-conception, to 8–10 mg/kg on days 7–14 days post-conception, and 20 mg/kg on day 15. The literature further provides strong links between cyclophosphamide and a wide spectrum of teratogenic embryopathy, particularly if the drug was administered during the first trimester of pregnancy [16].

There is also very little correlation between the maternal-LD_{50} and the fetal-TD/LD_{100} within the same species, and the correlation ratio between the maternal LD_{50} and the fetal TD/LD_{100} is different for different embryotoxic substances. This is

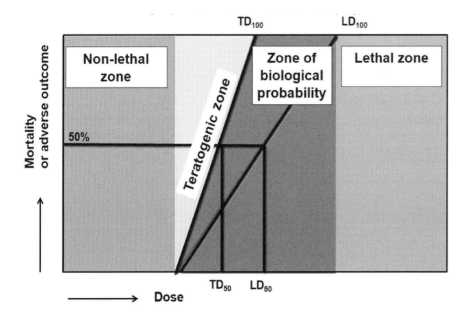

Figure 4.3 Dose response chart for developing fetus

Table 4.1 Maternal LD_{50} and fetal TD/LD_{100} in rat for various substances

Agent	Maternal LD_{50} mg/kg	Fetal TD/LD_{100} mg/kg	Correlation ratio
Antibiotics			
• Actinomycin D	0.4	0.3	1.3
• Mitomycin	3.0	3.0	1
• Streptonigrin	0.4	0.2	2
Antimetabolites			
• Azaserine	100	3	33
• 6-Mercaptopurine	250	25	10
• 6-Mercaptopurine riboside	2000–3000	50	50
• Thioguanine	350	12	29
• Thioguanine riboside	200–400	15	20
• 5-Fluorouracil	230	30	8
• Methotrexate	17	0.5	34
Alkylating agents			
• Cyclophosphamide	40	15	3
• Chlorambucil	24	6	4
• Busulfan	60	18	3

particularly evident for the antimetabolites tested where the correlation ratio ranges from 8 for 5-fluorouracil to 50 for 6-mercaptopurine riboside. Minor changes to the chemical formula can also result in significant changes in the correlation ratio: the ratio for 6-mercaptopurine was 10, a figure that is in marked contrast to that of 6-mercaptopurine riboside (Table 4.1) [17].

In addition to being species specific and variable with differing gestational age, the fetal-TD/LD_{100} can have multifactorial influences that range from the genetic makeup of the individual to the presence or absence of player substances. The teratotoxic effect of cyclophosphamide has been shown to be reduced by the conjoint administration of folic acid, vitamin A and vitamin E [18]. This multifactorial influence is best exemplified by the teratotoxic effects of excessive vitamin A ingestion. Vitamin A excess alone increases the risk of fetal anomalies characterized by exencephaly and cleft palate. The effect of vitamin A is potentiated by the administration of dexamethasone, which thus serves to decrease the TD/LD_{100} of vitamin A. In contrast, the conjoint administration of vitamin B appears to be protective, serving to increase the TD/LD_{100} of vitamin A. Genetic predispositions may also contribute towards enhancing the teratogenic effects of administered drugs. Acetaminophen used in the first trimester of pregnancy is associated with a risk of developing gastroschisis. Studies have suggested a link between gastroschisis development and the genetic variation in SULT1A3/4 in the human species [19]. Studies in humans relating specific genetic syndromes causing characteristic features with similar characteristic drug-induced embryopathies have indicated potential genetic phenocopies with embryopathies reported with use of thalidomide, warfarin, angiotensin-converting enzyme (ACE) inhibitors, fluconazole, leflunomide, mycophenolate and mofetil. It appears that the phenocopies are caused be mutation of genes that encode the main target for the teratotoxin [20].

4.4 Teratotoxic Physical Agents

Exogenous chemical substances are not the only significant teratogenic substances the fetus is potentially exposed to. The experiences following the development of radiation for diagnostic procedures and nuclear warfare emphasized the potential adverse roles played by exogenous physical agents on the developing fetus. Physical agents generally refer to frequencies of the electromagnetic spectrum that have properties affecting individual cell development. The electromagnetic spectrum involves a range of frequencies of radiation that generate different photon energies. The higher the frequency of radiation, the greater is the energy provided. The high-end part of the spectrum includes those frequencies causing ionizing radiation in the form of high ultraviolet, x-ray and gamma ray wavelengths. These provide energy levels sufficient to release electrons and create electrically charged ions within the tissue, causing intracellular chemical reactions. At high levels of exposure, these can constitute a health hazard, causing radiation sickness, DNA damage and malignant transformation. In the developing fetus, the cellular damage caused by the electrically charged ions can contribute to developmental abnormalities.

The effects of radiation damage on the developing fetus have been elucidated from experimental animal studies, diagnostic and therapeutic radiation observations in humans, and nuclear irradiation effects following use of the atomic bomb and nuclear power plant accidents. The risks from electromagnetic radiation is dependent on the magnitude of the dose and the stage of pregnancy. Depending on the gestational age at exposure, radiation effects can include embryonic death, leading to miscarriages and intrauterine deaths; neural tube development abnormalities, leading to microcephaly, mental retardation and neurobehavioural disorders; congenital abnormalities; intrauterine growth retardation; and late-onset infertility and increased cancer risks.

Studies have suggested that the fetal irradiation dose threshold causing fetal long-term sequelae is in the region of 100 milligray units (mGy) [100 mGy = 10 rads = 10 000 mrem]. The risks seem to be negligible with a dose of 50 mGy, and unclear in significance between doses of 50–100 mGy. To put dosages in perspective, an abdominal x-ray provides a fetal irradiation dose of 1.5–2.6 mGy, whereas an abdominal CT scan provides 8–30 mGy [21]. Natural background ionization radiation at sea level amounts to about 0.27 mGy units per year, with higher levels being absorbed at higher altitudes (0.34–1.66 mGy at about 2000 m above sea level). Flight crews can be exposed to an additional 0.2 to 5.0 mGy per year depending on the number, duration and altitude of flights flown per year [22]. The airport walk-through 'full-body' x-ray scanners use a very low-energy and low-intensity ionizing radiation that should not penetrate the skin. Thus, exposure to the developing fetus is minimal, if any. The airport walk-through metal detectors operate by generating a low-intensity magnetic field using non-ionizing waves that is disrupted and triggers an alarm if a metal object interrupts the field. The non-ionizing field generated by these scanners is therefore considered to be safe in pregnancy [23].

If the use of ionizing electromagnetic radiation during pregnancy is essential for diagnostic or therapeutic purposes, then the ALARA principle (as low as reasonably achievable) should be foremost. Exposure should ideally be delayed to the second trimester, preferably to after 18 weeks of gestation when brain development has occurred. Measures should be taken to attempt to reduce the exposure dose and potential fetal irradiation through photon leakage and scatter from the radiation source. This may be achieved through the use of suitable lead-protective aprons, though this may be difficult in the late third trimester. Pregnant healthcare workers who are potentially regularly exposed to ionizing radiation should reduce their level of potential exposure by being particularly vigilant in using protective risk-reducing principles. All healthcare institutions should have easily available radiation safety standard operating procedures for their pregnant staff. The employee should wear an additional abdominal badge to the regular collar badge to monitor fetal exposure. Because the effects are cumulative, the employee at risk should make every effort to reduce unnecessary exposure by wearing protective lead aprons and moving away from the source during exposure. Simply doubling the distance between the radiation source and the operator reduces the exposure fourfold. Radiation scatter can be reduced by colimiting the radiation beam using metal diaphragms interposed in the beam path. The aim should be to ensure that the fetus receives less than 5 mGy of radiation over the entire pregnancy [24].

The opposite end of the electromagnetic spectrum includes non-ionizing low-frequency waves that are used for anything from radio and TV broadcasting to cell phones, radars and microwave ovens. During pregnancy, exposure to these waves is generally through the use of diagnostic ultrasound and Doppler studies. Low-frequency radiation does not sufficiently have the intensity needed to directly damage biological tissue. However, exposure to wavelengths over 100 kHz promotes intracellular molecular vibrations that with prolonged exposure can cause a rise in cellular temperature. The mechanical and thermal effects can be measured as specific indices often displayed on screen. While it has generally been assumed that this thermal effect is benign, studies have suggested that non-ionizing radiation may have the capability of causing disturbances at the cellular level, resulting in delayed adverse health effects in the developing fetus, including neural tube defects, early fetal loss and cardiovascular malformations. In light of these concerns, a number of professional societies have issued guidelines for ultrasound use especially during pregnancy. Since diagnostic ultrasound scanning is reportedly safe when the thermal and mechanical indices are less than 1.0, operators should continually use settings to keep these indices as low as is consistent with obtaining a useful diagnostic scan. Since the thermal effect is further dependent on the exposure duration, examination time should also be kept to a minimum. The ALARA principle should always be kept in mind. There is no place for unnecessary scans during pregnancy performed simply for the sole purpose of producing souvenir photographs or videos. Judicious use of ultrasound should be made when scanning particularly thermal-sensitive regions including the embryo before the eighth week of pregnancy, the neural tube derivatives of the fetus, and the eye at any gestational age. The recommended thermal index (TI) and mechanical index (MI) settings for obstetric scanning should be 0.7 and 0.3, respectively, provided an image suitable for diagnosis is obtained. Higher TI and MI settings can only be used provided scanning time is significantly curtailed. There is no place in obstetric scanning for using TI and MI settings greater than 3.0 and 0.7, respectively. The TI and MI levels used by dedicated fetal Doppler heart monitors are sufficiently low to present no risk even when used for extended periods. The cellular thermal effects generated by ultrasound scanning are augmented in febrile patients with a temperature >37°C [25]. Animal studies have suggested that prolonged high fever resulting from a pyrexia-causing infection or prolonged sauna use may also act as a physical teratogen linking hyperthermia to neural tube malformations, abdominal wall defects, eye defects, cardiac malformations and limb deformities [26]. A meta-analysis of three birth cohorts involving 3089 five-year-old children has suggested lower general cognitive performance scores with increasing maternal prenatal cell phone use [27].

Magnetic resonance imaging is another diagnostic tool using non-ionizing electromagnetic waves. MRI during pregnancy is generally believed to be safe for the fetus in the second or third trimester. Exposure to MRI during the first trimester was also shown to present no particular risk to the developing fetus; however, the use of gadolinium to enhance the MRI image at any time during pregnancy was associated with an increased risk of rheumatological, inflammatory or infiltrative skin conditions and for perinatal deaths [28, 29].

4.5 Discussion

In the book *Epidemics* attributed to Hippocrates, it is stated that 'the physician must … have two special objects in mind with regard to disease, namely, to do good and to do no harm' – the *primum non nocere* principle. This principle becomes even more important when managing pregnant women where the investigative procedure and/or the therapeutic option may irreparably harm the developing fetus. The healthcare professional must remain vigilant and judiciously use his or her investigative and therapeutic armamentarium basing decisions on evidence-based medicine and absolute need. It is safer to assume that any substance administered to the pregnant woman has the potentiality of being harmful in some way to the developing fetus in the short- or long-term period. Such an attitude will avoid unnecessary prescriptions that could potentially be harmful. In 2015, the FDA revised its criteria for Pregnancy and Lactation Risk Information Labelling requiring a narrative summary, instead of the previous risk categories use, in the hope that a narrative summary of the risks of a drug during pregnancy and lactation would provide more meaningful information for clinicians to allow them to make an evidence-based benefit-risk assessment [30].

References

1. Curtin F, Schulz P. Assessing the benefit: risk ratio of a drug – randomized and naturalistic evidence. *Dialogues Clin Neurosci.* 2011;**13**(2):183–90.

2. Vargesson N. Thalidomide-induced teratogenesis: History and mechanisms. *Birth Defects Res C Embryo Today.* 2015;**105**(2):140–56.

3. Götz F, Thieme S, Dörner G. Female infertility–effect of perinatal xenoestrogen exposure on reproductive functions in animals and humans. *Folia Histochem Cytobiol.* 2001;**39**(Suppl 2):40–3.

4. Wilson RD, Davies G, Désilets V, et al. The use of folic acid for the prevention of neural tube defects and other congenital anomalies. *J Obstet Gynaecol Can.* 2003;**25**(11):959–73.

5. Ornoy A. Embryonic oxidative stress as a mechanism of teratogenesis with special emphasis on diabetic embryopathy. *Reprod Toxicol.* 2007;**24**(1):31–41.

6. El Hachem H, Crepaux V, May-Panloup P, et al. Recurrent pregnancy loss: current perspectives. *Int J Womens Health.* 2017;**9**:331–45.

7. Sugiura-Ogasawara M, Ozaki Y, Suzumori N. Management of recurrent miscarriage. *J Obstet Gynaecol Res.* 2014;**40**(5):1174–9.

8. Martin KL. Nutritional and metabolic requirements of early cleavage stage embryos and blastocysts. *Hum Fertil.* 2000;**3**(4):247–54.

9. Eckert JJ, Fleming TP. The effect of nutrition and environment on the preimplantation embryo. *Obstet Gynaecol.* 2011;**13**:43–8.

10. Chen CH, Xirasagar S, Lin CC, et al. Risk of adverse perinatal outcomes with antithyroid treatment during pregnancy: a nationwide population-based study. *BJOG.* 2011;**118**(11):1365–73.

11. Polańska K, Jurewicz J, Hanke W. Smoking and alcohol drinking during pregnancy as the risk factors for poor child neurodevelopment – A review of epidemiological studies. *Int J Occup Med Environ Health.* 2015;**28**(3):419–43.

12. Savona-Ventura C, Sammut M, Sammut C. Pethidine blood concentrations at time of birth. *Int J Gynecol Obstet.* 1991;**36**:103–7.

13. Iqbal MM, Sobhan T, Ryals T. Effects of commonly used benzodiazepines on the fetus, the neonate, and the nursing infant. *Psychiatric Services.* 2002;**53**(1):39–49.

14. Chinedu E, Arome D, Ameh FS. A new method for determining acute toxicity in animal models. *Toxicol Int.* 2013;**20**(3):224–6.

15. McColl JD. Drug toxicity in the animal fetus. *Appl Ther.* 1967;**9**(11):915–17.

16. Rengasamy P. Congenital malformations attributed to prenatal exposure to cyclophosphamide. *Anticancer Agents Med Chem.* 2017;**17**(9):1211–27.

17. Murphy ML. Teratogenic effects in rats of growth inhibiting chemicals, including studies on thalidomide. *Clin Proc Child Hosp Dist Columbia.* 1962;**18**:307–22.

18. Ma A, Xu H, Du W, Liu Y. Effect of folic acid and supplemented with vitamin A and vitamin E on depressing teratogenesis induced by cyclophosphamide. *Wei Sheng Yan Jiu.* 2001;**30**(6):343–6.

19. Adjei AA, Gaedigk A, Simon SD, Weinshilboum RM, Leeder JS. Interindividual variability in acetaminophen sulfation by human fetal liver: implications for pharmacogenetic investigations of drug-induced birth defects. *Birth Defects Res A Clin Mol Teratol.* 2008;**2**(3):155–665.

20. Cassina M, Cagnoli GA, Zuccarello D, Di Gianantonio E, Clementi M. Human teratogens and genetic phenocopies. Understanding pathogenesis through human genes mutation. *Eur J Med Genet.* 2017;**60**(1):22–31.

21. Needleman S, Powell M. Radiation hazards in pregnancy and methods of prevention. *Best Pract Res Clin Obstet Gynaecol.* 2016;**33**:108–16.

22. UNSCEAR. *Sources and Effects of Ionizing Radiation.* Vol. 1 of *UNSCEAR 2008 Report to the General Assembly.* New York: United Nations; 2011.

23. Wu D, Qiang R, Chen J, et al. Possible overexposure of pregnant women to emissions from a walk-through metal detector. *Phys Med Biol.* 2007;**52**(19):5735–48.

24. Shaw P, Duncan A, Vouyouka A, Ozsvath K. Radiation exposure and pregnancy. *J Vascular Surgery.* 2011;**53**(Suppl 15):28S–34S.

25. Safety Group of the BMUS. Guidelines for the safe use of diagnostic ultrasound equipment. *Ultrasound.* 2010;**18**:52–9.

26. Cockroft DL, Trevor New DA. Effects of hyperthermia on rat embryos in culture. *Nature.* 1975;**258**:604–6.

27. Sudan M, Birks LE, Aurrekoetxea JJ, et al. Maternal cell phone use during pregnancy and child cognition at age 5

years in 3 birth cohorts. *Environ Int.* 2018;**120**:155–62.

28. Bulas D, Egloff A. Benefits and risks of MRI in pregnancy. *Semin Perinatol.* 2013;**37**(5):301–4.

29. Ray JG, Vermeulen MJ, Bharatha A, Montanera WJ, Park AL. Association between MRI exposure during pregnancy and fetal and childhood outcomes. *JAMA.* 2016;**316**(9):952–61.

30. FDA. Content and format of labeling for human prescription drug and biological products; Requirements for pregnancy and lactation labeling. *Federal Register.* 2014;**79**(233):72064–103.

Chapter 5

Genetics in Fetomaternal Medicine

Jennifer Allison

Over the past 160 years there have been many relevant break-throughs and discoveries allowing the features that underlie both common and rare genetic conditions to be understood. The father of modern genetics, Gregor Mendel, provided an early recognition of human genetic variability using basic modes of inheritance after studying *Pisum sativum*, the common pea plant, in 1865 [1]. In 1953, James Watson and Francis Crick went on to describe the double helix structure of DNA [2]. This was then followed by the discovery of sequence reactions by Sanger and Coulson [3] and the polymerase chain reaction technique by Mullis et al [4], which in turn helped make genome sequencing possible. The Human Genome Project was then completed on 21 October 2004, supplying the nucleotide sequence of all chromosomes [5].

5.1 Structure of the Genome

The body is made up of millions of cells, each cell containing a complete copy of a person's genetic material, known as a genome. A gene is a hereditary component which can be passed to children from their parents. To be able to understand both normal and abnormal inheritance patterns, one must first have an understanding of the deoxyribonucleic acid (DNA) nucleotide structure. DNA is a long-chain double-stranded molecule made of four nucleotides or bases: adenine (A), a purine base that pairs with thymine on the opposite strand; guanine (G), a purine base that pairs with cystosine; thymine (T), a pyrimidine base that pairs with adenine; and cytosine (C), a pyrimidine base that pairs with guanine [6]. A codon (a sequence of three nucleotide bases) represents a particular amino acid, thus a series of bases code for a protein or a polypeptide, with either an enzymatic or structural role [6]. These long chains of DNA are packaged into the cell nucleus as chromosomes.

Clinical genetics studies how these components interact, alter and change to cause different diseases. The double strands of DNA can separate, thus allowing recombination, resulting in normal variation and disease in humans [7]. Anomalies in these recombinations can result in deletions and duplications, also known as copy number variants (CNVs) [7], either as large-scale rearrangements, point mutations or expanding trinucleotide repeats. Examples of syndromes resulting from these include the following:

1. DiGeorge = 22q11.2 deletion [6]
2. Hereditary motor and sensory neuropathy type 1A = duplication of PMP22 on chromosome 17 [6]
3. Prader-Willi = 15q11.2-q13 paternal deletion [7]

4. Haemophilia A = intron 22 inversion [6]
5. Cri-du-chat = 5p deletion [8]

5.2 Cell Division

5.2.1 Meiosis

Meiosis is the process by which the primordial germ cells, specific to the ovary and testes, give rise to gametes, which have n (23) chromosomes (haploid), from their 2n (46) chromosomes (diploid) [7]. Meiosis occurs in two parts as meiosis I and meiosis II. A significant difference between female and male gamete development is the point in life when meiosis commences, and the time taken to complete. In males this takes around 64 days, commencing at puberty and continuing throughout a man's reproductive life [7]. In females, oogenesis commences in utero then stops during prophase I, usually by 8 months' gestation [7]. Meiosis I resumes at puberty, and each month one or more oocytes resume the reduction division, with meiosis I being completed at the time of ovulation [7], when meiosis II starts, but then unless fertilized it halts at metaphase [7].

5.3 Error in Meiosis

The aim of meiosis is to reduce the 2n content of DNA in the primordial germ cell to 1n in the mature gamete, allowing the restoration of 2n when a single sperm fertilizes the mature ovum [7]. If the DNA is not acquired in equal amounts from the sperm and egg, then there is an impact on human development, cell function and organ function, in all of which DNA is involved, resulting in miscarriage, developmental delay and birth defects [7].

5.3.1 Triploidy

Triploidy occurs in around 2–3% of conceptions and is one of the most common causes of fetal loss [9]. It can occur due to various mechanisms, including errors in meiosis. Examples include:

– Primary oocyte being fertilized
– One egg being fertilized by two sperms, resulting in a diandric conception
– Nondisjunction meiosis I or meiosis II in either the sperm or egg
– Secondary oocyte with retained first or second polar body being fertilized

5.3.2 Nondisjunction

Nondisjunction is an error in meiosis, resulting in gametes with either too many or too few chromosomes, known as aneuploidy [7].

There are three different forms of nondisjunction [10]:

- Failure of homologous chromosomes to separate during meiosis I
- Failure of sister chromatids to separate during meiosis II
- Failure of sister chromatids to separate during mitosis

When mitotic nondisjunction occurs in cell lines intended to form placental mesenchyme and/or trophoblast, placental mosaicism occurs, resulting in a discrepancy between the genetic makeup of the cells in the fetus and the cells of the placenta. Although this usually results in having no impact on fetal development, it can on occasion impact fetal growth.

5.3.3 Trinucleotide Repeats

Repetitive sequences of the same three nucleotides are known as trinucleotide repeats. Classic trinucleotide repeat disorders are:

- Fragile X syndrome (CGG repeat)
- Huntington's disease (CAG repeat)
- Myotonic dystrophy (CTG repeat)

Trinucleotide expansion during gametogenesis across generations, known as anticipation, results in more severe symptoms often at an earlier age of onset [7].

5.4 Examples of Error in Meiosis

5.4.1 Turner Syndrome – X Monosomy

Turner syndrome is the only known survivable monosomy in humans, occurring due to the absence of one partial or complete copy of the X chromosome in either some or all of the cells in the body.

5.4.2 Down Syndrome – Trisomy 21 (T21)

Trisomy 21 is found in about 1 in 800 births, with the risk increasing with maternal age. The life expectancy is about 60 years [7].

Down syndrome is usually caused by nondisjunction, which results in an embryo with three copies of chromosomes 21. Ninety-five per cent of T21 cases are due to nondisjunction wherein a pair of 21 chromosomes fails to separate in the reproductive cells prior to conception and as the embryo develops, the extra chromosome is replicated in every cell of the body [7].

Translocation accounts for around 4% of cases of Down syndrome [7]. In this situation, the total numbers of chromosomes remain at 46; however, a full or partial copy of chromosome 21 attaches to another chromosome, usually chromosome 14. This extra chromosome 21 causes the characteristics of Down syndrome.

In 1% of cases of T21, a diagnosis of mosaicism is made, in which there is a mixture of two types of cells, some containing 46 chromosomes and others containing 47 chromosomes (an extra chromosome 21) [7]. Individuals with mosaicism of T21 tend to have fewer characteristics of Down syndrome than those with other types.

All three types of Down syndrome are genetic conditions; however, only 1% of all cases of Down syndrome have a hereditary component. Mosaicism and T21 (nondisjunction) do not have a hereditary component; however, one third of cases with translocation causing Down syndrome has a hereditary component [7].

5.4.3 Edwards Syndrome – Trisomy 18

Trisomy 18 (T18), also known as Edwards syndrome, occurs in about 1 in 5000 live births. It is more common in pregnancy since many affected fetuses do not survive to term [11]. T18 is associated with intrauterine growth restriction, small abnormally shaped head, overlapping fingers, small jaw and mouth, cardiac defects and larger choroid plexus cysts [12]. The 5–10% of children with T18 who do live past their first year often have severe intellectual disability [11].

The majority of cases of trisomy 18 result from having three copies of chromosome 18 in each cell of the body rather than two copies, with around 5% of people with trisomy 18 in some but not all cells, known as mosaicism [11]. Very rarely, part of the long arm (q) of chromosome 18 attaches (translocates) to another chromosome; therefore, these individuals have two copies of chromosome 18 with the additional extra chromosome 18 material on another chromosome [11]. This is known as partial trisomy 18 and the severity of the condition depends on the length of the additional chromosome 18 that has translocated [13].

Most cases of trisomy 18 occur as random events, where an error in cell division (nondisjunction) results in an extra chromosome 18 within a reproductive cell, which, if this cell is involved in the genetic makeup of the child, will result in trisomy 18 in each of those body's cells. Although mosaic trisomy 18 is also a random event, at this point in cell division during early embryonic development, partial trisomy 18 can be inherited. In an unaffected parent, they may be carrying a balanced translocation of chromosome 18 with another chromosome, which carries an increased risk of their offspring having partial trisomy 18 [11].

5.4.4 Patau Syndrome – Trisomy 13

Trisomy 13 (T13), also known as Patau syndrome, is one of the few trisomies identified in live-born fetuses [14] and occurs in around 1 in 16 000 newborns [15]. T13 is associated with brain and/or spinal cord abnormalities, cardiac defects, microphthalmia (poorly developed eyes), hypotonia (weak muscle tone), cleft lip with or without cleft palate and extra digits [16]. Due to these abnormalities, many children live for only a few days to weeks, with only 5–10% living beyond 1 year of age [15].

Most cases of T13 occur as a consequence of nondisjunction during cell division and are not inherited [14]. More than 91% of cases of T13 are maternal in origin, with the extra chromosome mainly occurring due to an error in meiosis I; however, in around 37% of cases the error occurs during meiosis II [14]. In most cases, T13 results from having three copies of chromosome 13 in each cell of the body, although it can also occur when part of chromosome 13 translocates to another chromosome, resulting in two normal copies of chromosome 13 with an additional copy attached to another chromosome [14].

5.4.5 Fragile X Syndrome

Fragile X syndrome is a trinucleotide repeat disorder of CGG sequence, located in the 5′ untranslated region of the *FMR1* gene in the X chromosome [7], resulting in inherited intellectual disability. A repeat size of less than 45 is stable, individuals with an expansion of 45–59 are at risk of ataxia syndrome (males) and premature ovarian failure (females) [7], while those with a greater than 200 CGG repeats have fragile X syndrome [7].

5.5 Single Gene Disorders

A pattern of inheritance that applies to disorders caused by a single gene defect was first described by Gregor Mendel (1822–1884) [17]. As previously mentioned, a gene is a hereditary component which is passed to children from their parents. They are inherited in pairs, with one of each pair inherited from each parent [17]. An allele (a variant form of a given gene) is one of a pair of genes that act in a dominant or recessive manner, this impacting on how the disorder is inherited, discussed further below.

5.5.1 Autosomal Dominant Inheritance

With autosomal dominant inheritance, the disorder is transmitted by both sexes and affects males and females equally. An affected person is usually heterozygous for the disorder, as it is rare, and in certain cases lethal, to be homozygous [17]. There are few noteworthy situations [17]:

– Age-dependent penetrance
   Some disorders do not become apparent until adult life – for example, Huntington's disease – and if the gene carrier dies before the condition was apparent, then there may be the appearance of a 'skipped generation'.
– Reduced penetrance
– Variable expression
   There are many disorders that show a difference in expression between and within families, where mildly affected parents have severely affected children and vice versa.
– New mutations
   In many severe conditions, the majority of cases have parents who are unaffected, and the disorder is a new mutation. Disorders such as achondroplasia, with a high mutation rate, have also been shown to have an increasing incidence with increasing paternal age.
– Germ-line mosaicism
   If the mutation is carried in some but not all of the gonadal cells (germ-line mosaicism), the child may be affected but the oparents appear unaffected, such as in cases of tuberous sclerosis.

– Anticipation
   Where the sex of the affected parent influences the phenotype in the child, for example, in congenital myotonic dystrophy following maternal rather than paternal transmission of the mutation.
– Imprinting
   Where a small proportion of genes exhibit epigenetic silencing, for example, the *UBE3A* gene, 15q11, in Angelman syndrome.

5.5.2 Autosomal Recessive Inheritance

An autosomal recessive disorder will have been inherited from a mutation in the same gene from both parents, who are heterozygous for the disorders (unaffected carriers). If the disorder is rare, the risk of recurrence in the family is low unless there is consanguinity [17]. This mutation that the parents carry may be the same and the child is homozygote for the mutation, for example both parents carrying the DF508 mutation in the cystic fibrosis gene [17]. Alternatively, the parents may carry different mutations in the same gene and the child is compound heterozygote for the mutation, for example, one parent carries the G551D and the other DF508 in the cystic fibrosis gene [17].

5.5.3 X-Linked Disorder Inheritance

The majority of these disorders are recessive and often if a female has a mutation in one copy of an X-linked gene, the other X chromosome will carry a normal copy and therefore she will be unaffected [17]. However, if a male was to inherit an X-linked mutation (from their mother) they will be affected. There is also the possibility of a new mutation as seen in autosomal dominance inheritance [17].

X-linked disorders can be dominant or semi-dominant and the female carriers will have clinical signs and symptoms, such as seen in fragile X mental retardation syndrome. In some cases of X-linked dominant disorders, such as Rett syndrome, almost all the affected patients are female as these conditions demonstrate male lethality [17].

5.6 Example of a Single Gene Disorder

5.6.1 Cystic Fibrosis

Cystic fibrosis (CF) is one of the UK's most common inherited conditions, affecting 1 in 2500 live births. It is an autosomal recessive disease, which means for a baby to be born with CF both their mother and father have to be carriers of the faulty gene. If both parents are carriers, then the child has:

A 25% chance of being born with cystic fibrosis.

A 50% chance of being a carrier like their parent, therefore unaffected.

A 25% chance of being free from the condition – neither affected nor a carrier.

CF is a multisystem disease affecting the body's ability to move salt and water into and out of cells of the respiratory system, gastrointestinal system, sweat glands and reproductive system in males. This is due to the mutation in a single large gene on chromosome 7 that encodes the CF transmembrane conductance regulator (CFTR) protein, which regulates the activity of sodium and chloride channels of the epithelial surface of these systems [17].

Prenatal screening is offered to relatives (and partners) of a person diagnosed with CF or if an echogenic bowel is seen in the second-trimester ultrasound scan. Whenever a carrier of CF is detected, carrier testing is possible for the carrier's relatives and partners in a cascade fashion. However, as the test for common mutations only detects 90–95% of mutations, there is a risk of false negative results, although the statistical likelihood of this is less than 1 in 250 [18].

There are more than 2000 mutations of the CF gene discovered; however, in the UK, delta F508 accounts for the majority of the cases, with a further 49 mutations accounting for more than 95% of the total UK mutations in Caucasian patients [18]. These mutations are split into different categories:

Class I – Shortened CFTR protein (7%)

Class II – CFTR protein is not transported, for example, delta F508 (85%)

Class III – CFTR protein is not regulated (<3%)

Class IV – Reduced chloride conductance due to altered protein channel (<3%)

Class V – Reduction in amount of CFTR produced (<3%) [18]

Due to the complex genetics, for example, with some of the rarer mutations only being associated with an isolated feature of the disease (R117 H mutation linked with congenital absence of the vas deferens) [17], it is important to have detailed multidisciplinary pre-test counselling, as well as to discuss further management if a positive diagnosis is made. During these counselling sessions, the possibility of pre-implantation genetic diagnosis using in vitro fertilization (IVF) techniques are explained, thus allowing an embryo free of CF to be implanted in the womb. The use of chorionic villi sampling (CVS) and amniocentesis for antenatal diagnosis, along with the risks associated with these tests, is explained, with the options of continuing or ending the pregnancy discussed at these times.

CF is still an onerous condition; however, the quality and length of life for people with CF have improved with recent new developments in treatment, with expectant survival up to 30–40 years. Although there is no cure at present, new generations of medications that target specific mutations are being developed and research into gene therapy is ongoing [18].

5.7 Screening for Genetic Disorders

Traditionally, certain populations have an increased frequency of specific disease-associated genetic variants; however, as populations have become more ethnically and racially diverse, screening for a panel of disorders is now offered to all individuals regardless of their ethnicity to allow individuals to gain understanding and information that will aid their management decisions [19].

5.7.1 Criteria for Implementing Screening Tests

Wilson and Junger mentioned the following gold standard criteria for decision making about screening in the World Health Organization report as follows [20]:

- The condition sought should be an important health problem.
- There should be an accepted treatment for patients with recognized disease.
- Facilities for diagnosis and treatment should be available.
- There should be a recognizable latent or early symptomatic stage.
- There should be a suitable test or examination.
- The test should be acceptable to the population.
- The natural history of the condition, including development from latent to declared disease, should be adequately understood.
- There should be an agreed policy on whom to treat as patients.
- The cost of case-finding (including diagnosis and treatment of patients diagnosed) should be economically balanced in relation to possible expenditure on medical care as a whole.
- Case-finding should be a continuing process and not a 'once and for all' project.

5.7.2 Principle of Screening Tests

There are four main methods used to evaluate screening tests [17]:

1. Sensitivity – percentage of the total number of diseased or affected people identified by the test.
2. Specificity – proportion of all those who did not have the disease and tested negative.
3. Positive predictive value (PPV) – percentage of all those who tested positive who actually had the disease.
4. Negative predictive value (NPV) – percentage of those who did not have the disease who had a negative screening test result.

As screening tests improve the sensitivity increases as the false positive rate decreases.

Within the UK, antenatal screening occurs for the following:

- T21: combined test in the first trimester and quadruple test in the second trimester
- T13 & T18: combined test in the first trimester
- T13, T18, T21: NIPT as second line screening in first and second trimester
- Screening for haemoglobinopathy
- Fetal anomaly: ultrasound scan between 18+0 weeks and 20+6 weeks

– Infections: hepatitis B, syphilis, rubella, human immunodeficiency virus

5.8 Invasive Prenatal Diagnosis

5.8.1 Chorionic Villus Sampling (CVS) and Amniocentesis

CVS and amniocentesis are the most common invasive prenatal diagnostic tests currently used in the UK. CVS is performed transabdominally or transcervically after 11+0 weeks' gestation, where trophoblastic cells are removed from the placenta. Amniocentesis meanwhile is performed by transabdominal aspiration of amniotic fluid from the uterine cavity at or beyond 15+0 weeks' gestation.

Amniocentesis or CVS is usually undertaken for increased risk of fetal aneuploidy, which may be derived from a screening test such as the first-trimester combined test, second-trimester biochemistry, previous fetus affected by aneuploidy, abnormal ultrasound findings or family history of aneuploidy [21]. They may also be undertaken due to maternal transmittable infectious disease, increased risk for a known genetic or biochemical disease of the fetus and, in certain circumstances, maternal request [21].

Complications associated with CVS and amniocentesis vary from pain, bleeding and infection to rupture of membranes, fetal injury and fetal loss. For women undergoing CVS, the additional risk of fetal loss in comparison with controls have been reported to vary between 0.2% and 2%. While the risk of vaginal bleeding is 10% of CVS cases, the risks of membrane rupture and infection are rare [21].

In women undergoing amniocentesis, the risk of membrane rupture is 1–2% and the additional risk of fetal loss in comparison to controls has been reported from 0.1–1%, with fetal injury being rare events [21]. However, a systematic review of literature and updated meta-analysis by Salomon et al [22] has recently shown that the procedure-related risks of miscarriage after CVS and amniocentesis are lower than previously thought, with the risk appearing to be negligible when the interventions are compared to control groups of the same risk profile [22].

5.9 Cytogenetic Testing

5.9.1 Karyotype

Karyotype can be verified from the fetal cells obtained by CVS or amniocentesis, either after direct analysis or after cell culture with chromosomal Giemsa staining (G-banding) [7], where every chromosome has a unique pattern. Light microscopy is used to see the stained chromosomes, where large deletions or rearrangements (5 to 10 Mb) can be detected. However, molecular cytogenetic technology such as fluorescence in situ hybridization (FISH) and chromosomal microarray analysis (CMA) is required for higher resolution or more specific testing.

5.9.2 Fluorescence In Situ Hybridization (FISH)

FISH is a useful tool in diagnosing or confirming syndromes that are caused by microdeletions of segments of chromosomal material, such as 22q11.2 deletion syndrome. Denatured DNA sequences which have been labelled with a fluorescent dye are hybridized onto denatured chromosomes that have already been immobilized onto a slide, with the chromosomes then seen with a wavelength of light that excites the fluorescent dye [7].

FISH probes, which are fluorescence-labelled DNA sequences that are hybridized to a known location on a specific chromosome, are fairly short, which allows the number and location of specific DNA sequences to be determined [7]. Although FISH does not detect cytogenetic abnormalities such as rare aneuploidies, mosaics and translocations [23], it can detect aneuploidies caused by monosomies, complete trisomies, triploidy and trisomies associated with Robertsonian translocations [7]. Therefore, at present FISH analysis is not used as a primary screening test on all genetic amniocenteses due to its inability to detect uncommon trisomies, mosaicism, structural rearrangements and marker chromosomes [24].

5.9.3 Chromosomal Microarray Analysis (CMA)

CMA, with a greater than 100-fold resolution than traditional G-banding karyotyping, gives the ability to survey the entire genome and identify submicroscopic deletions and duplications (CNVs), as well as the chromosomal abnormalities detected by conventional cytogenetic techniques [25].

A microarray tends to be made from a postage-stamp-sized thin slice of glass or silicon on which threads of synthetic nucleic acids are arrayed, with sample probes added to the chip and matches read by an electronic scanner [7].

There are three common microarray platforms used for genome assessment:
1. Array comparative genomic hybridization (CGH)

    Two genomic libraries are mixed and hybridized to make a panel of reference oligonucleotides across the genome. This platform is then used to compare a patient's genome with that of a normal control, with the result expressed as a comparative intensity between the patient and control [26].
2. Pure single nucleotide polymorphism (SNP) array

    Probes are chosen from DNA locations that are known to vary by a single base pair; the patient's DNA is then hybridized to the array and result obtained from the absolute intensity of signal from bound DNA fragments [7]. A result of greater than or less than two alleles at any given tested locus symbolizes a gain or loss of genetic material in that region [7]. Pure SNP array allows the determination of paternity, zygosity, degree of consanguinity and maternal cell contamination [27].
3. Combination platform, using both oligonucleotides and SNPs

    This combination platform has the advantage of SNP information with a reduced background noise [7].

With microarray technology, clinicians and genetic counsellors must continue with reasonable caution when offering and interpreting microarray analysis, as genetic variant recognition may surpass the ability of interpretation [28]. Skilled genetic counselling is therefore needed to help patients decide what to do with the results of previously unreported rare variants with unknown phenotypes and genetic variants of uncertain significance which may be identified [7].

5.10 Non-Invasive Prenatal Screening/ Testing (NIPS/T)

During pregnancy, the mother's blood contains a mix of cfDNA (DNA fragments that are free-floating and not within cells) from her cells and cells from the placenta. These small fragments are normally made up of fewer than 200 DNA base pairs, having resulted from the breakdown of cells and release of contents into the bloodstream.

In 2008, two studies described NIPT for trisomy 21 by sequencing cell-free DNA (cfDNA) in maternal plasma [29, 30]. They implied that the test could reduce the number of unnecessary invasive procedures, as it only requires a maternal blood test and it was found to have a very low false positive rate. By taking blood from the pregnant mother and analyzing the cfDNA from the placenta, it is possible to detect genetic abnormalities without harming the fetus. False positive and false negative NIPS/T results can occur for a number of reasons, such as true fetal mosaicism, confined placental mosaicism, organ transplant, maternal neoplasm, maternal fibroids, co-twin demise, maternal chromosomal deletion and laboratory error [7].

In a pregnancy, where 10% of the cfDNA is fetal, a woman carrying a trisomy 21 fetus would likely have 1.05 times more DNA from chromosome 21 fragments [7]. By sequencing millions of fragments, identifying their chromosomal origin and quantifying their relative proportion, it is possible to distinguish this difference and predict trisomy 21 [7]. NIPT has since been developed to provide detection for not only trisomy 21 but also for other common aneuploidies using targeted sequencing, shotgun sequencing and SNP-based sequencing of cfDNA [31].

NIPS/T has been used to screen for trisomy 13, 18 and 21 over the past few years and although the statistics for detection of these aneuploidies in a high-risk population are better than any other standard screening method, it is not yet diagnostic [7]. Its efficacy in the general, low-risk population has not yet been established and there are concerns which have been raised regarding its performance in routine clinical practice [31]. A 2016 systematic review and meta-analysis found that the sensitivity of NIPS/T in a combined high-risk cohort of 10 000 pregnancies for trisomy 13 was 95%, trisomy 18 was 93% and trisomy 21 was 97% [32], while the positive predictive values were 87%, 84% and 91% for trisomy 13, 18 and 21, respectively [32]. In comparison, the low-risk pregnancy predictive values of NIPS/T fell to 49%, 37% and 82% for trisomy 13, 18 and 21, respectively [32]. However, a study by Zhang et al [31], which looked at NIPT for trisomies in 146 958 pregnancies, alludes that there is no statistical difference between low-risk and high-risk groups in detecting trisomy 21, thus suggesting it is appropriate to offer NIPS/T as a routine screening test for fetal trisomies 13, 18 and 21 [31]. Scotland is now using NIPT as second line screening for pregnancies with a higher chance result from a primary screen in the first or second trimester since 28 September 2020, whilst England introduced NIPT screening in 2018.

References

1. Miko I. Gregor Mendel and the principles of inheritance. *Nature Education*. 2008;**1**(1):134.

2. Watson JD, Crick FH. Molecular structure of nucleic acids: a structure for deoxyribose nucleic acid. *Nature*. 1953;**171**(4356):737–8.

3. Sanger F, Coulson AR. A rapid method for determining sequences in DNA by primed synthesis with DNA polymerase. *J Mol Biol*. 1975;**94**(3):441–8.

4. Mullis K, Faloona F, Scharf S, et al. Specific enzymatic amplification of DNA in vitro: the polymerase chain reaction. *Cold Spring Harb Symp Quant Biol*. 1986;**51**:263–73.

5. International Human Genome Sequencing Consortium. Finishing the euchromatic sequence of the human genome. *Nature*. 2004;**431** (7011):931–45.

6. Kumar B, Alfirevic Z. *Fetal Medicine*. Cambridge: Cambridge University Press; 2016.

7. Resnik R, Lockwood CJ, Moore TR, et al. *Creasy & Resnik's Maternal-Fetal Medicine. Principles and Practice*, 8th ed. Philadelphia: Elsevier; 2019.

8. Cerruti Mainardi P. Cri du chat syndrome. *Orphanet J Rare Dis*. 2006;**1** (1):33.

9. Wick JB, Johnson KJ, O'Brien J, et al. Second-trimester diagnosis of triploidy: a series of four cases. *AJP Rep*. 2013;**3** (1):37–40.

10. Simmons D, Sunstad P, Michael J. *Principles of Genetics*, 4th ed. New York: Wiley;2016.

11. NIH Genetics Home Reference. *Trisomy 18*. https://ghr.nml.nih.gov/condition/trisomy-18.

12. Bronsteen R, Lee W, Vettraino IM, Huang R, Comstock CH. Second-trimester sonography and trisomy 18. *J Ultrasound Med*. 2004;**23**(2):233–40.

13. Boghosian-Sell L, Mewar R, Harrison W, et al. Molecular mapping of the Edwards syndrome phenotype to two non contiguous regions on chromosome 18. *Am J Hum Genet*. 1994;**55**(3): 476–83.

14. Hall HE, Chan ER, Collins A, et al. The origin of trisomy 13. *Am J Med Genet A*. 2007;**143A**(19):2242–8.

15. NIH Genetics Home Reference. *Trisomy 13*. https://ghr.nml.nih.gov/condition/trisomy-13.

16. Parker MJ, Budd JL, Draper ES, Young ID. Trisomy 13 and trisomy 18 in a defined population: epidemiological, genetic and prenatal observations. *Prenat Diagn*. 2003;**23** (10):856–60.

17. Kumar B, Alfirevic Z. *Fetal Medicine.* Cambridge: Cambridge University Press; 2016.

18. Cystic Fibrosis Trust. What is cystic fibrosis. Family Genetic Testing: the family cascade screening programme for cystic fibrosis. Cystic Fibrosis factsheet – August 2015. www .cysticfibrosis.org.uk.

19. American College of Obstetricians and Gynecologists. Practice bulletin no.162: prenatal diagnostic testing for genetic disorders. *Obstet Gynecol.* 2016;127:e108.

20. Wilson JMG, Junger G. Principles and practice of screening for disease. Public Health Papers No. 34. Geneva: World Health Organization; 1968. http://whql ibdoc.who.int/php/WHO_PHP_34 .pdf.

21. Ghi T, Sotiriadis A, Calda P, et al. ISUOG practice guidelines: invasive procedures for prenatal diagnosis. *Ultrasound Obstet Gynecol.* 2016;48:256–68.

22. Salomon LJ, Sotiriadis A, Wulff CB, Odibo A, Akolekar R. Risk of miscarriage following amniocentesis or chorionic villus sampling: systematic review of the literature and updated meta-analysis. *Ultrasound Obstet Gynecol.* 2019;54(4). DOI: 10.1002/ uog.20353.

23. Lo YM, Corbetta N, Chamberlain PF, et al. Presence of fetal DNA in maternal plasma and serum. *Lancet.* 1997;350:485–7.

24. Evans MI, Goldberg JD, Horenstein J, et al. Selective termination for structural, chromosomal, and Mendelian anomalies: international experience. *Am J Obstet Gynecol.* 1999;181:893–7.

25. Dugoff L, Norton ME, Kuller JA. The use of chromosomal microarray for prenatal diagnosis. *Am J Obstet Gynecol.* 2016;215:B2–9.

26. Snijders AM, Nowak N, Segraves R, et al. Assembly of microarrays for genome-wide measurement of DNA copy number. *Nat Genet.* 2001;29 (3):263–4.

27. Beaudet AL, Belmont JW. Array-based DNA diagnostics: let the revolution begin. *Annu Rev Med.* 2008;59: 113–29.

28. Yatsenko SA, Davis S, Hendrix NW, et al. Application of chromosomal microarray in the evaluation of abnormal prenatal findings. *Clin Genet.* 2013;84(1):47–54.

29. Fan HC, Blumenfeld YJ, Chitkara U, Hudgins L, Quake SR. Noninvasive diagnosis of fetal aneuploidy by shotgun sequencing DNA from maternal blood. *Proc Natl Acad Sci USA.* 2008;105:16266–71.

30. Chiu RW, Chan KC, Gao Y, et al. Noninvasive prenatal diagnosis of fetal chromosomal aneuploidy by massively parallel genomic sequencing of DNA in maternal plasma. *Proc Natl Acad Sci USA.* 2008;105:20458–63.

31. Zhang H, Gao Y, Jiang F, et al. Non-invasive prenatal testing for trisomies 21, 18, 13: clinical experience from 146 958 pregnancies. *Ultrasound Obstet Gynecol.* 2015;45 (5):530–8.

32. Taylor-Phillips S, Freeman K, Geppert J, et al. Accuracy of non-invasive prenatal testing using cell-free DNA for detection of Down, Edwards and Patau syndromes: a systematic review and meta-analysis. *BMJ Open.* 2016;6(1): e010002. DOI: 10.1136/bmjopen-2015-010002.

Chapter

6

Bleeding in Early Pregnancy

Kahyee Hor & Tahir A. Mahmood

6.1 Introduction

Early pregnancy encompasses the first 12 weeks of pregnancy – also known as the first trimester. Vaginal bleeding (PV bleeding) in early pregnancy is one of the most common gynaecological presentations, affecting between 7 and 21% of all pregnancies [1].

The main causes of PV bleeding in early pregnancy include 1) miscarriage, 2) ectopic pregnancy and 3) gestational trophoblastic disease. This chapter will discuss the background, presentation, investigations and management of miscarriage. Other less common causes of PV bleeding in pregnancy include cervical or vaginal lesions.

6.2 Epidemiology and Aetiology

The World Health Organization (WHO) defines *miscarriage* as the expulsion of a fetus weighing 500 g or less at less than 22 'completed' weeks of gestation. In the UK, it is estimated that approximately 25% of pregnancies end with a miscarriage [2]. Most miscarriages occur in the first trimester, and only 4% of miscarriages occur in the second trimester.

The underlying cause of the majority of cases of early miscarriages is not known. However, there are factors associated with an increased risk of miscarriages. These risk factors can be divided into three categories – maternal, paternal and genetic factors – and are summarized in Table 6.1.

The major cause of early miscarriages is chromosomal abnormalities, which contribute to approximately 40–50% of spontaneous early miscarriages [3]. Eiben et al [4] undertook an early study on cytogenetic abnormalities in miscarriages between 5 and 25 weeks' gestation using chorionic villus sampling (CVS). This study showed that 54.1% of pregnancies under 12 weeks' gestation demonstrated chromosomal abnormalities. The majority of the abnormalities in all the miscarriages in this study were due to trisomy (62.1%), of which the three most prevalent were due to chromosomes 16 (21.8%), 22 (17.9%) and 21 (10%). Other abnormalities included triploidy (12.4%) and monosomy X (10.5%).

Increased maternal age is an established risk factor for early miscarriages. A large register linkage study performed in Denmark by Nybo Andersen et al [5] demonstrated that the risk of spontaneous miscarriage was increased with increasing maternal age. This relationship was independent of potential confounding factors including parity and previous obstetric history. Women at 42 years of age have approximately a 50% risk of spontaneous miscarriage, compared with 8.7% at 22 years old. Another study [6] showed that the risk of early

Table 6.1 Factors associated with increased risk of miscarriage

Maternal factors	Genetic factors	Paternal factors
• Maternal age • Previous history of miscarriage • Maternal body mass index (BMI) (low and high) • Infection • High caffeine consumption • Alcohol intake • Smoking • Heavy PV bleeding (in pregnancy)	Chromosomal abnormalities	Paternal age

miscarriage is almost doubled in women older than 35 years compared with those between 25–29 years old (odds ratio (OR) 1.98, 95% confidence interval (CI) 1.01–3.98, p=0.047).

This increase in miscarriage risk could be associated with the increased incidence of chromosomal abnormalities seen with increasing maternal age. A multicentre study [7] of singleton pregnancies have shown that women between 35–39 years have a 4-fold risk of having a pregnancy with chromosomal abnormality (adjusted OR 4.0, 95% CI 2.5–6.3, p<0.001). This risk is increased further in women greater than 40 years of age (adjusted OR 9.9, 95% CI 5.8–17.0, p<0.001).

Another recognized risk factor for early miscarriages is a history of miscarriage(s). Nybo Andersen et al [5] have shown that nulliparous women who have had one previous miscarriage in the preceding 10 years have a 12.4% risk of spontaneous miscarriage, compared with 8.9% if they have not had a miscarriage previously. Importantly, this study identified that this risk increases with the number of previous miscarriages with a risk of miscarriage as high as 44.6% if a woman has had three or more previous miscarriages. A similar finding has been reported by Maconochie et al [8] using a UK population-based case control study, whereby those with one previous miscarriage had an adjusted OR of 1.65 (95% CI 1.27–2.13). This risk increased further in those with three or more miscarriages (adjusted OR 3.87, 95% CI 2.29–6.54).

Other maternal risk factors for early miscarriage include smoking [9], high caffeine intake [8, 10], alcohol intake [11], low [12] and high body mass index (BMI) [13] and infection [14]. Heavy PV bleeding in early pregnancy has also been shown to be an important risk factor in several studies [1, 6].

Table 6.2 Classification of different types of miscarriages

Type of miscarriage	Clinical features	US features
Threatened miscarriage	• PV bleeding with/without abdominal pain • Cervical os closed	• Intrauterine gestational sac with fetal pole and fetal heart activity
Missed miscarriage	• May be completely asymptomatic	• Gestational sac diameter >20 mm without any identifiable fetus; or • Absence of fetal heart activity when crown–rump length ≥7 mm
Incomplete miscarriage	• May present with bleeding and/or abdominal pain • Cervical os usually open	• Products of conception still visible in uterine cavity
Complete miscarriage	• Usually associated with cessation of PV bleeding and/or abdominal pain • Some may describe loss of pregnancy symptoms (e.g. nausea) • Cervical os usually closed	• Empty uterus

The main paternal factor associated with miscarriage is paternal age at conception [8]. The risk of first trimester miscarriage was significantly increased in men greater than 45 years at the time of conception (adjusted OR 1.64, 95% CI 1.08–2.47). Further, de La Rochebrochard and Thonneau [15] demonstrated that this risk is dramatically increased when combined with advanced maternal age with an adjusted odds ratio of 6.73 (95% CI 3.50–12.95) of miscarriage when the mother was between 35 and 44 years of age and the father was between 40 and 64 years of age. Other paternal factors including paternal smoking and alcohol intake did not appear to have any impact on risk of early miscarriage [8, 15].

6.3 Pathology

The diagnosis of early miscarriage can be challenging for the attending clinician or midwife. The main investigation to identify a miscarriage is ultrasonography (US), and 'early pregnancy loss' is the 'ultrasound definition of intrauterine pregnancy with reproducible evidence of lost foetal heart rate activity and/or failure of increased crown–rump length over one week, or persisting presence of empty sac, at less than 12 weeks' gestation' [16].

There are four types of miscarriages – threatened, missed, incomplete and complete miscarriage, which are described in Table 6.2.

There are various terminologies used when reporting findings and describing clinical events associated with early miscarriage. Some of these terms are historical and poorly defined including *missed abortion* and *blighted ovum*. In order to improve consistency and clarity, the European Society of Human Reproduction and Embryology (ESHRE) Special Interest Group for Early Pregnancy issued an updated list of common terms and their definitions [16]. The relevant terms from this list have been included in Table 6.3.

6.4 Clinical Features

Patients in early pregnancy presenting with PV bleeding should be assessed clinically and offered further investigations

Table 6.3 The ESHRE classification for early pregnancy

Term	Definition
Biochemical pregnancy loss	Pregnancy not located on scan associated with falling serum or urine human chorionic gonadotropin (hCG) (cf. pregnancy of unknown location)
Empty sac	Gestation sac without structures or minimal embryonic debris, without heart rate activity To replace: 'anembryonic pregnancy' and 'early embryonic demise'
Foetus	Ultrasound-based definition to include foetal heart activity and/or crown–rump length >10 mm To replace: 'embryo'
Missed / Spontaneous / Threatened miscarriage	To replace: 'missed abortion', 'spontaneous abortion' and 'threatened abortion' respectively

including serum human chorionic gonadotropin (hCG) measurement and ultrasonography.

PV bleeding in early pregnancy is a distressing symptom for the patient and is one of the common presenting complaints in women presenting with an early miscarriage. A prospective study undertaken at a primary care setting reported that PV bleeding at 20 weeks' gestation or less affected 21% of the pregnancies recorded over the 2-year period [17]. Of these pregnancies, 57% (67 out of 117 pregnant women with PV bleeding) ended with a miscarriage.

Another study [6] performed in a tertiary unit reported an adjusted OR of 18.88 (95% CI 13.88–25.69, p<0.001) for early miscarriage in women presenting with moderate to heavy PV bleeding. The amount of bleeding was defined as equal to or heavier than menstrual bleeding for moderate and heavy PV bleeding, respectively.

In order to investigate the pregnancy outcome among women presenting with PV bleeding in very early pregnancy, Harville et al [18] followed up 151 women with 'clinical pregnancies', defined as pregnancies lasting ≥6 weeks from the last menstrual period (LMP), until 8 weeks from their LMP. They have shown that only 9% of these women had ≥1 day of PV bleeding, which was generally reported as 'light'. Notably, only 14% of those with PV bleeding miscarried, while 9% of those without bleeding had a miscarriage. This study suggests that the gestational age at the time of PV bleeding, as well as the amount of bleeding, may influence the risk of miscarriage, with those who are in very early pregnancy and have 'light' PV bleeding having a lower risk of miscarriage compared to those who are further on and presenting with moderate to heavy PV loss.

Abdominal pain may or may not be present with miscarriage and indeed, the presence of abdominal pain is not associated with an increased risk of miscarriage [6].

Table 6.4 describes a list of key information which should be elicited from the history which will guide subsequent investigation and management.

The spectrum of the severity of PV bleeding associated with early miscarriage is varied and can range from anywhere between no bleeding, mild PV spotting to heavy PV loss with clots. Therefore, it is essential to assess these patients to ensure they are clinically stable. Baseline observations should be obtained, including blood pressure, pulse, respiratory rate and temperature.

Speculum examination and pelvic examination will help the clinician evaluate the amount of bleeding, assess the cervical os and size of the uterus, as well as identify any tissue that may be passed PV. When considering other potential differential diagnoses, physical examination will aid in eliciting cervical tenderness, and a mass/fullness or pain in the ovarian fossa which may suggest an ectopic pregnancy.

6.5 Investigations

As described above, the primary tool for investigation when a patient presents with PV bleeding and suspected miscarriage is ultrasonography. The purpose of ultrasonography is two-fold – to confirm the location of the pregnancy and assess viability.

A transabdominal (TA) ultrasound examination should be performed while the patient has a full bladder and is lying in a supine position. This will allow for assessment of possible uterine or other pelvic pathology, including fibroids. This should be followed by a transvaginal (TV) ultrasound examination, which is preferable for investigating the location and viability of early pregnancies. However, not all women will find this acceptable. In this situation, TA US will be the only option and the patient should be made aware of its limitations. The patient should be advised that diagnosis of a miscarriage can be challenging, and that a single ultrasound scan (both TA and TV) may not be sufficient. Figure 6.1 describes the US findings and recommended follow-up.

Table 6.4 A list of key information which should be collected at history taking

History	
Last menstrual period	This will allow for estimation of gestational age
Past obstetric and gynaecological history	The most relevant information includes previous history of miscarriages, as well as previous live births. A history of ectopic pregnancy and/or pelvic inflammatory disease would increase the risk of an ectopic pregnancy.
Contraception use	The use of intrauterine device or previous tubal ligation increases the risk of ectopic pregnancy
Symptoms	
Bleeding	Onset, severity, presence of clots or tissue
Abdominal pain	May or may not be present with miscarriage. If unilateral pelvic pain is described, suspect ectopic pregnancy. Other causes include ovarian causes and surgical causes including appendicitis
Shoulder tip pain	This is often due to diaphragmatic irritation secondary to intra-peritoneal bleeding, and is highly suggestive of a ruptured ectopic pregnancy
Bloatedness	This could be a 'pregnancy-related' symptom, but can also be due to intra-peritoneal bleeding
Fainting/collapse	This may give an indication of the severity of bleeding

US findings should be complemented by a thorough history, clinical examination and, if required, serum hCG levels. This is particularly important if an intrauterine gestational sac is not visible and the location of the pregnancy is unknown as described in Figure 6.2. Further, clinicians and other healthcare professionals managing patients in early pregnancy should be cautious when diagnosing a complete miscarriage in the absence of a previous scan confirming an intrauterine pregnancy. This is due to the possibility of an undiagnosed ectopic pregnancy, and these women should always be advised to contact EPAS or gynaecology emergency services if they have any concerns, and they should be advised regarding symptoms to look out for including abdominal pain, bleeding or collapse.

6.6 Differential Diagnosis

The main differential diagnosis when a patient presents with PV bleeding and a positive pregnancy test, and unknown gestation is ectopic pregnancy. A thorough history and examination, supplemented by further investigations with ultrasonography (TV or TA) and serum hCG, will aid diagnosis.

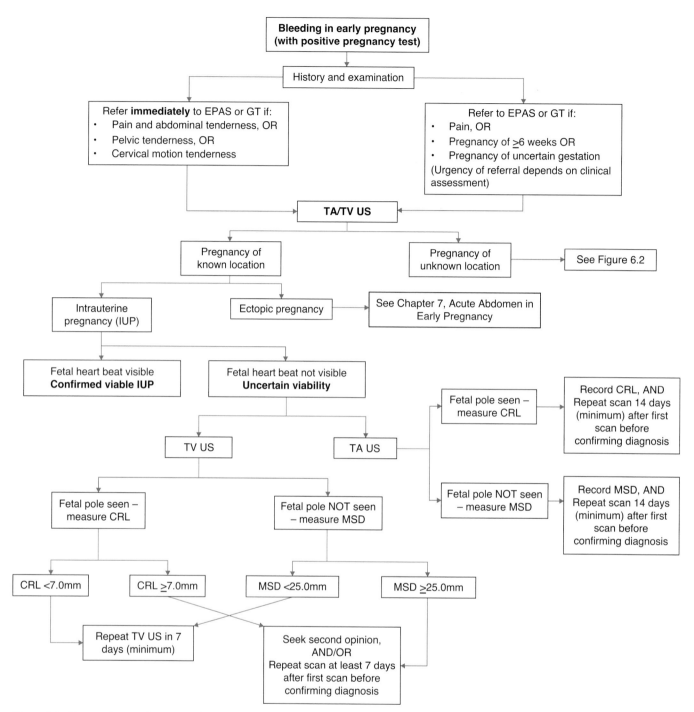

Figure 6.1 Diagram showing diagnosis and management of patient with bleeding in early pregnancy [19].
CRL: Crown–rump length; EPAS: Early pregnancy assessment services; GT: Gynaecology triage; MSD: Mean gestational sac diameter

Determining whether a pregnancy of unknown location is an ectopic pregnancy or a miscarriage can be challenging, particularly if the gestation is unknown. In this situation, it is pertinent that appropriate follow-up is organized with local early pregnancy services, and the patient has access to a 24-hour service for advice and medical attention.

Other differential diagnoses which should be considered are molar pregnancy, heterotrophic pregnancy (a rare condition where an ectopic pregnancy may be present with an intrauterine pregnancy), as well as cervical or vaginal lesions.

6.7 Clinical Management

The initial management of a patient who presents with PV bleeding in early pregnancy, irrespective of the diagnosis, depends on their clinical presentation. Patients who present with severe pain or bleeding, collapse or demonstrate signs of shock should be admitted for inpatient management. The majority of patients who present with PV bleeding in early pregnancy, in the absence of concerning symptoms including collapse and shoulder tip pain, can be managed as an

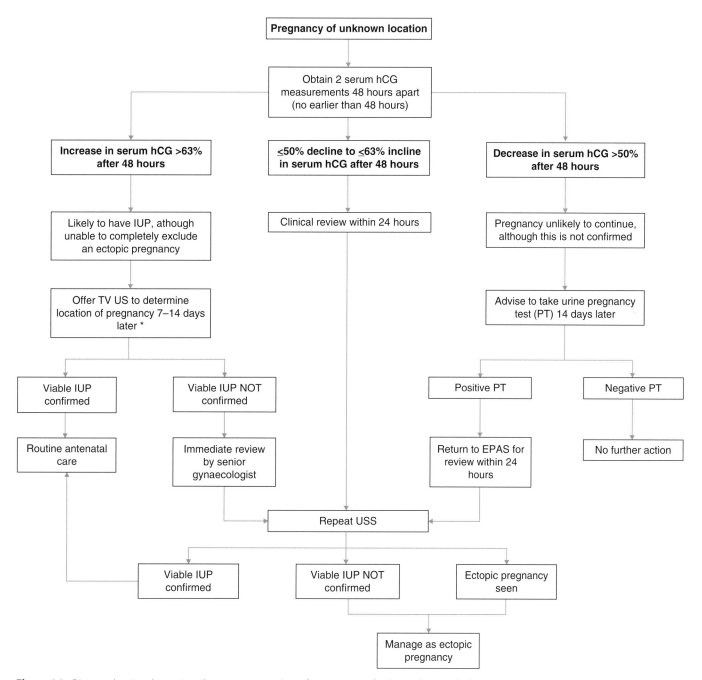

Figure 6.2 Diagram showing diagnosis and management pathway for pregnancy of unknown location [19].
* Consider offering an earlier scan for patients with serum hCG ≥1500 IU/L. IUP: Intrauterine pregnancy; USS: Ultrasound scan

outpatient through follow-up with EPAS. These women should be given contact details for emergency services and be advised to seek medical attention if their symptoms worsen.

6.7.1 General

Patients who have a 'threatened miscarriage' (i.e. present with PV bleeding but have a confirmed viable IUP) can be advised to continue with routine antenatal care if their bleeding has settled. Those who continue to bleed for more than 14 days, or if the bleeding deteriorates, should be reviewed [19].

If possible, tissue from the miscarriage should be sent for histology to confirm the pregnancy and exclude molar pregnancy and ectopic pregnancy (but will not exclude a heterotrophic pregnancy). The patient should be made aware of the options for disposal of remains of the pregnancy. The Human Tissue Authority has issued guidance for the sensitive disposal of pregnancy remains, and have advised that the option of returning the remains to the patient should be offered [20].

The National Institute for Health and Care Excellence (NICE, UK) recommends that patients who are rhesus negative should be offered anti-D immunoglobulin prophylaxis (250

IU) if they are undergoing surgical treatment for their miscarriage [19]. It does not recommend routine anti-D prophylaxis for patients with threatened or complete miscarriage, or those who receive medical treatment for miscarriage.

The British Society for Haematology subsequently produced a guideline on the administration of anti-D immunoglobulin [21]. They recommend maternal blood group and antibody screen to check rhesus D and anti-D antibody status. Patients with complete miscarriage or mild PV bleeding at <12 weeks' gestation do not require anti-D prophylaxis as the risk of fetal-maternal haemorrhage is very small. However, if the patient is <12 weeks pregnant and presents with a history of recurrent episodes of heavy PV bleeding, or associated with abdominal pain, anti-D prophylaxis (250 IU) should be offered. Investigation for fetal-maternal haemorrhage (with Kleihauer–Betke test) is not required for patients less than 20 weeks' gestation.

Patients who are between 12 and 20 weeks' gestation and are known to be rhesus D negative but have not previously been sensitized are advised to receive anti-D prophylaxis (250 IU) within 72 hours of a sensitizing event [21]. Sensitizing events include threatened/incomplete/complete miscarriage and PV bleeding. In cases of recurrent PV bleeding between 12 and 20 weeks' gestation, repeated doses of anti-D prophylaxis (250 IU) at 6-weekly intervals should be considered.

The options for management of miscarriage include expectant, medical and surgical. The patient should be encouraged and supported to make her own decision with regards to management, unless there is a clinical indication for medical or surgical intervention. It has been shown that those who were given the choice had a better health-related quality of life [22].

6.7.2 Expectant Management

Expectant management following confirmation of a miscarriage does not involve any treatment and allows the patient to await natural resolution of the miscarriage. The NICE guidance has recommended this method as the first line management option for the first 7 to 14 days following confirmation of an early miscarriage [19]. It has been shown that this duration is sufficient for complete passage of remaining products of conception in majority of patients who opt for expectant management. Figure 6.3 describes the management pathway for patients undergoing expectant management as recommended by NICE.

When counselling patients regarding expectant management, they should be made aware of the risks and benefits associated with this option. Luise et al [23] reported 52% of incomplete miscarriages resolved within 7 days, and by the end of 14 days, this figure increased to 84%. Therefore, expectant management potentially avoids the need for hospital admission. However, it should be noted that compared with patients who opt for elective surgical management of miscarriage, those who are managed expectantly have an increased risk of incomplete miscarriage (relative risk (RR) 3.98, 95% CI 2.94–5.38) where there are residual products of conception in utero after 14 days, necessitating emergency surgical intervention [24]. Although only 1.4% of patients undergoing expectant management required blood transfusion, they are at a higher risk of this compared with

those managed surgically (RR 6.45, 95% CI 1.21–34.42) [24]. There is no difference in the risk of infection between all 3 methods of management [24, 25].

There are several circumstances when patients may be advised alternative management options. These include risk of haemorrhage, particularly if the miscarriage occurred in late first trimester or a known history of haemoglobinopathy, or if there are signs of infection. Further, patients who are unable to receive blood products in the event of a haemorrhage should also be offered medical or surgical treatment. It is important to consider the patient's past obstetric history, specifically if there is a past history of stillbirth, miscarriage or haemorrhage, and offer alternative management options appropriately.

6.7.3 Medical Management

The main agent used in the medical management of *early miscarriage* is prostaglandin (e.g. misoprostol or gemeprost). Occasionally this is used in combination with an anti-progesterone (e.g. mifepristone).

The Comparative Effectiveness of Pregnancy Failure Management Regimens (PreFaiR) trial compared the outcomes between patients with early miscarriage who were randomly assigned to receive pre-treatment with 200 mg of oral mifepristone prior to receiving 800 µg of vaginal misoprostol, or to receive 800 µg vaginal misoprostol alone [26]. The primary outcome measure was successful expulsion of the gestational sac (determined by US) following one dose of misoprostol within the 4 days of treatment. They reported a significantly higher rate of successful outcome in the group with mifepristone pre-treatment compared with those who received misoprostol alone (83.8% vs. 67.1%, p<0.001). By the end of the 30-day follow-up period, pre-treatment with mifepristone remained superior in achieving successful resolution of the miscarriage, and is associated with a lower risk of requiring further surgical intervention.

Mifepristone is not routinely used in the medical management of early miscarriage, and at present, NICE do not recommend prescribing mifepristone to patients with missed miscarriage or incomplete miscarriage [19].

Both gemeprost and misoprostol are synthetic prostaglandin E1 analogues which soften the cervix and enable cervical dilation, as well as stimulate uterine contractions. Misoprostol is the preferred treatment option for medical management of miscarriage as it causes fewer side effects, and is more cost-effective than gemeprost [27].

NICE recommends that patients with *missed or incomplete miscarriage* are offered vaginal misoprostol [19]. However, it can also be given orally if this is the patient's preferred choice. A randomized controlled trial by Pang et al [28] reported no difference in efficacy when patients with incomplete miscarriage were given 800 µg of misoprostol either orally or vaginally. However, this study identified a higher incidence of gastrointestinal side effects (diarrhoea) among patients who received the drug orally vs. vaginally (65.3% vs. 13.6%, p<0.01). Figure 6.4 describes the medical management of patients using misoprostol as recommended by NICE.

A Cochrane review [29] compared medical management of miscarriage with expectant management and did not identify any difference in achieving complete miscarriage, nor the need for unplanned surgical intervention. This review also compared medical vs. surgical management of miscarriage and reported a higher risk of unplanned surgical intervention in the group that received medical treatment (average RR 5.03, 95% CI 2.71–9.35).

6.7.4 Surgical Management

Indications for surgical management of miscarriage are included in Table 6.5.

The two surgical methods are 1) manual vacuum aspiration in an outpatient setting under local anaesthetic, and 2) surgical management under general anaesthetic. Both these options are

associated with less bleeding and involve a shorter duration to achieve resolution of the miscarriage [25]. However, patients should be advised of the attending risks associated with these surgical procedures.

The Royal College of Obstetricians and Gynaecologists (RCOG) recently published an updated guideline [30] for clinicians when counselling patients regarding surgical management of early miscarriage. The overall risk of a serious complication associated with this procedure is 6%. Bleeding can occur for up to 2 weeks; however, heavy bleeding is uncommon. Patients who have ongoing PV bleeding for more than 2 weeks or have very heavy bleeding should be advised to seek medical attention for further investigation to exclude retained products of conception.

Surgical management of miscarriage is associated with a risk of pelvic infection (3% risk of infection in the first 14 days following treatment [25]); however, studies have reported that the rates of infection are similar between the expectant, medical and surgical management [24, 25]. At present there are no conclusive data to confirm whether administration of prophylactic antibiotics in patients undergoing surgical management of miscarriage will reduce the risk of infection. Nevertheless, some units (in the UK) recommend that patients undergoing surgical management are prescribed azithromycin and/or metronidazole, even in the absence of proven pelvic infection or chlamydia infection.

Table 6.5 Indications for surgical management of miscarriage

- Patient's choice
- Unsuccessful expectant or medical management
- Evidence of ongoing heavy PV bleeding +/– clinical signs of shock
- Contraindications for medical management of miscarriage (e.g. on anticoagulants)
- Evidence of intrauterine infection
- Suspected molar pregnancy

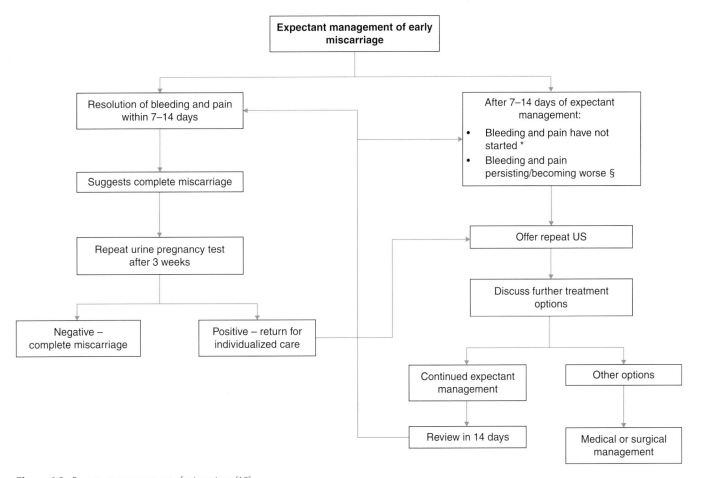

Figure 6.3 Expectant management of miscarriage [19].
*Miscarriage unlikely to have started. §Miscarriage likely to be incomplete.

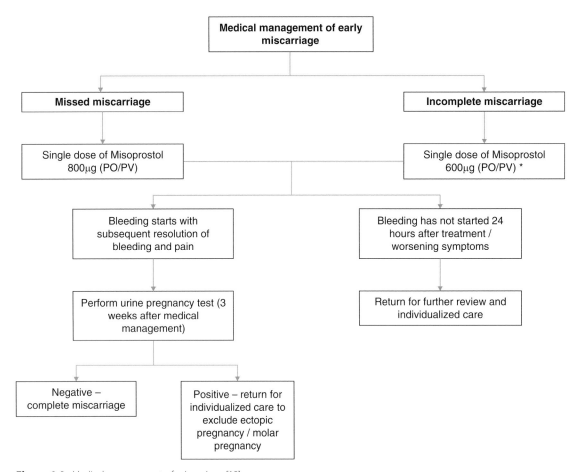

Figure 6.4 Medical management of miscarriage [19]
*Can offer 800 μg of misoprotol to allow alignment of treatment protocols for missed and incomplete miscarriage. PO: oral; PV: vaginal

A large multicentre randomized controlled trial [31] has recently been undertaken to assess the effects of administration of doxycycline and metronidazole vs. placebo in women undergoing surgical management of early miscarriage, and the results of this study are currently awaited. Although the centres recruited in this trial are primarily from low-income countries, the results will nevertheless be useful to inform national and international health governing bodies about the health and economic risks and benefits associated with the use of antibiotics in this group of patients.

There is a risk of retained products of conception following surgical evacuation of the uterus, and this is reported to affect approximately 4% of patients undergoing this procedure [30]. Nevertheless, it should be noted that the risk of retained tissue remains lower than both expectant and medical management of miscarriage.

Uterine perforation is an uncommon but severe risk associated with surgical management of miscarriage. This complication is estimated to occur in approximately 0.1% of patients undergoing surgical management [32]. Most of the patients with this complication can be managed conservatively with a period of inpatient observation +/– administration of antibiotic prophylaxis, without the need for further intervention. However, a small proportion of these patients – particularly those with deterioration of symptoms including bleeding and

abdominal pain – may require further intervention in the form of laparoscopy or laparotomy, depending on the severity of the complication and availability of surgical expertise.

Cervical trauma is another uncommon complication associated with surgical management of miscarriage. Cervical priming is thought to reduce the risk of uterine injury and cervical trauma during this procedure. This is common practice in many centres offering abortion services [33]. A large randomized controlled trial by the WHO was performed to investigate the role of cervical priming with misoprostol prior to first trimester abortion [34]. This study has shown that administration of misoprostol can make this an overall safer procedure by potentially reducing the incidence of incomplete abortions. However, it did not report a difference in the risk of uterine or cervical trauma. Further, a Cochrane review [35] on cervical ripening prior to surgical management of first trimester miscarriage showed that although this additional step reduces the need for manual dilation of the cervix, there is no conclusive evidence that it reduces the risk of uterine or cervical trauma.

Finally, surgical management of miscarriage is associated with a risk of uterine adhesions, although the true incidence of this condition is not determined as most patients can be asymptomatic. The RCOG guidance has suggested that the risk of uterine adhesions was 16.3–18.5% following surgical management of miscarriage [30].

6.7.5 Other Methods

It has been suggested that reduced levels of circulating progesterone are linked to miscarriage; however, the evidence on the use of progestogens to reduce the risk of miscarriage is inconclusive. A recent Cochrane review [36] has reported that administration of progesterone might reduce the risk of miscarriage in patients with a history of recurrent miscarriage. However, the authors are cautious with interpreting the findings of this meta-analysis due to the average quality of the studies included and the heterogeneity in the patients included (average RR 0.69, 95% CI 0.51–0.92). The use of progesterone in reducing the risk of miscarriage, particularly those without a history of previous miscarriage, therefore requires further research with standardized trial protocols.

6.7.6 Psychological Impact

PV bleeding in early pregnancy can be a difficult time for the patient, as well as her family. The attending healthcare professional should consider the psychological impact of miscarriage on the patient and her family and offer advice and support in a sensitive and objective manner.

Patients can be directed to support networks (see below) for further information and additional support. Referral to counselling services should be considered if this was felt to be appropriate. Further, close liaison with the patient's general practitioner or family doctor is crucial, and the patient should be offered early contact with EPAS in future pregnancies.

Useful websites/resources for healthcare professionals and patients:

- RCOG Patient Information Leaflet: www.rcog.org.uk/globa lassets/documents/patients/patient-information-leaflets/pre gnancy/pi-bleeding-and-or-pain-in-early-pregnancy.pdf
- The Association of Early Pregnancy Units: www.aepu.org.uk
- Tommy's: www.tommys.org
- Miscarriage Association: www.miscarriageassociation.org.uk

6.8 Key Guidelines Relevant to the Topic

- Ectopic pregnancy and miscarriage: diagnosis and initial management. National Institute for Health and Care Excellence (NICE) [19]
- Surgical management of miscarriage and removal of persistent placental or foetal remains. Consent Advice No. 10 (Joint with AEPU). Royal College of Obstetricians and Gynaecologists (RCOG) [30]
- Guidance on the disposal of pregnancy remains following pregnancy loss or termination. Human Tissue Authority (HTA) [20]
- BCSH guideline for the use of anti-D immunoglobulin for the prevention of haemolytic disease of the foetus and newborn. British Society for Haematology [21]

References

1. Sapra K, Joseph,K, Galea S, et al. Signs and symptoms of early pregnancy loss: a systematic review. *Reprod Sci.* 2017;**24**(4):502–13.

2. Tommy's. Miscarriage statistics. 2018. Website. www.tommys.org/our-organisation/charity-research/preg nancy-statistics/miscarriage. Accessed 10 September 2018.

3. van den Berg M, van Wely M, Goddijn M. Genetics of early miscarriage, *Biochim Biophys Acta.* 2012;**1822**(12):1951–9.

4. Eiben B, Bartels I, Bahr-Porsch D, et al. Cytogenetic analysis of 750 spontaneous abortions with the direct-preparation method of chorionic villi and its implications for studying genetic causes of pregnancy wastage. *Am J Hum Genet.* 1990;**47**:656–63.

5. Nybo Andersen A, Wohlfahrt J, Christens P, Olsen J, Melbye, M. Maternal age and fetal loss: population based register linkage study. *BMJ.* 2000;**320**:1708.

6. Gracia C, Sammel M, Chittams J, et al. Risk factors for spontaneous abortion in early symptomatic first-trimester pregnancies. *Obstet Gynecol.* 2005;**106**(5):993–9.

7. Cleary-Goldman J, Malone F, Vidaver J, et al. Impact of maternal age on obstetric outcome. *Obstet Gynecol.* 2005;**105**(5):983–90.

8. Maconochie N, Doyle P, Prior S, Simmons R. Risk factors for first trimester miscarriage – results from a UK-population-based case-control study. *BJOG.* 2007;**114**(2):170–86.

9. Pineles B, Park E, Samet J. Systematic review and meta-analysis of miscarriage and maternal exposure to tobacco smoke during pregnancy. *Am J Epidemiol.* 2014;**179**(7):807–23.

10. Weng X, Odouli R, Li D. Maternal caffeine consumption during pregnancy and the risk of miscarriage: a prospective cohort study. *Am J Obstet Gynecol.* 2008;**198**(3):279.

11. Avalos, L, Roberts S, Kaskutas, L, Block G, Li D. Volume and type of alcohol during early pregnancy and the risk of miscarriage. *Subst Use Misuse.* 2014;**49**(11):1437–45.

12. Arck P. Early risk factors for miscarriage: a prospective cohort study in pregnant women. *Reprod Biomed Online.* 2008;**17**(1):101–13.

13. Metwally M, Ong K, Ledger W, Li T. Does high body mass index increase the risk of miscarriage after spontaneous and assisted conception? A meta-analysis of evidence. *Fertil Steril.* 2008;**90**(3):714–26.

14. Giakoumelou S, Wheelhouse N, Cuschieri K, et al. The role of infection in miscarriage. *Hum Reprod Update.* 2016;**22**(1):116–33.

15. de la Rochebrochard E, Thonneau P. Paternal age and maternal age are risk factors for miscarriage: results of a multicentre European study. *Hum Reprod.* 2002;**17**(6):1649–56.

16. Farquharson RG, Jauniaux E, Exalto N, on behalf of ESHRE Special Interest Group for Early Pregnancy. Updated and revised nomenclature for description of early pregnancy events. *Hum Reprod.* 2005;**20**(11):3008–11.

17. Everett C. Incidence and outcome of bleeding before 20th week of pregnancy: prospective study from general practice. *BMJ.* 1997;**315**:32.

18. Harville E, Wilcox A, Baird D, Weinberg C. Vaginal bleeding in very early pregnancy. *Hum Reprod.* 2003;**18**(9):1944–7.

19. National Institute for Health and Care Excellence (NICE). Ectopic pregnancy and miscarriage: diagnosis and initial management (Clinical Guideline 154). 2012.

20. Human Tissue Authority UK (HTA). Guidance on the disposal of pregnancy remains following pregnancy loss or termination. 2015.

21. Qureshi H, Massey E, Kirwan D, et al. BCSH guideline for the use of anti-D immunoglobulin for the prevention of haemolytic disease of the fetus and newborn. *Transfus Med.* 2014;**24**(1):8–20.

22. Wierenga-de Waard M, Hartman E, Ankum W, et al. Expectant management versus surgical evacuation in first trimester miscarriage: health-related quality of life in randomised and non-randomised patients. *Hum Reprod.* 2002;**17**(6):1638–42.

23. Luise C, Jermy K, May C, et al. Outcome of expectant management of spontaneous first trimester miscarriage: observational study. *BMJ.* 2002;**324**:873.

24. Nanda K, Lopez L,. Grimes D, Peloggia A, Nanda G. Expectant care vs. surgical treatment for miscarriage. *Cochrane Database Syst Rev.* 2012 Mar; **2012**(3).

25. Trinder J, Porter R, Vyas S. Management of miscarriage: expectant, medical or surgical? Results of randomised controlled trial (miscarriage treatment (MIST) trial). *BMJ.* 2006;**332**:1235.

26. Schreiber C, Creinin M, Atrio J, et al. Mifepristone pretreatment for the medical management of early pregnancy loss. *N Engl J Med.* 2018;**378**:2161–70.

27. Saraswat L, Ashok P, Mathur M. Medical management of miscarriage. *Obstet Gynaecol.* 2014;**16**:79–85.

28. Pang M, Lee T, Chung T. Incomplete miscarriage: a randomised controlled trial comparing oral with vaginal misoprostol for medical evacuation. *Hum Reprod.* 2001;**16**(11):2283–7.

29. Kim C, Barnard S, Neilson J, et al. Medical treatments for incomplete miscarriage. *Cochrane Database Syst Rev.* 2017 Jan; **2017**(1).

30. Royal College of Obstetricians & Gynaecologists (RCOG), Surgical Management of Miscarriage and Removal of Persistent Placental or Fetal Remains (Consent Advice 10. Joint with AEPU). 2018.

31. Lissauer D, Wilson A, Daniels J, et al. Prophylactic antibiotics to reduce pelvic infection in women having miscarriage surgery – the AIMS (Antibiotics in Miscarriage Surgery) trial: study protocol for a randomised controlled trial. *Trials.* 2018;**19**:245.

32. Amarin Z. Badria L. A survey of uterine perforation following dilatation and curettage or evacuation of retained products of conception. *Arch Gynecol Obstet.* 2005;**271**(3):203–6.

33. Cameron S. Recent advances in improving the effectiveness and reducing the complications of abortion. *F1000 Research.* 2018;7.

34. Meirik O, Huong NTM, Piaggio G, Bergel E, von Hertzen H, on behalf of the WHO Research Group on Postovulatory Methods of Fertility Regulation. Complications of first-trimester abortion by vacuum aspiration after cervical preparation with and without misoprostol: a multicentre randomised trial. *Lancet.* 2012;**379**(9828):1817–24.

35. Webber K, Grivell R. Cervical ripening before first trimester surgical evacuation for non-viable pregnancy. *Cochrane Database Syst Rev.* 2015 Nov; **2015**(11).

36. Hass D, Hathaway T, Ramsey P. Progestogen for preventing miscarriage in women with recurrent miscarriage of unclear etiology. *Cochrane Database Syst Rev.* 2018 Oct; **2018**(10).

Chapter 7

Acute Abdomen in Early Pregnancy

David K. Gatongi, Shittu Akinola Saheed & Tahir A. Mahmood

7.1 Introduction

Acute abdomen describes severe abdominal pain usually of less than 24 hours' duration that may require emergency surgery. This is a very common presentation in the gynaecology services. In the pregnant patient the underlying cause may be pregnancy related or non-pregnancy related. Assessment and diagnosis are often challenging due to the influence of pregnancy on maternal physiology and the very wide range of differential diagnoses [1]. Abdominal pain is a very common symptom in pregnancy that most often resolves without much intervention. This observation may make the clinician complacent and therefore less suspicious of more serious or life-threatening underlying pathology. Diagnostic evaluation is further complicated by altered reference ranges of laboratory tests. A multidisciplinary team approach is essential to facilitate an efficient diagnostic workup as well as ensuring the most effective treatment is initiated without undue delay.

The gynaecologist is also faced with the need to reconcile the benefits to the mother and the potential safety concerns of the diagnostic tests and treatment on the fetus. The objective for the clinician is to identify the potential cause and implement effective intervention in a timely fashion in order to optimize outcome [2]. The interests of the mother should always override those of the fetus. The CEMACH report for 2003–2005 revealed many pitfalls in the assessment of pregnant women with abdominal pain leading to maternal mortality [3].

7.2 Anatomical and Physiological Changes of Pregnancy That May Create Diagnostic Challenges

Pregnancy is associated with anatomical and physiological changes that can cause abdominal pain, and often these may cause diagnostic uncertainty [4, 5]. The stretching of the round ligaments, which occurs as a normal benign process, may sometimes cause sufficient pain that may be severe enough to mimic acute abdomen. Nausea and vomiting are common symptoms in early pregnancy that usually resolve during the second trimester. These same symptoms are common in pathologies presenting with an acute abdomen. Underlying pathology should, however, be suspected when nausea and vomiting are associated with fever and changes in bowel habits. Furthermore, the enlarging uterus may make it difficult to carry out physical examination by affecting the normal position of abdominal organs and delaying peritoneal signs. Peritoneal irritation is also decreased as a result of the laxity of the abdominal wall which normally occurs during pregnancy. Compression of the urinary tract by the uterus causes hydroureter and hydronephrosis hence mimicking nephrolithiasis.

Aortocaval compression caused by the enlarged uterus may result in hypotension, making the interpretation of blood pressure readings less easy when the patient is in the supine position. When this happens in patients with an acute abdomen, it may mimic internal bleeding from an acute disease process. The high maternal blood level of progesterone in pregnancy lowers the tone of the lower oesophagus, reduces bowel motility, delays emptying of gallbladder and reduces ureteric tone. These effects underlie the pathogenesis of gastrointestinal and urological pathologies that can present acutely. White blood cell count increases in pregnancy and haemoglobin levels decrease in pregnancy due to the changes that take place in blood volume, causing what is termed the 'physiological anaemia of pregnancy'. Renal and liver functions tests are also normally affected by pregnancy. These biochemical pregnancy changes should be considered when interpreting laboratory results.

7.3 Pathogenesis of Acute Abdomen

Acute abdominal pain is generated through different mechanisms depending on the organ system and the pathological process involved. Free blood in the peritoneal cavity causes peritoneal irritation, resulting in pain sensation. The most common causes of intra-abdominal haemorrhage in early pregnancy is ruptured ectopic pregnancy resulting in haematoperitoneum and attendant acute pain [6]. The perforation of an abdominal viscus, commonly the bowel, discharges the contents into the peritoneal cavity, resulting in chemical peritoneal irritation and pain. This typically results in pain which starts at the site of perforation but quickly spreads and becomes generalized. Infection rapidly sets in. A ruptured appendix following appendicitis is a classical example of ruptured viscus and is not uncommon during pregnancy [7, 8].The classical signs of rebound tenderness, rigidity and reduced bowel sounds are present as well as tachycardia, pyrexia and hypotension due to sepsis. When intra-abdominal organs experience ischaemia, acute pain is a common presentation. Typically, the patient presents with a severe sudden onset of abdominal pain which generally is out of proportion with other clinical signs. This is the common presentation in torsion of ovarian cyst [9] or mesenteric venous thrombosis. Excessive spasms of abdominal viscera result in colicky abdominal pain that has crescendos, becoming very severe and then diminishing. This is most

55

typically seen in ureteric obstruction, bowel obstruction and biliary colic.

7.4 Epidemiology and Aetiology

About 2% of pregnant mothers require surgery for non-obstetric reasons. The underlying cause of acute abdomen may be pregnancy related or non-pregnancy related [5]. Possible causes are summarized in Table 7.1.

7.5 Gynaecological Causes

7.5.1 Ectopic Pregnancy (EP)

Ectopic pregnancy (EP) describes the implantation of a pregnancy outside the endometrial cavity. The majority of these pregnancies implant in the fallopian tubes. Other less common sites are the ovary, cervix, interstitium and abdomen. EP occurs in about 1% of spontaneous conception and is associated with recurrence rates of 10%. EP is a significant cause of maternal morbidity and mortality, contributing to about 5% of maternal deaths.

Table 7.1 Common causes of acute abdomen in early pregnancy

A: Pregnancy-related causes

	Miscarriage
	Ectopic pregnancy
	Round ligament haematoma
	Abruptio placentae
	Rupture of pregnant uterus

B: Non-pregnancy-related causes

Gynaecological causes	Ovarian cyst accident torsion, haemorrhage or rupture
	Degeneration of fibroid
	Torsion of the uterus
	Pelvic inflammatory disease
	Ovarian hyperstimulation syndrome
Gastrointestinal causes	Appendicitis
	Peptic ulcer disease
	Inflammatory bowel disease
	Intestinal obstruction
	Peritonitis
Genitourinary causes	Cystitis
	Pyelonephritis
	Urolithiasis
	Hydronephrosis
Hepatobiliary causes	Acute cholecystitis
	Acute pancreatitis
	Acute fatty liver of pregnancy
	Hepatitis
Vascular causes	Mesenteric vein thrombosis
	Vasculitis
	Aneurysm rupture
Medical causes	Lower lobe pneumonia
	Pulmonary embolism
	Sickle cell crisis

Patients with EP can present with no abdominal pain or with a dramatic picture of acute abdominal pain. The latter is commonly due to rupture of the EP, leading to intra-abdominal haemorrhage and causing peritoneal irritation. More frequently, EP presents with non-specific unilateral low abdominal pain which may be associated with vaginal bleeding. Other non-specific symptoms of diarrhoea and vomiting may also be present, further confusing the clinical picture [6, 10]. The patient may be tachycardic and hypotensive due to the pain or the intra-abdominal haemorrhage. There is low abdominal tenderness on examination. The abdomen may be distended if massive haemorrhage has occurred. Abdominal tenderness with rigidity and guarding due to peritoneal irritation is found on examination in these patients.

Diagnosis is clinched by a high index of suspicion in a pregnant patient presenting with abdominal pain. Transvaginal ultrasound reveals the absence of an intrauterine pregnancy and the presence an adnexal mass or adnexal gestation sac with or without fetal pole. In cases where ultrasound is inconclusive, correlation with serum βhCG may aid the diagnosis. Discriminatory levels of βhCG vary between laboratories; however, at a level of 1500 IU/L or above, an intrauterine gestation sac should be identifiable. If this is not visualized, this is highly suggestive of EP [11, 12]. Management of EP presenting with acute abdomen with suspicion of rupture or the presence of haemodynamic instability is laparoscopy. This serves both a diagnostic and therapeutic role. Salpingectomy is the preferred surgical intervention. Medical management of EP is reserved for patients with minimal pain or asymptomatic haemodynamically stable patients [10, 11].

7.5.2 Miscarriage

Miscarriage affects about 15% of pregnancies and presents as a continuum of several clinical entities. These conditions include missed, threatened, inevitable, incomplete, complete or septic miscarriage [10, 12]. With the exception of a missed miscarriage, which is asymptomatic, the cardinal presenting symptoms are vaginal bleeding and pain. The pain associated with a miscarriage is due to uterine contractions and the release of prostaglandins and inflammatory mediators form the decidual breakdown. The patient may have a high pulse rate and low blood pressure due to pain and bleeding. A vasovagal response sometimes occurs due to cervical distension by products of conception causing bradycardia and hypotension. Patients with septic miscarriage will be pyrexial. Where infection has spread to the fallopian tubes and pelvic cavity, overt signs of peritonitis are present. There is low abdominal tenderness on examination, and the uterus may be palpable consistent with the gestation age. Vaginal bleeding is present on examination, and the cervix may be open. Products of conception may be visible through the cervix. In a septic miscarriage, an offensive vaginal discharge will be present.

Diagnosis is made by ultrasound and the clinical examination findings. Pelvic ultrasound shows a viable intrauterine pregnancy in threatened miscarriage. Non-viable pregnancy products of conception will be identified on ultrasound in cases of inevitable, incomplete and septic miscarriage. The finding of an open cervix with products of conception in the cervical canal confirms an incomplete miscarriage. The definitive management of patients presenting with acute abdomen due to miscarriage is uterine evacuation. This is best carried out by surgical evacuation of the uterus in patients who are haemodynamically unstable. Medical management is an alternative for haemodynamically stable patients [12, 13].

7.5.3 Ovarian Cyst Torsion

Ovarian masses are found in up to 8.8% of pregnancies. The majority of these are unilateral functional corpus luteal and follicular cysts which tend to resolve by the 16th week of pregnancy. Hyperstimulated bilateral cystic enlarged ovaries are commonly found following assisted conception. Benign dermoid cysts are the most common neoplastic tumours found during pregnancy. Malignant tumours are less common [14]. The majority of these ovarian masses are asymptomatic and are usually identified during routine early pregnancy scanning. Torsion of ovarian cysts is more common in cysts measuring over 5 cm in diameter. Torsion results in ovarian ischaemia causing severe abdominal pain. It occurs more frequently in the right ovary compared to the left. Torsion is found in 2–15% of patients undergoing emergency surgery for adnexal masses. About 10–22% of ovarian torsion cases occur during pregnancy [9]. Typically, acute torsion presents with acute pelvic pain associated with nausea and vomiting. However, in the majority of patients, the presentation is subacute with long-standing history of low abdominal pain of sudden onset which resolves over a short period of time. This is due to repeated torsion and spontaneous detorsion. Torsion can also be precipitated by intercourse. On examination, patients are tachycardic and may have a low-grade pyrexia due to a systemic inflammatory response to the ovarian ischaemia. There is a generalized low abdominal tenderness with localized guarding and rebound tenderness. Adnexal tenderness and an adnexal mass may be palpated during vaginal examination.

Pelvic ultrasound is the imaging modality of choice for diagnosing ovarian cysts. The ultrasound appearance of ovarian torsion is very variable and unfortunately there are no distinctive diagnostic ultrasound features. Usually the ovary is enlarged compared to the contralateral ovary. The diagnosis of ovarian torsion is based on the clinical history, examination findings, ultrasound features and a high index of clinical suspicion. Ovarian torsion is a gynaecological emergency requiring urgent surgery due to the risk of ovarian ischaemic necrosis. The goal of surgery is timely detorsion and cystectomy. Oophorectomy should be avoided even where the ovary appears dark blue or black, as up to 80% of cases treated conservatively show follicular activity on follow-up. A laparoscopic approach is preferred to laparotomy. The choice of surgery is dependent on the availability of a trained laparoscopic surgeon and the size of the cyst [9, 15].

7.5.4 Ovarian Cyst Rupture and Haemorrhage

Bleeding into a cyst or rupture of a cyst causes acute pelvic pain. These two events may be spontaneous but sometimes they may follow minor trauma or intercourse. Bleeding is usually self-limiting and is confined to the cyst [1]. However, rupture of the cyst may lead to substantial intraperitoneal haemorrhage with haemodynamic instability. History and ultrasound imaging will aid diagnosis. In haemodynamically stable patients, conservative management with observation and analgesia will be sufficient. In patients where intra-abdominal haemorrhage results in haemodynamic instability, laparoscopy and cystectomy are the treatments of choice.

7.5.5 Degeneration of Fibroid

Fibroids are found in 10.7% of pregnancies during the first trimester and are the most common solid adnexal masses. The majority of fibroids are asymptomatic and are commonly identified during a routine pregnancy ultrasound scan. About 1 in 500 pregnant women are admitted to hospital due to a fibroid-related complication [14, 16]. Acute abdominal pain caused by fibroids is usually due to red degeneration or torsion of a pedunculated fibroid. Pain resulting from degeneration or torsion may be associated with nausea, vomiting and low-grade pyrexia. Torsion and necrosis occur in pedunculated fibroids. Any cystic changes in fibroids seen on ultrasound are suggestive of red degeneration. Symptomatic treatment with analgesia and antiemetics is the management of choice for red degeneration and torsion. Surgical intervention is reserved for when conservative management is not effective especially for fibroid torsion [17].

7.6 Non-Gynaecological Causes

7.6.1 Acute Appendicitis

Acute appendicitis is the most common cause of acute abdomen in pregnancy, being present in 1:500–2000 pregnancies. Pregnancy does not increase the overall incidence of acute appendicitis, but the overall severity of the condition may be increased. It is slightly more commonly seen in the second trimester. Maternal mortality is highest when the condition occurs during the third trimester due to a delay in diagnosis and refusal of laparotomy. A negative laparotomy of 35% is acceptable. Complications include peritonitis, sepsis, and perforation in about 25% of cases. Fetal complications are mainly due to the onset of preterm labour which occurs in 1–2% of uncomplicated cases and 25% in perforated cases. Fetal demise is rare. The diagnosis is clinical. Symptoms include periumbilical to right iliac fossa pain, fever, nausea and vomiting. Pain may be located in the right upper quadrant (RUQ). The anatomical alteration of the caecum caused by the enlarged uterus may shift the position of the appendix, placing the site of maximum tenderness at a higher level than expected in the non-pregnant state. Clinical signs include focal tenderness, rebound and guarding. Leukocytosis is normal in pregnancy. However, a raised neutrophil count and C-reactive protein (CRP) level suggest infection.

Ultrasound examination is often non-specific, but can rule out other differentials. It may show mural thickening and peri-appendiceal fluid. Magnetic resonance imaging (MRI) is helpful where ultrasound is inconclusive. Computed tomography (CT) scan of the abdomen is a better diagnostic modality but exposes the fetus to radiation. Management is surgical removal of the appendix. Surgery can be through open laparotomy or laparoscopy. A laparoscopic appendicectomy is now an acceptable procedure even in the third trimester. A 15 mm Hg pneumoperitoneum is well tolerated by the fetus. Palmer's point Veress needle entry has been described as suitable, but the open Hanson technique is generally recommended [18].

7.6.2 Acute Cholecystitis

Acute cholecystitis is the second most common cause of acute abdomen in pregnancy, occurring with an incidence of 1–8:10 000 pregnancies. More than 90% are caused by the presence of gallstones. Symptoms include prolonged RUQ pain, vomiting, fever, tachycardia and leukocytosis. Murphy's sign is less commonly elicited in pregnancy. The liver function tests may be slightly out of normal range. Alkaline phosphatase level assessment is of no diagnostic use, as it is normally increased in pregnancy. Jaundice suggest choledocholithiasis, i.e. blockage of the bile duct with stones. Ultrasound will detect 95% of gallstones and is diagnostic if additionally gallbladder thickening and pericholecystic fluid are seen [18]. Endoscopic retrograde cholangiopancreatography is an option to help establish the diagnosis using techniques to reduce fetal radiation dose.

The initial management is primarily supportive with intravenous fluids, nasogastric tube, antibiotics and analgesics as indicated. Morphine should be avoided since it induces spasm of the sphincter of Oddi. Cholecystectomy is indicated if patient is unresponsive to supportive management. The operation is best done in the second trimester. Surgical management can be through open laparotomy or laparoscopy. This being more readily undertaken during pregnancy to reduce the risks of gallstone pancreatitis, miscarriage and preterm labour. Fetal loss increases by 10–60% in gallstone pancreatitis [19, 20]

7.6.3 Acute Pancreatitis

Acute pancreatitis has a documented incidence of 1:1–3000 pregnancies. It occurs most commonly in the second half of pregnancy and the puerperium, though 19% of cases of acute pancreatitis are reported to occur in the first trimester. The commonest causes are gallstones and alcohol; however, surgery, viral infections, drugs and trauma are also causative. Pregnancy has no effect on the clinical presentation. The main symptoms include epigastric pain radiating to the back and shoulders, nausea, vomiting and fever. The clinical signs include mid-abdominal tenderness, guarding with rebound tenderness, hypoactive bowel sound and tympany. Serum amylase and lipase levels are key in making a diagnosis but are not prognostic. Ultrasound may show cholelithiasis and bile duct dilation. Grading systems are more complex to use during pregnancy [18].

Management is supportive and includes nil per oral, nasogastric tube insertion, intravenous fluids and analgesia (pethidine and tramadol). Pancreatitis in pregnancy is often mild and responsive to medical therapy. Multidisciplinary involvement is crucial in severe cases as radiological, surgical intervention, nutritional support in the form of total parenteral nutrition and intensive care unit (ICU) care may all be indicated. Pregnancy should not delay the performance of a CT scan of the abdomen to establish the diagnosis or undertaking surgery if this becomes necessary. Endoscopic sphincterotomy can be performed during pregnancy with minimal fetal radiation exposure. Pregnancy complications of acute pancreatitis include miscarriage and preterm labour in later pregnancy. The condition is associated with a maternal mortality in more than 10% of the complicated cases [20].

7.6.4 Nephrolithiasis

Nephrolithiasis in pregnancy has a documented incidence of 1:200–2000 pregnancies. The clinical significance of the condition is a predisposition to stimulating the onset of preterm labour. Hypercalciuria causes 50% of cases, especially in the last two thirds of pregnancy. Symptoms include flank pain radiating to the groin, fever, nausea and vomiting, haematuria and renal angle tenderness. Microscopic haematuria occurs in 75% of cases. Ultrasound is the initial investigation, but may miss partial blockage. Physiological ureteric dilation (<2 cm), especially on right side, affects interpretation. Pathological dilation is characterized by the absence of a visible jet of urine. Intravenous urogram (IVU) may be required but this involves a high radiation dose. Unenhanced helical CT is the gold standard for diagnosis outside pregnancy. Conservative management includes the administration of intravenous fluids, antibiotics and analgesics. Sixty-four to eighty-four per cent of cases respond to conservative management. The urologist should be involved in the management of these cases. Uncontrolled pain, single functioning kidney, sepsis or onset of preterm labour indicates the need for intervention which includes a percutaneous nephrostomy or a ureteric stent changed every 6 weeks. Extracorporeal shock wave lithotripsy is not recommended in pregnancy. Ureteroscopy using holmium laser is an option in pregnancy for stones <1 cm and without the association of sepsis [18].

7.6.5 Bowel Obstruction

Bowel obstruction is the third most common cause of acute abdomen in pregnancy with an incidence of 1:1500–16 000 pregnancies. It is most common in the third trimester. Intra-abdominal adhesions are the commonest cause. Volvulus is more common in pregnancy because of rapid change in the size of the uterus and displacement of bowel. Hernias are rare and should be suspected in patients who have had gastric bypass surgery. Intussusception is also not uncommon. The associated abdominal pain is periodic, mimicking labour. Vomiting is variable. There is complete cessation of stool and flatus passage. The examination reveals the classic distended tender abdomen with high-pitch bowel sound the exception in pregnancy. Rebound tenderness, fever and tachycardia may occur later. There is leukocytosis, haemo-concentration and electrolyte abnormality. An erect abdominal x-ray is needed to establish the diagnosis despite the radiation risks to the fetus. This will show characteristic dilated bowel loops with air-fluid levels. Ultrasound can also show this. MRI can help to characterize the site and degree of obstruction. Bowel obstruction is associated with a fetal-maternal mortality of 26% and 6%, respectively. While partial cases will respond to nasogastric tube insertion, intravenous fluids and electrolyte correction, a quarter of cases will require laparotomy with a midline abdominal incision for surgical resection [21, 22].

7.6.6 Peptic Ulcer Disease (PUD)

Gastroesophageal reflux disease (GERD) affects 45–80% of pregnant women due to raised intra-abdominal pressure, displacement and relaxation of the lower oesophageal sphincter and abnormal oesophageal motility. Peptic ulcer disease (PUD) is uncommon because of reduced gastric acid secretion and increased mucus secretion associated with pregnancy. The general incidence of peptic ulcer is 1:4500 as compared with 1:1000 during pregnancy. Clinical features include epigastric discomfort or pain, nausea, emesis, anorexia, regurgitation and haematemesis. While the symptoms of duodenal ulcer are relieved by food, food worsens those associated with a gastric ulcer. Chest x-ray with an abdominal shield would show air under diaphragm, though this can be absent in 10–20% of cases of perforation. Management should include lifestyle modification and use of antacids, H2-receptor blockers and the proton pump inhibitor omeprazole. One should consider deferring *Helicobacter pylori* eradication until after pregnancy because of possible teratogenic effect of some of the medications used in the treatment regime. Esophagogastroduodenoscopy may be indicated for diagnosis. Surgery for PUD is best delayed until after pregnancy, but surgery may be indicated if the patient's condition becomes unstable since the fetus tolerates maternal hypotension poorly. In advanced pregnancy, caesarean section may be needed before surgery for bleeding or perforation [21].

7.6.7 Spontaneous Intra-abdominal Haemorrhage

Spontaneous intra-abdominal haemorrhage is rare. Causes include rupture of the liver or splenic capsule, or ruptured aneurysms or uterine vessels plexus. Clinical presentation includes abdominal pain and haemorrhagic shock. Doppler auscultation or cardiotocography should be performed to assess fetal well-being. Investigations include a total blood count, liver function tests, renal function tests and a clotting profile. Blood should be crossmatched and made available. Management includes early resuscitation, multidisciplinary input and exploratory laparotomy [18].

7.6.8 Rectus Sheath Haematoma

A rectus sheath haematoma occurs as a result of rupture of the inferior epigastric artery or rectus muscle. It may follow a bout of coughing or after abdominal trauma in late pregnancy, especially in women on anticoagulation therapy. It presents with a large unilateral, painful swelling. The condition may mimic any abdominal condition including placental abruption. Ultrasound shows a sonolucent heterogeneous mass that can also be visualized on CT scan and on MRI. Management is generally conservative but may require operative exploration [18].

7.6.9 Psychological Cause

A psychological cause is a diagnosis by exclusion. It is more common in women with known psychosocial problems. Reporting a high number of ailments during antenatal care is common [18].

7.6.10 Other Causes of Acute Abdomen

It is not possible to discuss all the possible causes in detail. Other causes and their management are summarized in Table 7.2.

7.7 Clinical Assessment

The diagnostic approach for pregnant patients presenting with acute abdominal pain is similar to that of the non-pregnant patient. With a pregnant patient presenting with acute abdominal pain, the clinician is faced with a multipronged challenge. There is the need to make a diagnosis and initiate timely intervention, while safeguarding the well-being of the mother and the fetus. A systematic approach including thorough history, examination and investigations will lead to a diagnosis. Multidisciplinary consultation with other medical and surgical specialties supports the diagnostic process as well as appropriate treatment [23].

7.7.1 History and Physical Examination

A detailed targeted history is crucial in identifying the potential cause or organ system involved. The location of pain is vital, as it carries a clue to the organ system likely to be involved as well as guiding the type of imaging required. This is summarized in Table 7.3. During history taking, it is important to establish the onset, duration, nature and severity of pain. Pain of acute sudden onset indicates possibility of ruptured viscus or ectopic pregnancy. A relationship of pain to meals, bowel motion, vomiting and nausea is suggestive of a bowel cause. Other characteristics of pain such as radiation and aggravating and relieving factors are also helpful. The past medical, gynaecological and surgical history is important, especially where there was pain reported before the pregnancy. A history of pre-existing ovarian cyst or fibroid is useful, as these may cause acute pain. Dysuria, frequency of micturition or haematuria points to a urinary system source of pain. Presence of vaginal discharge or bleeding would suggest a septic miscarriage.

A general examination focusing on vital signs is essential. Pyrexia indicates a potential infective cause. Presence of tachycardia, tachypnoea and hypotension is a worrying trio found in

Table 7.2 Other causes of acute abdomen in pregnancy and their management

Disease	Signs and Symptoms	Investigations	Management
Pyelonephritis	Flank pain radiating to the groin (and tenderness) and fever	Urine dipstick. Culture (blood and urine) and renal ultrasound	Analgesics and antibiotics
Inflammatory bowel disease	Diffuse abdominal pain, vomiting, diarrhoea, passage of mucus and rectal bleeding, weight loss	Inflammatory markers, sigmoidoscopy and colonoscopy	Involve gastroenterologists, steroids and immune modulators
Strangulated hernia	Bulge with redness and severe pain, and features of bowel obstruction		Involve surgeons and treat bowel obstruction
Gastroenteritis	Diffuse abdominal cramps, diarrhoea and vomiting	Stool for culture	Fluids, home management if possible, isolation
Hepatitis	Right upper abdominal pain and jaundice	Liver function test, serology, ultrasound	Involve hepatologist. Management depends on cause
Intra-abdominal haemorrhage	Rare. Ruptured liver capsule, splenic or aortic artery aneurysm causes haemorrhagic shock and abdominal pain	FBC, group and crossmatch, check fetal compromise	Resuscitation and surgical management
Pelvic vein thrombosis	Iliac vein thrombosis, groin tenderness, leg swelling and pyrexia	Doppler ultrasound, venogram, thrombophilia screen	Involve haematologist, anticoagulation, may require filter in IVC
Pneumonia (right lower lobe)	Right upper quadrant pain, and respiratory symptoms	Blood gases. CXR, inflammatory markers and sputum cultures	Antibiotics may require O_2 and HDU support. Involve respiratory physician
Trauma (including domestic violence)	History not consistent with injury (domestic violence), trauma and bruising	Check injuries, assess pregnancy, check rhesus status, Kleihauer–Betke test	Treatment depends on extent of injury. Involve social services to ensure safety

CXR: Chest x-ray; FBC: Full blood count; HDU: High-dependency unit; IVC: Inferior vena cava

patients who are very unwell or likely to quickly deteriorate. If the patient is pale, there may be intra-abdominal haemorrhage. Abdominal examination aims at establishing the location of the pain, guarding, rigidity and rebound tenderness. The latter is a sign of peritoneal irritation. A tender pelvic mass suggests the possibility of ovarian cyst or fibroids. In the presence of pelvic pain, vaginal bleeding or discharge, vaginal examination is essential. Bimanual pelvic examination is carried out to evaluate for the presence of adnexal or pelvic masses. The cervix should be checked for any abnormality, dilation or discharge. Rectal examination is an important component of the physical examination when a patient presents with rectal bleeding or other symptoms suggestive of anorectal pathology [24].

7.7.2 Laboratory Investigations

Laboratory investigations are non-specific, and their interpretation is confounded by the physiological changes that occur in pregnancy. The choice of laboratory investigations is guided by the suspected organ system involved but, where this is unclear, a series of investigations may be carried out as screening tests. Repeat laboratory tests are useful for monitoring response to treatment or development of complications. A total blood count will show the presence of a low haemoglobin where there is haemorrhage; while a high white cell count suggests

the presence of infection. Urinalysis and urine culture will aid in the diagnosis of urinary infection or urolithiasis. C-reactive protein (CRP) is a non-specific inflammatory marker which is usually elevated in sepsis. In cases where sepsis is suspected, blood culture may help identify the responsible organism and guide the use of antibiotics. Renal and liver function tests assess for any renal and hepatic compromise. Blood grouping and clotting studies are useful in patients with haemodynamic instability or those who may need surgery. Arterial blood gas and lactate levels should be done in septic patients to assess tissue perfusion [24].

7.7.3 Imaging

Imaging in patients with acute pain in pregnancy is vital in helping to reach a diagnosis. Concerns about fetal risks of teratogenesis, miscarriage and childhood cancers from ionizing radiation remains a common concern among clinicians and parents alike. This often delays diagnosis and treatment, eventually leading to less favourable patient outcome [25, 26].

7.7.3.1 Ultrasonography

Ultrasound is the most common imaging modality used in assessing pregnant patients as it uses no ionizing radiation. It is safe for the fetus and helpful in diagnosing most common

Table 7.3 The location of pain and possible organ system involved

Location for pain	Possible organ involved	Possible pathology
Right hypochondrial region	Liver, kidney, hepatic flexure of colon, gallbladder	Hepatitis, cholecystitis, hepatic rupture or haemorrhage, HELLP syndrome, severe pre-eclampsia
Epigastric region	Stomach, pancreas, aorta, heart	Gastric ulcer, pancreatitis, aortic dissection/rupture, myocardial infarction
Left hypochondrial region	Splenic flexure of colon, spleen	Colitis, splenic infarction, rupture and haemorrhage
Left lumbar region	Left kidney, descending colon	Pyelonephritis, renal/ureteric, inflammatory bowel disease
Right lumbar region	Right kidney, ascending colon	Pyelonephritis, renal/ureteric calculi, inflammatory bowel disease
Umbilical region	Pancreas, transverse colon, appendix, uterus	Pancreatitis, mesenteric lymphadenitis, early stage of appendicitis, uterine rupture, abruption placenta
Right iliac region	Right tube and ovary, appendix, caecum	Ectopic pregnancy, tubo-ovarian abscess, ovarian cyst accident, appendicitis, caecal diverticulitis
Left iliac region	Sigmoid colon, left fallopian tube and ovary	Inflammatory bowel disease, ectopic pregnancy, ovarian cyst accident, tubo-ovarian abscess
Suprapubic region	Bladder, uterus	Bladder stone/infection, uterine scar dehiscence
Generalized	Any intraperitoneal organ	Early stage of visceral peritoneal irritation

HELLP: Haemolysis, elevated liver enzymes, low platelet count

causes of abdominal pain in pregnancy. Ultrasound is useful in the evaluation of suspected miscarriage, ectopic pregnancy, appendicitis, cholecystitis, nephrolithiasis and ovarian and uterine pathology [16].

7.7.3.2 Radiography and Computed Tomography (CT)

Due to safety concerns, the use of ionizing radiation should be kept to the absolute minimum necessary to aid diagnosis. Fortunately, fetal ionizing radiation exposure during single radiological investigations are minimal. Radiation doses of less than 50 mGy have not been shown to be associated with fetal risks. Before resorting to abdominal CT scan investigation, a risk-benefit analysis should be taken after discussion with the radiologist. A CT scan may be considered in situations where MRI and ultrasound are not helpful in establishing a diagnosis. Chest x-ray (CXR) exposes the patient to minuscule levels of radiation and should not be withheld if deemed to be helpful in patent evaluation and diagnosis. Erect CXR may demonstrate gas under the diaphragm in bowel perforation. Ventilation-perfusion scans and CT pulmonary angiography may be relevant if chest symptoms evident are suggestive of pulmonary embolism. Electrocardiogram may show myocardial infarction [26, 27].

7.7.3.3 Magnetic Resonance Imaging (MRI)

Magnetic resonance imaging (MRI) has no ionizing radiation and has not been linked with fetal harm. Although no adverse effect on fetal well-being has been documented, the American National Council on Radiation Protection and Measurements board advises against the use of MRI in the first trimester. MRI can aid in diagnosing acute appendicitis, cholecystitis, bowel obstruction and ovarian pathology. In patients presenting with acute abdominal pain, MRI is commonly used where ultrasound has not been helpful in making a diagnosis [28].

7.8 Clinical Management

7.8.1 General and Medical Management

After taking the initial history and performing physical examination and laboratory tests, supportive therapy should be commenced. Initial resuscitative measures like calling for assistance, relieving pain and administering oxygen and intravenous fluids may have to be taken before undertaking a more detailed history and examination. Standard approach should be to ensure a patent airway and respiratory system. Oxygen by mask should be provided where needed. Intravenous access should be established, followed by infusion of crystalloid intravenous fluids to support the cardiovascular system. As these patients are in pain, parenteral opiate analgesics should be made available. Other associated symptoms such as nausea and vomiting should be treated appropriately. Insertion of an indwelling urinary catheter should be considered where assessment of hourly urinary output is deemed necessary or where urinary retention occurs. The use of a modified early obstetric warning system (MEOWS) chart will help identify the acutely ill and deteriorating patient [29, 30].

7.8.2 Surgical Management

Multidisciplinary input should be sought from other specialties as appropriate before undertaking surgical intervention. Patient counselling and relevant consent should be obtained. Laparoscopy is increasingly used in the evaluation or treatment of acute abdomen in pregnancy. Laparoscopy is generally safe and can be performed on pregnant women patients during any trimester without appreciably increased risk to the mother or fetus. Clearly, only suitably trained and experienced surgeons should undertake laparoscopic surgery. Trocar location needs adjustment based on uterine size. Because of carbon dioxide exchange in the peritoneal cavity and concern over the effect of acidosis on the fetus, the use of capnography during laparoscopy in the pregnant patient is recommended. Advantages of laparoscopy over laparotomy include shortened hospital stay, less need for narcotics, earlier tolerance of oral intake and minimized manipulation of the uterus [31, 32, 33].

7.9 Conclusion

Acute abdomen is a common presentation during pregnancy. It is essential that all gynaecologists are familiar with the range of possible causes. Diagnosis is made difficult by the physiological changes that occur normally during pregnancy. A systematic approach involving history taking, examination and investigation including appropriate imaging will help in making a diagnosis. Initial resuscitative measures, pain relief and ensuring a competent respiratory system should be undertaken. Fetal radiation concerns should not delay imaging, as radiation exposure is minuscule. Consultation with other surgical and medical specialties as well as discussion with radiologists will enhance a multidisciplinary input. There should be no delay in surgical intervention where this is indicated. Laparoscopic surgery is the preferred approach where suitably qualified and experienced surgeons are available.

References

1. Chandraharan E, Arulkumaran S. Acute abdomen and abdominal pain in pregnancy. *Obstet Gynaecol Reprod Med.* 2008;**18**(8):205–12.

2. Sivanesaratnam V. The acute abdomen and the obstetrician. *Best Pract Res Clin Obstet Gynaecol.* 2000;**14**(1):89–102.

3. CEMACH. *Saving Mothers' Lives: Reviewing Maternal Deaths to Make Motherhood Safer – 2003–2005.* London: CEMACH; 2007.

4. Skubic JJ, Salim A. Emergency general surgery in pregnancy. *Trauma Surg Acute Care Open.* 2017;**2**(1): e000125.

5. Yeomans ER, Gilstrap LC. Physiologic changes in pregnancy and their impact on critical care. *Crit Care Med.* 2005;**33**: S256–8.

6. Madhra M, Otify M, Horne AW. Ectopic pregnancy. *Obstet Gynaecol Reprod Med.* 2017;**27**(8):245–50.

7. Weston P, Moroz P. Appendicitis in pregnancy: how to manage and whether to deliver. *Obstet Gynaecol.* 2015;**17**:105–10.

8. Aggenbach L, Zeeman GG, Cantineau AE, Gordijn SJ, Hofker HS. Impact of appendicitis during pregnancy: no delay in accurate diagnosis and treatment. *Int J Surg.* 2015;**15**:84–9.

9. Huang C, Hong MK, Ding DC. A review of ovary torsion. *Ci Ji Yi Xue Za Zhi.* 2017;**29**(3):143–7.

10. Elson CJ, Salim R, Potdar N, Chetty M, Ross JA, Kirk EJ, on behalf of the Royal College of Obstetricians and Gynaecologists. Diagnosis and

management of ectopic pregnancy. *BJOG.* 2016;**123**:e15–e55.

11. The National Institute for Health and Care Excellence (NICE). Ectopic pregnancy and miscarriage: diagnosis and initial management. Clinical guideline [CG154]. U.K.: NICE;2012. www.nice.org.uk/guidance/CG154.

12. Sagili H, Divers M. Modern management of miscarriage. *Obstet Gynaecol.* 2007;**9**:102–8.

13. Al-Memar M, Kirk E, Bourne T. The role of ultrasonography in the diagnosis and management of early pregnancy complications. *Obstet Gynaecol.* 2015;**17**(3):173–81.

14. Alalade A, Maraj H. Management of adnexal masses in pregnancy. *Obstet Gynaecol.* 2017;**19**(4):317–25.

15. Damigos E, Johns J, Ross J. An update on the diagnosis and management of ovarian torsion. *Obstet Gynaecol.* 2012;**14**(4):229–36.

16. Woodfield CA, Lazarus E, Chen KC, Mayo-Smith WW. Abdominal pain in pregnancy: diagnoses and imaging unique to pregnancy – review. *AJR Am J Roentgenol.* 2010 **194**(1):238–44.

17. Currie A, Bradley E, McEwen M, Al-Shabibi N, Willson PD. Laparoscopic approach to fibroid torsion presenting as an acute abdomen in pregnancy. *JSLS.* 2013;**17**(4):665–7.

18. Stone K. Acute abdominal emergencies associated with pregnancy. *Clin Obstet Gynaecol.* 2002;**45**:553.

19. Dhupar R, Smaldone GM, Hamad GG. Is there a benefit to delaying cholecystectomy for symptomatic

gallbladder disease during pregnancy? *Surg Endosc.* 2010;**24**:108–12.

20. Mali P. Pancreatitis in pregnancy: etiology, diagnosis, treatment, and outcomes. *Hepatobiliary Pancreat Dis Int.* 2016;**15**:434–8.

21. Longo SA, Moore RC, Canzoneri BJ, Robichaux A. Gastrointestinal conditions during pregnancy. *Clin Colon Rectal Surg.* 2010; **23**:80.

22. Perdue PW, Johnson HW, Stafford PW. Intestinal obstruction complicating pregnancy. *Am J Surg.* 1992;**164**:384–8.

23. Pinas-Carrillo A, Chandraharan E. Abdominal pain in pregnancy: a rational approach to management. *Obstet Gynaecol Reprod Med.* 2017;**27** (4):112–19.

24. Shervington JP, Cox C, Abdominal pain in pregnancy: diagnosis, surgery and anaesthesia. *Obstet Gynaecol.* 2000;**2**:17–22.

25. Casciani E, De Vincentiis C, Mazzei MA, et al. Errors in imaging the pregnant patient with acute abdomen. *Abdom Imaging.* 2015 Oct;**40** (7):2112–26.

26. Groen RS, Bae JY, Lim KJ. Fear of the unknown: ionizing radiation exposure during pregnancy. *Am J Obstet Gynecol.* 2012;**206**:456–62.

27. Jain C. ACOG Committee Opinion No. 723: Guidelines for Diagnostic Imaging During Pregnancy and Lactation. *Obstet Gynecol.* 2019;**133** (1):186.

28. Baron KT, Arleo EK, Robinson C, Sanelli PC. Comparing the diagnostic performance of MRI

versus CT in the evaluation of acute nontraumatic abdominal pain during pregnancy. *Emerg Radiol.* 2012;**19**:519–25.

29. Khandelwal A, Fasih N, Kielar A. Imaging of acute abdomen in pregnancy. *Radiol Clin North Am.* 2013;**51**(6):1005–22.

30. Kilpatrick CC, Orejuela FJ. Management of the acute abdomen in pregnancy: a review. *Curr Opin Obstet Gynecol.* 2008;**20**(6):534–9.

31. Al-Fozan H, Tulandi T. Safety and risks of laparoscopy in pregnancy. *Curr Opin Obstet Gynecol.* 2002;**14**:375–9.

32. Kilpatrick CC, Monga M. Approach to the acute abdomen in pregnancy. *Obstet Gynecol Clin North Am.* 2007;**34**:389–402.

33. Taylor D, Perry RL. Acute abdomen and pregnancy. eMedicine. 2014. https://emedicine.medscape.com/article/195976-overview#a12.

Gestational Trophoblastic Disease

Patrick Chien, Lesley McMahon, Anne Chien & Leigh Jenkins

8.1 Introduction

Gestational trophoblastic disease (GTD) is due to the abnormal and uncontrolled proliferation of the trophoblastic cells in a pregnancy. It encompasses a spectrum of conditions from benign hydatidiform mole to invasive mole and malignant choriocarcinoma and the rarer forms of placental site trophoblastic tumour (PSTT) and epithelioid trophoblastic tumour (ETT). The malignant forms of the disease, i.e. choriocarcinoma, PSTT and ETT, are collectively known as gestational trophoblastic neoplasia (GTN).

Hydatidiform moles tend to be localized within the uterus and can exist in two variants: partial, whereby there is evidence of fetal cells present, or complete, with absence of any fetal cells. Both forms of hydatidiform moles are incompatible with a viable pregnancy.

Choriocarcinoma exists in either a gestational (derived from gestational tissue) or non-gestational variant (derived from pluripotent germ cells in the gonads or in association with poorly differentiated somatic carcinomas) [1]. The genotype of the cells of gestational choriocarcinoma will contain paternal chromosome complement [2] and can be derived from a previous pregnancy, irrespective of whether this was a normal term pregnancy, miscarriage, termination or a previous hydatidiform mole [1].

The prognosis for all forms of GTD tends to be good, with cure rates for hydatidiform moles being almost 100% with the appropriate follow-up and/or chemotherapy treatment and in excess of 90% for the malignant spectrum of choriocarcinoma, PSTT and ETT in the UK [3].

8.2 Epidemiology and Aetiology

The incidence of GTD is low in the UK and Europe with the incidence of partial and complete hydatidiform mole being 3 per 1000 and 1–3 per 1000 pregnancies, respectively [3]. For choriocarcinoma, the incidence in the Western world is 1 per 50 000 pregnancies [4]. Both PSTT and ETT are even rarer, presenting in 1 in 50 000–100 000 pregnancies [5].

There is significant geographic variation and also ethnic differences in the incidence of GTD. The disease is far more common in Eastern countries (China, Japan, Hong Kong, Taiwan), South East Asia (Malaysia, Singapore, Indonesia, Philippines) and South Asia such as India. It is relatively less common in Latin American countries, North America and Europe.

There is considerable inaccuracy in the incidence of reported GTD cases as the presence of this disease may be unnoticed in some patients and also undiagnosed or misdiagnosed in others due to its rarity [6].

The precise aetiology of GTD is unknown but involves the uncontrolled proliferation of trophoblastic cells either from an existing pregnancy or from dormant cells from a previous pregnancy.

8.3 Pathogenesis/Pathophysiology

The two variants of hydatidiform moles are also distinguished by differences in the genetic composition.

Partial moles tend to exist as androgenetic triploids (3n) of 69 chromosomes, with two sets of paternal and one set of maternal chromosomes. Therefore, not all triploid conceptions are partial moles, as digynic triploids will contain two sets of maternal and one set of paternal chromosomes. The vast majority of partial moles arise via fertilization of a single ovum by two sperm (dispermy).

Complete moles generally have a diploid (2n) DNA content of 46 chromosomes, where both sets of chromosomes are paternally inherited. Approximately 25% of hydatidiform moles are complete moles, with the majority (90%) having a 46,XX karyotype, the remaining 10% show a 46,XY karyotype. It is believed 20% of complete moles arise via dispermic fertilization where two sperm, or a diploid sperm, fertilize an empty, anucleate, egg (i.e. will contain heterozygous paternal alleles). In around 80% of cases it is believed a single sperm may fertilize an empty egg, with the male pronucleus dividing to form a diploid nucleus (and containing homozygous paternal alleles). Only XX zygotes would exist, as YY zygotes would lack essential X chromosome genes required for further development. More recently it has been suggested that postzygotic diploidization of an initially triploid conceptus is another mechanism to generate complete androgenetic diploids and may be more common than the natural occurrence of anucleate eggs; however, this does not explain the 4:1 frequency of homozygous versus heterozygous androgenetic moles [7].

For gestational choriocarcinoma, the genotype may be identical to that from a previous pregnancy and it is presumed that some of the cells from this pregnancy remained within the uterus and remained dormant until, for some unknown reason, it then became malignant in nature [1].

8.4 Pathology [including clinical staging where relevant]

In an early normal conception, the cellular nuclei within the trophoblastic tissue are located in a polarized distribution, i.e. growth from one edge of the villous. In both partial and complete hydatidiform moles, this nuclear polar distribution

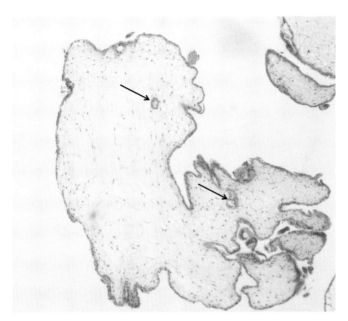

Figure 8.1 Histopathological features of partial hydatidiform mole – highly irregular villous contours with trophoblast pseudo-inclusions (arrows)

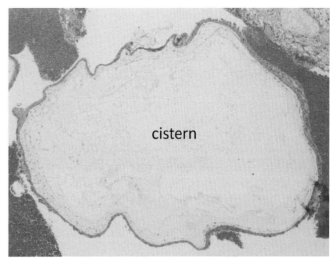

cistern

Figure 8.2 Histopathological features of complete hydatidiform mole – cistern formation

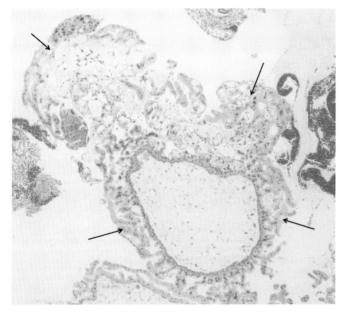

Figure 8.3 Histopathological features of complete hydatidiform mole – circumferential trophoblast hyperplasia (arrows)

is lost with the cellular nuclei being seen throughout the trophoblastic tissue in a circumferential fashion.

With partial hydatidiform moles, cistern formation is less intense with demonstration of villous scalloping and presence of inclusion bodies (Figure 8.1). Stromal blood vessels tend to contain nucleated (fetal) red blood cells.

Complete hydatidiform moles are characterized by the presence of large central, fluid-filled cistern formations (Figure 8.2) within the chorionic villi and circumferential villous trophoblastic formation (Figure 8.3). Nuclear debris within the stroma, known as stromal karyorrhexis, may be

present and any stromal blood vessel will contain non-nucleated red blood cells, i.e. maternal red cells. Secondary villous budding may also be present.

Although there is usually a marked histological difference between partial and complete hydatidiform moles in the latter part of the first trimester, these differences can be less obvious and difficult to be confidently diagnosed by a general pathologist in earlier gestation. In such cases, the use of p57 immunohistological staining for a maternally expressed (paternally imprinted) gene known as p57(KIP2) or CDKN1 C located at 11p15.4 may be useful. Lack of expression is associated with absence of maternal alleles and hence more likely to represent a complete molar phenotype [8]. Evidence of positive staining in the villous stromal cells and cytotrophoblast does not exclude or confirm a partial mole or distinguish this from a normal hydropic miscarriage.

Choriocarcinoma is an extremely aggressive trophoblastic tumour appearing grossly as a haemorrhagic and necrotic tumour mass within the endometrium typically with extensive myometrial infiltration. It can also arise at sites of ectopic pregnancy such as the cervix or fallopian tube. This has a biphasic growth pattern composed of highly atypical mononuclear and syncytiotrophoblastic (multinucleated) cells which express human chorionic gonadotropin (hCG) [8]. Chorionic villi are absent. Around half of gestational choriocarcinomas arise after a prior complete mole [9].

PSTT originates from the implantation site trophoblast presenting as a solid circumscribed mass in the endomyometrium which may show deep myometrial invasion. The tumour is composed of large mononuclear cells and lesser numbers of multinucleated cells which split the smooth muscle fibres [10]. These cells express human placental lactogen (hPL) [8]. This tumour does not arise in the context of a concurrent gestation but can mimic a non-neoplastic exaggerated implantation site, and this difficult diagnosis requires expert pathological opinion (Figure 8.4).

Table 8.1 FIGO GTD prognostic scoring system (2000)

Score	0	1	2	4
Age (years)	<40	≥40	-	-
Interval from index pregnancy (months)	<4	4–6	7–12	>12
Pre-treatment serum hCG (IU/L^{-1})	$<10^3$	10^3–10^4	10^4–10^5	$>10^5$
Largest tumour size (including uterus) (cm)	<3 cm	3–4 cm	≥5 cm	
Site of metastasis	Lung	Spleen Kidney	Gastrointestinal tract Brain	Liver
Number of metastases	-	1–4	5–8	>8
Previous failed chemotherapy	-	-	Single drug	≥2 Drugs

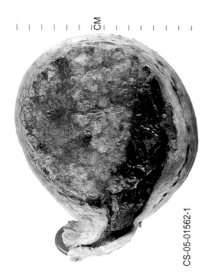

CM

CS-05-01562-1

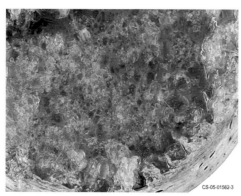

CS-05-01562-3

Figure 8.4 Macroscopic appearance of complete hydatidiform mole. A black and white version of this figure will appear in some formats. For the colour version, please refer to the plate section.

ETT arises from chorionic type trophoblast and around half originate in the cervix, typically as a circumscribed mass. In contrast with PSTT, the tumour has an expansile pushing border and is composed of mononuclear cells with scattered multinucleate giant cells [11].

Irrespective of whether the disease is a benign molar pregnancy or malignant carcinoma, all GTD requiring chemotherapy (see below) is staged in the same manner using the 2000 FIGO prognostic scoring system (Table 8.1) [12]. In this scoring system, there are 8 domains (patient's age, nature of the antecedent pregnancy, time interval (months) from index pregnancy, pre-treatment serum hCG (IU/L^{-1}), largest tumour size (cm) including that in the uterus, site of metastasis, number of metastasis and number of drugs in previous failed chemotherapy) that are used to give a score ranging from 0 to 4. Some of the domains, such as the site of metastasis, have a score of 0 for lung disease,

whereas the score is 4 for the presence of liver or brain metastasis, indicating the pulmonary nodules have less prognostic significance compared to cerebral or liver lesions. In general, cases of choriocarcinoma will score higher than that of hydatidiform moles, as the pre-treatment serum hCG is higher and distant metastases tend to be larger in size and numbers.

8.5 Clinical Features

Hydatidiform moles tend to present with vaginal bleeding in the first trimester of pregnancy. In some cases, patients have severe hyperemesis gravidarum due to the high levels of hCG. Rarer modes of clinical presentation include pre-eclampsia, hyperthyroidism and respiratory failure. There may also be evidence of a uterine size which is larger than the gestational age and theca lutein ovarian cysts.

Table 8.2 Confirmed hydatidiform moles in Scotland (2014)

	Complete	Partial	Total
Age (years)	30 (15–53)	29 (15–43)	
Gestation at diagnosis (weeks)	8 (5–16)	6 (4–21)	
Pregnancy outcome			
Surgical evacuation	58*	50 (72%)	108 (82%)
Medical evacuation	3(5%)	12 (17%)	15[+] (11%)
Spontaneous miscarriage	1 (1.5%)	7 (10%)	8 (6%)
Live birth**	1 (1.5%)	0(0%)	1 (1%)
Suspicion of mole before histology			
Yes	44 (72%)	18 (26%)	62 (47%)
No	12 (20%)	48 (70%)	62 (47%)
Not known	5 (8%)	3 (4%)	8 (6%)

Note: Continuous variables described as mean (range)
*3 patients require chemotherapy
**Twin pregnancy
[+]5 patients (1 complete and 4 partial moles) require a further surgical evacuation of uterus

It is not uncommon that the patient is initially thought to have a non-viable intrauterine pregnancy on pelvic ultrasound scan and then undergoes an evacuation of uterus without a suspicion of a hydatidiform mole until the diagnosis is subsequently made histologically [13]. This tends to be the case for partial hydatidiform mole, as complete moles tend to have the classical snowstorm appearance on ultrasound scan and appear macroscopically to have the typical vesicular appearance (Figure 8.4) and hence are more likely to be suspected without histology.

Table 8.2 shows that the data from Scotland in 2014 indicate that only 62 (47%) out of 132 histologically confirmed hydatidiform moles were suspected from a pelvic ultrasound scan prior to the evacuation of uterus being performed. As expected, the detection rate by ultrasound scanning was higher with complete hydatidiform mole (44/61 cases; 72%) compared to partial mole (18/69 cases; 26%). The data therefore support the importance of ensuring that there is histological examination performed on the products of conception from a non-viable pregnancy in order to avoid missing a diagnosis of a hydatidiform mole. The current trend to manage non-viable pregnancies medically outside a hospital setting may result in some of these cases being performed without any microscopic assessment of the pregnancy if the patient aborts the pregnancy at home.

It is also important to be aware that both hydatidiform moles and primary choriocarcinoma can also be present in an ectopic tubal pregnancy [13]. For this reason, it is important to be mindful when treating a pregnancy of unknown location (PUL) with systematic methotrexate for a presumed ectopic pregnancy on the possibility of these diagnoses, as there will be no histological evidence available to confirm the diagnosis.

Some cases of choriocarcinoma can be preceded with a previous hydatidiform molar pregnancy, especially a complete mole. Choriocarcinoma tends to present with vaginal bleeding either as abnormal menstrual bleeding or shortly after childbirth [13]. It can also present as a distant metastasis at sites stated previously and only diagnosed following histological examination of the metastatic nodule and/or finding an elevated serum hCG [13].

PSTT presents with irregular vaginal bleeding months or years after a normal pregnancy, miscarriage or, rarely, after a hydatidiform mole. The uterus is usually enlarged and although the serum hCG can be elevated, it is seldom as high as that found in choriocarcinoma [14]. PSTT can be associated with elevated hPL and β_1-glycoprotein (SP-1) [14].

8.6 Investigations

A semi-quantitative urine pregnancy test will confirm the presence of hCG. For suspected hydatidiform moles, it is not necessary to quantify the serum or urine level of hCG at this stage, as there is a wide variation with this measurement both in normal and molar pregnancies.

Blood investigations such as haemoglobin level, serum thyroid-stimulating hormone (TSH), urea and electrolytes should be performed. The patient should also be monitored for any evidence of early pre-eclampsia and respiratory failure.

A pelvic ultrasound scan is required to confirm or refute fetal viability and also to exclude a multiple pregnancy. The presence of a snowstorm appearance will provide evidence of a complete hydatidiform mole. Occasionally, the presence of multiple cystic lesions on the placental bed in the presence of a fetal echo may lead to a suspicion of a partial hydatidiform

Table 8.3 Referrals and registrations of GTD for Scotland (April 2017 – March 2018)

Health board	Referral	Registrations	Confirmed moles	Non-molar referrals	Non-molar registrations
Tayside	24	7	6	15	1
Grampian	47	29	27	16	2
Lothian	22	13	12	7	1
Highland	16	7*	5	10	1
Lanarkshire	26	13	12	13	1
Ayrshire	6	8	8	0	0
GG & Clyde	30	19**	17	11	1
Fife	31	15	14	18	1
Forth Valley	7	3	3	4	0
Dumfries	1	1	1	0	0
Borders	1	3	3	0	0
Western Isles	0	0	0	0	0
Orkney Isles	0	0	0	0	0
Shetland Isles	0	0	0	0	0

*Denotes registration for 1 postnatal follow-up with molar pregnancy managed outside the UK
**Denotes 1 patient with PSTT

mole. The presence of a viable intrauterine pregnancy will eliminate the possibility of a molar pregnancy unless there has been a multiple pregnancy present.

Serum measurement of hCG is usually not required until there is histological confirmation of a hydatidiform mole (see below). A chest x-ray is also not required unless the urine or serum hCG follow-up is abnormal after the evacuation of uterus.

For choriocarcinoma, PSTT and ETT, the diagnosis may be suspected with an elevated serum hCG.

8.7 Differential Diagnosis

The diagnosis of a hydatidiform mole, choriocarcinoma, PSTT or ETT is essentially made histologically. Due to the rarity of the disease, the most difficult task for the pathologist is to distinguish between a hydropic miscarriage and a partial hydatidiform mole [6]. This task is especially made more difficult with hydatidiform moles being managed at an earlier gestation within the first trimester of pregnancy, as the histological features between these two entities are less pronounced [13]. For example, the diagnosis of all suspected hydatidiform moles in Scotland is centralized to a single centre in Dundee. All cases of possible GTD following histological examination by a pathologist in all Scottish hospitals will routinely have the tissue blocks and slides sent to Dundee, whereby the slides are then re-examined by a national pathologist. We deliberately encourage pathologists working in any Scottish hospital to refer cases suspicious of GTD to this centralized service to ensure no cases of GTD are missed. From April 2017 to March 2018, we received 211 referrals

from all the different regional health boards in Scotland of which only 108 (51%) cases were confirmed GTD (Table 8.3).

On receipt of the tissue blocks in Dundee, we also routinely perform flow cytometry in order to ascertain the ploidy status of the pregnancy [15]. Occasionally, fluorescent in situ hybridization (FISH) may be required if there is an equivocal result with flow cytometry, or if there is limited amount of fetal material present in the tissue block [15]. In cases of diploidy, we routinely perform p57 immunohistological staining, absence of which is used to indicate the lack of maternal genes associated with a complete mole (stain negative) versus a non-molar pregnancy with both a maternal and paternal (biparental) chromosome complement (stain positive) [13].

Equivocal immunohistochemical staining and absence of clearly defined pathological features may hinder diagnosis. Further specialized testing can include genetic analysis to determine allele inheritance pattern. In some countries, this is routinely performed and considered to be the gold standard to diagnosing GTD [16].

DNA is extracted from fetal and maternal tissue which has been carefully microdissected from placental tissue blocks. Polymorphic short tandem repeats of DNA sequences can be amplified in a multiplex manner, and comparison of fetal and maternal markers allows interpretation of allele inheritance, in addition to ploidy status. Genotyping will identify complete homozygous moles, complete heterozygous moles, diandric triploidy (partial hydatidiform mole), digynic triploidy, and biparental inheritance. Interestingly, we have shown, amongst others, that genotyping can identify various atypical presentations of molar pregnancy including biparental/andro-genetic mosaics, and a twin pregnancy with presence of a complete mole and a normal biparental pregnancy [17].

These additional genotyping investigations may increase the diagnostic turnaround time, which may in turn be a source of anxiety and distress for patients. We have therefore employed the selective strategy of only genotyping cases where first line analysis of histology (including second histological examination by the national pathologist), flow cytometry/FISH and p57 immunohistochemistry remains equivocal.

8.8 Clinical Management

8.8.1 General

The mainstay of management is to perform a surgical evacuation of uterus in order to obtain tissue for diagnosis and also to obtain a cure by removing all the tissue within the uterus [13]. If the condition is suspected preoperatively, surgical evacuation is preferred rather than medical evacuation [18]. Although there have been reports of successful cure with medical evacuation using mifepristone and misoprostol, the experience with this treatment is less promising. Out of 15 hydatidiform moles treated with a medical evacuation, 5 (33%) of these patients required a subsequent surgical evacuation of uterus (see Table 8.2).

It is important to be aware that the uterus tends to be larger than expected for the gestational age and hence the operative blood loss may be higher than expected. It is therefore crucial that such patients are crossmatched for possible red blood cell transfusion and that the procedure is performed under ultrasound guidance by an experienced surgeon, to ensure that all tissue is removed without uterine perforation [13].

If a molar pregnancy is confirmed, the women are offered enrolment in a follow-up programme, which monitors urinary or serum hCG concentration, using a specialized radioimmunoassay (RIA). The programme ensures that the presence of persistent disease or the development of further malignant phenotypes, such as choriocarcinoma, can be detected at an early stage, allowing opportunity for timely and more successful treatment options. In the UK since 1973, this follow-up is centralized to centres at Dundee, Sheffield and London, all of which employ hCG testing using this specialized RIA (UK-RIA).

Why is there a need for a specialized form of hCG RIA? It is well documented that different variants and fragments of the hCG molecule known as isoforms exist in greater amounts in GTD cases compared to a normal pregnancy. These include isoforms with cleaved peptide bonds in one of the loops of the β-subunit ('nicked' hCG), free β-subunits and glycosylation variants (hyperglycosylated hCG) [19]. Often a raised level of the free β-subunit in serum is indicative of poor prognosis. The choice of assay used to quantify hCG in GTD is therefore extremely important due to the presence of a potentially heterogeneous population of hCG. An assay for monitoring hCG levels in GTD patients must recognize all potential isoforms of the protein [13, 15]. The use of inappropriate immunoassays

can lead to erroneous results, especially if the primary antibody with the immunoassay is not capable of detecting all the hCG species. Therefore, if such hCG isoforms go undetected, a false negative result may be obtained.

The UK-RIA employs a unique rabbit polyclonal primary antibody, which has been shown to detect different isoforms of hCG, currently undetected by commercial assays. This assay is considered the gold standard for quantifying serum and urinary hCG in GTD patients, detecting all forms of hCG in as near an equimolar fashion as possible [20].

Serum or urine hCG is initially measured 4 weeks post-surgical evacuation of uterus. Urine is the preferred specimen, as these non-invasive samples are easily collected, whilst serum samples require collection by a trained medical or nursing professional and attendance at an early pregnancy assessment unit or GP surgery. Normal urinary and serum hCG levels are <25 IU/24 hr^{-1} and <5 IU/L^{-1}, respectively. If the initial hCG level is normal, hCG measurement is then repeated every 4 weeks; otherwise, the measurements are performed every 2 weeks. Any patients with rising hCG values over 2 consecutive samples or static values over 3 consecutive weeks will require treatment with chemotherapy. A very high initial hCG measurement (>20 000 IU/24 hr^{-1}) will also indicate that chemotherapy is required [4]. Some centres outside the UK employ standardized hCG regression lines to decide on whether chemotherapy is required [21]. This has the potential advantage of commencing chemotherapy earlier based on a lesser number of hCG measurements.

For complete hydatidiform moles, provided the first normalized hCG measurement is within 56 days of surgery, the follow-up is calculated as 6 months from the date of the surgical evacuation of uterus. Otherwise, the 6-month follow-up period is calculated from the date of the first normalized hCG measurement.

During this follow-up period, patients should avoid any pregnancy as it would be impossible to determine whether the increased hCG levels are due to the new pregnancy or from residual trophoblastic tissue from the previous pregnancy. In such cases, the follow-up would be suspended.

Most patients with a hydatidiform mole are keen to conceive again as soon as the molar pregnancy has been successfully evacuated. The risk of requiring chemotherapy for a complete hydatidiform mole is 14%, whereas that for a partial hydatidiform mole is only 1.2% [3]. Therefore, the follow-up period for a partial molar pregnancy has recently been shortened to only 2 consecutive normal hCG measurements, with the initial sample also obtained at 4 weeks following the evacuation of uterus.

During this follow-up period, patients will require contraception to avoid unintentional pregnancies. All forms of contraception can be employed (including the combined oral contraception pill), although the insertion of the intrauterine contraceptive device should be avoided until hCG levels have normalized.

We no longer undertake postnatal hCG monitoring after each subsequent pregnancy unless the patient has had more than one previous hydatidiform mole or required chemotherapy [22].

8.8.2 Medical

All Scottish patients with GTD and choriocarcinoma requiring chemotherapy are referred to Charing Cross, London. Out of the 108 cases of GTD diagnosed in Scotland between April 2017 and March 2018, there were only 4 such patients. Given the small number of patients requiring chemotherapy, it is considered more appropriate for such patients to be treated in London where the increased patient numbers provide deliberate attention and focus to specialized treatment of the disease in order to achieve the best possible clinical outcome.

Such patients will require a pre-treatment serum hCG measurement, CT of thorax, abdomen and pelvis and MRI of brain [15] as part of the staging process. A uterine artery Doppler waveform analysis is also performed, as patients with an increased uterine artery blood flow tend to have a poorer prognosis [23]. Patients are staged using the 2000 FIGO prognostic scoring system as describe above. A score of 0–6 is considered to be low risk requiring monotherapy, whereas a score >6 indicates high risk with the need for polytherapy [13].

Monotherapy is usually undertaken with systematic methotrexate 50 mg intramuscularly on days 1, 3, 5, 7, and on alternate days with folinic acid 15 mg orally rescue to avoid methotrexate side effects of mouth ulcers, sore eyes and pleuritis, i.e. days 2, 4, 6, 8 [24]. Myelosuppression tends to be the main side effect of this treatment and it is generally well tolerated by patients. Treatment is repeated every 2 weeks. Alternatively, actinomycin-D can be used as a single agent [13]. The efficacy of the treatment is monitored using serum hCG measurements and provided hCG levels fall, treatment is continued until the serum hCG <5 IU/L^{-1}. A further 3 consolidation doses of chemotherapy are administered before treatment is discontinued. In the presence of metastasis, the treatment is also monitored with further subsequent imaging of these lesions.

The standard polytherapy regimen is to employ etoposide, methotrexate, actinomycin-D alternating with cyclophosphamide and vincristine (EMA-CO) [25]. The treatment is monitored with serum hCG measurements as above. This treatment is associated with more adverse effects of nausea, vomiting, alopecia and myelosuppression. If there is lack of a clinical response, then the combination treatment with etoposide, methotrexate, actinomycin-D alternating with etoposide and cisplatin (EMA-EP) or paclitaxel and cisplatin alternating with etoposide and cisplatin (TP-EP) or paclitaxel and cisplatin alternating with paclitaxel and etoposide (TP-TE) or gemcitabine, paclitaxel, ifosfamide and cisplatin (gem-TIP) may be used instead [13].

More recently, in patients who are resistant to the above agents, immunotherapy with the anti-programmed cell death protein 1 inhibitor drug pembrolizumab has been used successfully to achieve remission in patients with choriocarcinoma, PSTT and ETT [26]. Patients receiving this treatment are only considered to benefit if expression of programmed cell death ligand 1 (PD-L1) within the tumour cells is detected by positive immunohistochemistry staining [26].

Gestational choriocarcinomas tend to respond favourably to chemotherapy. However, non-gestational variants tend to respond less well and are associated with a poorer prognosis [27]. The primary sites for non-gestational choriocarcinoma include lung, cervix, endometrium, breast, bladder and gastrointestinal tract [27].

PSTT and ETT tend to have variable responses to chemotherapy compared to hydatidiform moles and gestational choriocarcinoma [13]. As these tumours have varying hCG levels, it can also be difficult to monitor the progress of any chemotherapy treatment.

Following remission with chemotherapy for hydatidiform moles and choriocarcinoma, such patients will be on hCG follow-up for 10 years with the advice to avoid a pregnancy for 12 months after completion of chemotherapy and normal hCG surveillance during this period [13].

8.8.3 Surgical

The use of repeat second evacuation of uterus for hydatidiform mole may be useful to avoid chemotherapy in low-risk GTD and serum hCG <5000 IU/L^{-1} [28].

Hysterectomy may also be used to treat hydatidiform moles, especially when there is uncontrolled uterine bleeding and future fertility preservation is not required. In general, it is easier to treat with chemotherapy given the excellent therapeutic response and the high cure rate.

Salvage hysterectomy in patients with persistent disease localized to the uterus which is resistant to chemotherapy may also be employed in selected cases [14].

Surgical resection of residual metastatic nodules (pulmonary lobectomy, liver resections) and neurosurgery for cerebral metastatic lesions following chemotherapy may be required in order to achieve a cure for some patients [14].

Because PSTT and ETT are less chemosensitive, hysterectomy is the main treatment employed [13]. An alternative option is to perform a laparotomy in order to undertake a radical localized excision of the nodule within the uterus and then repair the uterine defect using a modified Strassman procedure [29].

8.8.4 Special Circumstances [e.g. in presence of pregnancy]

This risk of having a second molar pregnancy after a previous hydatidiform mole is approximately 1% [30]. This risk is increased further if patients have had more than one previous hydatidiform mole [30].

Women with mutations in both alleles of either *NLRP7* or *KHDC3L* are predisposed to recurrent hydatidiform moles [31]. Unfortunately at the current moment, the only manner in achieving a normal conception without a molar pregnancy is through donor oocytes and in vitro fertilization (IVF) treatment [15].

In a twin pregnancy, the coexistence of a normal twin and hydatidiform mole is also possible. In these cases, there is a significant risk of early pregnancy loss or antenatal complications such as preterm delivery and pre-eclampsia associated with the normal twin [32]. The risk of developing GTN is also increased to 27–46% [13]; however, approximately 57% of cases will achieve a successful delivery [32]. With appropriate counselling and appropriate obstetric surveillance, such pregnancies can therefore be allowed to continue instead of being terminated [32].

8.9 Sequelae of Disease and Treatment – Prognosis

The vast majority (90%) of patients with hydatidiform moles and gestational choriocarcinoma will be cured with chemotherapy [4]. Furthermore, most of these patients will conceive again and have a live birth [33].

There is controversial evidence as to whether there is risk of patients developing subsequent tumours from the chemotherapy treatment received for their GTD [33]. It is likely, however, that menopause occurs earlier by a few years following their chemotherapy [33].

The key to this favourable prognosis for such patients with GTD is the centralization of the diagnosis, monitoring with a specialized hCG immunoassay and treatment at specialized centres [13].

8.10 Key Messages

- Due to the rarity of the disease, centralization of the diagnosis, hCG monitoring with a specialized immunoassay for follow-up and multidisciplinary treatment of GTD are essential to achieve excellent survival rates.
- Pregnancy tissue from non-viable pregnancies should be routinely examined histologically for GTD.
- It is useful to have a second, independent pathology review with additional tests such as flow cytometry, FISH, p57 immunohistological staining and genotyping to obtain an accurate and definitive diagnosis.
- The overall survival rate from GTD is 90%, and the vast majority of patients can still conceive again.

References

1. Jia N, Chen Y, Tao X, et al. A gestational choriocarcinoma of the ovary diagnosed by DNA polymorphic analysis: a case report and systematic review of the literature. *J Ovarian Res.* 2017;**10**:46.

2. Savage J, Adams E, Veras E, Murphy KM, Ronnett BM. Choriocarcinoma in women: analysis of a case series with genotyping. *Am J Surg Pathol.* 2017;**41**:1593–1606.

3. Seckl MJ, Sebire NJ, Berkowitz RS. Gestational trophoblastic disease. *Lancet.* 2010;**376**:717–29.

4. Seckl MJ, Fisher RA, Salerno G, et al. Choriocarcinoma and partial hydatidiform moles. *Lancet.* 2000; **356**: 36–9.

5. Hassadia A, Gillespie A, Tidy J, et al. Placental site trophoblastic tumour: clinical features and management. *Gynecol Oncol.* 2005;**99**:603–7.

6. Vang R, Gupta M, Wu LSF, et al. Diagnostic reproducibility of hydatidiform moles: ancillary techniques (p57 immunohistochemistry and molecular genotyping) improve morphologic diagnosis. *Am J Surg Pathol.* 2012;**36**:443–53.

7. Hoffner L, Surti U. The genetics of gestational trophoblastic disease: a rare complication of pregnancy. *Cancer Genet.* 2012;**205**:63–77.

8. Fukunaga M, Ushigome S. Malignant trophoblastic tumors: immunohistochemical and flow cytometric comparison of choriocarcinoma and placental site trophoblastic tumors. *Hum Pathol.* 1993;**24**:1098–1106.

9. Bagshawe KD, Golding PR, Orr AH. Choriocarcinoma after hydatidiform mole. Studies related to effectiveness of follow-up practice after hydatidiform mole. *Br Med J.* 1969;**3**(5673):733–7.

10. Baergen RN, Rutgers J, Young RH. Extrauterine lesions of intermediate trophoblast. *Int J Gynecol Pathol.* 2003;**22**:362–7.

11. Fadare O, Parkash V, Carcangiu ML, Hui P. Epithelioid trophoblastic tumour: clinicopathological features with an emphasis on uterine cervical involvement. *Mod Pathol.* 2006;**19**:75–82.

12. Ngan HY, Bender H, Benedet JL, et al. Gestational trophoblastic neoplasia, FIGO 2000 staging and classification. *Int J Gynecol Obstet.* 2003;**83**:175–7.

13. Ngan HY, Seckyl MJ, Berkowitz RS, et al. Update on the diagnosis and management of gestational trophoblastic disease. *Int J Gynecol Obstet.* 2018;**143**(Suppl 2):79–85.

14. Hancock BW, Newlands ES, Berkowitz RS. *Gestational Trophoblastic Disease.* London: Chapman & Hall Medical; 1997.

15. Mangili G, Lorusso D, Brown J, et al. Trophoblastic disease review for diagnosis and management: a joint report from the International Society for the Study of Trophoblastic Disease, European Organisation for the Treatment of Trophoblastic Disease, and the Gynecologic Cancer InterGroup. *Int J Gynecol Cancer.* 2014;**24**(9 Suppl 3):S109–16.

16. McConnell TG, Murphy KM, Hafez M, Vang R, Ronnett BM. Diagnosis and subclassification of hydatidiform moles using p57 immunohistochemistry and molecular genotyping: validation and prospective analysis in routine and consultation practice settings with development of an algorithm approach. *Am J Surg Pathol.* 2009;**33**:805–17.

17. Lewis GH, DeScipio C, Murphy KM, et al. Characterisation of androgenetic/biparental mosaic/chimeric conceptions, including those with a molar component: morphology, p57 immunohistochemistry, molecular genotyping, and risk of persistent gestational disease. *Int J Gynecol Pathol.* 2013;**32**:199–214.

18. Tidy JA, Gilliespie AM, Bright N, et al. Gestational trophoblastic disease: a study of mode of evacuation and subsequent need for treatment with chemotherapy. *Gynecol Oncol.* 2000;**78**:309–12.

19. Cole LA. hCG, its free subunits and its metabolites. Roles in pregnancy and trophoblastic disease. *J Reprod Med.* 1998;**43**:3–10.

20. Sturgeon CM, Berger P, Bidart JM, et al. Differences in recognition of the 1st WHO International Reference Reagents for hCG-related isoforms by diagnostic immunoassays for human chorionic gonadotropin. *Clin Chem.* 2009;**55**(8):1484–91.

21. Lybol C, Sweep FC, Ottevanger PB, Massuger LF, Thomas CM. Linear regression of post evacuation serum human chorionic gonadotropin concentrations predicts postmolar gestational trophoblastic neoplasia. *Int J Gynecol Cancer.* 2013;**23**:1150–6.

22. Earp K, Hancock BW, Short D, et al. Do we need post-pregnancy human chorionic gonadotrophin screening after previous molar pregnancy to identify patients with recurrent gestational trophoblastic disease? *Eur J Obstet Gynecol Reprod Biol.* 2019;**234**:117–19.

23. Agarwal R, Strickland S, McNeish IA, et al. Doppler ultrasonography of the uterine artery and the response to chemotherapy in patients with gestational trophoblastic tumours. *Clin Cancer Res.* 2002;**8**:1142–7.

24. McNeish IA, Strickland S, Holden L, et al. Low-risk persistent gestational trophoblastic disease: outcome after initial treatment with low-dose methotrexate and folinic acid from 1992 to 2000. *J Clin Oncol.* 2002;**20**:1838–44.

25. Alazzam M, Tidy J, Osborne R, et al. Chemotherapy for resistant or recurrent gestational trophoblastic neoplasia. *Cochrane Database Syst Rev.* 2012;**2012**(12). DOI: 10.1002/14651858.CD008891.pub3.

26. Ghorani E, Kaur B, Fisher RA, et al. Pembrolizumab is effective for drug resistant gestational trophoblastic neoplasia. *Lancet.* 2017;**390**;2344–5.

27. Stockton L, Green E, Kaur B, De Winton E. Non-gestational choriocarcinoma with widespread metastases presenting with type 1 respiratory failure in a 39-year-old female: case report and review of the literature. *Case Rep Oncol.* 2018;**11**:151–8.

28. Osborne R, Filiaci V, Schink JC, et al. Second curettage for low-risk nonmetastatic gestational trophoblastic neoplasia. *Obset Gynecol.* 2016;**128**:535–42.

29. Chiofalo B, Palmara V, Laganà AS, et al. Fertility sparing strategies in patients affected by placental site trophoblastic tumour. *Curr Treat Options Oncol.* 2017;**18**:58.

30. Sebire NJ, Fisher RA, Foskett M, et al. Risk of recurrent hydatidiform mole and subsequent pregnancy outcome following complete or partial hydatidiform molar pregnancy. *BJOG.* 2003;**110**:22–6.

31. Fallahian M, Sebire NJ, Savage PM, Seckl MJ, Fisher RA. Mutations in *NLRP7* and *KHDC3L* confer a complete hydatidiform mole phenotype on digynictriploid conceptions. *Hum Mutation.* 2013;**34**:301–8.

32. Sebire NJ, Foskett M, Paradinas FJ, et al. Outcome of twin pregnancies with complete hydatidiform mole and healthy co-twin. *Lancet.* 2002;**359**:2165–6.

33. Seckl MJ, Sebire NJ, Fisher RA, et al. Gestational trophoblastic disease: ESMO Clinical Practice Guidelines for diagnosis, treatment and follow-up. *Ann Oncol.* 2013;**24**(Suppl 6):vi39–vi50.

Chapter 9

Hyperemesis Gravidarum

Jone Trovik, Hedvig Nordeng & Åse Vikanes

9.1 Introduction

Nausea and vomiting (NVP) together form one of the most common symptoms of early pregnancy, affecting approximately 70% of all women, with symptoms resolving for 90% before 20 weeks [1]. For 0.8–3.2% of women, NVP is so severe that it causes metabolic disturbances and is then further defined as hyperemesis gravidarum (HG) [2]. Hyperemesis is at present the leading cause for hospitalization during early pregnancy and is associated with negative health effects for mothers and children, short and long term, physically as well as psychologically [3]. The socio-economic costs include sick leave, and the level of healthcare provided (rather than medication costs) is the most cost-driving part of treatment [4].

9.1.1 Definition

Hyperemesis gravidarum is generally defined as extreme and persistent nausea and vomiting in pregnancy, causing metabolic disturbances such as dehydration, weight loss and electrolyte/nutritional deficiencies. This is a diagnosis of exclusion and any other disease should not cause the nausea/vomiting.

Hyperemesis gravidarum is a syndrome diagnosis since at present there is not one specific, uniformly accepted definition including definite measure of nausea/vomiting, a set amount of weight loss, whether ketonuria or any other lab test is mandatory. This hampers comparison of studies using different inclusion criteria [5]. The Pregnancy-Unique Quantification of Emesis and Nausea (PUQE) is the best-validated disease-specific questionnaire related to NVP. This three-tier questionnaire giving scores from 3–15 also includes a fourth general well-being question and has been translated and validated in several languages. High PUQE scores correlate with reduced nutritional intake, reduced quality of life (low well-being score), stopping iron/vitamin supplements and risk of hospitalization [6, 7].

A PUQE score of 13–15 identifies severe NVP/HG as opposed to mild NVP with scores of 4–6 (Figure 9.1).

The International Classification of Disease (ICD, 10th edition) separates ICD code O21.0: uncomplicated hyperemesis gravidarum, with a debut before the end of the 22nd week of gestation, from ICD code O21.1: complicated hyperemesis gravidarum with metabolic disturbances.

9.2 Aetiology

The aetiology of hyperemesis remains unknown, but is considered a multifactorial disease wherein genetic, hormonal and environmental factors are contributing [8].

9.2.1 Human Chorionic Gonadotropin (hCG)

Human chorionic gonadotropin (hCG) exists in five common forms with different biological functions, where the β-unit is common for all forms. Human chorionic gonadotropin induces angiogenesis in the uterine tissue to secure fetal nutritional supply and thus growth. The highest incidence and intensity of hyperemesis seems to coincide with the time of peaking hCG levels, and pregnancy-related conditions where hCG levels are raised; such as multiple, molar, and pregnancies with female fetuses [8]. Several meta-analyses have shown conflicting results regarding the aetiology and pathogenesis of hyperemesis and hCG levels; thus, it remains speculative as to whether hyperemesis is associated with increased levels of specific isoforms of the hormone.

9.2.2 Thyroid Hormones

Human chorionic gonadotropin and thyroid-stimulating hormone (TSH) have structural similarities leading to hCG stimulating thyrotrophic activity. During pregnancy, TSH levels fall when hCG levels peak, while circulating levels of T3 and T4 remain elevated [8]. Gestational transient hyperthyroidism (GTT) is observed in 60% of hyperemesis patients. As hCG levels decline during the second trimester, so do the elevated levels of thyroid hormones.

9.2.3 Oestrogen

Hyperemesis has been associated with both increased and reduced levels of oestrogen [8]. Studies have reported that hyperemesis is more common among women with high body mass index (BMI), among primiparous women and when the fetus is female; pregnancies where oestrogen levels are additionally raised.

9.2.4 Maternal Factors

Both high and low BMI have been associated with increased risk of hyperemesis, as has low maternal age [9]. Country of birth is strongly related to hyperemesis; women born in South East Asia and sub-Saharan Africa seem to be at highest risk [2]. Several studies have reported a reduced risk of hyperemesis among smokers. Recent systematic reviews and meta-analyses have confirmed *Helicobacter pylori* as a risk factor for the condition [8].

9.2.5 Genetic Factors

There is a high recurrence risk for women who experience hyperemesis in their first pregnancy – an absolute risk increase

PUQE form:

Pregnancy-Unique Quantification of Emesis and Nausea

Circle the answer that best suits your situation for the last 24 hours.

1. On average in a day, for how long do you feel nauseated or sick to your stomach?

> 6 hours	4-6 hours	2-3 hours	≤1 hour	Not at all
5 points	4 points	3 points	2 points	1 point

2. On average in a day, how many times do you vomit or throw up?

≥ 7 times	5-6 times	3-4 times	1-2 times	Not at all
5 points	4 points	3 points	2 points	1 point

3. On average in a day, how many times have you had retching or dry heaves without bringing anything up?

≥ 7 times	5-6 times	3-4 times	1-2 times	Not at all
5 points	4 points	3 points	2 points	1 point

Total score (sum of replies to 1, 2 and 3): mild NVP ≤6; moderate NVP 7-12; severe NVP ≥13.

Quality of life question:
On a scale of 0-10, how would you rate your well-being:_____
0 (worst possible), 10 (as good as you felt before pregnancy)

Figure 9.1 Pregnancy-specific questionnaire PUQE; measuring severity of nausea and vomiting

from 0.7% to 15.2% – and the condition is known to aggregate in families. If the mother of the pregnant woman had hyperemesis, the woman has a threefold increased risk herself [10]; while a change in paternity does not infer a significant effect on the incidence or recurrence risk of hyperemesis. Recently genes *GDF15* and *IGFBP7*, both involved in placentation, appetite and cachexia, were found to be associated with hyperemesis [11].

9.3 Clinical Features

Anamnestic information is the cornerstone in diagnosing hyperemesis; laboratory tests are used to determine the extent of metabolic consequences and to exclude other diseases.

As stated, the severity of NVP can be assessed using the three-tier questionnaire PUQE. After antiemetics/hospital treatment for hyperemesis, PUQE scores have been shown to decrease to levels comparable to those of healthy pregnant women [7]. Thus the effect of treatment could be monitored using the PUQE score; persisting high scores should prompt changes in treatment regimens such as increased dosage or added antiemetics.

Dehydration is estimated by reduced urine outputs and dry conjunctivae/oral mucosa. It is also important to question the woman regarding her nutritional intake and her ability to take recommended pregnancy vitamin supplements. Symptoms of severe undernutrition include a weight loss >5% from pre-pregnant weight and a feeling of general malaise, tiredness or dizziness.

9.4 Investigations

General examination should include measurements of blood pressure, pulse and weight. Ultrasound examination is warranted to identify a multifetal or molar pregnancy. Although the presence of hyperemesis is generally associated with significant reduced risk of miscarriage, visualizing a vital pregnancy could have a psychological beneficial effect on the woman's outlook for the pregnancy.

Laboratory tests should include estimation of the haemoglobin, haematocrit, electrolytes, thyroid tests and liver enzymes.

Urine dipstick analysis should be carried out to identify the presence of a urinary infection or diabetes. Positive ketones correlate to low glucose intake. Serum prealbumin is correlated to protein intake during the last 48 hours.

9.5 Differential Diagnosis

A wide range of conditions causing nausea and vomiting accidental to pregnancy should be excluded: gastroenteritis; appendicitis; urinary infection; hepatitis; pancreatitis; endocrine diseases such as diabetes and hyperthyroidism; neurological or vestibular diseases causing dizziness and vomiting; and psychiatric conditions such as anorexia nervosa and eating disorders.

9.6 Clinical Management

9.6.1 General

Treatment of nausea in pregnancy depends on the severity of the woman's symptoms, hydration status, concomitant conditions and the impact of NVP on her quality of life and daily functioning. Appropriate counselling, support and advice about safe and effective treatment are essential for women with NVP and hyperemesis [1, 12].

Mild NVP (PUQE <7 with no complications) can be self-managed in the community with support of first line healthcare professionals. Women with mild to moderate NVP should receive advice about dietary and lifestyle changes, and prescribed an antiemetic if needed. Early intervention can serve as pre-emptive treatment in women with a prior history of hyperemesis or in women presenting with mild to moderate symptoms. This may prevent progression to hyperemesis gravidarum thus reducing the impact on the woman's quality of life and daily functioning [12–15].

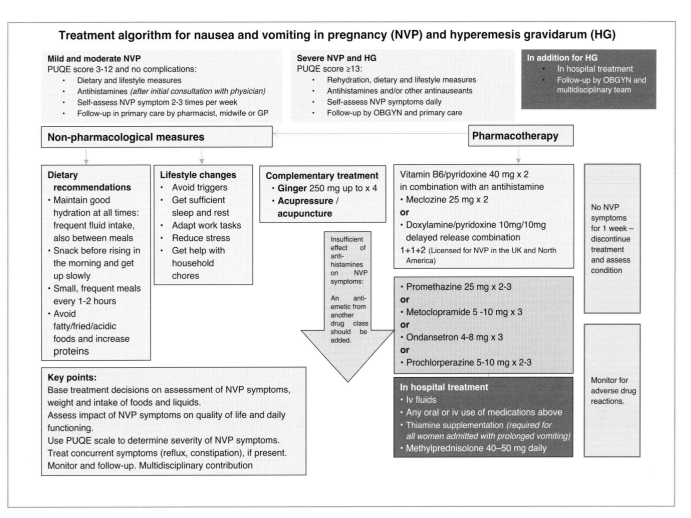

Figure 9.2 Flow chart of suggested antiemetic regimens

Women with moderate–severe NVP and hyperemesis require antiemetics. Combination therapy, adding on antiemetics from groups having different effects rather than changing from one medication to another, should be used in women who do not respond to a single antiemetic (Figure 9.2).

- Inpatient or hospital ambulatory management should be considered if there is:
  - severe nausea and vomiting (PUQE score ≥13) despite oral antiemetics
  - signs of dehydration, electrolyte deficiencies or metabolic complications due to low nutrition such as ketonuria and/or weight loss (>5% of body weight)
  - confirmed or suspected chronic or acute co-morbidity (e.g. infections, epilepsy, diabetes, mental health disorders)
  - a psychosocial situation that merits hospital treatment

In general, level of care is the most important factor regarding cost of treatment [4]. Thus, if medication therapy reduces the level of NVP effectively, avoiding hospitalization will add to societal cost-effectiveness. Rehydration and enteral and parenteral therapy may be administered on an outpatient basis. Different organizational settings (regions/hospitals/healthcare systems) may plan care differently. Patients' individual needs and preferences should be taken into consideration when planning treatment [1], including preparing an individualized management plan when specialist/secondary-level care is given.

Our recommendations are generally consistent with that of national Nordic or international guidelines [13–17] and on recent literature reviews [1, 4, 18].

9.6.2 Non-Pharmacological Treatment

Lifestyle and dietary recommendations include eating small, frequent meals (1- to 2-hour intervals between meals/snacks), since an empty or very full stomach may worsen the nausea. A snack (e.g. dry biscuits) before rising slowly out of bed in the morning may be useful. Spicy, odorous, high-fat, acidic and very sweet foods should be avoided, and substituted with protein-rich, bland, salty, soft, low-fat and/or dry, crunchy foods. Lying down after eating should be avoided.

It is recommended to drink 2 litres of fluid in a 24-hour period, consumed in several small portions, minimum 30 minutes before/after solid food to avoid a full stomach. Cold and clear fluids are better tolerated.

The woman should be advised to get plenty of sleep and rest, avoid stress, reduce her workload and to ask for help from family and friends with daily chores.

The scientific bases for this advice are mainly based on cohort studies of patients reporting personal preferences. Very few randomized controlled studies (RCTs) evaluating different food/lifestyle interventions exist.

For women with severe NVP/HG, lifestyle and dietary changes alone will not be sufficient.

9.6.3 Complementary Treatment

9.6.3.1 Ginger

Ginger is considered a complementary treatment for women with mild–moderate NVP. The exact mechanism of action against nausea is unclear [14]. In most scientific studies, dried ginger root powder in doses up to 250 mg four times daily was found to alleviate NVP symptoms[4], and no harmful fetal effects have been demonstrated. Danish authorities, however, advise pregnant women against using more than 1 g daily, as there are no safety studies regarding this. Ginger can aggravate heartburn and is not a suitable treatment for more pronounced nausea.

9.6.3.2 Acupuncture and Acupressure

A recent literature review concluded that women with mild symptoms might benefit from acupuncture or acupressure [4]. Overall, acupressure may reduce symptoms of nausea and retching in women with mild–moderate symptoms, but data are limited and inconclusive [4].

Some women experience relief from nausea by acupressure on pressure point P6 (Neiguan): 20–30 minutes of pressure on the inside of the forearm approximately two finger widths from the wrist. Bracelets or bands that provide a light, continuous pressure at this point are sold commercially.

9.6.3.3 Vitamin B6 (Pyridoxine)

Vitamin B6 in some women alleviates symptoms of nausea, often in combination with an antihistamine. The usual dosage is 1 tablet of 40 mg morning and evening. A recent literature review suggested that there was evidence that vitamin B6 was superior to placebo in women with mild to severe NVP [4].

9.6.4 Pharmacological Treatment

The proportion of pregnant women who use pregnancy-related medication varies considerably between different countries, from approximately 15% in Norway and England to over 30% in the United States [19]. The most commonly used anti-nauseants are antihistamines, metoclopramide and ondansetron (Table 9.1).The decision to initiate pharmacological treatment depends not only on the severity of symptoms, but also on how strongly the nausea affects the woman's well-being, quality of life and daily activities. In general, treatment with antiemetic medications is indicated in women with moderate emesis (PUQE scores 7–12). In severe NVP/HG (PUQE score ≥ 13), in addition to antiemetics, hospital treatment will most often be

Table 9.1 Medication used for treatment of NVP and hyperemesis

Medication group	Substance (brand name*)	Recommended dosage
Antihistamines (H$_1$-receptor blockers)	Meclozine (Postafen®)	25 mg x 1–2 times daily.
	Promethazine (Phenergan®)	25 mg at bedtime. Max. 25 mg x 2–3 times daily.
	Doxylamine 10 mg / pyridoxine 10 mg delayed-release tablets (Xonvea® in the UK)	Initial dosage: 2 tablets at bedtime. Max dosage: 1 + 1 + 2 Unlicensed, prescription by specific request.
Dopamine D$_2$ antagonists	Metoclopramide (Afipran®)	10 mg x 3 times daily. If needed for long-term use (>5 days), alternative medications should be used due to risk of neurological side effects.
	Prochlorperazine (Stemetil®)	5–10 mg x 2–3 times daily. Not recommended close to delivery due to potential blood pressure drop.
	Chlorpromazine (Largactil®)	10 mg x 2–3 times daily. Unlicensed, prescription by specific request. Avoid use in third trimester due to potential neurological adverse drug reactions in the newborn.
5HT$_3$-antagonist	Ondansetron (Zofran®)	4–8 mg x 2 times daily. IM: 4 mg x 2 times daily Preferably used after the first trimester.
Corticosteroids	Methylprednisolone	Oral: Prednisolone 50 mg once daily for 2–3 days. Discontinuation over 1–2 weeks. IV: Methylprednisolone 20 mg x 2 times daily for 3 days with discontinuation over 1–2 weeks. Preferably used after the first trimester.

*Giving examples of some brand names does not imply a recommendation to use specific brands over others.

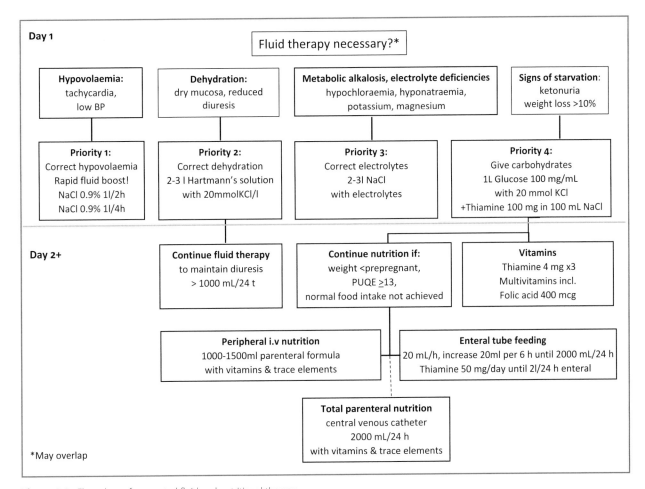

Figure 9.3 Flow chart of suggested fluid and nutritional therapy

required for intravenous rehydration and correction of electrolyte disturbances (Figure 9.3).

There are several antiemetics that can be safely used by pregnant women. The various drugs recommended for the treatment of nausea are shown in Table 9.1.

Important: Anti-nauseants should be taken as a daily prescription and not on an as needed basis. Combinations of different antiemetics should be used in women who do not respond to a single antiemetic (see Figure 9.2). Discontinuation of antiemetic treatment can be tried after the 16th gestational week as NVP symptoms resolve for most women by this time. Some women, however, might require antiemetic treatment throughout pregnancy.

9.6.4.1 Evidence of Efficacy

A recent review of both randomized and non-randomized controlled trials concluded that antihistamines and metoclopramide were superior to placebo in mild NVP. Ten milligrams doxylamine succinate combined with 10 mg pyridoxine hydrochloride delayed-release tablets were more effective than placebo, and ondansetron was more effective at reducing nausea than doxylamine in combination with pyridoxine. Promethazine was as effective as metoclopramide, while ondansetron was more effective than metoclopramide for severe NVP/HG [4]. A recent

Cochrane meta-analysis including only RCTs, however, concluded that there is insufficient evidence to recommend one drug over another. These authors recommended considering side effect profile, medication safety and healthcare costs when selecting one antiemetic over another [18]. In light of these findings, women with NVP or HG in a prior pregnancy should be asked about adverse reactions and response to previously prescribed antiemetic therapies.

9.6.4.2 Antihistamines

Antihistamines are the first line medications against NVP. These drugs block histamine-H_1 receptors in the vomiting centre, which communicate with the chemoreceptor trigger zone (CTZ). They have been used for decades among thousands of women with NVP, with the majority of evidence indicating no harmful effect on the fetus. Most of the research on antiemetics in pregnancy encompasses the older so-called first generation antihistamines, such as doxylamine, promethazine and meclizine. No antihistamines have been approved for use in NVP in the Nordic countries, in contrast to other countries such as the UK, the Netherlands, Switzerland, the United States and Canada. Antihistamines are often recommended in combination with vitamin B6 (pyridoxine). In 2018, the delayed-release tablets containing doxylamine 10 mg / pyridoxine 10 mg in combination was licensed for use against NVP in the UK. The most common side effect of antihistamines is sedation and patients should be cautioned against driving while under their influence.

9.6.4.3 Metoclopramide

Metoclopramide has a good safety profile regarding the fetus but is considered as second line therapy due to risk of extrapyramidal effects for the woman. In 2013, the European Medicines Agency published a public health communication stating that metoclopramide should be used for a maximum of 5 consecutive days to reduce the risk of neurological side effects. Since extrapyramidal side effects usually occur within 24–48 hours after initiation of metoclopramide, pregnant and other patients taking metoclopramide should be informed of possible side effects. The US Food and Drug Administration (FDA) allows metoclopramide to be used for a maximum of 21 days.

9.6.4.4 Dopamine Antagonists

Dopamine D_2 antagonists affect the vomiting centre and have been used for a number of years against nausea. There is no evidence that use of these agents is harmful to the fetus during the first trimester [17]. Some guidelines warn against use in the third trimester due to the risk of neurological side effects in neonates and the risk of maternal hypotension (prochlorperazine) [15].

9.6.4.5 Ondansetron

In Europe ondansetron is generally reserved for those cases where treatment with other antiemetics has not given sufficient efficacy (third line). Interestingly, ondansetron is the most commonly used antiemetics among pregnant women suffering from NVP/HG in the United States [19]. Studies have yielded conflicting results with respect to a possible small increased risk of cardiac malformations (for first trimester use), and some sources mention the possibility of prolonged QT-time as a side effect in the woman.

9.6.4.6 Corticosteroids

As an aim to achieve anabolism and as an adjunctive to other antiemetics, a short course of glucocorticoids has been added to the patient's current regimen for treatment of refractory cases where standard therapies have failed. Studies regarding antiemetic effect are contradictory. Preferably glucocorticoids should be administered after the first trimester despite newer studies showing no increased risk for the developing fetus [13, 14, 18].

9.6.5 Concurrent Gastrointestinal (GI) Symptoms

Many pregnant women with nausea will also be afflicted with heartburn, acid reflux and/or constipation, and frequently report burping, belching, stomach pain, indigestion, regurgitation and/or a sensation of having a lump at the back of the throat. Heartburn and acid reflux have been shown to correlate with increased severity of NVP. Healthcare professionals should therefore ask about and ensure adequate treatment of concurrent gastrointestinal (GI) symptoms. Anti-reflux medications such as aluminum hydroxide with alginate are safe during pregnancy. However, as part of their mechanism is to form a protective upper layer of acidic gastric content, they are deemed less suitable for patients who are mainly bedridden or who are hospitalized.

9.6.5.1 Antacids

Antacids (e.g. calcium carbonate up to 1 g per day) and H_2-blockers (e.g. ranitidine 150 mg x 1–2 per day) or a proton pump inhibitor (e.g. omeprazole 20 mg x 1–2 per day) may be required. These medications are considered safe during pregnancy. Studies from the Canadian Motherrisk group have shown that treatment of dyspepsia reduced NVP symptoms as determined by reduced PUQE scores. Probiotics can be used against indigestion.

9.6.5.2 Thrombosis Prophylaxis

Hyperemesis patients have increased risk of thrombosis. Women hospitalized will mostly be bedridden; in such a setting, thrombosis prophylaxis is recommended. The risk of thrombosis is much higher among women with BMI >30, and the risk rises incrementally with higher BMI. The prophylaxis may be given as subcutaneous low molecular heparin.

9.6.6 Fluid Therapy

A PUQE score of ≥13 should definitely merit assessment of a woman's general condition, amount of weight loss, ketonuria and signs of dehydration and the need for hospital care may be considered. Rehydration/parenteral nutritional supplementation or tube feeding may be implemented as outpatient treatment, depending on the woman's medical and psychosocial condition, her personal preferences and local hospital organization.

If the woman shows signs of hypovolaemia (low blood pressure, tachycardia), fluid should be infused rapidly at rate of 1000 mL every 2 hours. A normal daily fluid intake is 2 L; to correct dehydration at least 3 L/24 h is needed. (See Figure 9.3.) Sodium chloride 0.9% contains more than daily recommendations of sodium and chloride if >2 L is given, thus Hartmann's solution is more physiological in correcting an isotonic fluid deficit. A total of 60 mmol potassium/24 h is needed; thus, 20 mmol KCl should be added for each litre of intravenous fluid. Electrolyte measurements will guide in type of fluids given. In the presence of low sodium or chloride, then saline is best given; while for other electrolyte deficiencies, the appropriate electrolytes should be added. Severe hyponatraemia (<120 mmol/L) should be corrected slowly to avoid the rare, but potentially severe, complication of pontine myolysis. Rehydration should be continued to achieve a daily urine output of at least 1000 mL.

9.6.7 Nutritional Therapy

A maternal daily caloric intake of 2000 kcal is needed during the first trimester of pregnancy. Women suffering from hyperemesis have very low nutritional intakes; the higher the PUQE score, the less oral intake there is, and as a group hospitalized hyperemesis patients eat less than half of their daily energy recommendations [7]. Maternal pregnancy weight gain is the strongest correlate with fetal weight gain. A maternal pregnancy weight gain less than 7 kg correlates with increased risk of small for gestational age (SGA) babies [20]. Thus, measures to help a woman achieve sufficient nutritional intakes are likely to be beneficial. Providing 1 litre of dextrose 100 mg/mL IV will ensure 460 kcal in addition to any oral intake. There is only one RCT comparing 50 mg/mL dextrose to 0.9% saline for hyperemesis patients but even this lower glucose dose was found beneficial in relieving nausea scores and to be better than saline alone [4].

Thiamine (vitamin B1) should be given when parenteral nutrition (including dextrose infusion) is instituted to reduce the risk of refeeding syndrome. For women with continuous vomiting and very low food intake >2 weeks, parenteral infusion of 200 mg thiamine in 100 mL NaCl is recommended before the onset of a glucose infusion. Pregnant women are generally recommended supplementation of folic acid 400 mg during first trimester; this should be continued, either alone or as multivitamin tablets.

If antiemetics and fluids are not sufficient to reduce nausea (evaluated by PUQE scores) and thus increase oral food intake to normal (evaluated by simple food frequency charts) or restored nutritional status (regain lost weight, no ketonuria and normal prealbumin levels), further nutritional therapy would be needed.

Parenteral nutritional supplementation (1000 mL = 1000 kcal of standard manufactured parenteral solutions) may be given by peripheral venous line. However, vitamins and trace elements need to be specifically added before the infusion is started. Otherwise, severe vitamin deficiencies may occur. This can become sufficiently severe to cause a maternal death.

Enteral tube feeding is an alternative to parenteral nutrition. A jejunal tube could be placed by gastroscopy [20]; this potentially carries less risk of regurgitation (vomiting) of the nutritional solution than one may get from a gastric tube [21]. Tube feeding carries considerable less risks than total parenteral feeding needing a central venous catheter (thrombosis, pneumothorax, phlebitis and sepsis); thus, tube feeding is preferred when prolonged nutritional therapy is needed. The commercial enteral solutions are 'complete' regarding vitamins and trace elements if a daily dose of 2 L is achieved.

Tube feeding may be administered at home, as the patient may handle the equipment herself. Parenteral nutrition is generally more expensive than enteral feeding and will require administration by health personnel (infusion/home care nurse); thus this is mostly given in hospital settings, increasing the cost of this treatment even further.

In a Dutch randomized controlled study with tube feeding starting at first day of hospital admission for hyperemesis (n=59) compared to intravenous rehydration alone (n=59), the authors did not find significant different short- or long-term outcomes [21]. However, a Norwegian hospital cohort study [20] found that 108 women with failed primary interventions (fluid rehydration and partial IV parenteral supplementation) when receiving jejunal tube feeding started to regain weight and achieved similar total maternal and fetal weight gain until delivery as those not needing enteral treatment.

9.6.8 Psychosocial Support

Several studies have documented hyperemesis patients reporting lack of support and understanding from their healthcare providers, adding to their hopelessness and low quality of life [1, 12]. Providing patients with valid disease information and proper medical treatment may also reduce their psychological burden. In general, patients being able to choose treatment modalities (such as inpatient versus outpatient) will increase their satisfaction with treatment. Actively asking for and acknowledging any side effects or failed previous treatment options and seeking the woman's own preferences regarding treatment options may contribute to her coping. Psychological counselling may be needed, and there is some evidence that this may contribute to improved outcome [1].

9.7 Consequences of Hyperemesis

For the majority of patients, the hyperemesis symptoms will recede, well-being and feeding will improve and women will deliver a healthy, normal weight baby at term. However, there are possible risks that should be acknowledged.

9.7.1 Consequences for the Offspring

9.7.1.1 Short Term

Reduced Fetal Growth and Gestational Length

A systematic review by Veenendaal et al concluded that offspring are at increased risk of low birthweight, preterm birth (PTB) and being born SGA [22]. Substantial heterogeneity across the studies concerning both methodology and the applied definition of hyperemesis made the meta-analyses challenging. Two studies have reported increased risk of SGA with insufficient maternal pregnancy weight gain (<7 kg) [20].

Apgar Score

Hyperemesis have been reported to be associated with increased risk of low Apgar score, while the Veenendaal review [22] did not find such an association. A recent study from the UK including more than 8 million pregnancies reported that the offspring to hyperemetic mothers were more likely to undergo resuscitation or neonatal intensive care, although the absolute increased risks were low [3].

Coagulopathy

Fetal intracranial haemorrhage due to hyperemesis-induced vitamin K deficiency has been described as well as vitamin K deficient embryopathy [1].

Fetal death

Several studies have found a lower risk of fetal loss during the first trimester in women suffering from hyperemesis as compared to non/less emetic pregnancies [16, 17]. However, the proportion of hyperemesis patients choosing to terminate the pregnancy have been reported as high as 10–15% [1]. In spite of increased risk of SGA, several studies have reported no increased risk of fetal death after hyperemesis pregnancies [3, 22].

9.7.1.2 Long Term

Cancer

Although two small British studies have reported a slightly increased risk of leukaemia or testicular cancer, a large Scandinavian registry-based study concluded that hyperemesis was not associated with increased cancer risk in offspring, and that the positive association to lymphoma found could be due to chance and needs to be further explored [23].

Lower Insulin Sensitivity, Higher Fasting Blood Glucose and Blood Pressure

A recent study by Ayyavoo et al reported a 20% reduced insulin sensitivity, higher fasting insulin and cortisol, and lower levels of IGF-1 among pre-pubertal children of hyperemetic mothers [24]. Grooten et al found that early pregnancy weight loss, primarily as a manifestation of hyperemesis, was associated with increased blood pressure in offspring at 5–6 years of age [25].

9.7.2 Consequences of Hyperemesis for the Mother

9.7.2.1 Short Term

Weight Loss and Hospitalization

Patients with hyperemesis are reported to be at increased risk of extreme weight loss during pregnancy, defined as >15% of pre-pregnant weight. Women are recommended to gain 10–15 kg during pregnancy (given a normal BMI), while hyperemesis may result in a high net weight loss. Women suffering from hyperemesis are at increased risk of sick leave and hospitalization in pregnancy [3, 4].

Metabolic Disturbances

Ketonuria is an indicator of catabolic activity in the adipose tissue, particularly when carbohydrate energy intake is low. A recent meta-analysis could not confirm the degree of ketonuria to correspond to severity of hyperemesis, in terms of hospital (re)admissions [8]. Hypokalaemia is a marker for significant dehydration and has been reported as an independent risk factor for acute operative delivery among hyperemesis patients. Case-reports have described hyperemesis-induced hypokalaemia to cause maternal cardiac arrest and accompanying extreme weight loss (35 kg!) led to severe maternal rhabdomyolysis. Maternal undernutrition may cause vitamin K deficiency, which may induce coagulopathy. Increased risk of gestational anaemia has also been reported in hyperemesis pregnancies.

Thromboembolic Complications

Pregnancy is a hypercoagulable state. Dehydration and immobilization during hyperemesis may further contribute to the increased risk of thrombosis in pregnancy and after delivery described in a population-based British cohort study [3].

Disorders of the Thyroid

The risk of gestational transient thyrotoxicosis (GTT) is increased among hyperemesis patients. For the majority of patients, GTT is self-limiting and does not require treatment.

Neurological Complications

Left untreated, hyperemesis may cause severe damage to the central and peripheral nervous system [1]. Wernicke's encephalopathy is caused by thiamine deficiency, and is characterized by ataxia, nystagmus and ophthalmoplegia. Central pontine myelinolysis has also been described in hyperemesis patients, due to too rapid correction of hyponatraemia.

Psychological Disorders

In general, women experiencing hyperemesis have no significantly different prior psychiatric diagnosis/premorbid personalities as compared to non-hyperemetic women, but women with a prior history of depression have approximately a 50% increase in risk for developing hyperemesis compared to those without. Anxiety and depression are reported to be more common among hyperemesis patients than pregnant women without extreme nausea [1]. Several studies have shown that hyperemesis had a negative psychosocial impact on women's lives including changing their childbearing plans and abstaining from further pregnancies [12]. Women with hyperemesis had increased risk for emotional distress from the second trimester but it receded by 18 months postpartum. Hyperemetic women also had higher post-traumatic stress symptoms up to 2 years after birth.

Placental Dysfunction Disorders

Several studies have described increased risk of pre-eclampsia in hyperemesis pregnancies, including a large Swedish study which concluded that women with protracted hyperemesis (second trimester) have more than a doubled risk of pre-eclampsia and a threefold increase in risk of placental abruption compared to women without hyperemesis [26].

9.7.2.2 Long Term

Autoimmune Disease

Studies using Danish register data have reported that hyperemesis was associated with increased risk of autoimmune disease (relative risk (RR) 1.41, 95% confidence interval (CI) 1.30–1.51) [27]. The specific risk regarding rheumatoid arthritis has been conflicting, one study showing increased risk, another not finding this association.

Recurrence Risk of Hyperemesis

Based on data from the Norwegian Birth Registry, Trogstad et al reported in a large cohort study that women with hyperemesis in their first pregnancy had more than a 26-fold increased risk of hyperemesis in their second pregnancy [28]. The risk of recurrence in subsequent pregnancies is currently reported to vary between 15% and 80% [1].

Cancer

Two studies have report reduced breast cancer risk after hyperemesis, one even describing that severity of NVP was inversely associated with breast cancer risk. In contrast, a more recent British study reported that hyperemesis was associated with an increased risk of HER-2-enriched tumours, but not with other subtypes of breast cancer [29]. Another study from Scandinavian cancer registries found hyperemesis to be inversely associated with overall cancer risk, but positively associated with thyroid cancer (absolute risk reduction (aRR), 1.45) [30].

Cardiovascular Disease (CVD)

Two recent studies based on Norwegian registry data reported no consistent evidence of increased risk for cardiovascular disease (CVD) subsequent to hyperemesis gravidarum pregnancies [31].

9.8 Key Messages

Hyperemesis gravidarum is a condition characterized by extreme and persistent nausea and vomiting in pregnancy with negative health effects for mothers and children:

- Hyperemesis causes reduced fluid and food intake, low quality of life and need for sick leave and hospital treatment.
- Maternal malnourishment includes dehydration, electrolyte deficiencies, low total energy intake as well as specific vitamin deficiencies.
- Treatment of hyperemesis should include antiemetics to reduce nausea, correction of fluid and electrolyte deficiencies as well as nutritional therapy.
- Psychosocial support includes acknowledgement of the emotional as well as the physical burden of this disease.
- Without adequate treatment, there is increased risk of adverse pregnancy outcomes, such as maternal thromboembolic complications and fetal SGA.

9.9 Key Guidelines Relevant to This Topic

RCOG. *The Management of Nausea and Vomiting of Pregnancy and Hyperemesis Gravidarum*, RCOG Green-top Guideline No 69. London: Royal College of Obstetricians and Gynaecologists; 2016. www.rcog.org.uk/en/guidelines-research-services/guidelines/gtg69/

"ACOG Practice Bulletin No. 189: Nausea and Vomiting of Pregnancy." *Obstet Gynecol.* 2018 Jan;131(1):e15-e30.

"Emesis & Hyperemesis Gravidarum." In *Nordic Guidelines Obstetrics and Gynecology.* Copenhagen, Denmark: NFOG; 2014. www.nfog.org/files/guidelines/7%20NGF%20Obst%20hyperemisis%20Vikanes.pdf

References

1. Dean CR, Shemar M, Ostrowski GAU, Painter RC. Management of severe pregnancy sickness and hyperemesis gravidarum. *BMJ.* 2018 Nov **30**;363: k5000.

2. Vikanes A, Grjibovski AM, Vangen S, Magnus P. Variations in prevalence of hyperemesis gravidarum by country of birth: a study of 900,074 pregnancies in Norway, 1967–2005. *Scand J Public Health.* 2008 Mar;**36**(2):135–42.

3. Fiaschi L, Nelson-Piercy C, Gibson J, Szatkowski L, Tata LJ. Adverse maternal and birth outcomes in women admitted to hospital for hyperemesis gravidarum: a population-based cohort study. *Paediatr Perinat Epidemiol.* 2018 Jan;**32**(1):40–51.

4. O'Donnell A, McParlin C, Robson SC, et al. Treatments for hyperemesis gravidarum and nausea and vomiting in pregnancy: a systematic review and economic assessment. *Health Technol Assess.* 2016 Oct;**20**(74):1–268.

5. Koot MH, Boelig RC, Van't Hooft J, et al. Variation in hyperemesis gravidarum definition and outcome reporting in randomised clinical trials: a systematic review. *BJOG.* 2018 Nov;**125**(12):1514–21.

6. Koren G, Piwko C, Ahn E, et al. Validation studies of the Pregnancy Unique-Quantification of Emesis (PUQE) scores. *J Obstet Gynaecol.* 2005 Apr;**25**(3):241–4.

7. Birkeland E, Stokke G, Tangvik RJ, et al. Norwegian PUQE (Pregnancy-Unique Quantification of Emesis and nausea) identifies patients with hyperemesis gravidarum and poor nutritional intake: a prospective cohort validation study. *PLoS One.* 2015;**10**(4):e0119962.

8. Niemeijer MN, Grooten IJ, Vos N, et al. Diagnostic markers for hyperemesis gravidarum: a systematic review and metaanalysis. *Am J Obstet Gynecol.* 2014 Aug;**211**(2):150e1–15.

9. Vikanes A, Grjibovski AM, Vangen S, et al. Maternal body composition, smoking, and hyperemesis gravidarum. *Ann Epidemiol.* 2010 Aug;**20**(8):592–8.

10. Vikanes A, Skjaerven R, Grjibovski AM, et al. Recurrence of hyperemesis gravidarum across generations: population based cohort study. *BMJ.* 2010;**340**:c2050.

11. Fejzo MS, Sazonova OV, Sathirapongsasuti JF, et al. Placenta and appetite genes *GDF15* and *IGFBP7* are associated with hyperemesis gravidarum. *Nat Commun.* 2018 Mar 21;**9**(1):1178.

12. Heitmann K, Nordeng H, Havnen GC, Solheimsnes A, Holst L. The burden of nausea and vomiting during pregnancy: severe impacts on quality of life, daily life functioning and willingness to become pregnant again – results from a cross-sectional study. *BMC Pregnancy Childbirth.* 2017 Feb 28;**17**(1):75.

13. Shehmar M, Maclean M, Nelson-Piercy C, Gadsby R, O'Hara M. *The Management of Nausea and Vomiting of Pregnancy and Hyperemesis Gravidarum*,RCOG Green-top Guideline No 69. London: Royal College of Obstetricians and Gynaecologists; 2016.

14. Bulletins-Obstetrics CoP. ACOG Practice Bulletin No. 189: nausea and vomiting of pregnancy. *Obstet Gynecol.* 2018 Jan;**131**(1):e15-e30.

15. Vikanes Å, Trovik J, Tellum T, et al. Emesis & hyperemesis gravidarum. In *Nordic Guidelines Obstetrics and Gynecology.* Copenhagen, Denmark: NFOG; 2014.

16. Quinlan JD. Nausea and vomiting in pregnancy. In *BMJ Best Practice.* London, UK: BMJ; 2018.

17. Smith JA, Fox KA, Clark S. Nausea and vomiting of pregnancy: treatment and outcome. In Barss VA, ed. *UpToDate*; 2019.

18. Boelig RC, Barton SJ, Saccone G, et al. Interventions for treating hyperemesis gravidarum: a Cochrane systematic review and meta-analysis. *J Matern*

Fetal Neonatal Med. 2018 Sep;**31**(18):2492–505.

19. Lupattelli A, Spigset O, Twigg MJ, et al. Medication use in pregnancy: a cross-sectional, multinational web-based study. *BMJ Open.* 2014 Feb 17;**4**(2):e004365.

20. Stokke G, Gjelsvik BL, Flaatten KT, et al. Hyperemesis gravidarum, nutritional treatment by nasogastric tube feeding: a 10-year retrospective cohort study. *Acta Obstet Gynecol Scand.* 2015 Apr;**94**(4):359–67.

21. Grooten IJ, Koot MH, van der Post JA, et al. Early enteral tube feeding in optimizing treatment of hyperemesis gravidarum: the Maternal and Offspring outcomes after Treatment of HyperEmesis by Refeeding (MOTHER) randomized controlled trial. *Am J Clin Nutr.* 2017 Sep;**106**(3):812–20.

22. Veenendaal MV, van Abeelen AF, Painter RC, van der Post JA, Roseboom TJ. Consequences of hyperemesis gravidarum for offspring: a systematic review and meta-analysis. *BJOG.* 2011 Oct;**118**(11):1302–13.

23. Vandraas KF, Vikanes AV, Stoer NC, et al. Hyperemesis gravidarum and risk of cancer in offspring, a Scandinavian registry-based nested case-control study. *BMC Cancer.* 2015 May 13;**15**:398.

24. Ayyavoo A, Derraik JG, Hofman PL, et al. Severe hyperemesis gravidarum is associated with reduced insulin sensitivity in the offspring in childhood. *J Clin Endocrinol Metab.* 2013 Aug;**98**(8):3263–8.

25. Grooten I, Painter R, Pontesilli M, et al. Weight loss in pregnancy and cardiometabolic profile in childhood: findings from a longitudinal birth cohort. *BJOG.* 2014;**2011**(12):22.

26. Bolin M, Akerud H, Cnattingius S, Stephansson O, Wikstrom AK. Hyperemesis gravidarum and risks of placental dysfunction disorders: a population-based cohort study. *BJOG.* 2013 Apr;**120**(5):541–7.

27. Jorgensen KT, Nielsen NM, Pedersen BV, Jacobsen S, Frisch M. Hyperemesis, gestational hypertensive disorders, pregnancy losses and risk of autoimmune diseases in a Danish population-based cohort. *J Autoimmun.* 2012 May;**38**(2–3):J120–8.

28. Trogstad LI, Stoltenberg C, Magnus P, Skjaerven R, Irgens LM. Recurrence risk in hyperemesis gravidarum. *BJOG.* 2005 Dec;**112**(12):1641–5.

29. Wright LB, Schoemaker MJ, Jones ME, Ashworth A, Swerdlow AJ. Breast cancer risk in relation to history of preeclampsia and hyperemesis gravidarum: prospective analysis in the Generations Study. *Int J Cancer.* 2018 Aug 15;**143**(4):782–92.

30. Vandraas KF, Grjibovski AM, Stoer NC, et al. Hyperemesis gravidarum and maternal cancer risk, a Scandinavian nested case-control study. *Int J Cancer.* 2015 Sep 1;**137**(5):1209–16.

31. Fossum S, Halvorsen S, Vikanes AV, et al. Cardiovascular risk profile at the age of 40–45 in women with previous hyperemesis gravidarum or hypertensive disorders in pregnancy: A population-based study. *Pregnancy Hypertens.* 2018 Apr;**12**:129–35.

Pre-Conception Care

Chu Chin Lim & Tahir A. Mahmood

10.1 Introduction

Pre-conception care is defined as 'any intervention provided to women and couples of childbearing age, regardless of pregnancy status or desire, before pregnancy, to improve health outcomes for women, newborns and children' [1]. All women hoping to conceive are considered as potential candidates for such a consultation.

The objectives of prenatal care are as follows:

1. Provide generic information to all women about lifestyle changes and healthy living interventions which could have a modifiable effect on the outcomes of their pregancies.
2. Counsel women with underlying chronic medical conditions, as regards the effect of pregnancy on their own health, the course of pregnancy and health of the newborn.
3. Counsel women at increased risk of adverse pregnancy outcome secondary to metabolic or chromosomal disorders.
4. Advise women in planning pregnancy who had an adverse outcome in the past.

10.2 Provide generic information to all women about lifestyle changes, and healthy living interventions which could have a modifiable effect on the outcomes of their pregnancies

Initial enquiries involve ascertaining general overall well-being, social habits, modifiable factors and carry out an assessment of risk factors. This information will inform a targeted pre-conception management plan:

1. Is she currently taking an appropriate dose of folic acid to reduce her risk of a neural tube defect (NTD)?
2. Is she up to date with her cervical cancer screening?
3. Is she a smoker and had she been advised to stop smoking?
4. How many units of alcohol does she consume each week? Does she get involved in binge drinking?
5. Does she use any illicit drugs?
6. Does she have immunity to rubella?
7. Does she have a definite history of chickenpox or shingles?
8. Has she been taking over-the-counter medicines, vitamins or herbal remedies?
9. Is she overweight or obese? And does she understand that a body mass index (BMI) >30 kg/m^2 increases risks for her and the baby during pregnancy?
10. Does she have a chronic health problem; what are her current medications?
11. Is she aware whether her current medications are safe to continue during her planned pregnancy?

10.2.1 Advice on Folic Acid

A Cochrane systemic review [2] has found that the intake of peri-conceptional folic acid starting at least 1 month before conception to 12 weeks of pregnancy is associated with reduced incidence of neural tube defects (NTD) and recurrence. All potential couples embarking on a planned pregnancy need to be risk assessed for their individualized risk of conceiving a child with an NTD. Women who are at a normal risk for an NTD should take folic acid 400 micrograms daily prior to conception and should continue until the 12th week of pregnancy. Women at high risk of an NTD as identified in Table 10.1 should take folic acid 5 mg daily and should continue this until the 12th week of pregnancy.

10.2.2 Smoking, Alcohol Consumption and Illicit Drug Use

All women should be advised to stop smoking and a referral to smoking cessation services should be made. Nicotine replacement therapy is not routinely recommended.

Alcohol consumption in the first 3 months of pregnancy may be associated with an increased risk of miscarriage. Getting drunk and binge drinking may be harmful to the unborn infant. Women should be informed there is no safe lower limit of alcohol during pregnancy. Most recent studies have reported adverse effect of drinking even at lower amount of intake. Therefore, they should be advised 'no alcohol during pregnancy'.

Table 10.1 Risk factors for neural tube defects

Either partner with NTD	Previous pregnancy affected by an NTD
Family history of NTD	Women on anti-epileptic medication
Women with coeliac disease, diabetes, haemoglobinopathies and obesity	

The fetus is particularly vulnerable to the harmful effects of drugs; therefore, women who have a history of substance misuse should be referred to specialist services.

10.2.3 Obesity

Women who are overweight or obese are at an increased risk of adverse pregnancy outcomes compared to women who are not overweight [3, 4]. The increased risk is modest in women who are overweight but incrementally increases with higher BMI, and therefore is significantly higher in people who are grossly obese, in particular among women with a BMI of over 40 kg/m^2.

Adverse pregnancy outcomes associated with obesity include:

- gestational diabetes, pre-eclampsia, venous thromboembolism and prematurity
- induced labour, instrumental delivery and shoulder dystocia
- caesarean section, anaesthetic complications and wound infections
- congenital anomalies (Table 10.2),
- stillbirth, macrosomia and neonatal death.
- problems initiating or maintaining breastfeeding

There is intergenerational effect of maternal obesity during pregnancy on the future health of the newborn. These children are at an increased risk of developing obesity and metabolic disorders in childhood.

Women should be advised to continue to undertake moderate activity during pregnancy. In 2009, the US Institute of Medicine (IOM) provided specific recommendations on the ideal gestational weight gain. A meta-analysis based on the IOM recommendation showed gestational weight gain below the recommendations was associated with a higher risk of a small baby and preterm birth. Gestational weight gain above the recommendations was associated with a higher risk of a large baby and caesarean delivery. There are no UK guidelines on recommended weight gain ranges during pregnancy, and there is great variability in the amount of weight pregnant women can gain during pregnancy. Women should be encouraged to eat a healthy and balanced diet, and be informed that energy needs do not significantly change during the first 6

months of pregnancy. During the last 3 months of pregnancy, women may need an additional 200 calories per day.

10.2.4 Immunization

Women planning pregnancy should be tested for immunity to rubella. Maternal immunity to rubella prevents acquiring an infection which can cause fetal death or congenital rubella syndrome. The measles, mumps and rubella (MMR) combined vaccine is now used for women of childbearing age, as a single vaccine for rubella is not available. Women should be advised to use effective contraception to avoid becoming pregnant for 1 month after receiving rubella-containing vaccine.

Immunity to varicella is tested if there is no definite history of chickenpox or shingles and the woman is deemed at high risk, such as healthcare workers who may come into direct contact with infected patients and healthy and susceptible close contacts of immunocompromised patients. Vaccination is offered if the test is negative, as immunization prevents fetal and maternal harm if varicella is contracted during pregnancy.

10.2.5 Hepatitis B Vaccine

Hepatitis B vaccine is offered to women if they are at high risk of contracting the disease. These include:

- Intravenous drug users
- Those having multiple sexual partners
- Those with chronic renal or liver disease
- Those who are in close contact with people with hepatitis B

10.3 Counsel women with underlying chronic medical conditions, as regards the effect of pregnancy on their own health, the course of pregnancy and health of the newborn

10.3.1 Chronic Medical Disorders

Women with chronic medical problems should be advised to plan for a pregnancy with careful consideration for an optimal outcome. Pre-conception care in these women involves:

- review of the current status of the clinical condition,
- assessment of possible impact of pregnancy on disease,
- effect of disease on the pregnancy outcome,
- type of antenatal care required, and
- review of current medications and their impact on the newborn [5, 6].

Most women with chronic medical disorders are classified as having a high-risk pregnancy and should be advised to attend for specialized hospital care at combined antenatal multidisciplinary clinics. These women will need serial growth monitoring of the fetus, and an anaesthetic risk evaluation for pain relief during labour and delivery should be made. Table 10.3 summarizes effects of various medical disorders on pregnancy.

Table 10.2 Congenital anomalies associated with pre-pregnancy obesity (described with odds ratios) [3]

Congenital anomaly	Odds ratio
Neural tube defects	1.87
Heart defects	1.30
Cleft palate and cleft lip	1.20
Cleft palate	1.23
Anorectal atresia	1.48
Hydrocephaly	1.68
Limb reduction abnormalities	1.34

Table 10.3 Effect of various medical conditions and their treatments on the fetus

Neurological	
1. Epilepsy	Risk of major fetal anomaly from antiepileptic
2. Multiple sclerosis	Overall rate of progression of disability is not altered by pregnancy

Cardiac Disease	
1. Congenital heart defects	Risk of fetus with congestive heart disease (CHD)
2. Artificial heart valves	Risk of anticoagulation
3. Chronic hypertension	Increase risk of pre-eclampsia

Renal Disease	
1. Moderate renal disease	May accelerate during pregnancy
2. Severe renal disease	Fertility issue, worsening of renal function in pregnancy
3. Renal transplant patient	Increase risk of miscarriage. High risk of graft complication if poor pre-conception graft function
4. Patient on dialysis	Subfertility issue. Poor erythropoietic function necessitate blood transfusion in pregnancy

Respiratory Disease	
1. Asthma	Increased risk of preterm delivery, low birthweight and congenital malformation
2. Cystic fibrosis	Safe in mild disease. Pregnancy is not recommended in women with pulmonary hypertension, cor pulmonale and poor pregnancy lung function
3. Restrictive lung disease	Poor pregnancy lung function is associated with poor pregnancy outcome

Haemoglobinopathies	
a. Thalassaemia	
1. Alpha-thalassaemia carriers	Anaemic during pregnancy
2. 3-Alpha-thalassaemia (HbH disease)	Chronic haemolytic anaemia
3. Homozygous alpha-thalassaemia	Associated with severe pre-eclampsia, macrosomia baby and bulky placenta
4. Beta-thalassaemia minor (beta-thalassaemia trait)	Need to rule out folic deficiency
5. Beta-thalassaemia major	Pregnancy is rare with serious complications
b. Sickle cell disease	Increase risk of intrauterine growth retardation, premature delivery and miscarriage. Increase risk of sickle cell crises

10.3.1.1 Liver Disease

This comprises a varied number of conditions as listed here.

Viral Hepatitis B (HBV): Maternal–neonatal transmission for hepatitis B usually occurs at delivery but may also be transplacental. Without the use of preventive measures, almost 90% of these babies will become chronically infected with hepatitis B at birth. Antiviral therapy (lamivudine, tenofovir) during the third trimester of pregnancy in high-risk women with chronic HBV infection reduces the viral load in the mother and may decrease the risk of perinatal transmission.

A woman with hepatitis B should be advised that her newborn child will require a first dose of hepatitis B vaccine and one dose of hepatitis B immunoglobulin (HBIG) within the first 12 hours of life. This will ensure that the newborn has a 95% chance of being protected against a lifelong hepatitis B infection. The infant will require additional doses of hepatitis B vaccine at 1 and 6 months of age to provide complete protection.

In women with cirrhosis associated with severe hepatic impairment, pregnancy should be discouraged.

Liver transplants: Pregnancy should be postponed for 1.5 to 2 years after transplantation. Management includes continuing immunosuppressive drugs throughout pregnancy which will affect intrauterine fetal growth.

10.3.1.2 Inflammatory Bowel Disease (IBD)

Women with inflammatory bowel disease (IBD) should be encouraged to conceive during the periods of disease remission. Aminosalicylates (sulfasalazine, mesalzine), oral and rectal steroids, azathioprine, and 6-mercaptopurine are safe to use during pregnancy. Etanercept, infliximab and adalimumab are probably safe in the second and third trimesters and during breastfeeding. Pregnancy has little effect on the course of IBD. Elective caesarean section is recommended for women with perianal Crohn's disease or with stomas.

10.3.1.3 Mental Health Issues

Common mental health conditions encountered include:

- Depression
- Bipolar disorder
- Schizophrenia

A woman with mental health problems should be assigned a mental health nurse/community psychiatric nurse (CPN) who will contribute to the woman's care throughout pregnancy. These women should be advised to seek advice from a specialist before planning pregnancy, preferably at the pre-pregnancy clinic.

Tricyclic antidepressants in therapeutic doses have been reported to be safe in pregnancy. The data on selective serotonin reuptake inhibitors (SSRIs) have shown a small increase in septal valvular defects if taken during the first trimester and persistent pulmonary hypertension if taken beyond 20 weeks. There is an association between antidepressants and poor neonatal adaptation syndrome which presents with irritability, difficulty feeding, hypoglycaemia, sleep disturbance, persistent crying and, in extreme cases, seizures. Monoamine oxidase inhibitors (MAOIs) and other antidepressants such as duloxetine, mianserin, reboxetine and trazadone are not recommended for use in pregnancy, as limited data are available on their safety in pregnancy.

Women with bipolar disorder and on anti-epileptic drugs are considered to be at high risk of conceiving a child with a neural tube defect and should be prescribed with folic acid 5 mg daily until the 12th week of pregnancy. Referral to a psychiatrist is recommended to assess and manage the potential risks to both mother and fetus when a woman is taking valproate, carbamazepine, lithium or lamotrigine, and alternative antipsychotic drugs should be considered.

A woman with schizophrenia needs psychiatric review of her medication before embarking on pregnancy.

A plan should be in place to deal with a postnatal flare-up or attack of severe postpartum psychosis. It should be noted that newborn babies of these mothers may experience withdrawal symptoms; therefore, a close coordination with neonatology team is desirable.

10.3.1.4 Metabolic Disorders

The care of women with metabolic disorders is covered in other chapters.

10.3.2 Chronic Medical Conditions

10.3.2.1 Epilepsy

Epilepsy is a common neurological condition in reproductive-aged women. All women taking anti-epileptic drugs (AEDs) should be referred to a specialist for review of epilepsy treatment before becoming pregnant to discuss the relative risks and benefits of adjusting their medication. Women should continue using effective contraception until a full assessment by the specialist has taken place and should not stop taking their medication unless otherwise directed by the specialist.

Control of epilepsy should be optimized prior to pregnancy with the lowest dose of the most effective treatment to provide best seizure control. Polytherapy should be avoided if possible. Women who have been seizure free for more than 2 years may wish to discontinue AEDs prior to conception and for the first trimester. This decision should only be taken following discussion with a neurologist. In most women, pregnancy does not affect the frequency of seizures; the risk of seizures is highest during the postpartum period.

Women taking AEDs are at high risk of conceiving a child with a neural tube defect, and should be prescribed a higher dose of folic acid (5 mg daily) pre-conceptually and continue until the 12th week of pregnancy. The risk of a major fetal malformation in pregnancy is 2%. This risk increases up to threefold in

a woman who is taking one anti-epileptic drug. Sodium valproate has been associated with a significantly higher risk of malformations than carbamazepine or lamotrigine [5]. The newer anti-epileptic levetiracetam, gabapentin and tiagabine are not teratogenic in animals. Vigabatrin and topiramate are teratogenic and should not be used in pregnancy.

Most parents with epilepsy do not have children with epilepsy, and the chances of inheriting epilepsy are generally low. The risk for any child developing epilepsy by the age of 20 is around 1% (1 in 100), and the risk may increase to around 2–5% (2 to 5 in 100) for most children of parents with epilepsy.

10.3.2.2 Multiple Sclerosis (MS)

The course of multiple sclerosis (MS) during pregnancy is extremely variable, and a decrease in relapse rate is most marked in the third trimester, whilst relapses are common in the first 3 months postpartum, settling to pre-pregnancy levels by 10 months after delivery. The overall rate of progression of disability is not altered by pregnancy. Beta interferon and glatiramer are avoided in pregnancy, and steroids can be safely used in acute relapses.

10.3.2.3 Cardiac Disease

Cardiac disease and its implications have been described in Chapter 28.

10.3.2.4 Artificial Heart Valves

Women with metal prosthetic heart valves must continue full anticoagulation throughout pregnancy. All women should be counselled prior to pregnancy regarding the potential risk to themselves and the fetus. Continuation of warfarin affords the mother the lowest risk of thrombosis; however, for the fetus, warfarin is associated with an increased risk of teratogenesis, miscarriage, stillbirth and intracerebral bleeding. High-dose low molecular weight heparin is safe for the fetus but is associated with a higher risk of thrombosis for the pregnant woman compared to warfarin. Advice regarding anticoagulation should be tailored to the individual woman with regard to both her previous medical and obstetric histories.

Women should continue using effective contraception until a full assessment by the cardiologist has taken place and to continue her medication unless otherwise advised by the cardiologist.

10.3.2.5 Chronic Hypertension

Chronic hypertension is associated with an increased risk of pre-eclampsia, placental abruption, small for gestation infants and increased neonatal morbidity and mortality. It is recommended that women with a history of hypertension should be reviewed by a cardiac specialist prior to becoming pregnant. This is to rule out an undiagnosed secondary hypertension due to renal artery stenosis, Conn's syndrome, pheochromocytoma, coarctation of aorta or Cushing's syndrome which can deteriorate rapidly during pregnancy.

It has been recognized that angiotensin-converting enzyme (ACE) inhibitors are associated with congenital malformations, intrauterine growth retardation, hypoglycaemia, kidney disease and premature delivery. Angiotensin II receptor antagonists (AIIRAs) are associated with congenital malformations. ACE inhibitors and AIIRAs are therefore contraindicated for women embarking on pregnancy.

The drugs with the most safety data are methyldopa, beta-blockers (labetalol, metoprolol, propranolol) and hydralazine. If these drugs are ineffective, then a modified-release preparation of nifedipine may be considered as a second-line alternative. However, the manufacturer recommends that this should not be used before the 20th week of pregnancy.

Pre-eclampsia complicates 25% of pregnancies in women with pre-existing hypertension. The incidence is higher if there is associated renal insufficiency, hypertension of 4 years' or more duration, and a history of hypertension in previous pregnancies.

Low-dose aspirin (75 mg daily) should be commenced before 12 weeks of pregnancy and continued throughout the pregnancy in cases of chronic hypertension with renal disease, diabetes or with a history of previous early-onset pre-eclampsia or recurrent pre-eclampsia.

10.3.2.6 Renal Disease

Renal disease during pregnancy is associated with risk of prematurity, intrauterine growth retardation and accelerated deterioration in maternal renal function. This has been discussed at length in the Chapter 32, Kidney Diseases in Pregnancy. All women with chronic kidney disease should be seen by the renal physician as part of pre-conception counselling. Assessment of pre-conception renal function, proteinuria and blood pressure enables accurate counselling and provides a baseline with which to compare trends during pregnancy.

Low-dose aspirin should be considered from the first trimester especially in those with associated hypertension.

10.3.2.7 Renal Transplant

Women who have had a renal transplant should be advised to wait 1.5–2 years after the transplant, allowing graft function to stabilize with maintenance levels of immunosuppressive drugs, thus minimizing the risk to the fetus. Pregnancy should be encouraged only if creatinine is stable at or below 200 micromol/L. The specialist may also need to review the dosage and the requirement for immunosuppressant medication (mycophenolate is contraindicated in pregnancy). Among those women who become pregnant and do not miscarry before 12 weeks, there is a 95% chance of a successful outcome. The poorer the graft function is at conception, the higher the risk of complications and deterioration in graft function.

Pregnancy has no adverse long-term effect on renal allograft or survival in women with baseline creatinine levels of <100 micromol/L, whereas renal graft survival is only 65% at 3 years if creatinine is more than 130 micromol/L.

Immunosuppressive drugs are maintained at pre-pregnancy levels. Women should be reassured of the relative safety of these drugs, as reduction or cessation of immunosuppressive therapy may provoke rejection. Cyclosporin, azathioprine and tacrolimus appear safe for use in pregnancy, whereas mycophenolate mofetil is generally contraindicated.

10.3.2.8 Pregnancy in Dialysis Patients

The chance of a successful pregnancy is low with both types of dialysis. Anaemia is worsened by pregnancy and transfusion requirements increase. Erythropoietin and iron infusions can be safely used. The dialysis requirement might increase markedly. The aim should be to maintain pre-dialysis urea at less than 15–20 mmol/L.

10.3.2.9 Respiratory Disease

Asthma

Treatment of controlled asthma requires little modification in pregnancy. The risks from uncontrolled asthma are much greater than the risk from asthma treatment during pregnancy. In poorly controlled asthma, there are increased risks of preterm delivery, low birthweight and congenital malformations. Women with severe asthma and those in whom asthma is poorly controlled should be referred to a chest physician to ensure adequate control and monitoring. Steroid tablets can be used as normally prescribed in the pre-conception period and during pregnancy. Prednisolone is the preferred oral corticosteroid as it is extensively metabolized by placental enzymes and only a minimal amount crosses the placenta. Prolonged exposure to prednisolone increases the risk of intrauterine growth retardation.

There are sufficient safety data available for long-acting and short-acting beta2-agonists, inhaled corticosteroids, antimuscarinic bronchodilators, cromones and theophylline and leukotriene receptor antagonists to recommend their use during pregnancy.

Cystic Fibrosis (CF)

Cystic fibrosis (CF) is the commonest autosomal recessive disorder in the UK, with a carrier rate of 1 in 25 in Caucasians. Increasing numbers of children with CF are surviving into adulthood. Pregnancy is safe in mild disease with a forced expiratory volume in 1 second (FEV1) >70–80% predicted. However, pregnancy is not recommended in women who have associated pulmonary hypertension, cor pulmonale or FEV1 <30–40% predicted. Infection with *Burkholderia cepacia* may be associated with a rapid deterioration in lung function, and recent acquisition or deteriorating lung function in the presence of this organism is also a contraindication to pregnancy.

Women should be screened for diabetes, because mucus blocks the ducts of the pancreas, reducing the production of insulin. Such a couple should be seen at the prenatal genetic counselling clinic. Once pregnancy is achieved, a multidisciplinary team input including an obstetrician, anaesthetist, neonatologist, pulmonary physician, specialist physiotherapist and specialist midwives at a tertiary unit will be required.

Severe Restrictive Lung Disease

Women with severe lung disease tolerate pregnancy better than women with severe cardiac insufficiency because of greater reserve in respiratory function. If the forced vital capacity (FVC) is >11, a successful pregnancy is usually possible. Women with the underlying cause of respiratory insufficiency, significant hypercapnia or hypoxia, pulmonary hypertension and cor pulmonale should be counselled regarding less favourable pregnancy outcomes.

Women with kyphoscoliosis who have Harrington rods inserted may preclude regional anaesthesia, and liaison with the obstetric anaesthetist is important.

10.3.2.10 Genetic Haemoglobinopathies
Genetic haemoglobinopathies are discussed in Chapter 31.

10.3.2.11 Thalassaemia
Women with thalassaemia should be referred for haematological assessment and their partner should also be tested.

Alpha-thalassaemia carriers (alpha-thalassaemia trait): the woman may become anaemic particularly if she is a carrier of two defective genes.

3-Alpha-thalassaemia (HbH disease): the woman will have chronic haemolytic anaemia and may require transfusion.

Homozygous alpha-thalassaemia (Bart's haemoglobin hydrops syndrome): this is more common in South East Asia, and pregnancy is associated with severe, sometimes life-threatening, pre-eclampsia.

Beta-thalassaemia minor (beta-thalassaemia trait) (symptomless carriers):if iron stores are depleted, the woman may need oral iron supplements during pregnancy. Most women with beta-thalassaemia are not usually iron deficient; therefore, before giving iron supplements it is important to check serum ferritin levels first and to see whether there is no other cause of anaemia such as folic acid deficiency.

Beta-thalassaemia major (homozygous beta-thalassaemia): pregnancy is rare in these women and is likely to have serious complications. These women need specialist reproductive endocrinological referral if they wish to become pregnant.

10.3.2.12 Haemolytic Anaemia
Women with haemolytic anaemia, including those with haemoglobinopathies, need extra folate supplementation from early pregnancy continued throughout pregnancy.

10.3.3 Safety of Prescription Medicine in Pregnancy
A cohort study in 81 975 pregnant women from the UK general practice research database showed that 65% of participants received one or more prescriptions in the 3 months before and 10 weeks after conception, of which 7% of prescriptions were under category 'X' drugs of the US Food and Drug Administration (FDA) (with potential teratogenic risk that outweighs maternal benefit). Table 10.4 summarizes various medications which women might be taking when they are planning to conceive. Because of their adverse effects, an alternative must be considered in the prenatal period. Preconception advice should be given on safety grounds. Advice on teratogenicity is available from the *British National Formulary* and the UK National Teratology Information Service.

10.4 Counsel women at increased risk of adverse pregnancy outcome secondary to metabolic or chromosomal disorders

10.4.1 Prenatal Diagnosis
Prenatal diagnosis is considered appropriate when the risk of a baby being affected by the disorder is high. This will offer choices to the woman regarding future management of her current pregnancy. She may wish to consider termination of an affected pregnancy or follow a conservative approach to continue with her affected pregnancy. The following groups of couples should be offered prenatal diagnosis:

1. A couple who are both carriers of a recessively inherited genetic disorder, where the chances of having an affected pregnancy are one in four.
2. When the woman is a carrier, then the risk of an affected pregnancy will depend on the prevalence of the disorder in a population. For certain high-prevalence disorders, the risk of an affected pregnancy may be high enough to justify offering prenatal diagnosis even when the carrier status of the man cannot be established.
3. For couples who would not consider late termination of pregnancy, it is important to refer them to a specialist fetal medicine team as early as possible during the first trimester of pregnancy. This will allow time for testing of the father of the baby (if necessary) and prenatal diagnosis testing prior to termination.

Prenatal diagnosis [7] can be carried out from 12 weeks of pregnancy onwards.

10.4.2 Sickle Cell Disease
All women with a sickle cell disease should be referred to a haematologist for assessment and monitoring pulmonary hypertension. (See Chapter 31 for further reading.)

Genetic counselling and screening of the partner are important. The risk of the baby's having HbSS is 50% if the partner has sickle cell trait.

The mother should be advised to take folic acid 5 mg for life irrespective of pregnancy. She should be advised to continue using adequate contraception until she has been fully assessed by a haematologist and a cardiologist. An echocardiogram should be performed to ensure there is no underlying cardiac anomaly.

10.4.3 Bleeding Disorders
Von Willebrand disease (vWD): This is the most commonly inherited bleeding disorder and is usually autosomal dominant. Close collaboration with the haematology team, ascertaining the subtype of vWd and whether the disease responds to desmopressin is important in the pre-conception period. Aspirin and NSAIDs should not be given to women with vWD.

Haemophilias A and B are rare X-linked disorders. Prenatal screening may be used to sex the fetus. Chorionic

Table 10.4 Drugs that need review during perinatal period

Drug	Potential teratogenic risk	Alternative to consider
ACE inhibitors and angiotensin receptor blockers	Increase risk of neurological, cardiac and skull abnormalities, fetal renal function impairment and oligohydramnios.	Nifedipine, labetalol, or methyldopa. Consider pre-pregnancy conversion to amlodipine in women with pre-pregnancy hypertension
Antidepressants: SSRIs and lithium	Defects associated with SSRIs are septal defects and neural tube defects; the absolute risk is low, and the risk is highest for paroxetine and lower for sertraline. Lithium is associated with cardiac abnormalities, but the absolute risk is low.	For many women already on an SSRI, sertraline may be the best option, but alternatives (tricyclic antidepressants) can be considered.
Antibiotics	Tetracycline can cause dental discoloration. Risk of malformations with trimethoprim (folate antagonist)	Consider penicillin or cephalosporins for long-term prevention of urinary tract infection.
Non-steroidal anti-inflammatory drugs (NSAIDs)	Can cause premature closure of ductus arteriosus if used in the 3rd trimester	Avoid use in 3rd trimester and consider other analgesics, such as paracetamol or codeine.
Warfarin	Cartilage defects, skeletal defects, brain defects and eye anomalies in the 1st and 2nd trimesters; associated with intracranial haemorrhage in the 3rd trimester	Consider low molecular weight heparin – liaise with a secondary care specialist before conversion.
Antiepileptics	Valproate carries the highest risk of impaired neurocognitive development and fetal malformations such as neural tube defects. Phenytoin can cause fetal hydantoin syndrome (microcephaly, intrauterine growth restriction and mental disability).	Liaise with a secondary care specialist before conversion. Consider lamotrigine or levetiracetam for women with epilepsy or alternative mood stabilizers for women with bipolar disorder.
Cytotoxins	Alkylating drugs, anthracyclines, cytotoxic antibiotics, vinca alkaloids (such as etoposide) have been shown to be teratogenic and mutagenic in animal studies. Antimetabolites (such as methotrexate) have been shown to be toxic in animal studies.	Effective contraception is needed during treatment; ensure adequate folic acid supplementation. Advise a woman planning to conceive to stop these drugs only after discussion with her hospital specialist.
Immunosuppressants	Mycophenolate mofetil is teratogenic and it causes microtia, low-set ears and other congenital malformations.	Effective contraception is needed before treatment, during treatment, and for 6 weeks after discontinuation of treatment.
Isotretinoin	Has a teratogenic effect in animal studies.	Effective contraception is needed for at least 1 month before starting treatment, during treatment, and for at least 1 month after stopping treatment.
Statins	Congenital anomalies have been reported in animal studies; decreased synthesis of cholesterol possibly affects fetal development.	Avoid in pregnancy; effective contraception is needed during treatment and for 1 month afterwards.

villus sampling can confirm an affected male fetus. Carriers should have factor VIII or IX level measured in early pregnancy and again after delivery.

10.4.4 Venous Thromboembolism (VTE)

All women with a personal or immediate family history of venous thromboembolism (VTE) for both inherited and acquired thrombophilia should be assessed. Both inherited and acquired thrombophilia increase the risk of venous thrombosis in pregnancy, and may also be partly responsible for recurrent intrauterine fetal demise and intrauterine growth retardation. Thromboprophylaxis, either in the first trimester or postpartum, may be required. All women receiving warfarin therapy and planning a pregnancy should be referred to a specialist for advice on whether warfarin should be stopped or replaced by heparin, depending on the woman's degree of risk of VTE.

Women with a history of deep vein thrombosis or pulmonary embolism in association with pregnancy, surgery or the

Table 10.5 The age-related risk of Down syndrome

Age of mother	Risk
20 years	1:1500
30 years	1:800
35 years	1:270
40 years	1:100
45 years and over	1:50 and greater

Table 10.6 Most common genetic disorders requiring referral for testing

Genetic disorder	Condition
Dominantly inherited disorders	Neurofibromatosis
	Tuberous sclerosis
	Huntington's disease
	Adult polycystic disease
	Marfan's syndrome
	Achondroplasia
Recessively inherited disorders	Haemoglobinopathies
	Cystic fibrosis
	Tay–Sachs disease
	Gaucher's disease
	Congenital adrenal hyperplasia
	Friedrich's ataxia
	Spinal muscular atrophy
X-linked disorders	Duchenne's muscular dystrophy
	Fragile X syndrome
	Haemophilias A and B
	Glucose-6-phosphate dehydrogenase deficiency

combined contraceptive pill should be considered at especially high risk of recurrence during pregnancy whether or not an underlying thrombophilia has been detected.

10.4.5 Advice for Older Women on Risks of Chromosomal Abnormality

Older women planning pregnancy should be warned about the risks of chromosomal abnormalities, such as Down syndrome (Table 10.5). The risk increases with maternal age and is higher following a previously affected pregnancy.

There is no pre-conception test that can predict whether a couple will conceive a baby with a chromosomal abnormality such as Down syndrome. Antenatal screening tests can estimate the likelihood of a pregnant woman carrying a baby with Down syndrome. Definitive diagnostic test for Down syndrome is offered to pregnant women at high risk. This can be established by amniocentesis, chorionic villus sampling (CVS) or fetal blood sampling. The risk of miscarriage is 1% with amniocentesis and is slightly higher with CVS carried out after 15 weeks of gestation. Early amniocentesis is not a safe alternative to second trimester amniocentesis because of increased pregnancy loss (7.6% compared with 5.9%). Early amniocentesis has a higher incidence of talipes when compared with CVS (RCOG Green-top Guideline No 8, *Amniocentesis and Chorionic Villus Sampling*).

10.4.6 Genetic Disorders

See Table 10.6. Referral for genetic screening and counselling is essential if the woman:

- Has a personal or family history of an inherited genetic disorder.
- Has had a previous pregnancy affected by an inherited genetic disorder.
- Is an Ashkenazi Jew (for Tay–Sachs disease).

10.4.7 Consanguineous Marriage

The indications for screening for a specific genetic disorder are determined by enquiring which region of the world the couple originates from, and their personal and family history. Inter-cousin marriage increases the risk of a couple having a child with a genetic disorder, but it does not alter the indications for screening.

Prenatal diagnosis testing is offered to women who may consider termination of an affected pregnancy when they are known to be a carrier of a recessively inherited genetic disorder and:

o the father of the baby is known to be a carrier for the same disorder

o the carrier status of the father is unknown and cannot be established

- **Cystic Fibrosis (CF):**

All women with CF are homozygous, and all offspring will be carriers of the CF gene. Determination of the carrier status of the partner is important, as the risk of a child being born with CF is 50% if father is heterozygous for the gene.

10.5 Advise women in planning pregnancy who had an adverse outcome in the past

Pre-pregnancy counselling for the following conditions have been discussed at length in individual chapters. Women with a previous pregnancy outcome should be advised to attend consultant delivered clinic for focused antenatal care meeting their individual needs.

1- Previous stillbirth

2- Previous traumatic birth injury

3- Previous caesarean section and wish to discuss mode of delivery

4- Previous 3rd–4th degree perineal tears

5- Previous major abruptio placentae and intrauterine death (IUD)

10.6 Points to Remember

- Folic acid 5 mg is advised until the 12th week of pregnancy in women at high risk of conceiving child with NTDs. Women with haemoglobinopathies should continue high-dose folic acid throughout the pregnancy.
- Women with pulmonary hypertension, an aortic aneurysm, severe aortic stenosis, symptomatic ventricular dysfunction or dilated aortic root >4.5 cm should be advised against becoming pregnant.
- Women planning pregnancy should ideally aim to achieve a pre-conception glycosylated haemoglobin (HbA1c) value of less than 42 mmol/mol (<6.1%), and should be advised to avoid pregnancy if the HbA1c is above 86 mmol/mol (10%).
- Newborn babies of hepatitis B positive mothers should receive their first dose of hepatitis B vaccine and one dose of hepatitis B immune globulin (HBIG) within 12 hours of life followed by vaccinations at 1 and 6 months.
- Plasma creatinine and estimated glomerular filtration rate are two important factors in chronic kidney disease that determine maternal and fetal outcome.
- Immunosuppressive drugs – prednisolone, azathioprine, cyclosporin and tacrolimus – used for organ transplant patients are safe and can be continued in pregnancy. Mycophenolate mofetil and sirolimus (rapamycin) are contraindicated and pregnancy should be delayed for at least 3 months from stopping the medication.
- Women on long-term steroids need parenteral steroids during labour and should be screened for gestational diabetes.

References

1. Bhutta ZA, Dean SV, Imam AM, Lassi ZS. A systematic review of preconception risks and interventions. Karachi, Aga Khan University, 2011. http://globalresearchnurses.tghn.org/site_media/media/articles/Preconception_Report.pdf
2. Dean S, Bhutta Z, Mason EM, et al., eds. Care before and between pregnancy. In *Born Too Soon: Global Action Report on Preterm Birth*. New York: World Health Organization; 2012.
3. Stothard KJ, Tennant PWG, Bell R, Rankin J. Maternal overweight and obesity and the risk of congenital anomalies, a systematic review and meta-analysis. *JAMA.* 2009;**301**(6).
4. Lim CC, Mahmood T. Obesity and pregnancy. *Best Pract Res Clin Obstet Gynaecol.* 2015;**29**(3):309–19.
5. Nelson-Piercy C, ed. *Handbook of Obstetric Medicine*, 4th ed. London: Informa Healthcare; 2010.
6. NICE. *Guidance on Pre-Conception – Advice and Management*, NICE Quality Statement 7, revised in August 2017.
7. RCOG. *Amniocentesis and Chorionic Villus Sampling*, Green-top Guideline No 8. London: Royal College of Obstetricians and Gynaecologists, 2010.

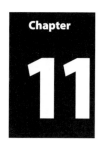

Chapter 11

Ultrasound Scanning in the First Trimester of Pregnancy

Juriy W. Wladimiroff

11.1 Introduction

The objective of this chapter is to provide information on embryonic and early fetal development in the first trimester of pregnancy.

The first trimester refers to the period of pregnancy which starts with establishing embryonic viability (cardiac activity) and ends at 13+6 weeks.

The term *embryo* is used up to 10 weeks of gestation, followed by the term *fetus*, as organogenesis is near completion by that time.

With further improvement of ultrasound equipment and increasing scanning expertise, first trimester ultrasound has become standard in early pregnancy care. Next to fetal presence, location, viability, number, age and risk of chromosomal abnormality based on fetal nuchal translucency (NT) thickness measurement, assessment of fetal anatomy has become an important part of the first trimester examination. This is further highlighted by the introduction of non-invasive prenatal testing (NIPT) by cell-free fetal DNA determination in maternal blood.

11.2 Basic Recommendations for Training

In order to provide high-quality ultrasound scans, proper training is essential.

The International Society of Ultrasound in Obstetrics & Gynaecology (ISUOG) Education Committee has laid down basic quality recommendations for training in obstetric ultrasound in the first trimester of pregnancy [1].

The trainee should be taught about the following:

- Basic physical principles of diagnostic ultrasound including biological, thermal and non-thermal effects of pulsed and continuous ultrasound;
- First trimester ultrasound features of normal early pregnancy: description of the intrauterine gestational sac, yolk sac and embryo;
- Early pregnancy biometry e.g. crown–rump length (CRL) and mean gestational sac diameter (MSD);
- Chorionicity and amnionicity in multiple pregnancies;
- How to recognize fetal viability and criteria used to diagnose definitive non-viability (miscarriage);
- Diagnosis of tubal and non-tubal ectopic pregnancy and the principle of a pregnancy of unknown location;
- How to interpret serum human chorionic gonatotropin (hCG) levels and progesterone in the event of a pregnancy of unknown location;

- Ultrasound features of molar pregnancy;
- Gross fetal malformations that can be recognized during the first trimester;
- Association between thickened nuchal translucency and fetal chromosomal anomalies (at the end of the first trimester).

During practical training, the following aspects of obstetric ultrasound should be learnt:

- Recognize the features of an intrauterine pregnancy (gestational sac, yolk sac and embryo);
- Recognize fetal viability and non-viability;
- Adequately measure mean MSD, embryonic/fetal CRL and fetal biparietal diameter (BPD) / fetal head circumference (HC) (if applicable);
- Establish the presence of multiple gestation and, if so, determine chorionicity;
- Understand how to calculate or correct gestational age estimation from crown–rump length measurements;
- Recognize the features of an extra-uterine (ectopic) pregnancy;
- Understand the concept of a pregnancy of unknown location and how to interpret serum biochemistry to assign risks.

11.3 Ultrasound Equipment Requirements

To conduct an optimal first trimester scan, ultrasound equipment should display the following facilities:

- Real-time, grey-scale two-dimensional (2D) imaging;
- Trans-abdominal (3–10 MHz curvilinear) and transvaginal (3–12 MHz) transducers;
- Freeze-frame and zoom options;
- Electronic callipers;
- Printing and storage of images;
- Acoustic power output controls.

High-frequency transvaginal ultrasound is the preferred method for studying embryonic/fetal development during the first trimester of pregnancy, particularly in the presence of maternal obesity (body mass index (BMI) >30 kg/m^2). However, there may be situations where transabdominal ultrasound will present a better image.

11.4 Safety of Diagnostic Ultrasound

The issue of safety of diagnostic ultrasound is particularly relevant in the first trimester of pregnancy. Acoustic outputs (thermal index (TI) and mechanical index (MI)) of current diagnostic ultrasound equipment is low and, therefore, considered safe during embryonic and early fetal development. Higher acoustic output is provided by Doppler equipment when there is a clinical indication. The most recent ISUOG safety statement on the use of Doppler ultrasound in first trimester pregnancy [2] states the following:

> Pulsed Doppler (spectral, power and color flow imaging) ultrasound should not be used routinely, but may be used for clinical indications such as to identify fetal cardiac abnormalities or to refine risks for trisomies.

When performing Doppler ultrasound, the displayed TI should be ≤1.0 and exposure time should be kept as short as possible (usually no longer than 5–10 min) and should not exceed 60 min.

When using Doppler ultrasound for research, teaching and training purposes, the displayed TI should be ≤1.0 and exposure time should be kept as short as possible (usually no longer than 5–10 min) and should not exceed 60 min. Informed consent should be obtained.

In educational settings, discussion of first trimester pulsed or colour Doppler should be accompanied by information on safety and bio-effects (e.g. TI, exposure times and how to reduce output power).

When scanning maternal uterine arteries in the first trimester, there are unlikely to be any fetal safety implications as long as the embryo/fetus lies outside the Doppler ultrasound.

Before conducting an ultrasound examination, some general questions need to be answered:

– When was the last menstrual period?
– Has a pregnancy test been performed?
– Are there any current symptoms?
– Have serum human chorionic gonatotropin levels been measured?
– Is there a previous pregnancy history?

11.5 Usefulness of First Trimester Ultrasound

A first trimester ultrasound scan may provide information on:

– The presence, location and duration of a pregnancy;
– Viability of the embryo/early fetus;
– Embryonic/ fetal size and growth;
– Monochorionic or dichorionic twin pregnancy;
– Normal or abnormal early fetal anatomy/chromosome pattern.

To gather the above information, the following sonographic features and their development have to be identified and measurements performed.

11.5.1 Sono-Anatomic Development

The presence of an intrauterine gestational sac is the earliest sonographic evidence of an intrauterine pregnancy. A thickened

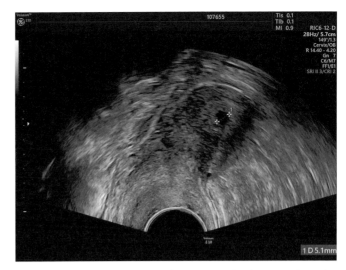

Figure 11.1 Intrauterine gestational sac at 4+ weeks of gestation (2+mm).

endometrium in itself is not an earlier pregnancy sign, as it is also found in the late luteal phase of the menstrual cycle.

Using transvaginal ultrasound, a gestational sac presents itself as a circular transonic area corresponding to the inner amniotic and outer chorionic cavity surrounded by a thick bright ring representing invading chorionic villi and underlying decidual reaction as early as 4+ weeks of gestation when its greater diameter is 2 mm. It increases 1.0–1.2 mm per day (Figure 11.1).

The fetal pole (embryo), yolk sac and cardiac activity become visible from 5 weeks of gestation. Embryo and yolk sac are situated close to the wall of the gestational sac. The yolk sac presents itself as a small circular structure within the chorionic cavity (Figure 11.2) and is situated outside the amniotic cavity after seven weeks of gestation. The wall of the yolk sac becomes thinner during week 9–11 and degenerates by 12–13 weeks of gestation.

The embryo is approximately 1–2 mm long when first detected by ultrasound. In the beginning it increases in length by about 1 mm per day. Applying transabdominal ultrasound, embryo and yolk sac will appear 1 week later.

Embryonic heart rate is about 80–100 beats per minute (bpm) at the end of the fifth week of gestation and increases to 140–160 bpm at seven weeks and 170–175 bpm at nine weeks followed by a drop to 140–150 bpm at 12–13 weeks of gestation.

Anatomical differentiation becomes visible at seven weeks together with the appearance of embryonic movements. At this early stage, these movements are difficult to classify. All types of movements emerging after eight weeks of gestation are specific and closely resemble those observed in preterm and full-term newborn infants [3].

The amniotic membrane and cavity become more distinct. More detailed aspects of embryonic development appear in the following weeks (Figure 11.3).

At 8 weeks, the choroid plexus becomes visible as echogenic areas in the lateral ventricles in the roof of the fourth ventricle.

At 9–10 weeks a physiological midgut herniation may be seen which should have disappeared by 11–12 weeks (Figure 11.4).

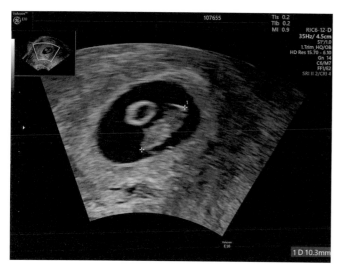

Figure 11.2 Gestational sac with embryo and yolk sac at 7 weeks of gestation. Crown–rump length (CRL) 10 mm.

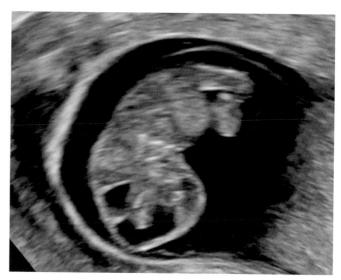

Figure 11.3 Embryo displaying development of cerebral ventricles (CRL = 20 mm) at 8+ weeks of gestation.

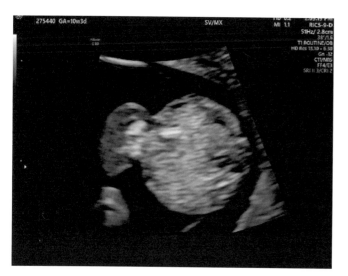

Figure 11.4 Physiological midgut herniation at 10 weeks of gestation.

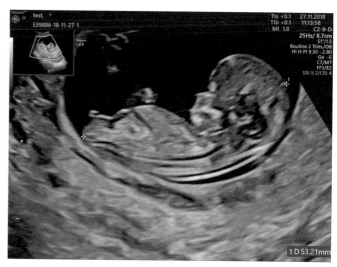

Figure 11.5 Calliper placement for fetal crown–rump length measurement (53 mm) at 12 weeks of gestation

11.5.2 Measuring the Embryo/Early Fetus

11.5.2.1 Measuring the Gestational Sac

Measurement of maximum longitudinal (L), transverse (T) and anteroposterior (AP) diameter (mm) of the fluid-filled space of the gestational sac allows calculation of mean sac diameter (MSD): L + T + AP/3. The MSD measures about 10 mm at 5 weeks. Its clinical importance of estimating gestational age is limited to 4–5 weeks of gestation.

11.5.2.2 The Crown–Rump Length

Gestational age can be determined with considerable accuracy by measurement of the crown–rump length (CRL) as soon as the embryonic pole becomes visible. The measurement can be performed by transvaginal and transabdominal ultrasound. The biological variability in size is small and growth is fast.

The CRL predicts gestational age with an error of 3 days from 7 to 10 weeks and of 5 days from 10 to 13 weeks of gestation. The optimal time for measuring the CRL is between 8 and 12 weeks. The CRL diagram published by Robinson in 1975 is still widely used for the evaluation and dating of early pregnancy [4]. Measurement of the CRL becomes inaccurate after 12–13 weeks or beyond 84 mm due to flexing of the fetal head and body.

To establish a reliable estimation of gestational age from a CRL measurement, the following sonographic imaging conditions should be met [5] (Figure 11.5):

A midline sagittal section of the whole embryo or fetus should be obtained, ideally with the embryo or fetus oriented horizontally on the screen. An image should be magnified sufficiently to fill most of the width of the ultrasound screen, so that the measurement line between crown and rump is at about 90° to the ultrasound beam. Electronic linear callipers should be used to measure the fetus in a neutral position (i.e. neither flexed nor hyperextended). The end points of crown and rump should be defined clearly. Care must be taken to avoid inclusion of structures such as the yolk sac. In order to ensure that the fetus is not flexed, amniotic fluid should be visible between the fetal chin and chest. However, this may be difficult to achieve at earlier gestations (around 6–9 weeks) when the embryo or fetus is typically hyperflexed. In this situation, the actual measurement represents the neck–rump length, but it is still termed the CRL. In very early gestations it is not usually possible to distinguish between the cephalic and caudal ends and a greatest length measurement is taken instead (see Figure 11.2).

Based on data from transvaginal ultrasound measurements, the following normal gestational age-related CRL ranges may serve as a guidance:

5.0 – 5+6 weeks: 0 – 3 mm;

(fetal heart rate should be visible at a CRL >2 mm).

6.0 – 6+6 weeks: 4 – 8 mm;

7.0 – 7+6 weeks: 9 – 14 mm;

8.0 – 8+6 weeks: 15 – 22 mm;

9.0 – 9+6 weeks: 23 – 31 mm;

10.0 – 10+6 weeks: 32 – 42 mm;

11.0 – 11+6 weeks: 43 – 54 mm;

12.0 – 12+6 weeks: 55 – 66 mm;

13.0 – 13+6 weeks: 67 – 79 mm.

In a systematic review of fetal crown–rump lengths charts [6], considerable heterogeneity and limitations have been reported for CRL equations for estimating gestational age. Papageorghiou et al [7] in the context of the Intergrowth-21st Project, carried out CRL measurements using strict protocols and quality-control measures in healthy well-nourished women with singleton pregnancies at low risk of fetal growth impairment in urban areas in eight geographically diverse countries.

11.5.2.3 The Fetal Biparietal Diameter/Head Circumference, Upper-Abdominal Circumference and Femur Length

The fetal biparietal diameter (BPD) and fetal head circumference (HC) (Figure 11.6) may be measured as from 10 weeks of gestation, but only becomes accurate to determine gestational age when the CRL is above 80 mm. The BPD and HC are measured in a horizontal plane at right angles to the fetal body axis. Callipers are placed at the outer border of the parietal bones at the level of the thalamus for measurement of the BPD and at the frontal and occipital bone using the ellipse facility for measurement of the HC. Some measure the BPD from the proximal outer border to the distal inner border. The cavum septi pellucidi, used as a landmark for BPD and HC measurements later in pregnancy, is not always visible at the end of the first trimester. HC probably is more accurate for determining gestational age than BPD.

The fetal upper abdominal circumference (AC) is measured at right angles to the fetal body axis below the heart at the level of the fetal stomach (Figure 11.7). Measurement of the fetal femur length is shown in Figure 11.8.

11.5.3 Normal Early Fetal Anatomy (11–14 weeks)

From 11 weeks of gestation, placental size and texture can be established. The developing fetus presents with much more anatomical detail. A large number of fetal anatomical structures can now be reliably assessed [8]. To give a few examples:

Head: cranial bones, midline falx; choroid plexus, ventricles;

Face: eyes; nasal bone; lips; mandible; profile;

Spine: vertebrae with overlying skin;

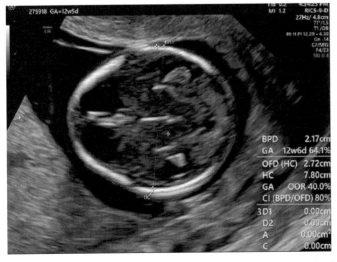

Figure 11.6 Transverse cross section through the fetal brain at 12+ weeks of gestation for measurement of the fetal biparietal diameter (BPD = 21.7 mm) and fetal head circumference (HC = 78 mm).

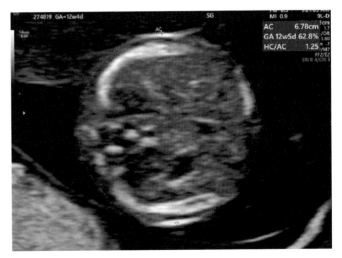

Figure 11.7 Transverse cross section through the fetal upper abdomen at 12+ weeks of gestation for measurement of the fetal upper abdominal circumference (AC = 67.8 mm). Spine at 9 o'clock; stomach visible as an echolucent round structure.

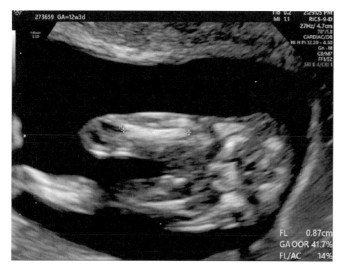

Figure 11.8 Full length of the fetal femur at 12+ weeks of gestation for measurement of femur length (FL = 8.7 mm).

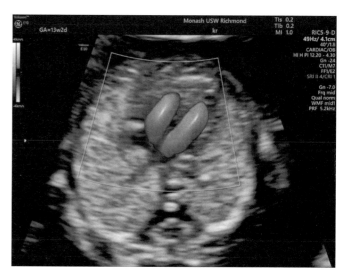

Figure 11.9 Fetal cardiac 4-chamber view at 13 weeks of gestation. Fetal spine posterior. Colour Doppler demonstrating blood flow from the left atrium into the left ventricle and from the right atrium into the right ventricle. Red = blood flow towards the ultrasound transducer. A black and white version of this figure will appear in some formats. For the colour version, please refer to the plate section.

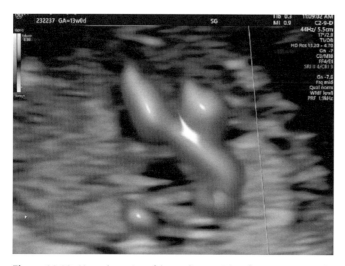

Figure 11.10 Normal crossing of the cardiac arterial outflow representing the ascending aorta and pulmonary artery at 13 weeks of gestation. Blue = blood flow away from the ultrasound transducer. A black and white version of this figure will appear in some formats. For the colour version, please refer to the plate section.

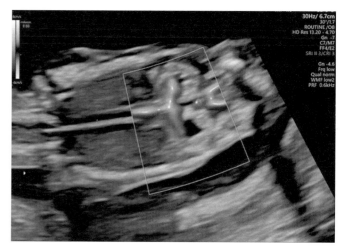

Figure 11.11 Fetal kidneys at 12 weeks of gestation. Note the colour Doppler images of the fetal descending aorta and branching of the renal arteries and common iliac arteries. A black and white version of this figure will appear in some formats. For the colour version, please refer to the plate section.

Chest: lungs; heart: 4-chamber view and arterial outflow tract (Figures 11.9 and 11.10);

Abdomen: stomach; kidneys (Figure 11.11); urinary bladder; abdominal wall;

Extremities: four limbs, hands and feet (Figure 11.12).

11.5.4 Monochorionic and Dichorionic Twin Pregnancy

Twin pregnancy is associated with an increased risk of perinatal mortality and morbidity. Chorionicity should preferably be established between 10 and 14 weeks of gestation. The pregnancy loss rate in monochorionic twins is about 5-fold higher compared to dichorionic twins. Main reasons for the high loss rate in monochorionic twins are the consequences of twin-twin

transfusion syndrome (TTTS) and selective growth restriction. Accurate determination of chorionicity is, therefore, essential to identify twin pregnancies at risk. The most accurate markers of chorionicity are the combination of placenta number with the use of the membrane T-sign indicating monochorionicity or the lambda sign (or when two separate placentas are present) indicating dichorionicity [9] (Figure 11.13). In dichorionic diamniotic twins, the fetuses are separated by a thick layer of fused chorionic membranes with two thin amniotic layers on each side, giving the appearance of a 'full lambda', compared with only two thin amniotic layers separating the two fetuses in monochorionic twins (T-sign) [10]. As pregnancy progresses into the second trimester, regression of the human chorion frondosum leads to gradual loss of the lambda sign. It is,

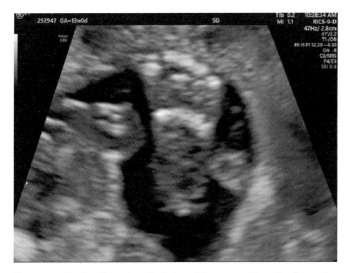

Figure 11.12 Fetal footprints displaying all five toes at 13 weeks of gestation. A black and white version of this figure will appear in some formats. For the colour version, please refer to the plate section.

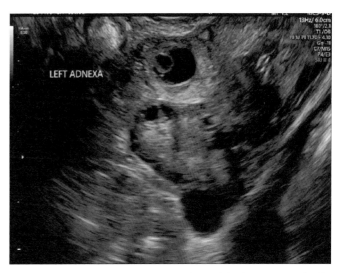

Figure 11.14 Ectopic pregnancy situated in the left adnexa at 7 weeks of gestation.

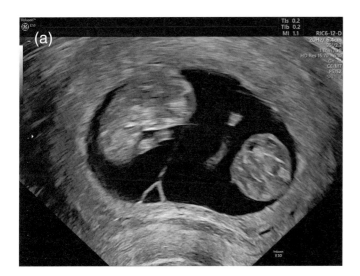

Figure 11.13 Monochorionicity (a) and dichorionicity (b) in a twin pregnancy at 11 weeks of gestation. Note the absence of placental tissue between the membranes in (a). Note the presence of lambda sign and placental tissue between the membranes in (b).

therefore, that the assignment of chorionicity is restricted to the first trimester. Dias et al [9] correctly assigned chorionicity by ultrasound in 99.8% at 11–14 weeks of gestation. They established a sensitivity of 100% and a specificity of 99.8% for determining monochorionicity. In rare cases, a mono-amniotic monochorionic twin pregnancy will be seen.

11.5.5 Complications of Early Pregnancy

The following complications can be recognized:

- Abnormal pregnancy location;
- Miscarriage;
- Gestational trophoblastic disease;
- Uterine abnormalities and adnexa masses;
- Abnormal embryonic/early fetal anatomy;
- First trimester screening for pre-eclampsia.

11.5.5.1 Abnormal Pregnancy Location

Ectopic Pregnancy

The prevalence of ectopic pregnancy is nearly 2%. Early diagnosis is essential as the condition is associated with maternal morbidity and mortality. Risk factors include previous tubal surgery, a previous ectopic pregnancy and intrauterine death (IUD). The diagnosis of an ectopic pregnancy is based on a positive visualization of an extra-uterine pregnancy by ultrasound (Figure 11.14). In case of an empty uterine cavity, beta hCG serum levels should be determined. If above the discriminatory level of 1500 IU/L, the presence of an ectopic pregnancy should be suspected. In about 10%, a living ectopic pregnancy will be found. Very occasionally, the combined presence of an intrauterine and extra-uterine pregnancy may exist. Ultrasound (transvaginal scan = TVS) is an accurate diagnostic test for ectopic pregnancy. Kirk et al [11] reported an overall sensitivity of TVS to detect ectopic pregnancy of 98.3%.

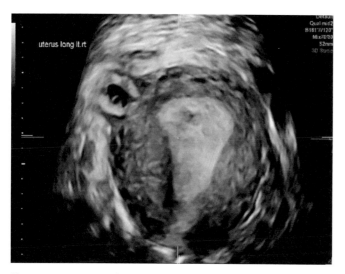

Figure 11.15 Interstitial pregnancy at 8 weeks of gestation.

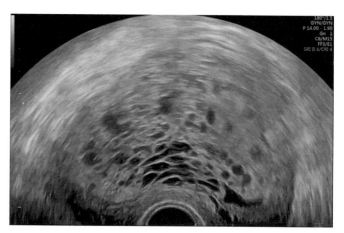

Figure 11.16 Complete hydatidiform mole. Note the so-called snowstorm appearance.

Interstitial and Cervical Pregnancy

In interstitial pregnancy, the gestational sac is located outside the endometrial cavity and surrounded by a thin myometrial layer within the interstitial region (Figure 11.15). A timely diagnosis is essential in order to avoid acute life-threatening bleeding. In cervical pregnancy, the uterus is empty. The gestational sac is implanted below the level of the uterine arteries. The cervix is barrel shaped. Also here, a timely diagnosis is essential for the aforementioned reason.

11.5.5.2 Miscarriage

Miscarriage is the loss of a pregnancy during the first 23 weeks. There is considerable variation in guidelines regarding the diagnosis of miscarriage [12–14]. In the current chapter, the focus is on the first 13 weeks.

The 2006 Royal College of Obstetricians and Gynaecologists (RCOG) guidelines use an empty sac with a mean gestational sac diameter (MSD) of 20 mm or more or lack of cardiac activity with an embryo of 6 mm or more as a miscarriage. The American College of Radiologists 2009 guidelines use an empty sac with a CRL >5 mm without cardiac activity as a miscarriage. The Society of Gynaecologists of Canada considers an early embryonic demise as certain when MSD >16 mm without an embryo on a transvaginal scan. All above recommendations come from small studies. Abdallah et al [12] demonstrated that using an empty sac with MSD >20 mm, there would be one viable pregnancy in every 200 cases classified as a miscarriage. In view of the inter-observer variability in MSD and CRL measurements, it was proposed the cut-off level for classification as a non-viable pregnancy should be: an empty sac with an MSD of 25 mm or more or a CRL of 7 mm or more with no heart activity [12].

Most guidelines state a repeat scan in 7–10 days is required when pregnancy is of uncertain viability. It is commonly accepted that a lack of MSD or CRL growth is a feature of miscarriage. Again, one has to be aware of the fact that there is a significant variation in the accuracy of CRL and MSD measurement. Failure to visualize a yolk sac or embryo on a repeat scan is considered a feature of miscarriage [14].

11.5.5.3 Gestational Trophoblast Disease

Gestational trophoblast disease displays a spectrum from benign hydatidiform mole (molar pregnancy) to choriocarcinoma.

A distinction should be made between complete and partial hydatidiform moles.

Complete Hydatidiform Mole

The incidence of complete hydatidiform mole is 1:700 [15]. A complete hydatidiform mole is characterized by vaginal bleeding in the presence of an enlarged uterus and raised serum beta hCG levels, usually >2.5 multiples of the median (MoM) and will increase as pregnancy advances. The latter will lead to ovarian hyperstimulation and, in some cases, to the development of theca lutein cysts. The detection rate of complete hydatidiform mole is about 95% [16]. Ultrasound examination reveals the so-called snowstorm appearance: a uterine cavity with multiple echodense and echolucent structures of variable size in the absence of an embryo/fetus (Figure 11.16).

Partial Hydatidiform Mole

Partial hydatidiform mole is characterized by the presence of an embryo/fetus and molar degeneration of the placenta. The latter is enlarged with multiple cystic structures on ultrasound examination. In the case of triploid partial moles (69,XXX or 69,XXY), there is a clear association with major fetal anomalies or severe intrauterine growth restriction. The incidence is 1:1500–2000 [15]. The overall detection rate is about 20% [16]. The detection rate of incomplete hydatidiform mole varies between 20 and 49%.

Choriocarcinoma

Choriocarcinoma may develop after a molar pregnancy, a miscarriage or an apparently normal pregnancy. On ultrasound examination it may be difficult to differentiate between choriocarcinoma and hydatidiform mole.

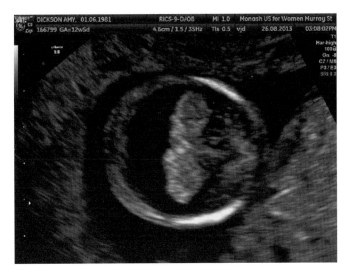

Figure 11.17 Alobar holoprosencephaly at 12+ weeks of gestation.

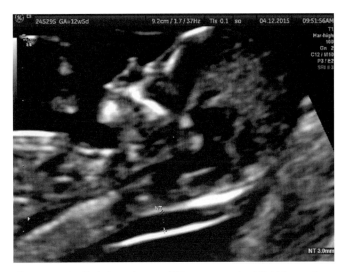

Figure 11.18 Nuchal translucency (NT) scan measuring NT thickness of 3.0 mm at 12+ weeks of gestation. A large fetal profile in neutral position and clear of amnion. Callipers 'on to on'.

Adnexal Masses

The incidence of adnexal pathology in the first trimester is 0.2–6%.

11.5.5.4 Abnormal Fetal Anatomy

A much more detailed sonographic description of normal fetal anatomy at 11–14 weeks of gestation has led to the identification of an increasing number of fetal structural abnormalities being diagnosed during this early period in pregnancy (Figure 11.17) including a range of fetal cardiac defects such as atrioventricular septal defect (AVSD), hypoplastic left heart syndrome (HLHS), tetralogy of Fallot and single ventricle. A comprehensive overview of early detection of fetal structural defects has been presented by Springhall et al [8].

Karim et al [17] conducted a systematic review of publications in the period 1991–2014 reporting on screening for fetal structural anomalies by ultrasound examination in the first trimester. They found 41% of all anomalies and 53% of major anomalies detected in a low-risk group. The use of standardized anatomical protocols increased the detection rate of fetal anomalies.

Screening for chromosomal anomalies is carried out by measurement of fetal nuchal translucency (NT) (Figure 11.18) in combination with maternal age, human chorionic gonadotropin (hCG) and pregnancy-associated plasma protein-A (PAPP-A), in a combined test [17]. Combined screening for Down syndrome should be offered at 11 to 13+6 weeks with a detection rate of 90% at a screen positive rate of 2%. A positive screening test is expressed by increased fetal nuchal translucency (NT=3.5 mm or more), raised PAPP-A and reduced free beta-human chorionic gonadotropins (hCG).

In a recent study [19], it was demonstrated that assessment of a combination of maternal age, fetal nuchal translucency, hCG and PAPP-A resulted in a detection rate of 90%, 97% and 92%, respectively, for trisomies 21, 18 and 13, as well as >95% of cases of monosomy X and triploidies, and >50% of other chromosomal abnormalities at a false positive rate of 4%.

Next to increased fetal nuchal translucency thickness (3.5 mm or more), other ultrasound markers such as absence of the nasal bone, reversed A-wave in the ductus venosus and tricuspid regurgitation are observed in about 60, 65 and 55% of fetuses with trisomy 21 as opposed to 2.6, 3.2, and 0.9% of euploid fetuses [18]. An increased fetal nuchal translucency is also associated with a raised risk of miscarriage, intrauterine death and fetal structural anomalies, in particular fetal cardiac abnormalities. In the absence of an abnormal fetal chromosome pattern, a fetal nuchal translucency of 3.5–4.4 mm and NT of >6.5 mm is associated with 20% and 80% adverse outcome, respectively.

As mentioned earlier, another development complementing the search for first trimester aneuploidy is the development of cell-free DNA screening [20]. However, the measurement of fetal nuchal translucency will continue to play a role, as increased nuchal translucency may indicate the presence of chromosomal anomalies which cannot be detected by cell-free DNA screening [17].

11.5.5.5 First Trimester Screening for Pre-Eclampsia

Both transvaginal and transabdominal Doppler examination of the maternal uterine arteries at 11+0 to 13+6 weeks of gestation is a useful tool for predicting early-onset pre-eclampsia (PE) (Figure 11.19). In normal pregnancy, the impedance to blood flow in the maternal uterine arteries decreases as pregnancy progresses, reflecting trophoblast invasion of the spiral arteries. The process is completed at around 18 weeks of gestation. In cases of abnormal placentation, the uterine artery impedance remains high.

It was recently shown that combined screening by maternal factors, uterine artery pulsatility index (PI), mean arterial pressure and placental growth factor (PlGF) predicted 90% of early PE, 75% of preterm PE, and 41% of term PE at a screen-positive rate of 10% [21].

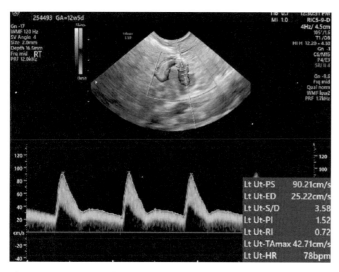

Figure 11.19 Maternal uterine artery waveform recording using colour Doppler ultrasound at 12+ weeks of gestation. A black and white version of this figure will appear in some formats. For the colour version, please refer to the plate section.

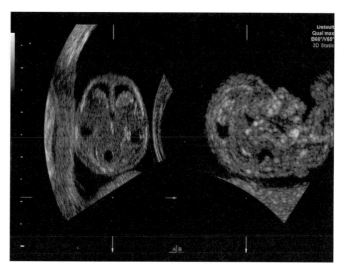

Figure 11.21 3D sonographic image of fetal cerebrum at 11 weeks of gestation. Axial (*left*) and sagittal (*right*) section demonstrating telencephalon, diencephalon and mesencephalon.

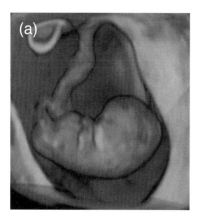

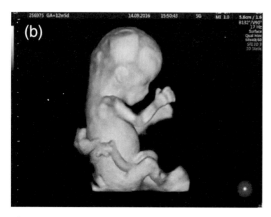

Figure 11.20 3D sonographic image of an embryo/fetus at 9 weeks (a) and at 12+ weeks (b) of gestation.

11.6 Three- and Four-Dimensional Ultrasound in First Trimester Pregnancy

The application of three-dimensional (3D; static) and four-dimensional (4D; movement in time) ultrasound has provided further insight in early pregnancy development. Both modalities are mainly achieved by a mechanical 3D transducer with a rapid acquisition from 1.5 to 40 volumes per second (Figure 11.20).

Trophoblast volume was calculated by subtracting gestational sac volume from total volume of pregnancy using 3D Virtual Organ Computer-aided Analysis (VOCAL™). Trophoblast volumes of pregnancies ending in miscarriage were significantly smaller than were those of pregnancies that resulted in live birth. Trophoblast growth in pregnancies ending in miscarriage was also reduced compared with that in pregnancies resulting in live birth [22]. Another example of 3D ultrasound imaging in the first trimester is the detailed development of embryonic/fetal cerebral ventricles (Figure 11.21).

11.7 Conclusions

In early first trimester pregnancy, an ultrasound scan will establish the presence, location, viability and duration of a pregnancy; embryonic size and growth; and whether it is a single or multiple pregnancy.

At 10–13 weeks of gestation, an ultrasound scan will provide reliable information on the day of delivery ('dating' scan); establish chorionicity in the presence of a multiple pregnancy; identify the majority of major fetal structural abnormalities; and improve Down syndrome screening.

Acknowledgements

I am greatly indebted to:

– Dr Torbjorn Eggebo and Dr Aurora Roset, National Center for Fetal Medicine, Trondheim University Hospital, Trondheim, Norway for providing figures 1–3; 5, 13 a and b, 16 and 20 a;

- Dr Simon Meagher, Dr Maria Maxfield, and Dr Sujatha Ganesan: Monash Ultrasound for women, Monash IVF, Monash University, Melbourne Victoria, Australia for providing figures 4, 6–12, 14,15, 17–19, 20 b;

- Dr SC Husen, Dr M Rousian, Prof RPM Steegers-Theunissen, Department of Obstetrics & Gynaecology, Erasmus University Medical Centre, Rotterdam, The Netherlands for providing Figure 11.21.

References

1. ISUOG Educational Committee recommendations for basic training in obstetric and gynaecological ultrasound. *Ultrasound Obstet Gynecol.* 2014;**43**:113–16.

2. Salvesen K, Lees C, Abramovicz J, et al. ISUOG statement on the safe use of Doppler in the 11 to 13+6 week fetal ultrasound examination. *Ultrasound Obstet Gynecol.* 2011;**37**:625–8.

3. De Vries JIP, Visser GHA, Prechtl HFR. The emergence of fetal behaviour, I. Qualitative aspects. *Early Hum Dev.* 1982;7:301–22.

4. Robinson HP, Fleming JEE. A critical evaluation of sonar 'crown-rump length' measurements. *Br J Obstet Gynaecol.* 1975;**82**:702–10.

5. Salomon LJ, Alfirevic Z, Bilardo CM, et al. ISUOG Practice Guidelines: performance of first-trimester fetal ultrasound scan. *Ultrasound Obstet Gynecol.* 2013;**41**:102–13.

6. Napolitano R, Dhami J, Ohuma EO, et al. Pregnancy dating by fetal crown-rump length: systematic review of charts. *Br J Obstet Gynaecol.* 2014;**121**:556–65.

7. Papageorghiou AT, Kennedy SH, Salomon IJ, et al. International standards for early fetal size and pregnancy dating based on ultrasound measurement of crown-rump length in the first trimester of pregnancy. *Ultrasound Obstet Gynecol.* 2014;**44**:641–8.

8. Springhall EA, Rolnik DL, Reddy M, et al. How to perform a sonographic morphological assessment of the fetus at 11–14 weeks of gestation. *Australian J Ultrasound Med.* 2018;**21**:125–37.

9. Dias T, Arcangeli T, Bhide A, et al. First-trimester ultrasound determination of chorionicity in twin pregnancy. *Ultrasound Obstet Gynecol.* 2011;**38**:330–2.

10. Khalil A, Rodgers M, Baschat A, et al. ISUOG Practice Guidelines: role of ultrasound in twin pregnancies. *Ultrasound Obstet Gynecol.* 2016;**47**:247–63.

11. Kirk E, Papageorghiou AT, Condous G, et al. The diagnostic effectiveness of an initial transvaginal scan in detecting ectopic pregnancy. *Hum Reprod.* 2007;**22**:2824–8.

12. Abdallah Y, Daemen A, Kirk E, et al. Limitations of current definitions of miscarriage using mean gestational sac diameter and crown-rump length measurements: a multicentre observational study. *Ultrasound Obstet Gynecol.* 2011;**38**:497–502.

13. Al-Memar M, Kirk E, Bourne T. The role of ultrasonography in the diagnosis and management of early pregnancy complications. *Obstet Gynaecol.* 2015:**17**:173–81.

14. Thilaganathan B. The evidence base for miscarriage diagnosis: better late than never. *Ultrasound Obstet Gynecol.* 2011;**38**:487–8.

15. Benson CB, Genest DR, Bernstein MR, et al. Sonographic appearance of first trimester hydatidiform moles. *Ultrasound Obstet Gynecol.* 2000,**16**:188–91.

16. Kirk E, Papageorghiou AT, Condous G, Bottomley C, Bourne T. The accuracy of first trimester ultrasound in the diagnosis of hydatidiform mole. *Ultrasound Obstet Gynecol.* 2007;**29**:70–5.

17. Karim JN, Roberts NW, Salomon LJ, Papageorghiou AT. Systematic review of first-trimester ultrasound screening for detection of fetal structural anomalies and factors that affect screening performance. *Ultrasound Obstet Gynecol.* 2017;**50**:429–41.

18. Kagan KO, Staboulidou I, Cruz J, Wright D, Nicolaides KH. Two-stage first-trimester screening for trisomy 21 by ultrasound assessment and biochemical testing. *Ultrasound Obstet Gynecol* .2010;**36**;542–7.

19. Santorum M, Wright D, Syngelaki A, Karagioti S, Nicolaides KH. Accuracy of first-trimester combined test in screening for trisomies 21, 18, and 13. *Ultrasound Obstet Gynecol.* 2017;**49**:714–20.

20. Salomon IJ, Alfirevic Z, Audibert F, et al. ISUOG consensus statement on the impact of non-invasive prenatal testing (NIPT) on prenatal practice. *Ultrasound Obstet Gynecol.* 2014;**44**:122–3.

21. Tan MY, Syngelaki A, Poon LC, et al. Screening for pre-eclampsia by maternal factors and biomarkers at 11–13 weeks' gestation. *Ultrasound Obstet Gynecol.* 2018;**52**:186–95.

22. Reus AD, El-Harbachi H, Rousian M, et al. Early first-trimester trophoblast volume in pregnancies that result in live birth or miscarriage. *Ultrasound Obstet Gynecol.* 2013;**42**:577–84.

Chapter 12

Prenatal Diagnostic Techniques

Guttorm Haugen & Vasilis Sitras

12.1 Introduction

Prenatal diagnosis provides the pregnant woman and her partner with information on possible fetal chromosomal aberrations and heritable genetic diseases. Genetic counselling should be provided to the couple with information on the technical procedure, predictive values, risk estimates, expected and unexpected results and management options. Prenatal diagnosis is typically performed early in pregnancy to give the couple the possibility to consider termination of pregnancy. The policy on prenatal diagnosis varies throughout Europe depending on tradition and national legislation, resulting in inconsistent use of the different screening and invasive methods.

The most common congenital cause of mental disability in humans is Down syndrome (DS), caused by having three rather than two copies of chromosome 21 (trisomy 21). Therefore, the present screening tests focus on the detection of trisomy 21, but may also detect other aneuploidies such as trisomies 13 and 18. The fetal nuchal translucency scan provides information on structural anomalies, and cell-free fetal DNA (cfDNA) in maternal blood may be used to determine fetal sex and rhesus genotype.

Amniocentesis and chorionic villus sampling (CVS) are invasive tests developed to obtain fetal cells or placental tissue used for diagnostic cytogenetic analyses. The use of both these tests has decreased during the last decades due to the introduction of first trimester scan and cfDNA to screen for fetal chromosomal diseases. However, in the era of these sensitive screening techniques, the invasive tests are still necessary to confirm or exclude the diagnosis of fetal chromosomal aberrations and to diagnose monogenetic diseases.

12.2 Non-Invasive Prenatal Testing (NIPT)

On the one hand, screening programmes aim to identify healthy individuals within a selected population that are at risk of developing a disease. On the other hand, diagnostic tests aim to assess individuals with symptoms of a disease or to follow its progress. In fact, screening tests look for risk markers of disease, not the disease itself, meaning that some individuals with risk markers will never develop the disease (false positive test). Furthermore, not all individuals who will develop the disease have risk markers (false negative test). Importantly, the accuracy of a screening test depends on the prevalence of the disease in the population.

Therefore, knowledge of the principles and performance characteristics of screening tests is mandatory in order to understand the prenatal screening techniques for fetal chromosomal aneuploidy. The definitions of screening test performance along with a simple numerical example are shown in Table 12.1.

12.2.1 Ultrasound and Biochemical Screening Markers for Chromosomal Abnormalities during the First and Second Trimesters of Pregnancy

The chance of giving birth to a baby with Down syndrome (DS) increases with maternal age. This is probably due to increased occurrence of non-disjunction of the ovum during meiosis in older women. Indeed, the chance of having a baby with DS increases 10-fold from 30 to 40 years of age (from 1/1000 to 1/100). Therefore, maternal age was the first marker of DS and screening has been traditionally offered to women above 35 years. In 1992, a strong association of DS with increased nuchal translucency (NT) was found and a novel screening marker was established [1]. NT is a fluid-filled space in the fetal neck measured with ultrasound between 11 to 13+6 weeks' gestation (embryonic crown–rump length 38–84 mm). The combination of NT and maternal age will detect approximately 75% of fetuses with DS, with a 5% false positive rate (FPR); meaning that 5% of women without an affected fetus will receive a high-risk test result. Moreover, several reports showed that increased NT above the 99th centile or 3.5 mm is associated with other fetal chromosomal abnormalities (trisomy 13, trisomy 18, Turner syndrome, triploidy), stillbirth and structural abnormalities, mainly congenital heart defects [2]. Therefore, fetuses without chromosomal/genetic abnormalities and NT ≥3.5 mm should be offered detailed echocardiography later in pregnancy.

In order to increase screening performance, several other ultrasound and biochemical markers were introduced to first trimester screening for fetal aneuploidy. Ultrasound markers include absent or hypoplastic nasal bone, tricuspid valve regurgitation (present during at least half of the systole and with a velocity above 60 cm/s) and reversed wave during atrial contraction (a-wave) in the ductus venosus. First trimester biochemical markers are human chorionic gonatotropin (hCG), which is elevated, and pregnancy-associated plasma protein-A (PAPP-A), which is lower in pregnancies affected with DS. Importantly, some maternal characteristics (ethnicity, body weight and diabetes mellitus) and use of assisted reproduction techniques influence the concentration of biochemical markers and should therefore always be

Table 12.1 Definitions of screening test performance

	Affected individuals (1000) Prevalence (1000/100 000 = 1%)	Unaffected individuals (99 000)	Total individuals tested Population (100 000)
Test POSITIVE	True positive (990)	False positive (1000) False positive rate (1000/99 000 = 1%)	Positive Predictive Value (proportion of truly positive results) (990/1990 = 49.75%)*
Test NEGATIVE	False negative (10) False negative rate (10/1000 = 1%)	True negative (98 000)	Negative Predictive Value (proportion of truly negative results) (98 000/98 010 = 98.99%)**
	Sensitivity or Detection rate (990/1000 = 99%)	Specificity (correctly negative) (98 000/99 000 = 98.99%)	

*Positive predictive value (PPV) means that if a healthy person is tested positive or high-risk, there is 49.75% chance that he/she will develop the disease, i.e. only 1 out of 2 persons who are screened at high-risk will develop the disease.
**Negative predictive value (NPV) means that if a healthy person is tested negative or low-risk, there is 98.99% chance that he/she will never develop the disease, i.e. almost all individuals with low-risk tests will remain healthy.
(Recommended bibliography: Making sense of screening; a guide to weighing up the benefits and harms of health screening programmes; Sense about Science; https://senseaboutscience.org/wp-content/uploads/2016/11/Makingsenseofscreening.pdf)

integrated in the screening algorithm. In general, the combination of maternal age with hCG and PAPP-A will detect 7 out of 10 pregnancies affected by DS, with a 5% FPR [3]. Currently, the combination of first trimester ultrasound combined with serum markers (hCG and PAPP-A) and maternal age will detect 9 out of 10 pregnancies with DS for a fixed 5% FPR, and represents the best first trimester screening method involving ultrasound [4]. Since prevalence of DS increases with maternal age, for high-risk populations the combined first trimester test has a detection rate for DS of 85–100%, whereas in unselected populations the detection rate falls.

The accuracy of first trimester combined tests for the detection of trisomy 18 and trisomy 13 is lower, but these fetuses are often growth restricted and have structural malformations, aiding in counselling women to perform further diagnostic tests.

12.2.2 Soft Markers at Second Trimester Ultrasound Scanning for Fetal Aneuploidy

During the *second trimester anomaly scan*, between 18–22 weeks' gestation, some '*soft*' *markers for fetal aneuploidy* can be detected. These are normal anatomical signs but are significant because they increase the risk for fetal aneuploidy.

These increase the likelihood of trisomy 21:
- increased nuchal fold,
- presence of echogenic intracardiac focus,
- echogenic bowel,
- short femur
- and short humerus

This increases the likelihood of trisomy 18:
- the presence of choroid plexus cysts

However, none of these soft markers has been validated as screening tools for trisomies. Moreover, biochemical markers of DS measured between 15 and 21 weeks' gestation, such as hCG, alpha fetoprotein (AFP), unconjugated oestriol (uE3) and inhibin A (IHA) have been used as double, triple or quadruple tests, but have lower screening performance [4].

12.2.3 Cell-Free Fetal DNA (cfDNA)

The first report on the presence of cfDNA from male fetuses in the maternal plasma was published in 1997 [5]. In fact, during the course of normal human pregnancy fetal cells and cfDNA of placental origin are shed into the maternal blood circulation. Based on these sources of placental (syncytiotrophoblast) DNA that corresponds in most cases to fetal DNA, scientists put efforts to establish methods for NIPT. However, the fact that fetal cells are difficult to isolate from the maternal plasma and can persist from previous pregnancies left the quest for NIPT to cfDNA, which is cleared from the maternal circulation shortly after delivery and is easier to identify. Initially, cfDNA testing has been used for fetal rhesus D genotyping and gender determination in case of X-linked diseases. Beginning in 2011, NIPT for fetal aneuploidies by cfDNA has been commercially available and there has been a rapid development of various laboratory techniques, driven primarily by the biotechnology industry. The initial efforts focused on the detection of trisomy 21, but have subsequently developed rapidly to the detection of other trisomies, sex chromosome aneuploidies and, more recently, for selected microdeletion and microduplication syndromes.

Currently there are three main commercially available approaches for cfDNA analysis: mass parallel shotgun sequencing (MPSS), targeted massively parallel sequencing (TMPS) and single nucleotide polymorphism (SNP) [6]. All approaches are based on sequencing and counting specific regions of all or selected chromosomes (genomic loci) or SNPs and compare the relative amount of these regions with expected normal counts. For example, the proportion of genomic loci belonging to chromosome 21 will be relatively higher in cases where the fetus has DS, compared to a reference dataset provided by pregnancies with euploid fetuses. Therefore, several laboratory steps involving sophisticated techniques and bioinformatics analyses are necessary in order to provide results. Thus, several sources of error exist and should be considered before the interpretation of cfDNA test results [7]. The main limitation is the ratio of placental to total (placental and maternal) cell-free DNA in the maternal circulation, called 'fetal fraction'. Shedding of apoptotic placental/fetal DNA starts at around 5–7 weeks at low rates and increases throughout gestation, counting on average for 10% of the total free DNA in the maternal circulation. The higher the fetal fraction the more accurate NIPT is to differentiate aneuploid from euploid fetuses. From 10 weeks' gestation onwards the fetal fraction is in general sufficient to produce an informative test result. Common causes of low fetal fraction are maternal obesity (due to increased maternal blood volume and adipocyte cfDNA release) and early gestational age (due to lower placental volume and shedding). Less often, maternal thromboembolic disorders, heparin use and vitamin B12 deficiency have been associated with low fetal fraction. Moreover, it has been shown that fetal fraction is inherently higher in cases of trisomy 21, while in cases of trisomy 18 and trisomy 13 placental apoptosis is decreased with reduced fetal fraction. Moreover, inconclusive results, due to low fetal fraction or technical problems such as failed sequencing, are shown to be associated with fetal aneuploidy. In fact, approximately 4.1% (range 0.8–12.6%) of cfDNA tests fail to provide results for various reasons [8]. Another important aspect is that the origin of cfDNA is placental and not fetal. In 1–2% of placentas with confined mosaicism, erroneous 'fetal triploidy' can result by NIPT. Moreover, maternal chromosomal abnormality, malignancy and organ transplantation may affect the maternal cfDNA fraction, which is commonly used as reference, leading to false positive NIPT results. Further, a cfDNA positive test result does not specify whether the trisomy is due to translocation, in which case specific genetic counselling along with maternal and paternal karyotypes should be obtained in order to estimate the recurrence risk.

Despite all these limitations, cfDNA has demonstrated robust performance characteristics as a screening test for the detection of fetal aneuploidy. A large validation multicentre study, funded by a private healthcare company, confirmed that cfDNA has excellent detection rate (100%) and specificity (99.9%) for DS, with very low FPR of 0.06%, compared to 5% for first trimester combined (standard) screening. The PPV for the unselected population was 80.9%, compared to 3.4% for standard screening. Importantly, 3% of women were excluded from final analysis due to lack of results on cfDNA testing, because of low or not measured fetal fraction and assay failure [9]. Furthermore, in a meta-analysis of 35 validation studies, screening by cfDNA in maternal blood in singleton pregnancies

could detect 98% of fetuses with trisomy 18 and 99% of trisomy 13, at a combined FPR of 0.13% [10]. Similarly, another meta-analysis has shown that both MPSS and TMPS are sensitive and highly specific methods for the detection of trisomy 21, 18, 13 and sex chromosome aneuploidies in high-risk pregnancies [11].

Given its accuracy, NIPT using cfDNA has been introduced in clinical practice in several countries, aiming to reduce the need for invasive procedures and eventually the miscarriage risk associated with these procedures. However, the ideal clinical implementation of prenatal testing techniques depends on several aspects that are peculiar to each country, society and healthcare system.

The possible clinical application of cfDNA as screening tool for fetal aneuploidy includes three scenarios: 1. Universal screening as first line screening; 2. offered only to selected high-risk pregnancies; and 3. second line test (contingency) after first trimester combined screening stratification. In this scenario, pregnancies at low-risk following first trimester combined screening would need no follow-up, women at high risk would be offered invasive diagnostic test, whereas women with intermediate risk would be offered cfDNA. Using this strategy, the number of invasive diagnostic procedures for high-risk cfDNA results has decreased considerably [12]. Due to possible false positive results, a positive result by cfDNA should generally be confirmed by an invasive diagnostic technique.

Nevertheless, some principles regarding cfDNA testing for screening of fetal aneuploidy should be followed. Ultrasound is recommended before obtaining maternal blood for cfDNA testing in order to estimate gestational age, to confirm the number of viable fetuses and to exclude major fetal structural abnormalities. All these aspects may affect the a priori aneuploidy risk and specific genetic counselling is warranted. For example, in the case of a fetus with NT ≥3.5 mm or major malformations, the woman could opt directly for a diagnostic invasive procedure to perform conventional cytogenetic techniques or high-resolution chromosomal microarray techniques to investigate for pathogenic copy number variations [13]. Moreover, the chance of carrying a fetus with malformations or microdeletion syndromes is not associated with maternal age and, therefore, ultrasound and/or invasive diagnostic testing should be offered rather than cfDNA.

12.2.4 Non-Invasive Prenatal Diagnostics in Multiple Pregnancies

The number of multiple pregnancies has increased during the last decades because of delayed maternal age at childbearing and increased use of assisted reproductive techniques. Multiple gestations are in general at increased risk of miscarriage and structural abnormalities compared to singleton pregnancies. Prenatal diagnosis is more complicated and depends on the number of fetuses, chorionicity (number of placentas) and zygosity (referring to genetic characteristics of the fetuses) that are difficult to determine. In fact, the definite diagnosis of zygosity can only be made by DNA fingerprint, after birth or by invasive prenatal procedures. Ultrasound, on the other hand, can aid in the differentiation of chorionicity/zygosity. For example, dichorionic twins (two separate placentas) of opposite gender will carry an individual risk of aneuploidy because they are dizygotic. Monozygotic twins, with rare exceptions, will carry the same risk of aneuploidy. However, concordance of structural malformations (both twins affected) even in monozygotic twins is uncommon. Interestingly, twins carry a lower risk of DS compared to singleton pregnancies [14].

In general, the accuracy of NIPT techniques is lower for multiple compared to singleton pregnancies, because any method containing serum analytes (hCG and PAPP-A) or cfDNA in the maternal blood will provide a single risk calculation for the entire gestation. The median values of serum analytes in twin pregnancies are about twice those in singleton pregnancies. Screening for fetal aneuploidy by NT measurement alone in dichorionic pregnancies will provide fetus-specific risk calculations, with similar accuracy as for singleton pregnancies. Moreover, chromosomal discordant twins will probably have additional ultrasonographic markers of aneuploidy, ensuring the correct identification of the aneuploid twin. For monochorionic twins, the average of two individual NT measurements is used to calculate the risk for the entire pregnancy. Increased NT in the recipient twin can be an early sign of twin-to-twin transfusion syndrome, resulting in higher false positive rates in aneuploidy screening. Although the absence of nasal bone as biophysical marker of DS in twin pregnancies may increase the detection rate of the test, it has been evaluated only in one study and should be further evaluated. Combined first trimester biochemical and NT screening has lower accuracy (lower detection rates and higher FPR) for twin compared to singleton pregnancies, with the lowest detection rates in dichorionic pregnancies, but is currently the best option for prenatal aneuploidy screening.

For cfDNA techniques the total fetal fraction is generally higher (18%) in twin compared to singleton pregnancies, due to the presence of additional placental tissue. The test failure rate (no result) is reported to be similar to singletons. Moreover, zygosity may affect screening performance as dizygotic twins are genetically discordant and do not contribute equally to the fetal fraction. Screening tests using SNP approaches might allow the determination of zygosity. A screen positive (high-risk) test result does not differentiate the affected twin. In conclusion, although preliminary data indicate that cfDNA methods have promising results and good performance for screening of fetal aneuploidies in twin pregnancies, large prospective data are warranted. Currently, cfDNA is not recommended for screening in twin pregnancies [15].

In high-order multiple gestations, maternal age and NT measurement are the only methods of risk calculation for fetal aneuploidy.

12.3 Invasive Prenatal Testing

12.3.1 Amniocentesis

Amniocentesis has been the main invasive sampling method used in prenatal diagnosis. The procedure has also been performed on other indications such as evaluation of haemolytic anaemia, fetal lung maturity and congenital infections (cytomegalovirus (CMV), toxoplasmosis). Most amniocenteses for prenatal diagnosis are performed at mid-trimester from 15 gestational weeks (15+0 weeks) onwards. Amniocentesis before this gestational age (early amniocentesis) is associated with an increased miscarriage rate. The procedure is performed during continuous ultrasound guidance using a freehand technique or with a biopsy guide mounted on the ultrasound transducer. The aspirated volume is about 15–30 mL dependent on the required analyses [16]. It is recommended to remove the first 2 mL of amniotic fluid before the final sampling to avoid contamination of maternal cells. Needle size 20–22 gauge (G) is recommended. If more than two punctures are needed, a third puncture should be delayed for 24 hours [16].

Transplacental needle passage has been associated with an increased risk of complications, ultimately leading to spontaneous miscarriage [17]. However, others have suggested that transplacental sampling may reduce the risk of amniotic fluid leakage and miscarriage. The complication rate following placental needle passage has been related to needle size. A randomized study showed higher risk of intrauterine bleeding following transplacental needle insertion with a 22 G compared to a 20 G needle. The larger needle was associated with more immediate discomfort [18]. Overall, it is recommended to avoid the placenta when an alternative exists, particularly in Rh-negative women to prevent immunization.

12.3.2 Chorionic Villus Sampling

Chorionic villus sampling was established later than amniocentesis and recognized as a first trimester procedure. CVS was initially developed as a transcervical route using a flexible catheter with an internal obturator or by using biopsy forceps.

The catheter and obturator are bent into a slight curve. The catheter with obturator is inserted through the cervical canal into the chorion frondosum under continuous ultrasound guidance. The catheter is placed parallel to the long axis of the placenta and withdrawn slowly under continuous negative pressure.

The transabdominal technique is performed either as a single- or double-needle technique. Both are performed under direct ultrasound guidance either as a freehand technique or using an ultrasound transducer with biopsy guide depending on operator comfort and preference. The double-needle technique makes use of an outer trocar through which the thinner sampling needle is inserted. The trocar is inserted into the placental margin and the sampling needle inserted into the chorion frondosum. The advantage of this technique is the possibility of performing repeated sampling with the inner needle without a second puncture if the initial sampling was not adequate. The single-needle technique is supposed to be quicker and less uncomfortable.

The transcervical sampling method is supposed to be more technically challenging than the transabdominal method. Some centres advocate the possibility of offering both methods with an individual evaluation of which method to use dependent on placental location. The transcervical approach is preferable for placentas with posterior location and the transabdominal for those with fundal or anterior location. Finally, the method depends on the experience and preference of the operator [16].

Main general aspects of aseptic techniques should be followed both during amniocentesis and CVS.

12.3.3 Miscarriage Rate

Miscarriage is the major complication following invasive procedures. A Danish randomized trial including women between 25 and 34 years showed a miscarriage rate of 1.7% in those having an amniocentesis compared to 0.7% in the control group without amniocentesis [17]. More than 80% of the invasive tests were performed in gestational week 15 to week 17, and median time from amniocentesis to spontaneous abortion was 21.5 days. Later reviews have stressed that the estimated increase in miscarriage rate was imprecise with a wide 95% confidence interval (CI) of 0 to 2% [19].

The absolute miscarriage rate following chorionic villus sampling is supposed to be higher than that following mid-trimester amniocentesis. However, CVS is performed at an earlier gestational age. Due to the higher background risk for spontaneous abortion earlier in pregnancy, the total risk for miscarriage is comparable between the two methods [19]. In their Cochrane review, Alfirevic et al concluded that the miscarriage rate between transcervical and transabdominal approach was more or less equal, but with heterogeneity between the included studies [19]. The transcervical route may have more sampling failures due to increased technical demands.

Following the Danish randomized study on amniocentesis versus no procedure, systematic reviews and meta-analyses of observational studies have been published. However, they are hampered by the study heterogeneity concerning gestational age at sampling and follow-up time. Generally, they have demonstrated a lower miscarriage rate than that reported by Tabor et al [17]. Akolekar et al (2015) reviewed patient series including more than 1000 procedures published during 2000–2014. They reported a pooled weighted risk of miscarriage up to 24 weeks as low as 0.11% for amniocentesis and 0.22% for CVS above the background risk compared with pregnancies without invasive procedures [20].

For women with a high risk (above 1:250) for fetal trisomy 21 following first trimester screening, a recent randomized clinical trial showed similar miscarriage rates following immediate invasive testing procedure (CVS or amniocentesis) compared to invasive testing only for those with a positive cfDNA test. The miscarriage rate was 0.8% before gestational week 24 in both groups [21]. Although the authors concluded that the study was underpowered to detect clinically important differences in miscarriage rate between the two groups, the study questioned the common assumption of a reduced miscarriage rate following cfDNA test.

12.3.4 Other Complications

12.3.4.1 Talipes

Early amniocentesis and amniotic fluid leakage have been associated with the development of talipes, suggesting that a reduction in amniotic fluid volume might be a causal factor

[19]. Due to this possible causal mechanism and the increased frequency of miscarriage following early amniocentesis, the procedure should be avoided before gestational week 15.

12.3.4.2 Limb Reduction Defects

In 1991, cases with severe limb abnormalities following CVS were reported. These samplings were performed before 66 gestational days [22]. Later studies could not demonstrate an association between these defects and CVS, but it is a general agreement to avoid CVS prior to 10 weeks' gestation [19].

12.3.4.3 Neonatal Respiratory Difficulties

The Danish randomized study on mid-trimester amniocentesis showed a doubling of the incidence of neonatal respiratory problems following amniocentesis compared to the control group [17]. However, follow-up studies have not confirmed any long-term consequences. Among these studies, a Dutch study compared the long-term consequences for children at a mean age of 4–5 years following transcervical CVS or mid-trimester amniocentesis [23]. No differences were observed in the frequency of respiratory problems or in other health issues, and the results were comparable to register studies of the general population [23].

12.3.5 Invasive Sampling in Multiple Pregnancies

A meta-analysis on studies published between 1970 and 2010 on amniocentesis in twin pregnancies showed a pooled procedure related loss rate up to 24 gestational weeks of 3.5% (95% CI 2.6–4.7). In the seven studies that included a control group without amniocentesis the pooled odds ratio (OR) for fetal loss was 1.8 (95% CI 1.2–2.7) [24]. Thus, the miscarriage rate after amniocentesis most likely is increased above the baseline risk of pregnancy loss due to twin pregnancy. However, the exact miscarriage rate is still uncertain due to the heterogeneity of the studies concerning definition of fetal loss (one versus both) and underpowered sample size [24]. In another review the authors emphasized the lack of randomized studies on invasive procedures in twin pregnancies, but estimated an excess miscarriage risk of about 1% above the background risk both following amniocentesis or CVS in twin pregnancies [25]. For CVS they did not observe any difference in pregnancy loss following a transcervical versus transabdominal approach or between the single- or double-needle techniques. For both amniocentesis and CVS there was no difference in loss rate, dependent on single (from one fetus only) or double (from both fetuses) samplings. Monochorionic pregnancies generally have a higher loss rate than dichorionic pregnancies. The opinion varies concerning sampling from one or both twins.

12.3.6 Invasive Sampling in the Area of Non-Invasive Prenatal Test

Following the introduction of NIPT, the number of invasive diagnostic procedures has declined, raising concern on the effect of a reduced procedural volume on the proficiency of the physician and the trainee, as well as the cytogenetic laboratories with a possible effect on neonatal outcome [26].

A Danish registry study showed an inverse association between miscarriage rate and the number of procedures performed at each prenatal diagnostic centre [27]. The risk for miscarriage before week 24 was double (OR 2.2, 95% CI 1.6–3.1) in centres with fewer than 500 annual amniocenteses compared with centres with more than 1500 procedures. The risk following chorionic villus sampling was 40% higher in centres with 500 to 1500 samplings per year compared to those with more than 1500 procedures.

Some professional societies and boards have accordingly recommended a minimum number of invasive tests per year to maintain competency. For example The Royal College of Obstetricians and Gynaecologists recommend a minimum of 30 procedures per year based on the clinical experience of the guideline development group [28]. Another approach is to include simulator-based training in invasive procedures, and in a study using simulator-based teaching of trainees in amniocentesis electronic needle guidance improved the learning curve [29]. The authors stated that the training in amniocentesis was of concern for other invasive procedures as well: 'The technical approach is similar for all procedures: bringing a needle to a specific point on the ultrasound image' [29]. Further, they stated: 'All transabdominal invasive procedures in fetal medicine can be performed using the same technique aiming at different targets. Once the technique is acquired, it can therefore be applied to all invasive procedures.'

12.4 Key Points

- Prenatal screening tests are offered to pregnant women who wish to estimate the chance of having a child with chromosomal abnormality. Depending on the background maternal risk and the inherent performance of diverse prenatal screening tests, women should be counselled upon expected and unexpected results and management options.

- It should be made clear that there is no screening or diagnostic test that can predict the severity of problems a baby with DS, or other chromosomal/genetic abnormalities, will have.
- Genetic counselling including the risks, benefits and performance metrics (sensitivity, specificity, PPV and NPV) of prenatal diagnostic techniques should be offered to all pregnant women that consider to undergo prenatal screening or diagnostic tests.
- Decision making and clinical management of pregnancy should not be based on NIPT alone. Moreover, women should be aware that a negative (low-risk) NIPT result does not ensure a healthy baby.
- cfDNA techniques have high accuracy in the detection of common aneuploidies, but are currently not diagnostic.
- There are limited data on the cost-effectiveness of cfDNA in the general average-risk population.
- Invasive procedures carry a risk of miscarriage well below 1% in singleton pregnancies.
- Chorionic villus sampling should be performed starting from 10 gestational weeks and amniocentesis from 15 gestational weeks.
- There seems to be no increased risk of congenital malformations following amniocentesis or chorionic villus sampling performed after the recommended gestational age limits.

12.5 Key Guidelines Relevant to the Topic

ISUOG Practice Guidelines. *Invasive Procedures for Prenatal Diagnosis in Obstetrics* [16].

Royal College of Obstetricians and Gynaecologists (RCOG). *Amniocentesis and Chorionic Villus Sampling.* Green-top Guideline No 8. [28].

References

1. Nicolaides KH, Azar G, Byrne D, Mansur C, Marks K. Fetal nuchal translucency: ultrasound screening for chromosomal defects in first trimester of pregnancy. *BMJ.* 1992;**304**:867–9.

2. Makrydimas G, Sotiriadis A, Ioannidis JPA. Screening performance of first trimester nuchal translucency for major cardiac defects: a meta-analysis. *Am J Obstet Gynecol.* 2003;**189**:1330–5.

3. Alldred SK, Takwoingi Y, Guo B, et al. First trimester serum tests for Down´s syndrome screening. *Cochrane Database Syst Rev* 2015, Issue 11. Art. No.: CD011975. DOI: 10.1002/14651858. CD011975.

4. Alldred SK, Takwoingi Y, Guo B, et al. First trimester ultrasound tests alone or in combination with first trimester serum tests for Down's syndrome screening. *Cochrane Database Syst Rev.*, 2017, Issue 3. Art. No.: CD012600. DOI: 10.1002/14651858. CD012600.

5. Lo YMD, Corbetta N, Chamberlain PF, et al. Presence of fetal DNA in maternal plasma and serum. *Lancet.* 1997;**350**:485–7.

6. Dar P, Shani H, Evans MI. Cell-free DNA. Comparison of technologies. *Clin Lab Med.* 2016;**36**:199–211.

7. Bianchi DW, Chiu RWK. Sequencing of circulating cell-free DNA during pregnancy. *N Eng J Med.* 2018;**379**:464–73.

8. Rink BD, Norton ME. Screening for fetal aneuploidy. *Semin Perinatol.* 2016;**40**:35–43.

9. Norton ME, Jacobsson B, Swamy GK, et al. Cell-free DNA analysis for noninvasive examination of trisomy. *N Engl J Med.* 2015;**372**:1589–97.

10. Gil MM, Quezada MS, Revello R, Akolekar R, Nicolaides KH. Analysis of cell-free DNA in maternal blood in screening for aneuploidies: updated meta-analysis. *Ultrasound Obstet Gynecol.* 2015;**45**:249–66.

11. Badeau M, Lindsay C, Blais J, et al. Genomics-based non-invasive prenatal testing for detection of fetal chromosomal aneuploidy in pregnant women. *Cochrane Database Syst Rev.* 2017, Issue 11. Art. No.: CD011767. DOI: 10.1002/14651858.CD11767. pub2

12. Hui L, Hutchinson B, Poulton A, Halliday J. Population-based impact of noninvasive prenatal screening on screening and diagnostic testing for fetal aneuploidy. *Genet Med.* 2017;**19**:1338–45.

13. Vogel I, Petersen OB, Christensen R, et al. Chromosomal microarray as primary diagnostic genomic tool for

pregnancies at increased risk within a population-based combined first-trimester screening program. *Ultrasound Obstet Gynecol.* 2018;**51**:480–6.

14. Boyle B, Morris JK, McConkey R, et al. Prevalence and risk of Down syndrome in monozygotic and dizygotic multiple pregnancies in Europe: implications for prenatal screening. *BJOG.* 2014;**121**:809–20.

15. Bender W, Dugoff L. Screening for aneuploidy in multiple gestations. The challenges and options. *Obstet Gynecol Clin North Am.* 2018;**45**:41–53.

16. Ghi T, Sotiriadis A, Calda P et al. on behalf of the International Society of Ultrasound in Obstetrics and Gynecology. ISUOG Practice Guidelines: invasive procedures for prenatal diagnosis in obstetrics. *Ultrasound Obstet Gynecol.* 2016;**48**:256–68.

17. Tabor A, Philip J, Madsen M, et al. Randomised controlled trial of genetic amniocentesis in 4606 low-risk women. *Lancet.* 1986;**1**:1287–93.

18. Athanasiadis AP, Pantazis K, Goulis DG, et al. Comparison between 20 G and 22 G needle for second trimester amniocentesis in terms of technical aspects and short-term

complications. *Prenat Diagn.* 2009;**29**:761–5.

19. Alfirevic Z, Navaratnam K, Mujezinovic F. Amniocentesis and chorionic villus sampling for prenatal diagnosis. *Cochrane Database Syst Rev.* 2017, Issue 9. Art. No.: CD003252. DOI: 10.1002/14651858.CD003252.pub2.

20. Akolekar R, Beta J, Picciarelli G, Ogilvie C, D'Antonio F. Procedure-related risk of miscarriage following amniocentesis and chorionic villus sampling: a systematic review and meta-analysis. *Ultrasound Obstet Gynecol.* 2015;**45**:16–26.

21. Malan V, Bussières L, Winer N, et al. Effect of cell-free DNA screening vs direct invasive diagnosis on miscarriage rates in women with pregnancies at high risk of trisomy 21. A randomized clinical trial. *JAMA.* 2018;**320**:557–65.

22. Firth HV, Boyd PA, Chamberlain P, et al. Severe limb abnormalities after chorion villus sampling at 56–66 days' gestation. *Lancet.* 1991;**337**:762–3.

23. Schaap AHP, van der Pol HG, Boer K, Leschot NJ, Wolf H. Long-term follow-up of infants after transcervical chorionic villus sampling and after amniocentesis to compare congenital abnormalities and health status. *Pranat Diagn.* 2002;**22**:598–604.

24. Vink J, Fuchs K, D'Alton ME. Amniocentesis in twin pregnancies: a systematic review of the literature. *Prenat Diagn.* 2012;**32**: 409–16.

25. Agarwal K, Alfirevic Z. Pregnancy loss after chorionic villus sampling and genetic amniocentesis in twin pregnancies: a systematic review. *Ultrasound Obstet Gynecol.* 2012;**40**:128–34.

26. Warsof SL, Larion S, Abuhamad AZ. Overview of the impact of noninvasive prenatal testing on diagnostic procedures. *Prenat Diagn.* 2015;**35**:972–9.

27. Tabor A, Vestergaard CHF, Lidegaard Ø. Fetal loss rate after chorionic villus sampling and amniocentesis: an 11-year national registry study. *Ultrasound Obstet Gynecol.* 2009;**34**:19–24.

28. Royal College of Obstetricians and Gynaecologists (RCOG). *Amniocentesis and Chorionic Villus Sampling.* Green-top Guideline No 8. London, UK; 2010. www.rcog.org.uk /en/guidelines-research-services/guide lines/gtg8/

29. Nizard J, Duyme M, Ville Y. Teaching ultrasound-guided invasive procedures in fetal medicine: learning curves with and without an electronic guidance system. *Ultrasound Obstet Gynecol.* 2002;**19**:274–7.

Invasive Fetal Therapies

Catherine E. Aiken & Jeremy Brockelsby

13.1 Introduction

In recent years, there has been an upsurge of interest in therapeutic intervention for fetal benefit prior to delivery. The main drivers of the increasing tendency towards intrauterine intervention are improving imaging techniques, increasing confidence and experience of global centres with fetal therapies and wider developments in the field of minimally invasive surgery. The accelerating trend for trialling new fetal therapies means that careful consideration of the overall benefit of intrauterine intervention is required. Any therapy performed for fetal benefit during pregnancy inherently requires consideration of maternal risks, whereas delaying intervention until after delivery avoids maternal complications. Therapies performed after birth are also technically easier; the baby is larger, surgical access is easier and appropriate anaesthesia can be assured. An additional risk of fetal therapy is of provoking preterm delivery, and hence complicating a precarious clinical condition with the additional burden of prematurity. Even if preterm delivery does not occur, there is still the hurdle of delivery itself to be overcome after definitive therapy has been performed. In view of these significant advantages associated with post-delivery interventions, it is vital to ensure that the benefits of intervening for fetal benefit during pregnancy truly outweigh the risks.

Two distinct scenarios can be identified where there is clear justification for attempting intervention in utero. The first case is where the fetus will not survive until delivery without intervention. In this instance, the choice is made between premature delivery to facilitate therapy and therapy within the womb. This is the case for severe fetal anaemia with developing hydrops, where it is clear that the oxygen-carrying capacity of the fetus is insufficient to sustain life. In such cases, gestational age is the crucial factor determining the optimal strategy – the risk of undertaking intrauterine therapy is balanced against the risk of prematurity. At non-viable gestations, the balance of risk clearly favours fetal intervention, but with increasing gestation the balance will tip in favour of delivery as the risks of prematurity decrease.

The second scenario in which fetal therapy is clearly justified is when the course of fetal development would be irreversibly altered without intervention. This justification may apply particularly to organ systems where there are critical windows of development for organogenesis, for example in lung development, when the respiratory tree is canalized between 16 and 24 weeks. If such windows are missed, then they cannot be compensated by later interventions. There is therefore rationale to focus on developing therapies to target these particular systems in the womb. This contrasts with other developing organ systems and structures, which can be repaired at the end of intrauterine development with excellent cosmetic and functional results. An example of this type of anomaly is fetal talipes, which can be entirely corrected in the postnatal period, and for which it would be extremely difficult to justify attempting fetal therapy. There is also an intermediate group of conditions, which do not have an absolute developmental window during which it is critical for determining outcome, but which may result in significant additional loss of function if left uncorrected during fetal life. An example of this type of condition is open neural tube defects. In this case, there are concerns that long-term central nervous function is irreversibly worsened by exposure of the delicate spinal cord to the intrauterine environment, hence repairing the defect in utero could preserve function.

Fetal therapies in various forms have been in existence for as long as the fetus could be visualized and monitored within the womb. However, recent technological advances make this a particularly exciting time for this developing field. It is important to note that, at present, performing fetal therapy is appropriately limited to a relatively small number of expert centres. The conditions treated are generally rare, and experience in treating the fetus as a patient is limited by the incidence of treatable anomalies. Importantly, outcomes of fetal therapy do vary between centres [1]. Thus, concentration of expertise and experience in sub-specialist centres is critical to ensure that outcomes can be optimized for every family who seeks therapy.

This chapter will explore the therapies currently in clinical use in sub-specialist centres, and briefly review those that are currently under evaluation. We have deliberately concentrated on interventions to treat the fetus directly – placental interventions are covered elsewhere. Inevitably, with the pace of modern global research, practice changes quickly and thus the underlying principles of each fetal therapy are of more value to explore than the current technical details of performing each technique.

13.2 Fetal Anaemia

Fetal anaemia is one of the best-established indications for fetal therapy. Anaemia in the fetus can be the end result of a variety of different pathologies, including maternal infections (e.g. parvovirus B12) and fetal structural lesions that destroy red blood cells through turbulent flow (e.g. sacrococcygeal teratomas). However the most common cause is alloimmunization, which can be due to any of a wide range of maternal antibodies, each with differing propensities to provoke anaemia in the fetus [2].

In pregnancies where there is reasonable cause to suspect that fetal anaemia might develop, close monitoring is required [1]. In cases where maternal red cell alloimmunization is suspected, then the fetal risk can be determined through several methods including paternal genotyping (where paternity is certain), direct genotyping of the fetus, or indirect fetal genotyping via cell-free DNA (cfDNA) analysis. For fetuses at risk of anaemia from any cause, the optimal non-invasive method of detecting moderate or severe fetal anaemia is through serial measurements of the peak systolic velocity (PSV) in the fetal middle cerebral artery (MCA) [3]. Using trends in serially measured MCA PSV values rather than a single threshold value reduces the false positive rate to <5%. If the fetus is hydropic, or the MCA PSV rises to ≥1.5 multiples of the median (MoM), and the gestation is not sufficiently advanced to make delivery the optimal strategy (usually around 35 weeks [2]), then invasive fetal testing and therapy should be considered [4].

13.2.1 Fetal Cordocentesis and Red Cell Transfusion

Undertaking cordocentesis is a technically challenging procedure, which needs careful coordination between clinical services. The parents must be carefully counselled about the risks to the pregnancy, which include preterm labour, premature rupture of the membranes, worsening alloimmunization, fetal or maternal bleeding and fetal death. The risk of fetal complications from transfusion increases at lower gestational ages and in more severely anaemic fetuses. The parents must understand and agree with the clinician's assessment of the risk/benefit ratio of the procedure. As with any fetal therapeutic procedure, the pregnant woman must fully understand what the procedure entails, approximately how long the procedure will take and what she can expect to experience.

Preparations for cordocentesis of a viable fetus include steroid administration and availability of facilities to undertake an emergency caesarean delivery, should complications occur. Maternal blood should be sampled, and the haematocrit determined for comparison prior to the procedure. A means of rapidly testing fetal haematocrit from the sample obtained via cordocentesis is essential – this can be either through near-patient testing or a through prior discussion with the laboratory. Irradiated, O-negative, cytomegalovirus (CMV) negative, packed red blood cells (to limit volume required) must be available for immediate transfusion, and the volume calculated when the fetal haematocrit is known. The fetal puncture site is often chosen pragmatically, depending on the gestation, fetal lie, placental site and maternal body habitus. Cordocentesis can be performed at the site of the placental cord insertion, the umbilical cord insertion, the fetal hepatic vein or in a free loop of cord (Figure 13.1).

It is also possible to transfuse blood directly into the peritoneal cavity in a severely hydropic fetus, although this precludes sampling the fetal blood, is less effective at increasing haematocrit and is more like to be associated with complications. The intraperitoneal approach tends to be favoured at earlier gestations (<22 weeks [5]).

Following transfusion, close surveillance of the pregnancy is required. If the cause of the fetal anaemia is alloimmunization, then a fall in haematocrit of approximately 1% per day can be expected following transfusion. The risk of requiring repeat transfusion is therefore high, particularly if the initial transfusion is performed at an early gestation. Because of the rapid rate of haematocrit drop, and the desire to limit risk by performing as few transfusions as possible, transfusion to above the target haematocrit of 40–50% has been suggested, but this approach may carry other risks including polycythaemia and increased blood viscosity [6].

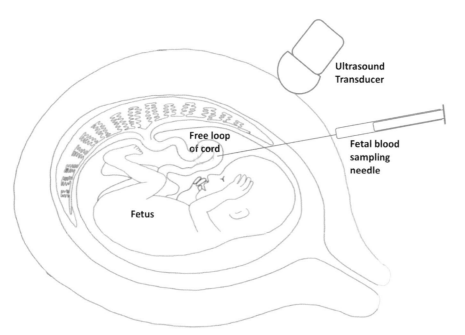

Figure 13.1 Schematic of cordocentesis sampling. Cordocentesis can be performed at the site of the placental cord insertion, the umbilical cord insertion, the fetal hepatic vein or as shown here in a free loop of cord. The site of the placenta and position of the fetus will determine the optimal site.

Perinatal survival of severe fetal anaemia is around 90% in otherwise structurally normal fetuses, although this appears to be lower in cases where parvovirus is the causative aetiology. The neonate must be carefully managed in the postnatal period, as complications such as anaemia from lack of reticulocytes, and hyperbilirubinaemia are likely, particularly if repeated transfusions have been required. The long-term prognosis for fetuses that undergo repeated intrauterine transfusion is less certain, although evidence suggests that the rate of serious neurodevelopmental impairment among survivors is around 5% [7].

13.3 Fetal Shunting

The accumulation of fluid in fetal body cavities is one of the most obvious anomalies seen on ultrasonography, and presents a relatively tractable problem that is potentially amenable to intrauterine therapy. It is considered that relieving the hydrostatic pressure of fluid accumulation in the body compartment may promote the development of the surrounding organ structures, hence the rationale for intervening in utero rather than waiting for postnatal intervention. The second rationale for intervening to remove fluid during prenatal life is to improve the chances of successful delivery and transition to postnatal life. Ascites reduction may facilitate vaginal delivery, which may be particularly important to preserve maternal health if the likely fetal outcome is known to be poor. Reduction of fluid in the pleural cavity may also be performed therapeutically prior to delivery to facilitate neonatal ventilation and lung expansion at delivery. If these procedures are performed for the specific purpose of improving delivery outcomes, then it is important that they are correctly timed just prior to planned delivery, as fluid can re-accumulate quickly depending on the aetiology.

13.3.1 Vesicocentesis and shunting

Approximately 2–3 in every 10 000 babies is delivered with evidence of lower urinary tract obstruction (LUTO) [8]. LUTO leads to progressive bladder wall thickening, hydronephrosis, and ultimately renal damage. There are multiple causative aetiologies, with the most common being posterior urethral valves. Other possible diagnoses include prune belly syndrome, urethral atresia, megacystis-microcolon-hyperperistalsis syndrome and cloacal malformations. The diagnosis of LUTO is usually made following ultrasound evidence of hydronephrosis, ureteric enlargement, oligohydramnios and bladder distension, often with bladder wall thickening and the characteristic 'keyhole sign' when posterior urethral valves are present. Untreated LUTO carries a poor prognosis, particularly if oligohydramnios is present [9]. For this reason, extensive research efforts have been made to develop successful intrauterine fetal therapy for the condition.

Diagnostic fetal urine sampling has been extensively evaluated to assess renal function in utero, and hence guide prognosis and management. A systematic review showed that while elevated urinary sodium and calcium were associated with poor postnatal renal function, no single electrolyte was sufficiently predictive of outcome to be of clinical utility as a test [10]. The optimal patient group who would benefit most from intervention in the context of LUTO remains unclear, despite the proposal of new staging systems based on renal tract appearance, amniotic fluid volume and fetal urinalysis [11].

If intervention is deemed appropriate, there are several possible options. Simple vesicocentesis can relieve pressure on the renal tract, with the intention of preserving renal function as far as possible. Placement of a vesico-amniotic shunt, using a pigtail catheter (Figure 13.2), has the additional advantage of replenishing the amniotic fluid and hence promoting

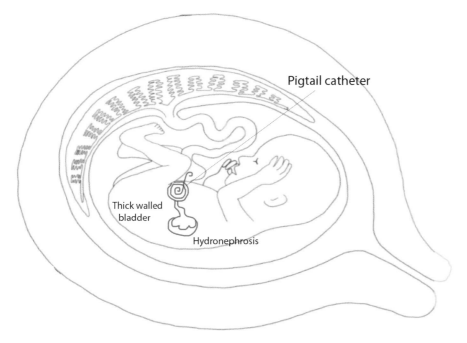

Figure 13.2 Vesico-amniotic shunt in situ. The pigtail catheter curls in the fetal bladder and drains freely into the surrounding amniotic fluid, reducing the back pressure on the kidney and increasing the amniotic fluid index.

Pigtail catheter

Thick walled bladder

Hydronephrosis

fetal lung development in addition to relieving pressure on the renal parenchyma. This technique is complicated by the relatively high incidence of shunt displacement, which occurs in up to 50% of cases[12]. Other potential complications include shunt blockage, premature rupture of the membranes, and preterm labour. Fetal cystoscopy is a further option, which offers the additional advantage of diagnosing and potentially treating the cause of LUTO. A 1–1.3 mm fetoscope is passed through a percutaneous trocar into the uterus and thence into the urethra. If posterior urethral valves are encountered, then laser ablation can be performed. After fetal cystoscopic treatment, obstruction due to posterior urethral valves is estimated to recur in around 20% of cases [13].

Despite much research effort and procedure development, the long-term outcomes for fetuses affected by LUTO remains poor. The only randomized trial to investigate the utility of vesico-amniotic shunting to relieve LUTO (the PLUTO trial [14]) could not conclusively show evidence of benefit to recommend shunting as the standard of care to improve outcomes. However, the most striking finding of the PLUTO trial was the very poor outcome associated with LUTO, regardless of therapy. Of the 24 babies born alive in the cohort, 50% died in the early neonatal period due to pulmonary hypoplasia, and there were only two survivors with normal renal function in early childhood. While fetal therapy for LUTO does show promise, it is essential that parents continuing pregnancies with this diagnosis are fully counselled regarding the likely outcomes in both the early and later postnatal period.

13.3.2 Thoracocentesis and Shunting

Fetal hydrothorax in the absence of other structural or genetic anomalies is a relatively rare and poorly understood condition [15]. Regardless of the underlying aetiology, factors associated with poor prognosis are bilateral effusions, mediastinal shift and fetal hydrops. Fetal intervention is normally based on the presence of mediastinal shift, cardiac compromise, developing hydrops, or a rapidly evolving clinical picture. There is little high-quality clinical evidence to guide the decision for intervention, but theoretically pulmonary hypoplasia is thought to be reduced by the reduction in fetal thoracic pressure that a shunt provides. The other main indication for fetal thoracocentesis is immediately prior to planned delivery, when postnatal lung inflation may be aided by prior reduction in the intrathoracic pressure. Fetal thoracocentesis is also described in macrocystic adenomatous lung disease, when a single enormous cyst may be decompressed in order to promote development of the normal lung tissue.

As with removal of fluid from other body compartments, the chest can be drained with single or repeated thoracocentesis, or a pleuro-amniotic shunt can be placed. There have also been reports of fetal pleurodesis, which is performed with a streptococcal derivative called Picibanil (OK-432). Unfortunately, there is a deficit of high-quality short- or long-term outcome data to guide management recommendations for management of fetal pleural effusions. However, the dismal prognosis associated with severe fetal pleural effusions means that many clinicians undertake such procedures after thorough counselling of the parents.

13.3.3 Congenital Diaphragmatic Hernia

The other major fetal chest anomaly where fetal therapy is also often considered in an attempt to promote normal lung development is congenital diaphragmatic hernia (CDH). CDH occurs in approximately 1:2500–3500 live births [16]. It is caused by a failure of fusion between the pleuroperitoneal folds and the septum transversum during the first trimester. The resulting defect allows the abdominal viscera to herniate into the thorax, which impairs growth and maturation of the developing lung buds, often leading to pulmonary hypoplasia and an associated poor development of the pulmonary vasculature. Congenital diaphragmatic hernia is a potentially operable anomaly postnatally, but neonatal survival depends on sufficient lung development in utero.

Fetal therapies have therefore been developed with the aim of increasing intrathoracic pressure and trapping lung fluid within the bronchial tree during gestation to promote canalization of the lung tissue. Several different forms of therapy have been attempted, but currently the most commonly performed procedure is fetal endoluminal tracheal occlusion (FETO) using balloons that were originally developed for interventional radiology procedures. This procedure is carried out under maternal regional anaesthesia and fetal analgesia. A balloon is placed endoscopically via the fetal trachea into the space between the vocal cords and the carina, and inflated. The balloon should be removed prior to delivery (by fetoscopy or ultrasound-guided puncture) in order to promote lung maturation during the final stages of gestation, but can be punctured at delivery if preterm or emergency delivery is required. Neonatologists have raised concerns about reports of difficulty in removing balloons in fetuses delivering unexpectedly in unprepared obstetric centres, and the possibility of fetal asphyxiation and death as a result. Concerns have also been raised about the possibility of long-term tracheal damage following FETO.

Patient selection is a very important aspect of offering any fetal therapy, and particularly so in CDH, where associated genetic and other structural anomalies are common. In 30–40% of fetuses with CDH there is an associated underlying condition; including 10% who have chromosomal anomalies and 30% with a major structural anomaly. The most commonly associated structural anomalies are congenital heart defects, which are present in around 20% of cases. Therefore, when counselling parents regarding the long-term prognosis after fetal therapy for CDH, it is vital that a detailed fetal phenotyping with genetic testing (usually via microarray analysis) and fetal magnetic resonance imaging (MRI) has been offered. Tracheal balloon placement is the subject of the global TOTAL trials, investigating whether FETO truly improves outcomes in moderate and severe lung dysplasia in left-sided isolated CDH. The Tracheal Occlusion To Accelerate Lung Growth (TOTAL) trials are still ongoing, but a recent systematic review and meta-analysis, mainly of observational studies, suggests that FETO may confer a survival advantage at both 30 days and 6 months of postnatal life.

13.3.4 Paracentesis

Isolated fetal ascites is a rare diagnosis, with a wide range of potential aetiologies. If diagnosed early in pregnancy (<24 weeks), it is generally associated with a poor prognosis [17]. The finding of fetal ascites merits an extensive prenatal workup of genetic and structural studies in order to counsel the parents as carefully as possible about expected outcomes.

Due to the relative ability of the abdominal cavity to distend without increasing intra-abdominal pressure, contrasting with the highly pressure-sensitive thorax, fetal ascites is less often considered for fetal therapy than pleural fluid accumulation. However, there are several specific scenarios when paracentesis may be considered. The first instance is where massive ascites occurs, and there is concern that fetal circulatory development is hampered by the large preload index. In this instance, paracentesis may reduce preload, promote fetal lung development and delay progression to fetal hydrops. The second instance is when delivery would be facilitated by prior reduction in abdominal circumference. A pre-delivery reduction in abdominal fluid volume may allow vaginal delivery or enable caesarean section to be safely performed via a lower segment transverse uterine incision rather than a classical incision. In this instance, the mother's future reproductive health is safeguarded, and the risk of future pregnancies is reduced. Predelivery reduction in intra-abdominal pressure may also mean that the newborn is more easily ventilated and stabilized postdelivery, which is particularly important if urgent surgical intervention needs to be considered. A further potential indication for performing fetal paracentesis may be to derive further diagnostic information about the aetiology of the ascites. This may be considered particularly if the parents would consider interrupting the pregnancy in the face of particular aetiologies, or if immediate neonatal management would be influenced by more certain diagnostic information.

13.3.5 Future Directions for Fetal Shunting

Recent technical advances in fetal therapy have reawakened an interest in whether the prognosis of significant fetal ventriculomegaly might be improved by placement of in utero shunts. Earlier experience with the technique suggested high procedure-related death rates, high postnatal infection risk and a significant risk of neurodevelopmental delay among survivors [18]. However, several research groups have recently begun to consider whether improved imaging techniques (particularly MRI of the fetal brain) could be used to improve outcomes by improving patient selection. There have also been advances in fetal surgery techniques, through development of other shunt placement procedures, and of shunt tubing design. This area requires further research and exploration of the risk/benefit ratio.

13.4 Ex-Utero Intrapartum Treatment (EXIT) Procedures

Many fetal conditions, particularly those involving the airway and fetal circulation, are stable whilst in utero but become life-threatening emergencies in the immediate neonatal period.

Oxygen delivery via the placental circulation during intrauterine life means that airway obstruction, for example from giant neck masses, congenital high airway obstruction syndrome (CHAOS), and severe micrognathia, is not problematic for the fetus. However, immediately after the umbilical cord is cut, the newborn is reliant on a patent airway for oxygen delivery. Ex-utero intrapartum treatment (EXIT) procedures are designed to take advantage of placental gas exchange whilst a patent airway is established, hence creating a controlled time-window for therapy and avoiding the critical neonatal emergency. If a patent airway cannot be established during the EXIT procedure itself then proceeding to resection or transferring the baby directly from placental circulation to extracorporeal membrane oxygenation (ECMO) may be possible. As with other fetal therapies, EXIT procedures require a highly engaged, experienced and coordinated multidisciplinary team, involving obstetricians, anaesthetists, operating department personnel, neonatologists and paediatric otorhinolaryngologists. The parents must be carefully counselled about the risks, and the possibility that the long-term outcome will be guarded even if the initial stabilization is successful. The maternal morbidity associated with EXIT procedures, and the implications for future pregnancies, must also be fully understood [19].

EXIT procedures are performed under general anaesthesia in order to prevent uterine contraction and adequate maternal blood pressure to maintain sufficient placental perfusion pressure for the procedure [19]. The uterine incision is carefully planned using ultrasound guidance to avoid the placenta edge and may need to be large and unusually placed. The edges of the uterine incision are secured with stapling or with a specially designed retractor to minimize maternal blood loss, to maintain a clear operating field and to help maintain placental blood flow. The baby is partially delivered via the hysterotomy with minimal handling of the umbilical cord, which should be kept perfused and free-floating as far as possible in order to prevent physiological spasm. The paediatric team then follow a pre-agreed algorithm (see Figure 13.3 for an example) in order to secure a definitive airway as rapidly as possible. As soon as the paediatric team are confident that the airway is secure and the baby can be ventilated, then delivery is completed and the umbilical cord cut. The placenta is delivered and the hysterotomy closed. The degree of uterine atony required for the procedure increases the risk of maternal haemorrhage, and uterotonics and crossmatched blood should be available. In the postoperative period, the mother is at increased risk of delayed wound-healing, infection and uterine dehiscence. The family are also likely to need considerable psychological support in the face of a major operation and potentially a very unwell or non-surviving neonate.

Outcomes reported for neonates following EXIT procedures are highly variable, depending primarily on the aetiology of the underlying condition. A recent systematic review suggests that the prognosis of fetal head and neck tumours is improved when EXIT procedures are available [20]. The long-term prognosis for fetuses in whom the airway lesion is purely structural is often good after definitive surgical repair. In fetal therapy centres with

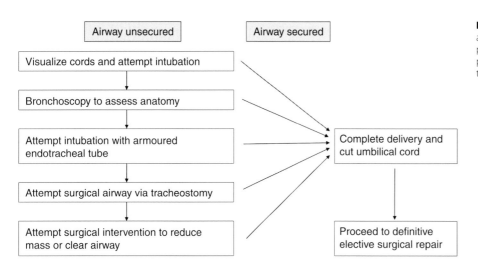

Figure 13.3 Example of airway securement algorithm for ex-utero intrapartum treatment (EXIT) procedure. The agreed steps to be followed in any particular case will depend on the precise nature of the fetal anomaly being treated.

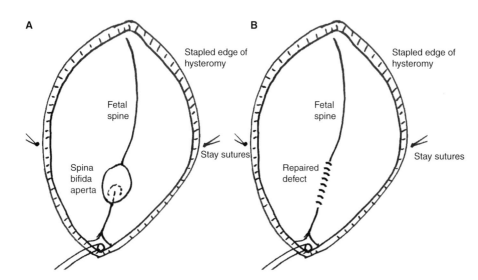

Figure 13.4 Schematic diagram of fetal spina bifida repair. (a) Fetal back exposed at the hysterotomy site prior to repair of lumbar myelomeningocoele. (b) After repair and prior to closure.

experienced and coordinated teams, these procedures are of benefit for well-selected and carefully counselled patients.

13.4.1 Spina Bifida Repair

Open fetal surgery can be undertaken for a variety of conditions, but the indication that has gained the most widespread acceptance is for open neural tube defects. Spina bifida aperta is one of the most common fetal anomalies, occurring in around 0.1 to 2 in 1000 pregnancies depending on the population. Postnatal repair is often successful, but long-term outcomes are poor, partially because of irreversible neural damage that has occurred in utero. The aim of fetal surgery for spina bifida is to repair the defect prior to prolonged exposure of the spinal nerves to the amniotic fluid or intrauterine trauma, and to limit the continual cerebrospinal fluid leak that increases hindbrain herniation [21].

Fetal spina bifida repair is usually performed between 19 and 25 weeks of gestation. Maternal general anaesthetic and

laparotomy are performed. A hysterotomy is then created and the edges stapled to limit blood loss and seal the membranes to the myometrium, as for an EXIT procedure. The fetus is then positioned at the hysterotomy site to allow surgical access to the defect (Figure 13.4). The exposed fetus remains intrauterine during the repair, but it is important to remember that it has no significant means of thermoregulation, and therefore careful attention to maternal heat loss is essential. Fetal echocardiographic monitoring during the surgery has been shown to be beneficial in monitoring fetal response. The main means of ensuring fetal anaesthesia and analgesia during the procedure are via maternal administration of volatile anaesthetic agents that readily cross the placenta, and by direct administration of intramuscular or intravenous opioids [22]. Towards the end of the interval for intervention, around 24 weeks and above, the fetus is potentially viable. In this instance, a detailed preoperative plan should be agreed with the parents and neonatologists in the event that fetal distress should become apparent during the procedure.

A randomized controlled trial (MOMS trial [23]) has demonstrated that prenatal repair of open spina bifida reduces requirement for ventriculoperitoneal shunting (and hence reduced shunt infection and revision) by 12 months of age and improves motor function by 30 months. In light of this evidence, fetal spina bifida surgery is becoming available at more expert fetal therapy centres worldwide, who are sharing expertise and experience to maximize outcomes.

Minimally invasive approaches to fetal spina bifida repair using patch repair, which avoids the need for maternal hysterotomy, are being developed but remain in early phases at present [24]. This approach holds promise, and is an important research goal to reduce the procedure-associated morbidity. Despite the improvements in prognosis for open neural tubes defects with fetal repair, there is still a need for better therapy. Open fetal spina bifida repair still carries a 40% risk of requiring a ventriculoperitoneal shunt, and fewer than half of children are walking independently by 30 months of age. Fetal repair also increases the risk of preterm delivery (average delivery gestation in the MOMS trial was 34 weeks), premature rupture of the membranes and amniotic fluid leak. Long-term follow-up of the children in the MOMS trial is planned but has yet to be reported. This will include assessing cognitive as well as motor functioning. Parents considering fetal spina bifida repair must also be carefully counselled about the maternal implications of the operation itself. When hysterotomy sites are inspected at the time of delivery by caesarean section, there is evidence of wound thinning in 25% and of partial or complete tissue edge separation in 10%. Implications for future pregnancies should be fully discussed with women who are considering this intervention.

13.4.2 Other Possibilities for Fetal Therapy

Fetal cardiac intervention has been evaluated as a developing therapy for specific forms of congenital heart disease in which an early intervention might improve the natural evolution of cardiac development during gestation. The forms of fetal heart disease that have currently been considered are severe aortic stenosis with evolving hypoplastic left heart syndrome (HLHS), pulmonary atresia with intact ventricular septum and evolving hypoplastic right heart syndrome, and HLHS with intact or highly restrictive atrial septum [25]. Particularly in severe aortic stenosis and pulmonary atresia, it has been suggested that if a valvuloplasty can be achieved in utero, then the chances of achieving postnatal biventricular repair should be increased. The approach to fetal aortic valvuloplasty is normally using a trocar passed via the maternal abdomen into the uterine cavity and into the apex of the fetal left ventricle. A guide wire is then introduced across the left outflow tract to enable inflation of a balloon in the annulus of the aortic valve. The balloon is normally inflated twice, and the flow checked using colour Doppler. The few case series for these techniques published thus far show promise in immediate survival and achievement of a biventricular circulation. However, considerable further evaluation is required to determine the optimal patient selection and to refine the technical aspects. There is also a need for careful study of the long-term outcomes compared to the outcomes of a conservative approach.

13.5 Conclusion

Given the potential of fetal therapies to do harm to mother and fetus, as well as to improve fetal outcomes, it is vital that new therapies are carefully evaluated in well-executed and adequately powered trials before becoming the standard of care. This is an extremely difficult research objective, particularly given the rarity of many of the fetal conditions that therapies are designed to combat. Recruitment of fetal therapy trial participants is limited by difficulties with accurate antenatal diagnosis for many conditions, by the preferences of many parents not to continue with pregnancies where the fetal prognosis is poor and by the high background rates of associated genetic anomalies and fetal loss. A further issue with fully disentangling the risk versus benefit balance of fetal therapies is that long-term outcomes should be the ultimate end-point by which therapeutic success is judged. Many fetal therapy trials are, for pragmatic purposes, designed and powered for intermediate primary outcomes that can be assessed at birth. However, the over-arching goal of fetal therapy is to promote neurologically and developmentally optimal survival into later childhood and adulthood. Without robust assessment of whether these end-points are truly reached, definitively advocating fetal therapies as a gold-standard of care remains a complex issue. Many of the fetal therapy trial examples discussed in this chapter show an improvement in intermediate end-points. A good example is the MOMS trial, which doubled the number of children with open spina bifida lesions who are walking independently at 30 months [23]. However, despite the promise this therapy holds, outcomes at follow-up to mid-childhood are yet to be determined. It is therefore important, despite excitement and enthusiasm for developing new invasive fetal therapies, to bear in mind the overall goal of improving the health of the child, and preserving the health of the mother, in the long term as well as in the neonatal period.

References

1. Society for Maternal-Fetal Medicine; Mari G, Norton ME, Stone J, et al. Society for Maternal-Fetal Medicine (SMFM) Clinical Guideline #8: the fetus at risk for anemia–diagnosis and management. *Am J Obstet Gynecol.* 2015 Jun;**212**(6):697–710.

2. Moise KJ. Fetal anemia due to non-Rhesus-D red-cell alloimmunization. *Semin Fetal Neonatal Med.* 2008 Aug;**13**(4): 207–14.

3. Mari G, Deter RL, Carpenter RL, et al. Noninvasive diagnosis by Doppler ultrasonography of fetal anemia due to maternal red-cell alloimmunization. Collaborative Group for Doppler Assessment of the Blood Velocity in Anemic Fetuses. *N Engl J Med.* 2000 Jan 6;**342**(1):9–14.

4. Moise KJ Jr., Argoti PS. Management and prevention of red cell alloimmunization in pregnancy: a systematic review. *Obstet Gynecol.* 2012 Nov;**120**(5):1132–9.

5. Fox C, Martin W, Somerset DA, Thompson PJ, Kilby MD. Early intraperitoneal transfusion and adjuvant maternal immunoglobulin therapy in the treatment of severe red cell alloimmunization prior to fetal intravascular transfusion. *Fetal Diagn Ther.* 2008;**23**(2):159–63.

6. Welch R, Rampling MW, Anwar A, Talbert DG, Rodeck CH. Changes in hemorheology with fetal intravascular transfusion. *Am J Obstet Gynecol.* 1994 Mar;**170**(3):726–32.

7. Lindenburg IT, Smits-Wintjens VE, van Klink JM, et al. Long-term neurodevelopmental outcome after intrauterine transfusion for hemolytic disease of the fetus/newborn: the LOTUS study. *Am J Obstet Gynecol.* 2012 Feb;**206**(2):141e1-8.

8. Malin G, Tonks AM, Morris RK, Gardosi J, Kilby MD. Congenital lower urinary tract obstruction: a population-based epidemiological study. *BJOG.* 2012 Nov;**119**(12):1455–64.

9. Hobbins JC, Romero R, Grannum P, et al. Antenatal diagnosis of renal anomalies with ultrasound. I. Obstructive uropathy. *Am J Obstet Gynecol.* 1984 Apr 1;**148**(7):868–77.

10. Morris RK, Quinlan-Jones E, Kilby MD, Khan KS. Systematic review of accuracy of fetal urine analysis to predict poor postnatal renal function in cases of congenital urinary tract obstruction. *Prenat Diagn.* 2007 Oct;**27**(10):900–11.

11. Ruano R, Sananes N, Wilson C, et al. Fetal lower urinary tract obstruction: proposal for standardized multidisciplinary prenatal management based on disease severity. *Ultrasound Obstet Gynecol.* 2016 Oct;**48**(4):476–82.

12. Kurtz MP, Koh CJ, Jamail GA, et al. Factors associated with fetal shunt dislodgement in lower urinary tract obstruction. *Prenat Diagn.* 2016 Aug;**36**(8):720–5.

13. Sananes N, Cruz-Martinez R, Favre R, et al. Two-year outcomes after diagnostic and therapeutic fetal cystoscopy for lower urinary tract obstruction. *Prenat Diagn.* 2016 Apr;**36**(4):297–303.

14. Morris RK, Malin GL, Quinlan-Jones E, et al. Percutaneous vesicoamniotic shunting versus conservative management for fetal lower urinary tract obstruction (PLUTO): a randomised trial. *Lancet.* 2013 Nov 2;**382**(9903):1496–506.

15. Yinon Y, Kelly E, Ryan G. Fetal pleural effusions. *Best Pract Res Clin Obstet Gynaecol.* 2008 Feb;**22**(1):77–96.

16. McGivern MR, Best KE, Rankin J, et al. Epidemiology of congenital diaphragmatic hernia in Europe: a register-based study. *Arch Dis Child Fetal Neonatal Ed.* 2015 Mar;**100**(2):F137-44.

17. Catania VD, Muru A, Pellegrino M, et al. Isolated fetal ascites, neonatal outcome in 51 cases observed in a tertiary referral center. *Eur J Pediatr Surg.* 2017 Feb;**27**(1):102–8.

18. Manning FA, Harrison MR, Rodeck C. Catheter shunts for fetal hydronephrosis and hydrocephalus. Report of the International Fetal Surgery Registry. *N Engl J Med.* 1986 Jul 31;**315**(5):336–40.

19. Taghavi K, Beasley S. The ex utero intrapartum treatment (EXIT) procedure: application of a new therapeutic paradigm. *J Paediatr Child Health.* 2013 Sep;**49**(9):E420-7.

20. Tonni G, Granese R, Martins Santana EF, et al. Prenatally diagnosed fetal tumors of the head and neck: a systematic review with antenatal and postnatal outcomes over the past 20 years. *J Perinat Med.* 2017 Feb 1;**45**(2):149–65.

21. Joyeux L, Danzer E, Flake AW, Deprest J. Fetal surgery for spina bifida aperta. *Arch Dis Child Fetal Neonatal Ed.* 2018 Nov;**103**(6):F589–F595.

22. Ferschl M, Ball R, Lee H, Rollins MD. Anesthesia for in utero repair of myelomeningocele. *Anesthesiology.* 2013 May;**118**(5):1211–23.

23. Adzick NS, Thom EA, Spong CY, et al. A randomized trial of prenatal versus postnatal repair of myelomeningocele. *N Engl J Med.* 2011 Mar 17;**364**(11):993–1004.

24. Graf K, Kohl T, Neubauer BA, et al. Percutaneous minimally invasive fetoscopic surgery for spina bifida aperta. Part III: neurosurgical intervention in the first postnatal year. *Ultrasound Obstet Gynecol.* 2016 Feb;**47**(2):158–61.

25. Gellis L, Tworetzky W. The boundaries of fetal cardiac intervention: Expand or tighten? *Semin Fetal Neonatal Med.* 2017 Dec;**22**(6):399–403.

Normal Fetal Growth and Fetal Macrosomia

Juriy W. Wladimiroff

Born either small or large for gestational age is associated with raised perinatal mortality and morbidity. Insight into normal fetal growth is a prerequisite for our understanding of abnormal fetal growth. Sonographic monitoring of fetal growth and size has contributed to a better perinatal outcome.

14.1 Normal Fetal Growth

Fetal growth is much determined by maternal characteristics, placental function and environmental factors. Trophoblast invasion of the spiral arteries in early pregnancy allows increasing blood flow to the developing fetus, ensuring adequate oxygen and nutrients supply and removal of waste products. Glucose is the main source of energy to the fetus. Insulin-like growth factor 2 plays an essential part in regulating fetal growth and amino acid transport.

14.1.1 Methods of Establishing Fetal Growth

14.1.1.1 Measurement of Symphyseal Fundal Height (SFH)

Symphyseal fundal height (SFH) measurement still plays an important role in daily obstetric care. This is particularly the case in parts of the world where no ultrasound equipment is available. The use of different measuring methodologies and reference charts makes the SFH measurement less sensitive for the assessment of fetal growth. SFH measurements are unreliable in the presence of maternal obesity and multiparity and should not be the method of choice when monitoring high-risk pregnancies. Diagnostic ultrasound is considered to be the method of choice in establishing normal and abnormal fetal growth.

14.1.1.2 Sonographic Determination of Fetal Growth

- To accurately determine fetal growth, one first has to know the exact gestational age;
- To accurately establish gestational age, one needs to resort to embryonic/fetal biometry;
- To accurately perform fetal biometry, one has to select and measure the appropriate fetal anatomic dimensions;
- Having measured the correct fetal anatomic dimensions, one has to conduct serial fetal biometric measurements to establish fetal growth.

Selecting the Appropriate Embryonic and Fetal Anatomical Dimensions

Traditionally, the preferred fetal parameters for establishing gestational age, fetal growth and size are the embryonic/fetal crown–rump length during the first trimester of pregnancy (see also Chapter 11, Ultrasound Scanning in the First Trimester of Pregnancy) and the fetal biparietal diameter (BPD) and head circumference (HC), fetal abdominal circumference (AC) and fetal femur length (FL) in the second and third trimesters of pregnancy.

It is essential the above fetal parameters are correctly measured. The fetal head is imaged well-magnified in a horizontal and oval position, demonstrating the midline representing the falx cerebri, interrupted anteriorly by the cavum septum pellucidum. The thalami and third ventricle are situated centrally on either side of the midline. The occipital horns of the lateral ventricles can be visualized posteriorly (Figure 14.1). The BPD measurement is taken from the outer table of the proximal skull to the outer table of the distal skull (outer-to-outer). Some measure from outer-to-inner. The HC is measured at the same level as the BPD using available trace callipers. The BPD shows linear growth of 3 mm per week between 14 and 28 weeks and 2 mm per week until term. The HC grows about 14 mm per week between 14 and 17 weeks and 5 mm per week near term [1].

The cross section for measurement of the fetal abdominal circumference should be presented as a well-magnified circular structure showing the echolucent stomach, spine and a short segment of the umbilical vein away from its entrance into the fetal abdomen (Figure 14.2). Usually, trace callipers are used to determine the AC. The AC demonstrates linear growth with a mean of 11–12 mm per week throughout pregnancy [1].

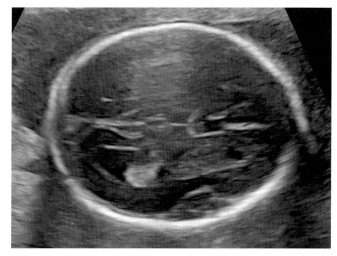

Figure 14.1 Second trimester ultrasound image for the measurement of the fetal head. Note the well-magnified and horizontal position of the head.

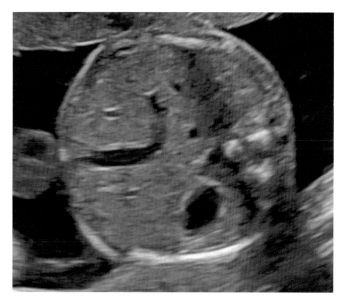

Figure 14.2 Second trimester ultrasound image for the measurement of the fetal abdomen. Note the well-magnified and circular cross-sectional shape of the abdomen and the short segment of the umbilical vein in the anterior third of the abdomen. The echolucent stomach is visible.

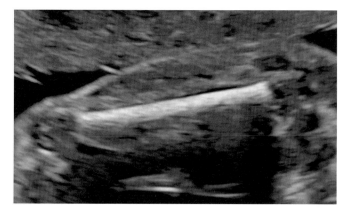

Figure 14.3 Second trimester ultrasound image for the measurement of the fetal femur length.

The fetal femur is presented in its full length by the ossified diaphysis; the trochanter becomes visible in later pregnancy (Figure 14.3). The measurement of the femur length should be carried out with the femur perpendicular to the ultrasound beam. The femur grows 3 mm per week from 14 to 27 weeks and 1 mm per week in the third trimester [1].

Determining Gestational Age

In pregnancies following an unknown menstrual history, irregular menstrual cycle or use of oral contraception, the exact gestational age may be unclear or even unknown. Knowledge of gestational age is important for various reasons: monitoring of fetal growth and size, timing of screening for chromosomal abnormalities in early pregnancy, prophylactic corticosteroid treatment for lung maturity in premature labour and timing of induction of labour or caesarean section.

Based on little variability in embryonic and fetal growth pattern in the first trimester of pregnancy, measurement of the embryonic/early fetal crown–rump length (dating scan) provides accurate information on gestational age and expected date of delivery. In early second trimester pregnancy, gestational age and expected date of delivery are best determined from measurement of the fetal BPD or HC. Longitudinally collected data from a large population-based cohort have demonstrated that pregnancy dating could be optimized using crown–rump length (CRL) from 20 to 65 mm and fetal BPD from 23 mm onwards [2]. However, pregnancy dating becomes increasingly unreliable after 21–22 weeks. Fetal abdominal circumference (AC) and femur length (FL) do not provide accurate information on gestational age.

Fetal Weight Estimation

Estimation of fetal weight may contribute to our understanding of normal and abnormal growth. Many methods of estimating fetal weight have been developed, ranging from a single biometric parameter to the combination of several parameters. Hadlock et al in 1985 produced a landmark paper on estimating fetal weight based on fetal head, body and femur measurements [3].

Most of the methods published advocate the use of multiple fetal ultrasound parameters which will affect accuracy. Errors in estimated fetal weight range between 10 and 15% on average, but may be as high as 25% [4]. Fetal weight prediction is particularly prone to error at the extremes of fetal weight with large-for-gestational age often being underestimated and small-for-gestational age often being overestimated. Possible explanations are variations in fetal tissue density and reduced amniotic volumes affecting the accuracy of the relevant fetal measurements. It has been suggested that fetal weight estimation could be further improved by adding fractional limb and/or fractional arm volume to conventional two-dimensional (2D) biometry [5].

Measurement methods and observer variability form a major contribution to systematic and random errors in fetal weight estimation [4]. To minimize variability in estimated weight measurements, it was suggested to average multiple fetal measurements, improve image quality, ensure uniform calibration of ultrasound equipment, careful design, refinement of measuring methods, and regular audit of measuring quality [4].

Recently, international estimated fetal weight standards were developed from a prospective, international, multicentre, population-based Fetal Growth Longitudinal Study and Interbio-21st Fetal Study, two components of the Intergrowth-21st Project. It concerned an assessment of estimated fetal weight, as adjunct to routine ultrasound biometry, from 22 to 40 weeks of gestation. It was advocated to evaluate fetal growth using separate biometric measures such as head and abdominal circumference, as well as estimated fetal weight instead of focusing on a single value [6]. Whereas, high-resolution magnetic resonance imaging (MRI) has been suggested to be accurate in determining fetal volume allowing reliable estimation of fetal weight [7], for daily clinical practice ultrasound is superior to all other methods of fetal weight estimation.

Birthweight has been studied in dichorionic and mono-chorionic twins and trichorionic triplets. It was demonstrated that the number of fetuses, the presence of a monochorionic placenta and gestational age were independently associated with birthweight with fetal number displaying the strongest effect [8].

Establishing Fetal Growth

Serial measurements of fetal BPD/HC, fetal AC and fetal FL in an individual fetus will establish its individual fetal growth and estimated fetal weight pattern. A multitude of fetal growth charts has been published. Yet, there is a wide variation of methodologies for the creation of these charts.

Basic issues in producing fetal growth charts are [9]:

- Sample selection and sample design;
- Statistical methods used;
- Assumption of a normal data distribution;
- The centiles change/do not change smoothly across gestation;
- To take account of change in variability with gestation;
- Verification that centiles are a good fit to the data.

In utero fetal growth studies have demonstrated that fetal growth is different in subsets of pregnancies with different maternal height and weight, smoking status, ethnic origin, parity and fetal sex. Gardosi et al [10] performed mathematical modelling which included the effects of above pregnancy characteristics to develop a customized birthweight standard. Customized fetal growth charts adjust for constitutional or physiological variation and exclude pathological factors that affect growth. Gardosi [11] proposed to determine individual growth potential rather than population-based standards, and to use estimated fetal weight rather than separate ultrasound measurements. Taking ethnicity into account may improve the accuracy of weight estimation [11]. Drooger et al [12] demonstrated variation of growth in different ethnic groups within the Dutch population, with some of the variation explained by maternal height and weight, age and parity. Fetal growth charts based on the same principles were constructed by Pang et al [13]. Customized charts appear to be more efficient in identifying pregnancies at risk of intrauterine fetal death (IUFD) compared with population-based charts. However, adding second trimester ultrasound biometric parameters to the customized model did not improve the prediction of IUFD compared with using maternal characteristics only [11]. An example of a population-based prospective cohort study is the Generation R study (Erasmus University Medical School, Rotterdam) which had been designed to identify early environmental and genetic determinants of growth, development and health. Reference curves for normal fetal growth as from 10 weeks of gestation onwards for fetal BPD, fetal HC and fetal AC and from 12 weeks onwards for fetal FL were constructed [2].

The issue of wide methodologies for the creation of fetal growth charts was further highlighted in a study evaluating the methodological quality of studies of fetal biometry using a set of predefined criteria of study design, statistical analysis and reporting methods [14]. Potential for bias was particularly noted for lack of a rigorous set of antenatal and fetal conditions which should be excluded from analysis; lack of ultrasound quality control measures as no study demonstrated a comprehensive quality assurance strategy; and lack of sample size calculation.

It became clear, there was a need for standardization of fetal growth assessment methodology. The World Health Organization (WHO) had produced international growth standards for infants and children up to the age of 5 years in 2006. Based on the same principle and methods, the Fetal Growth Longitudinal Study, as part of the Intergrowth-21st Project, aimed at developing international fetal growth and size standards [15]. Fetal growth was established taking fetal anthropometric measurements prospectively from 14+0 weeks of gestation until birth in a cohort of women at low risk of fetal growth restriction in eight geographically diverse countries in which most of the maternal health and nutritional needs were met and adequate antenatal care was provided. Based on >4300 pregnancies without major complications and delivery of live singletons without congenital abnormalities, the study generated international standards of fetal growth based on the primary ultrasound measures of fetal BPD, HC, AC, and FL according to gestational age. Within the same Intergrowth-21st Project, Cavallaro et al [16] made a distinction between *qualitative* control or visual assessment by sonographers of their images at eight different study sites based on specific criteria and *quantitative* assessment of measurement data by comparing the first, second and third ultrasound measurement in 20 000 ultrasound images from over 4000 fetuses at 14–41 weeks of gestation. Quality control monitoring turned out to be feasible and highly reproducible.

The need for the establishment of fetal growth charts for international use was also highlighted by the WHO. New fetal growth charts for common fetal measurements and estimated fetal weight were based on a longitudinal study of >1300 low-risk pregnancies from 10 countries (Argentina, Brazil, Democratic Republic of Congo, Denmark, Egypt, France, Germany, India, Norway and Thailand) that provided >8200 sets of ultrasound measurements [17]. The WHO fetal growth charts are intended to be used internationally based on low-risk pregnancies from populations in Africa, Asia, Europe and South America.

Fetal Growth and Obesity – – The increasing prevalence of maternal obesity emphasizes the need of establishing the association of maternal obesity with fetal growth. In a cohort study of pregnant women from 12 US healthcare institutions, it was demonstrated that fetal head circumference, humerus and femur length were significantly longer in the subset of obese women (body mass index (BMI) >30 kg/m^2) compared with non-obese women (BMI: 19–29.9). Fetal abdominal circumference was not greater in the obese cohort compared to the non-obese cohort, but was significantly larger than in fetuses of normal-weight women (BMI: 19.6–24.9). As from 32 weeks of gestation, estimated fetal weight in obese women was significantly higher than in non-obese women [18].

Fetal Growth in Twin Pregnancies – – Customized fetal growth charts have also been developed for twin pregnancies. Several studies have reported differences in fetal growth between singletons and twins. Based on population data from the USA National Centre for Health Statistics between 1995 and 2002, it was argued that plurality-specific fetal growth standards were needed [19]. This is supported by a more recent report demonstrating customized fetal growth charts designed specifically for twins to be more effective at identifying twin pregnancies at risk of poor fetal outcome [20].

14.2 Macrosomia

Fetal macrosomia is defined as a neonate with a birthweight at term above 4.5 kg. Occasionally, a gestational age-dependent definition, the 97th centile, is used. The prevalence in developed countries is 1.3–1.5% of all births for both definitions. Of all macrosomic fetuses, 5–10% are associated with maternal diabetes. Other risk factors are maternal obesity and family history [21]. In obese women (BMI: >30 kg/m^2), pre-pregnancy weight is the most important factor influencing birthweight. Even after adjustment for diabetes mellitus, obese women are 2–3 times more likely to give birth to a large-for-date infant [22].

14.2.1 Maternal and Fetal Risks of Macrosomia

Fetal macrosomia is associated with complications to both the mother and newborn. The emergency caesarean section rate is approximately 45% and the instrumental delivery rate 17% [23].

As for the newborn, there is an increased risk of shoulder dystocia which varies from 9 to 24%. Central nervous system injuries of the newborn have been seen following shoulder dystocia [24]. Another complication is brachial palsy injury, which in the presence of fetal macrosomia may be increased 18–21-fold when compared with the average incidence of 0.5–1.9 per 1000 in the general obstetric population. Other injuries as a result of fetal macrosomia are facial nerve injuries and fractures of the clavicle and humerus. Fetal growth above the 97th centile in the third trimester of pregnancy is associated with an increased risk of metabolic problems [25].

Complications to the mother are trauma to the bladder, perineum and anal sphincter. There is a strong correlation between fetal macrosomia and pelvic floor damage, development of anal and urinary stress incontinence and prolapse [21]. Particularly for sphincter damage, fetal macrosomia is a strong independent risk factor. There is a clear association between anal sphincter damage and maternal faecal incontinence. The incidence of anal sphincter injury following the delivery of a macrosomic fetus has been reported to be as high as 26%, with one third being symptomatic [26].

Vaginal birth may predispose to vaginal prolapse and urinary stress incontinence. This is even more so following the delivery of a macrosomic fetus. A clear association has been established between a large fetus, prolonged second stage and perineal nerve damage.

14.2.2 Fetal Weight Estimation and Macrosomia

Estimated fetal weight formulae are associated with large deviations when used in the macrosomic fetus. A literature review [27] demonstrated the post-test probability of sonographic-estimated fetal weight of >4000 g to identify a macrosomic newborn varied widely from 15 to 79%. Specific formulae for estimating the weight of the macrosomic fetus have been developed taking both fetal biometry and maternal height into account, resulting in improved detection rates of macrosomia [28].

14.3 Conclusions

Fetal growth is much determined by maternal characteristics, placental function and environmental factors. Sonographic parameters for establishing gestational age, fetal growth and size are the embryonic/fetal crown–rump length during the first trimester of pregnancy and the fetal biparietal diameter (BPD) and head circumference (HC), fetal abdominal circumference (AC) and fetal femur length (FL) in the second and third trimesters of pregnancy. Many methods of estimating fetal weight have been developed, ranging from a single biometric parameter to the combination of several parameters. Customized and population-based fetal growth charts have been developed. The need for standardization of growth curves has been emphasized. Customized fetal growth charts designed specifically for twins have shown to be more effective at identifying twin pregnancies at risk of poor fetal outcome. Fetal macrosomia which is defined as a neonate with a birthweight at term above 4.5 kg, is associated with complications to both the mother and newborn. Of all macrosomic fetuses, 5–10% are associated with maternal diabetes. Specific formulae for estimating the weight of the macrosomic fetus have been developed taking both fetal biometry and maternal height into account resulting in improved detection rates of macrosomia.

Acknowledgements

I am greatly indebted to Dr Daren Chaplin, Rosie Maternity, Addenbrooke's University Hospital, Cambridge, UK for Figures 14.1–14.3.

References

1. Stebbins B, Jaffe R. Fetal biometry and gestational age estimation. In Jaffe R, Bui TH, eds. *Textbook of Fetal Ultrasound*. Carnforth: Parthenon; 1999, pp 47–57.

2. Verburg BO, Steegers EAP, De Ridder M, et al. New charts for ultrasound dating of pregnancy and assessment of fetal growth: longitudinal data from a population-based cohort study. *Ultrasound Obstet Gynecol.* 2008;**31**:388–96.

3. Hadlock F, Harrist RB, Sharman RS, Deter RL, Park SK. Estimation of fetal weight with the use of head,body and femur measurements – a prospective study. *Am J ObstetGynecol.* 1985;**151**:333–7.

4. Dudley NJ. A systematic review of the ultrasound estimation of fetal weight. *Ultrasound Obstet Gynecol.* 2005;**25**:80–9.

5. Lee W, Balasubramaniam M, Deter RL, et al. New weight estimation models

using fractional limb volume. *Ultrasound Obstet Gynaecol.* 2009;**34**:556–65.

6. Stirnemann J, Villar J, Salomon LJ, et al. International estimated fetal weight standards of the Intergrowth-21st Project. *Ultrasound Obstet Gynecol.* 2017;**49**:478–86.

7. Uotila J, Dastidar P, Heinonen T, et al. Magnetic resonance imaging compared to ultrasonography in fetal weight and volume estimation in diabetic and normal pregnancy. *Acta Obstet Gynecol Scand.* 2000;**79**:255–9.

8. Papageorghiou AT, Bakoulas V, Sebire NJ, Nicolaides KH. Intrauterine growth in multiple pregnancies in relation to fetal number, chorionicity and gestational age. *Ultrasound Obstet Gynecol.* 2008;**32**:890–3.

9. Altman DG, Chitty LS. Design and analysis of studies to derive charts of fetal size. *Ultrasound Obstet Gynecol.* 1993;**3**:378–84.

10. Gardosi J, Mongelli M, Wilcox M. An adjustable fetal weight standard. *Ultrasound Obstet Gynecol.* 1995;**6**:168–74.

11. Gardosi J. Fetal growth: towards an international standard. *Ultrasound Obstet Gynecol.* 2005;**26**;112–14.

12. Drooger JC, Troe JWM, Borsboom GJJM, et al. Ethnic differences in prenatal growth and the association with maternal and fetal characteristics. *Ultrasound Obstet Gynecol.* 2005;**26**;115–22.

13. Pang MW, Leung TN, Sahata DS, Lau TK, Chang AMZ. Customizing fetal biometry charts. *Ultrasound Obstet Gynecol.* 2003;**22**:271–6.

14. Ioannou C, Talbot K, Ohuma E, et al. Systematic review of methodology used in ultrasound studies aimed at creating charts of fetal size. *BJOG.* 2012;**119**:1425–39.

15. Papageorghiou A, Ohuma EO, Altman DG, et al. International standards for growth based on serial ultrasound measurements: the Fetal Growth Longitudinal Study in the Intergrowth-21st Project. *Lancet.* 2014:**384**:869–79.

16. Cavallaro A, Ash ST, Napolitano R, et al. Quality control of ultrasound for biometry: results from the INTERGROWTH-21st Project. *Ultrasound Obstet Gynecol.* 2018;**52**:332.

17. Kiserud T, Benachi A, Hecher K, Piaggio G, Platt LD. The World Health fetal growth charts: concept, findings, interpretation, and application. *Am J Obstet Gynecol.* 2018, **218**(2):S619-S629.

18. Zhang C, Hediger ML, Albert PS, et al. Association of maternal obesity with longitudinal ultrasonographic measures of fetal growth: findings from the NICHD Fetal Growth Studies – Singletons. *JAMA Pediat.* 2018;**172**:24–31.

19. Joseph KS, Fahey J, Platt RW, et al. An outcome-based approach for the creation of fetal growth standards: do singletons and twins need separate standards? *Am J Epidemiol.* 2009;**169**:616–20.

20. Odibo AO, Cahill AG, Goetzinger KR, et al. Customized growth charts for twin gestations to optimize identification of small-for-gestational age fetuses at risk of intrauterine death.

Ultrasound Obstet Gynecol. 2013;**41**:637–42.

21. Campbell, S. Editorial: fetal macrosomia in need of a policy. *Ultrasound Obstet Gynecol.* 2014;**43**:3–10.

22. Ehrenberg HM, Mercer BM, Catalano PM. The influence of obesity and diabetes on the prevalence of macrosomia. *Am J Obstet Gynaecol.* 2004;**191**:964–968.

23. Kolderup LB, Laros RK Jr, Musci TJ. Incidence of persistent birth injury in macrosomic infants: association with mode of delivery. *Am J Obstet Gynecol.* 1997;**177**:37–41.

24. Iffy L, Brimacombe M, Appuzzio JJ, et al. The risk of shoulder dystocia related permanent fetal injury in relation to birth weight. *Eur J Obstet Gynecol Reprod Biol.* 2008;**136**:52–60.

25. Boney CM, Verma A, Tucker R, Vohr BR. Metabolic syndrome in childhood: association with birth weight, maternal obesity and gestational diabetes mellitus. *Pediatrics.* 2005;**115**:290–6.

26. Oberwalder M, Connor J, Wexner SD. Meta-analysis to determine the incidence of obstetric and sphincter damage. *Br J Surg.* 2003;**90**:1333–7.

27. Chauhan SP, Grobman WA, Gherman RA. Suspicion and treatment of the macrosomic fetus: a review. *Am J Obstet Gynecol.* 2005;**193**:332–46.

28. Hart NC, Hilbert A, Meurer B. Macrosomia: a new formula for optimized fetal weight estimation. *Ultrasound Obstet Gynecol.* 2010;**35**:42–4.

15.1 Introduction

Fetal haemolysis results from the breakdown of red blood cells secondary to immunoglobulin G (IgG) antibodies that pass from the mother through to the fetus resulting in anaemia and fetal hydrops which may result in intrauterine fetal death [1]. Fetal haemolysis is also known as haemolytic disease of the fetus and newborn (HDFN) and erythroblastosis fetalis. Historically, fetal haemolysis was almost synonymous with rhesus D (RhD) alloimmunization and was common until the late 1960s. Since crossmatching red blood cell transfusions for RhD and introduction of routine anti-D immunoglobin (anti-D Ig) prophylaxis in the 1970s, the spectrum of haemolytic disease of the fetus and newborn has changed dramatically [2].

There are a number of other red cell antibodies including anti-D Ig and anti-K Ig that are implicated in severe fetal haemolytic disease; these will be described in more detail in this chapter. There are many other antibodies that are unlikely to have a significant effect on the fetus but may result in neonatal anaemia or hyperbilirubinaemia. In addition, some antibodies will be more significant in the screening and provision of blood products for the mother, fetus or neonate [3].

15.2 Incidence and Epidemiology

Despite the success of the routine antenatal anti-D prophylaxis (RAADP) programme, RhD Ig remains the most commonly encountered antibody in pregnancy. The incidence of fetal haemolysis is variable through the world depending on ethnicity and the availability and uptake of anti-D Ig prophylaxis. In the UK, around 16% of women of childbearing age are RhD negative and around 10% of pregnancies are to RhD negative women carrying a RhD-positive fetus [4].The prevalence of rhesus antigens varies widely, from 0.3% in China to up to 15% in Caucasians in North America and Europe [5]. Despite a low uptake of anti-D Ig prophylaxis in low-income countries, the incidence of fetal haemolysis remains low, this is most likely due to the much lower prevalence of the RhD negative phenotype in these populations.

Before anti-D Ig became available, the incidence of RhD alloimmunization in RhD-negative women following two deliveries of RhD-positive, ABO-compatible infants was around 16%, and HDFN was a significant cause of morbidity and mortality. Following routine postpartum administration of anti-D Ig, the rate of alloimmunization decreased to around 2%. A further reduction in the sensitization rate to as low as 0.17% was then achieved by introducing routine antenatal prophylaxis during the third trimester of pregnancy [6].

Anti-c antibodies are rare but are associated with severe HDFN. In the majority of women, the presence of Anti-c Ig is associated with a prior blood transfusion. The exact incidence of fetal haemolysis with anti-c antibodies has not been determined. A review of 55 cases published in 2004 found that up to 25% of at risk fetuses developed severe haemolysis [7].

Anti-K Ig accounts for 10% of the cases of antibody-mediated fetal anaemia. A recent Canadian study calculated estimated anti-K Ig to be present in 0.1% of the antenatal population with blood transfusions again being implicated as the major sensitizing event leading to their development [8].

Haemolysis resulting from antibodies secondary to antigens to the ABO blood group system are reported in 2–3% of all births but severe cases are rare.

15.3 Blood Group Systems and Clinically Significant Antigens

The nomenclature involved in describing red cell antigens has evolved since the ABO blood group was first discovered by Landsteiner in 1900. Since then, several hundred red cell antigens have been identified, each belonging to one of over 30 blood group systems. The terminology is most likely complicated due the eponymous names assigned to antigens as they were discovered. In an effort to clarify the nomenclature, the International Society of Blood Transfusion (ISBT) has established an internationally agreed numerical system. This system is yet to have made its way into routine clinical practice. Additionally, incorrect use of the name of blood group systems when in fact referring to a specific antigen within that system is used in clinical practice. The most common example of this is referring to patients as being Rh (rhesus)negative or positive when referring to the D antigen status [9]. It is therefore important to understand the current nomenclature used for describing blood group systems and clinically significant antigens.

The antigens expressed by the red blood cell of an individual are determined by the pattern of inheritance from the parents. Any particular red cell antigen is expressed by an individual if he or she is heterozygous or homozygous for the gene responsible for its expression. This means that if the mother does not carry an antigen and the father does, then the likelihood of the baby carrying the antigen will be 100% if the father is homozygously positive and 50% if the father is heterozygously positive. Equally, if the baby is negative for the risky antigen, then there is no risk of fetal or neonatal haemolysis.

Table 15.1 The blood group systems and antibodies implicated in fetal and neonatal haemolysis

Blood group system (ISBT* number)	Major antigens / antibodies	Chromosome location	Antibodies implicated in severe HDFN
ABO (001)	A, B, A$_1$B, A$_1$	9	
MNS (002)	M,N,S, s, U	4	
Rh (004)	**D**, C, **E, c**, e	1	D, c, c+E,
Kell (006)	**K**, k, Kp^a	7	K
Duffy (008)	Fy^a, Fy^b	1	
Kidd (009)	Jk^a	18	
H (018)	H	19	

*ISBT: International Society of Blood Transfusion. Antigens/antibodies highlighted in bold are those known to cause severe HDFN [3, 9].

Anti-D, -c and -K are the main antibodies known to cause the majority of cases of severe anaemia, hydrops, jaundice or death of the fetus and newborn, but other antibodies have also been implicated in rarer cases of severe disease. Table 15.1 lists the majority of the red blood cell antibodies known to be implicated in fetal and neonatal haemolysis [3, 9].

Antibodies of the ABO blood group systems can cause mild to moderate anaemia and jaundice in the neonate and occasionally in the fetus. This is most likely when the mother has the blood group O, and therefore has both anti-A and anti-B antibodies while the fetus has the blood group A or B [3].

15.4 Risk Factors for the Development of Maternal Alloantibodies

The development of alloantibodies requires a sensitizing event. The larger the volume of blood encountered, the higher the risk of antibody formation, hence the most common sensitizing event is a blood transfusion where exposure to a foreign red cell antigen results in the formation of antibodies to antigens not expressed by the recipient. Routinely, blood is tested and matched for just ABO and RhD antigens; hence, blood transfusions can trigger the formation of other antibodies that are major contributors to fetal haemolysis such as anti-K (Kell blood group system) or anti-c and anti-E (Rh blood group system).

Fetomaternal bleeding results in fetal red blood cells entering the maternal circulation. In instances when the fetal red cells carry antigens not expressed by the mother, alloantibody formation is again triggered. Fetomaternal haemorrhage can occur at any stage of pregnancy as a result of miscarriage, ectopic pregnancy, amniocentesis, placental abruption, abdominal trauma or delivery. It can also occur without the presence of a recognized sensitizing event.

Even a minimal fetomaternal haemorrhage of 0.1 mL can lead to the formation of anti-D antibodies [10]. Spontaneous miscarriages have been shown to carry a 1.5–2% risk of alloimmunization in susceptible women, while the risk following surgical management is estimated as 4–5%. The risk of fetomaternal haemorrhage following chorionic villus sampling

Table 15.2 Sensitizing events that increase the risk of development of red cell antibodies

Sensitizing events

- Blood transfusion
- Early pregnancy
  - Spontaneous miscarriage
  - Surgical management of miscarriage
  - Termination
  - Ectopic pregnancy

- Events leading to fetomaternal haemorrhage
  - Amniocentesis
  - Chorionic villus sampling
  - Cordocentesis
  - In utero therapeutic procedures such as blood transfusion
  - Abdominal trauma
  - External cephalic version
  - Placental abruption
  - Delivery: normal, assisted or surgical
  - Intraoperative cell salvage

- Shared needles

(CVS) is 14%, whilst the risk following both amniocentesis and attempted external cephalic version has been estimated at around 2–6%. It is therefore recommended that each of these events should be covered by anti-D Ig.

Table 15.2 provides a list of sensitizing events [10].

Assisted reproductive techniques in themselves are not known to increase the risk of red cell alloimmunization; however, where a donor egg is used for a mother with a known alloantibody, it may be advisable to carry out fetal genotyping.

Following sensitization, subsequent exposure during a future pregnancy will elicit an antibody response.

15.5 Mechanism of Fetal Haemolysis

For fetal haemolysis to occur, the woman needs to be negative for a red cell antigen which is present in her partner and for

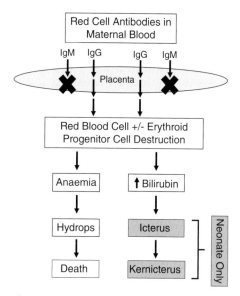

Figure 15.1 Pathophysiology of HDFN.

which she has been previously sensitized. In addition, the gene for the antigen is required to have been inherited by the fetus. For fetal haemolysis to occur, the antibody needs to be transported across the placenta. IgG antibodies are transported across the placenta, while IgM antibodies are not. This narrows the possibility of the antigen that can be implicated in the disease process.

IgG red cell antibodies are actively transported across the placenta (Figure 15.1). If the fetal red cells carry the corresponding antigen, the IgG antibody will bind to these antigens and cause destruction of the red cells. This process is known as haemolysis. Initially, the fetus may compensate for this by triggering erythropoiesis, which may result in hepatosplenomegaly. If the degree of haemolysis is extensive, the compensatory mechanisms are insufficient, and the fetus becomes anaemic. The anaemia causes the fetus to develop a hyperdynamic circulation, which results in cardiomegaly, fetal hydrops with the accumulation of fluid in the body cavities and skin, heart failure and eventually fetal death [11]. In addition, some antibodies such as anti-K result in a destruction of erythroid progenitor cells, hence resulting in an earlier anaemia without erythropoiesis. Red cell destruction also results in a hyperbilirubinaemia. Although in the fetus the bilirubin enters the maternal circulation and is cleared by the mother, in the newborn the immature liver is not able to sufficiently conjugate the bilirubin. In severe cases, hyperbilirubinaemia may lead to irreversible damage to the central nervous system [12].

15.6 Prevention

The prevention of HDFN plays a key role in reducing its incidence. The most notable reduction has been observed following the introduction of RAADP. The incidence can be further reduced by judicious use of blood transfusions in young women to avoid unnecessary sensitizing events. Where necessary, it has been suggested that extended matching of

blood prior to transfusion may also play a role in reducing the risk of fetal haemolysis. A Dutch Cohort Study (2016) showed that extended matching of blood in women needing repeated transfusions to include the C, c, E, K, and Jk^a will prevent alloimmunization to these antibodies [13].

All women should have their blood group and antibody status determined at booking and then checked again at 28 weeks of gestation to identify babies at risk of HDFN [3, 14].

15.6.1 Anti-D Prophylaxis

If postnatal anti-D prophylaxis is not given, 14% will develop anti-D antibodies within 6 months or during a subsequent pregnancy. In contrast, in those that receive anti-D prophylaxis, 1.8% will develop antibodies. This is likely due to iso-immunization during the pregnancy or transplacental haemorrhage at the time of delivery [5].

In RhD-negative women who are already sensitized and have developed anti-D antibodies, there is no benefit in the use of anti-D Ig prophylaxis and these women should be managed in accordance with the following recommendations: The American College of Obstetricians and Gynecologists (ACOG) practice bulletin *Prevention of RhD Alloimmunization* (2017) and the British Committee for Standards in Haematology (BCSH) guideline for the use of anti-D immunoglobulin for the prevention of HDFN (2013) both outline the recommended indications, timing and dosages for anti-D immunoglobulin administration following sensitizing events which are summarized below [6, 10].

15.6.1.1 Laboratory Testing

Routine testing for blood group and antibody screening should be carried out at booking and at 28 weeks of gestation.

Following sensitizing events in gestations below 20 weeks, maternal blood grouping and antibody screening should be performed to confirm the RhD and antibody status. Where new anti-D antibodies are detected, anti-D should be administered as indicated until confirmatory tests have established if these reflect the development of alloantibodies. Where the tests are unable to differentiate between passive anti-D Ig from previous anti-D Ig administration or from the development of alloantibodies, anti-D should be administered as normal. A test to confirm fetomaternal haemorrhage is not indicated at this gestation.

Following sensitizing events between 20 weeks' gestation and term, maternal blood group and antibody testing should be performed and interpreted as described above. In addition, a test should be carried out to quantify the amount of fetomaternal haemorrhage. If a fetomaternal haemorrhage of greater than 4 mL is detected, then a follow-up sample is required 48 to 72 hours after anti-D Ig administration to determine clearance.

15.6.1.2 Routine Antenatal Anti-D Ig Prophylaxis (RAADP)

For non-sensitized RhD-negative women, RAADP is recommended in the third trimester and following birth if the baby is found to be RhD positive. Third trimester prophylaxis can be administered as a large 1500 IU dose at 28 weeks or as two smaller doses of 500 IU each at 28 and 34 weeks of gestation.

Following delivery, the baby's RhD status should be confirmed using cord blood or a heel prick test. Where the baby is found to be RhD positive, a 500 IU dose of anti-D Ig should be administered. Maternal testing should also be carried out at least 30 minutes following delivery to screen for additional antibodies and to quantify any fetomaternal haemorrhage that may have occurred. Additional dosing may be required depending on the result.

15.6.1.3 Anti-D Ig Administration for Sensitizing Events <20 Weeks' Gestation

In line with both the ACOG and BCSH guidelines, anti-D Ig is offered to all non-sensitized RhD-negative pregnant women in the UK in the third trimester at about 28 weeks of gestation. Following delivery, cord blood is sent to determine the RhD antigen status of the baby and anti-D Ig is administered to the mother if the baby is RhD positive. Additionally, anti-D Ig is also offered to this group of women following a sensitizing event. This should ideally be administered within 72 hours, but in the presence of extenuating circumstances, some protection may be offered if anti-D Ig is administered within 10 days [6, 10].

Where minimal bleeding or complete spontaneous miscarriage occurs prior to 12 weeks' gestation and the uterus is not instrumented, the risk of fetomaternal haemorrhage is negligible and hence anti-D Ig is not recommended. There is, however, a significant risk of fetomaternal haemorrhage in the presence of an ectopic or molar pregnancy and termination or surgical management of miscarriage regardless of gestation, so in these cases a minimum dose of 250 IU of anti-D Ig should be offered. The same minimal dose of anti-D Ig should also be offered in cases where there is a heavy or recurrent bleed in an ongoing pregnancy prior to 12 weeks' gestation, especially in the presence of abdominal pain [6, 10].

In pregnancies between 12 to 20 weeks of gestation, 250 IU of anti-D Ig should be administered for all sensitizing events as discussed previously. In cases on ongoing vaginal bleeding at this gestation, 250 IU anti-D Ig should be administered a minimum of 6 weeks apart [6, 10].

15.6.1.4 Anti-D Ig Administration for Sensitizing Events from 20 Weeks' Gestation to Term

Women at 20 weeks or more of gestation who have been exposed to a potentially sensitizing event should receive a minimum of 500 IU anti-D Ig. This dosage should be administered regardless of timing of 28-week RAADP. Additional dosage may be needed if indicated by the fetomaternal haemorrhage quantification testing. If continued bleeding in pregnancy occurs but this is deemed to be the same sensitizing event on clinical grounds, 500 IU anti-D Ig dosage should be repeated after a minimum of 6 weeks. In these situations, testing for fetomaternal haemorrhage should be carried out at two-weekly intervals [6].

15.7 Management

Routine pre-pregnancy screening for red cell antibodies is not recommended; however, women known to have significant antibodies identified in a previous pregnancy or incidentally should be offered appropriate pre-pregnancy counselling depending on the maternal and/or fetal implications of the antibodies identified [3].

15.7.1 Paternal Bloods

Where clinically significant maternal red cell antibodies are detected, the paternal phenotype can be ascertained using serology. However, genotyping is required to determine whether he is homozygous or heterozygous for the *RHD* gene. If the father is homozygous, then all pregnancies are at risk. On the other hand, if the father is heterozygous, there is a 50% chance of the pregnancy being at risk. An alternative option would be to proceed to fetal genotyping using cell-free fetal DNA (see below), as this takes away any uncertainty that may arise from non-paternity.

15.7.2 Cell-Free Fetal DNA

Maternal blood can be used to detect cell-free fetal DNA (cffDNA) and determine D, C, c, E, e and K antigens expression. For other antigens, invasive testing using amniocentesis or CVS can be considered specially where the test is being carried out for another indication [15].

When carrying out cffDNA, it is important to recognize that the results are 95–98% accurate so there is a risk of missing small numbers of pregnancies at risk. Genotyping can take place from 16 weeks, except for K. The test for K antigen expression should be delayed until 20 weeks due to the risk of attaining a false negative test result [3].

Cell-free fetal DNA testing may be particularly useful in the presence of persistent bleeding following 20 weeks of gestation to try and avoid repeated doses of anti-D Ig being unnecessarily administered in the presence of a RhD-negative baby [6].

It has been postulated that cffDNA testing could also be used to avoid the use of anti-D Ig in those pregnancies that are not at risk. Currently around 40 000 women in England and Wales receive anti-D Ig unnecessarily as they carry a fetus that is RhD negative. Testing of cffDNA could help to establish the RhD status of the fetus and allow for targeted administration of anti-D Ig only to those RhD-negative women who are at risk. However, at present this test is not available to all RhD-negative patients in the absence of sensitization. A study conducted in the south-west of England and published in 2014 demonstrated that cffDNA testing allowed a 29% reduction in the administration of anti-D Ig dosages, which equated to 35% of women avoiding receiving unnecessary RAADP [16]. In addition, this study calculated the cost of performing the cffDNA test would be covered by the savings from reducing the use of anti-D Ig [17].

15.7.3 Antibody-Level Monitoring

Traditionally, antibody titration is used to determine clinically significant antibody levels using a double dilutional technique (1 in 2, 1 in 4, 1 in 8, etc.). The titre reported is the reciprocal of the highest dilution that gives a positive result. There is considered to be a significant rise when there is an increase in titre of more than one dilution (e.g. a previous titre of 4 rising to a titre of 16). Very careful attention to technique is necessary to ensure results are valid and reproducible [18].

Measuring concentrations of antibodies requires specific equipment and currently anti-D and anti-c are the only antibodies for which validated equipment is available to measure concentrations. These are reported as IU/mL in some countries, including the UK. All other antibody levels are established using a double dilution titration technique.

Anti-D, anti-c and anti-K Ig levels should be tested every four weeks until 28 weeks' gestation, then fortnightly until delivery. When other antibodies are detected at booking, the levels should be re-checked at 28 weeks and additional antibodies looked for, which may have developed. For rarer antibodies, set thresholds have not been established and individualized plans should be established with advice from the transfusion services.

An anti-D Ig level of less than 4 IU/mL is unlikely to cause fetal haemolysis. There is a moderate risk at levels between 4 IU/mL and 15 IU/mL, while levels above 15 IU/mL present a high risk of haemolysis [19].

The thresholds for anti-c levels implicated in HDFN are higher than for anti-D. Anti-c Ig levels of less than 7.5 IU/mL carry a low risk, levels between 7.5 IU/mL and 20 IU/mL a moderate risk and those above 20 IU/mL a high risk. These levels therefore dictate the recommendations for referral for more intensive monitoring as described below [20].

15.7.4 Referral to Fetal Medicine Specialist

The RCOG Green-top Guideline (2014) outlines a number of scenarios in which referral to a fetal medicine specialist are recommended [3]. These are described in more detail below.

• Previous history of a pregnancy affected by HDFN regardless of antibody titre levels.

Where there is a history of a previous pregnancy affected by HDFN, specialist review is required to determine the potential risks of recurrence in the current pregnancy and to make an individualized plan accordingly. The important features in the previous history that would point towards the need for close monitoring of the index pregnancy include a need for intrauterine transfusion, the gestation at which they were commenced, gestation at delivery and the need for exchange transfusions and phototherapy. The majority of clinicians are likely to carry out serial ultrasound monitoring even when antibody levels are low in such cases [3, 14].

• Signs of fetal anaemia on antenatal ultrasound scan.

If fetal anaemia is suspected on fetal ultrasound scan, namely a raised middle cerebral artery (MCA) peak systolic velocity (PSV) or signs of fetal hydrops, then urgent referral is recommended regardless of the antibody status.

• Presence of anti-K antibody or co-existing anti-E and anti-c antibodies, regardless of titre levels.

Where anti-K antibodies are present or where anti-E and anti-c antibodies coexist, fetal haemolysis is known to occur

even at very low titre levels; therefore, referral should be made at the time that the antibodies are detected [12].

• Anti-D levels of <4 IU/mL or anti-c levels of <7.5 IU/mL.

Anti-D Ig levels over 4 IU/mL and anti-c levels of over 7.5 IU/mL confer a risk of fetal anaemia, which makes referral to a fetal medicine specialist for regular ultrasound screening for signs of fetal anaemia necessary [3].

15.7.5 Ultrasound Monitoring

Historically, fetal anaemia in at risk pregnancies was quantified using amniocentesis and the analysis of the amniotic fluid. The amniotic fluid spectrophotometry was then performed to assess bilirubin levels via optical density. Due to the invasive nature of this test, pregnancies were exposed to the risk of miscarriage, preterm rupture of membranes and preterm labour.

This test has now been superseded by MCA PSV Doppler assessment, which is a non-invasive ultrasound assessment with reasonable sensitivity and specificity. A randomized controlled trial by Oepkes et al (2006) concluded that Doppler ultrasonography was 12% more sensitive and 9% more accurate when compared to the measurement of amniotic fluid optical density [21]. However, a systematic review by Pretlove et al (2009), which assessed the value of MCA PSV in the evaluation of fetal anaemia, identified that the positive and negative predictive values of MCA PSV Doppler are not ideal. It highlighted the need for the development of more accurate, non-invasive screening modalities [22]. However, in the absence of such established techniques, MCA PSV remains widely used as the gold standard test for predicting fetal anaemia in most developed and developing countries. Therefore, when a pregnancy is deemed to be at a moderate to high risk of developing haemolysis, established by prior history or antibody levels, the woman should be referred to a specialist able to screen for fetal anaemia MCA PSV Doppler as well as looking for other signs such as polyhydramnios, cardiomegaly, skin oedema and fetal hydrops.

At risk pregnancies should be screened with weekly ultrasound scans. An MCA PSV greater that 1.5 MoM (multiples of the median) is indicative of fetal anaemia with a sensitivity of 100% and a false positive rate of 12%. This finding should therefore trigger a prompt review by a specialist able to perform fetal blood sampling and intrauterine transfusion (IUT) if needed.

15.7.6 Fetal Blood Sampling / Intrauterine Transfusion (IUT)

Fetal blood sampling and IUT administration are highly specialized procedures. The woman should be adequately counselled regarding the risks and benefits of the procedure including the potential outcomes in the absence of the procedure to allow her to make an informed decision. The procedure should be performed in centres that have the requisite expert skills in fetal medicine and perinatal haematology.

Red cell preparations used for IUTs should be group O or ABO identical with the fetus; in addition, they should be negative for antigen corresponding to the mother's antibodies. Furthermore, the blood should ideally be K-negative, cytomegalovirus seronegative, less than 5 days old and transfused within 24 hours of irradiation. Ideally fetal blood sampling should only be performed once the appropriate blood is available. The fetal blood should be tested immediately and IUT performed at the same time if needed [3].

The thresholds for performing IUT following fetal blood sample results is variable between fetal medicine centres. It is generally agreed that IUTs should be performed if the fetal haemoglobin is four to five standard deviations below the mean/median for that gestational age or when there is a haemoglobin deficit of 5 g/dL or more. IUTs are performed under direct ultrasound guidance. The use of premedication, local or regional anaesthesia varies between centres [23]. Transfusion volumes depend on gestational fetoplacental blood volume, fetal haematocrit and donor haematocrit. Standardized nomograms along with perceived risk of cardiovascular overload are then used to decide on the volume to be transfused [24].

Various techniques can be used to perform an IUT. A Cochrane review published in 2012 found that there is a paucity of high-quality data from randomized controlled trials to guide clinicians in choosing an optimal technique [25]. The most common fetal puncture site for IUT is intrahepatic or at the level of the cord insertion. Less commonly 'free loops' of cord can be used but are associated with a higher complication rate. Intraperitoneal transfusions are used by some centres in combination with intrahepatic or transplacental techniques in an attempt to prolong the intertransfusion interval but they carry the disadvantage of a longer and higher risk procedure. In some cases, especially at earlier gestations, intravascular access may be limited, making intraperitoneal access the only option.

15.7.6.1 Outcome Following IUT

The overall perinatal survival following treatment IUT over the last 10 years has been reported between 88.9 and 100% [23]. Procedure-related complications include bleeding from fetal puncture site, infection, cord occlusion, fetal demise, preterm rupture of membranes, miscarriage and preterm birth. The risk profile has improved over the decades with increased expertise and better equipment. It is recommended that IUTs should be performed by those with enough activity to be performing around 10 procedures a year. The risks are found to be highest in earlier gestations, particularly in pregnancies at less than 22 weeks' gestation [23].

Long-term neurodevelopmental and cardiovascular outcomes of babies following IUT have been studied. The neurodevelopmental outcome appears to be related to the underlying indication for the IUT and the severity of fetal disease. For instance, the presence of severe fetal hydrops or parvovirus B19 associated with adverse long-term neurodevelopmental outcome. In contrast, where the anaemia is attributed to red cell alloimmunization, over 95% of children have a normal neurodevelopmental outcome [26]. A retrospective cohort study by Wallace et al (2017) compared the long-term cardiovascular outcome of those that had required an IUT to treat fetal anaemia to their non-anaemic siblings and found that cardiovascular development is altered in the exposed group and these changes persist through into adulthood. Adults that had been exposed to an IUT were found to have smaller, thicker-walled hearts and an unfavourable lipid profile when compared to their siblings [27].

15.7.7 Other Treatment Options

In view of the high risk of complications of IUTs, especially at earlier gestations, several non-invasive techniques have been investigated.

Intravenous immunoglobulin (IVIG) works by reducing or preventing fetal haemolysis rather than treating the fetal anaemia. Several mechanisms for this have been proposed including inhibition of antibody passage through the placenta to the fetus and a negative feedback on maternal antibody production. Various proposed treatment regimens for IVIG have been proposed. Most advocate starting its use from around 12 weeks' gestation with weekly administration, sometimes with a more intensive loading regime in the first week [23]. A Cochrane review published in 2013 found no randomized controlled trials but reported that several case series have suggested a beneficial role in delaying the onset of fetal anaemia requiring transfusion [28].

Therapeutic plasma exchange is another treatment modality that has been shown to reduce the risk of fetal haemolysis rather than treat fetal anaemia. It involves removing and replacing the mother's plasma with albumin-rich fluid. This involves passing the woman's blood through a separator, thus removing the maternal antibodies. This technique has been showed to decrease antibody titres by up to 75%. This technique had also been used and found to be beneficial in combination with IVIG [23].

Although both these non-invasive techniques show promise in the delay for need for IUT, further rigorous evaluation of both techniques is required and at present their use remains confined to severe early cases on an individualized basis.

15.8 Mode, Place and Timing of Birth

There is limited evidence to help guide decisions regarding mode, place and timing of birth. Both ACOG and RCOG guidelines suggest delivery at 37–38 weeks' gestation in cases where antibodies implicated in HDFN are present but have been stable throughout the pregnancy [3, 14]. In cases where an IUT has not been required but antibody levels are rising, an elective late preterm delivery may be justified. In cases requiring multiple transfusions, the risks associated with IUT need to be balanced against the potential sequelae of prematurity. Delivery is usually timed by taking into consideration the timing of the latest IUT, as it is preferable not to deliver a baby in a severely anaemic state. Decisions regarding delivery in these cases are complex and influenced by multiple factors. They should therefore be made in centres with experience in managing such cases in conjunction with the fetal medicine specialists, haematologists and neonatologists. An IUT in itself is not a contraindication to a vaginal delivery and usual obstetric factors should guide the chosen mode of delivery. Pregnancies complicated by such antibodies are considered high risk and continuous fetal monitoring is advisable in such cases.

15.9 Postnatal Management

Babies of all RhD-negative women should have cord blood sent to determine ABO and RhD typing to establish the need for postnatal RAADP. In addition, where maternal antibodies exist, cord blood should be subjected to the direct antiglobulin test (DAT) and haemoglobin and bilirubin levels checked. These additional tests are essential to help determine the degree of neonatal haemolysis and thus help to guide initial neonatal management.

The severity of disease at the time of delivery will determine the intensity of neonatal support required. Where possible, these babies should be delivered in a unit that has the appropriate facilities and expertise. Babies with severe HDFN resulting in hydrops may need immediate intervention at birth, such as the insertion of chest drains to allow the lungs to inflate. Following delivery, the babies should be closely monitored for

signs of anaemia and jaundice with particular attention to haemoglobin and bilirubin levels. If the bilirubin levels rise above the threshold level, phototherapy or exchange transfusions may become necessary.

15.10 Key Guidelines

Royal College of Obstetrics and Gynecologists (RCOG). *The Management of Women with Red Cell Antibodies during Pregnancy*. Green-top Guideline No 65, May 2014.

American College of Obstetricians and Gynecologists. *Prevention of RhD Alloimmunization*. ACOG Practice Bulletin 181. ACOG 2017.

American College of Obstetricians and Gynecologists. *Management of Alloimmunization during Pregnancy*. ACOG Practice Bulletin 192. ACOG 2018.

White J, Qureshi H, Massey E, et al. Guideline for blood grouping and red cell antibody testing in pregnancy. *Transfusion Med.* 2016;**26**:246–63. doi: 10.1111/tme.12299

Qureshi H, Massey E, Kirwan D, et al. BCSH guideline for the use of anti-D immunoglobulin for the prevention of haemolytic disease of the fetus and newborn. *Transfusion Med.* 2014;**24**:8–20. DOI:10.1111/tme.12091.

References

1. Chatziantoniou V, Heeney N, Maggs T, et al. A descriptive single-centre experience of the management and outcome of maternal alloantibodies in pregnancy. *Transfusion Med.* 2017;**27**:275–85. doi: 10.1111/tme.12430

2. Koelewijn JM, Vrijkotte TG, de Haas M, van der Schoot CE, Bonsel GJ. Risk factors for the presence of non-rhesus D red blood cell antibodies in pregnancy. *BJOG.* 2009;**116**(5):655–64. doi: 10.1111/j.1471-0528.2008.01984.x

3. Royal College of Obstetrics and Gynaecologists (RCOG). *The Management of Women with Red Cell Antibodies during Pregnancy*. Green-top Guideline No 65, May 2014.

4. Chilcott J, Lloyd Jones M, Wight J, et al. A review of the clinical effectiveness and cost-effectiveness of routine anti-D prophylaxis for pregnant women who are rhesus-negative. 2003. In *NIHR Health Technology Assessment Programme: Executive Summaries*. Southampton: NIHR Journals Library; 2003–. www.ncbi.nlm.nih.gov/books/NBK62211/

5. Zipursky A, Paul VK. The global burden of Rh disease. *Arch Dis Child Fetal Neonatal Ed.* 2011;**96**:F84–5.

6. Qureshi H, Massey E, Kirwan D, et al. BCSH guideline for the use of anti-D immunoglobulin for the prevention of haemolytic disease of the fetus and newborn. *Transfusion Med.* 2014; **24**:8–20. doi: 10.1111/tme.12091

7. Hackney DN, Fau KE, Fau RK, et al. Management of pregnancies complicated by anti-c isoimmunization. *Obstet Gynecol.* 2004;**103**(1):24–30.

8. Goldman M, Lane D, Webert K, Fallis R. The prevalence of anti-K in Canadian prenatal patients. *Transfusion.* 2015;**55**:1486–91. doi: 10.1111/trf.13151

9. Smart E, Armstrong B, Blood group systems. *ISBT Science Series.* 2009;**3**:68–92. doi: 10.1111/j.1751-2824.2008.00188.x

10. American College of Obstetricians and Gynecologists. *Prevention of RhD Alloimmunization*. ACOG Practice Bulletin 181. ACOG 2017.

11. de Haas M, Thurik F, Koelewijn J, Schoot C, Haemolytic disease of the fetus and newborn. *Vox Sang.* 2015;**109**:99–113. doi: 10.1111/vox.12265

12. Daniels G, Hadley A, Green CA. Causes of fetalanemia in hemolytic disease due to anti-K. *Transfusion.* 2003;**43**:115–16. doi: 10.1046/j.1537-2995.2003.00327.x

13. Evers D, Middelburg RA, de Haas M, et al. Red-blood-cell alloimmunisation in relation to antigens' exposure and their immunogenicity: a cohort study. *Lancet Haematol.* 2016;**3**(6):e284–92. https://doi.org/10.1016/S2352-3026(16)30019-9.

14. American College of Obstetricians and Gynecologists. *Management of Alloimmunization during Pregnancy*. ACOG Practice Bulletin 192. ACOG 2018.

15. Scheffer P, van der Schoot C, Page-Christiaens G, de Haas M. Noninvasive fetal blood group genotyping of rhesus D, c, E and of K in alloimmunised pregnant women: evaluation of a 7-year clinical experience. *BJOG.* 2011;**118**:1340–8. doi: 10.1111/j.1471-0528.2011.03028.x

16. Kent J, Farrell A, Soothill P. Routine administration of anti-D: the ethical case for offering pregnant women fetal *RHD* genotyping and a review of policy and practice. *BMC Pregnancy Childbirth.* 2014;**14**:87. doi: 10.1186/1471-2393-14-87

17. Soothill PW, Finning K, Latham T, et al. Use of cffDNA to avoid administration of anti-D to pregnant women when the fetus is RhD-negative: implementation in the NHS. *BJOG.* 2015;**122**:1682–6. https://doi.org/10.1111/1471-0528.13055

18. White J, Qureshi H, Massey E, et al. Guideline for blood grouping and red cell antibody testing in pregnancy. *Transfusion Med.* 2016;**26**:246–63. doi: 10.1111/tme.12299

19. Nicolaides KH, Rodeck CH. Maternal serum anti-D antibody concentration and assessment of rhesus isoimmunisation. *BMJ*. 1992, **304**:1155–6.

20. Kozlowski CL, Lee D, Shwe KH, Love EM. Quantification of anti-c in haemolytic disease of the newborn. *Transfusion Med*. 1995;**5**:37–42.

21. Oepkes D, Seaward G, Vandenbussche FP, et al. Doppler ultrasonography versus amniocentesis to predict anaemia. *N Engl J Med*. 2006;**355**:156–4. doi: 10.1056/NEJMoa052855

22. Pretlove S, Fox C, Khan K, Kilby M. Noninvasive methods of detecting fetal anaemia: a systematic review and meta-analysis. *BJOG*. 2009;**116**:1558–67. doi: 10.1111/j.1471-0528.2009.02255.x

23. Zwier C, van Kamp I, Oepkes D, Lopriore E. Intrauterine transfusion and non-invasive treatment options for hemolytic disease of the fetus and newborn – review on current management and outcome. *Expert Review of Hematol*. 2017;**10**(4):337–44. doi: 10.1080/17474086.2017.1305265.

24. Rodeck CH, Nicolaides KH, Warsof SL, et al. The management of severe rhesus isoimmunization by fetoscopic intravascular transfusions. *Am J Obstet Gyanecol*. 1984;**150**(6):769–74. https://doi.org/10.1016/0002-9378

25. Dodd JM, Windrim RC, van Kamp IL. Techniques of intrauterine fetal transfusion for women with red-cell isoimmunisation for improving health outcomes. *Cochrane Database Syst Rev*. 2012 Sep 12(9):CD007096. doi: 10.1002/14651858.CD007096.pub3

26. Lindenburg IT, Klink JM, Smits-Wintjens VE, et al. Long-term neurodevelopmental and cardiovascular outcome after intrauterine transfusions for fetal anaemia: a review. *Prenat Diagn*. 2013;**33**:815–22. doi:10.1002/pd.4152

27. Wallace AH, Dalziel SR, Cowan BR, et al. Long-term cardiovascular outcome following fetal anaemia and intrauterine transfusion: a cohort study. *Arch Dis Child*. 2017;**102**:40–45.

28. Wong KS, Connan K, Rowlands S, Kornman LH, Savoia HF. Antenatal immunoglobulin for fetal red blood cell alloimmunization. *Cochrane Database Syst Rev*. 2013 May 31(5):CD008267. doi: 10.1002/14651858.CD008267.pub2

Chapter 16

Antenatal Care of a Normal Pregnancy

Irene Hösli, Gwendolin Manegold-Brauer & Olav Lapaire

16.1 Definition of Antenatal Care and Purpose

Antenatal care (ANC) of a normal pregnancy is defined as the routine care of presumed healthy, pregnant women with a singleton uncomplicated pregnancy provided between conception and the onset of labour. A woman's health during her pregnancy is critical to the outcome of the pregnancy and may have a lifelong impact on her and her baby's health.

ANC is an opportunity to provide evidence-based information for use by clinicians and pregnant women to make decisions about screening and appropriate treatment in specific circumstances. For the woman, any intervention or treatment should have known benefits and be appropriate, accessible, of high quality and acceptable for her. She and her partner should be treated with respect and dignity and her views, beliefs and values in relation to her care should be sought and respected at all times [1].

The aim of the ANC is

- Optimal outcome for mother and child with a general reduction of maternal and perinatal morbidity and mortality
- Individual satisfaction and positive experience with pregnancy, delivery and postpartum period
- Early recognition of maternal/fetal conditions and appropriate treatment
- Adherence to efficacy, usefulness and cost-effectiveness

Although ANC is a core component of maternity care, both quality of care provision and rates of attendance vary widely between and within countries. For women, initial or continued use of ANC depends on a perception that doing so will be a positive experience.

The capacity of healthcare providers to deliver the kind of high-quality, relationship-based, locally accessible ANC depends on the provision of sufficient training and education, sufficient resources and staffing as well as the time to provide flexible personalized, private appointments that are not overloaded with organizational tasks [2].

ANC in its current form became the standard of care before any randomized controlled trials were conducted to prove efficacy concerning the number of ANC visits, the content of the care and the group providing the care.

16.2 Number of Antenatal Care Visits

The number of visits for ANC has developed without evidence of how many visits are necessary. In a Cochrane review, where

a reduced number of antenatal visits was compared with standard care, women were less satisfied with the reduced visits schedule and perceived the gap between visits as too long.

In high-income countries, there were no differences in perinatal mortality between women randomized to higher vs. reduced (eight visits) ANC visit groups, but low- and middle-income countries had significantly higher rates of perinatal mortality in women with a reduced ANC schedule (fewer than five) (RR 1.15; 95% CI 1.01 to 1.32) [3]. In a Finnish hospital register-based cohort under 1–5 visits or non-attendance of ANC was associated with social and health behavioural risk factors: unmarried status, lower educational level, young maternal age, smoking and alcohol use. There were significantly more low birthweight infants in under- and non-attenders (OR: with 95% CI): 9.18 (6.65–12.68) and 5.46 (3.90–7.65), respectively, more fetal deaths: 5.19 (2.04–13.22) and 12.05 (5.95–24.40), respectively, and more neonatal deaths: 10.03 (3.85–26.13) and 8.66 (3.59–20.86), respectively [4]. Contrariwise, more ANC visits may not necessarily mean better outcomes. In a retrospective cohort, low-risk women with more than 10 antenatal visits had higher rates of pregnancy interventions without improvement in neonatal outcomes [5]. The WHO recommends therefore a minimum of 8 contacts to reduce perinatal mortality and improve women's experience of care [6].

ANC visit schedule for uncomplicated pregnancies, recommended by the American College of Obstetricians and Gynecologists (ACOG), consists of an initial prenatal visit, followed by every 4–6 weeks until 28 weeks, every 2–3 weeks until 36 weeks, and then weekly until delivery. Historically, the majority of visits toward the latter part of pregnancy were to detect maternal and fetal complications and to avoid adverse outcomes, which were unpredictable during the first or even second trimester [7]. However, with the integration of diagnostic techniques such as ultrasound, Doppler, biochemical screening tests and detecting cell-free fetal DNA in maternal blood, the first trimester became more important in recent years with dating of pregnancy, detection of multiple pregnancies and detection of chromosomal and structural fetal disorders. Progress has been achieved in the field of early prediction and prevention of preeclampsia, the consequence of the disturbed or dysfunctional placentation. Nicolaides has coined this changing trend with the term 'Turning the Pyramid' and proposed reducing the number of visits to four in an uncomplicated pregnancy [8]. Earlier screening enables earlier identification and more focused follow-up of high-risk groups, but there needs to be a multidisciplinary team dealing with the pregnant women and explaining the often-complex information. There are no randomized data about the maternal or neonatal outcome and the perception of the pregnant women within this concept.

16.3 Provision of Care

Midwife-led continuity-of-care models, in which a known midwife or small group of known midwives supports a woman throughout the antenatal, intrapartum and postnatal continuum, are recommended for pregnant women with an uncomplicated pregnancy and in settings with well-functioning midwifery programmes [6, 9]. Specialists in obstetrics and gynaecology also offer antenatal care to healthy pregnant women. However, routine involvement of obstetricians in the care of women with an uncomplicated pregnancy at scheduled times does not appear to improve perinatal outcomes compared with involving obstetricians when complications arise [9].

16.4 Carrying Notes

Results from randomized controlled trials (RCTs) confirm that women carrying their own notes were more likely to feel in control (RR 1.56, 95% CI 1.18 to 2.06). More women in the case notes group want to carry their own notes in a subsequent pregnancy (RR 1.79, 95% CI 1.57 to 2.03). More women in the case notes group had operative deliveries (RR 1.83, 95% CI 1.08 to 3.12), and caesarean sections (RR 1.51, 95% CI 1.10 to 2.08). The results suggest that there are both potential benefits (increased maternal control and increased availability of antenatal records during hospital attendance) and harms (more operative deliveries). Importantly, all of the trials report

that more women in the case notes group would prefer to carry their antenatal records in another pregnancy [9].

Pre-conceptional visits: see Chapter 10, Section 3.
Physiological adaptation: see Chapter 2, Section 1.

16.5 Nutrition, Supplementation

Counselling about healthy eating, hygiene for food preparation and keeping physically active during pregnancy is recommended for pregnant women to stay healthy and to prevent excessive weight gain during pregnancy [6]. Several food pyramids guide pregnant women through their pregnancy and meet the requirement for most nutrients [10]. Figure 16.1 represents a food pyramid.

The key components of a healthy diet during pregnancy are appropriate weight gain; appropriate vitamin and mineral supplementation; avoidance of alcohol, tobacco and other harmful substances; and safe food handling. Figure 16.2 represents the recommended intake of vitamins according to the German-Austrian-Swiss (D-A-CH) guideline.

Recommended weight gain is between 11 and 16 kg, based on the pre-conceptional body mass index (BMI). There is an increase of 300–400 kcal/day after 12 weeks of pregnancy. Pregnancy is a risk factor for excessive weight gain, which increases future risks of cardiovascular disease and diabetes. According to the Institute of Medicine classification, recommendations are listed in Table 16.1.

Nutrition and lifestyle before and during pregnancy, lactation, infancy and early childhood have been shown to induce long-term effects on later health of the child, including the risk of common non-communicable diseases such as obesity, diabetes

Figure 16.1 Wider choice of food consumed by women during pregnancy irrespective of nutritional values.

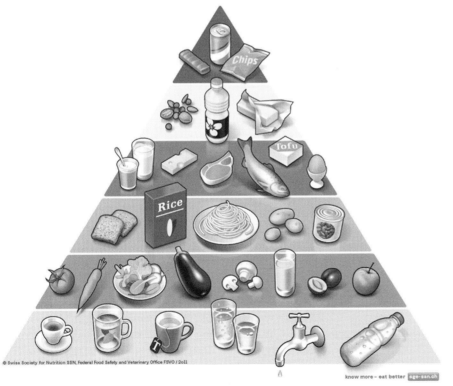

Table 16.1 Recommended weight gain according to pre-pregnancy BMI [11, 12]

BMI (kg/m^2)	Weight gain in kg
<18.5 (underweight)	12.5–18.0
18.5–24.9 (normal weight)	11.5–16.0
25.0–29.9 (overweight)	7.0–11.5
≥30.0 (obese)	5.0–9.0

and cardiovascular disease. This phenomenon is referred to as 'early metabolic programming of long-term health and disease' or 'developmental origins of adult health and disease' [13]. The 'fetal origins' hypothesis stands for the principle that the nutritional, hormonal and metabolic environment afforded by the mother may permanently programme the structure and physiology of her offspring. It is proposed that during the critical periods of growth, an insult caused by either maternal illness or change in the nutrients supplied to the fetus can interrupt the genetic programming for hormonal axes, causing an increased risk for diseases in adult life.

The risk for food-acquired infections like listeriosis, toxoplasmosis or salmonella infection can be reduced by avoiding raw unpasteurized milk or cheese and uncooked meals and meat, especially poultry.

Primary prevention measures such as washing hands and washing fruits and vegetables can help to avoid toxoplasmosis and cytomegaly virus.

16.6 Folic Acid

Folic acid alone or in combination with vitamins and minerals supplemented before conception and throughout the first 12 weeks prevents congenital neural tube defects (NTD) (e.g. anencephaly or spina bifida) based on RCTs [14]. For women with a low risk, the recommended dose is 400–600 micrograms folic acid per day, leading to a 93% decrease in NTD. For women with a high risk, e.g. with prior children with NTD or NTD herself, 4–5 mg/day for women are recommended (69% decrease in NTD). For women with a medium risk (e.g. diabetes mellitus, gastrointestinal malabsorption, bariatric surgery, liver or kidney disease or those on folic acid antagonist medication), the Canadian Society for Obstetrics and Gynaecology recommend 1 mg/day folic acid. Medications with a folic acid antagonist effect are anticonvulsant medications like phenytoin, phenobarbital, carbamazepine, valproate, metformin sulfasalazine or trimethoprim [15]. Folic acid, alone or in combination with vitamins and minerals, does not have a clear effect on other birth defects. National Institute for Care and Health Excellence (NICE) guidelines also recommend that women with higher BMI (usually regarded as >30) should be on 5 mg folic acid, especially in the pre-conceptual period.

16.7 Iron

As iron deficiency anaemia is the most common form of nutritional deficiency worldwide, the WHO recommends daily oral iron and folic acid supplementation with 30 mg to 60 mg of elemental iron and 400 μg (0.4 mg) of folic acid for pregnant women to prevent maternal anaemia, puerperal sepsis, low birthweight and preterm birth. The International Federation of Gynecology and Obstetrics (FIGO) recommend a continuous or intermittent iron supplementation (one to three times per week) of 30 mg per day starting at the first ANC visit or as soon as possible [12]. Authorities from high-income countries (e.g. NICE) recommend caution about routine iron supplementation as it does not benefit the mother's or the baby's health and may have unpleasant maternal side effects. The quality assurance committee of the Swiss Society of Obstetrics and Gynaecology recommends screening for iron-deficiency anaemia in every pregnant woman. This should be done by serum ferritin-level screening in the first trimester and regular haemoglobin checks at least once per trimester in order to supplement only iron-deficient or anaemic women [16].

16.8 Vitamin D

At the booking appointment, pregnant women should be informed about the importance for their own and their baby's health of maintaining adequate vitamin D stores during pregnancy and whilst breastfeeding. In order to achieve this, women should be advised to take a vitamin D supplement (10 micrograms of vitamin D per day). At risk for vitamin D deficiency are:

- women with darker skin (such as those of African, African–Caribbean or South Asian family origin)
- women who have limited exposure to sunlight, such as women who are housebound or confined indoors for long periods, or who cover their skin for cultural reasons [9]

16.9 Vitamin A

Excessive intake of vitamin A affects the embryo and is teratogenic or can provoke miscarriages at doses >25 000 IU/day. Maximum supplementation should be 5000 IU/day, certainly not >10 000 IU/day. Isotretinoin, a synthetic derivate of vitamin A, is used for treatment of severe acne and is one of the most potent human teratogens. Most supplements contain beta-carotene rather than retinol, and high beta-carotene intakes have not been related to birth defects. There is good evidence that antenatal vitamin A supplementation reduces maternal night blindness, and maternal anaemia for women who live in areas where vitamin A deficiency is common or who are HIV-positive. In addition, the available evidence suggests a reduction in maternal infection, but these data are not of a high quality [17].

16.10 Omega-3 Fatty Acids

Pregnant women should aim to consume two weekly portions of ocean fish, including oily fish such as mackerel, herring, sardines or salmon. Consumption of large predator fish (e.g. tuna, swordfish) should be limited. Women who do not achieve regular fish consumption should aim to achieve an

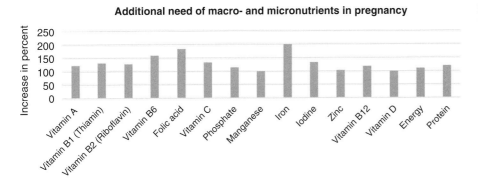

Figure 16.2 Vitamin and mineral requirements in pregnancy (@ University Hospital of Basel)

average total daily intake of at least 300 mg omega-3 docosahexaenoic acid (DHA) by taking a supplement providing at least 200 mg omega-3 DHA per day, in addition to the dietary DHA intake. Regular consumption of fish as well as supplementation of omega-3 long-chain polyunsaturated fatty acids (LC-PUFA) was found to reduce the risk of early preterm birth prior to 34 weeks of gestation [13, 18–20].

16.11 Iodine

Women who are planning pregnancy and those who are pregnant should supplement their diet with a daily oral multiple micronutrient supplement that contains 150 µg of iodine in the form of potassium iodide. Pregnant women should be encouraged to routinely use iodized salt (containing 95 µg of iodine per one-quarter teaspoon) if it is available [12]. Dietary supplementation with iodine alone may be indicated in women at risk of poor supply and insufficiency of these micronutrients [13]. Thyroid-stimulating hormone levels should be measured in women with a history of thyroid disease or symptoms of disease in pregnancy, although there is no evidence that universal testing during pregnancy improves outcomes compared to case reporting [21].

16.12 Calcium

Context-specific recommendations exist for calcium supplements in populations with low dietary calcium intake. In populations with low dietary calcium intake, daily calcium supplementation (1.5–2.0 g oral elemental calcium) is recommended for pregnant women to reduce the risk of pre-eclampsia. Zinc supplementation is only recommended in populations with a zinc deficiency [6]. There are no data for general supplementation as regards vitamins B6, E and C.

16.13 Multivitamins

A Cochrane review suggests a positive impact of multivitamin or multiple micronutrient (MMN) supplementation with iron and folic acid on several birth outcomes. MMN supplementation in pregnancy led to a reduction in babies considered low birthweight, and probably led to a reduction in babies considered small for gestational age. In addition, MMN probably reduced preterm births. No important benefits or harms of MMN supplementation were found for mortality outcomes (stillbirths, perinatal and neonatal mortality). These findings

may provide some basis to guide the replacement of iron and folic acid supplements with MMN supplements for pregnant women residing in low- and middle-income countries [22].

16.14 Caffeine Intake

For pregnant women with high daily caffeine intake (more than 300 mg per day), lowering daily caffeine intake during pregnancy is recommended to reduce the risk of pregnancy loss and low-birthweight neonates [6].

16.15 Alcohol, Tobacco and Other Drugs

Alcohol passes freely across the placenta and is a recognized teratogen with effects including a decrease in DNA synthesis, impaired cellular growth and differentiation, changes in placental function and decrease in glucose and amino acid transfer to the fetus. The minimum or threshold level at which alcohol begins to pose a significant threat to pregnancy is not known. It is therefore preferable that women avoid the intake of alcohol during pregnancy.

Pregnant women should be screened for tobacco use, and individualized, pregnancy-tailored counselling should be offered to smokers. Smoking cessation counselling and multi-component strategies are effective in decreasing the incidence of low-birthweight infants and preterm birth [23]

16.16 Exercise, Travel, Working

It is recommended that pregnant women engage in 30 minutes or more of moderate-intensity physical activity on most, and preferably all, days of the week [24]. High-quality evidence indicates that diet or exercise, or both, during pregnancy can reduce the risk of excessive gestational weight gain. Other benefits may include a lower risk of caesarean delivery, macrosomia and neonatal respiratory morbidity, particularly for high-risk women receiving combined diet and exercise interventions. Maternal hypertension may also be reduced. Exercise appears to be an important part of controlling weight gain in pregnancy [25].

16.17 Maternal and Fetal Well-Being

Standard elements of prenatal care include a routine physical examination (including pelvic examination) at the initial visit, maternal weight and blood pressure measurements at all visits, fetal heart rate auscultation after 10 to 12 weeks with a Doppler monitor and Leopold manoeuvres to assess fetal position by 36 weeks. Auscultation confirms fetal viability but there is no evidence of other clinical or predictive value.

A pelvic examination at the initial visit is useful in detecting reproductive tract abnormalities. Routine pelvimetry is not useful. Although promotion of breastfeeding is critical, there is no clear evidence to support clinical breast examinations. However, breast examinations may help to address proactively breastfeeding concerns or problems.

Although assessment of symphysis fundal height (SFH) and fetal heart tones at every visit is recommended in multiple guidelines, the effect on outcomes is not clear [9, 11]. However it is not recommended to abandon SFH, especially in low-income countries, where antenatal ultrasound is not available [6]. Daily fetal movement counting, such as with 'count-to-ten' kick charts, is only recommended in the context of rigorous research [6]. Routine antenatal cardiotocography is not recommended for pregnant women to improve maternal and perinatal outcomes [6].

16.18 Blood Pressure and Urine

Blood pressure measurement and urine analysis for protein should be carried out at each antenatal visit to screen for pre-eclampsia, and women should be counselled on warning signs of pre-eclampsia.

Blood pressure should be measured as outlined below:

- Remove tight clothing, ensure arm is relaxed and supported at heart level
- Use cuff of appropriate size
- Inflate cuff to 20–30 mm Hg above palpated systolic blood pressure
- Lower column slowly, by 2 mm Hg per second or per beat
- Read blood pressure to the nearest 2 mm Hg
- Blood pressure reading ends as disappearance of sounds (phase V) [9]

Urine testing does not reliably detect proteinuria in patients with early pre-eclampsia; trace glycosuria is unreliable for the detection of gestational diabetes and represent physiological change during pregnancy.

16.19 Asymptomatic Bacteriuria

Most international guidelines recommend screening and treatment for asymptomatic bacteriuria early in pregnancy. Asymptomatic bacteriuria complicates 2–7% of pregnancies [6, 9, 11]. However antibiotic treatment for women having significant bacteriuria likely reduces the incidence of pyelonephritis and low birthweight, but there is uncertainty about the magnitude of the effect and about the extent to which we can apply these results to asymptomatic populations and screening programmes [28].

16.20 Routine Antenatal Infection Screening

A survey was conducted among European Ministries of Health and equivalent bodies, including European Societies of Obstetricians and Midwives, in 2004. The guideline overview showed that only 3 out of 37 screening tests (blood pressure, blood group and rhesus factor) had been recommended in all 20 countries. The number of the provided laboratory tests ranged from 8 to 21.

Maternal infections in pregnancy may cause severe child morbidity. Vertically transmitted infections (e.g. cytomegalovirus (CMV), HIV, rubella, toxoplasmosis, syphilis or varicella) may lead to malformations, neurodevelopmental delay and long-term childhood consequences. Maternal genital infections may increase the risk for miscarriage or preterm birth (e.g. bacterial vaginosis) or cause neonatal infection by intrapartum transmission (e.g. group B streptococcal (GBS) infection or genital herpes). Hence, the main rationale for infection screening during pregnancy is to reduce fetal or neonatal infections by early treatment of the infected pregnant woman. Another justification might be to enhance targeted preventive measures during the current pregnancy (e.g. hygiene, caesarean section) or with regard to subsequent pregnancies (e.g. postpartum varicella or rubella immunization). In a comparison of different evidence-based guidelines, variation in direction pro or contra screening as well as differences in grading was shown.

Uniform recommendations were found for:
- Hepatitis B, asymptomatic bacteriuria, HIV, syphilis and rubella susceptibility.

Universal screening was not recommended for:
- Bacterial vaginosis, toxoplasmosis, hepatitis C and parvovirus.

Different opinions were observed for:
- Group B streptococcus, *Chlamydia trachomatis*, genital herpes and gonorrhoea screening [26].

16.21 Screening for Haematological Conditions Including Blood Grouping

Screening for iron-deficiency anaemia is recommended in every pregnant woman. This should be done by serum ferritin-level screening in the first trimester and regular haemoglobin checks at least once per trimester.

Women should be tested for blood group and rhesus D status in early pregnancy. Women should be screened for atypical red cell alloantibodies in early pregnancy and again at 28 weeks, regardless of their rhesus D status. If a pregnant woman is rhesus D-negative, consideration should be given to offering partner testing to determine whether the administration of anti-D prophylaxis is necessary. The risk of developing alloimmunization for an RhD-negative woman can be reduced from 1.5% to 0.2% with Rh0 (D) immune globulin given to non-sensitized women at 28 weeks and again within 72 hours after delivery if the infant has a RhD-positive blood group [11, 27].

In several countries (e.g., Denmark, the Netherlands, Sweden, England, France, Finland) fetal RHD determination is performed routinely in D-negative women and administration of antenatal anti-D immune globulin is avoided when an

RHD-negative fetus is identified. Over one third of D-negative women appropriately avoided antenatal anti-D immune globulin in large studies from Denmark and Sweden [28, 29].

Screening for sickle cell diseases and thalassaemia should be offered to all women as early as possible in pregnancy. A family origin questionnaire can be used to detect specific ethnic groups with increased risk for haematological conditions. The type of screening depends upon the prevalence [9].

16.22 Pap Screening

Papanicolaou smears (Pap test) should be obtained at the first antenatal visit if none has been documented during the last 12 months or based on Pap test history. A Pap test might be avoided if three consecutive normal Pap tests have been documented in the last three years before pregnancy [11].

Ultrasound scanning in the first trimester including noninvasive prenatal diagnosis and testing: see Chapter 11, Section 3 & Chapter 12, Section 3.

16.23 Screening for Gestational Diabetes

Hyperglycaemia in pregnancy is a global issue, as it increases risks for both the mother and child. There remains considerable disparity in clinical practice and national policies for this screening. The International Federation of Gynecology and Obstetrics (FIGO), the European Board and College of Obstetrics and Gynaecology (EBCOG) and the European Association of Perinatal Medicine (EAPM) recommend universal screening for gestational diabetes. However, even among advocates of universal testing there is a lack of uniformity in approach to testing methodology between the 50 g glucose challenge test followed by the 100 g oral glucose tolerance test (OGTT) or the 1-step 75 g OGTT, recommended by the International Association of Diabetes and Pregnancy Study Groups (IADPSG) [30].

According to NICE, screening for gestational diabetes using risk factors is recommended in a healthy population. At the booking appointment, the following risk factors for gestational diabetes should be determined: BMI above 30 kg/m^2, previous macrosomic baby weighing 4.5 kg or above, previous gestational diabetes, family history of diabetes (first-degree relative with diabetes), family origin with a high prevalence of diabetes: South Asian (specifically women whose country of family origin is India, Pakistan or Bangladesh), black Caribbean, Middle Eastern (specifically women whose country of family origin is Saudi Arabia, United Arab Emirates, Iraq, Jordan, Syria, Oman, Qatar, Kuwait, Lebanon or Egypt). Women with any one of these risk factors should be offered testing for gestational diabetes [9].

See also Chapter 27, Section 4
Screening for pre-eclampsia: Chapter 25, Section 4
Screening for preterm birth: Chapter 49, Section 5

16.24 Rubella, Varicella

Women should be screened for rubella immunity during the first prenatal visit, ideally before conception when vaccination is safe. All women who are nonimmune should be offered vaccination postpartum to prevent congenital rubella syndrome in subsequent pregnancies. Vaccination should not be given during pregnancy, but may be given during lactation. There is some evidence to support assessing the mother's varicella history at the first prenatal visit, with serologic testing for those with a negative history [11].

16.25 Vaccination for Pertussis, Influenza

Physicians should recommend that all pregnant women receive vaccination for influenza. Pregnant women may be at higher risk of influenza complications than the general population. Women should receive a diphtheria, tetanus and pertussis vaccine during each pregnancy. The best time for vaccination is between 27 and 36 weeks' gestation for antibody response and passive immunity to the fetus; however, the vaccine may be given any time during pregnancy [11].

16.26 Sexuality

Intercourse has not been associated with adverse outcome in pregnancy [9].

16.27 Domestic Violence

Healthcare professionals need to be alert to the symptoms or signs of domestic violence, and women should be given the opportunity to disclose domestic violence in an environment in which they feel secure. Domestic violence during pregnancy increases the risk of complications, such as spontaneous abortion, placental abruption, premature rupture of membranes, low birthweight and prematurity [11].

16.28 Depression Screening

The ACOG supports depression screening during pregnancy. Perinatal depression is underdiagnosed and complicates 10–15% of pregnancies, resulting in significant morbidity for the mother and infant. Complications include prematurity, low birthweight, neurodevelopmental delays and issues with maternal/infant bonding [11].

16.29 Oral Hygiene

Periodontal disease is associated with increased risk of preterm birth, and an oral examination is often included in the first prenatal visit [11].

16.30 Umbilical Cord Blood Donation

Umbilical cord blood contains potentially lifesaving stem cells that can be used for haematopoietic stem cell transplantations in the treatment of malignant and non-malignant haematological disorders. Today more than 40 000 transplants have been performed worldwide mainly in children or adults who lack an human leukocyte antigen-matched sibling or unrelated donor. During antenatal care, pregnant women should be informed about the option to donate umbilical cord blood, and the benefits and limitations of private and public umbilical cord blood banks should be discussed since they serve different purposes. While public umbilical cord blood banks store umbilical cord blood

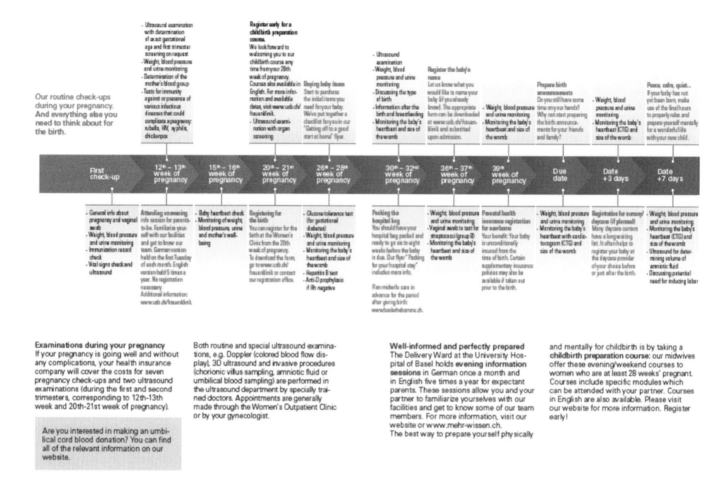

Figure 16.3 Journey through the pregnancy.

anonymously for allogeneic use, private umbilical cord blood mainly is stored for potential autologous use in regenerative medicine. Family-directed storage needs to be considered when there is a family member who has been diagnosed with a disease and might benefit from haematopoietic stem cell transplantation in the future. The information on banking options needs to be balanced, and it needs to be stressed that there is no current evidence to support private umbilical cord blood banking for the use in regenerative medicine. On the other hand, women need to be aware that only about every seventh eligible donor will have enough stem cells at delivery to be useful for a potential future transplantation and it will only be stored in a public bank if it meets all quality criteria and a minimum stem cell count [31]. At the same time, pregnant women need to be reassured that umbilical cord blood donation will not compromise obstetric or neonatal care and that during delivery there may be circumstances that preclude adequate and safe collection [32].

16.31 Initial Visit

Ideally, the first visit should occur before 12 weeks of pregnancy. Women should receive written protocols regarding the content of the visits, information about screening tests and the right of non-knowledge. Major aspects of the visit include history, counselling, physical examination and laboratory testing. According to the NICE clinical guideline, the content of the visits should include [9]:

First contact:
- folic acid supplementation
- food hygiene, including how to reduce the risk of a food-acquired infection
- lifestyle advice, including smoking cessation, and the implications of recreational drug use and alcohol consumption in pregnancy
- all antenatal screening, including screening for haemoglobinopathies
- the anomaly scan and screening for Down syndrome, as well as risks and benefits of the screening tests
- Comprehensive history, to identify women who may require additional care
- Information on prior pregnancies: outcomes of pregnancies and births (vaginal delivery, caesarean section, assisted vaginal birth, abortion, miscarriage, intrauterine fetal death, ectopic pregnancy, length of pregnancy in weeks, progress in labour, complications postpartum, child's weight and gender, fetal malformations)

At booking (ideally by 10 weeks):
- how the baby develops during pregnancy
- nutrition and diet, including vitamin D supplementation for women at risk of vitamin D deficiency
- exercise, including pelvic floor exercises
- place of birth

- pregnancy care pathway
- breastfeeding, including workshops
- participant-led antenatal classes
- further discussion of all antenatal screening
- discussion of mental health issues

Before 36 weeks:

- breastfeeding information, including technique and good management practices, that would help a woman succeed
- preparation for labour and birth, including information about coping with pain in labour and the birth plan
- recognition of active labour
- care of the new baby
- vitamin K prophylaxis
- newborn screening tests
- postnatal self-care
- awareness of 'baby blues' and postnatal depression
- information of umbilical cord blood donation

At 38 weeks:

- options for management of prolonged pregnancy

Figure 16.3 provides a detailed look at what to expect during a series of antenatal care visits.

16.32 Key Messages

Antenatal care (ANC) of a normal pregnancy is defined as the routine care of presumed healthy, pregnant women with a singleton uncomplicated pregnancy provided between conception and the onset of labour. The aim of the ANC is: optimal outcome for mother and child with a general reduction of maternal and perinatal morbidity and mortality; individual satisfaction and positive experience with pregnancy, delivery and postpartum period; early recognition of maternal/fetal conditions and appropriate treatment and adherence to efficacy, usefulness and cost-effectiveness. Ideally, the first visit should occur before 12 weeks of pregnancy and include confirmation of the intact pregnancy and information of the upcoming visits and measures. This include maternal and fetal well-being, routine antenatal infection screening, screening for haematological conditions including blood grouping, screening for gestational diabetes, appropriate weight gain, vitamin and mineral supplementation, avoidance of alcohol, tobacco and other harmful substances, and screening for violence and depression.

References

1. Moller AB, Petzold M, Chou D, Say L. Early antenatal care visit: a systematic analysis of regional and global levels and trends of coverage from 1990 to 2013. *Lancet Glob Health*. 2017;5(10):e977–83.

2. Downe S, Finlayson K, Tuncalp O, Gulmezoglu AM. Provision and uptake of routine antenatal services: a qualitative evidence synthesis. *Cochrane Database Syst Rev*. 2019 Jun 12;6(6): CD012392.

3. Dowswell T, Carroli G, Duley L, et al. Alternative versus standard packages of antenatal care for low-risk pregnancy. *Cochrane Database Syst Rev*. 2010 Oct 6 (10): CD000934.

4. Raatikainen K, Heiskanen N, Heinonen S. Under-attending free antenatal care is associated with adverse pregnancy outcomes. *BMC Public Health*. 2007; 7:268.

5. Carter EB, Tuuli MG, Caughey AB, et al. Number of prenatal visits and pregnancy outcomes in low-risk women. *J Perinatol*. 2016;36 (3):178–81.

6. WHO. *WHO Recommendations on Antenatal Care for a Positive Pregnancy Experience*. Geneva: WHO; 2016.

7. American Academy of Pediatrics. *Guidelines for Perinatal Care*. Elk Grove Village, IL: American Academy of Pediatrics; 2012.

8. Nicolaides KH. Turning the pyramid of prenatal care. *Fetal Diagn Ther*. 2011;29 (3):183–96.

9. NICE. *Antenatal Care for Uncomplicated Pregnancies*. Clinical Guideline CG 62. 2019.

10. Swiss Society for Nutrition. Swiss food pyramid. 2011. www.sge-ssn.ch/media/ sge_pyramid_E_basic_20161.pdf

11. Zolotor AJ, Carlough MC. Update on prenatal care. *Am Fam Physician*. 2014;89(3):199–208.

12. Good clinical practice advice: Micronutrients in the periconceptional period and pregnancy. *Int J Gynecol Obstet*. 2019;144(3):317–21.

13. Koletzko B, Godfrey KM, Poston L, et al. Nutrition during pregnancy, lactation and early childhood and its implications for maternal and long-term child health: the early nutrition project recommendations. *Ann Nutr Metab*. 2019;74(2):93–106.

14. De-Regil LM, Pena-Rosas JP, Fernandez-Gaxiola AC, et al. Effects and safety of periconceptional oral folate supplementation for preventing birth defects. *Cochrane Database Syst Rev*. 2015 Dec 14(12): CD007950.

15. Wilson RD, Genetics Committee, et al. Pre-conception folic acid and multivitamin supplementation for the primary and secondary prevention of neural tube defects and other folic acid-sensitive congenital anomalies. *J Obstet Gynaecol Can*. 2015;37 (6):534–52.

16. Breymann C, Honegger C, Hosli I, Surbek D. Diagnosis and treatment of iron-deficiency anaemia in pregnancy and postpartum. *Arch Gynecol Obstet*. 2017; 296(6):1229–34.

17. McCauley ME, van den Broek N, Dou L, Othman M. Vitamin A supplementation during pregnancy for maternal and newborn outcomes. *Cochrane Database Syst Rev*. 2015 Oct 27(10):CD008666.

18. Berti C, Cetin I, Agostoni C, et al. Pregnancy and infants' outcome: nutritional and metabolic implications. *Crit Rev Food Sci Nutr*. 2016;56 (1):82–91.

19. Koletzko B, Lien E, Agostoni C, et al. The roles of long-chain polyunsaturated fatty acids in pregnancy, lactation and infancy: review of current knowledge and consensus recommendations. *J Perinat Med*. 2008;36(1): 5–14.

20. Middleton P, Gomersall JC, Gould JF, et al., Omega-3 fatty acid addition during pregnancy. *Cochrane Database Syst Rev*. 2018;Nov 11: CD003402.

21. Spencer L, Bubner T, Bain E, Middleton P. Screening and subsequent management for thyroid dysfunction pre-pregnancy and during pregnancy for improving maternal and infant health. *Cochrane Database Syst Rev.* 2015 Sep 21(9):CD011263.

22. Keats EC, Haider B, Tam E, Bhutta ZA. Multiple-micronutrient supplementation for women during pregnancy. *Cochrane Database Syst Rev.* 2019 Mar 14;**3**(3):CD004905.

23. Lumley J, Chamberlain C, Dowswell T, et al. Interventions for promoting smoking cessation during pregnancy. *Cochrane Database Syst Rev.* 2009 Jul 8 (3):CD001055.

24. Artal R. Exercise in pregnancy: guidelines. *Clin Obstet Gynecol.* 2016;**59** (3):639–44.

25. Muktabhant B, Lawrie TA, Lumbiganon P, Laopaiboon M. Diet or exercise, or both, for preventing excessive weight gain in pregnancy. *Cochrane Database Syst Rev.* 2015 Jun 15(6):CD007145.

26. Piso B, Reinsperger I, Winkler R. Recommendations from international clinical guidelines for routine antenatal infection screening: does evidence matter? *Int J Evid Based Healthc.* 2014;**12**(1):50–61.

27. McBain RD, Crowther CA, Middleton P. Anti-D administration in pregnancy for preventing Rhesus alloimmunisation. *Cochrane Database Syst Rev.* 2013 Feb 28(9):CD000020.

28. Clausen FB, Steffensen R, Christiansen M, et al. Routine noninvasive prenatal screening for fetal RHD in plasma of RhD-negative pregnant women-2 years of screening experience from Denmark. *Prenat Diagn.* 2014;**34**(10):1000–5.

29. Wikman AT, Tiblad E, Karlsson A, et al. Noninvasive single-exon fetal RHD determination in a routine screening program in early pregnancy. *Obstet Gynecol.* 2012;**120**(2 Pt 1):227–34.

30. Hod M, Pretty M, Mahmood T. Joint position statement on universal screening for GDM in Europe by FIGO, EBCOG and EAPM. *Eur J Obstet Gynecol Reprod Biol.* 2018;**228**:329–30.

31. Manegold-Brauer G, Borer B, Bucher C, et al. A prenatal prediction model for total nucleated cell count increases the efficacy of umbilical cord blood banking. *Transfusion.* 2014;**54** (11): 2946–52.

32. ACOG Committee Opinion No. 771: Umbilical Cord Blood Banking. *Obstet Gynecol.* 2019;**133**(3): e249–53.

Chapter 17

Screening for High-Risk Pregnancy

Miroslaw Wielgoś & Przemyslaw Kosinski

There are several medical conditions, both maternal and fetal, which can influence the course of pregnancy or even the developing fetus. In the era of modern technology, high-tech ultrasound machines, sophisticated monitoring methods for both mother and her unborn child, it is not enough to deliver a live neonate. What is highly expected by all future parents is a delivery of a healthy baby with a very good prognosis. Therefore, it has to be acknowledged and appreciated that the role of an obstetrician or maternal-fetal specialist cannot be underestimated. General population screening of all pregnant women for medical conditions is essential to achieve this target; otherwise, it is not possible to select a group of pregnant women who require more detailed and watchful monitoring, special care or even targeted treatment. However, not only identification of pregnancies at increased risk for maternal or fetal morbidity and mortality is involved, but also health promotion, education and support for parents. Nowadays, it is possible to predict many severe medical conditions as early as in the first trimester of pregnancy. The awareness of a high-risk pregnancy may improve pregnancy outcomes or even be life-saving for a mother, her fetus or even both.

17.1 Multiple Pregnancy

The diagnosis of a multiple pregnancy usually brings much joy to the patient and her family, but at the same time a lot of concern for her obstetrician. This anxiety results from the awareness that the risk of complications in multiple pregnancy is much higher compared to a singleton pregnancy. This includes the high risk of preterm delivery, low birthweight and complications typical for monochorionic pregnancy. About 1 in 89 spontaneous conceptions results in the birth of twins. In some countries twins now occur once in every 30 pregnancies due to widespread introduction of reproductive techniques. It is recognized that mortality and the risk of complications such as cerebral palsy in twins may be up to seven times higher than in a singleton pregnancy [1]. Of spontaneously conceived twins, 55% are dizygotic, whereas 45% are monozygotic. The neonatal mortality rate in the case of monochorionic pregnancy is 2.5 times higher compared to dichorionic pregnancy [2]. Also, there is approximately a sevenfold higher risk of neurological complications in prematurely born monochorionic twins as compared to prematurely born dichorionic twins [3]. This fact suggests that chorionicity determines the risk of complications, and therefore the diagnosis of twin pregnancy and determining the chorionicity are essential. This can be achieved by the early

ultrasound scan or during routine first trimester scan. The presence of the lambda sign (for dichorionicity) or T sign (for monochorionicity) in the first trimester has been shown to be highly reproducible and accurate in determining chorionicity [4]. In monochorionic twin pregnancies the majority of the pregnancy losses will occur between the first and the second trimester [5]. The vast majority is a result of acute twin-to-twin transfusion syndrome, selective fetal growth restriction, and discordance for fetal anomalies [6]. Twin-to-twin transfusion syndrome (TTTS) and selective intrauterine growth restriction (sIUGR) have a different aetiology and clinical picture; however, the differential diagnosis is not always straightforward. In the case of TTTS, the cause is the presence of vascular anastomoses predominantly of the artery-to-vein (A-V) type. In this case, blood flows from the donor fetus to the recipient, initiating a number of adverse haemo-dynamic changes. In the case of sIUGR, the unequal division of trophoblast responsible for gas exchange is considered as the primary cause. The growth-restricted fetus has insufficient trophoblast surface. Another usual feature of sIUGR is the occurrence of marginal attachment of the umbilical cord. It was also observed that the greater the discordance between the placental surface between the fetuses, the greater the difference between birthweights of the neonates [7]. Selective IUGR is associated with a significant risk of intrauterine death and abnormal neurological development of both fetuses [5, 8, 9]. A complication typical of selective suppression of fetal growth is the intrauterine death of an abnormally growing fetus. Due to the unique angioarchitecture of the placenta, there is a risk of acute transfusion of large volumes of blood, which may result in a 25–30% risk of fetal death for the surviving twin. The risk of abnormal neurological development is as high as 30% [10]. The management of twin pregnancies is complex because the interests of both twins have to be taken into account. Depending on chorionicity, growth and Doppler studies should be monitored every two weeks for uncomplicated monochorionic twins and every four weeks in uncomplicated dichorionic twins. Ultrasound plays a key role in the surveillance of these pregnancies. A detailed description of multiple pregnancy can be found in Chapter 18, Multiple Pregnancy.

17.2 Fetal Aneuploidies

Aneuploidies are major causes of perinatal death and childhood disability. Consequently, the detection of chromosomal disorders constitutes the most frequent indication for invasive prenatal diagnosis. Nowadays, the first trimester scan between 11+0 and

Fetal Medicine

Table 17.1 Performance of first trimester screening for trisomy 21

Performance of different methods of screening for trisomy 21	Detection rate (%)	False positive rate (%)
Maternal age (MA)	30	5
MA + fetal nuchal translucency (NT)	75–80	5
MA + serum free β-hCG and PAPP-A	60–70	5
MA + NT + free β-hCG and PAPP-A (combined test)	85–95	5
Combined test + nasal bone or tricuspid flow or ductus venosus flow	93–96	3

Table 17.2 Second trimester ultrasound markers and their positive and negative likelihood ratios (LR) for trisomy 21

Second trimester ultrasound marker	Positive LR	Negative LR
Intracardiac echogenic focus	5.85	0.80
Ventriculomegaly	25.78	0.94
Increased nuchal fold	19.18	0.80
Echogenic bowel	11.44	0.90
Mild hydronephrosis	7.77	0.92
Short humerus	4.81	0.74
Short femur	3.72	0.80
Aberrant right subclavian artery	21.48	0.71
Absent or hypoplastic nasal bone	23.26	0.46

13+6 weeks allows for the assessment of ultrasound and biochemical markers for chromosomal disorders. In the last decades, the risk for aneuploidies was estimated based on maternal age with detection rate as low as 30%. The use of the first trimester ultrasound markers (nuchal translucency, nasal bone, ductus venosus and tricuspid regurgitation) combined with placental biochemical products – pregnancy-associated plasma protein-A (PAPP-A) and free β-hCG – allows for the screening for trisomy 21, trisomy 18 and trisomy 13 with high detection rate and low false positive rates. The performances of the different methods of screening for trisomy 21 are summarized in Table 17.1.

In screening for trisomy 21 by maternal age and serum free β-hCG and PAPP-A, the detection rate is about 65% with a false-positive rate of 5%. For the sake of the performance of screening it is better to take a blood sample at 9–10 weeks rather than at 13 weeks because the difference in PAPP-A between trisomic and euploid pregnancies is greater in earlier gestations [11, 12]. More information about the role of ultrasound in the first trimester can be found in Chapter 11, Ultrasound Scanning in the First Trimester of Pregnancy. There is also extensive literature on the association between aneuploidies and a wide range of second trimester ultrasound findings. Based on the presence or absence of second trimester ultrasound 'soft markers' and adjusted risk for trisomies calculated in the first trimester, it is possible to recalculate the risk during the second trimester. The positive and negative likelihood ratios of selected second trimester ultrasound markers for trisomy 21 are summarized in Table 17.2 [13].

Karyotyping should be offered in cases of high risk for trisomies or if ultrasound examination in the first or second trimester demonstrates major anatomical defects. In the case of intermediate risk for trisomy 21 in the absence of fetal abnormalities, cell-free fetal DNA test might be considered as prenatal screening for trisomy 21, trisomy 18, trisomy 13, and sex chromosome aneuploidies can be performed using next-generation sequencing of cell-free DNA (cfDNA) in the maternal circulation. The primary source of so-called fetal cfDNA in the maternal circulation is thought to be apoptosis of placental cells (syncytiotrophoblast). The concentration of fetal cfDNA

increases 0.1% per week from 10 weeks' gestation to approximately 20 weeks, and then increases more rapidly with a pace of 1% per week until term [14]. Cell-free DNA is the most sensitive screening option for aneuploidies, in particular trisomy 21 with the detection rate of >99% [15, 16]. The detection rates of trisomies 13 and 18 are also extremely high, but vary by trisomy and by methodology. Cell-free fetal DNA has very high sensitivity and specificity for Down syndrome, with slightly lower sensitivity for Edwards and Patau syndromes. However, it is not 100% accurate and should not be used as a final diagnosis for positive cases. Invasive procedures such as CVS or amniocentesis should be offered for patients who received positive cfDNA test results for trisomy [16].

17.3 Pre-Eclampsia

Incomplete placental invasion leads to oxidative stress, autoimmunity, platelet and thrombin activation, intravascular inflammation, endothelial dysfunction and an imbalance in angiogenesis and is strongly associated with most cases of early (<34 weeks) and severe pre-eclampsia (PE) [17]. On the other hand, the cases of PE developing after 34 weeks' gestation seems to be less related to defective placentation. The risk of pre-eclampsia is increased twofold to fourfold if a patient has a first degree relative with a medical history of the disorder and is increased sevenfold if pre-eclampsia complicated a previous pregnancy [18]. Multiple gestation is an additional risk factor; triplet gestation is a greater risk than twin gestation. Risk factors for pre-eclampsia are summarized in Table 17.3. However, due to the multifactorial aetiology of pre-eclampsia, the assessment of the personalized risk of PE based only on the medical history is insufficient. Therefore, biophysical and biochemical markers have been investigated for early identification of pregnant women at risk of pre-eclampsia. A combination of medical history, biophysical methods (ultrasound and mean arterial blood pressure (MAP) – measured on both arms at the same time (according to the Fetal Medicine Foundation recommendations)) and

Table 17.3 Risk factors for pre-eclampsia

- Advanced maternal age (older than 40 years)
- Black race
- Family history of pre-eclampsia
- Primiparity
- Previous pre-eclamptic pregnancy
- Chronic hypertension
- Chronic renal disease
- History of thrombophilia
- Multiple pregnancy
- In vitro fertilization
- Type 1 diabetes mellitus
- Type 2 diabetes mellitus
- Obesity
- Antiphospholipid syndrome
- Systemic lupus erythematosus

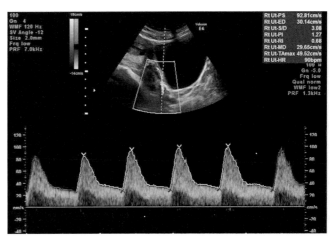

Figure 17.1 Transabdominal Doppler ultrasound examination of uterine artery in the first trimester. The peak systolic velocity should be >60 cm/s (here 92.81 cm/s) to verify that the uterine artery is being examined. A black and white version of this figure will appear in some formats. For the colour version, please refer to the plate section.

biochemical markers allows identification of pregnant women at high risk for PE [19, 20].

Modern screening for pre-eclampsia is based on maternal history, demographics and biomarkers [21]. Defective or partial placentation results in incomplete transformation of the spiral arteries and therefore increased resistance to uterine artery blood flow. Ultrasound can be used to assess the pulsatility index (PI) of the uterine arteries. Adherence to a standardized methodology is essential to ensure reproducible measurements. Therefore, regular certification and training is needed to achieve desired level of expertise and the adherence to a standardized protocol of examination is fundamental to minimize operator-dependent variability [22]. For the first trimester transabdominal assessment of uterine artery resistance, a midsagittal section of the uterus and cervix must be obtained and by gently tilting the probe sideways uterine artery can be visualized with high-velocity blood flow along the side of the cervix and uterus. The pulsed-wave Doppler sampling gate set at 2 mm should be positioned on either the ascending or descending branch of the uterine artery at the point closest to the internal cervical os, with an insonation angle <30° (Figure 17.1). The uterine artery blood flow assessment can also be performed with transvaginal probe, and both techniques have been precisely described previously [23, 24]. Increased PI is the most predictive Doppler index for PE [25]. Screening only by first trimester uterine artery PI >90th centile detects 48% of women who will develop early PE (7.9% false positive rate), 39.2% of cases of early fetal growth restriction (6.7% false positive rate) and 26.4% of cases of PE at any stage (6.6% false positive rate) [26, 27].

The 95th centile of mean uterine artery PI obtained using a transabdominal approach is about 2.35 measured between 11+0 to 13+6 weeks [24]. Considering there is a number of maternal factors that can influence uterine artery PI (ethnicity, body mass index (BMI), previous PE) an absolute numerical cut-off for uterine artery PI may not reflect accurately uterine artery resistance. Therefore, it has been suggested that first-trimester uterine artery PI should be expressed as multiples of the median (MoM) rather than absolute values [28]. The association between uterine artery PI and maternal BMI is not clear, but it has been suggested that the decreasing PI with increasing maternal BMI may be related to vasodilatory effect of increased levels of estrogens in these women [29, 30].Uterine artery 'notching' may be observed in around 50% of pregnant women at 11+0 to 13+6 weeks and therefore has a very low specificity for PE [24]. Alterations in a number of circulating antiangiogenic proteins (soluble fms-like tyrosine kinase 1 (sFlt1) and soluble endoglin) and proangiogenic proteins (placenta growth factor (PlGF) and vascular endothelial growth factor (VEGF)) have been evaluated as biomarkers for use in screening for pre-eclampsia [31, 32]. Combined screening including maternal factors, maternal mean arterial blood pressure, uterine artery Doppler and biochemical markers, such as placental growth factor (PlGF), has a better predictive value comparable to ultrasound alone and therefore should be offered for screening when available [26]. Given the superiority of combined screening, the use of Doppler cut-offs as a standalone screening modality should be avoided if combined screening is available.

Similar to the first trimester, in the second trimester, uterine artery pulsatility index may also be measured both transvaginally and transabdominally. Between 20 and 26 weeks the mean uterine artery PI was 1.07 with the transvaginal and 0.96 with the transabdominal approach [33]. Second trimester screening model based on uterine artery PI, maternal BMI, ethnic origin, previous obstetric history, smoking status, type of conception, medical history and mean arterial blood pressure (MAP) may detect as many as 100% of women who will develop early PE for a false positive rate of 10%; the sensitivity for late PE and gestational hypertension is 56.4% and 54.1%, respectively [34]. Although second trimester prediction of PE appears to be as sensitive as prediction in the first trimester, its value is limited by the lack of effective interventions at this gestational stage. It has been shown that in pre-eclampsia the concentration of sFlt1 starts to increase from the second trimester and the concentration of PlGF begins to decrease from the end of the first trimester [35]. The decrease in PlGF concentration and the increase in sFlt1 concentration advance the clinical symptoms of pre-eclampsia by 5 weeks. The sFlt1/PlGF ratio evaluated between 20 and 35 weeks' gestation allows pre-eclampsia to be excluded. If the test is positive, the risk of PE increases to 80%; if it is negative, then the risk of PE in the next 4 weeks is reduced to 7% [35, 36]. Multiple studies have shown that women who develop PE have, on average, higher mean arterial pressure [37], higher concentrations of maternal serum soluble fms-like tyrosine kinase-1 (sFlt1) [38] and alpha-fetoprotein (AFP) [39], and lower concentrations of pregnancy-associated plasma protein-A (PAPP-A) [40] and PlGF [41], along with higher resistance in the uterine arteries [42], compared with women who do not develop PE [26].

Selection of patients at increased risk of developing PE many weeks before the appearance of clinical symptoms allows for the implementation of pharmacological treatment. Meta-analyses of randomized studies have shown that acetylsalicylic acid (ASA) started before 16 weeks of gestation significantly reduces the risks of pre-eclampsia [43, 44]. The results of ASPRE study (Aspirin versus Placebo in Pregnancies at High Risk for Preterm Preeclampsia) have confirmed the effectiveness of ASA in reducing the number of patients with PE <34 weeks by 80% and <37 weeks by 63% [45]. The American College of Obstetricians and Gynecologists (ACOG) [46], the UK National Institute for Health and Care Excellence (NICE) [47] and the Society of Obstetricians and Gynaecologists of Canada (SOGC) [48], among others, are now recommending the administration of low-dose aspirin before 16 weeks to women at risk for pre-eclampsia [26].

17.4 Preterm Labour

Despite major progress in maternal-fetal medicine, the global number of cases of preterm labour is not decreasing and prematurity is still affecting more than 1 in 10 babies. Neonates born before 37 weeks of gestation are more likely to experience complications, not only soon after delivery but also various long-term health problems such as developmental disorders associated with prematurity. Babies born extremely prematurely are associated with a high mortality rate (10–15%) and a higher risk of cerebral palsy (5–10%). Neonatal conditions including respiratory distress syndrome (RDS), intraventricular haemorrhage (IVH), necrotizing enterocolitis (NEC) or sepsis are inversely associated with gestational age at birth [49]. Many recent publications describe how prematurity increases the risk of developing chronic diseases in adulthood. As many as 80% of preterm births are spontaneous, either due to spontaneous uterine contractions leading to cervical dilation and preterm labour (40–50%), or spontaneous preterm premature rupture of membranes (20–30%).The pathogenesis of spontaneous preterm delivery remains unknown. Some authors suggest there is no single trigger leading to initiation of the delivery, but a range of different causes initiating a cascade of biochemical and biophysical changes resulting in a start of labour. Romero et al underline there is a substantial difference in the mechanisms of term and preterm delivery. Preterm birth is a complex cluster of problems with a set of overlapping factors of influence. Both term and preterm birth

Table 17.4 Risk factors for preterm birth

Previous preterm delivery

Low socio-economic level

Multiple gestation

Polyhydramnios

Abdominal surgery during pregnancy

Uterine anomaly, leiomyomas

Preterm premature rupture of membranes

History of cervical surgery

Systemic infection, pyelonephritis, pneumonia

Bacteriuria

Fetal growth restriction

Smoking

share a common pathway composed of uterine contractility, cervical dilation and activation of the membranes, but preterm labour arises from pathological signalling and activation of one or more components of the common pathway of parturition [50]. In some cases, risk factors of preterm labour can be identified – the most recognized are listed in Table 17.4.

Preterm delivery by definition affects pregnancies between 22 and 37 weeks of gestation. In most patients, cervical dilation and effacement are assessed by digital examination or confirmed rupture of membranes. The traditional criteria for the diagnosis of preterm labour (painful uterine contractions accompanied by cervical change) lack precision, which as a result leads to overdiagnosis in as many as 40–70% of women diagnosed with preterm labour. Cervical dilation, effacement, consistency, position and station of the presenting part as determined by manual examination describe the stage of preterm birth. Clinical markers for high risk for imminent preterm delivery in women with symptoms include ruptured membranes, vaginal bleeding and cervical dilation beyond 2 cm. Unfortunately, vaginal examination and the use of the Bishop score (the most commonly used method to manually assess the cervix) are highly subjective.

In some cases, it may be useful to confirm threatening preterm delivery with a use of several diagnostic tests. One of such tests might be for example fetal fibronectin in vaginal discharge. Fetal fibronectin (fFN) is an extracellular matrix protein present at the decidual-chorionic interface. If the presence of fFN in vaginal discharge is present, disruption of decidual-chorionic interface due to subclinical infection or inflammation, abruption or uterine contraction is confirmed. A positive fFN test refers to an fFN concentration ≥50 ng/mL in cervicovaginal fluid and suggests that delivery is imminent within 7 to 10 days of testing with sensitivity and specificity 76.7% and 82.7%, respectively. Nevertheless, in most studies fFN has moderate accuracy for predicting preterm labour and the main potential role is likely to be reducing healthcare resource usage by identifying women not requiring intervention [51]. Another potential marker for increased risk of preterm labour is placental alpha-microglobulin-1 (PAMG-1) or phosphorylated insulin-like growth factor binding protein-1 (pIGFBP-1) in vaginal or cervical secretions. The positive result confirms disruption of the fetal membranes or imminent labour [52, 53].

The risk of spontaneous preterm birth is inversely related to the cervical length measured by transvaginal ultrasonography at 20–24 weeks' gestation [54, 55]. The risk of preterm labour before 35 weeks of gestation is about sixfold higher among women whose cervical length is less than the 10th percentile (25 mm) than that among women with a cervical length above the 75th percentile (40 mm). A systemic review also confirmed the risk of preterm birth before 34 weeks of gestation is 6.3 times greater for women whose cervical length is <25 mm, when the length was measured before 20 weeks of gestation, than for those whose cervical length is >25 mm [56].

Before the measurement, the patient needs to empty her bladder and should be placed in the dorsal lithotomy position. Transvaginal transducer is introduced in the anterior fornix of the vagina and a sagittal view of the entire length of the cervical canal should be obtained. Callipers should be used to measure the linear distance between the two ends of the glandular area around the endocervical canal [57] (Figure 17.2).

In women with a short cervix, administration of progesterone reduces the risk of spontaneous early preterm delivery by about 45% [58, 59]. However, progesterone is not as effective in women with cervical length less than 10 mm as it is in those with a length of 10–20 mm. Consequently, it may be preferable to measure cervical length in all patients to detect short cervix before the critical length of 10 mm is reached.

17.5 Serology and Laboratory Tests

When screening for high-risk pregnancy, it has to be acknowledged there are many other potential risks related to maternal health that need testing during pregnancy. Appropriate history, physical examination and laboratory studies can help identify pregnant women at increased risk of medical and pregnancy complications or fetal abnormalities. In many countries, routine antenatal visits are planned every few weeks and blood samples are taken at the first visit. By taking appropriate medical history and planning several blood tests, it is possible to screen for many potential pregnancy complications (Table 17.5). Early identification of such women gives the provider an opportunity to discuss these issues and their management with the patient and, in some cases, offer interventions to prevent or minimize the risk of an adverse outcome. Laboratory tests available for screening high-risk pregnancy are summarized in Table 17.6.

17.6 Summary

The major goal of prenatal care is to help ensure the birth of a healthy baby while minimizing risk to the mother. Despite

Table 17.5 Risk factors identified from medical history

Personal and demographic information

Past obstetric history

Infection history/exposure

Teratogen exposure

Risk assessment for heritable disorders

Risk assessment for substance abuse

Past surgical history

Travel to areas endemic for malaria, tuberculosis, Zika virus

Previous stillbirth

Previous small for gestational age

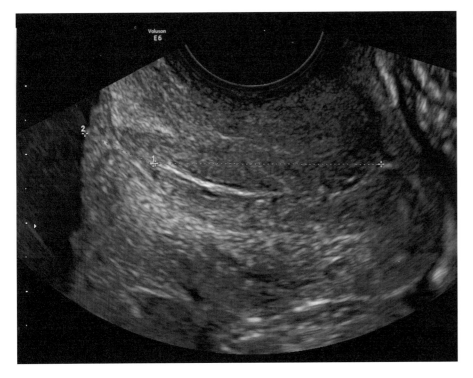

Figure 17.2 Transvaginal scan with the measurement of the length of cervical canal and cervical isthmus.

Table 17.6 Laboratory tests available for pregnant women useful in high-risk pregnancy screening

ABO and rhesus type and antibody screen*

Screening for rubella immunity

Screening for toxoplasmosis

Screening for varicella

Thyroid function screening

Diabetes screening (including OGTT)

Testing for syphilis, hepatitis B and C antigens, and chlamydia

Testing for HIV

Qualitative assessment of urine protein

Assessment for asymptomatic bacteriuria

Cervical cancer screening

OGTT: Oral glucose tolerance test
*RhD-negative women without alloantibodies should receive prophylactic anti(D)-immune globulin at 28 weeks and when clinically indicated to prevent alloimmunization

advances in maternal-fetal medicine and growing availability of hi-tech and sophisticated screening techniques for high-risk pregnancy, one must not forget to analyze gathered medical data in a holistic manner. Increasing complexity of specialization of care demands healthcare professionals to develop new skills to position a pregnant patient in the centre of medical care and resist the temptation of treating a patient as a collection of different and separate risks. A great focus should be made on the patient as a whole, because all medical conditions and complications interfere with each other. Above all described personalized risk evaluation and screening techniques in pregnancy, a global assessment of risk should cover: **personal risk profile** (age, ethnicity, parity, smoking, alcohol consumption, medical and obstetric history, conception method), **metabolic risk profile** (BMI, diabetes), **cardiovascular risk profile** (chronic conditions and measurement of arterial blood pressure) and **placental risk profile** (uterine artery Doppler studies and biochemical markers).

References

1. Sherer DM. Adverse perinatal outcome of twin pregnancies according to chorionicity: review of the literature. *Am J Perinatol.* 2001;**18**(1):23–37.

2. Dube J, Dodds L, Armson BA. Does chorionicity or zygosity predict adverse perinatal outcomes in twins? *Am J Obstet Gynecol.* 2002 Mar;**186**(3):579–83.

3. Adegbite AL, Castille S, Ward S, Bajoria R. Neuromorbidity in preterm twins in relation to chorionicity and discordant birth weight. *Am J Obstet Gynecol.* 2004 Jan;**190**(1):156–63.

4. Dias T, Arcangeli T, Bhide A, et al. First-trimester ultrasound determination of chorionicity in twin pregnancy. *Ultrasound Obstet Gynecol.* 2011 Nov;**38**(5):530–2.

5. Sebire NJ, Snijders RJ, Hughes K, Sepulveda W, Nicolaides KH. The hidden mortality of monochorionic twin pregnancies. *Br J Obstet Gynaecol.* 1997 Oct;**104**(10):1203–7.

6. Napolitano R, Thilaganathan B. Late termination of pregnancy and foetal reduction for foetal anomaly. *Best Pract Res Clin Obstet Gynaecol.* 2010 Aug;**24**(4):529–37.

7. Denbow ML, Cox P, Taylor M, Hammal DM, Fisk NM. Placental angioarchitecture in monochorionic twin pregnancies: relationship to fetal growth, fetofetal transfusion syndrome, and pregnancy outcome. *Am J Obstet Gynecol.* 2000 Feb;**182**(2):417–26.

8. Gratacos E, Carreras E, Becker J, et al. Prevalence of neurological damage in monochorionic twins with selective intrauterine growth restriction and intermittent absent or reversed end-diastolic umbilical artery flow. *Ultrasound Obstet Gynecol.* 2004 Aug;**24**(2):159–63.

9. Victoria A, Mora G, Arias F. Perinatal outcome, placental pathology, and severity of discordance in monochorionic and dichorionic twins. *Obstet Gynecol.* 2001 Feb;**97**(2):310–5.

10. Bejar R, Vigliocco G, Gramajo H, et al. Antenatal origin of neurologic damage in newborn infants. II. Multiple gestations. *Am J Obstet Gynecol.* 1990 May;**162**(5):1230–6.

11. Wright D, Kagan KO, Molina FS, Gazzoni A, Nicolaides KH. A mixture model of nuchal translucency thickness in screening for chromosomal defects. *Ultrasound Obstet Gynecol.* 2008 Apr;**31**(4):376–83.

12. Kagan KO, Wright D, Valencia C, Maiz N, Nicolaides KH. Screening for trisomies 21, 18 and 13 by maternal age, fetal nuchal translucency, fetal heart rate, free beta-hCG and pregnancy-associated plasma protein-A. *Hum Reprod.* 2008 Sep;**23**(9):1968–75.

13. Agathokleous M, Chaveeva P, Poon LC, Kosinski P, Nicolaides KH. Meta-analysis of second-trimester markers for trisomy 21. *Ultrasound Obstet Gynecol.* 2013 Mar;**41**(3):247–61.

14. Wang E, Batey A, Struble C, et al. Gestational age and maternal weight effects on fetal cell-free DNA in maternal plasma. *Prenat Diagn.* 2013 Jul;**33**(7):662–6.

15. Mackie FL, Hemming K, Allen S, Morris RK, Kilby MD. The accuracy of cell-free fetal DNA-based non-invasive prenatal testing in singleton pregnancies: a systematic review and bivariate meta-analysis. *BJOG.* 2017 Jan;**124**(1):32–46.

16. Iwarsson E, Jacobsson B, Dagerhamn J, et al. Analysis of cell-free fetal DNA in maternal blood for detection of trisomy 21, 18 and 13 in a general pregnant population and in a high risk population – a systematic review and meta-analysis. *Acta Obstet Gynecol Scand.* 2017 Jan;**96**(1):7–18.

17. Chaiworapongsa T, Chaemsaithong P, Yeo L, Romero R. Pre-eclampsia part 1: current understanding of its pathophysiology. *Nat Rev Nephrol.* 2014 Aug;**10**(8):466–80.

18. Duckitt K, Harrington D. Risk factors for pre-eclampsia at antenatal booking: systematic review of controlled studies. *BMJ.* 2005 Mar 12;**330**(7491):565.

19. Roberts L, Chaemsaithong P, Sahota DS, Nicolaides KH, Poon LCY. Protocol for measurement of mean arterial pressure at 10–40 weeks' gestation. *Pregnancy Hypertens.* 2017 Oct;**10**:155–60.

20. Tan MY, Syngelaki A, Poon LC, et al. Screening for pre-eclampsia by maternal factors and biomarkers at 11–13 weeks' gestation. *Ultrasound Obstet Gynecol.* 2018 Aug;**52**(2):186–95.

21. Baschat AA. First-trimester screening for pre-eclampsia: moving from personalized risk prediction to prevention. *Ultrasound Obstet Gynecol.* 2015 Feb;**45**(2):119–29.

22. Khalil A, Nicolaides KH. How to record uterine artery Doppler in the first trimester. *Ultrasound Obstet Gynecol.* 2013 Oct;**42**(4):478–9.

23. Tayyar A, Guerra L, Wright A, Wright D, Nicolaides KH. Uterine artery pulsatility index in the three trimesters of pregnancy: effects of maternal characteristics and medical history. *Ultrasound Obstet Gynecol.* 2015 Jun;**45**(6):689–97.

24. Martin AM, Bindra R, Curcio P, Cicero S, Nicolaides KH. Screening for pre-eclampsia and fetal growth restriction by uterine artery Doppler at 11–14 weeks of gestation. *Ultrasound Obstet Gynecol.* 2001 Dec;**18**(6):583–6.

25. Cnossen JS, Morris RK, ter Riet G, et al. Use of uterine artery Doppler ultrasonography to predict pre-eclampsia and intrauterine growth restriction: a systematic review and bivariable meta-analysis. *CMAJ.* 2008 Mar 11;**178**(6):701–11.

26. Sotiriadis A, Hernandez-Andrade E, da Silva Costa F, et al. ISUOG Practice Guidelines: role of ultrasound in screening for and follow-up of pre-eclampsia. *Ultrasound Obstet Gynecol.* 2019 Jan;**53**(1):7–22.

27. Velauthar L, Plana MN, Kalidindi M, et al. First-trimester uterine artery Doppler and adverse pregnancy outcome: a meta-analysis involving 55,974 women. *Ultrasound Obstet Gynecol.* 2014 May;**43**(5):500–7.

28. Poon LC, Nicolaides KH. Early prediction of preeclampsia. *Obstet Gynecol Int.* 2014;**2014**:297397.

29. Plasencia W, Maiz N, Bonino S, Kaihura C, Nicolaides KH. Uterine artery Doppler at 11 + 0 to 13 + 6 weeks in the prediction of pre-eclampsia. *Ultrasound Obstet Gynecol.* 2007 Oct;**30**(5):742–9.

30. Resnik R, Killam AP, Battaglia FC, Makowski EL, Meschia G. The stimulation of uterine blood flow by various estrogens. *Endocrinology.* 1974 Apr;**94**(4):1192–6.

31. Kusanovic JP, Romero R, Chaiworapongsa T, et al. A prospective cohort study of the value of maternal plasma concentrations of angiogenic and anti-angiogenic factors in early pregnancy and midtrimester in the identification of patients destined to develop preeclampsia. *J Matern Fetal Neonatal Med.* 2009 Nov;**22**(11):1021–38.

32. Kosinski P, Bomba-Opon D, Biskupski Samaha RB, Wielgos M. Suitable application of selected biochemical and biophysical markers during the first trimester screening. *Neuro Endocrinol Lett.* 2014;**35**(6):440–4.

33. Ferreira AE, Mauad Filho F, Abreu PS, et al. Reproducibility of first- and second-trimester uterine artery pulsatility index measured by transvaginal and transabdominal ultrasound. *Ultrasound Obstet Gynecol.* 2015 Nov;**46**(5):546–52.

34. Onwudiwe N, Yu CK, Poon LC, Spiliopoulos I, Nicolaides KH. Prediction of pre-eclampsia by a combination of maternal history, uterine artery Doppler and mean arterial pressure. *Ultrasound Obstet Gynecol.* 2008 Dec;**32**(7):877–83.

35. Agrawal S, Cerdeira AS, Redman C, Vatish M. Meta-analysis and systematic review to assess the role of soluble fms-like tyrosine kinase-1 and placenta growth factor ratio in prediction of preeclampsia: the SaPPPhirE Study. *Hypertension.* 2018 Feb;**71**(2):306–16.

36. Zeisler H, Llurba E, Chantraine F, et al. Soluble fms-like tyrosine kinase-1-to-placental growth factor ratio and time to delivery in women with suspected preeclampsia. *Obstet Gynecol.* 2016 Aug;**128**(2):261–9.

37. Tayyar A, Krithinakis K, Wright A, Wright D, Nicolaides KH. Mean arterial pressure at 12, 22, 32 and 36 weeks' gestation in screening for pre-eclampsia. *Ultrasound Obstet Gynecol.* 2016 May;**47**(5):573–9.

38. Tsiakkas A, Mendez O, Wright A, Wright D, Nicolaides KH. Maternal serum soluble fms-like tyrosine kinase-1 at 12, 22, 32 and 36 weeks' gestation in screening for pre-eclampsia. *Ultrasound Obstet Gynecol.* 2016 Apr;**47**(4):478–83.

39. Bredaki FE, Matalliotakis M, Wright A, Wright D, Nicolaides KH. Maternal serum alpha-fetoprotein at 12, 22 and 32 weeks' gestation in screening for pre-eclampsia. *Ultrasound Obstet Gynecol.* 2016 Apr;**47**(4):466–71.

40. Spencer K, Cowans NJ, Nicolaides KH. Low levels of maternal serum PAPP-A in the first trimester and the risk of pre-eclampsia. *Prenat Diagn.* 2008 Jan;**28**(1):7–10.

41. Khalil A, Maiz N, Garcia-Mandujano R, Penco JM, Nicolaides KH. Longitudinal changes in maternal serum placental growth factor and soluble fms-like tyrosine kinase-1 in women at increased risk of pre-eclampsia. *Ultrasound Obstet Gynecol.* 2016 Mar;**47**(3):324–31.

42. O'Gorman N, Tampakoudis G, Wright A, Wright D, Nicolaides KH. Uterine artery pulsatility index at 12, 22, 32 and 36 weeks' gestation in screening for pre-eclampsia. *Ultrasound Obstet Gynecol.* 2016 May;**47**(5):565–72.

43. Roberge S, Bujold E, Nicolaides KH. Aspirin for the prevention of preterm and term preeclampsia: systematic review and metaanalysis. *Am J Obstet Gynecol.* 2018 Mar;**218**(3):287–93 e1.

44. Bujold E, Roberge S, Nicolaides KH. Low-dose aspirin for prevention of adverse outcomes related to abnormal placentation. *Prenat Diagn.* 2014 Jul;**34**(7):642–8.

45. Rolnik DL, Wright D, Poon LC, et al. Aspirin versus placebo in pregnancies at high risk for preterm preeclampsia. *N Engl J Med.* 2017 Aug 17;**377**(7):613–22.

46. ACOG Committee Opinion No. 743 Summary: low-dose aspirin use during pregnancy. *Obstet Gynecol.* 2018 Jul;**132**(1):254–6.

47. Redman CW. Hypertension in pregnancy: the NICE guidelines. *Heart.* 2011 Dec;**97**(23):1967–9.

48. Lausman A, McCarthy FP, Walker M, Kingdom J. Screening, diagnosis, and management of intrauterine growth restriction. *J Obstet Gynaecol Can.* 2012 Jan;**34**(1):17–28.

49. Treyvaud K. Parent and family outcomes following very preterm or very low birth weight birth: a review. *Semin Fetal Neonatal Med.* 2014 Apr;**19**(2):131–5.

50. Romero R, Espinoza J, Kusanovic JP, et al. The preterm parturition syndrome. *BJOG.* 2006 Dec;**113** Suppl 3:17–42.

51. Deshpande SN, van Asselt AD, Tomini F, et al. Rapid fetal fibronectin testing to predict preterm birth in women with symptoms of premature labour: a systematic review and cost analysis. *Health Technol Assess.* 2013 Sep;**17**(40):1–138.

52. Wing DA, Haeri S, Silber AC, et al. Placental alpha microglobulin-1 compared with fetal fibronectin to predict preterm delivery in symptomatic women. *Obstet Gynecol.* 2017 Dec;**130**(6):1183–91.

53. Ting HS, Chin PS, Yeo GS, Kwek K. Comparison of bedside test kits for prediction of preterm delivery: phosphorylated insulin-like growth factor binding protein-1 (pIGFBP-1) test and fetal fibronectin test. *Ann Acad Med Singapore.* 2007 Jun;**36**(6):399–402.

54. To MS, Skentou CA, Royston P, Yu CK, Nicolaides KH. Prediction of patient-specific risk of early preterm delivery using maternal history and sonographic measurement of cervical length: a population-based prospective study. *Ultrasound Obstet Gynecol.* 2006 Apr;**27**(4):362–7.

55. Celik E, To M, Gajewska K, Smith GC, Nicolaides KH, Fetal Medicine Foundation Second Trimester Screening G. Cervical length and obstetric history predict spontaneous preterm birth: development and validation of a model to provide individualized risk assessment. *Ultrasound Obstet Gynecol.* 2008 May;**31**(5):549–54.

56. Honest H, Bachmann LM, Coomarasamy A, et al. Accuracy of cervical transvaginal sonography in predicting preterm birth: a systematic review. *Ultrasound Obstet Gynecol.* 2003 Sep;**22**(3):305–22.

57. Greco E, Lange A, Ushakov F, Calvo JR, Nicolaides KH. Prediction of spontaneous preterm delivery from endocervical length at 11 to 13 weeks. *Prenat Diagn.* 2011 Jan;**31**(1):84–9.

58. Fonseca EB, Celik E, Parra M, Singh M, Nicolaides KH, Fetal Medicine Foundation Second Trimester Screening G. Progesterone and the risk of preterm birth among women with a short cervix. *N Engl J Med.* 2007 Aug 02;**357**(5):462–9.

59. Hassan SS, Romero R, Vidyadhari D, et al. Vaginal progesterone reduces the rate of preterm birth in women with a sonographic short cervix: a multicenter, randomized, double-blind, placebo-controlled trial. *Ultrasound Obstet Gynecol.* 2011 Jul;**38**(1):18–31.

Multiple Pregnancy

Andrii V. Tkachenko, Asma Khalil & Iryna Tepla

18.1 Introduction

Multiple pregnancy is a high-risk pregnancy. The antenatal care of these pregnancies is often complicated and intrapartum care may be technically challenging and require a skilled and xperienced clinician. Women with multiple pregnancies have increased risk of adverse outcomes for both mother and fetuses during the pregnancy and childbirth, such as an increased risk of miscarriage, anaemia, hypertensive disorders, haemorrhage, operative delivery, caesarean section (CS) and postnatal complications. Maternal mortality is 2.5 times higher in multiple births than in singletons [1], and there is an increased risk of preterm birth, pre-eclampsia, prelabour rupture of membranes (PROM), placental abruption, other placental abnormalities (including placenta praevia), gestational diabetes, pyelonephritis, postpartum haemorrhage, etc. The hospital admission rate of such patients is six times greater than in singleton pregnancies [2]. Multiple pregnancy is associated with a sixfold increase in the risk of preterm birth, which is the leading cause of infant mortality and long-term mental and physical disability, including cerebral palsy, learning difficulties and chronic lung disease [1]. All these potential complications provide the incentive for doctors to learn more about multifetal pregnancy to enable them to provide optimal clinical care to such patients in accordance with the best available evidence and standards of care.

18.2 Epidemiology

Within the past 40 years there has been an increase in the frequency of multiple pregnancies. This rise is primarily associated with more frequent use of fertility treatment methods: induction of ovulation, stimulation of superovulation in assisted reproductive technology (ART) programmes, including in vitro fertilization (IVF) and transfer of several blastocysts at a time. Up to 24% of successful IVF procedures result in multiple pregnancies. Twinning rates are higher in European countries, Canada and Australia than in East Asian countries. Among Asian and Middle East countries, twinning rates are similar (5.5–8.9 per 1000 births) except in Israel, which is higher (9.7–17.4 per 1000 births). Among Western countries, the twinning rate was highest in Ireland until 1984; since then, the highest rates were observed in the Netherlands and Denmark. The last few years have seen the beginning of a decline in the proportion of twin deliveries in several countries, including the Netherlands, Germany, Norway, Finland, Switzerland, England and Wales. In the UK, multiple births currently account for 2–3% of live births [1]. According to

PERISTAT data, the median multiple pregnancy rate in Europe is 16.7 per 1000 maternities [3]. However, this rate varies considerably from over 19 per 1000 women in Ireland, Germany, Slovenia, Spain and Cyprus to under 14 per 1000 women in Romania, Slovakia, Poland, Greece, Finland and Lithuania. The increase in multiple births represents an important public health issue because of its large socio-economic, physical and psychological impact [4].

18.3 Aetiology

Many factors are linked to having a multiple pregnancy; they are traditionally divided into spontaneous and iatrogenic. Iatrogenic twins or higher-order pregnancies are a consequence of ARTs such as: ovulation-stimulation medicine and IVF. Moreover, there are some risk factors associated with an increased rate of *spontaneous* multiple pregnancies:

- Older age (women over the age of 35);
- Race (low prevalence between 2 and 7 per 1000 deliveries, in Hawaii, Japan and Taiwan; intermediate between 9 and 20 per 1000 maternities, in most countries in North Africa, America, Asia, Oceania and Europe; high prevalence, 20 per 1000 and higher, represented mostly by African countries, especially Nigeria, Seychelles, Transvaal and Zimbabwe [5];
- Family history

Other possible contributing factors remain unknown or poorly evaluated. For instance, the use of pesticides and food additives, growth promoters in agriculture and animal husbandry, or increased environmental pollution in general may play a role. Further studies are needed to allow significant conclusions concerning these factors to be drawn, in particular comparisons between countries and regions with marked variation in these environmental factors [4].

18.3.1 Origin of Twins

Based on the origin, there are two types of twins: monozygotic (MZ) and dizygotic (DZ). Monozygotic twins occur when only one oocyte was fertilized by one sperm; splitting into two independently developing embryos occurs later, at the stage of crushing a blastocyst. In such circumstances fetuses have inherited the same set of chromosomes and genes, are the same sex and are called homologous or identical twins. Dizygotic twinning occurs when two separate oocytes are released during the same menstrual cycle (a multiple ovulation event) and then are fertilized by two sperms of the same or different partners. Superfecundation is a type of multiple fertilization in which two oocytes are fertilized by sperm from two different partners within the same ovulatory period. Superfetation, which is a quite rare biological phenomenon, is a condition in which a second oocyte is released and fertilized in a woman already pregnant (the father might be the same or different). Genetically and phenotypically, DZ twins are like ordinary siblings; they can be same sex or different sex [5].

18.3.2 Chorionicity of Twins

Knowing the zygosity of multiples is key when it is necessary to assess the risk of inheritance by offspring of a chromosomal or genetic disorder present in one or both parents. Chorionicity refers to the type of placentation; from the clinical point of view, this is the most important determinant of the risk of twin-specific complications and their antenatal management. Multiples can be either monochorionic (MC), when the same placenta is shared by two or more fetuses, or dichorionic (DC), trichorionic (TC), etc., if each fetus has a separate placenta, amniotic sac, outer membrane and other extra-embryonic structures correspondingly.

18.3.2.1 Chorionicity and Amnionicity of DZ Twins

It is essential to understand that DZ twins can result only in a DC diamniotic (DCDA) twin pregnancy (Figure 18.1). DZ twins constitute around 80% of all twin pregnancies [6]. It is difficult to determine zygosity routinely as it is not routinely tested.

18.3.2.2 Chorionicity and Amnionicity of MZ Twins

Monozygotic twins can develop into either MC or DC twin pregnancies, depending on the separation (splitting) (Figure 18.1). In the case of DC twins, each fetus will have its own amniotic sac, so the pregnancy will be DCDA, irrespective of the zygosity. Monochorionic twin pregnancies may have separate or a common amniotic sac, so will be classified as MC diamniotic (MCDA) or MC monoamniotic (MCMA).

As mentioned, in MZ twins the number of placentas (chorions) depends on the timing of separation (splitting), i.e. the stage when the cells divide into two or more embryos (Figure 18.1). If separation occurs in the first 3 days after conception, it will develop into a DCDA twin pair; between 4–8 days, it will result in MCDA twins; between 8–13 days, MCMA twins; later than 13 days, conjoined twins. Monozygotic twins are always genetically identical, but their growth and phenotype may vary depending on the characteristics of the sharing parts of placenta, placentation itself and the presence of specific complications (see below). Monozygotic twins comprise up to 30% of all twin pregnancies [6]. The incidence of MC pregnancy remains relatively constant (1:250 of all pregnancies) unlike DC, which is influenced by race, heredity, maternal age, parity and medically assisted conception [7].

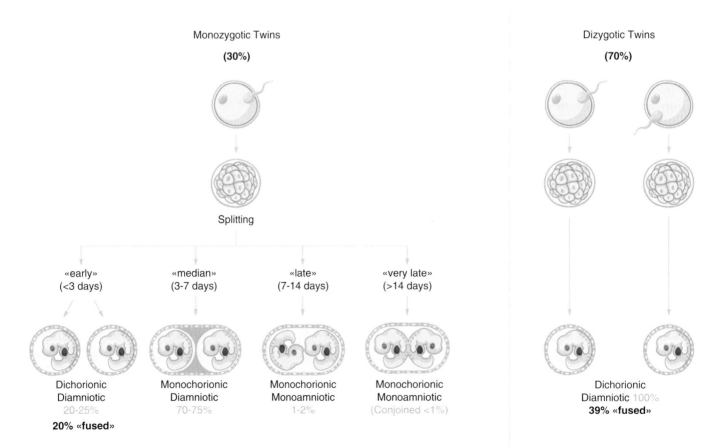

Figure 18.1 Chorionicity of MZ and DZ twins.

18.3.3 Placentation of Multiples

All DZ twins and up to 25% of MZ twins result in DCDA twin pregnancies, which are clinically the least complicated type of multiple pregnancies. Depending on the characteristics of implantation and further placental development, DCDA placentas may be either separately located in the uterus or adjacent/fused (but still functionally separate). Differential diagnosis between DCDA twins with fused placentas and MCDA twins might not be easy even for someone experienced in obstetric ultrasound, and sometimes requires expert fetal medicine evaluation. At the same time, about 75% of MZ twins develop the MC type of placentation, with either separate (MCDA) or shared (MCMA) amniotic sacs. The phenomenon of conjoined twins (Siamese twins) is extremely rare, with an incidence ranging from 1:49 000 to 1:189 000 births, with an unexplained higher prevalence in south-west Asia and some African countries. All MC (thus MZ) twins represent high obstetric risk pregnancies, and the greatest risk of perinatal complications, prematurity and antenatal demise occur in MCMA and MCDA multiples.

18.4 Diagnosis of Chorionicity and Amnionicity

Chorionicity should be determined between 11+0 and 13+6 weeks using the membrane thickness at the site of insertion of the amniotic membrane into the placenta, identifying the T sign or lambda sign (ultrasound image), and the number of placental masses visualized using ultrasound [1, 8]. The twins are separated by a thick layer of fused chorionic membranes in DCDA pregnancies, with two thin amniotic layers, one on each side, giving the appearance of a 'full lambda' (Figure 18.2), compared to only two thin amniotic layers separating the two fetuses in MCDA twin pregnancies (the T sign) (Figure 18.3).

Chorionicity can be challenging after 14 weeks and is best determined using the same ultrasound signs, in particular counting of the membrane layers, and noting discordant fetal sex. The reliability of the number of placental masses is poor, as DC placentas are commonly adjacent to each other, appearing

as a single mass, and 3% of MC twin pregnancies have two placental masses on ultrasound, which does not preclude the presence of vascular anastomosis [9]. It has been shown that a combination of ultrasound features, rather than a single one, is more accurate [1, 8].

If it is not possible to determine chorionicity by transabdominal ultrasound scan, transvaginal scan should be attempted. If it is still not possible to determine chorionicity, a second opinion should be sought from a tertiary referral centre. If the tertiary centre is uncertain about the chorionicity, it is recommended to treat the pregnancy as MC [1, 8].

The absence of the inter-twin membrane and the presence of cord entanglement are ultrasound signs of monoamnionicity. The former is best confirmed by transvaginal scan. Cord entanglement is almost universal in MCMA twin pregnancies and can be demonstrated using colour and pulsed-wave Doppler ultrasound. Using pulsed-wave Doppler, two distinct arterial waveform patterns with different heart rates are seen within the same sampling gate [10].

18.5 Pathology

It is already well proven that fetuses, newborns and babies from women with multiple pregnancies have much higher rate of adverse outcomes than singletons, including intrauterine fetal demise, stillbirth, preterm birth, low birthweight, growth restriction, congenital anomalies, neonatal and infant mortality and neurodevelopmental delay [3].

18.5.1 Specific Complications of Multiple Pregnancies

18.5.1.1 Twin-to-Twin Transfusion Syndrome

Twin-to-twin transfusion syndrome (TTTS) or feto-fetal transfusion syndrome (FFTS), also called twin oligohydramnios-polyhydramnios sequence (TOPS), is a potentially severe complication specific to MC pregnancy. TTTS is associated with increased risk of fetal/neonatal morbidity and mortality,

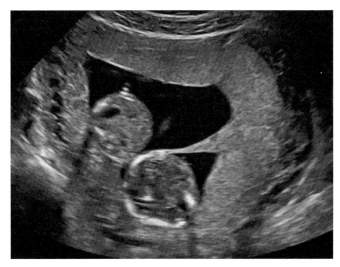

Figure 18.2 The 'lambda sign' seen in DCDA twin pregnancies.

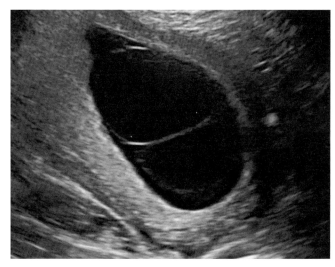

Figure 18.3 The 'T sign' seen in MCDA twin pregnancies.

especially when it occurs at a pre-viable gestation. Children who survive are at increased risk of cardiac, neurological and neurobehavioural disorders. Reported current incidence of TTTS is 1:40 to 1:60 twin pregnancies overall, affecting from 9% to 15% of MCDA and around 6% of MCMA twin pregnancies [11, 12]. It usually manifests at the beginning or in the middle of the second trimester, thus serial ultrasound diagnostic evaluations every 2 weeks starting from 16 weeks of gestation for the early detection of TTTS is recommended [2].

Pathophysiology of TTTS is based on the imbalance of blood flow through the placental vascular anastomosis between fetuses, which are always present in cases of MC placentation. This could be initially be due to mono-directional arteriovenous (AV) anastomoses shunting the blood via the intraplacental circulation from one fetus to another, or acquired imbalance of blood circulation between fetuses with predominant outflow from one fetus to the other. This can occur despite an adequate morphological structure of the intraplacental vascular system and initially balanced bidirectional blood flow. In both cases, unbalanced blood flow between fetuses through the placental vascular anastomosis leads to hypovolaemia of one fetus (donor) and hypervolaemia in the other (recipient). In addition to the hypovolaemia, the donor suffers from anaemia, oliguria, oligohydramnios, growth restriction and body compression due to the polyhydramnios in the sac of the recipient. As well as polyhydramnios, the recipient suffers from hypervolaemia, polyuria and cardiovascular insufficiency. In the most severe cases, congestive heart failure can result in systemic oedema and hydrops fetalis, and intrauterine death of one or both fetuses (Figure 18.4).

The main method for diagnosing TTTS is ultrasound examination, when the following criteria must be fulfilled: MCDA twin pregnancy with polyhydramnios (maximum

vertical pocket <18 weeks: ≥6 cm; 18–20 weeks: ≥8 cm; >20 weeks: ≥10 cm) in one sac and oligohydramnios (MVP ≤ 2 cm) in the other [13]. Staging of TTTS is usually according to the Quintero system [14].

Staging of TTTS:

- Stage 1: MCDA twins with oligohydramnios (MVP ≤ 2 cm) and polyhydramnios (MVP ≥8 cm)
- Stage 2: Absent (empty) bladder in donor
- Stage 3: Abnormal Doppler ultrasonography findings in one or both fetuses (presence of one or more of the following: umbilical artery absent or reversed diastolic flow; ductus venosus absent or reversed diastolic flow; or umbilical vein pulsatile flow)
- Stage 4: Hydrops of the recipient fetus
- Stage 5: Death of one or both twins.

It is important to differentiate TTTS from selective fetal growth restriction (sFGR), fetal growth discordance, chromosomal abnormalities and genetic diseases, structural disorders and infectious conditions, which may affect one or both twins and also lead to abnormal volume of amniotic fluid in one or both sacs and disproportion in fetal growth. TTTS in MCMA twins is a far less common complication in comparison to MCDA gestations. TTTS in MCMA gestations is associated with polyhydramnios in the single sac shared by both fetuses and discordant bladder sizes. As stated in the International Society of Ultrasound in Obstetrics and Gynecology (ISUOG) Clinical Practice Guidelines, MCDA twin pregnancies with inter-twin amniotic fluid discordance which does not fulfil the 8 cm/2 cm criterion (in other words, it falls within the 'normal' range), and normal umbilical artery Doppler measurements, are associated with a favourable outcome (93% overall survival) and a low risk (14%) of progression to severe TTTS. However, it is recommended for these pregnancies to be followed up on a weekly basis, to ensure that there is no progression to TTTS [8].

There are several options for treatment of TTTS depending on the stage, available facilities and the skills of medical providers:

- Laser ablation of abnormal vascular anastomosis is the treatment of choice for TTTS at 16–26 weeks' gestation (Quintero stage II and above);
- Conservative treatment (or just observation) with close surveillance is a common management option for Quintero stage I. Some centres advocate laser surgery as the treatment of choice in these cases;
- Serial amnioreduction (with or without septostomy) after 26' weeks of gestation or if laser ablation is not possible;
- Intrauterine selective feticide (if the gestation is less than 22 weeks, TTTS is likely to result in the demise of one fetus, and other options are not possible);
- Preterm delivery after a course of steroids in case of TTTS after 26–28 weeks' gestation.

In a systematic review of the management of stage 1 (Quintero) TTTS pregnancy, the overall survival rate for twins with TTTS stratified for stage and first-choice treatment was similar for those

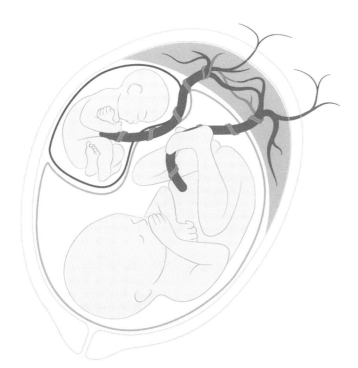

Figure 18.4 Twin-to-twin-transfusion syndrome (TTTS) in MCDA twins.

undergoing laser therapy or conservative management (85% and 86%, respectively), but was somewhat lower for those undergoing amnioreduction (77%) [15]. If during conservative management of Quintero stage I polyhydramnios continues to increase or the cervix becomes shorter, it is considered an indication to proceed to fetoscopy and laser ablation. The recurrence rate of TTTS after fetoscopy with laser treatment is up to 14%, likely to be secondary to missed anastomosis during the ablation procedure. The risk of recurrent TTTS is reduced by the use of the Solomon technique in comparison to selective laser ablation of anastomosis [12]. Selective feticide is a last resort in severe TTTS. Rarely parents make the difficult decision to sacrifice one fetus to give the other (co-twin) a chance to survive or to avoid cerebral disorders. The other option in cases of severe TTTS in the third trimester (26 weeks of gestation and more) is consideration of planned delivery by preterm CS after a course of steroids.

18.5.1.2 Twin Anaemia Polycythaemia Sequence (TAPS)

Twin anaemia polycythaemia sequence (TAPS) is another complication specific to MC twinning. TAPS can be considered as an atypical chronic form of TTTS or it can occur as a consequence of TTTS managed by laser ablation. The incidence of laser TAPS following laser treatment ranges between 2 and 13% [16, 17].

Pathophysiology of TAPS is similar to what happens in the case of TTTS; the imbalance of blood flows through the vascular anastomosis between MCDA/MCMA fetuses results in the development of anaemia of one twin and polycythaemia in the other, without measurable discordance in amniotic fluid volume in their sacs. In contrast to TTTS, in TAPS the presence of a small number of minuscule arteriovenous anastomoses in which diameters are less than 1 mm is more typical. These anastomoses may cause the slow blood transfusion from the donor to the recipient, leading to anaemia of the donor and polycythaemia in the recipient. As the result of the persistent blood transfusion through AV anastomoses, highly discordant haemoglobin (Hb) levels between twins is possible at birth.

Until now, only little evidence exists to guide the management of TAPS. There is a consensus that treatment of patients with TAPS should be individualized. Prenatal diagnosis should be made by evaluation of MCA Doppler velocity in both twins. The criteria for the diagnosis of TAPS in the prenatal period is based on the finding of discordant MCA Doppler indices, including MCA PSV (peak systolic velocity) >1.5 multiples of the median (MoM) in the donor, suggesting fetal anaemia, and MCA PSV <1.0 MoM in the recipient, suggesting polycythaemia. Additional findings such as differences in placental echo-density and thickness may aid diagnosis. A bright, thickened part of the placenta is associated with the donor and an echolucent thin part associated with the recipient [8]. The postnatal diagnosis of TAPS is easier and based on the finding of chronic anaemia in the donor and polycythaemia in the recipient, with the difference in haemoglobin concentration >8 g/dL, reticulocyte count ratio in one twin >1.7 and/or presence of small vascular anastomoses in the MC placenta (Table 18.1) [8].

The outcome of TAPS varies depending on the stage, parental choice and feasibility of surgical treatment. Earlier (mild) stage will usually result in the birth of two live neonates with discordant haemoglobin levels. Severe TAPS may result in intrauterine death (IUD) of one or both fetuses.

The management options for TAPS include the following:

- Conservative management with close surveillance
- Early delivery after a course of steroids
- Laser ablation of small AV vascular anastomoses
- Intrauterine blood transfusion for the anaemic fetus and intrauterine infusion to dilute the blood in the polycythaemia fetus.

Conservative management is common practice for TAPS, especially for stage 1 and 2. The one possibility to prevent post-laser TAPS is the use of Solomon technique during fetoscopic laser surgery [12]. For identification of TAPS, it is mandatory to measure the MCA PSV for both fetuses during the follow-up of TTTS cases treated by laser surgery and from 20 weeks of

Table 18.1 Antenatal and postnatal staging of twin anaemia polycythaemia sequence (TAPS)

Stage	Antenatal staging	Postnatal staging: intertwin Hb diff (g/dL)
1	Donor MCA-PSV >1.5 MoM, recipient MCA-PSV <1.0 MoM, no other signs of fetal compromise	>8.0
2	Donor MCA-PSV >1.7 Mom, recipient MCA-PSV <0.8 MoM, no other signs of fetal compromise	>11.0
3	MCA-PSV flow – look at stage 1 or 2 and cardiac compromise in donor (UA-AREDF, UV pulsatile flow, or DV increased or reversed flow)	>14.0
4	Hydrops of donor twin	>17.0
5	Death of one or both fetuses, preceded by TAPS	>20.0

AREDF: absent or reversed end-diastolic flow; DV: ductus venosus; Hb: haemoglobin; MCA: middle cerebral artery; MoM: multiples of the median; PI: pulsatility index; PSV: peak systolic velocity; UA: umbilical artery; UV: umbilical vein.

gestation every 2 weeks in uncomplicated MC twin pregnancies [8].

18.5.1.3 Twin Reversed Arterial Perfusion Sequence (TRAP)

Twin reversed arterial perfusion sequence (TRAP) or acardiac twinning is a rare complication of MC twin pregnancies. The prevalence is around 2.6% of MC twin pregnancies and 1 in 95 000 to 11 000 of all pregnancies [18]. This condition may also be considered similar to TTTS, but it is a most severe form.

Pathophysiology of TRAP is due to the presence of initially abnormally formed arterio-arterial (AA) anastomoses between twins' circulations, which exist mostly along the placental surface. In addition, a range of related vascular atypia and other morphological abnormalities, such as direct umbilical artery to umbilical artery communications that bypass the chorionic plate, have been described. Veno-venous (VV) anastomoses may also be present, but are haemodynamically less significant [19, 20]. In TRAP sequence, a normal fetus (pump twin) perfuses in a cardiac mass (a cardiac co-twin). The pump twin maintains its normal fetal circulatory pattern, but a portion of its cardiac output passes through AA anastomoses, then flows retrograde into one or both umbilical arteries and the systemic circulation of the acardiac twin, thus creating 'reversed' circulatory perfusion. An acardiac twin usually does not have an upper body or head and is not viable.

Among treatment options for TRAP, there is only one that will prevent the demise of the pump twin, namely termination of the acardiac twin. Invasive techniques, such as cord coagulation, cord ligation, photocoagulation, radiofrequency ablation of the anastomoses or intrafetal laser ablation, can be performed for cessation of blood flow in the acardiac co-twin. The survival rate of the pump fetus is around 80%. It is generally recognized that without treatment, the pump twin is at risk of developing heart failure, polyhydramnios, preterm birth and IUD. Some authors recommend minimally invasive techniques at 12–14 weeks, which may increase the survival rate for the normal fetus [12].

18.5.1.4 Growth Discordance and Small-for-Gestational-Age, Selective Fetal Growth Restriction (sFGR)

Growth discordance is a frequent finding among multiple gestations. The pregnancy outcomes depend more on the gestation and birthweight at delivery than on the degree of growth discordance. Birthweight (BW) discordance is associated with an increased risk of adverse outcomes such as stillbirth, neonatal death, preterm birth, respiratory distress and admission to the neonatal intensive care unit [21]. Twenty-five per cent birthweight discordance is an indication for referral to tertiary level fetal centre [8]. In comparison to European Guidelines, the American College of Obstetricians and Gynecologists consider that a difference in estimated fetal weight (EFW) in the range 15–25% should be termed fetal growth discordance [2]. When the EFW of one or both fetuses is less than the 10th centile, it should be termed small for gestational age (SGA).

EFW discordance of twins should be calculated using the following formula:

$$\frac{(Weight\ of\ larger\ twin\ -\ weight\ of\ smaller\ twin)}{Weight\ of\ larger\ twin} \times 100$$

The sFGR is conventionally defined as a condition in which one fetus has an EFW <10th centile and the inter-twin EFW discordance is ≥25% (Good Practice Principles, GPP). A discordance cut-off of 20% seems acceptable to distinguish pregnancies at increased risk of adverse outcome. Such phenomenon can be detected in multiples with different types of placentation (MC and DC) but more often affects MC twin couples with higher rate of unfavourable perinatal consequences. Classification of sFGR in MC twins depends on the pattern of end-diastolic velocity (EDF) of the umbilical artery Doppler of the smaller fetus (GPP) [8] (Figure 18.5).

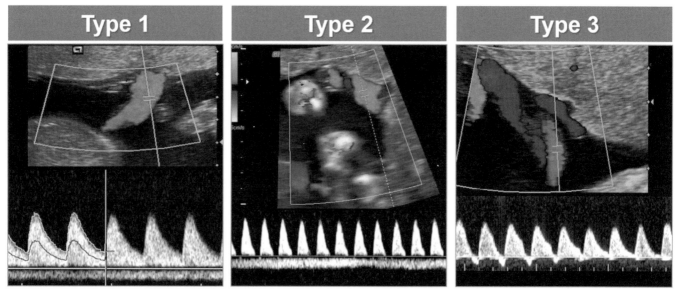

Figure 18.5 Classification of selective fetal growth restriction (sFGR) in MC twins. A black and white version of this figure will appear in some formats. For the colour version, please refer to the plate section.

Classification of sFGR in MC twins:

- Type I: EDF positive. Survival rate for both fetuses is 90%; in utero mortality rates of up to 4%.
- Type II: AREDF (absent or reversed end-diastolic flow). Both fetuses are at risk of adverse outcome; for the growth-restricted fetus the risk is IUD and for both fetuses, there is a risk of very preterm delivery. IUD of either twin occurs in up to 29% and the risk of neurological sequelae is up to 15% in those born prior to 30 weeks.
- Type III: EDF cyclical/intermittent changes from positive to AREDF. The demise of the smaller fetus is unpredictable, and there is a high risk of neurological morbidity in the larger surviving twin. The risk of sudden death of the growth-restricted fetus is 10–20%, even in cases in which ultrasound features have been stable, with the associated rate of neurological morbidity in the surviving larger twin up to 20% (EVIDENCE LEVEL: 2++).

Currently, the charts used to monitor fetal growth in twin pregnancies are the same as those used for singletons. However, there is a reduction in fetal growth in twins compared with singleton pregnancies, particularly in the third trimester. This suggests that twin-specific growth charts should be used for documenting and monitoring growth in twin pregnancies. Compared with the Southwest Thames Obstetric Research Collaborative (STORK) chorionicity-specific twin charts, the customized and non-customized singleton charts classified prenatally as small for gestational age (SGA) more liveborn fetuses. However, the three charts classified as SGA a similar proportion of stillborn cases. These results suggest that these twin charts could safely reduce unnecessary medical intervention in twin pregnancies [22].

Among treatment options for sFGR in MC twins is planned preterm birth, laser ablation of the placenta or cord occlusion of the growth-restricted fetus. MC twin pregnancies affected by sFGR should be assessed by Doppler once a week. In DC twins, sFGR should be managed similar to singletons. This group of women should undergo ultrasound assessment with fetal Doppler (umbilical artery and MCA) every two weeks at

least. Treatment should be performed by skilled medical providers in special centres with relevant experience [8].

18.5.1.5 Intrauterine Fetal Death (IUFD) or Single Intrauterine Fetal Demise (sIUFD)

The incidence of single intrauterine fetal demise (sIUFD) is 3.7–6.8% of all twin pregnancies. Death of one co-twin is a severe complication of an already complicated pregnancy and should be managed in special centres with relevant experience. Death of one fetus may occur in any trimester; the reasons are variable. Fetal demise may be caused by complications related to chorionicity (MC-specific complications) or any pathological conditions that can affect any pregnancy (multiple or singleton). Severe complications, such as brain, kidney or gastrointestinal injury, may occur in the surviving MC co-twin after demise of the other co-twin. Single intrauterine fetal demise may also occur in DC pregnancies, but its incidence is much lower in comparison to MC twins, and the risk of adverse outcomes for the survivor is much less, most commonly the risk of preterm birth [23, 24].

The risk of adverse outcomes of sIUFD in multiples depends on the gestational term at which fetal death occurs, the chorionicity and the cause of death (Figure 18.6). The demise of one twin in MC pregnancy causes disruption in the circulation. From the pathophysiological point of view, the sudden fall of blood pressure (vascular resistance) in the dead twin leads to acute haemodynamic imbalance between the fetuses, thus leading to a loss of blood from the surviving fetus into the dead fetus. This is considered the main reason for brain injury, neurological deficit and disorders of other systems causing adverse perinatal and postnatal outcomes in the surviving twin. The existence of major placental vascular anastomoses is thought to be the mechanism of life-threatening hypovolaemia of the co-twin following sIUFD [25].

Vanishing twin is a well-known phenomenon, first described by Stoeckel in 1945 [26]. The incidence is 21–30% of multifetal gestations [27]. This condition occurs in the first trimester and does not usually cause any significant harm to the surviving twin. It is unknown whether anastomoses between the chorions are

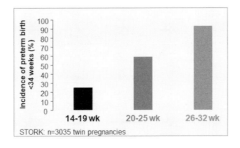

Figure 18.6 Consequences of sIUD depending on chorionicity and term of incident.

	Monochorionic twins	Dichorionic twins
Death of co-twin	15%	3%
Preterm delivery	68%	54%
Postnatal brain abnormalities	34%	16%
Neurological abnormalities	26%	2%

The incidence of preterm birth <34 weeks is higher if the sIUD occurs later in the second half of pregnancy

already formed at this early gestation. The recognized incidence of vanishing twin increased when ultrasound assessment was implemented as a standard of pregnancy care, leading to the appreciation that far more twins are conceived than are born. The predominant factors leading to this condition are severe chromosomal abnormalities and implantation failure. Clinically, it often manifests as painless vaginal bleeding. In the case of DC twins, no negative consequences for the surviving embryo has been demonstrated, and there is no apparent effect on pregnancy duration or outcomes. In the case of MC twins, early onset of IUGR might be observed more commonly.

In all clinical cases of sIUFD in MC twin pregnancy, a thorough assessment of fetal well-being should be carried out. If there are no other indications for urgent delivery, such as fetal distress of the surviving twin or severe obstetric complication, conservative management might be considered with close monitoring of the surviving co-twin by ultrasound with fetal Doppler (umbilical artery and MCA). Antenatal corticosteroids should be administered, and planned delivery should be considered at 34–36 weeks [8].

18.5.2 Non-Specific Complications of Multiple Pregnancies

Women carrying twins also have a higher risk of obstetric and perinatal complications – conditions which may also affect singleton pregnancies but occur significantly more frequently in multiple gestations. These include miscarriage, preterm birth, PROM, placental abruption and abnormalities of placentation (including placenta praevia), gestational anaemia, pyelonephritis, gestational diabetes, pre-eclampsia and hypertensive disorders, dystocia of labour and postpartum haemorrhage [28]. The principal pregnancy complications leading to perinatal mortality and morbidity are preterm birth, fetal growth restriction and congenital anomalies.

18.5.2.1 Maternal Complications

Women with multiple pregnancy are at greater risk of maternal complications during pregnancy in comparison to women carrying singletons and need closer monitoring by healthcare professionals. There is a higher incidence of anaemia; full blood count should be performed at 20–24 weeks of gestation and iron supplementation commenced if necessary. This test should be repeated at 28 and 34 weeks of gestation. To help identify among all women carrying multiples those at particularly increased risk of hypertensive disorders, the following risk factors should be taken into account:

- First pregnancy;
- Age 40 years or older;
- Pregnancy interval of more than 10 years;
- Body mass index (BMI) of 35 kg/m^2 or more at first visit;
- Family history of pre-eclampsia.

For women with these risk factors, low-dose aspirin (75–120 mg daily) should be prescribed starting from 12 weeks of gestation and continued until the end of pregnancy [29].

18.5.2.2 Preterm Birth

Multiple pregnancies carry a higher risk of both spontaneous and iatrogenic preterm birth due to the high incidence of maternal and fetal complications. Over 50% of twins and triplets are born before 37 weeks of gestation. Prematurity is the biggest challenge for multiple pregnancies; more than 15–20% of admissions to neonatal intensive care units are for preterm twins and triplets [29].

The following criteria may be used for the prediction of spontaneous preterm birth:

- Cervical length ≤ 25 mm is the cut-off commonly used in the second trimester [8];
- Obstetric history [1].

Preterm birth is associated with considerably higher morbidity and mortality and use of healthcare resources. For the prevention of spontaneous preterm birth in singletons several interventions have been investigated, such as bed rest at home or in hospital, intramuscular or vaginal progesterone, cervical cerclage and oral tocolytics. Unfortunately, there is no high-quality evidence that any of these interventions are effective in the prevention of preterm birth in multiple pregnancies. Thus, according to National Collaborating Centre for Women's and Children's Health multiple pregnancy guidelines, none of these methods should be routinely used in twins [29].

18.6 Management of Twin Pregnancy

All twin pregnancies should undergo ultrasound assessment between 11+0 to 13+6 weeks of gestation, when the crown–rump length (CRL) measurement should be between 45 and 84 mm. There is still some debate around which fetus (the larger or smaller) should be used for determining gestational age. The most widespread practice is to use the biometry (CRL) of the larger twin. If the woman presents after 14 weeks of gestation, the larger head circumference should be used for estimation of the term of gestation [1]. For dating of twins conceived by IVF, the oocyte retrieval date or the embryonic age from the day of fertilization should be used. Ultrasound assessment of chorionicity and amnionicity in twin pregnancy implies the determination of the membrane thickness at the site of insertion of the amniotic membrane into the placenta, identifying the T sign or lambda sign (Figures 18.2, 18.3), as well as estimation of the number of placental masses (see above). It is important to identify and record amnionicity and chorionicity in the first trimester, because in later pregnancy it may be technically difficult or even impossible. If estimation of the number of placentas and clarification of the amnionicity of twins is not clear, referral to a tertiary-level centre for expert ultrasound assessment is recommended.

For the management of multiple gestations, it is very important to label fetuses carefully, starting from early gestation.

Labelling of fetuses may include:
- The site in the uterus in relation to laterality (left/right or upper/lower);

- Detection of the cord insertion into the placenta relative to the placental edges and membrane insertion;
- Definition of fetal sex, if it is visible and parents agree to it being disclosed.

All information about fetuses should be clearly documented for further follow-up and management. It is recommended that as many fetal features as possible are used to enable their accurate identification at subsequent ultrasound assessments.

Twin pregnancy monitoring with ultrasound:
- Women with uncomplicated MC twin pregnancy should undergo routine ultrasound assessment in the first trimester (11+0 to 13+6 weeks) and every 2 weeks starting from 16 weeks of gestation for the early diagnosis and assessment of specific complications (such as TTTS and TAPS).
- Complicated MC twins should be scanned more frequently, but the number of scans depends on the type of complication(s) and their severity.
- Women with uncomplicated DC twins should have ultrasound examination in the first trimester (11+0 to 13+6 weeks); a detailed anatomy scan should be performed in the second trimester (20–21 weeks) and every 4 weeks thereafter.
- Complicated DC twins will be assessed by ultrasound examination more frequently, depending on the fetuses' well-being, pathological findings and their severity.

All ultrasound scans should include the following:
- Biometry of both fetuses;
- Evaluation of amniotic fluid volume for both twins by measuring the deepest vertical pocket (DVP) in each twin to detect the development of TTTS (in case of MC multiples);
- Umbilical artery Doppler for both twins (starting from 20 weeks of gestation);
- Calculation of EFW discordancy (at every scan starting from 20 weeks of gestation);
- MCA PSV should be measured in MC twin pregnancies to detect the development of TAPS.

It is well-recognized that multifetal pregnancies are at increased risk of congenital anomaly. The prevalence of fetal anomalies in twins is 406 per 10 000 twins in comparison to 238 per 10 000 singletons [30]. Detailed ultrasound assessment in the first and second trimesters is therefore necessary. All twins should be offered first trimester screening for chromosomal abnormalities, which can be along with the combined test (nuchal translucency thickness (NT), free beta-human chronic gonadotropin (β-hCG) and pregnancy-associated plasma protein-A (PAPP-A) levels) or combination of maternal age and NT measured between 11+0 and 13+6 weeks of gestation. It is important to remember that the risk of trisomy in MC twins should be calculated per pregnancy rather than per fetus, because both twins have an identical karyotype, so the risk is averaged for both fetuses. In DC twin pregnancies, the risk is calculated per fetus, because these twins might have different karyotypes in more than 90% of cases. Women with a history of or at high risk of chromosomal abnormalities

should be referred to a fetal medicine specialist to define the best screening strategy and possibly to undergo invasive prenatal diagnostic testing (amniocentesis, chorion villus sampling, cordocentesis). Cell-free fetal DNA or non-invasive prenatal screening (NIPT) is fetal genetic testing on a maternal blood sample which carries no risk for the mother or fetuses. NIPT screens only for trisomies 21, 18, 13, but not for other genetic conditions, birth defects or pregnancy complications. These tests could be used in twin pregnancy and in the not so distant future potentially might be recommended for screening for chromosomal abnormalities.

18.7 Delivery of Twin Pregnancy

18.7.1 Gestation at Delivery for Twin Pregnancies

The optimal timing of birth for women with an otherwise uncomplicated twin pregnancy is uncertain, with clinical support for both elective delivery at 37 weeks and for expectant management (awaiting the spontaneous onset of labour) [31]. Cincotta and colleagues retrospectively reviewed data from Queensland, Australia, over a 10-year period in 6328 women with a twin pregnancy, to establish the gestational age-specific stillbirth risk for both twins and singleton gestations [32]. On the basis of this information, the authors concluded that the gestation-specific rise in stillbirth rate seen in singletons from 40 weeks occurs in twins from 36 weeks' gestation onwards. Based on retrospective information obtained from almost 89 000 infants born to women with a multiple pregnancy in Japan, Minakami and Sato have suggested that the lowest risk of perinatal death in multiple pregnancies at 38 weeks' gestation corresponded to that observed in singleton pregnancies at 43 weeks' gestation [33].

18.7.1.1 Gestation of Delivery for DC Twins

Early birth at 37 weeks' gestation compared with ongoing expectant management for women with an uncomplicated twin pregnancy does not appear to be associated with an increased risk of harms. Furthermore, there may be possible benefits in earlier birth (including a reduction in infants being born small for gestational age). The findings of no increased risk of harms with birth at 37 weeks' gestation is consistent with the NICE recommendations advocating birth for women with a DC twin pregnancy at 37+0 weeks' gestation [1].

Table 18.2 summarizes the current recommendations for the optimal timing of delivery for twins in relation to chorionicity and the presence of specific complications. This analysis is based on the most recent Cochrane reviews, ISUOG, ACOG, RCOG guidelines and NICE statements[1, 2, 8].

There is much variation in the intrapartum management of twin pregnancies worldwide. Three potential modes of delivery are possible: vaginal (VB) of both twins (VB–VB), caesarean section (CS) for both twins (CS–CS), and VB of the first and CS of the second twin (VB–CS). Decisions regarding the mode of delivery are based mainly on the gestational age and the presentation of the first twin. The ACOG recommends VB for vertex–vertex (V/V) twin gestations, unless specific contraindications

Table 18.2 Optimal timing of delivery for different types of twin pregnancies

Gestational age	32	33	34	35	36	37
Type of twins						
DCDA (uncomplicated)						✓
DCDA (sFGR with normal fetal Doppler)					✓	✓
MCDA (uncomplicated)					✓	
MCDA (treated TTTS)			✓			
MCDA (sFGR I)			✓	✓	✓	
MCMA	✓	✓	✓			
MCDA (sFGR II)	✓					
MCDA (sFGR III)	✓					

exist [2]. For pregnancies with the first twin in a non-vertex (NV) presentation, CS is now widely preferred [28]. The mode of delivery for vertex/non-vertex (V/NV) twins remains controversial. Caesarean section has been advocated based on reports of increased perinatal mortality and lower Apgar scores for second twins in breech presentation delivered vaginally. However, many of these reports date from the 1970s, when fetal heart rate monitoring and ultrasound were not routine. The ACOG noted the lack of evidence for advocating a specific route of delivery for NV second twins weighing less than 1500 g, but stated that vaginal birth is reasonable for infants weighing more than 1500 g when criteria for vaginal birth are met. The updated recommended management of the V/NV presentation considers the possibility of a vaginal birth, but also highlights the increased risk of emergency CS, especially where there is a large size discordance [34].

References

1. NICE. *Multiple Pregnancy: Antenatal Care for Twin and Triplet Pregnancies.* Clinical Guideline CG129. 2011. http://dx.doi.org/10.1016/j.rcl.2013.07.010%0Ahttps://www.nice.org.uk/guidance/cg129

2. American College of Obstetricians and Gynecologists; Society for Maternal-Fetal Medicine. Practice Bulletin No 144: multifetal gestations: twin, triplet, and higher-order multifetal pregnancies. *Obstet Gynecol.* 2014;**123**(5):1118–32. http://content.wkhealth.com/linkback/openurl?sid=WKPTLP:landingpage&an=00006250-201405000-00040

3. European Perinatal Health Report [Internet]. Available from: www.europeristat.com

4. Pison G, D'Addato A V. Frequency of twin births in developed countries. *Twin Res Hum Genet.* 2006;**9**:250–9.

5. Hoekstra C, Zhao ZZ, Lambalk CB, et al. Dizygotic twinning. *Hum Reprod Update.* 2008;**14**(1):37-47.

6. Bręborowicz GH, Malinowski W. *Atlas ciąży wielopłodowej.* Poznań: Ośrodek Wydawnictw Naukowych; 2008.

7. Manso P, Vaz A, Taborda A, Silva IS. [Chorionicity and perinatal complications in twin pregnancy: a 10 years case series]. *Acta Med Port.* 2011;**24**:695–8.

8. Goya M, Carreras E, Cabero L. Re: ISUOG Practice Guidelines: role of ultrasound in twin pregnancy. *Ultrasound Obstet Gynecol.* 2016;**48**(5):669-70.

9. Lopriore E, Sueters M, Middeldorp JM, et al. Twin pregnancies with two separate placental masses can still be monochorionic and have vascular anastomoses. *Am J Obstet Gynecol.* 2006;**194**:804–8.

10. Lewi L, Devlieger R, De Catte L, Deprest J. Assessment of twin gestation. In Coady AM, Bower S, eds. *Twining's Textbook of Fetal Abnormalities*, 3rd ed. London: Churchill Livingstone, Elsevier Ltd; 2015.

11. Martin JA, Hamilton BE, Sutton PD, et al. Births: final data for 2005. *Natl Vital Stat Rep.* 2007;**56**:1–103.

12. Slaghekke F, Kist WJ, Oepkes D, et al. Twin anemia-polycythemia sequence: diagnostic criteria, classification, perinatal management and outcome. *Fetal Diagn Ther.* 2010;**27**:181–90.

13. Khalil A. Modified diagnostic criteria for twin-to-twin transfusion syndrome prior to 18 weeks' gestation: time to change? *Ultrasound Obstet Gynecol.* 2017;**49**:804–5.

14. Quintero RA, Morales WJ, Allen MH, et al. Staging of twin-twin transfusion syndrome. *J Perinatol.* 1999;**19**:550–5.

15. Khalil A, Cooper E, Townsend R, Thilaganathan B. Evolution of stage 1 twin-to-twin transfusion syndrome (TTTS): systematic review and meta-analysis. *Twin Res Hum Genet.* 2016;**19**:207–16.

16. Habli M, Bombrys A, Lewis D, et al. Incidence of complications in twin-twin transfusion syndrome after selective fetoscopic laser photocoagulation: a single-center experience. *Am J Obstet Gynecol.* 2009;**201**:417.e1–417.e7.

17. Robyr R, Lewi L, Salomon LJ et al. Prevalence and management of late fetal complications following successful selective laser coagulation of chorionic plate anastomoses in twin-to-twin transfusion syndrome. *Am J Obstet Gynecol.* 2006;**194**:796–803.

18. van Gemert MJC, van den Wijngaard JPHM, Vandenbussche FPHA. Twin reversed arterial perfusion sequence is more common than generally accepted. *Birth Defects Res A Clin Mol Teratol.* 2015;**103**:641–3.

19. Steffensen TS, Gilbert-Barness E, Spellacy W, Quintero RA. Placental pathology in trap sequence: clinical and

pathogenetic implications. *Fetal Pediatr Pathol.* 2008;**27**:13–29.

20. van Gemert MJC, Ross MG, Nikkels PGJ, Wijngaard JPHM van den. Acardiac twin pregnancies part III: Model simulations. *Birth Defects Res Part A Clin Mol Teratol.* 2016;**106**:1008–15.

21. D'Antonio F, Khalil A, Dias T, Thilaganathan B. Weight discordance and perinatal mortality in twins: Analysis of the Southwest Thames Obstetric Research Collaborative (STORK) multiple pregnancy cohort. *Ultrasound Obstet Gynecol.* 2013;**41**:643–8.

22. Kalafat E, Sebghati M, Thilaganathan B, et al. Predictive accuracy of Southwest Thames Obstetric Research Collaborative (STORK) chorionicity-specific twin growth charts for stillbirth: a validation study. *Ultrasound Obstet Gynecol.* 2019;**53**:193–9.

23. Hillman SC, Morris RK, Kilby MD. Co-twin prognosis after single fetal death. *Obstet Gynecol.* 2011;**118**:928–40.

24. D'Antonio F, Thilaganathan B, Dias T, Khalil A, Southwest Thames Obstetric Research Collaborative (STORK). Influence of chorionicity and gestational age at single fetal loss on risk of preterm birth in twin pregnancy: analysis of STORK multiple pregnancy cohort. *Ultrasound Obstet Gynecol.* 2017;**50**:723–7.

25. *Prognosis for the Co-Twin Following Intrauterine Single-Twin Death.* Swiss Society of Neonatology; 2016 [Internet]. Available from: www .wikipedia.org.

26. Landy H. The vanishing twin: a review. *Hum Reprod Update.* 1998;**4**:177–83.

27. Sampson A, de Crespigny LC. Vanishing twins: the frequency of spontaneous fetal reduction of a twin pregnancy. *Ultrasound Obstet Gynecol.* 1992;**2**(2):107-9.

28. A.C.O.G., S.M-F.M. ACOG Practice Bulletin No. 144: multifetal gestations: twin, triplet and higher order multifetal pregnancies. *Obstet Gynecol.* 2014;**123**:1118–32.

29. National Collaborating Centre for Women's and Children's Health. *Multiple Pregnancy: The Management of Twin and Triplet Pregnancies in the Antenatal Period.* London: RCOG Press; 2011.

30. Glinianaia SV, Rankin J, Wright C. Congenital anomalies in twins: a register-based study. *Hum Reprod.* 2008;**23**:1306–11.

31. Dodd JM, Crowther CA, Haslam RR, Robinson JS. Elective birth at 37 weeks of gestation versus standard care for women with an uncomplicated twin pregnancy at term. *Obstet Gynecol Surv.* 2012;**67**:675–6.

32. Cincotta R, Flenady V, Hockey R, King J. Mortality of twins and singletons by gestational age: a varying coefficient approach. Perinatal Society of Australia and New Zealand, 5th Annual Congress: 2001; Canberra, Australia. 2001. p. 22.

33. Minakami H, Sato I. Reestimating date of delivery in multifetal pregnancies. *JAMA.* 1996;**275**:1432–4.

34. Twin and triplet pregnancy: NICE guideline DRAFT. March 2019.

Chapter 19

Intrauterine Growth Restriction

George J. Daskalakis, Panos Antsaklis, Maria Papamichail & Aris J. Antsaklis

19.1 Introduction

Intrauterine growth restriction (IUGR) refers to diminished fetal growth during intrauterine life and is defined as decreased fetal growth. However, what needs to be clarified is that IUGR does not refer to just small fetal size, but to smaller size than what this particular fetus was genetically programmed to be. So IUGR refers to a fetus that is genetically programmed to reach a specific weight, but for some reason it fails to reach this weight. There is generally a main underlying pathological cause that is responsible for this clinical condition, such as genetic or environmental factors [1]. IUGR is a common obstetric complication that remains a leading cause of neonatal and fetal mortality and morbidity. It alters the antenatal care regimen, increasing antenatal visits, ultrasound examinations and admissions to the hospital. The incidence of IUGR varies from 7–24% in different studies and this broad range reflects, on one hand, the multifactorial nature of IUGR and, on the other hand, it results from the lack of a homogeneous universal definition, something that leads to different diagnostic criteria being used antenatally and, as a result, different detection rates. As mentioned, IUGR refers to a decrease in the rhythm of fetal growth, caused usually by underlying pathological reasons, so that the fetus is unable to reach its growth potential, making the IUGR fetus at risk of developing complications such as fetal hypoxia and acidosis. There are ethnic, racial and individualized variations that must be taken into account when examining a fetus before classifying it as IUGR. A diagnosis of IUGR is classically made antenatally; however, in some cases the diagnosis is made only after birth, especially in pregnancies with poor or complete lack of antenatal care. Prompt recognition of IUGR fetuses is of utmost importance, as there is an increased risk of perinatal morbidity and mortality. Identification and appropriate management of these cases can reduce this risk and improve their outcome [2–4].

19.1.1 Epidemiology and Aetiology

Intrauterine growth restriction (IUGR) is one of the most frequent obstetric complications, affecting up to 10–15% of all pregnancies, with some studies ranging from 7–24% [1–3]. The diagnosis of IUGR in most cases is done antenatally and the detection of an IUGR fetus aims to introduce better obstetric management and consequently better fetal outcomes. However, there are still cases where the diagnosis of IUGR is made only after delivery, either because these cases are clinically missed during the antenatal period, or else because of the lack of proper antenatal care in areas of low socio-economic status or in developing countries [4–5].

The reported incidence of IUGR is different in different countries, reflecting the variation of IUGR among many ethnicities, the absence of a homogeneous definition of IUGR, which leads to different diagnostic criteria, and the differences in screening strategies for IUGR in various healthcare systems. It appears, however, that IUGR cases seem to be more common in the so-called resource-limited, developing countries when compared to developed countries. The incidence of IUGR in the low-resource developing countries may actually be greater than that reported, since in these countries with lower socio-economic status, many deliveries take place in a non-hospital or domiciliary environment and thus have poor birth records. The incidence of IUGR at term is reportedly twice as high in developing countries (20%) compared to the developed countries (10%) [1–3].

Intrauterine growth restriction is considered to be a major obstetric problem because it remains one of the main contributors to both intrauterine and neonatal mortality, with female fetuses being more prone to develop IUGR [4]. IUGR may be caused by fetal, placental and maternal factors (Table 19.1) [5]. In up to 40% of cases, the underlying cause cannot be identified. When a specific cause is identified, IUGR is generally associated with a genetic underlying condition (30%) or with intrauterine environmental factors [6, 7].

19.1.2 Maternal Factors

Extremes of reproductive age appear to contribute to an increased risk of IUGR, being more commonly associated with a young maternal age. Advanced maternal age has also been related to IUGR, but to a lesser extent than the very young mother. An epidemiologic study including more than 1700 pregnancies aged under 25 years showed that young age alone was not a risk factor for IUGR but rather the association was the generally more disadvantaged socio-economic environment that adolescent pregnancies are more likely to be associated with. Maternal race has also been correlated to IUGR. However, it is not clear whether the increased risk for IUGR is directly related to the maternal ethnic origins or whether it is due to the fact that some ethnic groups are more likely to come from a low socio-economic stratum. Both extremes of age and ethnicity are further associated with other risk factors for IUGR including lack of proper antenatal care, undernourishment, iron deficiency and anaemia of pregnancy, substance abuse (illicit drugs) and alcoholism. Undernourishment, such as may occur

158

Table 19.1 Causes & risk factors of IUGR

Fetal genetic abnormalities	- 5–20% of IUGR Include: aneuploidy, uniparental disomy, single gene mutations (e.g. IGF1, IGF2, IGF1R), partial deletions or duplications, ring chromosome, and aberrant genomic imprinting, syndromes (e.g. Russell–Silver, Smith–Lemli–Opitz).
Fetal infection	- 5–10% of IUGR Includes: CMV, toxoplasma, rubella, varicella zoster, malaria, syphilis and herpes simplex.
Fetal structural anomaly	The frequency of IUGR is related to both the type and number of anomalies.
Multiple gestation	IUGR is associated with: • An inability of the environment to meet the nutritional needs of multiple fetuses. • Pregnancy complications more common in multiple gestations (e.g. pre-eclampsia, twin-to-twin transfusion). • Placental and umbilical cord anomalies more common in multiple gestations (e.g. velamentous cord insertion).
Ischaemic placental disease	Cause of IUGR, pre-eclampsia, placenta abruption.
Confined placental mosaicism (CPM)	- 10% of idiopathic IUGR. - One-third of IUGR associated with placental infarction and decidual vasculopathy. Refers to chromosomal mosaicism in the placenta but not in the fetus. The severity of IUGR associated with CPM depends upon the chromosomes involved, the proportion of mosaic cells and the presence of uniparental disomy.
Gross cord and placental abnormalities	Include: single umbilical artery, velamentous umbilical cord insertion, marginal cord insertion, bilobate placenta, circumvallate placenta, placental haemangioma, placental mesenchymal dysplasia.
Maternal genetic factors	• Women who were growth-retarded at birth have an increased risk of IUGR in their offspring. • Women with an IUGR fetus are at high risk of recurrence which increases with increasing numbers of IUGR deliveries.
Maternal medical and obstetric conditions	IUGR is associated with diminished uteroplacental-fetal blood flow and/or oxygen delivery. Include: pre-eclampsia, chronic hypertension, abruption placenta, chronic kidney disease, pregestational diabetes mellitus, systemic lupus erythematosus and antiphospholipid syndrome, cyanotic heart disease, chronic pulmonary disease, severe chronic anaemia, sickle cell disease, uterine malformations, heavy first trimester antepartum bleeding, pre-pregnancy radiation therapy to the pelvis, misuse of alcohol, cigarettes, and/or drugs (e.g. heroin, cocaine).
Teratogens and other environmental factors	Include: medications (warfarin, anticonvulsants, antineoplastic agents, and folic acid antagonists), alcohol, tobacco, air pollution, exposure to radiation.
Assisted reproductive technologies	
Low pre-pregnancy weight, poor gestational weight gain, malabsorption, poor nutritional status	
Residing in high altitude	
Short inter-pregnancy interval	
Extremes of maternal age	
Abnormal maternal biochemical markers for Down syndrome screening	Include: low pregnancy-associated plasma protein-A (PAPP-A), low beta-human chorionic gonatotropin (hCG), high alpha-fetoprotein (AFP)

in cases of poor weight gain in pregnancy and/or low pre-pregnancy weight, has also been correlated to IUGR, reflecting the importance of proper nutrition during pregnancy. No specific nutritional deficiencies have been particularly linked with the predisposition for IUGR [8–10].

Intrauterine growth restriction is also associated with chronic hypoxia of the developing fetus. Women living in high-altitude areas are at increased risk of having an IUGR fetus. Smoking is also one of the strongest antenatal risk factors for contributing to IUGR, causing a 3.5-fold increase in the risk for IUGR and it has been responsible for almost 20% of all the at-term cases of low birthweight (LBW). Women should be advised about the harmful effects of smoking during pregnancy and also that risk becomes greater the more cigarettes they smoke per day and the longer they smoke throughout pregnancy, especially during the third trimester of pregnancy. Smoking cessation in pregnancy decreases the risk of an LBW fetus by almost 17% [11, 12].

Other behavioural risk factors for IUGR are alcohol consumption (related to the amount and duration of that consumption), substance abuse (especially illicit drugs such as heroin and cocaine) and the use of some medications (such as warfarin, anticonvulsants, antineoplastic agents, folic acid antagonists and teratogenic agents). Pre-pregnancy counselling is very important for those women exposed to these agents so that they can be screened and advised properly in order to restrict the use of these agents during pregnancy or change their medication accordingly [13, 14].

Maternal disorders that contribute to IUGR include vascular and renal disease (chronic renal failure, renal transplantation), hypertensive disorders, systematic connective tissue disorders, autoimmune diseases (systemic lupus erythematosus (SLE)) and some acquired thrombophilias such as the antiphospholipid syndrome, pre-existing diabetes and anaemia (e.g. severe anaemia, sickle cell anaemia). Also, some cardiac diseases (cyanotic congenital heart disease, heart failure), maternal malnutrition and gastrointestinal conditions (e.g. Crohn's disease, ulcerative colitis) have been related to IUGR. A previous history of IUGR further increases the risk of recurrence in a next pregnancy by up to 25%. Women who were themselves born as IUGR babies carry a 2-fold increase in their risk of carrying an IUGR fetus themselves; and finally, a short inter-pregnancy interval between two pregnancies and having a pregnancy after assisted reproductive techniques (ARTs) also increase the risk of IUGR [15].

19.1.3 Fetal Factors

Fetal factors that increase the risk of IUGR are mainly genetic-chromosomal abnormalities, congenital malformations and congenital infections. Genetic abnormalities have been strongly associated with IUGR, particularly with so-called early-onset IUGR, being reportedly responsible for up to 20% of these cases. The classical trisomies, such as 21, 18, 13 and 16, are also very often related to IUGR, with trisomy 18 being the more characteristic type of chromosomal abnormality related with the more severe types of IUGR. Autosomal abnormalities, including Wolf–Hirschhorn syndrome, cri du chat and other ring chromosome structural abnormalities, have been associated with IUGR. More rare chromosomal abnormalities such as uniparental disomy, as well as sex chromosomal abnormalities such as Turner syndrome (45,XO), have also been associated with IUGR [6, 12, 16].

Congenital infections are a well-established but not very common cause for IUGR. Viral infections, affecting both the mother and fetus, most significantly cytomegalovirus (CMV) and rubella, can lead to IUGR. The classical protozoan infections of pregnancy, like toxoplasmosis and syphilis, and some

bacterial infections, mainly listeriosis, have also been documented to cause IUGR [10, 11, 16, 17].

Congenital malformations such as cardiac defects are the most common abnormalities related to IUGR, but other structural abnormalities affecting the gastrointestinal tract (particularly gastroschisis) and the urogenital system, as well as the presence of a single umbilical artery, have been related to IUGR [12, 16, 17].

Multiple pregnancies have a much higher risk for IUGR when compared to singleton pregnancies with a difference that can be up to 10–15 times higher in multiple pregnancies. The possibility of IUGR depends on the type of chorionicity, which usually also increases the risk for umbilical cord variations, such as velamentous cord insertion or single umbilical artery, and placental sharing, which can lead to twin-to-twin transfusion syndrome and selective IUGR. High multiple pregnancies are at greater risk of IUGR fetuses, with the risk increasing with the number of fetuses [11, 12, 16, 17].

19.1.4 Placental Factors

It is a well established that placental insufficiency is the most common cause that leads fetuses to be smaller than expected for their gestational age. There is no clear understanding of the mechanism of how placental insufficiency leads to IUGR. It is suspected that through a defective placental circulation an environment of inadequate fetal nutrition is formed, leading to growth restriction of the fetus. In animal studies, a reduction of the size of the placenta is directly related to the risk of developing IUGR, and in general the placenta of the IUGR fetus is considerably smaller compared to the placental size of fetuses with normal weight. The role of the placenta in the cause of IUGR is also shown by cases of so-called abnormal placentation (e.g. placenta accreta), which also carry an increased risk of IUGR. Some rarer clinical situations that have been related to IUGR include placental tumours, (e.g. chorioangioma), chronic villitis, placental infarctions, fetal vessel thrombosis and chronic placental abruptions. Increased concentration of C4d and chronic villitis have been associated with reduced placental weight and perfusion, fetal acidaemia, fetal growth restriction, pre-eclampsia and preterm birth [11, 12, 16–20].

19.2 Classification

According to the traditional classification, IUGR fetuses are divided into asymmetrical and symmetrical types, based on the ratio of head and abdominal circumference. Asymmetrical IUGR is the most common type, accounting for 70–80% of all IUGR cases. It usually presents during the third trimester of pregnancy and is caused by malnutrition of the fetus resulting from uteroplacental insufficiency. The typical presentation of these fetuses is the clinical observation of a normal estimated fetal weight and measurements until the third trimester of pregnancy, followed by a decline in the fetal growth with the abdominal circumference being the only or the most prominent abnormal measurement [13, 14, 16, 20, 21].

Symmetrical IUGR on the other hand is less common accounting for about 20–30% of all IUGR cases. The deterioration of fetal growth in the symmetrical IUGR starts earlier in pregnancy when compared to the asymmetrical IUGR fetuses, even before the third trimester. The causes of symmetrical IUGR are usually not related directly to malnutrition due to placental insufficiency, but rather they are more likely to originate from genetic abnormalities and congenital infections. Ultrasound characteristic of symmetrical IUGR is that all fetal measurements are small and more or less to the same degree. When comparing the two types of IUGR in terms of postnatal outcome, asymmetric IUGR has a better prognosis [22].

A decreased fetal size is always a finding that should elicit concern as it has been related with an increased risk of poor perinatal outcome. Many times however, there is a confusion whether one is dealing with a fetus which is constitutionally meant to be small anyway called small for gestational age (SGA), or with a fetus which is smaller than it should be and is therefore growth restricted (IUGR). IUGR fetuses pose a higher possibility to be stressed in utero, either during the antepartum or intrapartum period. They carry an increased risk of stillbirth and, in general, a poorer perinatal outcome. IUGR is associated with a decrease in the fetal growth, which is seen as a drop in the estimated fetal weight centile. This is followed by alterations in the Doppler waveforms, which show gradual haemodynamic redistribution, as a result of fetal adaptation to malnutrition, which may lead to hypoxia. In comparison to the SGA fetuses, there are no obvious markers that would represent fetal adaptation to an abnormal environment. Since the SGA fetuses do not have an increased risk for a bad perinatal outcome, while IUGR fetuses do, the distinction between these two clinical conditions is of great importance. On one hand we would like to decrease unnecessary interventions in SGA fetuses which are misdiagnosed for IUGR; while on the other hand, true IUGR fetuses require correct timing of delivery, ideally after lung maturation has been achieved, to decrease the risk of a poor neonatal outcome. So, the differential diagnosis between these two conditions is a great challenge in perinatal medicine and is based on fetal growth charts and Doppler studies [22, 23].

The traditional way of assessing the well-being of IUGR fetuses and differentiating from SGA has been the use of Doppler studies, mainly the umbilical artery Doppler (UAD) measurements. Abnormal Doppler waveforms (an absent or a reversed end-diastolic wave) when applied to IUGR fetuses is related to a worse perinatal outcome, and the management of these fetuses according to the UAD result can improve their outcome. The disadvantage of UAD is that although it has a very good sensitivity in detecting severe cases of IUGR, it has a poor role as a screening tool for IUGR and fails to identify IUGR cases at an early stage. As such, it has a poor role in detecting the so-called late-onset IUGR cases. Latest studies show that even SGA fetuses cannot be considered as completely normal when compared to fetuses with normal growth. These do carry a higher risk for a worse perinatal outcome. Umbilical artery Doppler cannot be used as a single factor to assess these fetuses, but other parameters should be included in the assessment. These include growth curves throughout gestation, amniotic fluid volume assessments and Doppler parameters including uterine artery Dopplers, first trimester ultrasound assessments and PAPP-A levels when available. Another useful parameter that has been widely used the last few years is the cerebroplacental ratio (CPR) calculated by dividing the pulsatility index (PI) of the middle cerebral artery (MCA) by the PI of the umbilical artery. Cerebroplacental ratio has the advantage that it can detect even subtle changes in placental resistance, and it can further detect earlier mild reductions of vascular resistance of the fetal brain. This makes CPR more sensitive to identify hypoxia than each individual parameter alone and it also shows better correlation with the perinatal outcome [14]. When the CPR or the umbilical artery is used in combination with the uterine artery Dopplers, the detection rate of a poor perinatal outcome is increased. Finally, an estimated fetal weight below the 3rd centile is a standalone strong risk factor of a poor perinatal outcome. In conclusion an abnormal CPR or uterine artery Doppler PI or an estimated fetal weight (EFW) <3rd centile suggests a strong likelihood of a poor perinatal outcome. These parameters should be taken into consideration when assessing an IUGR fetus and trying to differentiate it from an SGA fetus, at least until other biomarkers that characterize placental disease are introduced into clinical practice for the detection of IUGR [13, 16, 19, 21, 22].

The typical classification divides growth restriction into two subgroups: the 'early-onset' IUGR and the 'late-onset' IUGR. The cut-off week has been determined as the 32nd week of gestation, as fetuses that present growth restriction before this timeline are in a higher risk for perinatal complications [2]. Additionally, there is evidence suggesting that early-onset and late-onset IUGR have different pathophysiology patterns.

19.2.1 Early-Onset IUGR

'Early-onset' IUGR is responsible for 30% of all the fetuses with growth restriction, while the 50% of them is also associated with pre-eclampsia [3]. Moreover, disorders affecting the vascular system, such as chronic renal disease and systemic connective tissue disorders, are highly associated with early-onset IUGR. Placental insufficiency in early-onset IUGR is found to be more severe, resulting to fetal hypoxia earlier in pregnancy. When the villous vascular area is reduced by more than 30%, the resistance in the umbilical artery increases [5]. The measurement reflecting this pathway is the abnormal Doppler waves of the umbilical artery [4]. Histologically, when the placentas of fetuses that had presented early-onset growth restriction are examined, massive lesions are detected. In addition, a characteristic defective spiral artery remodelling and fibrinoid necrosis is present. The pathogenesis originates from the fact that the spiral arteries failed to achieve an effective trophoblastic invasion, resulting in abnormal villous vessels and reduction of the cross-sectional vascular area. The final consequence is reduced placental perfusion [5–9, 16, 18].

19.2.2 Late-Onset IUGR

As mentioned above, late-onset IUGR presents in the third trimester of pregnancy and after the 32nd week of gestation. Late-onset IUGRs occur more commonly than early-onset IUGRs and are responsible for the majority (70%) of all IUGR fetuses. In contrast to early-onset IUGR, late-onset IUGR is associated with maturation insufficiency of the placental villi, rather than surface area reduction resulting in reduced perfusion of gas and nutrients to the fetus. This is translated into hypoxia and therefore to a decreased impedance of the middle cerebral artery, when MCA is evaluated by pulse-wave Doppler [7]. Histologically, the placentas of fetuses that had presented with late-onset growth restriction have no identifiable lesions; or, in cases where lesions are present, these are small and without any clinical significance [5–9, 16, 18].

The difference between the two type of IUGRs, apart from the different time during pregnancy that they present, is that umbilical artery Doppler is becoming abnormal in early-onset IUGR, while the MCA impedance follows. For late-onset IUGR, this pattern is transverse.

19.3 Management of the IUGR Fetus

As the mortality and morbidity of the fetus developing intrauterine growth restriction are high, correct and accurate management is the key for reducing perinatal risk [1]. The aim of antenatal screening for IUGR is the early identification of IUGR fetuses or fetuses at risk to develop IUGR. However, there is to date no clear evidence that such a policy improves significantly the outcome of these cases, and this is one of the reasons why there is no consensus regarding the method of antenatal monitoring of IUGR cases and the optimal time of delivery. Many tests and methods have been used for the surveillance of the SGA fetus including ultrasound evaluation of fetal biometry, Doppler assessment of the most significant fetal vessels, cardiotocography, biophysical profile and clinical examination. This surveillance supplements the personal and family history of the couple (both mother and father) focusing on possible risk factors for IUGR, maternal characteristics such as pre-pregnancy weight and height, weight gain during pregnancy, smoking, blood pressure and antenatal blood results, including first trimester biochemical markers such as PAPP-A. The main aim of the fetal monitoring is to detect timely changes in fetal Doppler studies before the development of fetal acidaemia. Therefore, interventions should be made accurately and prior to severe, non-reversible organ damage or even intrauterine fetal death [2–7, 16, 20, 22].

Ultrasound assessment is the most significant tool for optimizing the perinatal outcome in IUGR fetuses. However, what is even more important is accurate dating of the pregnancy and for that it is essential to know, whenever possible, the last menstrual period and preferably the crown–rump length (CRL) from the first trimester ultrasound scan. During the second trimester of pregnancy, estimation of fetal weight should be made by the classical ultrasound measurements, such as abdominal circumference (AC), head circumference

(HC), biparietal diameter (BPD) and femur length (FL), and ideally serial ultrasound assessments should be made every 2–3 weeks, with AC having the higher specificity and negative predictive value for the detection of IUGR. More specifically, in a high-risk population, Doppler assessment of the umbilical artery should be the main measurement for the SGA surveillance, as it has been found that it can reduce perinatal morbidity and mortality, in addition to the need for labour induction and caesarean section [2]. This is because fetal compromise can be detected in a timely manner and interventions can be made quickly. In IUGR fetuses of all gestational ages, it is reasonable to perform an ultrasound scan every 2–3 weeks. However, if the fetus is severely growth restricted or the end-diastolic flow of the umbilical artery is absent or reversed, the fetus should be monitored more frequently [2]. Biophysical profile (BPP), is thought to be a good method that reflects fetal acid-base status; for IUGR it has a specific pattern of changes, with reactivity being the first parameter that disappears, the fetal breathing movements next, followed by a reduction in fetal movement and fetal tone and finally a decrease in the amount of amniotic fluid [2–7, 16, 20, 22].

The algorithms of management for fetuses with IUGR according to their gestational age (24–34 weeks and 34–38 weeks of gestation) are shown in Figure 19.1 and Figure 19.2. As mentioned above, before any evaluation of the fetus is carried out, it is essential to perform a complete assessment of the maternal status and evaluate for maternal co-morbidities. Also, the method of fetal assessment should be uniform. According to the Royal College of Obstetricians and Gynaecologists, cardiotocography and amniotic fluid volume have to be a part of the complete fetal approach of the IUGR fetus and they should not be used as individual measurements [2]. Ideally, amniotic fluid volume should be assessed by evaluating the deepest vertical pocket, as it has been shown that the evaluation of the amniotic fluid volume can help to confirm the diagnosis of the placental insufficiency [1]. Concerning early IUGR fetuses, the biophysical profile cannot predict accurately fetal acidaemia and it should not be used as a standalone method for fetal surveillance [2]. In addition, in preterm fetuses complicated with IUGR, MCA Doppler evaluation has limited prediction value for fetal distress, especially when the Doppler evaluation of the umbilical artery is normal. Therefore, it should not be used as a single measurement to decide upon delivery. Ductus venosus (DV) is another fetal vessel that has an important role in surveillance of the IUGR fetus, as cardiac compromise can be suspected from a retrograde a-wave. For preterm fetuses with abnormal umbilical artery waves, DV Doppler assessment should be the diagnostic tool for delivery planning [1–3, 6, 16, 20–24].

In term IUGR fetuses (after the 32nd week of gestation), MCA becomes a greatly significant tool for fetal monitoring, especially when umbilical artery Doppler studies are normal. More specifically, MCA PI below the 5th centile is highly associated with neonatal metabolic acidosis (pH <7.15). As a result, when the umbilical artery Doppler assessment is normal but MCA PI is extremely low, delivery should be scheduled [2]. Regardless of the gestational age, intensive surveillance,

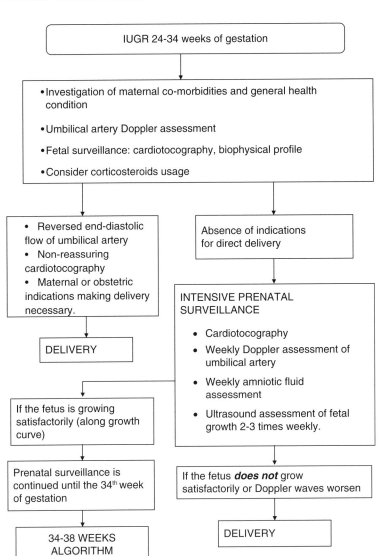

Figure 19.1 *Management of early-onset IUGR in second trimester.*

maternal hospitalization or, in extreme cases, delivery has to be considered if the fetus ceases its growth, amniotic fluid volume decreases and fetal movements are getting diminished or absent [1–3, 5, 6, 16, 20].

19.3.1 Antenatal Management

When delivery is indicated and the fetal age is between the 24th and 36th week of gestation, the mother should receive a single course of antenatal corticosteroids. There is evidence proving that 12 mg of betamethasone intramuscularly accelerates fetal lung maturation. As a result, neonatal death rates and morbidity are reduced [2, 3]. Additionally, neonates that had presented intrauterine growth restriction are very likely to be delivered prematurely. As cerebral palsy is a very common and severe complication of prematurity, IUGR fetuses are at a high risk for developing neurological disorders. The usage of magnesium sulphate when the fetus is going to be delivered before the 30th week of gestation, is found to have neuroprotective action and could have the potential to reduce cerebral palsy rates in preterm neonates [2, 3, 5, 6, 16, 20–24].

19.3.2 Delivery Management

19.3.2.1 Delivery Timing

Where delivery is concerned, gestational age is the factor with the most critical role and the higher predicting value for neonatal survival [2]. Baschat [22] came to the conclusion that when a fetus develops intrauterine growth restriction before the 33th week of gestation, gestational age was the most significant determinant for total survival. If the Doppler assessment of the umbilical artery reveals a reverse or absent end-diastolic flow before the 32nd week of gestation, delivery should be planned when the DV Doppler becomes abnormal, when pulsations are present in the umbilical vein or if the fetus reaches the 30–32th week of gestation [1, 2]. For term SGA fetuses presenting abnormal MCA Doppler assessment, delivery should be planned not later than the 37th week of gestation, as the possibilities for adverse outcomes are getting higher after that timeline [2]. For fetuses small for their gestational age, but with normal Doppler evaluation, delivery should be planned at the 37th week of gestation or beyond, with the expert opinion of a senior obstetrician [2, 25–28].

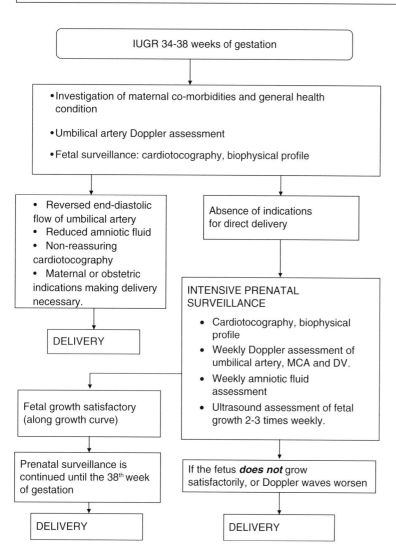

Figure 19.2 Management of IUGR pregnancy in third trimester.

19.3.2.2 Mode of Delivery

Although caesarean section is very common among fetuses complicated with intrauterine growth restriction, it should be reserved only for fetuses with absent or reversed end-diastolic flow on the umbilical artery. A caesarean section is the choice for these fetuses, as there are not any clinical trials comparing different modes of delivery for such situations. Induction of labour is recommended for small-for-gestational-age fetuses with normal Doppler assessment. In addition, induction of labour can also be a choice for fetuses with abnormal umbilical artery waves, but with present end-diastolic velocities [28–31].

Regardless of the timing of delivery, the fetal heart should be monitored continuously as soon as uterine contractions begin [2]. If the fetus develops heart rate decelerations, or fetal compromise and acidaemia is suspected, emergency caesarean section has to be the choice of delivery.

19.4 Identification of the Cause of the IUGR Fetus

19.4.1 Management and Prevention

Several trials and articles have proved that placental insufficiency is the most common cause responsible for intrauterine

growth restriction. Recent evidence suggests that in women with previous history (i.e. IUGR or pre-eclampsia), or having risk factors for placental insufficiency, low-dose aspirin use should be recommended, with the first aspirin dose being ideally given between the 12th and 16th weeks of gestation and continued until the 36th week [1] (level of evidence I-A). Additionally, as mentioned above, intrauterine growth restriction and pre-eclampsia are two disorders associated with uteroplacental vascular insufficiency. Therefore, women whose pregnancy is complicated with intrauterine growth restriction are at a high risk for developing severe pre-eclampsia; therefore, they should be monitored closely (level of evidence II-1). In contrast, antithrombotic factors, such as heparin, are not recommended, as the evidence provided so far is insufficient.

Nevertheless, some other factors have the potential to lead to an IUGR fetus and they need to be evaluated, if indications are present. For example, for fetuses small for gestational age with structural anomalies and normal uterine artery Doppler, karyotype evaluation is recommended. Moreover, infections – mainly from CMV, rubella and toxoplasma – can also lead to IUGR. Serological screening detecting antibodies for these organisms is recommended. In populations where malaria and syphilis are met with high prevalence, immunological evaluation should be extended [2–5, 25–31].

19.5 Conclusion

Intrauterine growth restruction is a clinical condition that is common in pregnancy and it is a well-recognized risk factor that increases perinatal morbidity and mortality. Classically, we divide IUGR fetuses into two categories, symmetrical and asymmetrical, depending on the ultrasound measurements, the gestational age of detection and the possible aetiology of IUGR. These fetuses are at increased risk for both short- and long-term complications, and for that reason it is essential in modern obstetrics that IUGR fetuses or fetuses at increased risk to develop IUGR are detected promptly and managed appropriately. One of the most basic interventions is to try and modify risk factors that affect the maternal influence (e.g. smoking, nutrition) and optimize the maternal health. Also, through a complete medical and family history high-risk women for IUGR should be identified and a further screening for high-risk cases could be done by performing uterine artery Doppler, especially as evidence shows that early initiation of low-dose aspirin in high-risk cases can reduce the risk of IUGR. It is also important to clarify distinct dating criteria, ideally through a first trimester ultrasound, and establish a clear definition of growth restriction, one that could differentiate SGA and IUGR, as the definition of small fetal size remains controversial and complex. The common practice is that, when a fetus with an EFW <10th centile is identified, the obstetrician should be alert for the possibility of IUGR and a comprehensive ultrasound examination should be performed, including the assessment of the amniotic fluid and the placenta, the plotting of the fetal growth measurements on specific growth charts and Doppler studies of both the umbilical artery and middle cerebral artery. These observations can help in the diagnosis and differentiation of IUGR and SGA. Evidence show that application of umbilical artery Doppler and serial ultrasound scans in diagnosed IUGR fetuses does improve their perinatal outcome so that early diagnosis and management reduce perinatal mortality; while on the other hand correct diagnosis of IUGR and differentiation from SGA or normally grown fetuses (e.g. due to wrong dating) reduce the possibility of unnecessary interventions.

References

1. Lausman A, Kingdom J; Maternal Fetal Medicine Committee. Intrauterine growth restriction: screening, diagnosis and management. *J Obstet Gynaecol Can.* 2013;**35**(8):741–8.

2. *The Investigation and Management of the Small-for-Gestational-Age Fetus*, Green-top Guideline No 31. London: Royal College of Obstetricians and Gynaecologists, 2002.

3. Ebbing C, Rasmussen S, Godfrey KM, Hanson MA, Kiserud T. Redistribution pattern of fetal liver circulation in intrauterine growth restriction. *Acta Obstet Gynecol Scand.* 2009;**88** (10):1118–23.

4. David LS, Cherian AG, Beck MM. Management of intrauterine growth restriction. *Curr Med Issues.* 2017;**15**:271–7.

5. Bloom S, Cunningham FG, Leveno KJ, et al. Fetal-growth disorders. In *Williams Obstetrics*, 24th ed. New York: McGraw-Hill Education; 2014.

6. Baschat AA, Cosmi E, Bilardo CM, et al. Predictors of neonate outcome in early-onset placental dysfunction. *Obstet Gynecol.* 2007;**109**:253–61.

7. American College of Obstetricians and Gynecologists. *Intrauterine Growth Restriction*. Practice Bulletin no. 12, 2000. www.acog.org.

8. Sharma D, Shastri S, Farahbakhsh N, Sharma P. Intrauterine growth restriction – part 1. *J Matern Fetal Neonatal Med.* 2016 Dec;**29**(24): 3977–87.

9. Suhag G, Berghella V. Intrauterine growth restriction (IUGR): etiology and diagnosis. *Curr Obstet Gynecol Rep.* 2013;**2**(2):102–11.

10. Srinivas M, Deepak M. Intrauterine growth retardation: a review article. *J Neonatal Biol.* 2014;**3**(3):1–11.

11. Figueras F, Gratacós E. Update on the diagnosis and classification of fetal growth restriction and proposal of a stage-based management protocol. *Fetal Diagn Ther.* 2014;**36**:86–98.

12. Reeves S, Galan HL. *Fetal Growth Restriction. Maternal-Fetal Evidence Based Guidelines*, 2nd ed. London: Informa Health Care; 2012. pp. 329–44.

13. Alfirevic Z, Stampalija T, Gyte GML. Fetal and umbilical Doppler ultrasound in high-risk pregnancies. *Cochrane Database Syst Rev.* 2010;**1**:CD007529.

14. Berghella V. Prevention of recurrent fetal growth restriction. *Obstet Gynecol.* 2007;**110**(4):904–12.

15. Figueras F, Gardosi J. Should we customize fetal growth standards? *Fetal Diagn Ther.* 2009;**25**:297–303.

16. Mandruzzato G, Antsaklis A, Botet F, et al. WAPM. Intrauterine restriction (IUGR). *J Perinat Med.* 2008;**36**(4):277–81.

17. Sharma D, Shastri S, Sharma P. Intrauterine growth restriction: antenatal and postnatal aspects. *Clin Med Insights Pediatr.* 2016 Jul 14;**10**: 67–83.

18. Rizzo G, Arduini D. Intrauterine growth restriction: diagnosis and management. A review. *Minerva Ginecol.* 2009 Oct;**61**(5):411–20.

19. Unterscheider J, Daly S, Geary MP, et al. Definition and management of fetal growth restriction: a survey of contemporary attitudes. *Eur J Obstet Gynecol Reprod Biol.* 2014 Mar;**174**:41–5.

20. Baschat AA, Hecher K. Fetal growth restriction due to placental disease. *Semin Perinatol.* 2004 Feb;**28**(1):67–80.

21. Wada N, Tachibana D, Kurihara Y, et al. Alterations in time intervals of ductus venosus and atrioventricular flow velocity waveforms in growth-restricted fetuses. *Ultrasound Obstet Gynecol.* 2015 Aug;**46**(2):221–6.

22. Baschat AA. Pathophysiology of fetal growth restriction: implications for diagnosis and surveillance. *Obstet Gynecol Surv.* 2004 Aug;**59**(8):617–27.

23. Turan OM, Turan S, Gungor S, et al. Progression of Doppler abnormalities in intrauterine growth restriction. *Ultrasound Obstet Gynecol.* 2008 Aug;**32**(2):160–7.

24. Mari G, Picconi J. Doppler vascular changes in intrauterine growth restriction. *Semin Perinatol.* 2008 Jun;**32**(3):182–9.

25. Pardi G, Marconi AM, Cetin I. Placental-fetal interrelationship in

IUGR fetuses– a review. *Placenta.* 2002 Apr;**23** Suppl A:S136–41.

26. Alberry M, Soothill P. Management of fetal growth restriction. *Arch Dis Child Fetal Neonatal Ed.* 2007 Jan;**92**(1):F62-7.

27. Lee VR, Pilliod RA, Frias AE, et al. When is the optimal time to deliver late preterm IUGR fetuses with abnormal umbilical artery Dopplers? *J Matern Fetal Neonatal Med.* 2016 Mar;**29**(5):690–5.

28. Figueras F, Gratacos E. An integrated approach to fetal growth restriction. *Best Pract Res Clin Obstet Gynaecol.* 2017 Jan;**38**:48–58.

29. Baschat AA. Fetal growth restriction – from observation to intervention. *J Perinat Med.* 2010 May;**38**(3):239–46.

30. Maulik D, Mundy D, Heitmann E, Maulik D. Umbilical artery Doppler in the assessment of fetal growth restriction. *Clin Perinatol.* 2011 Mar;**38**(1):65–82.

31. Thompson JL, Kuller JA, Rhee EH. Antenatal surveillance of fetal growth restriction. *Obstet Gynecol Surv.* 2012 Sep;**67**(9):554–65.

20 Fetal Origin of Adult Disease

Johann Craus

Undernutrition and overnutrition in early life are both associated with a greater occurrence of chronic disease that will manifest themselves decades later in adulthood.

Pedersen [1] in 1954 published his work where he noted that infants of diabetic mothers were born bigger, fatter and more oedematous than those born to biochemically normal pregnant women. These infants were later noticed to be more at risk of developing obesity, type 2 diabetes mellitus (T2DM), hypertension and hyperlipidaemia [2].

David Barker and his team published epidemiological data in the 1980s where they showed an association between under nutrition in utero and development of hypertension, cardiovascular disease, T2DM and obesity. The 'Barker hypothesis' led to the concept of Developmental Origins of Health and Disease (DOHaD) [3–5].

20.1 Background

The Hertfordshire longitudinal study linked suboptimal in utero fetal growth with cardiovascular disease, obesity, hypertension, insulin resistance and impaired glucose tolerance in adult women and men. The Hertfordshire study traced 5654 men born during 1911–1930. Men with the lowest birthweight and body weight at one year of age had the highest death rates from cardiovascular disease. The study also showed that whilst increased body weight at 1 year of age was protective, an increased body weight in adult life had the opposite effect of predisposing towards a diabetic tendency. In the study, low birthweight and reduced growth in the first year of life were shown to be associated with abnormalities of glucose and insulin metabolism [6].

In the Helsinki Birth Cohort study 13 345 men and women born during 1934–1944 and 7086 people born during 1924–1933 in Helsinki showed the same trend as that reported in the Hertfordshire study [7].

In utero, a fetus that is suffering from uteroplacental insufficiency or from a poor nutrition will divert resources at its disposal towards brain development and to promote survival, the so-called brain-sparing effect.

20.2 Fetal Growth

One theory behind the hypertension observed in the association studies mentioned above is that fetuses that were undernourished in utero during the critical period of nephrogenesis, would have developed a reduced number of nephrons. The number of nephrons in each kidney that each fetus has is in proportion to the body size. A second theory is that an undernourished baby may develop a 'thrifty' genotype to ensure that blood glucose concentrations are maintained to ensure optimal brain development at the expense of other organs. The fetus gives precedence to brain development over organs such as muscle, kidneys and lungs. The latter organs do not have priority in utero since renal and lung function are performed by the corresponding maternal organs. A third theory between low birthweight and development of later disease is that low birthweight babies are more prone to adverse environmental stimuli and are known to have a more heightened response to stress. The Pro12Pro polymorphism of the peroxisome proliferator-activated receptor (PPAR)-Υ is known to be associated with insulin resistance, diagnosed by an elevated fasting insulin level. The effect of this gene was determined by body weight at birth, and the effect of the Pro12Pro polymorphism of the PPAR-Υ was only noted amongst men and women in the Helsinki study who had a low birthweight [7].

Two natural epidemiological studies, the Dutch famine study of 1944–1945 and the Leningrad famine study between 1941 and 1994, show that apart from the long-term effect of in utero nutritional deficiencies, the timing of the exposure is important. The effects of nutritional deficiency in utero will differ according to when the fetus will be exposed. The metabolic programming will differ in the effects that it will have on the fetus and eventually the adult human being.

The Dutch famine occurred in 1944–1945 in the German-occupied Netherlands in the densely populated western provinces north of the great rivers, at the end of World War II. Approximately 4.5 million people were affected and as many as 18 000 to 22 000 were reported to have died. These were mostly elderly men. Many people survived because of the soup kitchens. The famine occurred during a relatively short period and the daily nutritional intake of pregnant women was reduced to about 400 to 1000 calories a day. The timing during pregnancy of this nutritional deficiency was associated with different birthweights and subsequent development of adult disease. Infants who in mid- or late gestation suffered from nutritional restriction were lighter at birth, whereas those who underwent the nutritional restriction in early gestation had normal birthweights. The former group had reduced glucose tolerance, whereas the latter group of in utero exposure showed a more atherogenic lipid profile and a higher body mass index (BMI).

Conversely, the Leningrad hunger period spanned a period of 872 days, during which German troops imposed a prolonged military blockade against the Russian city of Leningrad on the

Eastern Front in World War II. It was one of the longest and most destructive sieges in history. Fetuses subjected to the famine did not demonstrate increased rates of insulin resistance, dyslipidaemia, hypertension or coronary artery disease (CAD). This observation was in marked contrast to observations noted in the Dutch famine study [8].

In utero nutrition deprivation promotes physiological adaptive changes in utero aiming towards a compensatory adaptive mechanism, ensuring survival of the malnourished fetus. These adaptive mechanisms will affect the pancreas, liver and blood vessels, amongst other organs [9]. In the concept of developmental plasticity, a single genotype (the 'thrifty' genotype) being influenced by different environmental stimuli in utero will produce different phenotypes (the 'thrifty' phenotype). This concept rests on a theory that specific developmental windows exist in utero whereby an organism is 'plastic' or 'receptive' to its environment. The adaptive changes that the fetus undergoes in utero are in order to preserve neurodevelopment and promote survival and to prepare the fetus for extrauterine life. Whilst these changes are adaptive and ensure survival in utero, they may be maladaptive in adult life and lead to the development of obesity, T2DM and cardiovascular disease. This will occur if the adaptive changes that occurred due to an altered uterine environment mismatch the environment postnatally [8]. In the study of the Leningrad famine, the fetuses adapted well to the nutritional deficiency that was experienced in uterine life. This adaptation prepared the infants well for a nutritional deficiency in extrauterine life. The long exposure of the famine lasting for the whole gestation in utero could have a role rather than a short period of nutritional deprivation, as occurred during the Dutch famine. In the latter group, the Dutch babies exhibited a form of compensatory growth after birth where there was a mismatch between the nutritional deficiency in utero and the extrauterine life. In today's modern world, the mismatch concept applies as well, whereby a growth-restricted fetus won't be well adapted to live in a world where energy-rich foods and a sedentary lifestyle predominate. Children in developed countries spend less time in active play and spend more time playing sedentary computer games. In the USA, obesity has more than doubled amongst children and teenagers. The incidence of obese adolescents rose from 5% in 1976–1980 to 17.6% in 2003–2006. Insulin resistance, CAD, hypertension and dyslipidaemia are associated with T2DM. The latter is now a global epidemic, affecting in excess of 170 million people and the prevalence is expected to double by 2030 [8].

20.3 Infant and Childhood Growth

The Hertfordshire study recorded data on body size at 1 year of age with no further data collected afterwards. The Helsinki Birth Cohort was set up to ascertain how childhood growth patterns would modify the effect of birth and infant size on later disease manifestation in adult life. The birth records of 13 345 men and women who were born in one of the two public maternity hospitals in Helsinki and attended child welfare clinics were recorded. The birth records included birthweight,

length, head circumference and the gestational age calculated from the maternal last menstrual period. The maternal height, weight and 4 pelvic diameters (the external conjugate, intercristal, interspinous and intertrochanteric) were recorded. Serial measurements were done on children with an average of 11 measurements of height and weight from birth to 2 years of age and a further six measurements from 2 to 11 years. Data from the Helsinki study show that adults who are most at risk of coronary heart disease (CHD) are those individuals who after 2 years of age had the most rapid increase in BMI, rather than those who were overweight at any particular point in time. Individuals with the highest risk were children who had the lowest birthweight but the highest BMI at 11 years of age. All these observations point out that CHD, T2DM and hypertension are independently linked with both pre- and postnatal growth.

The theory behind a low birthweight, being thin at 2 years of age and later having CHD is that these babies lack muscle mass. This deficiency will continue into adulthood, as after 1 year of age there is very little cell replication in striated muscle. A rapid weight gain after this period will lead to a higher fat-mass-to-muscle-mass ratio. This could explain the insulin resistance in adults who as babies were noted to have a low birthweight, low BMI at 2 years of age and a high BMI at 11 years of age.

The weight gain during the first 6 months of life is important in the setting of insulin resistance. Those babies who have a poor weight gain in infancy and are of low BMI at 2 years of age seem to experience an early 'adiposity rebound'. Physiologically children around 6 years of age experience an increase in BMI. Children who experience a poor weight gain in infancy and have a low BMI at 2 years of age will have the physiological rise in BMI earlier in life at around 4 or 5 years of age. This early BMI rise will cause a predisposition for these individuals to have a higher BMI in childhood and in adult life.

It is known that low birthweight and high BMI in adulthood are both associated with hypertension and T2DM that leads to CHD. In the Helsinki Birth Cohort study a subpopulation study of 2003 people showed that two different patterns of early growth heralded the development of hypertension in adulthood. The first pattern noted was that a low birthweight and a low weight gain in infancy were succeeded by a rapid gain in BMI in childhood. This led to the development of the metabolic syndrome, a body composition with low muscle-mass-to-fat-mass ratio and CHD. In the other pattern of growth, a sluggish growth in utero and during childhood was followed by a continued small body size so that at 11 years of age the children were short and thin. This is the same pattern of growth that led to cerebrovascular disease. This pattern of growth led to the atherogenic lipid profile, which may result from sluggish pre- and postnatal liver growth. The hepatocyte is an important regulator of lipid metabolism, and findings from numerous studies point out that set points for non-HDL cholesterol metabolism are set in response to fetal nutrition and liver growth in utero. The high cholesterol of breast milk during infant feeding challenges the baby's cholesterol metabolism, and this may modify the set points of cholesterol metabolism during liver growth. On the other hand, the set points for HDL cholesterol metabolism does not seem to be related to the prenatal growth; they are established during infant feeding [7].

Those infants who are formula fed will experience a more disturbing challenge to their lipid profile set points due to the fact that formula feeding has a higher lipid content than human milk as well as being associated with childhood obesity. Human milk contains cholesterol and the brain-building omega-3 fatty acid docosahexaenoic acid (DHA), which is important in relation to the developing brain. These two key components are not present in formula milk. Human breast milk also contains lipase, which is an important aid in lipid metabolism [10].

20.4 The Intergenerational Growth Relationship

In the Helsinki study, there were routine measurements of the maternal pelvis. A small maternal pelvis is a sign of poor nutrition during childhood, especially of vitamin D, as the soft bones that result from the poor mineralization will result in smaller pelvic diameters. The external conjugate diameter is the most affected, and is known as a flat pelvis. It is the distance from the fifth lumbar vertebrae to the front of the pubic bone. The forces exerted on the pelvis when the child starts to stand up on its feet will tend to flatten the pelvis from front to back. In the Helsinki study, a quarter of mothers had a flat pelvis, a sign of poor nutrition in the mother herself during her infancy. These mothers' offspring were noted to have an increased risk of hypertension and stroke. Other studies have replicated this finding and confirmed the association of a flat maternal pelvis and increased stroke in their children in adulthood. One theory to explain this finding is that women with a flat pelvis who suffered poor nutrition in childhood had impaired vascular development in the brain during its rapid development both before and after birth. In another study, mothers with a flat pelvis were more likely to deliver infants who developed hypertension and narrow carotid arteries in adulthood.

Poor and inadequate nutrition in infancy will lead to the impairment of protein metabolism. Mothers with a low rate of protein synthesis will have offspring with a reduced linear growth and are small at birth. A very important time to establish a proper and adequate protein metabolism in infancy is during weaning. A maternal flat pelvis may therefore be a harbinger of a low rate of maternal protein synthesis, which will jeopardize the fetal growth of the next generation and lead to the setting of a lipid profile that favours atherosclerosis, hypertension and stroke [7].

20.5 Assessing Fetal-Growth-Restricted Babies

The problem in assessing fetal growth restriction in utero is that most data are gathered by relying only on biophysical parameters such as fetal weight at birth. The problem using this approach is the failure to correctly identify the fetal-growth-restricted baby from the one who is genetically small, being born to small parents. In the fetal-growth-restricted baby a poor maternal diet or placental insufficiency does not allow the fetus to attain its proper growth potential. This will lead to metabolic consequences for the baby both in the short and long term. On the other hand, a small baby who is genetically determined to be small will not suffer from the deleterious consequences of growth restriction. Other authors in the literature have utilized short stature to assess fetal growth restriction. However, using this parameter will lead to the same problem described with birthweight. Individuals of short stature who are genetically determined will reduce the strength of the association between stature or fetal weight as a measure of fetal growth restriction and investigated outcomes such as blood pressure, obesity and dyslipidaemia.

Da Silva Ferreira et al [11] took into consideration that a growth-restricted baby will adapt to poor resources by shunting nutrients for brain development rather than for linear growth invested in skeletal and muscle growth. This adaptation aims at neuroprotection ('brain-sparing effect') in favour of other organs less high up in the fetal 'hierarchy' of organ importance. Therefore, babies born suffering from growth restriction would have preserved head size at the expense of height. Da Silva Ferreira et al from this perspective tried to construct a new anthropometric method that relates head circumference to stature in order to be able to better identify the growth-restricted fetus. In 2014–2015 Da Silva Ferreira et al studied 3109 women from Alagoas, one of the poorest Brazilian states, where food insecurity is 34.7% prevalent. Alagoas is considered to be one of the poorest Brazilian states, with the worst social indicators such as illiteracy rates, hazardous infrastructure of basic sanitation services and high inequality in socio-economic conditions. In 1989 chronic undernutrition in preschool children in Alagoas was more than seven times higher than that observed in Santa Catarina, one of the states in the southern region of Brazil which boasts greater social and economic development. Anthropometric data gathered from this population were height, weight, waist and occipitofrontal circumference.

The head to height index (HHI) was created to reveal the disproportion between the head size and the respective height. A good cut-off may be a good indicator to highlight nutritional disorders that occurred in utero and in early postnatal life. The value corresponding to the 75th centile was the most appropriate for the projected objective, as it presented the best compromise between sensitivity and specificity, the largest area under the ROC curve and the highest correlation coefficient. Values above the 75th centile were assigned as high HHI.

In the study by Da Silva Ferreira et al [11], there were no associations between short stature and obesity, high blood pressure, hypercholesterolaemia and hypertriglyceridaemia. However, the same parameters were associated with high HHI, indicating that this parameter is more predictive than short stature in assessing the risk of malnutrition affecting children in adulthood. While short stature may be simply due to genetic determination, body disproportionality is due to metabolic adaptations [11].

20.6 Pubertal Growth

In utero exposure to maternal sex hormones has been linked with the pathogenesis of breast cancer. Breast stem cells form at around 6 weeks of gestation. The placenta is able to break 90% of maternal sex steroid, but at 6 weeks of gestation the placenta does not offer this function. If a female embryo is exposed to high concentrations of maternal serum oestradiol, the breast stem cells may be predisposed to develop breast cancer later in life.

At puberty, a woman's sex hormone profile is established. The skeleton of pubertal girls is characterized by a rapid expansion of the distance between the iliac crests, the intercristal diameters. The enlarged iliac crests tend to be rounded. They are measured by the difference between the intercristal diameter and the interspinous diameter (the distance between the anterior superior iliac spines). The changes described are dependent on adequate nutrition and under the control of oestrogens. A high level of circulating oestrogens at puberty may cause a large intercristal diameter due to a greater-than-normal expansion of the iliac crests, which may persist throughout adulthood.

In the Helsinki Birth Cohort, 300 women were diagnosed with breast cancer. A large maternal intercristal diameter was associated with a high risk of having a breast cancer diagnosed in one of the daughters. The maternal intercristal diameter is proportionally related to the risk of breast cancer. This may be due to the fact that excessive maternal sex steroids may cause genetic instability in differentiating breast cancer stem cells in the offspring.

Ovarian cancer was also correlated in women whose mothers had broad hips. This association was noted with a masculine type of maternal pelvis with large intertrochanteric and interspinous diameters. Maternal early menarche was also associated with each measure of the maternal pelvis to an increased risk of ovarian cancer in their female offspring. It has been hypothesized that ovarian cancer may be caused by exposure to maternal sex steroid hormones at an early gestation. In the fetal ovary the aromatase present may lead to maternal androgens being converted to oestrogens. Mothers who had an early menarche may have higher circulating androgens. Since neither breast nor ovarian cancer was linked to maternal height, the theory is that a maternal sex hormone environmental milieu that promotes the two cancers is the result of poor nutrition and growth in early childhood, followed by a 'catch up' in pre-pubertal growth.

20.7 Adult Body Weight

The maternal diet and nutrient and fat stores in her body and the placenta's ability to transfer nutrients from mother to fetus will affect and determine the fetal nutrition in utero. It is well known that the fetal size is related to maternal size. Large mothers have large babies and vice versa due to genetic restraints and genetic potential accordingly. The mother's current body size influences the effects of the baby's body size on later disease. Mothers with a high BMI and short stature below 158 cm in pregnancy who had a baby with a low ponderal index

at birth were associated with the highest risk of later development of coronary artery disease. The effect noted was limited to those women who had a height under 158 cm. Thus, programming of adult coronary heart disease was affected by the maternal lifetime nutrition, as denoted by her height, as well as her current nutrition, indicated by her BMI.

The maternal body size will have an impact on the effects of the placenta on later disease. The placenta exerts a major role on fetal programming, with big babies having big placentas. The effect of the placenta on the fetus is related to its size. Barker et al [3] found that both the shape and the size of the placenta predict the later development of cardiovascular disease. It was noted that hypertension developed if the placenta was small, but this association was only noted in short women who were under 160 cm, the median height of the cohort population. The association between the maternal BMI and placental size with later development of adult disease may mirror the relationship between her body's BMI and the concentrations of nutrients in her bloodstream. These changes may also reveal the effects of the mother's BMI on the transport of nutrients across the maternal-fetal interface of the placenta.

20.8 Epigenetics

20.8.1 Phenotype Induction

The phenotype of the infant is induced to change, and these changes persist throughout the lifespan of the infant. This implies a stable change to the gene transcription that results in altered activities of metabolic and homeostatic control pathways. In experimental models with rats, feeding the pregnant mother a protein-restricted diet resulted in reduced expression of 11β-hydroxysteroid dehydrogenase type 2 and increased expression of the glucocorticoid receptor in the liver, lung, kidney and brain of the offspring during fetal, neonatal and adult life. In the hepatocyte, increased glucocorticoid receptor activity will result in upregulation of phosphoenolpyruvate carboxykinase expression and activity, leading to an increased ability for gluconeogenesis [12]. Lipid metabolism is also affected by maternal protein restriction in pregnancy and/or during lactation. The offspring of these mothers will have increased triglycerides and non-esterified fatty acid concentrations [13].

20.8.2 Regulation of Transcription

Maternal malnutrition may exert its long-term genetic changes in the newborn through altered epigenetic regulation. Epigenetic processes are critical in controlling which genes are switched on at a particular point in time for transcription. This alteration in epigenetic regulation may exert profound phenotypic effects. These processes alter gene expression without alteration in the DNA sequence. The major epigenetic processes are DNA methylation, histone modification and microRNAs. DNA methylation is the process that is best understood; however, new evidence is emerging of the importance of the two other processes (Figure 20.1).

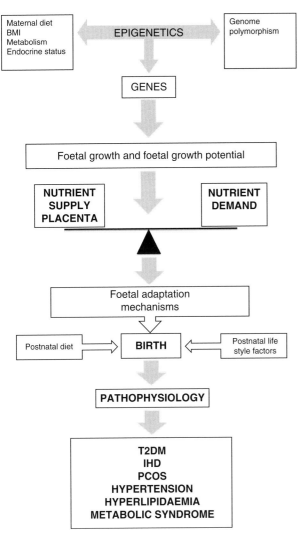

Figure 20.1 Interaction between the maternal in utero environment, the genetic makeup and epigenetics.

20.8.2.1 DNA Methylation

Methylation is a covalent binding of a chemical methyl group to the cytosine (C) base in the DNA code, specifically at the CpG (cytosine-phosphate-guanine) dinucleotides [14]. Cytosine residues present in the CpG dinucleotides are targets for DNA methylation in eukaryotic cells. DNA methylation is associated with transcriptional silencing such as the inactive X chromosome. DNA hypomethylation is associated with gene activity and transcriptional activity. The transcriptional silencing is achieved by either inhibiting the binding of transcription factors or by engaging proteins that specifically bind to methylated CGs (methyl-CG-binding proteins such as MeCP2). These can further recruit histone deacetyltransferases (HDACs) and corepressors [15].

DNA methylation is a common modification in eukaryotic genomes. It is considered a stable epigenetic phenomenon that is transmitted through DNA replication and cell division. DNA methylation requires the activity of methyltransferases [14]. There are two groups of DNA methyltransferases. DNMT1 copies DNA methylation patterns between cell

generations during replication. This is known as maintenance methylation. DNMT3a and DNMT3b are responsible for de novo DNA methylation [16]. DNA methylation established during development and in neonatal and infant life plays crucial roles in cell- and tissue-specific gene expression and genomic imprinting. Genomic imprinting is an epigenetic phenomenon in which the expression of a gene copy is limited on its parent of origin. Normally paternal *IGF2* and maternal *H19* genes are expressed. DNA methylation is responsible for silencing maternal *IGF2* and paternal *H19*. It is normal that with age a gradual hypomethylation occurs.

20.8.2.2 Histone Modification

In eukaryotic cells, genomic data are packed together with histones, special proteins, to form chromatin. The nucleosome is the basic building block of chromatin, and this consists of around 147 base pairs of DNA wrapped around an octamer of histone proteins. The octamer is composed of an H3-H4 tetramer bordered on each side by an H2A-H2B dimer. The core histones are tightly packed; the NH_2-terminal tails can be changed by histone-modifying enzymes, resulting in acetylation, methylation, phosphorylation, sumoylation or ubiquitination. These changes are crucial in the access of transcription machinery to the DNA strands. These changes are important as well for replication, recombination and chromosomal organization.

Histone deacetyltransferases can remove acetyl groups, whilst histone acetyl transferases (HATs) can add acetyl groups to lysine residues on histone tails. HAT activity and increased histone acetylation relate with increased gene transcription. Lysine residues on histone tails are positively charged and this can bind negatively charged DNA to form a condensed structure with low transcriptional activity. At first it was thought that histone acetylation removed these positive charges, thus causing the chromatin structure to relax and therefore facilitate the transcriptional machinery to access DNA. Nonetheless, different models have been proposed, including the histone code hypothesis. This hypothesis proposes that multiple histone modifications act together to regulate transcription. Histone acetylation can also attach bromodomain proteins and these act as transcriptional activators.

Histone methylation can result in either transcriptional activation or inactivation, depending on the degree of methylation and the specific lysine and/or arginine residues modified. These processes are mediated by histone methyltransferases and histone demethylases [15]. Histone methylation is considered to be more stable and longer lasting than acetylation. Protein arginine methyltransferase (PRMTs) are accountable for either mono- or dimethylation of arginine residues most often associated with gene activation [17].

Studies in monozygotic twin pairs have shown that DNA methylation and histone acetylation patterns differed more strongly in older twin pairs than in younger twin pairs. This proves that DNA methylation increases with environmental effect. The more marked the difference between DNA methylation and histone acetylation patterns the more marked the life history differences between the two cohorts will be [18]. Consumption of a high maternal calorific diet leading to obesity can epigenetically alter chromatin structure via covalent modifications of histones [19].

20.8.2.3 Micro-RNAs

Micro-RNAs are a group of short, about 22-nucleotide, non-coding regions of RNA. They have been implicated in the epigenetic regulation of gene expression by silencing of target genes or target mRNA degradation by binding to the 3'-untranslated region of target mRNAs. Micro-RNA can induce chromatin remodelling. Micro-RNAs provide a rapid but reversible means of gene regulation, which allows the cell to adapt to environmental stimuli without changing the DNA structure itself. They have been found to be negative regulators in various pathways targeting signalling molecules, transcription factors and numerous other enzymes and proteins. Micro-RNAs can also affect chromatin-modifying enzymes, resulting in epigenetic modifications affecting gene expression. Histone modifications and changes in chromatin structure could also affect transcription and expression of micro-RNAs. Thus, micro-RNAs may themselves be epigenetically regulated. They have been identified as playing key roles in proliferation, differentiation and development and in cancer, whereby they may act as oncogenes or proto-oncogenes. Micro-RNAs also play a role in insulin secretion, cholesterol biosynthesis, fat metabolism and adipogenesis, critical steps in the pathophysiology of diabetes [14, 17].

Gene expression and regulation are regulated by the conjoint effect of DNA methylation, histone modification and micro-RNA.

20.9 Diethylstilboestrol: Intrauterine Exposure and Long-Term Effects in Humans

Diethylstilboestrol (DES) is a recognized transplacental teratogen and carcinogen that was formulated in 1933. It was prescribed to two million women in the USA alone between the late 1930s and the early 1970s [20, 21]. There are estimates that the drug was given to up to 5–10 million people [22]. It is a synthetic oestrogen that was prescribed to pregnant women in the prevalent but unfounded belief that it prevented spontaneous abortion. In the early 1950s, four clinical trials reported that there was no evidence of efficacy, and its use started to decline [23]. Its use was discontinued after a strong association was reported with vaginal clear cell adenocarcinoma after in utero exposure [20]. In clinical and experimental studies, it was later shown that in utero exposure to this oestrogenic compound during critical periods of organogenesis resulted in disruption of the differentiation of oestrogen target organs. In humans and experimental animals, reproductive organs that appear to be at particular risk for being affected by these developmental abnormalities are the ovaries, fallopian tubes, uterus, cervix and vagina in females. In males the testes, epididymis and the prostate are affected by these developmental

abnormalities. Diethylstilboestrol exposure has been shown to affect bone and the immune system, with an increased prevalence of autoimmune diseases being noted [24]. The US National Cancer Institute (NCI) DES Combined Cohort Follow-up Study showed elevated relative risks of 12 adverse health outcomes including reproductive tract anomalies, infertility, pregnancy complications, cervical intraepithelial neoplasia and vaginal clear cell adenocarcinoma. Adverse pregnancy outcomes include miscarriage, preterm delivery, stillbirth, ectopic pregnancy and neonatal death [23]. Female fetuses exposed in utero before the 7th week of gestation had more than a 20-fold greater risk of developing clear cell vaginal adenocarcinoma than those exposed after the 16th week of gestation [24].

A mother, carrying a female fetus, is denoted as the future second generation, whereas the ovaries of the fetus in utero are referred to as the third generation. In utero exposure to DES may induce epigenetic alterations of the primordial germ cells in the developing female fetus ovaries, affecting the health outcomes of the next generations. Many studies have proven epigenetic changes in prenatally DES-exposed animals as well as an increased frequency of reproductive tract tumours in the next generation offspring. One study has shown that this 'transgenerational effect' extends into the fourth generation, pointing towards a true epigenetic transmission of epigenetic alterations. A fourth generation transmission suggests epigenetic alterations, as the fourth generation was not exposed to DES in utero. This raises concerns about the same transgenerational effect in those DES exposed fetuses in utero.

20.10 Conclusion

The DES case reports even though being now history sends an important message. Herbst and colleagues in 1970 reported seven cases of clear cell vaginal adenocarcinoma. These were seen at the Massachusetts General Hospital in Boston, which was a hospital with a high prevalence of DES use by pregnant women [25]. This high prevalence was due to George and Olive Smith, two enthusiastic advocates of DES use in 1940. The use of DES in other areas was far less prevalent. Therefore, the identification of this strong carcinogen required two unlikely events. The first was an unusual high prevalence of the use of the drug in a concentrated area and secondly the recognition of the unusual cancer cluster by alert physicians. If this connection had gone unnoticed no DES cohorts would have been identified, no screening for DES would have occurred and the teratogenic as well as the poor reproductive potential of these women would have gone unnoticed [24].

Exposure in utero may have short- and long-term effects on the developing fetus. More research is necessary in this area as the association between an exposure and onset of disease occurring four decades later will remain elusive unless vigilant physicians and observers establish the link. The effect of the environment and its effects on epigenetics make the establishment of an association more difficult due to the variable nature of the exposure.

References

1. Pedersen J. Weight and length at birth of infants of diabetic mothers. *Acta Endocrinol (Copenh)*. 1954 Aug 1;**16**(4):330–42.

2. Frienkel N. Banting Lecture 1980. Of pregnancy and progeny. *Diabetes*. 1980;**29**(December 1980): 1023–35.

3. Barker DJP, Bull A, Osmond C, Simmonds S. Fetal and placental size and risk of hypertension in adult life. *Br Med J*. 1990 Apr **8**(301):259–62.

4. Barker DJ, Osmond C, Winter PD, Margetts B, Simmonds S. Weight in infancy and death from ischaemic heart disease. *Lancet*. 1989 Sep 9;**334**(8663):577–80.

5. Barker DJP, Osmond C, Kajantie E, Eriksson JG. Growth and chronic disease: findings in the Helsinki Birth Cohort. *Ann Hum Biol*. 2009 Jan 1;**36**(5):445–58.

6. Barker DJP. *Fetal & Infant Origins of Adult Disease*. London: British Medical Journal; 1992.

7. Barker DJP, Osmond C, Kajantie E, Eriksson JG. Growth and chronic disease: findings in the Helsinki Birth Cohort. *Ann Hum Biol*. 2009 Oct 9;**36**(5):445–58.

8. Calkins K, Devaskar SU. Fetal origins of adult disease. *Curr Probl Pediatr Adolesc Health Care*. 2011 Jul;**41**(6):158–76.

9. Barker DJP, Godfrey KM, Gluckman PD, et al. Fetal nutrition and cardiovascular disease in adult life. *Lancet*. 1993 Oct 4;**341**(8850):938–41.

10. Kries R von, Koletzko B, Sauerwald T, et al. Breast feeding and obesity: cross sectional study. *BMJ*. 1999 Jul 17;**319**(7203):147–50.

11. Da Silva Ferreira H, Xavier AF Jr, Assunção ML de, et al. Developmental origins of health and disease: a new approach for the identification of adults who suffered undernutrition in early life. *Diabetes Metab Syndr Obes*. 2018;**11**:543–51. www.dovepress.com/developmental-origins-of-health-and-disease-a-new-approach-for-the-ide-peer-reviewed-article-DMSO

12. Bertram CE, Hanson MA. Animal models and programming of the metabolic syndrome. *Br Med Bull*. 2001;**60**:103–21.

13. Burdge GC, Phillips ES, Dunn RL, Jackson AA, Lillycrop KA. Effect of reduced maternal protein consumption during pregnancy in the rat on plasma lipid concentrations and expression of peroxisomal proliferator–activated receptors in the liver and adipose tissue of the offspring. *Nutr Res*. 2004 Aug 1;**24**(8):639–46.

14. Jang H, Serra C. Nutrition, epigenetics, and diseases. *Clin Nutr Res*. 2014 Jan 1;**3**(1):1–8.

15. Ling C, Groop L. Epigenetics: a molecular link between environmental factors and type 2 diabetes. *Diabetes*. 2009 Dec 1;**58**(12):2718–25.

16. Clouaire T, Stancheva I. Methyl-CpG binding proteins: specialized transcriptional repressors or structural components of chromatin? *Cell Mol Life Sci CMLS*. 2008;**65**(10):1509–22.

17. Villeneuve LM, Natarajan R. The role of epigenetics in the pathology of diabetic complications. *Am J Physiol-Ren Physiol*. 2010 Jul;**299**(1): F14–25.

18. Fraga MF, Ballestar E, Paz MF, et al. Epigenetic differences arise during the lifetime of monozygotic twins. *Proc Natl Acad Sci*. 2005 Jul 26;**102**(30):10604–9.

19. Aagaard-Tillery KM, Grove K, Bishop J, et al. Developmental origins of disease and determinants of chromatin structure: maternal diet modifies the primate fetal epigenome. *J Mol Endocrinol*. 2008 Aug 1;**41**(2): 91–102.

20. Titus L, Hatch EE, Drake KM, et al. Reproductive and hormone-related outcomes in women whose mothers were exposed in utero to diethylstilbestrol (DES): A report from the US National Cancer Institute DES Third Generation Study. *Reprod Toxicol*. 2019 Mar;**84**: 32–8.

21. Walker BE, Haven MI. Intensity of multigenerational carcinogenesis from diethylstilbestrol in mice. *Carcinogenesis*. 1997 Apr;**18**(4):791–3.

22. Diethylstilbestrol. *Rep Carcinog Carcinog Profiles*. 2011;**12**:159–61.

23. Hoover RN, Hyer M, Pfeiffer RM, et al. Adverse health outcomes in women exposed in utero to diethylstilbestrol. *N Engl J Med*. 2011 Oct 6;**365**(14):1304–14.

24. Swan SH. Intrauterine exposure to diethylstilbestrol: long-term effects in humans. *APMIS*. 2001;**109**(S103): S210–22.

25. Herbst AL, Scully RE. Adenocarcinoma of the vagina in adolescence. A report of 7 cases including 6 clear-cell carcinomas (so-called mesonephromas). *Cancer*, 1970;**25**:745–757.

Antepartum Haemorrhage

Neela Mukhopadhaya

21.1 Definition

Antepartum haemorrhage (APH) is defined as any bleeding from the genital tract after 24+0 weeks of pregnancy until the delivery of the baby.

21.2 Background

Antepartum haemorrhage occurs in 3–5% of pregnancies and this has remained constant. The MBRRACE-UK maternal report 2017 has shown a small but worrying increase in the number of women dying from haemorrhage in relation to abnormally invasive placentation; however, this increase is not statistically significant [1]. Obstetric haemorrhage encompasses both antepartum and postpartum bleeding. The causes of APH include: placenta praevia, placental abruption and local causes (e.g. bleeding from the vulva, vagina or cervix). If a cause for APH cannot be determined, it is described as 'unexplained APH'. The severity of bleeding can vary from spotting to a major haemorrhage and should be managed accordingly.

21.3 Causes

- In placenta praevia, the placenta lies within the lower uterine segment.
- In placental abruption, premature separation of the placenta leads to painful vaginal bleeding and fetal distress.
- Local causes include cervical lesions such as polyps, ectropion, vaginal lesions and show (blood-stained mucous discharge in early labour or after a membrane sweep). Early cervical cancer/suspicious lesions on the cervix may cause a significant APH and must be borne in mind.
- The majority of minor bleeding in pregnancy can be attributed to unexplained causes.
- Vasa praevia is a condition in which the bleeding is massive and is mainly of fetal origin. The bleeding usually arises from the fetal blood vessels that traverse through the membranes overlying the internal os. Once the membranes rupture, there is bleeding from these vessels.

21.4 Clinical Presentation

Most patients present with vaginal bleeding in pregnancy which can be of any severity:

- Spotting – staining, streaking or blood spotting noted on underwear or sanitary protection.
- Minor haemorrhage – blood loss <50 mL that has settled

- Major haemorrhage – blood loss of 50–1000 mL, with no signs of clinical shock
- Massive haemorrhage – blood loss greater than 1000 mL and/or signs of clinical shock

A detailed history should be obtained with particular focus on some key symptoms which will help make a diagnosis and help to plan management.

- Pain – Any bleeding associated with continuous pain should indicate an abruption unless ruled out. Other causes of a painful APH are preterm labour, urinary tract infections and unexplained causes.
- Amount of bleeding – Any major haemorrhage needs admission and urgent intervention particularly if the baby is compromised.
- Fetal assessment – Gestation, growth, fetal movements and fetal heart assessment are all important factors.

21.5 Examination

- Maternal observations include full detailed general observations including pulse, blood pressure (BP), temperature, capillary refill, urinary output, consciousness and skin turgor (pale, cold, clammy skin suggests a shock).
- A maternal examination includes an abdominal and vaginal assessment. A soft nontender abdomen generally rules out an abruption. A hard and tender uterus is typically suggestive of an abruption. Irregular tightening may suggest a labour or a minor abruption and requires a further observation. A speculum examination is mandatory to rule out local causes, assess the cervix, rupture of membranes and assess the amount of blood loss; and where indicated a vaginal assessment should take place (once a placenta praevia is ruled out).
- A fetal assessment includes an abdominal palpation for assessment of gestation and growth, and a Doppler heartbeat is auscultated. Further assessment is usually with a CTG (cardiotocograph) and, if needed, an ultrasound scan can be done for growth, fluid volume and Dopplers (only if the mother is stable).

21.6 Investigation

The level of investigation will depend on the severity of bleeding.

Minor bleeding: All women with spotting or minor bleeding should be observed for at least 24–48 hours after the bleeding has ceased.

- A full blood count (FBC) and a 'group and save' (G&S) sample should be taken.
- A Kleihauer–Betke test to quantify the fetomaternal haemorrhage (FMH) may be needed.
- All women with any history of bleeding and with an Rh-negative blood group will require anti-D prophylaxis.

Major or massive haemorrhage: All women with major or massive haemorrhage will require the following:

- FBC, G&S, crossmatch four units of red blood cells (RBCs)
- Liver function tests (LFTs), urea and electrolyte (U&Es) blood test, coagulation profile
- Intake/output chart
- Ultrasound scan to exclude placenta praevia if this has not been done previously (ultrasound scan has a poor specificity and sensitivity to diagnose an abruption)

21.6.1 Fetal Assessment

- Cardiotocograph for fetal monitoring after 26+0 weeks of gestation. Any signs of fetal distress with an ongoing major or massive APH will indicate delivery.
- Fetal heart auscultation in gestations less than 26 weeks, but a multidisciplinary team (MDT) approach with a neonatologist, anaesthetist and an obstetrician is indicated where a baby is well grown based on mortality and morbidity outcomes and a discussion with the mother.
- Diagnosis of vasa praevia is often difficult if not indicated from a previous scan, and tests available to distinguish fetal from maternal blood are often either not feasible or poorly sensitive. Delivery has to be expedient in such cases, as fetal mortality rates are quite high.

21.7 Antenatal Management

The mainstay of management is hospitalization: All women with any vaginal bleeding should be hospitalized for observations.

- If no further bleeding occurs after a minor bleed for 24–48 hours, women can be discharged with information and follow-up plans. Where other maternal or fetal risk factors exist, an individualized care plan should be made.
- Women with ongoing minor bleeding should be admitted for observations, bloods and investigations. They need regular monitoring. (Figure 21.1 summarizes management plans at different stages of pregnancy according to the examination findings.)

21.8 Antepartum Monitoring

- Daily bloods may be indicated in ongoing bleeding.
- Continuous or twice daily CTG should be done for fetal well-being.
- Growth scan, fluid volume and Dopplers should be done at 2- to 4-week intervals as there is a risk of intrauterine growth restriction (IUGR) and small for gestational age (SGA) babies in this group of women.
- Maternal monitoring with regular observations should be plotted on a modified early obstetric warning system (MEOWS) chart and fluid intake/output chart.
- Watching pads may be used for bleeding (most units weigh them to accurately assess the amount of blood loss).
- Steroids should be considered for those with gestation of 24+0 and 34+6.
- Tocolysis can be used if the bleeding stops or is minimal and delivery is not imminent. If a woman is stable and needs a transfer to another unit for availability of neonatal cots, tocolysis may be used. Where there is ongoing bleeding, tocolysis should not be considered as this increases bleeding and hypotension in the mother, particularly if calcium channel blockers like nifedipine are used.
- Keep the woman on the consultant-led delivery suite or on the antenatal ward, depending on the assessment.
- Anti-D 500 µg IM should be given to all women who present with bleeding irrespective of the prophylactic dose. They should also have a Kleihauer–Betke test to identify an FMH greater than 4 mL of red blood cells, in which case additional anti-D Ig should be given as required. In the non-sensitized rhesus D-negative woman, in the event of recurrent vaginal bleeding after 20+0 weeks of gestation anti-D Ig should be given at a minimum of 6-weekly intervals.

21.9 Intrapartum Care

21.9.1 Maternal

- Frequent observations should be done, as there is a risk of maternal collapse with concealed abruption. This should include abdominal palpation and monitoring of blood loss.
- Intravenous (IV) access should be instituted and fluids should be given.
- Bloods including FBC, clotting, U&Es and LFTs (crossmatch if Hb is low or falling).
- Prophylaxis for thromboembolism with thromboembolic deterrent (TED) stockings may be needed.
- Analgesia: Discussion with a consultant anaesthetist should take place. The choice of analgesia will depend on the maternal observations, Hb and platelet levels and clotting.

    Regional analgesia/anaesthetic is the recommended if safe. General anaesthesia (GA) may be needed in an emergency.

- If there is a high risk of maternal postpartum haemorrhage (PPH), then active management of the third stage of labour should take place as there is a high risk of bleeding postpartum. Use oxytocin and ergometrine (but not in women with hypertension).

21.9.2 Fetal Monitoring

- Continuous fetal heart rate monitoring in labour is recommended in patients with ongoing APH or preterm labour.

Time and mode of delivery

Mother is unstable		• Resuscitate the mother • Immediate delivery by caesarean section even if the fetus is premature or dead

Figure 21.1 A summary of various factors influencing management plan at different stages of pregnancy. CTG: cardiotocograph; HELLP: haemolysis, elevated liver enzymes, low platelet count; IOL: induction of labour; PPH: postpartum haemorrhage

Fetus shows signs of distress on CTG		**Extremely preterm 24-26 weeks** • MDT approach with a clear documented discussion with neonatologist, anaesthetist, obstetrician and the mother regarding outcomes • Discussion of fetal monitoring, mode of delivery should be considered including the risks and complications • Expectant management if both mother and fetus improve • Deliver if mother unstable

Fetus is dead and mother is stable		• Aim for vaginal delivery if feasible • Caesarean section may be indicated based on history and findings (previous caesarean sections/malpresentation of the fetus/HELLP/bleeding etc • Risk of PPH for mother

No maternal or fetal compromise		• Consider expectant management • Prophylactic single course steroids • If <37 weeks can wait and watch with close monitoring on fetal growth • If >37 weeks consider IOL if there is ongoing bleeding or fetal growth restriction • > 37 weeks with placenta praevia deliver by elective caesarean section

- Where there has been one episode of APH and none thereafter in a woman in term labour with a well-grown fetus, there is no evidence that continuous monitoring will benefit. Intermittent auscultation is sufficient.

21.10 Postpartum Care

21.10.1 Maternal
- There is a risk of secondary PPH.
- Check Hb- blood transfusion and iron supplementation as appropriate.
- Thromboprophylaxis
- Debrief
- Postnatal depression
- Follow-up with midwife

21.10.2 Neonate
- Usually neonatologists will be present at delivery.

- Provide neonatal support if fetus is preterm, IUGR or distressed.
- In cases of vasa praevia, there may be a need for blood transfusion.

21.11 Placenta Praevia

21.11.1 Definition
In placenta praevia, the placenta is inserted wholly or partially in the lower uterine segment. Previous classification of the grades of placenta praevia was based on the findings of the transabdominal ultrasound scan at the routine 20 weeks' anomaly scan. The estimated incidence of placenta praevia at term is 1 in 200 pregnancies [2].

Grade 1 or minor: when the lower end of placenta is in the lower uterine segment.

Grade 2 or marginal: when the lower edge of the placenta reaches the internal os.

Grade 3 or partial: when the placenta partially covers the internal os.

Grade 4 or complete: when the placenta covers the internal os completely.

With the greater precision, safety and wide use of transvaginal ultrasound and better resolution and accuracy in determining the location of placenta, a different classification system recommended by the American Institute of Ultrasound in Medicine is used [3].For pregnancies greater than 16 weeks of gestation, the placenta should be reported as 'low lying' when the placental edge is less than 20 mm from the internal os, and as normal when the placental edge is 20 mm or more from the internal os on transabdominal sonography (TAS) or transvaginal sonography (TVS). This has a better correlation with the maternal and perinatal outcomes of pregnancy [4]. The following placental conditions will be discussed below.

In placenta accreta, the placenta lies in the lower uterine segment and the villi are adherent to the myometrium with various degrees of invasiveness. Due to the lack of standardization in the classification at both radiological examination and at histopathological review, the incidence can vary from 1:300 to 1:2000 [3, 5].

In placenta increta, the villi penetrate deeply into the uterine myometrium down to the serosa.

In placenta percreta, the villous tissue perforates through the entire uterine wall and may invade the surrounding pelvic organs, such as the bladder.

21.11.2 Risk Factors

The main risk factors are the following:

- Prior caesarean delivery. A systematic review and meta-analysis of 22 studies including over 2 million deliveries indicated that the incidence of placenta praevia increases from 10 in 1000 deliveries with one previous caesarean delivery to 28 in 1000 with three or more caesarean deliveries [6]. The odds ratio (OR) was 1.47 (95% confidence interval (CI) 1.44–1.51) for placenta praevia, 1.96 (95% CI 1.41–2.74) for placenta accreta, and 1.38 (95% CI 1.35–1.41) for placental abruption [7].
- Interval after the index pregnancy. Cohort studies have also reported that a second pregnancy within 1 year of a caesarean section is associated with an increased risk of placenta praevia (risk ratio (RR) 1.7, 95% CI 0.9–3.1) [8].
- Pregnancies resulting from assisted reproductive techniques (ARTs). A 2017 meta-analysis showed an increased incidence of placenta praevia following ART conception (OR 2.67, 95% CI 2.01–3.34) [9].
- Maternal smoking. A 2017 meta-analysis on the impact of maternal smoking on placental position (OR 1.42, 95% CI 1.30–1.50) has found an increased risk of placenta praevia [10].
- Maternal age. Advanced maternal age has been also associated with a slight increase in the risk of placenta

praevia (OR 1.08, 95% CI 1.07–1.09), but this effect may be due to parity [11].

21.11.3 Clinical Presentation

Patients often present with a painless bleeding after 20 weeks' gestation which may be unprovoked or after sexual intercourse. A definitive diagnosis is based on the ultrasound scan of the placenta located in the lower segment overlying the internal os completely or partially.

21.11.4 Diagnosis

- Routine transabdominal scan at 20 weeks includes placental localization. For pregnancies at more than 16 weeks of gestation, the term 'low-lying placenta' should be used when the placental edge is less than 20 mm from the internal os on TAS or TVS.
- If the placenta is thought to be low lying (less than 20 mm from the internal os) or praevia (covering the os) at the routine fetal anomaly scan, a follow-up ultrasound examination including a TVS is recommended at 32 weeks of gestation to diagnose persistent low-lying placenta and/or placenta praevia. After 32 weeks of gestation, around 50% of the remaining placenta praevia will resolve, with no further changes after 36 weeks of gestation [12].
- Transvaginal sonography (TVS) improves the accuracy and precision of placental localization, particularly when the placenta is low lying. This is particularly so in women who are obese, in posterior placentas and in women who have fibroids. It is safe to perform unless a woman is actively bleeding. Overall, TVS has a high accuracy in predicting placenta praevia in women suspected of having a low-lying placenta on TAS in the second and early third trimesters (positive predictive value of 93.3%, negative predictive value of 97.6% and false negative rate of 2.33%), with a sensitivity of 87.5% and a specificity of 98.8% [13].
- Cervical length measured during a TVS can predict outcomes. A short cervical length (<3.5 cm) at 32 weeks may predict a preterm delivery and risk of PPH. Compared with women with a long cervical length, women with a short cervical length (less than 25 mm) have an RR of 7.2 (95% CI 2.3–22.3) for massive haemorrhage during caesarean section for placenta praevia [14].

21.12 Management

21.12.1 Antenatal Care

- Women with a diagnosis of placenta praevia should be seen by a consultant or an appropriately experienced person.
- They should be counselled about the risks of haemorrhage and preterm delivery and a plan for emergency delivery should be documented clearly after a discussion with the woman. The risk of massive haemorrhage together with the possibility of needing a blood transfusion has been estimated to be approximately 12 times more likely in caesarean section

for placenta praevia than in caesarean delivery for other indications [15].

- Where necessary, use iron supplementation to prevent and/or treat anaemia. Similarly to uncomplicated pregnancies, women with placenta praevia should be screened for anaemia and investigated if their haemoglobin levels are outside the normal UK range (110 g/L at first visit and 105 g/L at 28 weeks of gestation).
- The need for transfusion of blood and blood products should be discussed and documented.
- Women with atypical antibodies form a particularly high-risk group, and the care of these women should involve discussions with the local haematologist and blood bank.
- The need for transfer to a specialist unit should be discussed.
- Women should be advised to go to the hospital if they experience any bleeding or pain. There is no evidence in better outcomes with hospitalization and hence patients should be provided with outpatient care if the bleeding stops and advised to stay within proximity of the hospital and with a companion.
- When they are admitted to the hospital, a venous thromboembolism (VTE) risk assessment should take place to decide on thromboprophylaxis on an individualized risk basis.
- There is no role for cervical cerclage in reducing the bleeding in women with placenta praevia.
- A single course of antenatal corticosteroids for fetal lung maturity should be considered in women between the gestation of 34+0 and 35+6. Where a preterm delivery is anticipated it can be given before 34 weeks. The 2016 RCT has found that the administration of betamethasone to women with a singleton pregnancy at risk for late preterm delivery (34+0 to 36+5 weeks of gestation) significantly reduces the rate of neonatal respiratory complications [16].
- Tocolysis should be used only to administer steroids or transfer the woman to an appropriate unit with neonatal care. Where there is a need to deliver because of fetal or maternal concerns, there is no evidence that tocolysis will be beneficial.
- Four-weekly growth scans from 28 weeks should take place to monitor fetal growth.

21.12.2 Planning for Delivery

- Women with a low-lying placenta or placenta praevia with a history of bleeding or other risk factors should be delivered between 34+0 to 36+5 weeks of gestation. An individualized care plan should be instituted.
- In women with uncomplicated placenta praevia, delivery should be planned between 36+0 and 37+0 weeks. As the gestation period lengthens, there is an increasing risk of haemorrhage.
- Caesarean section is the recommended mode of safe delivery in these women. Although vaginal delivery is not usually recommended in UK practice, in women with a third trimester asymptomatic low-lying placenta the mode of delivery should be based on the clinical background, the

woman's preferences, and supplemented by ultrasound findings, including the distance between the placental edge and the fetal head position relative to the leading edge of the placenta on TVS.

21.12.3 Consent

- It is important to have a detailed and open discussion with the woman and her partner about the risks associated with delivery with placenta praevia. Besides the risks of a caesarean section (infection, damage to bowel, bladder, blood vessels, thromboembolism, cut to the baby), the specific risks of haemorrhage requiring additional procedures including a hysterectomy should be discussed.
- The risk of a major obstetric haemorrhage (MOH) is high and so is the need for transfusion of blood and blood products.

21.12.4 Delivery

- A senior obstetrician/consultant should be present during the caesarean section. Placenta praevia may be complicated with the need for internal manoeuvres due to breech or transverse lie, hence an experienced operator should perform the procedure.
- Regional anaesthetic is safe but there is a chance of converting to GA in case of a MOH.
- Rapid infusion and fluid warming equipment should be ready in theatre.
- Cell salvage is recommended for women where the anticipated blood loss is great enough to induce anaemia, in particular, in women who would decline blood products.
- Blood should be crossmatched and kept ready for transfusion as per hospital policy. Most hospitals recommend four units to be crossmatched when the Hb is normal.
- Interventional radiology should be alerted in cases of major placenta praevia and/or where placenta accreta is suspected.

The six elements considered to be reflective of good care are [17]:

- Consultant obstetrician planning and directly supervising delivery.
- Consultant anaesthetist planning and directly supervising anaesthesia at delivery.
- Blood and blood products available.
- Multidisciplinary involvement in preoperative planning.
- Discussion and consent, including possible interventions (such as hysterectomy, leaving the placenta in situ, cell salvage and interventional radiology).
- Local availability of a level 2 critical care bed.

21.12.5 Surgical Approach

- In preterm caesarean section, placental localization with ultrasound in theatre helps in planning the incision.
- Consider a vertical skin incision on extreme preterm caesareans where there may be a transverse lie.
- If the placenta is transacted during incision, the cord should be clamped to avoid fetal blood loss.

- Use pharmacological measures first when there is a haemorrhage but surgical techniques should be resorted to quickly to avoid excessive blood loss. Balloon tamponade, uterine and vaginal packing, B-Lynch suture, vertical compression sutures and suturing an inverted lip of the cervix over the bleeding placenta bed should be considered in quick succession.
- Interventional radiology where available should be used for prophylactic uterine artery catheterization.
- Early recourse to hysterectomy should be considered when medical and other surgical measures fail.

21.13 Diagnosis of Morbidly Adherent Placenta

- Women who have had a caesarean delivery and a persisting placenta praevia at 32 weeks are at a higher risk of a placenta accreta.
- Increased vigilance for an antenatal diagnosis and planning of delivery can reduce maternal morbidity and mortality.
- Consider an MRI scan where an ultrasound scan has not confirmed an accreta but there remains a high suspicion.

21.13.1 Placenta Accreta Spectrum

The major risk factors for placenta accreta spectrum are similar to that of placenta praevia.

- History of accreta in a previous pregnancy
- Previous caesarean delivery
- Repeated endometrial curettage, manual removal of the placenta, postpartum endometritis or myomectomy has been associated with accreta placentation in subsequent pregnancies. This risk rises as the number of prior caesarean sections increases. Overall, the OR for placenta accreta spectrum after previous uterine surgery is 3.40 (95% CI 1.30–8.91) [18].
- Higher incidence is also seen in women with bicornuate uterus, adenomyosis, submucous fibroids and myotonic dystrophy [5].
- Caesarean section scar implantation can lead to a morbidly adherent placenta if the pregnancy continues. Due to the increasing number of caesarean sections and early ultrasound diagnosis of scar pregnancies, this is a definitive risk factor.

21.13.2 Diagnosis

When performed by an experienced operator, ultrasound remains highly diagnostic for the placenta accreta spectrum. Women who have had a previous caesarean section with an anterior low-lying placenta should have an ultrasound screening for placenta accreta spectrum. In a recent systematic review and meta-analysis of women with previous caesarean and a placenta praevia, the sensitivity, specificity and OR of ultrasound diagnosis of placenta accreta was as high as 97.0% (95% CI 93.0–99.0), 97.0% (95% CI 97.0–98.0), 228.5 (95% CI 67.2–776.9), respectively [19]. Typical ultrasound findings are loss of retroplacental sonolucent zone, thinning or disruption of the serosa/bladder interface and the presence of exophytic structures into the bladder. 'Moth-eaten' appearance on grey ultrasound suggest placental lacunae and the appearance of large blood vessels supplying the lacunae are characteristic ultrasound signs of placenta accrete spectrum [19]. Colour Doppler with vascular lakes with turbulent flow with a systolic velocity of >15 cm/s and numerous vessels joining the uterine serosal border on three-dimensional colour Doppler are diagnostic.

The role of MRI scan in diagnosis of placenta accreta spectrum is still debatable. It should be considered where the ultrasound scan findings are inconclusive with a high clinical suspicion. MRI is safe but the long-term safety to the baby is yet to be proven. The new RCOG recommendation [18, 20] is that MRI can complement an ultrasound scan in assessing the depth and lateral invasion of the placenta, especially in a posterior placenta. The typical features are uterine bulging, heterogenous signal intensity within the placenta and disorganized placental vasculature with disrupted uteroplacental interface.

21.13.3 Planning Delivery in Women with Placenta Accreta Spectrum

- All women with a placenta accreta spectrum should be cared for in a specialist centre with experience in managing these patients.
- In the absence of risk factors for preterm delivery in women with placenta accreta spectrum, planned delivery at 35+0 to 36+6 weeks of gestation provides the best balance between fetal maturity and the risk of unscheduled delivery.
- The availability of blood and blood products, adult and neonatal intensive care, vascular surgeons, interventional radiology and a team experienced in complex pelvic surgery are mandatory within such specialist centres.
- A clear, documented plan of delivery and in case of an emergency should take place after discussions with the woman including the risk of a caesarean hysterectomy and blood transfusion.

21.13.4 Consent

- This should include the general risks like infection, damage to lower urinary tract, bowel and thromboembolism. The risk of haemorrhage is extremely high and all the additional procedures such as tamponade, B-Lynch sutures, packing, uterine artery embolization should be discussed and documented.
- The risk of a caesarean hysterectomy, cell savage and blood transfusion should be discussed.

21.13.5 Surgical Approach in Placenta Accreta

- The choice of surgical technique will depend on the position of the placenta, the depth of invasion and the parametrial extension of the placenta accreta spectrum as assessed by ultrasound and/or MRI before delivery. It also depends on the visual assessment of the uterus at the time of surgery and the presenting clinical symptoms and amount of bleeding.

- In all cases it is advisable to avoid entry through the placenta. This may indicate an ultrasound scan in theatre for placental localization and a vertical skin incision or a higher transverse incision.
- Caesarean hysterectomy with the placenta in situ should be considered if there is difficulty in separating the accreta from the placenta bed.
- When the extent of the placenta accreta is limited in depth and surface area, and the entire placental implantation area is accessible and visualized, uterus-preserving surgery may be considered. A partial myometrial resection can be performed in certain cases.
- Ureteric stenting prior to surgery is only indicated when the urinary bladder is involved and should not be routinely performed as they have their own inherent risks. A urologist should be involved.

21.13.6 Surgical Management in Women with Placenta Percreta

- In cases of percreta, there is a better outcome after a hysterectomy and hence uterus-preserving techniques may not work. The risk of peripartum complications and the need for a secondary hysterectomy should be discussed with the woman and documented.
- The following standard approaches have been described in cases of percreta [17, 21].

  1) Primary hysterectomy after delivering the fetus, without any attempts to remove the placenta.
  2) Entry into the uterus without disturbing the placenta, delivery of the fetus and leave placenta in situ. This may be considered as a uterus-preserving procedure in women desiring future fertility.
  3) Entry into the uterus without disturbing the placenta, delivery of the fetus and remove part of the uterine wall with the placenta and repair the uterine musculature, as in an open myomectomy.
  4) Entry into the uterus without disturbing the placenta, delivery of the fetus and leave placenta in situ followed by an elective secondary hysterectomy after 7 days.

- Women with placenta percreta have a higher risk of maternal and neonatal mortality and morbidity.
- No clear recommendations can be made due to lack of robust evidence in the management.
- When the placenta is left in situ, follow-up plans with ultrasound scans and emergency admission if there was bleeding or infection should be carefully explained to the woman.
- There is still no clear evidence in treating women with methotrexate when the placenta has been left is situ [22]. Women should be warned of the risks of chronic bleeding, sepsis, septic shock, peritonitis, uterine necrosis, fistula

formation, injury to adjacent organs, acute pulmonary oedema, acute renal failure, deep venous thrombosis and pulmonary embolism.
- Interventional radiology is being used more regularly in centres dealing with morbidly adherent placentas. There is merging evidence that this may have a benefit in reducing perioperative blood loss. Various techniques have been used such as including intraoperative internal iliac artery and/or postoperative uterine artery embolization, internal iliac artery or abdominal balloon occlusion. Abdominal balloon occlusion has been increasingly used in China. Although promising for the future, the methodology of these studies is very heterogeneous with no data on the diagnosis of the different grades of villous invasion and variable confounding factors, such as placental position and number of previous caesarean deliveries [23].
- The value of prophylactic placement of balloon catheters in the iliac arteries in cases of placenta accreta has been more controversial. This is mainly because of the higher risks of complications than embolization, including iliac artery thrombus or rupture, and ischaemic nerve injury [24].
- If placenta accreta is found before or after the delivery of baby during an elective caesarean section, where mother and baby are stable, caesarean section should be delayed or maternal uterus and abdomen closed and the mother should be transferred to a specialist unit.

21.14 Placental Abruption

21.14.1 Risk Factors

- Previous abruption is the most predictive risk factor. A large observational study from Norway reported a 4.4% incidence of recurrent abruption (adjusted OR 7.8, 95% CI 6.5–9.2) [25].
- Recurrence of abruption is reported in 19–25% of women who have had two previous pregnancies complicated by abruption [26].
- Other risk factors are pre-eclampsia, fetal growth restriction, non-vertex presentations, polyhydramnios, advanced maternal age, multiparity, low body mass index (BMI), pregnancy following assisted reproductive techniques, intrauterine infection, premature rupture of membranes, abdominal trauma (both accidental and resulting from domestic violence), smoking and drug misuse (cocaine and amphetamines) during pregnancy [27].
- First trimester bleeding increases the risk of abruption later in the pregnancy. A retrospective cohort study from Denmark found that threatened miscarriage increases the risk of placental abruption from 1.0% to 1.4% (OR 1.48, 95% CI 1.30–1.68) [28].
- There is a small increased risk with maternal thrombophilias particularly heterozygous factor V Leiden and prothrombin gene mutation (20210A)

21.14.2 Prevention and Managing Future Pregnancies

- Postpartum debriefing and planning for future pregnancy are important.

- Screening for maternal thrombophilia is recommended.
- Where risk factors exist, women should be encouraged to lose weight and stop smoking, and help with cocaine and amphetamine misuse should be offered.
- There is no clear evidence that either aspirin or low molecular weight heparin reduces the risk of abruption in women with thrombophilia.
- There is no good evidence that folic acid supplementation reduces risk of abruption.

21.15 Vasa Praevia

21.15.1 Definition

In vasa praevia, the fetal vessels traverse through the membranes over the internal cervical os and they are unprotected by placental tissue or umbilical cord. The prevalence is quoted as 1:1200–1:5000. It is usually diagnosed during labour when a vaginal examination takes place or an artificial rupture of membranes is performed. It can be diagnosed by the detection of pulsating vessels or dark bleeding which is fetal in origin. When bleeding, the risk of fetal mortality is as high as 60% despite an emergency caesarean delivery. However, improved survival rates of over 95% have been reported where the diagnosis has been made antenatally by ultrasound followed by planned caesarean section [2].

21.15.2 Types

There are two types of vasa praevia. Type 1 can be secondary to a velamentous insertion of the cord in a single or bilobed placenta. In type 2, the fetal vessels run through the membranes between succenturiate lobes or accessory lobes of the placenta.

21.15.3 Risk Factors

- Placental anomalies increase the risk of vasa praevia. A systematic review and meta-analysis of the association among placental implantation abnormalities (including placenta praevia, placenta accreta, vasa praevia, velamentous cord insertion) and preterm delivery in singleton gestations have found a perinatal death rate random effect pooled risk ratio of 4.52 (95% CI 2.77–7.39) for vasa praevia [4].
- Low-lying placenta in the second trimester forms a risk factor.
- Multiple pregnancy associated with IVF can increase the risk of vasa praevia (incidence of 1:300). Disturbed orientation of the blastocyst may be a possible explanation, although it is poorly understood.
- Coexistence of velamentous insertion of the cord and the vasa praevia is reported between 2 and 6% of cases.

21.15.4 Clinical Presentation

It is not feasible to diagnose vasa praevia clinically in the absence of any bleeding. The main indicators to suspect vasa praevia are the following:
- Dark red bleeding after amniotomy
- Pulsations felt on vaginal examination during labour

- Direct visualization of fetal vessels on amnioscopy is rarely observed and is only possible with a dilated cervix.
- Fetal heart rate abnormalities due to compression of the vessels as the presenting part advances may raise a suspicion.

At the current moment, there is no specific diagnostic test for vasa praevia.

There is insufficient evidence to support universal screening for vasa praevia. The accuracy and practical application of the screening model cannot be to interpolated into the pregnant population. Also, there is no management protocol that can be followed if vasa praevia is diagnosed.

A second trimester grey scale ultrasound with Dopplers is the mainstay of diagnosis. Transvaginal Doppler scan has improved the accuracy of greyscale imaging in diagnosing vasa praevia by demonstrating flow and fetal vascular waveforms on pulsed Doppler through at least one aberrant vessel. Vasa praevia has been defined as a vessel running in the free placental membranes within 2 cm of the cervix. The ultrasound definition of 'within 2 cm from the internal cervical os' was modelled after the existing definitions for low-lying placentas [29] and will vary with gestational age, in particular during the third trimester when the lower segment of the uterus forms. There is limited information regarding the actual safe distance that a vasa praevia needs to be from the internal os to be confident that there is no risk for vessel rupture during labour and delivery.

No accurate diagnostic tests exist in clinical practice to differentiate maternal from fetal blood. Additionally, when bleeding from vasa praevia occurs, delivery should be expedient to avoid an adverse fetal outcome.

21.15.5 Management

When diagnosed antenatally, the presence of vasa praevia should be confirmed in the third trimester. Fifteen per cent of cases resolve in the third trimester and a caesarean can be avoided. If confirmed in the third trimester, a prelabour caesarean section between 34 and 36 weeks has the best outcome. Data on the use of TVS cervical length measurements in the management of vasa praevia are limited, and the role of cervical cerclage is unknown [30]. There may be a role for laser ablation in utero. Antenatal steroids should be used based on the gestation.

When vasa praevia is diagnosed in labour or when bleeding, a category 1 caesarean delivery should take place, with the neonatal team present to resuscitate and transfuse baby is necessary. There is a risk of maternal haemorrhage, as with any other cases of antepartum haemorrhage, and because vasa praevia is associated with placental anomalies.

21.16 Conclusion

Antepartum haemorrhage is a commonly encountered condition in maternity units. It can present with an abruption, placenta praevia, vasa praevia or bleeding of indeterminate origin. Cases should be managed based on the condition of the mother and the fetus. Morbidity and mortality rates for both mother and baby are high. Delivery by caesarean section can lead to complications and a senior team should be available. Where resources are not available, women should be stabilized and transferred to a specialist unit if time permits.

References

1. Knight M, Nair M, Tuffnell D, et al. eds., on behalf of MBRRACE-UK. *Saving Lives, Improving Mothers' Care: Lessons Learned to Inform Maternity Care from the UK and Ireland Confidential Enquiries into Maternal Deaths and Morbidity 2013–15.* Oxford: National Perinatal Epidemiology Unit, University of Oxford; 2017.

2. Silver RM. Abnormal placentation: placenta previa, vasa previa and placenta accreta. *Obstet Gynecol.* 2015;**126**:654–68.

3. Reddy UM, Abuhamad AZ, Levine D, Saade GR; Fetal Imaging Workshop Invited Participants. Fetal imaging: executive summary of a joint Eunice Kennedy Shriver National Institute of Child Health and Human Development, Society for Maternal-Fetal Medicine, American Institute of Ultrasound in Medicine, American College of Obstetricians and Gynecologists, American College of Radiology, Society for Pediatric Radiology, and Society of Radiologists in Ultrasound Fetal Imaging Workshop. *J Ultrasound Med.* 2014;**33**:745–57.

4. Vahanian SA, Lavery JA, Ananth CV, Vintzileos A. Placental implantation abnormalities and risk of preterm delivery: a systematic review and metaanalysis. *Am J Obstet Gynecol.* 2015;**213**:S78–90.

5. Jauniaux E, Jurkovic D. Placenta accreta: pathogenesis of a 20th century iatrogenic uterine disease. *Placenta.* 2012;**33**:244–51.

6. Klar M, Michels KB. Cesarean section and placental disorders in subsequent pregnancies–a meta-analysis. *J Perinat Med.* 2014;**42**:571–83.

7. Marshall NE, Fu R, Guise JM. Impact of multiple cesarean deliveries on maternal morbidity: a systematic review. *Am J Obstet Gynecol.* 2011;**205**(262.):e1–8.

8. Downes KL, Hinkle SN, Sjaarda LA, Albert PS, Grantz KL. Previous prelabor or intrapartum cesarean delivery and risk of placenta previa. *Am J Obstet Gynecol.*2015;**212**(669):e1–6.

9. Karami M, Jenabi E, Fereidooni B. The association of placenta previa and associated reproductive techniques: a meta-analysis. *J Matern Fetal Neonatal Med.* 2017;**284**:47–51.

10. Shobeiri F, Jenabi E. Smoking and placenta previa: a meta-analysis. *J Matern Fetal Neonatal Med.* 2017;**30**:2985–90.

11. Rosenberg T, Pariente G, Sergienko R, Wiznitzer A, Sheiner E. Critical analysis of risk factors and outcome of placenta previa. *Arch Gynecol Obstet.* 2011;**284**(1):47–51.

12. Leerentveld RA, Gilberts EC, Arnold MJ, Wladimiroff JW. Accuracy and safety of transvaginal sonographic placental localization. *Obstet Gynecol.* 1990;**76**:759–62.

13. Weis MA, Harper LM, Roehl KA, Odibo AO, Cahill AG. Natural history of placenta previa in twins. *Obstet Gynecol.* 2012;**120**:753–8.

14. Mimura T, Hasegawa J, Nakamura M, et al. Correlation between the cervical length and the amount of bleeding during cesarean section in placenta previa. *J Obstet Gynaecol Res.* 2011;**37**:830–5.

15. *Blood Transfusions in Obstetrics.* Green-top Guideline No 47. London: Royal College of Obstetricians and Gynaecologists, 2015.

16. Gyamfi-Bannerman C, Thom EA, Blackwell SC, et al.; NICHD Maternal–Fetal Medicine Units Network. Antenatal betamethasone for women at risk for late preterm delivery. *N Engl J Med.* 2016;**374**:1311–20.

17. Publications Committee, Society for Maternal-Fetal Medicine, Belfort MA. Placenta accreta. *Am J Obstet Gynecol.* 2010;**203**:430–9.

18. Fitzpatrick KE, Sellers S, Spark P, et al. Incidence and risk factors for placenta accreta/increta/percreta in the UK: a national case-control study. *PLoS One.* 2012;**7**:e52893.

19. Jauniaux E, Bhide A. Prenatal ultrasound diagnosis and outcome of placenta previa accreta after cesarean delivery: a systematic review and meta-analysis. *Am J Obstet Gynecol.* 2017;**217**:27–36.

20. *Placenta Praevia and Placenta Accreta: Diagnosis and Management,* Green-top Guideline No 27a. London: RCOG; 2018

21. Wright JD, Silver RM, Bonanno C, et al. Practice patterns and knowledge of obstetricians and gynecologists regarding placenta accreta. *J Matern Fetal Neonatal Med.* 2013;**26**:1602–9.

22. Sentilhes L, Ambroselli C, Kayem G, et al. Maternal outcome after conservative treatment of placenta accreta. *Obstet Gynecol.* 2010;**115**:526–34.

23. Wang YL, Duan XH, Han XW, et al. Comparison of temporary abdominal aortic occlusion with internal iliac artery occlusion for patients with placenta accreta - a non-randomised prospective study. *Vasa.* 2017;**46**:53–7.

24. Bishop S, Butler K, Monaghan S, et al. Multiple complications following the use of prophylactic internal iliac artery balloon catheterisation in a patient with placenta percreta. *Int J Obstet Anesth.* 2011;**20**:70–3.

25. Rasmussen S, Irgens LM. Occurrence of placental abruption in relatives. *BJOG.* 2009;**116**:693–9.

26. Tikkanen M. Etiology, clinical manifestations, and prediction of placental abruption. *Acta Obstet Gynecol Scand.* 2010;**89**:732–40.

27. Pariente G, Wiznitzer A, Sergienko R, et al. Placental abruption: critical analysis of risk factors and perinatal outcomes. *J Matern Fetal Neonatal Med.* 2010;**24**:698–702.

28. Lykke JA, Dideriksen KL, Lidegaard O, Langhoff-Roos J. First trimester vaginal bleeding and complications later in pregnancy. *Obstet Gynecol.* 2010;**115**:935–44.

29. Bronsteen R, Whitten A, Balasubramanian M, et al. Vasa previa: clinical presentations, outcomes, and implications for management. *Obstet Gynecol.* 2013;**122**:352.

30. UK National Screening Committee. *Screening for Vasa Praevia in the Second Trimester of Pregnancy. External Review Against Programme Appraisal Criteria for the UK National Screening Committee (UK NSC).* London: UK NSC; 2017.

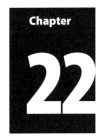

Chapter 22

Obstetric Care of Migrant Populations

Apostolos M. Mamopoulos, Ioannis Tsakiridis & Apostolos P. Athanasiadis

22.1 Introduction – Epidemiology

Migration is defined as movement into a country with the intent to settle; refugees are a subgroup of people who are unable or unwilling to return to their country of origin because of persecution or a well-founded fear of persecution due to their race, religion, nationality, membership of a particular social group or political opinion, and who have been granted refugee status by the host country. Each year, millions of women flee their homelands to escape local crises across the globe. War, genocide, persecution and natural disasters may be the major causes of migration, often without the option of returning back home. It is estimated that about 44 000 people are forcibly made to migrate every day [1]. Populations in developed countries comprise a considerable and growing proportion of migrants and descendants of migrants with a great proportion of births from foreign-born women. To date, European data on the health of migrants and their descendants are incomplete and show contradictory results.

In general, migrants face many challenges, particularly in terms of socio-economic conditions, since they tend to have higher rates of unemployment and work in occupations that are less advantaged than natives in the host countries. On the contrary, migrants may benefit from the reported 'healthy migrant effect', since individuals who are able to migrate are younger and healthier than their non-migrating counterparts or non-migrants. Additional problems for the migrant women include accessing the healthcare system and being adequately prepared to follow clinical regimens as they are recommended by their healthcare providers.

22.2 Ethnicity-Related Issues

22.2.1 Migrant Lifestyle

Women comprise 50% of the refugee population, 25% of whom belong to the reproductive age group. Compared to non-migrant women, pregnant migrants have behavioural issues (e.g. tobacco and alcohol abuse), worse physical health (e.g. body mass index (BMI), gestational diabetes (GDM)) and higher maternal mortality. Migrants are varied not only in terms of geographic region of origin or ethnicity, but also in terms of their migration history: therefore, identifying populations at risk of perinatal health problems entails distinguishing specific subgroups. Regarding migrants' housing, different patterns in home-building are adopted, depending on the country of origin, country of destination and the period of migration, as well as the historical, economic and social contexts around migration. Housing may affect pregnancy care, since it may be overcrowded and filthy.

ELFE (Etude Longitudinale Francaise Depuis l'Enfance) is a national French birth cohort study that examined health outcomes and behaviours of migrant populations [2]. Data for this study were collected by trained investigators via standardized face-to-face interviews and self-reported questionnaire, while medical records were also assessed. Migrants' regions of origin were North Africa, Turkey, sub-Saharan Africa, Eastern Europe and Asia. Compared to non-migrants, women from sub-Saharan Africa were more likely to be overweight or obese, those from North Africa or Turkey had a higher likelihood of being overweight, whereas women from Eastern Europe and Asia were less likely to have high BMIs. Women from North Africa or Turkey, as well as those from Eastern Europe or Asia, were more likely to have GDM compared to non-migrant women.

Regarding alcohol and tobacco consumption, it appears that women progressively adopt the behavioural patterns prevalent in the host country, implicating that tobacco and alcohol use levels need to be monitored. Smoking is a harmful habit that should be clearly documented during pre-conception and antenatal period. It is estimated that the prevalence of smoking among pregnant women in Europe varies from 10% to 27%. The World Health Organization (WHO) advises pregnant women to abstain from cigarette use due to its well-known detrimental effects on maternal and fetal health [3] such as miscarriage, stillbirth, low birthweight, small-for-gestational-age infants, preterm birth, premature rupture of membranes, congenital anomalies, perinatal mortality and morbidity. Evidence from a single-centre experience in Greece showed that prevalence of smoking before pregnancy was significantly lower in migrants than local population, but migrant smokers tended to quit smoking in a lower rate than the Greek pregnant women [4]. Evidence from ELFE study in France showed that compared to the native-born, migrant women had lower levels of tobacco smoking (8.8 vs. 21.9%) and alcohol use (23.4 vs. 40.7%) [5]. Single parenthood was associated with alcohol consumption in migrants.

22.2.2 Dietary Habits and Traditional Regimens

Maternal nutrition during pregnancy seems to be of major importance, since it not only influences fetal growth and development but also sets a foundation for long-term maternal and child health. Since pregnancy is a situation of high nutrient and energy demands, the WHO has established certain guidelines and recommendations for intakes of various nutrients, in order to improve health outcomes and prevent deaths in women and their children [6]. The WHO also recommends that adults aged 18–64 years old should do at least 150 min of moderate or 75 min of vigorous physical activity per week [7]. Several studies on migrant populations show that migration is associated with changes in dietary and physical activity patterns [8]. Moreover, populations migrating from low- or middle-income to high-income countries tend to adopt less healthy dietary behaviours and engage in lower physical activity levels. Reasons for unhealthy diet include long work hours, pregnancy stress and lack of social support. Dietary and physical activity behaviours are often influenced by post-migration environments, culture, religion, and food or physical activity-related beliefs and perceptions. Some women believe that foods in high-income countries are healthier than their traditional foods, because they are less dense and contain less oil and sugar; on the contrary, other women feel that those foods are lacking in nutrients.

Evidence from a recently published systematic review [9] and framework synthesis showed that migrant pregnant women tend to get low levels of folate, calcium and iron; sodium intake was higher than recommended levels. A study from Sweden showed that migrants face anaemia more often than the host populations [10]. Deficiencies in multiple micronutrients reflect poor diets and are associated with pregnancy complications and haematological defects, which may increase the risk of haemorrhage and even death rates during pregnancy. A high sodium intake increases the risk of metabolic disorders and pregnancy complications such as pre-eclampsia.

The National Institute for Health and Care Excellence (NICE) [11] recommends that pregnant women (and those intending to become pregnant) should be informed that dietary supplementation with folic acid, before conception and throughout the first 12 weeks, reduces the risk of having a baby with a neural tube defect. The recommended dose is 400 micrograms per day. High-income countries have seen an increase in pre-conception folic acid uptake as a result of awareness campaigns, with increases from baseline 2.4–25.1% to post-campaign levels of 8.3–53.5% in Norway, the Netherlands, the UK, Israel and Australia [12]. Nevertheless, evidence from a study in Thailand [13], which is considered as a low-income country, showed that no significant improvement in pre-conception folic acid uptake (<2% uptake) was detected, even after an action plan to enhance pre-conception uptake. Since most pregnancies in this local community sample were reported to be unplanned, pre-conception folic acid uptake rates were low after the audit.

Some traditional practices known to be highly prevalent in pregnancy include geophagia, the ingestion of herbal medicines, medicinal plants or salt and the application of skin-lightening creams. Geophagia is defined as the ingestion of earth or soil-like substances, and it has been observed in up to 84% of pregnant women in African countries [14], while the worldwide prevalence is estimated to be 27.8%. Geophagia may be complicated by iron and zinc deficiency, intestinal obstruction or perforation, parasitic infestations and hypokalaemia.

The consumption of herbal medicines in pregnancy is a common practice worldwide, and half of the use reported takes place in the first trimester of pregnancy. The practice is more prevalent in women consuming alcohol and those from lower income households. The safety of herbal medicines in pregnancy is still unclear due to the limited number of studies, while hepatotoxicity has been reported in many cases after consumption. The traditional practice of eating kanwa, as well as consuming additional salt after delivery may lead to hypertension and peripartum cardiac failure, especially in women from Africa.

As for the use of skin-lightening creams during pregnancy, light skin colour is considered a sign of affluence and prosperity in some African communities. Those creams usually contain a high proportion of corticosteroids, mercury and hydroquinone. Studies have proven that prenatal and postnatal mercury exposure may cause permanent neurological damage to newborns, as well as birth defects. While prevalence rates of these practices have been described in pregnant women in their native communities, information on the rates of these practices in migrant women is lacking. Western health professionals have no experience on most of the traditional practices in pregnancy and must also be aware of the potential of non-disclosure of traditional practices by migrant women even with specific enquiry.

22.3 Antenatal Care

22.3.1 Antenatal Visits

Routine prenatal care is associated with reduced maternal mortality, since it provides women and their unborn children with access to various screening tests and interventions. WHO recommends at least four prenatal visits with a detailed list of recommended components of antenatal care both for developed as well as developing countries [15]. It is already proven that prenatal care rates tend to be lower for migrant populations. Migrant women of younger age, lower educational level and lower income are less likely to have five or more prenatal examinations. Refugee women tend to be younger when they get pregnant and are predominantly multiparous [16]. Several systematic reviews [17–19] reported that access to perinatal care was worse for migrant women and one study showed that most of them tended to attend their initial prenatal visit while in the second trimester [16]. The same study showed that longer residency in the host community, primiparity, having medical insurance, having partners with higher educational level and staying in the host community during pregnancy have a positive effect on receiving prenatal care. Another study showed that receiving prenatal care from the first trimester and/or achieving an adequate number of antenatal visits was more likely for those women that have achieved their pregnancy while residing in the host country and, especially so, for those who had already spent enough time there [20].

A three-centre experience study in Europe [21] found that the most frequent demand in all consultations of pregnant refugees was to receive a general check-up by a specialized obstetrician or midwife without reporting any specific complaints (almost half of the consultations). The most frequent reported symptoms that migrants presented with were abdominal pain, urinary tract infections, skin rash and itching. More than half of the consultations were because of general pregnancy-related medical demands for check-ups or nutritional supplements, one fourth due to pain-related problems, 20% due to infections and 20% because of other, less frequent complaints.

22.3.2 Barriers to Antenatal Care

Midwives, usually of female gender, can play a crucial role in the proper initiation and uptake of antenatal care and there is, nowadays, abundant evidence to highlight that effect. It is proven that a poor relationship between a pregnant woman and her midwife may also lead to poor obstetric outcomes for the former [22]. Moreover, a study in the UK [23] assessed the midwife–woman relationships and found that the involvement of the women's family members in maternity care may influence midwife–woman relationships, especially when it comes to competing advice about pregnancy and postnatal practices. Muslim culture and religion have also influenced midwife–woman relationships through midwives' perceptions of the role of faith in determining pregnancy outcomes. Midwives expressed concerns that such beliefs downplayed the role of antenatal care and voiced anxieties regarding their professional and legal accountability for decisions made by women in terms of their engagement in care. The lack of lone contact with migrant women is also highlighted as a concern by midwives, who suggested that the presence of male partners not only negated the possibility of conducting routine enquiry but also prevented the establishment of a good midwife–woman relationship. What's more, it may prevent the woman from revealing crucial information such as problems with domestic violence that appear to be more frequent in certain populations, especially under abnormal circumstances such as being an immigrant in a foreign country.

Late or non-attendance at antenatal appointments is seen by midwives to be one of the biggest influences on their relationships with women and could also be an early warning sign for in-house problems. Unfamiliarity with local systems seems to be the main reason for that phenomenon. Lack of knowledge and awareness of services, difficulties in navigating the local healthcare system, lack of information about appointments, language and communication problems, access to translation services and lack of documented postnatal follow-up seem to be major problems. A systematic review of systematic reviews [24] mentioned that migrant women's experiences of care included negative communication, discrimination, poor relationships with health professionals, cultural clashes and negative experiences of clinical intervention. Data on the reliance on interpreters represented an inadequacy of service provision, leading the way to adoption of body language and facial expressions in order to express the maternal concerns. Hence, there was mentioned a need for more consistent professional interpreting support for migrants, including integrated services, continuity of competent interpreters and improvement of health professionals' knowledge when interpreting services were required. Additional data for asylum seekers and refugees demonstrated complex obstetric issues, sexual assault, offspring mortality, unwanted pregnancy, poverty, social isolation and experiences of racism, prejudice and stereotyping within perinatal healthcare.

Other migrants report social problems as barriers to the prenatal care; poverty, safe housing, unemployment, lack of health insurance and lack of childcare have also been reported. The rates of homelessness and poor social support tend to be high in refugee women. At the same time, the ability to achieve a healthy pregnancy following resettlement may be influenced in part by the structure and makeup of the social networks that surround them during pregnancy. Barriers in social support networks due to refugee resettlement is a concern for women in the context of pregnancy and childcare. Women may be at risk for losing access to connections they had in their country of origin that would be important sources of help, advice and emotional support during pregnancy, childbirth and beyond. As previously introduced by a US study, which was conducted using the Norbeck Social Support Questionnaire (a validated survey instrument that considers support in three categories – affect, affirmation and aid – and was used to measure social support) [25], migrant pregnant women with a secondary resettlement within the USA were more likely to report a 'high support' network compared to participants who resettled directly from Nepal.

Cultural issues seem to be another major problem for migrant women. Lack of cultural acceptability for health, local beliefs about woman and fear of stigma in some countries, lack of the early understanding of possible mental disorders, fears of losing the fetus, preference of female health providers due to religious (especially for Muslims) and traditional reasons exist among migrants. Migrant women usually lack understanding about Western medicine and care and they feel pressurized, while sometimes also being labelled as non-compliant.

22.3.3 Physical Health Issues and Screening in Pregnancy

As already mentioned, according to the ELFE study, higher rates of overweight and GDM among migrants have been reported. Explanations for this may include nutritional factors, stressful events, change in lifestyle habits and differences in screening rates. Health professional awareness of this may facilitate appropriate screening; culturally appropriate GDM education and management would be expected to have benefits for both maternal and neonatal health. According to NICE [26], all women with risk factors (BMI above 30 kg/m^2, previous macrosomic baby weighing 4.5 kg or above, previous gestational diabetes, family history of diabetes, minority ethnic family origin with a high prevalence of diabetes) should be offered testing for GDM during the booking appointment. As for the hypertensive disorders during pregnancy, a systematic review and meta-analysis of epidemiological studies suggested that migrant populations have lower risk for pregnancy-related hypertension, compared to their non-migrant counterparts [27]. This could be probably explained again by the 'healthy migrant effect' or because of their multiparity.

Regarding screening for infections, NICE [11] mentions that screening for syphilis should be offered to all pregnant women at an early stage in antenatal care because treatment of syphilis is beneficial to the mother and baby. Evidence from a retrospective observational study [28], showed that migrants from humanitarian source countries had high rates of tuberculosis (0.4%) and syphilis (2.5%). A retrospective study [29] in Australia evaluated maternal health and pregnancy outcomes in refugee women who gave birth at a single metropolitan maternity centre. It showed that refugees from African countries were often younger than 20 years old, lived in relatively socio-economic disadvantaged geographic areas and needed an interpreter more commonly. In addition, female genital mutilation, vitamin D insufficiency, syphilis and hepatitis B were also generally more common among that group. Unplanned birth before arrival at the hospital (3.6%) was particularly high in the North African refugee group. In addition, toxoplasmosis is a worldwide endemic disease caused by *Toxoplasma gondii* and infection during pregnancy can cause congenital infection and manifest as mental retardation and blindness in the infant. Nevertheless, NICE [11] and the American College of Obstetricians and Gynecologists [30] state that routine antenatal serological screening for toxoplasmosis should not be offered because the risks of screening may outweigh the potential benefits. Data from a cross-sectional study in Spain [31] found a higher seroprevalence of infection of *Toxoplasma gondii* in migrant women, compared to the native population. Furthermore, migrants are at risk for insufficient vaccination against diseases such as rubella and varicella, which can lead to profound and fatal outcome in the neonates. In addition, it has been proven that significant differences exist in vaginal colonization patterns among pregnant women of different ethnic groups, with the highest rates of potentially pathogenic organisms observed in black women.

Concerning HIV infection, NICE [11] recommends that pregnant women should be offered screening for HIV infection early in antenatal care because appropriate antenatal interventions can reduce mother-to-child transmission of HIV infection. As estimated, there has been a substantial increase in the number of HIV-infected women reported as pregnant to the UK's National Study of HIV in Pregnancy and Childhood (the UK and Ireland's national surveillance programme for HIV in pregnancy and childhood): a 17-fold increase, from 82 in 1990 to over 1400 per year in 2006; approximately 80% of pregnancies reported recently as HIV infected were in women born in sub-Saharan Africa. Data from Canada [16] have also shown that refugee women were more likely to be HIV-positive (3.6%) than controls.

22.3.4 Mental Health Problems

Mental health disorders during the perinatal period appear to be common in studies of the developed countries with a prevalence of about 28% [32] among pregnant women (high-risk pregnancies) and 27.5% for the postpartum women in the general population; prevalence of antenatal depression among migrant women is reported to be 12–45%. Although definitive evidence of benefit is limited, the US Preventive Services Task Force, the American College of Obstetricians and Gynecologists, the Royal Australian and New Zealand College of Obstetricians and Gynaecologists, and the National Institute for Health and Care Excellence recommend routine screening for depressive symptoms during the perinatal period [33–36]; unfortunately, this approach is not universally adopted as a routine.

Mental disorders during pregnancy, especially antenatal depression, are associated with adverse outcomes for both the mother and the fetus. Prevalence of mental disorders is reported to be higher among lower socio-economic groups. Since migrant pregnant women are more likely to belong to low economic groups, worse perinatal outcomes are probably expected for these populations. Refugee and asylum-seeker women are found to have higher levels of mental disorders, not only because they are more likely to have experienced traumatic life events, but also because insecure migrant status itself and the asylum process can cause great anxiety. Low social support, minority ethnicity, low socio-economic status, lack of proficiency in host country language and refugee or asylum-seeking status all put migrant populations at increased risk of perinatal mental disorders. Anderson et al reported also that anxiety and post-traumatic stress disorder were higher among migrants [37]. Several systematic reviews reported that perinatal mental health disorders were more frequent in migrant women than in women from host countries [37, 38], with postnatal depression being the most frequently reported disorder.

22.4 Postpartum Care

During the postpartum period, some studies report positive experiences among migrants regarding the breastfeeding support in hospital, but on the contrary, sometimes migrant women are less positive about the care they receive; they report that health professionals discuss their care with them less frequently than they do with women from host countries. Other reports mention poor experiences of care and pain management and prescription of medications that are inappropriate for them in terms of cultural beliefs. The maternity ward during postpartum hospital discharge presents an ideal opportunity to provide contraception counselling and to initiate use of contraceptive methods, even during the early postpartum period. As compared to permanent residents, migrant women have a higher unmet need for contraception and experience increased levels of unintended pregnancies. It is highlighted that migrants are usually at risk of sexual victimization and that many women are forced to pay for their migration through prostitution or are subject to brutal sexual exploitation and torture along their journey. Hence, it is of major importance to note that contraceptive counselling and access to free contraceptive methods with relevant social support of such services seems to be an effective approach for promoting early use of contraception, decreasing the unmet need for contraception and the incidence of postpartum unintended pregnancies. One study in China showed that promoting awareness of free family planning services and ensuring access to these services, including among unmarried women, is vital for reducing the high level of unintended pregnancies among rural-to-urban migrant women.

22.5 Maternal and Perinatal Morbidity and Mortality

Several systematic reviews reported data on maternal mortality among migrant women [18, 39]. Lack of care and late initiation of pregnancy care are linked to increased risk of perinatal mortality and women of refugee background have a greater risk of perinatal mortality than women born in resettlement countries. Between 2011 and 2013, the estimated mortality rate for white women in UK was 7.8 per 100 000 maternities, while the same rate for black women was more than triple, at 28.3 per 100 000 maternities, and was also significantly higher for both Pakistani and Bangladeshi women, 15.9 and 14.7, respectively. Moreover, Pedersen et al [39] reported increased risk for maternal mortality among migrant women, especially due to hypertensive disorders, deep vein thrombosis and pulmonary embolism. Moreover, this meta-analysis showed that the risk of dying during or after pregnancy is almost double in migrant women in Western European countries compared to indigenous born women, corresponding to an absolute additional risk of nine maternal deaths per 100 000 deliveries among migrant women per year. Additionally, migrants tend to have a higher risk of dying from direct rather than from indirect causes. The increased risk of death among migrant women may be due in part to increased incidence of different diseases and pre-pregnancy health problems (migrants, especially from subtropical Africa, tend to be more often anaemic, malnourished, grand multipara and hypertensive).

As for the offspring mortality, Gissler et al [40] reported an increased risk of stillbirth, perinatal, neonatal and infant mortality in migrant women in Europe compared with women from the same host countries: mothers of African ethnicity were twice as likely to have a stillbirth than mothers of European ethnicity and women of Asian ethnicity had up to 64% higher stillbirth rates than their European counterparts. Particular migrant groups tend to have increased neonatal mortality rates due to raised preterm birth rates, excess deaths from congenital anomalies and hereditary metabolic diseases. In addition, for other migrants, mainly from Africa, the increased risk for intrapartum and neonatal deaths was associated with suboptimal antenatal care related to insufficient fetal surveillance for fetal growth restriction, inadequately given corticosteroids or surfactants and delay in contact with healthcare.

22.6 Conclusions

Pregnant women of migrant origin have particular health needs and should benefit from a medical follow-up addressing those needs. Early pregnancy care provides an opportunity to improve maternal health, connect women with social support and monitor maternal risk factors for adverse pregnancy outcomes. Given the high proportion of births that occur among migrant women, in terms of public health, strengthening existing positive health behaviours and preventing deleterious ones during pregnancy in this population may add a substantial population impact. Studies show that refugees who resettle near or with their families tend to face improved integration with the community of resettlement compared to individuals who do not. Improving their connections and their social networks in the host country may improve the pregnancies and the labour experiences in general.

22.7 Key Messages

- Migrants must have easy access to host countries' health system.
- Migrant pregnant women should be able to fully understand their rights and entitlements.
- A professional interpreter should be provided for all appointments, preferably via face-to-face contact, during and after childbirth.
- Information points should be accessible for all migrants 24 hours a day.
- Healthcare providers' sex should be taken into consideration upon availability. The role of midwife should be upgraded and highlighted since it is easier to establish a discrete and confidential relationship.
- Emotional support, appropriate training and supervision to all staff working with migrant pregnant women should be provided in order to successfully overcome the language, cultural and financial barriers.
- Evidence-based national guidelines should be adopted, based on different ethnic groups, religious and dietary factors.

References

1. United Nations High Commissioner for Refugees. (n.d.). Figures at a glance. www.unhcr.org/en-us/figures-at-a-glance.html.

2. El-Khoury Lesueur F, Sutter-Dallay AL, Panico L, et al. The perinatal health of immigrant women in France: a nationally representative study. *Int J Public Health*. 2018;**63**(9):1027–36.

3. Papoulidis I, Oikonomidou E, Orru S, et al. Prenatal detection of TAR syndrome in a fetus with compound inheritance of an RBM8A SNP and a 334kb deletion: a case report. *Mol Med Rep*. 2014;**9**(1):163–5.

4. Tsakiridis I, Mamopoulos A, Papazisis G, et al. Prevalence of smoking during pregnancy and associated risk factors: a cross-sectional study in northern Greece. *Eur J Public Health*. 2018;**28**(2):321–5.

5. Melchior M, Chollet A, Glangeaud-Freudenthal N, et al. Tobacco and alcohol use in pregnancy in France: the role of migrant status: the nationally representative ELFE study. *Addict Behav*. 2015;**51**:65–71.

6. World Health Organization. *Good Maternal Nutrition the Best Start in Life.* Copenhagen, Denmark: World Health Organization; 2016.

7. World Health Organization. *Global Recommendations on Physical Activity for Health.* Geneva, Switzerland:World Health Organization; 2010, pp. 34–58.

8. Osei-Kwasi HA, Powell K, Nicolaou M, Holdsworth M. The influence of migration on dietary practices of Ghanaians living in the United Kingdom: a qualitative study. *Ann Hum Biol.* 2017;**44**(5):454–4.

9. Ngongalah L, Rankin J, Rapley T, et al. Dietary and physical activity behaviours in African migrant women living in high income countries: a systematic review and framework synthesis. *Nutrients.* 2018;**10**(8)pii: E1017.

10. Essen B, Hanson BS, Ostergren PO, Lindquist PG, Gudmundsson S. Increased perinatal mortality among sub-Saharan immigrants in a city-population in Sweden. *Acta Obstet Gynecol Scand.* 2000;**79**(9):737–43.

11. National Institute for Health and Care Excellence (NICE). *Antenatal Care for Uncomplicated Pregnancies.* Clinical Guideline. 26 March 2008.

12. Rofail D, Colligs A, Abetz L, Lindemann M, Maguire L. Factors contributing to the success of folic acid public health campaigns. *J Public Health (Oxf).* 2012;**34**(1):90–9.

13. Stevens A, Gilder ME, Moo P, et al. Folate supplementation to prevent birth abnormalities: evaluating a community-based participatory action plan for refugees and migrant workers on the Thailand-Myanmar border. *Public Health.* 2018;**161**:83–9.

14. Fawcett EJ, Fawcett JM, Mazmanian D. A meta-analysis of the worldwide prevalence of pica during pregnancy and the postpartum period. *Int J Gynaecol Obstet.* 2016;**133** (3):277–83.

15. Simkhada B, Teijlingen ER, Porter M, Simkhada P. Factors affecting the utilization of antenatal care in developing countries: systematic review of the literature. *J Adv Nurs.* 2008;**61** (3):244–60.

16. Kandasamy T, Cherniak R, Shah R, Yudin MH, Spitzer R. Obstetric risks and outcomes of refugee women at a single centre in Toronto. *J Obstet Gynaecol Can.* 2014;**36** (4):296–302.

17. Alhasanat D, Fry-McComish J. Postpartum depression among immigrant and arabic women: literature review. *J Immigr Minor Health.* 2015;**17**(6):1882–94.

18. Gagnon AJ, Zimbeck M, Zeitlin J, et al. Migration to western industrialised countries and perinatal health: a systematic review. *Soc Sci Med.* 2009;**69**(6):934–46.

19. Balaam MC, Akerjordet K, Lyberg A, et al. A qualitative review of migrant women's perceptions of their needs and experiences related to pregnancy and childbirth. *J Adv Nurs.* 2013;**69** (9):1919–30.

20. Zong Z, Huang J, Sun X, et al. Prenatal care among rural to urban migrant women in China. *BMC Pregnancy Childbirth.* 2018;**18**(1):301.

21. Dopfer C, Vakilzadeh A, Happle C, et al. Pregnancy related health care needs in refugees – a current three center experience in Europe. *Int J Environ Res Public Health.* 2018;**15** (9):pii: E1934.

22. Cantwell R, Clutton-Brock T, Cooper G, et al. Saving mothers' lives: reviewing maternal deaths to make motherhood safer: 2006–2008. The Eighth Report of the Confidential Enquiries into Maternal Deaths in the United Kingdom. *BJOG.* 2011;**118** Suppl 1:1–203.

23. Goodwin L, Hunter B, Jones A. The midwife–woman relationship in a South Wales community: Experiences of midwives and migrant Pakistani women in early pregnancy. *Health Expect.* 2018;**21**(1):347–57.

24. Heslehurst N, Brown H, Pemu A, Coleman H, Rankin J. Perinatal health outcomes and care among asylum seekers and refugees: a systematic review of systematic reviews. *BMC Medicine.* 2018;**16**(1):89.

25. Norbeck JS, Lindsey AM, Carrieri VL. The development of an instrument to measure social support. *Nurs Res.* 1981;**30**(5):264–9.

26. National Institute for Health and Care Excellence (NICE). *Diabetes in Pregnancy: Management from Preconception to the Postnatal Period.* NICE Guideline. 25 February 2015.

27. Mogos MF, Salinas-Miranda AA, Salemi JL, Medina IM, Salihu HM. Pregnancy-related hypertensive disorders and immigrant status: a systematic review and meta-analysis

of epidemiological studies. *J Immigr Minor Health.* 2017;**19**(6):1488–97.

28. Gibson-Helm ME, Teede HJ, Cheng IH, et al. Maternal health and pregnancy outcomes comparing migrant women born in humanitarian and nonhumanitarian source countries: a retrospective, observational study. *Birth.* 2015;**42**(2):116–24.

29. Gibson-Helm M, Teede H, Block A, et al. Maternal health and pregnancy outcomes among women of refugee background from African countries: a retrospective, observational study in Australia. *BMC Pregnancy Childbirth.* 2014;**14**:392.

30. American College of Obstetricians and Gynecologists. Practice bulletin no. 151: Cytomegalovirus, parvovirus B19, varicella zoster, and toxoplasmosis in pregnancy. *Obstet Gynecol.* 2015;**125** (6):1510–25.

31. Ramos JM, Milla A, Rodriguez JC, et al. Seroprevalence of *Toxoplasma gondii* infection among immigrant and native pregnant women in Eastern Spain. *Parasitol Res.* 2011;**109** (5):1447–52.

32. Dagklis T, Papazisis G, Tsakiridis I, et al. Prevalence of antenatal depression and associated factors among pregnant women hospitalized in a high-risk pregnancy unit in Greece. *Soc Psychiatry Psychiatr Epidemiol.* 2016;**51**(7):1025–131.

33. NICE. *Antenatal and Postnatal Mental Health. Clinical Management and Service Guidance.* London: National Institute of Health and Clinical Excellence; 2014.

34. The Royal Australian and New Zealand College of Obstetricians and Gynaecologists. *Perinatal Anxiety and Depression.* 2015.

35. American College of Obstetricians and Gynecologists. *Screening for Perinatal Depression.* Committee Opinion Number 630. May 2015. Reaffirmed 2016.

36. Siu AL, USPST, Bibbins-Domingo K, et al. Screening for depression in adults: US Preventive Services Task Force recommendation statement. *JAMA.* 2016;**315**(4):380–7.

37. Anderson FM, Hatch SL, Comacchio C, Howard LM. Prevalence and risk of mental disorders in the perinatal period among migrant women: a systematic review and meta-analysis. *Arch Womens Ment Health.* 2017;**20** (3):449–62.

38. Fellmeth G, Fazel M, Plugge E. Migration and perinatal mental health in women from low- and middle-income countries: a systematic review and meta-analysis. *BJOG.* 2017;**124**(5):742–52.

39. Pedersen GS, Grontved A, Mortensen LH, Andersen AM, Rich-Edwards J. Maternal mortality among migrants in Western Europe: a meta-analysis. *Matern Child Health J.* 2014;**18**(7):1628–38.

40. Gissler M, Alexander S, MacFarlane A, et al. Stillbirths and infant deaths among migrants in industrialized countries. *Acta Obstet Gynecol Scand.* 2009;**88**(2):134–48.

Chapter 23

Care of Women with Previous Adverse Pregnancy Outcome

Manjiri Khare & Gauri Karandikar

23.1 Introduction

Pregnancies with previous adverse outcomes present unique challenges to healthcare professionals caring for them. They are a heterogeneous group that includes adverse outcomes for mother, fetus and/or baby. Adverse outcome of pregnancy may include miscarriage, stillbirth, preterm delivery, fetal growth restriction, congenital anomalies, intrapartum stillbirths, birth asphyxia, birth trauma, neonatal morbidity and neonatal mortality. These could be a result of antenatally known factors, intrapartum events or neonatal complications. Adverse pregnancy events may have long-term implications for the health of the surviving babies/children and mothers.

Miscarriage, stillbirth and neonatal death are significant life-changing and tragic events for couples and the families involved. The maternal adverse outcomes may have significant impact on the physical, mental, psychological and emotional well-being of the mother, as well as the partner and other family members. This also causes the couple to encounter increased anxiety and emotional concerns for planning a future pregnancy.

Almost 3 million families are affected by third trimester stillbirths each year. The global stillbirth rates have not shown a significant decline despite improvements in maternal healthcare, hence adverse maternal and neonatal outcomes remain a major challenge to healthcare providers and policy makers. The contributing reasons why there has been no decline can be attributed to a variety of factors. Adverse pregnancy outcome itself can be multifactorial in aetiology and there are wide variations between the causes in the developed and developing countries making it a challenge to the healthcare providers worldwide. There has been a lack of global initiatives and interventions towards the cause of reducing global stillbirths; however, this is changing [1]. Inadequate postmortem investigation and lack of agreed guidelines for classification of causes of death lead to poor support in determining the aetiology. The true estimate of adverse pregnancy outcomes related to stillbirths may be difficult to assess due to underreporting of earlier losses in particular from the developing countries. There is insufficient evidence to form changes in clinical practice to improve care prior to and during subsequent pregnancies following stillbirth [2].

Enhanced screening and early birth (due to iatrogenic preterm delivery) have contributed to improving the live birth chances for some of the groups of women that would have been at a higher risk for stillbirth, but have also been associated with iatrogenic complications and increased operative interventions for the mothers.

The chapter will address the management of pregnancies following previous adverse outcomes including antepartum and intrapartum stillbirth, early neonatal death, neonatal morbidity due to known antepartum or intrapartum causes.

23.2 Defining Adverse Birth Outcomes

There is heterogeneity in the definitions used for adverse outcomes in the literature.

The International Statistical Classification of Diseases and Related Health Problems (10th revision) have used the following definitions [1]:

- **Miscarriage** – pregnancy loss before 22 completed weeks of gestation
- **Early fetal death** – fetal death occurring at 22 weeks or more of gestation or at fetal weight of 500 g or more or body 25 cm or more in length
- **Late fetal death** – fetal death occurring after 28 weeks' gestation or with birthweight of at least 1000 g or body 35 cm in length
- **Term stillbirth** – fetal death occurring between 37 and 40 weeks of gestation. (Limitations – Birthweight was given more priority over gestational age; however, gestational age threshold is a better predictor of viability than birthweight and estimation of gestational age is comparatively more feasible than the birthweight. Hence, birthweight and gestational age thresholds do not appear to give equivalent results.)
- **Intrapartum stillbirth** – diagnosed when the fetal death is diagnosed intrapartum after fetal heart rate has been determined at the onset of labour
- **Early neonatal death** – the death of a newborn within the first seven days after delivery
- **Congenital anomalies** – birth defects (sometimes life threatening) that occur during fetal development and present as deviations from the normal development
- **Traumatic birth** – injuries sustained during the birth process, often neurologic in manifestation (e.g. hypoxic-ischaemic encephalopathy, brachial plexus paralysis)
- **Adverse perinatal outcome** – composite outcome including stillbirth, neonatal death and major neonatal morbidity such as hypoxic-ischaemic encephalopathy; intracranial haemorrhage; retinopathy of prematurity; necrotizing enterocolitis
- **Preterm birth** – birth <37 weeks [3]

In the UK, the following definitions are used:

Miscarriage is defined as pregnancy loss before 24 weeks.

Stillbirth is a baby born after 24 weeks who did not breathe or show signs of life.

Neonatal death is defined as death of a baby in the first 28 days of life.

Perinatal mortality includes stillbirths and deaths in the first 28 days of life.

23.3 Epidemiology

There is variation in the adverse pregnancy outcomes across the world [4]. Almost 98% of the 2.6 million stillbirths that occur worldwide each year occur in low- and middle-income countries, especially sub-Saharan Africa and South Asia. Even in high-income countries the stillbirth rate varies from 1.3 to 8.8 per 1000 live births [5].

Half of the stillbirths occur intrapartum and are mainly a result of lack of adequate intrapartum care and home deliveries. The stillbirth rates vary from 10% in developed countries to 59.3% in South Asia and other developing regions [5]. Congenital anomalies contribute to 7.4% of the stillbirths after 28 weeks. Ninety per cent of stillbirths in high-income countries can be associated with preventable lifestyle factors like obesity, smoking and sub-optimal antenatal care [5].

According to the UK Parliament's briefing "Infant Mortality and Stillbirth in the UK" (2016), 70% of the mortality in infants in 2014 in UK included infants who died in the neonatal period (i.e. in the first 28 days of life). In addition to prematurity and congenital anomalies, infections, hypoxia and trauma during birth were the main attributable reasons.

23.4 Risk Factors Associated with Adverse Pregnancy Outcome [6]

Categorizing the risk factors or causes of adverse pregnancy outcomes helps in better estimation of recurrence risk for the individual pregnancy and in creating an antenatal and intrapartum care plan [7]. The common maternal, fetal, placental causes or risk factors associated with stillbirths, neonatal loss or adverse perinatal outcomes are shown in Table 23.1.

23.5 Risk Assessment and Recurrence Risk

A systematic review in high-income countries regarding the recurrence risk of stillbirths, wherein over 3 million women were included in the study, revealed a fivefold recurrence risk in those with a previous stillbirth arising due to all causes [8]. However, accurate prediction of risk could be difficult as it may involve a variety of factors which could be responsible for the index loss.

Uteroplacental or maternal risk factors for stillbirth have a higher risk of recurrence of stillbirth. There is an increased risk of ischaemic placental disease in pre-eclampsia, intrauterine growth restriction, abruption and small for gestational age (SGA) in the subsequent pregnancy following a previous stillbirth. The risk of recurrence is eightfold in those with previous SGA babies or fetal growth restriction (FGR) births [8, 9]. The risk of stillbirth, preterm birth and FGR is elevated after a loss in one pregnancy, while it increases two- to threefold when prior adverse

Table 23.1 Maternal and fetal risk factors contributing to adverse outcome during pregnancy

Maternal

Maternal age >35 years
Overweight and obesity; pre-pregnancy body mass index greater than 30 kg/m^2
Adolescent pregnancy
Short inter-pregnancy interval
Social inequality
Ethnicity
Smoking
Alcohol
Substance misuse
Pre-existing medical conditions (e.g. diabetes, chronic hypertension, lupus, antiphospholipid antibodies)
Pregnancy-related medical complications (e.g. gestational diabetes mellitus, pre-eclampsia, obstetric cholestasis)
Previous stillbirth, neonatal death, adverse pregnancy outcome

FETAL

Low birthweight
Prematurity
Chromosomal and genetic abnormalities
Congenital anomalies
Multiple pregnancy
Post term pregnancy >42 weeks
Rhesus isoimmunization

PLACENTAL

Uteroplacental insufficiency
Placental abruption
Vasa praevia

outcomes are combined. These factors are interrelated and can be an independent risk factor for the other conditions [10]. Antepartum stillbirth in the first pregnancy is with associated higher incidence of ischaemic placental dysfunction rather than intrapartum loss [11, 12].

The risk of recurrence of preterm birth is 2.5- to 10.6-fold and almost 14-fold in preterm births less than 34 weeks of gestation [10]. Stillbirth or neonatal death due to congenital anomalies will depend on whether there is an underlying genetic or chromosomal cause. Those associated with genetic or chromosomal causes may have increased risk of recurrence. In cases where the reason is unclear or unexplained, the risk will be similar to that of the general population.

23.6 Management of Pregnancy with Previous Adverse Outcome

23.6.1 Investigations Following Previous Fetal or Neonatal Adverse Outcomes

It is important to offer investigations immediately following an adverse pregnancy outcome [13] to determine the cause of the loss or severe morbidity so the mother can be screened for any specific contributing factors to avoid risk of recurrence where this can be prevented or screened for in future pregnancies.

Investigations offered will depend on the circumstances of the adverse outcome. A genetic survey, an autopsy and in cases of fetal anomalies, microarray or cytogenetic studies of the fetus can be useful. Placental examination and placental histopathology conducted by a skilled perinatal pathologist is of great value in cases of abruption, in order to demonstrate any signs of infection and histological evaluation for fetal vascular occlusion, perivillous fibrin deposition that can suggest the possibility of placental factors responsible for the loss of pregnancy. Fetomaternal haemorrhage estimation should be done in those cases where indicated. Screening the mother for diabetes, haemoglobinopathies and autoimmune disorders may help to establish the cause. It is possible that in some cases, despite extensive investigations, a definitive diagnosis may not be given. It can in fact be reassuring to some couples that no obvious genetic or chromosomal cause was found, as this may reduce the risk of recurrence. For some couples, having a definitive cause for the outcome brings a sense of closure.

23.6.2 Postnatal Debriefing Following the Adverse Outcome

Honest and sensitive communication of findings following the investigations is an important aspect of care. The debriefing meeting should ideally be led by the lead clinicians involved in the care of the woman and her baby. The focus of the meeting will depend on the adverse outcome and individual circumstances. This should be an opportunity to discuss the clinical findings and answer any queries that the couple may have regarding the care. Findings should be explained in lay terms and a written summary should be sent to the parents. The baby should be addressed by their name if this is confirmed by parents in the meeting as well as in any correspondence sent to the parents. Plans for future pregnancy care and risks for recurrence should be discussed.

It is also important to review for depression and anxiety disorders commonly noticed in parents and the family associated with the outcome and to offer further support [14].

Healthcare professionals should receive training for breaking bad news and caring for bereaved families.

23.6.3 Inter-Pregnancy Interval and Pre-conception Health

Data regarding the inter-pregnancy interval suggest that most women conceived within one year following the stillbirth, which is due to the desire to fulfil their reproductive aspirations. Also, it is known to reduce the anxiety associated with the previous experience for some women. The studies that advocate longer interval between the pregnancies are correlated with the possibility that the chronic inflammatory pathology associated with the pregnancy may not resolve in the short interval or the maternal depletion hypothesis wherein the nutritional loss and maternal stress need optimal time to

recover [11]. However, there is no strong evidence to suggest the ideal time interval between the index and future pregnancy following an adverse outcome. It would be helpful if the woman was feeling physically, mentally and emotionally fit before embarking on the next pregnancy.

23.6.4 Care in Pregnancy after a Previous Adverse Outcome

The provision of antenatal care should be individualized based on the specific need and circumstances. The risk assessment at booking based on history, review of previous medical records when available and clinical assessment will decide the specific care plan during that pregnancy. In particular, if there is a need for referral to a specialist team or clinic or tertiary unit, this should be organized promptly to avoid delays in providing the level of care for that woman. The woman may have a preference for the clinicians involved due to her previous pregnancy experience and outcome and this should be respected and supported where possible. Multidisciplinary involvement to provide the expertise and support would include obstetricians, bereavement support midwives, specialist teams, neonatologists, psychologists, general practitioners, support workers and any other team members relevant to the specific needs of the individual woman and her family. Good communication between team members and the woman helps with providing continuity of care, trust and support.

23.6.5 Booking Visit

Every effort should be made to request the medical records / the details of the previous pregnancy/pregnancies with reference to the adverse outcome (Table 23.2). The emphasis should be on obtaining a thorough obstetric history and identifying risk factors (Table 23.3). This can be particularly challenging if patients have moved to another hospital/country for antenatal care in a subsequent pregnancy. An individualized care plan with referral to specialist clinics can offer better care through the pregnancy.

Care for women with a previous adverse outcome or previous maternal complications should be consultant led. The couple should be offered additional appointments for reassurance based on the antenatal care model in the local setting. This should include a discussion of the care plan regarding the pregnancy and investigations to be done and a time plan for these. The healthcare professionals should be sensitive and aware of the needs of the mother, especially those with heightened anxiety and around milestones or critical points when the adverse outcome may have occurred or triggered during the previous pregnancy, intrapartum or postpartum. These critical times may be documented and longer consultation time offered for open discussion of the issues and the concerns regarding these critical events [15, 16]. Additional clinic visits, reassurance scans and fetal monitoring during the periods of the previous adverse events may be offered depending on individual circumstances. This may not necessarily change the outcomes; however, it may help allay anxiety around critical time points in the pregnancy. Clear advice about the actions to be

Table 23.2 A guide to reviewing information from the previous adverse outcome

Time of occurrence of the adverse event – antepartum/
intrapartum/postpartum
Gestational age in case of antepartum events
Type of anomaly in fetus/stillbirth/fetal-growth-restricted baby/
early neonatal death
Birthweight of the baby
Maternal complications and associated intervention
Family history of genetic disorders, birth defects
Review results of cytogenetics, molecular genetics, microarray,
placental histology, fetal autopsy, infection screen
Review correspondence, discharge summaries from previous
adverse outcomes

Table 23.3 Antenatal screening and risk assessment at booking

Booking weight and height assessment (body mass index (BMI))
Ethnicity
Booking bloods include:
    Baseline full blood count
    Haemoglobinopathies
    Blood group and RH antibodies
    HIV screening
    Hepatitis screen

Offer first trimester combined screening for common trisomies
(21, 18, 13).
Discuss other available options including non-invasive prenatal
testing

Folic acid supplementation
Nutritional advice

Possible exposure to teratogens
Smoking cigarettes (CO monitoring should be offered to at-risk
women) and support for stopping smoking should be provided
Alcohol and substance abuse

Autoimmune disorders
Glucose intolerance
Thyroid disorders
Risk for hypertensive disorders

Screening for cervical and vaginal infections
Asymptomatic bacteriuria
Sexually transmitted infections

Mental health issues
Risk for domestic violence or sexual abuse
Discuss immunization

History of gynaecological cervical surgery (risk factor
for preterm birth)
Assisted conception

taken if there were any concerns about the pregnancy and contact numbers for support if required should be discussed.

23.6.6 Maternal Serum Screening Placental Biochemical Markers Associated with Adverse Outcome [17, 18]

Various placental biochemical markers have been studied as predictors of stillbirths or poor perinatal outcomes. The FASTER trial showed an increased rate of stillbirth and spontaneous loss prior to 24 weeks where the pregnancy-associated plasma protein-A (PAPP-A) was below the fifth percentile during a first trimester screening and where chromosomal abnormalities had been ruled out [19]. Evidence does suggest a negative predictive value where PAPP-A levels and Doppler flow studies are normal in predicting stillbirths due to placental causes, especially at less than 32 weeks. Also, a normal second trimester uterine artery Doppler pulsatility index (PI) reduces the risk of stillbirth to less than 0.03%.

Low levels of PAPP-A are associated with low levels of insulin-like growth factor, which plays a role in trophoblast invasion of the decidua. Low levels of PAPP-A (0.4–0.5 multiples of the median (MoM)) have also been associated with abnormal trophoblast invasion, which in turn is associated with pre-eclampsia and fetal growth restriction [17].

High levels of human chorionic gonadotropin (hCG) are associated with large placentas and fetal growth restriction.

Raised levels of alpha fetoprotein (AFP) have been associated with chorionic villitis and vascular lesions or thrombosis of the placenta. Mid-trimester amniotic fluid angiogenin levels, a marker of tissue ischaemia, is found to be altered in pregnancies with unexplained elevated AFP levels. Hence, it could be associated with adverse obstetric outcomes [19].

Placental growth factor (PlGF) is a vascular endothelial growth factor synthesized in villous and extravillous cytotrophoblast. It has functions of vasculogenesis and angiogenesis. Lower levels in the first trimester are predictive of early-onset pre-eclampsia.

23.6.7 Ultrasound for Screening and Surveillance

23.6.7.1 Dating Scan

Early confirmation of a viable pregnancy can provide reassurance and hope for an ongoing pregnancy. This will allow the confirmation of the viability of the pregnancy, dating the pregnancy, confirming number of fetuses and commencing aspirin in pregnancies where indicated, especially placenta-mediated pregnancy losses. First trimester combined screening, non-invasive prenatal testing and diagnostic testing options should be discussed if there is a previous history of chromosomal or genetic conditions.

Transvaginal cervical length screening from 12–14 weeks may be helpful in screening for those at risk of second trimester losses and preterm delivery. Further management plan for surveillance versus cervical cerclage will be decided based on previous obstetric history and individual circumstances.

23.6.7.2 Detailed Anatomy Scan

Referral to a specialist clinic and assessment by the fetal medical team may be necessary for some cases with a previous adverse outcome related to previous loss following congenital anomaly, chromosomal/genetic history in previous pregnancy or family history or unexpected or missed anomalies in previous pregnancy.

23.6.7.3 Serial Ultrasound for Fetal Growth, Amniotic Fluid Volume, Fetal Dopplers

Assessing for growth trajectory, amniotic fluid volume and fetal umbilical Doppler in high-risk pregnancies may provide reassurance to some couples, although this may not alter outcomes. Attending for additional scans may raise anxiety levels for some couples, and professionals need to be aware of the sensitivity around some landmark times during pregnancy when the previous adverse outcome may have occurred. Umbilical artery Dopplers provide additional assessment for women at high risk of stillbirths due to placental dysfunction or small-for-gestational-age fetus. Middle cerebral artery Doppler PI can be assessed along with the umbilical artery to identify fetal compromise after 34 weeks of gestation and reduce stillbirth risks by timely delivery for these babies. The type of fetal growth restriction early onset or late onset will influence decision making following findings of fetal Doppler abnormalities.

23.6.7.4 Uterine Artery Doppler

A failure of invasion of spiral arteries and subsequent placental dysfunction can be early predictors of issues arising due to uteroplacental disorders or hypertensive disorders. An abnormal second trimester uterine artery Doppler flow was associated with a 3–4 times risk of a stillbirth. Doppler flow studies in the third trimester also offer valuable data regarding fetal circulation and uteroplacental insufficiency.

23.6.7.5 Screening for Pre-eclampsia, Placental Dysfunction and Small for Gestational Age

Blood pressure (BP) monitoring, biochemical screening and Doppler flow studies can be used to screen and manage women with previous adverse pregnancy outcomes related to uteroplacental causes affecting mother and fetus.

23.6.8 Fetal Movements Awareness

Multiple episodes of reduced fetal movements in late pregnancy after 28 weeks are associated with increased risk of stillbirth. Especially in women with previous adverse outcomes, the anxiety levels are already high. Their concerns should be taken seriously by healthcare professionals. Computerized antepartum cardiotocogram is recommended for fetal monitoring following episodes of reduced fetal movement.

23.6.9 Medical Management

Treatment of any known cause and medical disorder, if any, is beneficial in reducing the recurrence risk. Managing pre-existing medical conditions that may have contributed to the previous adverse outcomes and involving physicians or obstetricians with expertise in management of medical disorder during pregnancy would form an essential part of the care.

Fetal growth restriction or women with early-onset or severe pre-eclampsia or in unexplained causes of poor earlier outcome of pregnancy have been associated with placental dysfunction.

The use of low-dose aspirin has been shown to be beneficial as a preventive measure and is found to be associated with improved birthweight when compared to placebo.

Recent evidence suggests that treatment with higher doses of aspirin (100–150 mg) beginning before 16 weeks of pregnancy and administered ideally at night improves the pregnancy outcome and reduces the recurrence risk in cases of fetal growth restriction and pre-eclampsia and may be considered for use in pregnancy complications arising out of placental dysfunction.

The use of low molecular weight heparin (LMWH) in the absence of established autoimmune disorders or thrombophilias has not been established. LMWH can be added to the treatment regime in cases of confirmed antiphospholipid syndromes and history suggestive of thromboembolism in the past. Ongoing assessment for risk of venous thromboembolism through the pregnancy and postpartum and need for prophylactic LMWH in high-risk cases should be instituted.

23.6.10 Delivery Considerations

There will be considerable anxiety about the timing and mode of delivery depending on the specific circumstances of the previous adverse outcome. Providing reassurance and support and involving parents in intrapartum care plans is crucial. Individualized care plans should be made based on timing of previous loss, intrapartum history and outcome and the safety considerations for vaginal birth versus need for elective caesarean section. Discussions for delivery plans should include preferences of the couple during labour for additional support with birthing partners and midwives.

23.6.11 Mode of Delivery

The stillbirth rates do increase after 39 weeks and hence elective induction of labour is advised by most clinicians in the pregnancy after an adverse outcome. 'Early term' gestation at 37 and 38 weeks does pose some risks related to premature births. The complications, especially where induction is planned at late prematurity or early term, need to be explained. The decision for induction of labour will depend on the choice of the mother after thorough counselling and weighing the risks and benefits. Early term induction may be offered to those at increased risk of perinatal death.

Intrapartum continuous fetal heart rate monitoring should be discussed and offered, especially if previous late fetal loss or intrapartum stillbirth had occured. Improvements in intrapartum care are essential for the reduction in intrapartum stillbirth rates.

Paediatric alert criteria should be in place for ensuring neonatal team and senior help available if there is risk of recurrence of previous adverse outcome or in particular if there had been issues related to intrapartum events needing resuscitation, neonatal condition at birth or neonatal unit admission.

23.6.12 Managing Mental Health and Psychosocial Aspects of Care

Anxiety, depression and post-traumatic stress disorders are commonly associated with adverse pregnancy outcomes. Prenatal depression has been associated with higher incidence of postnatal depressive symptoms. Higher levels of stress disorders have been correlated with increased incidence of obstetric, neonatal and postpartum complications. Many women refrain from attachment to their baby as a mechanism to cope with the loss and doubt their capacity to maintain a healthy pregnancy. This may in turn lead to disorganized attachment among infants born after an adverse outcome and adverse family consequences.

Antenatal care providers for patients with previous loss should offer a detailed session with the couple to discuss the gravity of the previous loss and the concerns regarding the possible relation with the present pregnancy. This would help in alleviating the anxiety and create a supportive environment and dialogue between the patient and the healthcare provider.

Psychosocial concerns must be taken into consideration. Acceptance from partners and society may vary, from a preference to hide or avoid sharing these events with their family or social circle to a complete support group available and acceptance of the event. The response from the partners may be of denial or an extra cautious approach and hence need to be addressed in the counselling and with an individualized approach. Perception towards stillbirths is varied, from pathological to belief systems, and so is the attitude of the society, the couple and the healthcare providers towards the event. Stillborn babies are perceived as a deceased child in some countries but less so in others. The level of support received and the attitude towards the event show wide variations between different high-income countries [20].

23.6.13 Befriender Groups and Support Groups

Bereaved parents who have achieved a healthy pregnancy following their loss and local support groups and healthcare professionals, including bereavement specialist midwives, can provide additional support during the pregnancy.

23.7 Key Messages

- Previous adverse pregnancy outcomes have a significant impact on the physical, mental and emotional health of the mother in subsequent pregnancies.
- The psychosocial aspects of management should be taken into consideration when planning care.
- Individualized care, multidisciplinary input when relevant and joint decision making with the woman and her partner will go a long way in the experience of these women during pregnancy and long term.
- Compassion, empathy, giving adequate time and listening to patient concerns and couples' anxiety after previous pregnancy adverse outcomes are important.
- Every effort to find the cause of the miscarriage, stillbirth or neonatal death will help with the counselling and management of risk in future pregnancies.
- Even when no cause is found following investigations for the loss, normal findings may be reassuring to some parents.
- Although there is no published good evidence for some of the clinical interventions offered to these women relating to timing and mode of delivery, based on clinical experience and of those involved, these plans will need to be individualized.
- Stillbirth has been taken as an indicator of progress in the sustainable developmental goals by the World Health Organization (WHO) [21], which is a step towards improvement in stillbirth rates and care for bereaved parents.

23.8 Key Guidelines for Further Reading

- SOGC clinical practice guidelines for managing pregnancy following previous stillbirth [22]
- RCOG guidelines for management of intrauterine fetal death and stillbirth [13]
- NICE Guideline NG121: *Intrapartum Care for Women with Existing Medical Conditions or Obstetric Complications and Their Babies*, March 2019

References

1. Lawn JE, Blencowe H, Waiswa P, et al. Stillbirths: rates, risk factors, and acceleration towards 2030. *Lancet.* 2016;**387**(10018):587–603. doi: 10.1016/S0140-6736(15)00837-5

2. Am W, Shepherd E, Middleton P, et al. Care prior to and during subsequent pregnancies following stillbirth for improving outcomes (Review) summary of findings for the main comparison. *Cochrane Database Syst Rev.* 2018;**2018**(12):CD012203. doi: 10.1002/14651858.CD012203.pub2

3. Van Dinter MC, Graves L. Managing adverse birth outcomes: helping parents and families cope. *Am Fam Physician.* 2012;**85**(9):900–4. www.ncbi.nlm.nih.gov/pubmed/22612185

4. Kramer MS. The epidemiology of adverse pregnancy outcomes: an overview. *J Nutr.* 2003;**133**(5 Suppl 2):1592S-6S. doi: 10.1093/jn/133.5.1592S

5. Frøen JF, Lawn JE, Heazell AEP, et al. *Ending Preventable Stillbirths: An Executive Summary for The Lancet's Series Ending Preventable Stillbirths.* 2016.

6. Flenady V, Koopmans L, Middleton P, et al. Major risk factors for stillbirth in high-income countries: a systematic review and meta-analysis. *Lancet.* 2011;**377**(9774):1331–40. doi: 10.1016/S0140-6736(10)62233-7

7. Reddy UM. Management of pregnancy after stillbirth. *Clin Obstet Gynecol.* 2010;**53**(3):700–9. doi: 10.1097/GRF.0b013e3181eba25e

8. Lamont K, Scott NW, Jones GT, Bhattacharya S. Risk of recurrent stillbirth: systematic review and meta-analysis. *Obstet Gynecol Surv.* 2015;**350**:h3080. doi: 10.1097/01.ogx.0000472120.21647.71

9. Baskaradoss JK, Geevarghese A, Al Dosari AAF. Causes of adverse pregnancy outcomes and the role of

maternal periodontal status – a review of the literature. *Open Dent J.* 2012;**6**(1):79–84. doi: 10.2174/1874210601206010079

10. Malacova E, Regan A, Nassar N, et al. Risk of stillbirth, preterm delivery, and fetal growth restriction following exposure in a previous birth: systematic review and meta-analysis. *Obstet Gynecol Surv.* 2018;**125**(2):183–92. doi: 10.1097/OGX.0000000000000574

11. Getahun D, Lawrence JM, Fassett MJ, et al. The association between stillbirth in the first pregnancy and subsequent adverse perinatal outcomes. *Am J Obstet Gynecol.* 2009;**201**(4):378.e1-6. doi: 10.1016/j.ajog.2009.06.071

12. Monari F, Pedrielli G, Vergani P, et al. Adverse perinatal outcome in subsequent pregnancy after stillbirth by placental vascular disorders. *PLoS One.* 2016;**11**(5):2–3. doi: 10.1371/journal.pone.0155761

13. *Late Intrauterine Fetal Death and Stillbirth Late Intrauterine Fetal Death and Stillbirth*, Green-top Guide No 55. London: Royal College of Obstetricians and Gynaecologists, 2010.

14. Gravensteen IK, Jacobsen EM, Sandset PM, et al. Anxiety, depression and relationship satisfaction in the pregnancy following stillbirth and after the birth of a live-born baby: a prospective study. *BMC Pregnancy Childbirth.* 2018;**18**(1):41. doi: 10.1186/s12884-018-1666-8

15. Côte-Arsenault D, Mahlangu N. Impact of perinatal loss on the subsequent pregnancy and self: women's experiences. *J Obstet Gynecol Neonatal Nurs.* 1999;**28**(3):274–82. doi: 10.1111/j.1552-6909.1999.tb01992.x

16. Robertson PA, Kavanaugh K. Supporting parents during and after a pregnancy subsequent to a perinatal loss. *J Perinat Neonatal Nurs.* 1998;**12**(2):63–71. doi: 10.1097/00005237-199809000-00007

17. Gagnon A, Wilson RD, Audibert F, et al. Obstetrical complications associated with abnormal maternal serum markers analytes. *J Obstet Gynaecol Canada.* 2008;**30**(10):918–32. doi: 10.1016/S1701-2163(16)32973-5

18. Metcalfe A, Langlois S, Macfarlane J, Vallance H, Joseph KS. Prediction of obstetrical risk using maternal serum markers and clinical risk factors. *Prenat Diagn.* 2014;**34**(2):172–9. doi: 10.1002/pd.4281

19. Lakhi N, Govind A, Moretti M, Jones J. Maternal serum analytes as markers of adverse obstetric outcome. *Obstet Gynaecol.* 2012;**14**:267–73. doi: 10.1111/j.1744-4667.2012.00132.x

20. Frøen JF, Cacciatore J, McClure EM, et al. Stillbirths: why they matter. *Lancet.* 2011;**377**(9774):1353–66. doi: 10.1016/S0140-6736(10)62232-5

21. Sustainable Development Goals. *Indicator and Monitoring Framework for the Global Strategy for Women's, Children's and Adolescents' Health (2016–2030).* Geneva, Switzerland: WHO; 2016.

22. Ladhani NNN, Fockler ME, Stephens L, Barrett JFR, Heazell AEP. No. 369 – Management of Pregnancy Subsequent to Stillbirth. *J Obstet Gynaecol Canada.* 2018;**40**(12):1669-83. doi: 10.1016/j.jogc.2018.07.002

23. NHS England. *Saving Babies' Lives: A Care Bundle for Reducing Stillbirth.* 2016.

24. NHS England. *Saving Babies' Lives Version Two: A Care Bundle for Reducing Perinatal Mortality.* March 2019.

Chapter 24

Preterm Prelabour Rupture of Membranes

Kamaleswari Camille Aiyaroo Thyne & Tahir A. Mahmood

24.1 Definition

Preterm prelabour rupture of membranes (PPROM) is defined as rupture of the membranes before 37 weeks' gestation. PPROM complicates only 2% of pregnancies but it is associated with 40% of preterm deliveries [1]. It is the single most common identifiable factor associated with preterm births. The latency period between rupture of membranes and labour tends to be inversely correlated with gestation, being longer with decreasing gestational age. The majority of pregnancies complicated by PPROM will deliver within a week of amniorrhexis.

The fetus carries a greater burden of morbidity and mortality than the mother. The associated significant fetal consequences typically result from the effects of prematurity, pulmonary hypoplasia and sepsis [1]. In addition to hypoplasia of the lungs, which promotes lethality, particularly when it occurs in the early mid-trimester, sustained oligohydramnios can also cause facial deformities and contracture deformities of the limbs. The other co-morbidities include gestational age-related respiratory distress syndrome, intraventricular haemorrhage and death. Infants born with sepsis have a mortality rate four times higher than non-infected babies. Prematurity-related morbidity varies with gestational age and is higher in the context of chorioamnionitis [1].

Infective morbidity resulting from ascending infection leads to chorioamnionitis and sepsis. This is the most significant maternal complication. Other complications include an increased incidence of retained placenta, postpartum endometritis and haemorrhage and surgical complications from operative abdominal and vaginal deliveries when therapeutic cessation of pregnancy is required. Both extreme prematurity and the higher prevalence of malpresentation in earlier gestations may require delivery via a vertical uterine incision (classical). This carries higher surgical morbidity for the index pregnancy and has obstetric implications for any subsequent pregnancies.

Intrauterine infection and premature rupture of membranes are risk factors for developing abruptio placentae [2]. Abruptio placentae can cause fetal hypoxic injury, iatrogenic and spontaneous prematurity, neonatal anaemia, death and a plethora of maternal complications which include anaemia, infection, acute kidney injury, complications from the transfusion of blood products and consumptive coagulopathy and shock resulting from massive ante- and postpartum haemorrhage [2]. There is a 5% risk of subsequent abruption following preterm membrane rupture.

24.2 Aetiology

The causative effect of PPROM appears to result from underlying pathological processes that incorporate infection and inflammation of the membranes, culminating in their disruption.

The strongest risk factors include a history of PPROM or preterm birth in a previous pregnancy, antepartum haemorrhage, ascending genital tract infection (often subclinical) and maternal smoking. However, most women will have no prior risk factors [1]. The effect of smoking is dose dependent and the increased risk is greatest at gestations below 28 weeks. The benefits of smoking cessation or even reduction should be emphasized to women who have had a past history of PPROM, as it is a modifiable risk factor.

Infection often appears to be a cause rather than a consequence of amniorrhexis. It is reasonable to assume that any risk factor implicated in the development of preterm labour may also cause PPROM. These would include pathological distention of the uterus (polyhydramnios, pregnancies of higher orders, congenital fetal anomalies that prevent swallowing, maternal diabetes) and some treatment procedures for cervical intraepithelial neoplasia. An increased risk is seen following excisional treatments of the cervix [3].

24.3 Assessment

This is a clinical diagnosis best achieved by taking an accurate history and performing a sterile speculum examination.

24.3.1 History

An accurate history can correctly identify the majority of cases. The enquiry should include
- Timing and nature of suspected rupture of membranes
- Colour of fluid
- Fetal movement pattern
- Presence or absence of abdominal pain/contractions and vaginal bleeding
- Feeling systemically unwell

24.3.2 Examination

- Temperature, pulse, blood pressure recorded on a modified early obstetric warning system (MEOWS) chart.
- Abdominal palpation to assess for tenderness, uterine activity, presentation, fetal lie and measurement of fundal height.

197

- Auscultation of fetal heart. Consider continuous cardiotocographic monitoring if the gestation is greater than 26 weeks.
- Sterile speculum examination to confirm the diagnosis. This is best performed after the mother has been lying supine for 20–30 minutes. Visualize the cervix and observe for fluid draining through the os or pooling of fluid in the posterior fornix. Ensure that the umbilical cord is neither presenting nor prolapsed. If fluid is not observed, consider performing the insulin-like growth factor binding protein-1 test or placental alpha-microglobulin 1 test of vaginal fluid if available [4].
- Digital vaginal examination should be avoided unless there is a strong suspicion of labour, as it is known to increase the incidence of an ascending infection, postpartum endometritis and neonatal infection and decrease the latency period before labour ensues.

24.3.3 Investigations

- Women should be observed for clinical signs of chorioamnionitis, which include maternal pyrexia and tachycardia, leukocytosis, offensive vaginal discharge and fetal tachycardia.
- High vaginal swab taken at the time of presentation for microscopy, culture and sensitivity.
- Bacteriological testing for group B streptococcus (GBS) is not recommended for women with preterm rupture of membranes [5].
- Cardiotocographic monitoring if over 28 weeks. Consider performing for gestations between 26 to 28 weeks.
- Ultrasound to confirm presentation.
- The role of the ultrasonic assessment of the amniotic fluid index is unclear; however a scan demonstrating oligohydramnios may be useful to support the diagnosis of PPROM [6].
- Baseline inflammatory markers – full blood count (FBC) and C-reactive protein (CRP).

24.4 Management

Delivery should be invoked immediately if there is evidence of compromise of the fetomaternal unit secondary to infection or abruption. The basis of expectant management is balancing the risk of an ascending infection by allowing the pregnancy to continue against the devastating consequences of delivering a premature baby.

24.4.1 No Clinical Signs of Chorioamnionitis

These patients are managed expectantly. The initial management is as an inpatient for the first 24–48 hours when the risk of delivery is highest. The maternal parameters are monitored 4 hourly and fetal monitoring performed twice daily. Erythromycin 250 mg is given orally 4 times a day for a maximum of 10 days or until the woman is in established labour, whichever is sooner. Erythromycin reduces the incidence of chorioamnionitis and neonatal infection rates as well as reducing the number of babies born within 48 hours [7]. The other benefits in short-term outcomes include prolongation of pregnancy, reductions in infection, need for surfactant, oxygen therapy and fewer babies with abnormal cerebral ultrasound before discharge from hospital should be balanced against a lack of evidence of benefit for others, including perinatal mortality and longer-term outcomes [8].

For those allergic to or unable to tolerate erythromycin, consider oral penicillin [4].

Corticosteroids should be administered for gestations between 24–34 weeks including women with diabetes mellitus, in whom the dosing of insulin may require adjustment or control with a sliding scale. Consider corticosteroids for gestations between 34 and 36 weeks after consultation with a senior clinician [4, 9]. **TOCOLYSIS is not recommended** [1]. There is no role for tocolysis in the absence of uterine activity but may be considered for those cases that require transfer to a neonatal unit that is equipped to manage the gestation of the neonate or for completion of the corticosteroid regime. This decision should be made by a senior clinician [1, 4].

If the clinical picture remains stable with no signs of labour or infection, subsequent management can be as an outpatient.

24.4.1.1 Long-Term Management

- Weekly HVS is no longer recommended [1]
- Women should check their own temperature at home, four times a day.
- Twice weekly review in the day bed setting where maternal observations will be checked and fetal monitoring performed.
- Weekly inflammatory markers (FBC, CRP) be performed to look for a rising trend.
- Ultrasound for growth assessment and umbilical artery Doppler be performed every 21 days. Fetal growth restriction may develop.
- Advise to contact the hospital if the temperature is elevated (>37.5°C), if the fluid becomes offensive or changes colour, if there has been a change in fetal movement pattern, if there is vaginal bleeding and if the woman feels unwell.
- These patients should have a review by their named consultant with a plan of care documented. This will include the timing of delivery and mode of delivery based on gestation, presentation and previous mode of delivery.
- Where there is no contraindication to continuing the pregnancy when PPROM occurs after 24+0 weeks' gestation, expectant management should be offered until 37+0 weeks' gestation. The timing of delivery should be individualized [6]. A recent Cochrane review showed that expectant management with careful monitoring is associated with better outcomes for the mother and baby [9].
- **For known GBS carriage, it may be beneficial to expedite delivery at more than 34 weeks' gestation** [5].

All preterm labourers should routinely be covered by intravenous (IV) antibiotics with regular benzylpenicillin irrespective of GBS status. For suspected penicillin allergy, a cephalosporin should be used and for those with a severe allergy to penicillin, vancomycin should be used [5].

24.4.2 Clinical Signs of Chorioamnionitis

- Maternal tachycardia and/or pyrexia
- Leukocytosis
- Uterine tenderness
- Offensive vaginal discharge or amniotic fluid
- Fetal tachycardia. Fetal tachycardia predicts 20–40% of clinical cases but it is a late sign.
- Note that inflammatory markers have a low sensitivity in predicting intrauterine infection.

These cases should be discussed with a senior clinician. **Conservative management is no longer appropriate.** Delivery should be expedited. Management will be the same as outlined in Chapter 50, Preterm Labour. The important points are listed below.

- Inform consultant obstetrician and neonatologist and charge midwife.
- In select cases, intrauterine transfer may be appropriate but decision to deliver should not be delayed for this purpose. The fetus can be delivered and stabilized prior to extrauterine transfer.
- Continuous fetal heart rate monitoring of gestations greater than 26 weeks but explain the potential difficulties in continuously monitoring a preterm labourer. Discuss and agree to a plan with the patient. Continuous monitoring if appropriate or intermittent auscultation may be considered.
- Normal fetal monitoring is reassuring, but an abnormal fetal heart rate pattern does not necessarily indicate fetal hypoxia or acidosis. Senior input is recommended.
- Magnesium sulphate given to mothers shortly before delivery reduces the risk of cerebral palsy and protects gross motor function in those infants born preterm. The effect may be greatest at early gestations and is not associated with adverse long-term fetal or maternal outcome [10].
- Magnesium sulphate for fetal neuroprotection is offered to gestations between 24+0 and 29+6 weeks and considered for gestations between 30+0 and 33+6 weeks. A 4 g loading dose is followed by a sustained infusion of 1 g per hour for 24 hours or until delivery, whichever is sooner [4].
- Mode of delivery – this will depend on the clinical circumstances, gestation and previous mode of delivery. Care must be individualized.
- Intrapartum antibiotic prophylaxis in accordance with local policy.
- Use of heat-preserving bags for delivery.
- Deferred cord clamping of at least 30 seconds but no longer than 3 minutes. The duration should be documented in the maternal notes for the purpose of deciphering paired cord blood gases.
- Placenta to be sent for histopathological analysis.

24.5 Special Considerations

The incidence of PPROM in twin pregnancies is higher but they generally follow the same management principles as singleton pregnancies. Monochorionic twin pregnancies have an added complexity and management should be made in consultation with a fetal medicine specialist.

The management of women with primary herpes simplex virus and human immunodeficiency virus (HIV) also warrants additional mention. The entire clinical picture needs to be considered, as these cases can be quite difficult to manage.

There is limited evidence to inform best obstetric practice when PPROM is complicated by primary herpes simplex virus infection; the management should be guided by the multidisciplinary team and will depend on the gestation when PPROM occurred. For immediate deliveries, the benefits of caesarean section will remain. For cases of initial expectant management, the recommendations are that the mother receives intravenous aciclovir 5 mg/kg 8 hourly. If delivery is indicated within 6 weeks of primary infection, caesarean section may still confer some benefit.

The risk of neonatal infection is low in the setting of recurrent genital herpes. Expectant management is appropriate for gestations under 34 weeks with the mother prescribed aciclovir 400 mg 3 times daily. For gestations beyond 34 weeks, the same management principles of PPROM will apply [11].

The management of women with HIV infection and ruptured membranes in gestations between 34 and 37 weeks is similar to management of cases beyond 37 weeks where delivery should be expedited with the addition of antibiotic chemoprophylaxis for group B streptococcus. The decision to augment labour or deliver by caesarean section will be determined by the viral load, previous mode of delivery and the presence of other obstetric co-morbidities. For those cases before 34 weeks, the optimal management is less clear, and cases should be discussed in the multidisciplinary setting. Steroids should be administered, and an uncontrolled viral load should be optimized [12].

24.5.1 Postdelivery

Review and discuss the events leading to delivery, allowing for any questions to be answered. Discuss and offer contraception.

In pregnancies following PPROM, women should be cared for by an obstetrician with an interest in preterm birth, ideally in the setting of a dedicated preterm birth clinic. Modifiable risk factors (eg smoking, respiratory diseases) should be addressed. There is evidence that screening for lower genital tract infections and midwife continuity throughout antenatal care are beneficial in preventing preterm birth [6]. Clinicians may offer these women genital tract screening for infection and/or serial transvaginal ultrasound scans to determine the cervical length, but the evidence to support these interventions is lacking[4].

References

1. *Preterm Prelabour Rupture of Membranes*, Green-top Guideline No 44. London: Royal College of Obstetricians and Gynaecologists, 2010.

2. *Antepartum Haemorrhage*, Green-top Guideline No 63. London: Royal College of Obstetricians and Gynaecologists, 2011.

3. *Reproductive Outcomes after Local Treatment for Preinvasive Cervical Disease*, Scientific Impact Paper No 21. London: Royal College of Obstetricians and Gynaecologists, 2016.

4. NICE Guideline NG25: *Preterm Labour and Birth*. November 2015.

5. *Prevention of Early-Onset Neonatal Group B Streptococcal Disease*, Green-top Guideline No 36. London: Royal College of Obstetricians and Gynaecologists, 2017.

6. *Care of Women Presenting with Suspected Preterm Prelabour Rupture of Membranes from 24+0 Weeks of Gestation*, Green-top Guideline No 73. London: Royal College of Obstetricians and Gynaecologist, 2019 https://doi.org/10.1111/1471-0528.15803

7. Broad-spectrum antibiotics for preterm, prelabour rupture of fetal membranes: the ORACLE I randomized trial. ORACLE Collaborative Group. *Lancet.* 2001;**357**(9261):979–94.

8. *Preterm Labour, Antibiotics and Cerebral Palsy*, Scientific Impact Paper No 33. London: Royal College of Obstetricians and Gynaecologists, 2013.

9. *Antenatal Corticosteroids to Reduce Neonatal Morbidity*, Green-top Guideline No 7. London: Royal College of Obstetricians and Gynaecologists, 2010.

10. *Magnesium Sulphate to Prevent Cerebral Palsy following Preterm Birth*, Scientific Impact Paper No 29. London: Royal College of Obstetricians and Gynaecologists, 2011.

11. *Genital Herpes in Pregnancy, Management*, Green-top Guideline No 30. London: Royal College of Obstetricians and Gynaecologists, 2007.

12. British HIV Association Guidelines for the Management of HIV in Pregnancy and Postpartum. 2018.

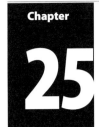

Chapter

25

Hypertensive Disorders in Pregnancy and Eclampsia

Anne Cathrine Staff & Ralf Dechend

25.1 Introduction: Why Are Hypertensive Disorders of Pregnancy Important?

Hypertensive disorders of pregnancy (HDP) remain a major obstetric challenge across the world. No other antenatal complication is both so common and dangerous for the mother and baby together. Hypertension is the commonest medical problem encountered in pregnancy, and affects 10–15% of all pregnancies. Hypertension in pregnancy is divided into pre-existing hypertension (chronic hypertension), gestational hypertension (previously named pregnancy-induced hypertension) and pre-eclampsia. Pre-eclampsia is the most severe HDP form, with great mortality and morbidity risk for the mother and offspring, especially in countries with inadequate antenatal care.

25.1.1 Major Cause of Maternal and Fetal Mortality and Morbidity

Pre-eclampsia/eclampsia is among the leading causes of maternal morbidity and mortality worldwide, and represents the most important antenatal complication of pregnancy, in terms of its incidence and combined short- and long-term effects on maternal and offspring health[1, 2]. The maternal mortality deaths are at least 50 000 [3] to 76 0000 [4] per year, while fetal and neonatal pre-eclampsia deaths are assumed to be at least 500 000 annually [4]. Pre-eclampsia is a major cause for intrauterine fetal death and stillbirth [5], and for small-for-gestational-age babies, as well as for iatrogenic premature delivery [6].

25.1.2 Great Global Differences in Pre-eclampsia Morbidity and Mortality

The rates of HDP and their subtypes are often poorly documented in low-income countries, which are lacking antenatal and obstetric registrations. The complications of pre-eclampsia are more often fatal in low-income countries, due to lack of adequate healthcare resources. Whereas the maternal mortality rates are now very low in high-income countries (0–1.8%), the mortality rates are up to 15% in developing countries [7], often due to eclampsia [3]. HDP is, however, still a great challenge also in high-income countries in Europe, where maternal deaths are closely monitored and classified in order to reduce mortality and morbidity to a minimum [8, 9].

25.2 Hypertensive Disorders of Pregnancy Classification and Epidemiology

25.2.1 Definition of Hypertension and Types of HDP

25.2.1.1 Hypertension

Hypertension is defined as systolic blood pressure (BP) ≥140 and/or diastolic BP ≥90 mm Hg [4]. Blood pressure should be rechecked to confirm true hypertension (within 15 minutes if severe BP with systolic BP ≥160 and/or diastolic BP ≥110) [4]. A validated BP device for pregnancy should be used, as well as adequate-sized cuffs (e.g. using a thigh cuff if upper arm is >44 cm in measurement to minimize overdiagnosis of hypertension) [10].

25.2.1.2 HDP Classification [4, 11]

Chronic hypertension is known hypertension before pregnancy or first diagnosed hypertension before 20 weeks' gestation. Chronic hypertension can be further divided into essential and secondary. Up to 25% will develop 'superimposed pre-eclampsia' [4] (see below).

Gestational hypertension is defined as 'hypertension arising after 20 weeks' gestation'. Up to 25% may progress to pre-eclampsia [4].

Pre-eclampsia is hypertension arising after 20 weeks' gestation (gestational hypertension) accompanied by ONE or MORE of the following new-onset signs after 20 weeks' gestation (in recognition of the syndromic nature of pre-eclampsia, proteinuria is no longer a mandatory requirement for a pre-eclampsia definition in many updated guidelines [4, 11]):

1) Proteinuria:

   o ≥0.3 g per 24 hours (time-consuming and rarely performed nowadays)

   o Spot urine protein/creatinine ratio >0.3 mg/mmol (equals >0.26 mg/mg)

   o ≥1+ proteinuria on urine dip stick test (acceptable if above tests are unavailable), preferably on at least two occasions

2) Evidence of maternal organ dysfunction, including one or more of the following:

   o Liver involvement (elevated transaminases, e.g. alanine aminotransferase (ALT) or aspartate aminotransferase (AST)) o Neurological complications (e.g. eclampsia, stroke, persistent visual scotomata)

o Haematological complications (thrombocytopenia, disseminated intravascular coagulation; haemolysis)

o Uteroplacental dysfunction (e.g. fetal growth restriction, stillbirth, abnormal fetal Doppler findings)[4, 10]. This feature is, however, not included as a criterion for diagnosing pre-eclampsia in most medical birth registries and many national clinical guidelines, such as the American College of Obstetricians and Gynecologists [11].

'Superimposed' pre-eclampsia upon chronic hypertension occurs when a pregnant woman with a chronic hypertension develops proteinuria or any of the other maternal syndromic features of pre-eclampsia presented above [4].

Pre-eclampsia Diagnosed before 20 Weeks' Gestation [12]

In some rare cases, such as in hydatidiform mole, maternal signs of pre-eclampsia may appear earlier than 20 weeks' gestation.

Pre-eclampsia with Severe Features

As pre-eclampsia is a complex medical syndrome, where maternal and fetal conditions can deteriorate rapidly, classifying pre-eclampsia into severe or mild disease is no longer recommended [4]. However, classifying pre-eclampsia with or without severe features is a sensible clinical approach.

Features of severe pre-eclampsia include [11]:

1) Systolic BP ≥160 or diastolic BP ≥110 mm Hg (on at least two occasions after rest)
2) Eclampsia (see below)
3) Maternal clinical symptoms and signs: epigastric pain, malaise, severe headache and/or other cerebral symptoms (irritability, visual disturbances, hyperreflexia), rapidly increasing oedema, and pulmonary oedema (dyspnoea, cyanosis)
4) Laboratory tests: proteinuria ≥3 g per 24 hours, concentrated urine with oliguria (<500 mL/24 hours), rapidly decreasing platelet count, signs of microangiopathic haemolytic anaemia (increasing lactate dehydrogenase (LD), decreasing haptoglobin), elevated liver enzymes (partial or complete HELLP syndrome development, see below)

HELLP (haemolysis, elevated liver enzymes, and low platelets) is defined by:

- Haemolysis: detected as low haptoglobin in serum (<0.2 g/L) and elevated bilirubin and/or elevated LD
- Liver affection: elevated ALT, AST and LD
- Low (by repeated measurements) platelets <100 x 10^9/L [11, 12]

In eclampsia, general maternal seizures occur during pregnancy, childbirth or during the first seven days after delivery, coexisting with pre-eclampsia or gestational hypertension (all degrees of severity) and where there are no other neurological causes for the seizures.

25.2.2 Risk Factors for Pre-eclampsia and Gestational Hypertension

Table 25.1 summarizes important risk factors for pre-eclampsia/gestational hypertension.

25.2.3 Epidemiology of HDP

The rate of hypertensive disorders of pregnancy varies across populations, typically affecting 10% of all pregnancies, but depending on presence of risk factors, as presented above, including rate of chronic diseases, parity and obesity. Chronic hypertension affects 1–5% [13], gestational hypertension 2–17%, and pre-eclampsia complicates about 2–5% of pregnancies [14–16]. These different categories of hypertension do not occur in isolation. Chronic hypertension is a major

Table 25.1 Risk factors for hypertensive disorders of pregnancy

Risk factor start	Increases risk for pre-eclampsia/gestational hypertension [12, 29, 30]
Pregestational factors	*Primiparity/primigravidity *High maternal age (>40 years) *Maternal overweight/obesity ≥35 kg/m² (risk increases, however, linearly from body mass index (BMI) 28 [47]) **Chronic hypertension (by definition not a risk factor for gestational hypertension) **Pregestational diabetes mellitus **Renal disease (incl. kidney transplantation) **Autoimmune diseases (e.g. systemic lupus erythematosus and antiphospholipid syndrome) Short pre-pregnancy intercourse time (with baby's biological father). *Long inter-pregnancy time (>10 years) Women of African (genetic) descent **Previous hypertensive disease in pregnancy, especially severe/early-onset pre-eclampsia (delivery prior to gestational week 34) and/or fetal growth restriction. *Pre-eclampsia in mother/sisters
Pregnancy factors	*Multiples and other pregnancies with large placentas (e.g. moles) [48] Fetal growth restriction (FGR) Gestational diabetes mellitus Uterine artery notch/elevated pulsatility index (PI) Low circulating level of placental growth factor (PlGF) Assisted reproductive techniques (ARTs)

** denotes high risk and * denoted moderate risk factors for pre-eclampsia according to NICE 2019 guidelines, when considering low-dose aspirin prophylaxis [35]

risk factor for pre-eclampsia (e.g. superimposed pre-eclampsia) and gestational hypertension may be an early sign of pre-eclampsia in some women. All three forms of hypertension increase the risk of fetal growth restriction (FGR).

Eclampsia is a rare form of pre-eclampsia, affecting 5 in 10 000 pregnancies in Scandinavia [17]. In developing countries, 16–70 of 10 000 pregnancies develop eclampsia [3], due to inadequate healthcare. In Scandinavia, eclampsia occurs during pregnancy in one third of the cases, whereas two thirds have their episodes during childbirth or during the first seven days after delivery [17].

The rates for pre-eclampsia seem to have declined in some high-income regions over the last two decades, such as in Northern Europe and Australia [18], despite high and increasing rates of obesity, an important risk factor for any type of HDP. Increasing trends for induced delivery of post-term deliveries, in order to avoid fetal death, may be an explanation for the reduced rate of late-onset pre-eclampsia, in addition to an increasing use of low-dose aspirin as prophylaxis for pre-eclampsia in women at increased risk (see Section 25.8.3 below).

25.3 Pathogenesis/Pathophysiology of Pre-eclampsia and Eclampsia

25.3.1 Two-Stage Placental Model for Pre-eclampsia [19–22]

Pre-eclampsia has long been recognized as a syndrome that requires the presence of placental tissue, but where maternal predisposition also plays a significant role. For pre-eclampsia (and gestational hypertension) development, a fetus is not needed (e.g. in complete hydatidiform mole), nor is a uterus (women with abdominal pregnancy may develop pre-eclampsia). Also, pre-eclampsia is cured after removal of the placenta, except in some rare cases of postpartum disease.

The maternal multi-organ distress features of pre-eclampsia derive from diffuse systemic vascular endothelial activation (excessive vascular inflammation), and include the classical signs of hypertension and proteinuria. Pre-eclampsia is often classified into early- and late-onset. Traditionally, clinicians simplify 'onset' and dichotomize into preterm/term delivery (< or ≥ gestational week 37) or into a very premature delivery/or not (< or ≥ gestational week 34) [23].

The classical '2-stage placental model of pre-eclampsia' was introduced in 1991 [19]. Stage 1 is the 'preclinical stage' (placental stage), which is secondary to a poor placentation, involving a shallow remodelling of maternal uteroplacental spiral arteries that supply the placenta with maternal blood. Poor placentation is common in early-onset pre-eclampsia, and is affected by multiple immunological factors, including certain combinations of fetal and maternal genotypes (affecting the interaction of fetal trophoblast and maternal uterine immune cells) [24], and non-optimal immune adaptation to the woman's partner (the baby's father).

Poor placentation leads to abnormal perfusion of the placenta. The cells covering the placenta villi (syncytiotrophoblasts)

then release pro-inflammatory stress signals into the maternal circulation. A systemic endothelial dysfunction follows these stress signals, involving an excessive maternal vascular inflammatory response in the whole body. This endothelial dysfunction is a key event for both the development of hypertension and leakage of protein through affected glomeruli (resulting in proteinuria) and the other potential widespread maternal features of the second stage of pre-eclampsia ('the clinical stage').

There are several stress/inflammatory signals from the placenta, including microvesicles from the syncytiotrophoblasts and dysregulated anti- and proangiogenic proteins. In 2003 proangiogenic (e.g. PlGF-placental growth factor) and anti-angiogenic factors (e.g. sFlt1-soluble fms-like tyrosine kinase receptor 1) of mainly placental origin in pregnancy were shown to contribute to the pre-eclampsia syndrome by inducing a systemic antiangiogenic state with endothelial dysfunction [25]. This discovery helped to link Stage 1 and 2 concepts.

Whereas the early-onset type of pre-eclampsia is linked to poor placentation and fetal growth restriction, maternal factors have been suggested to cause the late-onset disease, without a major placental impact, sometimes described as maternal pre-eclampsia [26]. As an alternative model, we have suggested that both pre-eclampsia forms (early- and late-onset) are the result of placental dysfunction (Stage 1) prior to development of its clinical signs (Stage 2), but that the causes of the placental malperfusion and its timing in pregnancy differ [20, 21]. The late-onset pre-eclampsia type has little or no evidence of poor placentation typical of early-onset disease (Figure 25.1, Pathway A), but may be secondary to an intraplacental cause of placental malperfusion (Figure 25.1, Pathway B), due to the growing placenta reaching its size limit, resulting in secondary malperfusion and a hypoxic placenta. Pathway B depicts what is seen in postmature or multiple pregnancies, where the size of the term placenta may restrict intervillous perfusion. The key feature of the revised model is therefore that placenta malperfusion (Stage 1) may arise from two placental causes: from poor placentation, but also from an undersupply due to the placenta outgrowing its limit.

According to this revised two-stage placental model of pre-eclampsia, the placenta is the cause of all cases of pre-eclampsia, whereas many maternal factors contribute to its pathophysiology. The model predicts that maternal predisposing factors may affect both pathways (A and B) leading to the first stage (placental dysfunction), as well as may accelerate the steps towards the second stage of the disease (clinical presentation with new-onset hypertension and proteinuria), such as priming the maternal systemic endothelium for placental stress factors.

This revised two-stage model of pre-eclampsia is consistent with the clinical presentations and risk factors of early- and late-onset pre-eclampsia (as presented in Table 25.1). The key to understanding the syndromic and unpredictable nature of pre-eclampsia is this excessive maternal vascular inflammatory response in the whole body, following stress signals from the placenta. This explains the potential widespread maternal features of the second stage of pre-eclampsia (the clinical stage), as any organ can be affected, until the dysfunctional placenta is removed.

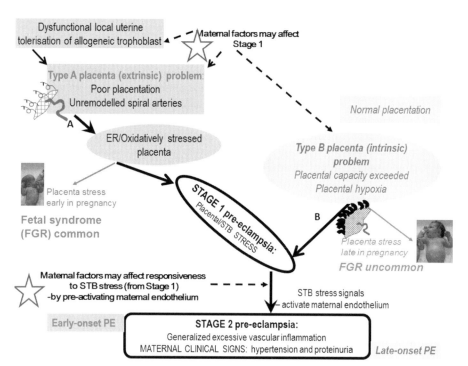

Figure 25.1 Revised two-stage pre-eclampsia (PE) model. Reprinted with approval from Springer [23].
All PE is dependent on placenta syncytiotrophoblast (STB) stress and maternal risk factors may impact on several levels and both stages.
Pathway A (associated with early-onset PE) illustrates the 'extrinsic' cause, and pathway B (associated with late-onset PE) illustrates the 'intrinsic' cause for placental malperfusion and dysfunction (STAGE 1), leading to the clinical recognized maternal syndrome of pre-eclampsia (STAGE 2).

25.3.2 How Can Placental Dysfunction Mediate Eclampsia?

The cause of eclamptic seizures is not known, but one theory is that the cerebrovascular changes are the same as in hypertensive encephalopathy, including loss of autoregulation of cerebral blood flow followed by hyperperfusion and development of cerebral oedema. Pre-eclampsia may have several adverse effects on the maternal brain, due to disruption of the blood–brain barrier, with posterior reversible encephalopathy syndrome (PRES) and maternal stroke as severe consequences [27]. Placenta stress factors are likely to mediate these cerebral effects.

25.3.3 Pre-eclampsia: A Primarily Cardiovascular Cause?

The placental model of pre-eclampsia has been challenged recently. It has been argued that pre-eclampsia represents the failure of the maternal cardiovascular system to adapt to pregnancy, and that placental dysfunction is a secondary feature [28]. This model does, however, not fit with several well-known pre-eclampsia risk factors, such as primiparity and change of partnership (i.e. immunological factors important for the placentation process), which fit better with the two-stage placental pre-eclampsia model.

25.4 Clinical Features of Pre-eclampsia [12, 29]

25.4.1 Women with Pre-eclampsia Often Lack Symptoms

Most women with any form of new-onset hypertension in pregnancy will not have any subjective symptoms. This emphasizes the importance of regular antenatal follow-up and screening (blood pressure and urine testing for proteinuria) in all pregnancies.

Some HDP women with affected placental dysfunction may sense reduced fetal movements, or even absent movement following fetal death. Women who have developed severe features of pre-eclampsia (see above) may also have clinical symptoms such as abdominal pain, typically epigastric or right upper quadrant pain (due to liver affection in pre-eclampsia). Nausea and vomiting (after gestational week 20, when hyperemesis gravidarum is uncommon) can also be first symptoms of severe pre-eclampsia. Severe headache or flashing lights might be observed by women prior to an eclamptic fit.

25.4.2 Clinical Maternal and Fetal Objective Signs That May Imply Development of Pre-eclampsia

- Reduced symphysis fundal height development (due to placental dysfunction and fetal growth restriction)
- Rapidly increasing maternal weight, with rapidly increasing and severe swelling of the face, fingers and legs (due to systemic vascular inflammation and oedema development)
- Measurement of hypertension (may develop prior to proteinuria), proteinuria (may develop prior to the hypertension), HELLP
- Convulsions (eclampsia)
- Fetal growth restriction (as assessed by ultrasound) or intrauterine death
- Abruptio placenta (associated with placental dysfunction and thereby pre-eclampsia)

25.5 Investigations [12]

Every pregnant woman should be informed about the risk of developing pre-eclampsia and gestational hypertension, and to seek healthcare professionals if they experience alarming symptoms like severe headache, vision problems (blurring and flashing before the eyes), subcostal pain, sudden swelling of face, hands or feet or decreased fetal movements [30]. Blood pressure measurement and urine testing for proteinuria or laboratory investigations (for other organ involvements) will diagnose HDP or not. Laboratory assessment of maternal circulating angiogenic proteins may help to rule out the diagnosis of pre-eclampsia before week 35 (see Section 25.5.3 below), and may represent an added diagnostic tool in women presenting with suspected pre-eclampsia, but lacking the required diagnostic clinical signs [31].

25.5.1 Monitoring for Maternal Disease Severity When Pre-eclampsia is Diagnosed

- BP measurements: frequency depending on clinical situation (method: see above, Section 25.2.1.1).
- Proteinuria: if present; no point in further testing of proteinuria, as proteinuria level lacks predictive information (exception: chronic renal disease where proteinuria may be used to assess severity of disease).
- Blood tests: Hb, platelets, AST/AL/LD, uric acid, creatinine. In severe pre-eclampsia and HELLP; additionally measure albumin, international normalized ratio (INR), fibrinogen, D-dimer, antithrombin and haptoglobin. In case of suspected acute fatty liver, additionally measure plasma glucose, leukocytes, triglycerides and total cholesterol.

Tight follow-up for development of any signs of severe pre-eclampsia features, as described above (Section 25.4), including rapidly increased weight gain, sudden headache and abdominal pain (especially upper right quadrant, as seen in liver involvement/HELLP).

25.5.2 Fetal Surveillance When Pre-eclampsia is Diagnosed

- The patient should be reminded about reporting any lack of fetal movements
- Cardiotocography (CTG), if possible with short time variability
- Ultrasound: fetal biometrics (assess asymmetrical growth and overall fetal growth), biophysical profile and Doppler blood flow examination (umbilical artery, possibly middle cerebral artery and ductus venosus in selected cases).

25.5.3 Ruling Out Pre-eclampsia with Placenta-Derived Biomarkers in Women with Suspected, but Not Confirmed Disease

The 2016 UK guidelines (www.nice.org.uk/guidance/dg23) recommend the use of two types of angiogenic blood tests (Elecsys immunoassay for the sFlt1/PlGF ratio, and the Triage PlGF test) to help rule out pre-eclampsia requiring delivery within the next 1–2 weeks, in women with suspected pre-eclampsia between 20 and 35 weeks' gestation [32, 33].

25.6 Differential Diagnoses of Severe HDP Features

The following conditions may present some features similar to those of HDP [12]:

- Renal disease
- Hepatitis (autoimmune and infectious)
- Gastroenteritis/gastritis/ulcer
- Bile disease /pancreatitis
- Worsening of systemic lupus erythematosus (SLE)
- Acute fatty liver of pregnancy (AFLP)
- Haemolytic uraemic syndrome (HUS)
- Thrombotic thrombocytopenic purpura (TTP), thrombocytopenia caused by autoimmunity
- Appendicitis/other causes of acute abdominal pain
- Migraine (if diagnosed first time in pregnancy)
- Infections, especially in renal involvement (e.g. hantavirus, cytomegalovirus)

It may be difficult to diagnose whether a patient with chronic hypertension also has developed pre-eclampsia (25% risk). A study suggested that circulating measurement of PlGF protein may be of value to discriminate renal and placental failure [34], which may have important clinical intervention consequences.

The differential diagnosis of eclampsia includes epilepsy or other diseases that can cause seizures in pregnancy (delirium, cerebral tumours, infections etc.).

25.7 Clinical Management

25.7.1 Pregnancies with HDP Need Dedicated Care

Pre-eclamptic women should be referred to an obstetric department for evaluation of maternal and fetal well-being. In pre-eclampsia without severe features (see Section 25.2.1.2) the woman may be followed up as an outpatient with a few days' interval [4, 11, 12], in an obstetric setting or by another healthcare professional trained in the management of HDP [35]. A similar approach is recommended for women with gestational hypertension who have high risk for developing pre-eclampsia. Women with chronic hypertension are often followed up in specialist care prior to pregnancy, and will often need a combination of obstetric and physician follow-up.

For a woman with HDP, and in particular pre-eclampsia, the clinical situation may change at short notice, and admittance to the obstetric department is required in pre-eclampsia with severe features to reduce maternal and fetal morbidity and to avoid mortality. Clinical continuity in follow-up is important after admission to the hospital.

25.7.2 Specific Pre-eclampsia Treatment is Lacking

The only cure for pre-eclampsia is at present delivery of the placenta (and therefore also the baby), although ongoing clinical studies are testing whether pregnancy may be prolonged by affecting placenta-mediated stress signals (e.g. by reducing circulating sFlt1), or by their effect on a stressed vasculature (e.g. statins).

The main maternal pharmacological approach to hypertensive disorders in pregnancy today is to use antihypertensives to reduce the risk for maternal hypertensive cerebral haemorrhage. There is, however, a trade-off between lowering maternal risk of cerebral haemorrhage and affecting placental circulation, and hence fetal growth, negatively. For the fetus, the main pharmacological approach is giving the expecting mother corticosteroids whenever premature iatrogenic delivery (prior to gestational week 34) is likely, in order to increase lung maturation and reduce fetal postnatal mortality and morbidity.

25.7.3 Antihypertensive Treatment in Pregnancy

In general, there is a lack of trials assessing optimal antihypertensive drug use in pregnancy. A recent Cochrane meta-analysis concluded that 'antihypertensive drug therapy for mild to moderate hypertension during pregnancy reduces the risk of severe hypertension. The effect on other clinically important outcomes remains unclear. If antihypertensive drugs are used, beta blockers and calcium channel blockers appear to be more effective than the alternatives for preventing severe hypertension. High-quality large sample-sized randomized controlled trials are required in order to provide reliable estimates of the benefits and adverse effects of antihypertensive treatment for mild to moderate hypertension for both mother and baby, as well as costs to the health services, women and their families' [36].

25.7.3.1 Blood Pressure Treatment in Women with Chronic Hypertension

Non-pregnant women using ACE (angiotensin-converting enzymes) inhibitors / angiotensin II-receptor blockers or other potentially teratogenic antihypertensive drugs are advised to change these drugs when they plan pregnancy, or at latest when pregnancy is confirmed. In some cases, women with chronic hypertension may be without medication for a period in the middle of pregnancy due to the physiological drop in blood pressure at this time of pregnancy.

The 2018 International Society for the Study of Hypertension in Pregnancy (ISSHP) guidelines recommend target blood pressure in the range of 110–140/80–85 mm Hg in pregnant women with chronic hypertension, and delivery at 39 weeks unless other indications exist (similar to those of pre-eclampsia, see below) [4].

25.7.3.2 Blood Pressure Treatment in Moderate and Severe Pre-eclampsia Prior to Delivery [12]

Blood pressure ≥150/100 mm Hg [30] is an indication for antihypertensive treatment. The purpose is to avoid maternal complications such as brain haemorrhage, hypertensive encephalopathy and seizures. The goal is not a normalization of the blood pressure, but achieving diastolic values around 80–100 mm Hg and a systolic BP <150 mm Hg. High systolic pressure increases the risk of cerebral haemorrhage. There is no evidence of a beneficial effect of lowering the blood pressure <150/100 mm Hg in pregnancy, except that this strategy gives less episodes of severe maternal hypertension [37], which is why ISSHP recently suggested a stricter blood pressure goal in pregnancy of 150/85, based on a randomized controlled trial (RCT) of non-proteinuric women with chronic or gestational hypertension [4].

A BP that is difficult to control may indicate worsening of the syndrome, and an overall assessment of indication for delivery is recommended.

25.7.3.3 First Line Antihypertensive Drugs Recommended in Pregnancy

Current US [11] and Norwegian [12] guidelines recommend three first line antihypertensives in pregnancy, whereas the UK NICE guidelines suggests labetalol as the single first line drug [30, 35]. The ISSHP 2018 recommendations include these three drugs as well as some others [4]. A recent published RCT performed in India demonstrated similar effects of oral regimens with labetalol, nifedipine and methyldopa in reducing blood pressure without causing maternal adverse events [38]. Methyldopa was, however, not sufficient as a single drug for obtaining the blood pressure goal in one fifth of the women. See the following list.

Labetalol (alpha- and beta blocker) orally 100 mg x 2, augmenting to 200 mg x 3–4. Max dose 500 mg x 4 [29]. Maximum plasma concentrations 1–2 hours after intake. Combination with nifedipine doses listed below is possible.
- Contraindication: asthma.
- Safe to use when breastfeeding

Nifedipine (calcium antagonist) (*slow release*) orally 10 mg x 2, augmenting to a maximum of 40 mg x 2. Effect after 45–60 minutes.

Depot tablets may be appropriate (but not suitable if acute BP is the aim, as max concentration is after 6–12 hours): 30 mg x 1, augmenting to 30 mg x 2.
- Safe to use when breastfeeding

Methyldopa orally 250 mg x 2–3. May be increased to 500 mg x 3. Max dose 1000 mg x 3 [29]. Effect after 3–8 hours, full effect after 12 hours. This drug is not suitable if acute BP reduction is the aim. If higher doses of methyldopa are needed, it may be useful rather to choose a combination with labetalol or nifedipine due to the risk of side effects (dry mouth, constipation, depression).
- Contraindication: depression.
- Safe to use when breastfeeding.

25.7.3.4 Contraindicated Antihypertensive Drugs in Pregnancy or Postpartum

ACE inhibitors (e.g. enalapril): Contraindicated in pregnancy, but can be used during the postpartum period [29], and is safe to use when breastfeeding.

Alpha-blockers (e.g. doxazosin): second line therapy in pregnancy. Contraindicated when breastfeeding (enalapril or prazosin should be used instead) [29].

25.7.3.5 Blood Pressure Treatment in Acute Hypertension [12]

Both oral labetalol and nifedipine are sufficiently fast acting and can be used for gradual lowering of blood pressure, possibly in combination with methyldopa. If this is not sufficient, intravenous (IV) treatment is recommended. Too rapid lowering of blood pressure should be avoided as it threatens the uteroplacental circulation and increases the risk of fetal intrauterine demise.

If oral therapy (see above for options, such as labetalol orally 200 mg, expected effect after about 30 minutes) is not tolerated because of nausea and vomiting, or there is an unstable BP and rapid rise in BP, labetalol can be administrated intravenously, either intermittent or as a continuous infusion:

– Labetalol loading dose intravenously: 20 mg intravenously and it is effective after 5–10 minutes. If suboptimal effect is seen after 10–15 minutes, then the dose may be increased to 40–50 mg IV. Maximum dose is 200 mg.
– Labetalol continuous infusion (1 mg/mL): Infusion start rate is 20 mL/hour, i.e. 20 mg/hour, which can be increased with 10 to 20 mL/hour about every 20–30 minutes until satisfactory BP control is achieved. Maximum infusion rate is 160 mL/hour.

25.7.3.6 Antihypertensive Treatment during Delivery [12]

Blood pressure increases during uterine contractions and especially during delivery of the baby. Women with severe pre-eclampsia who wish to deliver vaginally should be closely monitored, both during delivery and postpartum. Epidural is recommended in hypertensive women who wish to deliver vaginally, because of the beneficial antihypertensive effect. Platelet levels should be checked in advance to avoid spinal bleed (see below).

25.7.3.7 Antihypertensive Treatment Postpartum [12]

Maternal BP target should be lower than before delivery, e.g. 140/90 mm Hg, as there is no uteroplacental circulation. When choosing an antihypertensive drug postpartum, methyldopa should be discontinued first because of side effects (dry mouth, constipation, depression). Treatment could continue with labetalol or nifedipine, or as a combination.

If there is much oedema noted during postpartum, the significant quantities of liquid will be mobilized into the bloodstream and can contribute to pulmonary oedema; therefore, it may be appropriate to give furosemide in small doses postpartum. If symptoms of fluid overload are present, including dyspnoea and possibly reduced oxygenation, admission to an intensive care unit is almost always necessary.

25.7.4 Timing of Delivery in HDP

For pregnant women with chronic hypertension, the 2018 ISSHP guidelines recommend delivery at 39 weeks unless other reasons (similar to those of pre-eclampsia, see below) indicate earlier delivery [4].

These guidelines also recommend delaying delivery to term (39+6) in women with gestational hypertension, provided good control of blood pressure, reassuring fetal monitoring and no development of pre-eclampsia. For pre-eclampsia, ISSHP recommends delivery at 37 weeks (or earlier if repeated episodes of severe hypertension despite three antihypertensive agents, or development of severe features of pre-eclampsia, as well as non-reassuring fetal status) [4].

25.7.4.1 Timing of Delivery in Pre-eclampsia [12]

Delivery is the only final 'cure' for pre-eclampsia. The decision to deliver or not at any gestational age will be a balance between maternal and fetal well-being.

Pre-eclampsia <34 Weeks

The maternal and fetal condition is assessed from day to day. Especially in severe prematurity, a prolongation of the pregnancy is desired, if possible. The risk of extremely preterm infants must be continually balanced against the maternal risk by prolonging the pregnancy. Available randomized trials and observational studies indicate that expectancy may improve the neonatal outcome in pre-eclampsia before 34 weeks. Conditions that are not consistent with prolonging the pregnancy is: eclampsia, HELLP, or progressive or severe pre-eclampsia with severe clinical or pathophysiological deterioration (e.g. disseminated intravascular coagulation (DIC) development). Lung maturation of the fetus with corticosteroid injections to the mother (gestational week 23/24–34) increases fetal survival. In very early-onset pre-eclampsia (before 28–30 weeks), it is recommended to discuss delivery or expectancy with referral obstetric centres.

Pre-eclampsia 34 to 37 Weeks (late preterm)

A randomized controlled trial from 2015 [39] concluded that immediate delivery gave a non-significant reduction in maternal complications, but an increase in neonatal respiratory distress syndrome outcomes. A recent meta-analysis of individual patient data suggests, however, a maternal benefit also for this late preterm pre-eclampsia group in not prolonging the pregnancy, and that the risk for fetal adverse outcomes was not increased after gestational week 36 as compared to postponing delivery [40]. Whether planned delivery in late preterm uneventful pre-eclampsia is better than expectant management for the total maternal and fetal situation, is being addressed by the PHOENIX trial in a UK setting [41].

Pre-eclampsia ≥37 Weeks

According to a randomized trial from 2009 where women were either induced or treated with expectancy in gestational hypertension or mild pre-eclampsia, the induction group had better maternal outcomes without increased rates of caesarean sections. The study found no differences between the groups in neonatal outcome [42]. Many guidelines, therefore, suggest induction of labour from 37 weeks in order to prevent severe complications of pre-eclampsia.

Objective Signs of Severe Pre-eclampsia Features That Indicate Need for Delivery

Mother -- These are all signs indicating the need for delivery: high blood pressure (where it is difficult to control), eclampsia, thrombocytopenia (especially if rapid and sustained decreasing platelet number), severe/increasing liver involvement, pulmonary oedema, and creatinine elevation.

Fetus -- These are the signs indicating the need for delivery: pathological CTG, including pathological short-term variability (computer-assessed), oligohydramnios/severe fetal growth restriction/alarming Doppler findings (absent or reversed flow in umbilical artery, centralization in the middle cerebral artery and increased PI in ductus venosus).

25.7.5 Delivery Mode and Management in HDP [12]

Caesarean section versus vaginal delivery should be considered individually; many factors are to be taken into account (gestational age, maturity of the cervix, parity, severity of pre-eclampsia, fetal condition and the availability of obstetric and anaesthesiology resources). In pre-eclampsia without severe features, induction of labour is to be considered as first choice, unless contraindicated for other reasons.

If IV fluid is needed, pulmonary oedema may develop following much lower volume load than for other patient groups, and monitoring of the circulation must be considered.

Women with severe pre-eclampsia/HELLP with coagulation disorders should not receive thrombosis prophylaxis with low molecular weight heparin (LMWH) before the coagulopathy has improved and there is no clinical bleeding problem. In case of severe coagulopathy, consultation with a haematologist is recommended.

Spinal anaesthesia is first choice at caesarean section (CS) in women with rapidly increasing severity of pre-eclampsia and HELLP development (as long as the platelet count is not too low). Spinal anaesthesia confers less tissue trauma than epidural anaesthesia. If an epidural catheter is in place before the woman is diagnosed with reduced platelet count (as in HELLP), the catheter can be used also for epidural analgesia at CS. In women with increased risks during general anaesthesia (hypertension, obesity, difficult airway intubation), these risks must be weighed against the spinal anaesthesia risks (spinal haematoma) in women with HELLP and rapidly falling thrombocytes.

Before starting anaesthesia in women with severe pre-eclampsia, opioids should be administered (alfentanil, remifentanil, fentanyl) before intubation to avoid a potentially dangerous increase in blood pressure. A dedicated neonatal team should be present during CS and should be informed of opioids given to the mother which will have depressive effects on the newborn respiration.

25.7.6 Seizure Prophylaxis in Pre-eclampsia with Severe Features

In cases of rapidly developing pre-eclampsia with severe features, $MgSO_4$ seizure prophylaxis should be administered. The ISSHP 2018 recommendation suggests that women with severe hypertension and proteinuria should receive prophylaxis, as well as women with hypertension and neurological signs or symptoms [4], which is in line with clinical practice in Europe. It halves the risk of eclampsia and reduces the risk of maternal death (Magpie Trial) [43]. Clinical evaluation includes considering the severity and how quickly the condition worsens (threatening eclampsia). The initial dose is the same as eclampsia (see below) but the maintenance dose is halved (see eclampsia treatment). It is essential to monitor a woman treated with $MgSO_4$. The ISSHP recommends continuing with $MgSO_4$ infusion for seizures prophylaxis for 24 hours postpartum [4], although the evidence for its benefit is not conclusive .

25.7.7 Treatment of Eclampsia [12, 43]

- Free airways. Make sure the patient does not fall out of bed.
- Call for help (e.g. nurse/midwife, obstetrician, anaesthesiology personnel).
- Magnesium sulphate ($MgSO_4$) is the primary treatment of seizures in eclampsia. Some women will experience flushing symptoms due to vasodilation following $MgSO_4$ administration.

Diazepam 10–20 mg (IV or rectally) has not as good seizure control effect as $MgSO_4$ and will also affect the baby after delivery, but may be administered first, if $MgSO_4$ is not available. Start $MgSO_4$ as soon as it is available.

Magnesium sulphate loading dose (17.5 to 20 mmol) slowly IV (5–15 minutes).

Magnesium sulphate maintenance dose over 24 hours (4.6 mmol/h; maximum daily dose: 150 mmol).

If recurrent eclamptic episodes continues during $MgSO_4$ infusion (or after the infusion is discontinued), the loading dose of IV $MgSO_4$ (see above) is repeated (17.5 to 20 mmol, depending on body weight) over 5 minutes, and an hourly maintenance dose for the next 24 hours is given.

25.7.7.1 Control of MgSO₄ Therapy

Toxic side effects of $MgSO_4$ can be seen clinically as abolished patellar reflex, respiratory depression and decreased urinary output.

- The first 2 hours of $MgSO_4$ therapy: check patellar reflex and respiration every 10 minutes, later in 15- to 60-minute intervals.
- Measure hourly urinary output.
- If patellar reflexes are abolished: discontinue magnesium infusion. Observe the respiration rate. When the patellar reflex returns, restart the infusing with a reduced dose, if the respiration rate is normal.
- If respiration rate is <16 minute: discontinue the infusion. Give O_2 on mask. Secure free airways. If pronounced respiratory depression: administer antidote (see below).
- If respiratory arrest: intubate and ventilate immediately and administer antidote (see below).
- If decreased urinary output (<25 mL/h), when it is assumed secondary to magnesium effect, without other symptoms of

magnesium intoxication: reduce infusion rate to 0.5 g/h (2 mmol/h).

- Check serum levels of magnesium when needed. Therapeutic level is 2–4 mmol/L.
- Treatment with magnesium sulphate should be continued for 24 hours after eclamptic seizures either ante- or intrapartum as well as after postpartum eclamptic seizures.

Antidote to $MgSO_4$ therapy is calcium glubionate 10 mL. Calcium-Sandoz® (9 mg calcium glubionate/mL) is to be in the room and to be given slowly intravenously if needed.

Further follow-up of eclampsia includes the following:

- Manage blood pressure if necessary (see above).
- If the patient is not delivered prior to an eclamptic seizure and there is a fetal delivery indication, evaluate whether the stabilization/treatment of the mother can be combined with delivery. If this is not possible, the mother must have priority. A caesarean section is often necessary if vaginal delivery is not imminent.
- Intensive monitoring after an eclamptic seizure is necessary. Adequate laboratory services for follow-up/treatment of multi-organ affect is important. If such services are unavailable, the patient should after stabilization be transferred to a tertiary centre where such facilities exist.

25.7.8 Postpartum Follow-Up of Eclampsia and Pre-eclampsia When in Hospital [12]

It is recommended that the patient is evaluated neurologically after eclampsia, in order to exclude differential diagnoses. Avoid using nonsteroidal anti-inflammatory drugs (NSAIDs) as postpartum pain regimen as long as the woman has a poorly regulated hypertension, or oliguria, signs of poor kidney function or thrombocytopenia.

Debriefing of the clinical events with the involved doctors and midwives postpartum is recommended. If the woman has hypertension at the time of hospital discharge, then appointment for BP control is made either at the maternity ward or in the community health service/with another doctor.

25.7.9 Postpartum Control after HDP [12]

In most pre-eclamptic women, blood pressure normalizes within days to weeks after a delivery. Previously healthy women who have had pre-eclampsia and who still have elevated blood pressure when discharged from the maternity ward should receive regular follow-up by the health services until their blood pressure has normalized, alternatively checked for secondary hypertension if there is unresolved hypertension over many weeks. Women who continue to have proteinuria after delivery should be checked for renal disease. Women with pre-pregnancy cardiovascular or renal disease are recommended to continue attending check-ups whether the pregnancy was complicated by pre-eclampsia or not.

Consultation at the obstetric outpatient unit is recommended after 2–3 months following premature pre-eclampsia, eclampsia and HELLP, including a new review of the pregnancy, information and planning of next pregnancies. Further maternal follow-up and assessments should be considered in order to reduce long-term morbidity (see Section 25.9).

25.8 Pre-eclampsia Prediction and Prophylaxis

25.8.1 Pre-eclampsia Prediction

Early-onset pre-eclampsia is affected with placental dysfunction early in pregnancy (Stage 1), prior to development of the clinical stage (Stage 2), as shown in the revised two-stage model of pre-eclampsia (see Figure 25.1). Hence, women with early-onset disease often have a dysregulated circulating antiangiogenic biomarker pattern early in pregnancy (e.g. low PlGF and/or high sFlt1 and/or high sFlt1/PlGF ratio). This explains why early-onset clinical pre-eclamptic disease is easier to predict by dysregulated placenta-derived biomarkers at early stages of pregnancy than late-onset pre-eclampsia, as these proteins are biomarkers of placental dysfunction, not of pre-eclampsia per se [21]. A strategy of combining maternal risk factors, ultrasound findings at first trimester (uterine artery Doppler), maternal BP (mean arterial pressure) and PlGF concentration has been shown to be superior in pre-eclampsia prediction [44] compared to only using clinical maternal risk factors (as depicted in Table 25.1). The International Federation of Gynecology and Obstetrics (FIGO) has therefore recommended this model in 2019, but supports an abbreviated form in low-resource settings due to the costs of and restricted access to ultrasound and PlGF analyses. However, as the 2018 ISSHP guidelines summarize, 'no first or second trimester test or set of tests can reliably predict the development of all cases of preeclampsia; however, a combination of maternal risk factors, BP, PlGF, and uterine artery Doppler can select women who may benefit in particular from 150 mg/d of aspirin to prevent preterm but not term preeclampsia. ISSHP supports first trimester screening for preeclampsia when this can be integrated into the local health system although the cost-effectiveness of this approach remains to be established' [4].

25.8.2 Pre-eclampsia Prevention in a Next Pregnancy Following Pre-eclampsia

In the next pregnancy, women with previously early-onset pre-eclampsia, eclampsia or HELLP syndrome are at increased risk for pre-eclampsia again (10–40%, highest risk for the early-onset disease). Low-dose aspirin prophylaxis is recommended (see below). In subsequent pregnancies, these women should be followed up in collaboration with the obstetric department. Doppler examination of the uterine artery is recommended for groups with increased risks for pre-eclampsia and growth-restricted fetuses.

Before any pregnancy, it is recommended that risk factors for HDP are reduced to a minimum, including avoiding obesity and optimizing treatment of any chronic disease (e.g.

hypertension), as well as adhering to a healthy lifestyle (e.g. physical activity). The ISSHP recommends that pregnant women should exercise at least 3 days per week for an average 50 minutes using a combination of aerobic exercise and strength and flexibility training. This has been associated with less weight gain and reduced incidence of hypertensive disorders in pregnancy; there are no significant adverse effects of exercise in pregnancy [4].

25.8.3 Pre-eclampsia Prophylaxis with Aspirin or Calcium

The ISSHP recommends [4] that women with established strong clinical risk factors for pre-eclampsia are treated in the next pregnancy with low-dose aspirin (defined as 75 to 162 mg/day in RCTs). These risk factors include:

- Prior pre-eclampsia
- Chronic hypertension
- Pregestational diabetes mellitus
- Maternal body mass index >30 kg/m^2
- Antiphospholipid syndrome
- Receiving assisted reproductive techniques

The aspirin dosage recommendation in the UK and Norwegian guidelines were, until 2019, 75 mg daily, until delivery of the baby [12, 30]. This dosage is shown to be safe in regard to placental abruption and haemorrhage risk. The 2017 ASPRE trial [44] demonstrated that women screened at high risk for pre-eclampsia (by first trimester BP, maternal risk factors, uterine artery Doppler and maternal PlGF) benefitted from 150 mg/day of aspirin (taken in the evening from 11–14 weeks until 36 weeks of gestation) by significantly reducing the rate of preterm pre-eclampsia, though no risk reduction was seen in women with chronic hypertension. At present, the optimal low-dose aspirin dosage is debatable, as 150 mg (dosage tested only until week 36 in fear of haemorrhage complications if used to term) has not been tested against 75 mg (dosage proven safe until delivery also at term). In line with this, the 2019 UK (NICE) guidelines recommend from 2019 that pregnant women at high risk for pre-eclampsia (defined as having either one high-risk factor or at least two moderate-risk factors at first trimester, see Table 25.1) are advised to take 75–150 mg of aspirin daily until the birth of the baby [35].

The ISSHP also recommends that women with a low calcium intake (<600 mg/day) and at increased risk for pre-eclampsia, should receive a calcium supplementation (total dose of 1.2 to 2.5 g/day) [4].

25.9 Long-Term Complications after HDP

Women with previous HDP have increased risk for long-term complications, even if the hypertension and proteinuria disappeared after the delivery. The most investigated long-term health problems are cardiovascular, but increased risk of diabetes mellitus, kidney disease, hypothyroidism are also documented [12, 45]. Women with severe features of pre-eclampsia (e.g. posterior reversible encephalopathy syndrome (PRES),

eclampsia) also have an increased risk of transient cognitive disturbance, mental imbalance and depressive reactions. Increased risk of neurodegenerative disorders is also under closer investigation as long-term effects of pre-eclampsia.

25.9.1 Long-Term Maternal Cardiovascular Risk, Follow-Up and Prophylaxis [12, 45]

Women with a history of pre-eclampsia and hypertension in pregnancy have increased risk of future cardiovascular disease (CVD). In general, the risk of future CVD is more strongly associated with early-onset pre-eclampsia (and therefore early delivery) and with severe placental dysfunction (e.g. growth-restricted fetus or intrauterine fetal death).

For the time being, there are no quality-assured guidelines as to how women should be followed up after pre-eclampsia in order to prevent and detect future cardiovascular disease. Annual follow-up with a general practitioner, even in clinically apparently healthy women, starting at 3 months postpartum follow-up, is advocated by several clinicians, especially for women with previous severe pre-eclampsia. Women are recommended to discuss their history of pre-eclampsia at routine check-ups in the healthcare system, for instance at follow-up 6–12 weeks postpartum. A general practitioner can schedule a customized follow-up programme, taking into account the woman's general health and other cardiovascular risk factors, e.g. family history of CVD and diabetes, blood pressure level, smoking habits, level of physical activity, diet, concurrent diseases (e.g. diabetes), body mass index (BMI) and waist/hip ratio, blood lipids, fasting blood sugar or HbA1c (glycosylated haemoglobin).

Based on the evidence that is currently available, a healthy lifestyle is recommended for all women with previous pre-eclampsia in order to prevent cardiovascular disease. This recommendation includes a healthy physical activity and food intake, smoking avoidance and a healthy normal body weight (body mass index 19–25 kg/m^2). For the time being, there is no evidence for efficient preventive drugs for CVD in women with only previous pre-eclampsia as a risk factor, such as statins, acetylsalicylic acids etc.

25.10 Key Messages for Hypertensive Disease of Pregnancy

- Correct clinical handling of hypertensive disorders of pregnancy is vital to maternal and fetal survival and well-being.
- Placental dysfunction with excessive release of stress factors to the maternal systemic vasculature are key events for pre-eclampsia development, and maternal risk factors contribute to the pathophysiology at several levels.
- Antihypertensive therapy is essential for reducing maternal cerebral complications.
- Magnesium sulphate remains the best prevention and therapy for eclampsia.
- Pre-eclampsia prediction improves by measuring circulating placenta-derived PlGF.

- Pre-eclampsia prophylaxis with low-dose aspirin is recommended to women at high risk for pre-eclampsia.
- Women with previous HDP are at increased risk for future long-term disease, in particular cardiovascular disease, and should be offered follow-up.

25.11 Key Guidelines
25.11.1 HDP Guidelines
- UK/NICE (National Institute for Health and Care Excellence) 2019 clinical guideline 33: [46]
- ISSHP (International Society for the Study of Hypertension in Pregnancy): [4]
- Australian guidelines: [10]
- American College of Obstetricians and Gynecologists: [11]

- FIGO 2019 first trimester screening and prevention of pre-eclampsia guide: [2]

25.11.2 Lay-Person Information
- Pre-eclampsia brochure: https://legeforeningen.no/PageFiles/169991/Patient%20Information%20on%20Preeclampsia.PDF
- Book: Cowan J, Redman C, Walker I. *Understanding Pre-Eclampsia: A Guide for Parents and Health Professionals.* Watford: Clearsay Publishing; 2017.
- APEK (UK): https://action-on-pre-eclampsia.org.uk/learning/courses/hypertensive-disorders-of-pregnancy/
- Pre-eclampsia Foundation (USA): www.pre-eclampsia.org/health-information/about-pre-eclampsia

References

1. Mol BW, Roberts CT, Thangaratinam S, et al. Pre-eclampsia. *Lancet.* 2015; **387**: 999–1011.
2. Poon LC, Shennan A, Hyett JA, et al. The International Federation of Gynecology and Obstetrics (FIGO) initiative on pre-eclampsia: A pragmatic guide for first-trimester screening and prevention. *Int J Gynaecol Obstet.* 2019; **145** Suppl 1: 1–33.
3. Duley L. The global impact of pre-eclampsia and eclampsia. *Semin Perinatol.* 2009; **33**: 130–7.
4. Brown MA, Magee LA, Kenny LC, et al. Hypertensive disorders of pregnancy: ISSHP classification, diagnosis, and management recommendations for international practice. *Hypertension.* 2018; **72**: 24–43.
5. Lawn JE, Blencowe H, Pattinson R, et al. Stillbirths: where? when? why? how to make the data count? *Lancet.* 2011; **377**: 1448–63.
6. Sibai BM. Preeclampsia as a cause of preterm and late preterm (near-term) births. *Semin Perinatol.* 2006; **30**: 16–9.
7. Ghulmiyyah L, Sibai B. Maternal mortality from preeclampsia/eclampsia. *Semin Perinatol.* 2012; **36**: 56–9.
8. Nyflot LT, Ellingsen L, Yli BM, Oian P, Vangen S. Maternal deaths from hypertensive disorders: lessons learnt. *Acta Obstet Gynecol Scand.* 2018; **97**: 976–87.
9. van den Akker T, Bloemenkamp KWM, van Roosmalen J, Knight M. Classification of maternal deaths: where does the chain of events start? *Lancet.* 2017; **390**: 922–3.

10. Lowe SA, Bowyer L, Lust K, et al. SOMANZ guidelines for the management of hypertensive disorders of pregnancy 2014. *Aust N Z J Obstet Gynaecol.* 2015; **55**: e1–29.
11. Hypertension in pregnancy. Report of the American College of Obstetricians and Gynecologists' Task Force on Hypertension in Pregnancy. *Obstet Gynecol.* 2013; **122**: 1122–31.
12. Staff AC, Andersgaard AB, Henriksen T, et al. Chapter 28 Hypertensive disorders of pregnancy and eclampsia. *Eur J Obstet Gynecol Reprod Biol.* 2016; **201**: 171–8.
13. Bramham K, Parnell B, Nelson-Piercy C, et al. Chronic hypertension and pregnancy outcomes: systematic review and meta-analysis. *BMJ.* 2014; **348**: g2301.
14. Klungsoyr K, Morken NH, Irgens L, Vollset SE, Skjaerven R. Secular trends in the epidemiology of pre-eclampsia throughout 40 years in Norway: prevalence, risk factors and perinatal survival. *Paediatr Perinat Epidemiol.* 2012; **26**: 190–8.
15. Sibai BM. Diagnosis and management of gestational hypertension and preeclampsia. *Obstet Gynecol.* 2003; **102**: 181–92.
16. Saftlas AF, Olson DR, Franks AL, Atrash HK, Pokras R. Epidemiology of preeclampsia and eclampsia in the United States, 1979–1986. *Am J Gynecol.* 1990; **163**: 460–5.
17. Andersgaard AB, Herbst A, Johansen M, et al. Eclampsia in Scandinavia: incidence, substandard care, and potentially preventable cases. *Acta Obstet Gynecol Scand.* 2006; **85**: 929–36.

18. Roberts CL, Ford JB, Algert CS, et al. Population-based trends in pregnancy hypertension and pre-eclampsia: an international comparative study. *BMJ Open.* 2011; **1**: e000101.
19. Redman CW. Current topic: pre-eclampsia and the placenta. *Placenta.* 1991; **12**: 301–8.
20. Redman CW, Sargent IL, Staff AC. IFPA Senior Award Lecture: Making sense of pre-eclampsia – Two placental causes of preeclampsia? *Placenta.* 2014; **35** Suppl: S20-S5.
21. Redman CW, Staff AC. Preeclampsia, biomarkers, syncytiotrophoblast stress, and placental capacity. *Am J Obstet Gynecol.* 2015; **213**: S9-4.
22. Staff AC. The two-stage placental model of preeclampsia: an update. *J Reprod Immunol.* 2019; **134–135**:1–10.
23. Staff AC, Redman C. The differences between early- and late-onset preeclampsia. In Saito S, ed. *Preeclampsia.* Singapore: Springer; 2018. pp. 157–72.
24. Moffett A, Hiby SE. How does the maternal immune system contribute to the development of pre-eclampsia? *Placenta.* 2007; **28** Suppl A: S51–S6.
25. Maynard SE, Min JY, Merchan J, et al. Excess placental soluble fms-like tyrosine kinase 1 (sFlt1) may contribute to endothelial dysfunction, hypertension, and proteinuria in preeclampsia. *J Clin Invest.* 2003; **111**: 649–58.
26. Ness RB, Roberts JM. Heterogeneous causes constituting the single syndrome of preeclampsia: a hypothesis and its implications. *Am J Obstet Gynecol.* 1996; **175**: 1365–70.

27. Hammer ES, Cipolla MJ. Cerebrovascular dysfunction in preeclamptic pregnancies. *Curr Hypertens Rep.* 2015; **17**: 64.

28. Thilaganathan B. Pre-eclampsia is primarily a placental disorder: AGAINST: Pre-eclampsia: the heart matters. *BJOG.* 2017; **124**: 1763.

29. Nelson-Percy C. *Handbook of Obstetric Medicine.* London: CRC Press, Taylor and Francis Group; 2015.

30. Visintin C, Mugglestone MA, Almerie MQ, et al. Management of hypertensive disorders during pregnancy: summary of NICE guidance. *BMJ.* 2010; **341**: c2207.

31. Duhig KE, Myers J, Seed PT, et al. Placental growth factor testing to assess women with suspected pre-eclampsia: a multicentre, pragmatic, stepped-wedge cluster-randomised controlled trial. *Lancet.* 2019; **393**: 1807–18.

32. Chappell LC, Duckworth S, Seed PT, et al. Diagnostic accuracy of placental growth factor in women with suspected preeclampsia: a prospective multicenter study. *Circulation.* 2013; **128**: 2121–31.

33. Zeisler H, Llurba E, Chantraine F, et al. Predictive value of the sFlt-1: PlGF ratio in women with suspected preeclampsia. *N Engl J Med.* 2016; **374**: 13–22.

34. Bramham K, Seed PT, Lightstone L et al. Diagnostic and predictive biomarkers for pre-eclampsia in patients with established hypertension and chronic kidney disease. *Kidney Int.* 2016; **89**: 874–85.

35. National Institute for Health and Care Excellence (NICE). *Hypertension in Pregnancy: Diagnosis and Management.* NICE Guideline 133. 2019

36. Abalos E, Duley L, Steyn DW, Gialdini C. Antihypertensive drug therapy for mild to moderate hypertension during pregnancy. *Cochrane Database Syst Rev.* 2018; **10**: Cd002252.

37. Magee LA, von Dadelszen P, Rey E, et al. Less-tight versus tight control of hypertension in pregnancy. *N Engl J Med.* 2015; **372**: 407–17.

38. Easterling T, Mundle S, Bracken H, et al. Oral antihypertensive regimens (nifedipine retard, labetalol, and methyldopa) for management of severe hypertension in pregnancy: an open-label, randomised controlled trial. *Lancet.* 2019; **394**: 1011–21.

39. Broekhuijsen K, van Baaren GJ, van Pampus MG, et al. Immediate delivery versus expectant monitoring for hypertensive disorders of pregnancy between 34 and 37 weeks of gestation (HYPITAT-II): an open-label, randomised controlled trial. *Lancet.* 2015; **385**: 2492–501.

40. Bernardes TP, Zwertbroek EF, Broekhuijsen K, et al. Delivery or expectant management for prevention of adverse maternal and neonatal outcomes in hypertensive disorders of pregnancy: an individual participant data meta-analysis. *Ultrasound Obstet Gynecol.* 2019; **53**: 443–53.

41. Chappell LC, Green M, Marlow N, et al. Planned delivery or expectant management for late preterm pre-eclampsia: study protocol for a randomised controlled trial (PHOENIX trial). *Trials.* 2019; **20**: 85.

42. Koopmans CM, Bijlenga D, Groen H, et al. Induction of labour versus expectant monitoring for gestational hypertension or mild pre-eclampsia after 36 weeks' gestation (HYPITAT): a multicentre, open-label randomised controlled trial. *Lancet.* 2009; **374**: 979–88.

43. Duley L, Gulmezoglu AM, Henderson-Smart DJ, Chou D. Magnesium sulphate and other anticonvulsants for women with pre-eclampsia. *Cochrane Database Syst Rev.* 2010; **2010**(11): CD000025.

44. Rolnik DL, Wright D, Poon LC, et al. Aspirin versus placebo in pregnancies at high risk for preterm preeclampsia. *N Engl J Med.* 2017; **377**: 613–22.

45. Staff AC, Redman CW, Williams D, et al. Pregnancy and long-term maternal cardiovascular health: progress through harmonization of research cohorts and biobanks. *Hypertension.* 2016; **67**: 251–60.

46. NICE. *Hypertension in Pregnancy Overview.* NICE Pathways. 2017.

47. Egeland GM, Klungsoyr K, Oyen N, et al. Preconception cardiovascular risk factor differences between gestational hypertension and preeclampsia: Cohort Norway Study. *Hypertension.* 2016; **67**: 1173–80.

48. Laine K, Murzakanova G, Sole KB, et al. Prevalence and risk of pre-eclampsia and gestational hypertension in twin pregnancies: a population-based register study. *BMJ Open.* 2019; **9**: e029908.

Obesity and Metabolic Syndrome in Pregnancy

Aoife M. Egan & Fidelma P. Dunne

26.1 Definitions and Prevalence

The term *obesity* refers to an excess of body fat. As direct measurements of total body fat mass are complex, body mass index (BMI) is commonly used in clinical practice as an obesity index. BMI may be defined as a person's weight in kilograms divided by the square of her height in metres (kg/m^2). Table 26.1 outlines the BMI categories frequently used in clinical practice, with a BMI ≥30 mg/m² categorized as obesity [1]. Due to the multiple changes in body mass that take place during pregnancy, pregnant women are typically described based on their pre-pregnancy BMI.

In the USA, data from the National Health and Nutrition Examination Survey reveal an obesity prevalence of 36.5% among women aged 20–39 years, with prevalence even higher among non-Hispanic black and Hispanic women [2]. Worldwide obesity has nearly tripled since 1975; in 2016, 39% of adults aged 18 years and over were overweight and 13% were obese [3]. This dramatic increase in prevalence of obesity would suggest that environmental rather than genetic factors have a greater role in this pandemic. These figures place obesity as the most common healthcare problem in women of reproductive age. Unfortunately, maternal obesity is independently associated with multiple adverse pregnancy outcomes with data suggesting a threshold BMI of 28 kg/m² for when complication rates become significantly elevated [4, 5].

The metabolic syndrome typically refers to the presence of a group of risk factors for cardiovascular disease and type 2 diabetes mellitus. This syndrome has also been referred to as 'syndrome X', 'the deadly quartet', 'insulin-resistance syndrome' and 'the hypertriglyceridemic waist'. Although precise definitions vary, risk factors included in the metabolic syndrome are typically hypertension, dyslipidaemia, raised fasting glucose and central obesity [6]. Table 26.2 outlines commonly used criteria as proposed by a working group representing a number of major organizations in this field [6]. The variation in diagnostic criteria makes it difficult to obtain accurate prevalence data; however, it is estimated that 35.0–38.0% of adult women in the USA have metabolic syndrome [6]. While there is significant overlap between women with obesity and metabolic syndrome; the presence of the latter syndrome undoubtedly confers additional risk in pregnancy beyond that of obesity alone.

26.2 Pathophysiology

Adipose tissue is metabolically active, and excessive amounts can affect a number of biological pathways. In the setting of pregnancy, its effects are likely multifactorial involving insulin resistance, altered glucose and lipid metabolism and increased inflammation [7]. Throughout this chapter, clinical effects of obesity on both the mother and offspring will be discussed with reference to the causal mechanisms.

26.3 Maternal Effects

26.3.1 Before Pregnancy

In obese women, insulin resistance and hyperinsulinaemia along with decreases in sex hormone-binding globulin leads to hyperandrogenaemia. This hyperandrogenaemia leads to

Table 26.1 WHO classification of adults according to BMI [1]

Classification	BMI (kg/m²)	Risk of co-morbidities
Underweight	<18.5	Low (but risk of other clinical problems increased)
Normal Range	18.5–24.99	Average
Overweight:	≥25.00	Increased
Preobese	25.00–29.99	Moderate
Obese Class I	30.00–34.99	Severe
Obese Class II	35.00–39.99	Very severe
Obese Class III	≥40.00	

BMI: body mass index; WHO: World Health Organization

Table 26.2 Criteria for diagnosis of metabolic syndrome [6]

Any 3 of the following 5 criteria
1. Elevated waist circumference using population- and country-specific definitions
2. Fasting glucose ≥5.5 mmol/L (100 mg/dL) or Rx
3. Triglycerides ≥1.7 mmol/L (150 mg/dL) or Rx
4. HDL cholesterol: <1.0 mmol/L (40 mg/dL) (male), <1.3 mmol/L (50 mg/dL) (female) or Rx
5. ≥130 mm Hg systolic or ≥85 mm Hg diastolic or Rx

HDL: high-density lipoprotein; Rx: pharmacological treatment

granulosa cell apoptosis that is deleterious for ovarian function. Obese women also have increased peripheral aromatization of androgens to oestrogens with negative effects on gonadotropin secretion. Leptin is increased, and this also acts as a gonadotropin inhibitor. As a whole, these changes lead to disruptions in menstrual function, impair ovulation and have a negative impact on fertility. As a result, obese women have poorer reproductive outcomes in the setting of both natural and artificial conception. It should be noted that while oligomenorrhoea and hyperandrogenism are classically associated with polycystic ovarian syndrome (PCOS), obese women appear to have reduced fecundity even if diagnostic criteria for PCOS are not reached [8].

26.3.2 During Pregnancy

Obesity increases the risk of early pregnancy loss. To illustrate this point, a systematic review including 28 538 women with spontaneous conceptions found that 16.6% of obese women had ≥1 miscarriage. This compared to 11.8% of overweight women and 10.7% of women with a normal BMI [9]. Multiple studies have confirmed elevated miscarriage rates among obese women undergoing assisted conception compared to normal weight counterparts. It is possible that a poor endometrial environment relating to hormonal changes may be driving early pregnancy loss in obese women.

As outlined in Chapter 18, multi-fetal pregnancies are considered high risk and obese women are more likely to have a twin gestation. Reddy et al evaluated 51 783 pregnancies (561 twin pregnancies) in the Collaborative Perinatal Project [10]. This study included 12 hospitals in the USA between 1959 and 1966 (before the widespread use of fertility drugs). The authors found that there was a significant trend for increased risk of total twinning with increasing BMI. Despite adjusting for a number of factors including maternal race, age, parity and height, the odds of dizygous (but not monozygous) twinning with increasing BMI remained significant. Interestingly, there was also a significant trend for increased twinning with increased maternal height. The authors postulate that the association between dizygotic twinning and maternal weight may be related to elevated follicle-stimulating hormone levels which have been observed in obese mothers (similar to the situation that occurs when gonadotropins are used in the setting of fertility treatments).

Once pregnancy is established, obese mothers have an increased risk of developing a number of medical disorders. Maternal BMI is an independent risk factor for hypertensive disorders of pregnancy. This is exemplified by a 2011 prospective cohort study of 6902 mothers. The study revealed that compared to mothers with a normal weight, maternal obesity is associated with a higher first trimester systolic blood pressure (10.8 mm Hg, 95% confidence interval (CI): 9.44–12.17). Risks of pregnancy-induced hypertension and pre-eclampsia were also significantly increased among obese women [odds ratio of 4.67 (95% CI 3.07–7.09) and 2.49 (95% CI 1.29–4.78) respectively] [11]. Both conditions are strongly associated with a large increase in maternal and fetal morbidity and mortality

and long-term cardiovascular complications in the mother (Chapter 25). Women with metabolic syndrome enter pregnancy with already established hypertension. These women have the added complication of requiring pharmacological intervention throughout the entire pregnancy and are at even greater risk of developing superimposed pre-eclampsia.

Insulin and glucose homeostasis are key elements underlying the pathogenesis of a number of pregnancy complications for obese women. Insulin resistance increases sharply in the second and early third trimesters of pregnancy. Ideally, insulin production is sufficient to meet this challenge but if this response is inadequate gestational diabetes mellitus (GDM) develops. Obesity causes insulin resistance independent of pregnancy, and therefore in the obese gravida there is an exaggerated response with marked maternal hyperinsulinaemia and hyperglycaemia, which may or may not reach the cutoff for GDM [7]. Although accurate estimates for prevalence of GDM among obese women are lacking, one European study that assessed women with a BMI ≥29.0 kg/m^2 in early, mid- and late gestation, identified GDM in 39% [12].

In 1952 Jorgen Pedersen formulated the hyperglycaemia-hyperinsulinaemia hypothesis [13]. He described a process by which maternal hyperglycaemia leads to fetal hyperglycaemia with subsequent hypertrophy of fetal islet tissue and an increase in fetal utilization of glucose (Figure 26.1).

This results in a multitude of effects including fetal macrosomia, neonatal hypoglycaemia and poor long-term metabolic profiles. This hypothesis was largely based on observations in women with type 1 diabetes who had frank hyperglycaemia. However, subsequent work has demonstrated an increased risk of adverse outcomes with various degrees of glucose intolerance less severe than that in overt diabetes mellitus. The Hyperglycemia and Adverse Outcomes Study (HAPO) included 25 505 pregnant women at 15 centres in 9 countries and found strong, continuous associations of maternal glucose levels below those diagnostic of diabetes with increased birthweight and increased cord blood serum C-peptide levels [14]. Further evaluation of these participants revealed that relative to women without GDM and non-obese women, the odds ratio for birthweight >90th percentile for GDM alone was 2.19 (95% CI 1.93–2.47), for obesity alone it was 1.73 (1.50–2.00), and for both GDM and obesity it was 3.62 (3.0–4.32). Similar findings were observed for primary caesarean delivery and pre-eclampsia. These data suggest that while both maternal GDM and obesity are independently associated with adverse pregnancy outcomes, their combination has a greater impact than either one alone [15]. Long term, the development of GDM during pregnancy confers a substantially increased risk of type 2 diabetes and its associated complications in the mother. Of course, women with obesity and metabolic syndrome are at higher risk of established type 2 diabetes prior to pregnancy. Pregestational diabetes is associated with an even higher morbidity than GDM. This includes an elevated risk of congenital anomalies due to abnormal prevailing glucose levels throughout conception and the first trimester of pregnancy (Chapter 27).

It is likely that in the setting of obesity, nutritional factors other than glucose play a role in disordered fetal

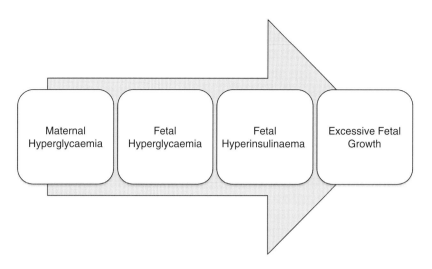

Figure 26.1 Impact of maternal hyperglycaemia (modified Pedersen Hypothesis) [13]

growth patterns. Accumulating evidence suggests that insulin resistance affects more than just glucose metabolism and is associated with increased free fatty acids and triglycerides particularly in the obese individual [16]. While the role of lipids in the regulation of fetal growth has not been examined as closely as glucose, several clinical studies have suggested that they make a significant contribution both in healthy and obese pregnancies. In this regard, it is considered normal for plasma triglyceride concentrations to increase up to fourfold in late gestation [17]. While this is well tolerated when baseline triglyceride levels are within normal range, severe hypertriglyceridaemia in pregnancy can result in pancreatitis and hyperviscosity syndrome, which can be life threatening [18]. This is of concern to women with metabolic syndrome as hypertriglyceridaemia is a defining factor.

Pregnancy itself is a risk factor for the development of venous thromboembolism (VTE), which may occur at any time during pregnancy but most cases occur in the first 6 weeks postpartum (Chapter 30). In the USA, a large nationwide inpatient sample revealed a 14% increase risk of overall VTE-associated pregnancy hospitalizations. Interestingly, between 1994–1997 and 2006–2009, the prevalence of hypertension and obesity doubled among all VTE-associated pregnancy hospitalizations. Although this study was not designed to assess causation, the findings are consistent with previous research identifying components of the metabolic syndrome as increasing the risk for pregnancy-associated VTE [19]. Additional medical complications that are more common in pregnancy and may be exacerbated by obesity include obstructive sleep apnoea, carpel tunnel syndrome and musculoskeletal pain.

At the time of delivery, obesity is again a concern. Due to increased rates of obstetric complications, obese women are more likely to have an induction of labour. Once induced, obese women are twice as likely to experience a failed induction of labour compared to their normal-weight counterparts. This was demonstrated in a population-based cohort study that found the rate of induction to be 28% in normal-weight women and a linear rise to 34% in class III obese women (BMI

≥40 kg/m^2). Failure rates ranged from 13% in normal-weight women to 29% in class III obese women [20].

Increasing pregravid BMI independently increases the risk for both elective and emergency caesarean delivery. In one prospective study, with each unit increase in pre-pregnancy or 27- to 31-week BMI, the odds of caesarean delivery increased by 7.0% and 7.8%, respectively [21]. Maternal obesity also reduces the chance of vaginal birth after caesarean delivery (VBAC), and BMI is a factor used in the various clinical calculators used to predict a successful VBAC and assist with delivery planning.

Finally, anaesthesia management is more complex in the setting of obesity. While the use of spinal or epidural anaesthesia is generally favoured to manage pain during delivery, these procedures are technically challenging due to obscured landmarks. Failed local analgesia will increase the need for general anaesthesia, particularly when an emergency caesarean delivery is necessary. This poses a significant risk due to difficult endotracheal intubation and postoperative atelectasis [22].

26.3.3 After Pregnancy

Postpartum haemorrhage, genital tract infection, urinary tract infection and wound infections are all more common in obese women. A study of over 287 213 pregnancies in the UK reported that the risk of these complications increases with the degree of obesity and persists after adjusting for other confounding demographic factors [23]. The increased rates of wound infection in this population have led providers to question the well-established practice of a transverse caesarean incision. While this procedure leads to a more visually appealing scar, a large panniculus overlying the wound can lead to poor healing with the need for additional intervention such as antibiotics or drain insertion. Although additional trial evidence is necessary, in the setting of significant abdominal obesity a vertical skin incision may confer some advantage [7].

26.3.4 Infant Outcomes

In 2009, Stothard et al completed a systematic review and meta-analysis of observational studies (number of studies included: 39 and 18, respectively) to assess and quantify the relationship between maternal overweight and obesity and the risk of congenital anomaly in the offspring. Although the absolute increase is likely to be small, maternal obesity was found to be associated with an increased risk of a range of structural abnormalities. These included: neural tube defects (OR 1.87; 95% CI 1.62–2.15), spina bifida (OR 2.24; 95% CI 1.86–2.69), cardiovascular anomalies (OR 1.30; 95% CI 1.12–1.51), septal anomalies (OR 1.20; 95% CI 1.09–1.31), cleft palate (OR 1.23; 95% CI 1.03–1.47), cleft lip and palate (OR 1.20; 95% CI 1.03–1.40), anorectal atresia (OR 1.48; 95% CI 1.12–1.97), hydrocephaly (OR,1.68; 95% CI 1.19–2.36) and limb reduction anomalies (OR 1.34; 95% CI 1.03–1.73) [24]. A number of explanatory mechanisms are proposed. As previously described, metabolic abnormalities including insulin resistance and hyperglycaemia can lead to abnormal fetal growth and development. A number of women included in these studies may have had undiagnosed or suboptimally treated diabetes in the first trimester of pregnancy when organogenesis takes place. Nutritional deficiencies, including folic acid and vitamin D deficiency, are more prevalent in the setting of obesity and this may be an underlying mechanism, particularly in the case of neural tube defects. Finally, as ultrasound scanning is technically more challenging in obese women, it is possible that early diagnosis and subsequent termination for fetal anomalies are less likely to occur. Of interest is the fact that this study found a negative association between obesity and gastroschisis – a condition known to be associated with low maternal age. The authors suggest that this may be explained by the fact that BMI increases with maternal age [24].

As described earlier in this chapter, maternal obesity is associated with fetal overgrowth leading to macrosomia (variably defined as a birthweight >4.0 or 4.5 kg) and large for gestational age (variably defined as a birthweight >90th – 97th centile). These infants are more likely to experience shoulder dystocia with or without brachial plexus injury and resultant Erb's palsy. Such complications can result in the need for significant medical intervention and long-term disability. These risks are heightened in the setting of concurrent maternal hyperglycaemia.

Of significant concern is a 2014 systemic review and meta-analysis revealing an association between even modest increases in maternal BMI and increased risk of fetal death, stillbirth and neonatal, perinatal and infant death. The authors included 38 studies with approximately 10 147 fetal deaths, 16 274 stillbirths, 4311 perinatal deaths, 11 294 neonatal deaths and 4983 infant deaths. The summary relative risk per 5-unit increase in maternal BMI for fetal death was 1.21 (95% CI 1.09–1.35; $I^2 = 77.6\%$; n = 7 studies); for stillbirth, 1.24 (95% CI 1.18–1.30; $I^2 = 80\%$; n = 18 studies); for perinatal death, 1.16 (95% CI 1.00–1.35; $I^2 = 93.7\%$; n = 11 studies); for neonatal death, 1.15 (95% CI 1.07–1.23; $I^2 = 78.5\%$; n = 12 studies); and for infant death, 1.18 (95% CI 1.09–1.28; $I^2 = 79\%$; n = 4 studies). A number of potential explanatory mechanisms were suggested by the authors including overt abnormalities such as gestational diabetes and pre-eclampsia. However, more subtle disturbances including increased inflammatory responses, vascular and

endothelial dysfunction and altered lipid metabolism may play a role. For example, hyperlipidaemia (present in obesity and metabolic syndrome) may reduce prostacyclin secretion and increase thromboxane production, and this can lead to a heightened risk of placental thrombosis with subsequent infarct and abruption [25]. On a more practical level, obese women may not notice reduced fetal movements as easily and so may be less likely to seek advice and intervention in a timely manner in the setting of fetal distress.

The adverse consequences of maternal obesity extend into adulthood for the offspring. It now appears that a plethora of neurodevelopmental and psychiatric disorders are associated with prenatal exposure to maternal obesity. These include, but are not limited to, the following: cognitive impairment, autism spectrum disorders, attention deficit hyperactivity disorder, anxiety, depression, schizophrenia and eating disorders [26]. While further studies are necessary, leading mechanisms include oxidative stress and inflammation-induced malprogramming; dysregulation of insulin, glucose and leptin signalling in the developing brain; and dysregulation of dopaminergic and serotonergic signalling with impaired reward circuitry. A longitudinal study of the northern Finland birth cohort for 1966 evaluated the associations between BMI and multiple factors including maternal BMI. The authors concluded that the heavier the mother is, the heavier the offspring will be from birth to 31 years of age [27]. Of course, the indirect environmental influence of nutritional status within the home is likely another significant contributor to these long-term effects.

26.4 Management

26.4.1 Before Pregnancy

Obese women with and without metabolic syndrome should receive appropriate counselling before pregnancy regarding the associated risks. Ideally, weight loss and optimization of comorbidities would take place prior to attempting pregnancy. Women should be reassured that most complications rise linearly with increasing weight; therefore, modest reductions in BMI can have positive clinical benefits.

Women should be provided access to specialist weight management programmes in a multidisciplinary setting to support weight loss pre-conceptually. Healthcare providers should appreciate that a 'one size fits all' approach is likely to fail, and each individual should be supported to identify personal barriers to weight loss and develop a weight loss programme that works best for their needs. There is no evidence that one approach should be favoured over another, and programmes may incorporate motivational interviewing, diet plans and exercise interventions. A number of weight loss medications are now available and are associated with modest weight reductions. Unfortunately, none of these compounds are suitable for use in pregnancy and reliable contraception should be used when they are prescribed in the pre-pregnancy setting [28]. Bariatric surgery, which includes banding, sleeve gastrectomy and gastric bypass procedures, results in a more significant weight loss as well as an improvement in obesity-related complications. It would appear that rates of outcomes such as gestational diabetes, pre-eclampsia, prematurity and extremes of birthweight are lower in women who become pregnant after having had bariatric surgery compared with pregnant women who are obese [29]. Nutritional deficiencies are frequent post-surgery, particularly following the malabsorptive bypass procedures, and pregnancy should be avoided until weight loss and serum nutrient levels have stabilized [30].

A full medication review should take place pre-conceptually and potentially teratogenic medications such as angiotensin-converting enzyme (ACE) inhibitors and statins should be discontinued. Satisfactory blood pressure control (<130/80 mm Hg) may be achieved with medications that are commonly used in pregnancy such as calcium channel blockers, beta-blockers and methyldopa. Dietary fat restriction is typically adequate to manage hypertriglyceridaemia; however, in more severe cases, nutritional fat supplements (medium chain triglycerides or omega-3-acid ethyl esters) or fibrates have been utilized with varying effects in pregnant women [18]. Ideally these would be prescribed under specialist supervision with a detailed discussion on risks and benefits of the treatment. This is particularly true with regard to use of fibrates in the first trimester of pregnancy where little clinical experience exists. For those women with abnormal glucose tolerance, metformin provides a good option to decrease hepatic glucose production and complement lifestyle interventions in optimizing glucose levels pre-pregnancy [31]. In all women, daily folic acid supplementation is recommended for at least one month before conception, and this should be continued through the first trimester of pregnancy. While the ideal dose of folic acid for obese women has been debated, a number of organizations including the Centre for Maternal and Child Enquiries and Royal College of Obstetricians and Gynaecologists in the UK recommend that all women with a BMI ≥30 kg/m² take 5 mg folic acid daily during this crucial time. In addition, they recommend that these same women take 10 micrograms of vitamin D supplementation daily during pregnancy and while breastfeeding [22].

26.4.2 During Pregnancy

26.4.2.1 General Advice

As described above, pre-conception counselling and management is ideal; however, women who present for the first time while pregnant should be given early opportunity to discuss risks and management strategies with an informed healthcare professional [22]. Medications and supplements should be reviewed to ensure they are suitable for pregnancy.

26.4.2.2 Measuring Weight

All women should have their height and weight measured at the initial antenatal visit and monitored throughout their pregnancy. Self-reported measures are not accurate. Collection of these simple measures will facilitate directed management as the pregnancy progresses.

The Institute of Medicine (IOM) guidelines for gestational weight gain (GWG) are summarized in Table 26.3 and a total weight gain of 5.0–9.1 kg (11–20 lb) is advised for obese women [32]. Remaining within these guidelines is challenging. One study of women with diabetes in pregnancy noted that there was excessive GWG in 59% and this was associated with higher odds for a large-for-gestational-age (LGA) infant (adjusted OR 2.01 (95% CI 1.24–3.25) in GDM; aOR 3.97 (95% CI 1.85–8.53) in pregestational diabetes). Among women with GDM specifically, excessive GWG was associated with an increased odds for gestational hypertension (aOR 1.72 (95% CI 1.04–2.85)) and treatment with insulin further increased the odds for LGA (aOR 2.80 (95% CI 1.23–6.38)) [33]. Clinical trials to limit GWG and improve pregnancy outcomes have been largely underwhelming. A meta-analysis of the effects of interventions in pregnancy on maternal weight and obstetric outcomes noted that dietary intervention resulted in the largest reduction in maternal GWG (3.84 kg, 2.45–5.22 kg) with improved pregnancy outcomes compared to other interventions. However, the rating of evidence for key outcomes such as pre-eclampsia and GDM was low [34]. Multiple studies have examined lifestyle approaches for GDM prevention with a large proportion focusing efforts on high-risk, obese women. Unfortunately, despite some individual trials revealing benefit; many more have not had positive outcomes, despite a significant reduction in GWG [35].

With weight loss or restricted weight gain during pregnancy, the risk of a small-for-gestational-age infant contrasts with potential benefits such as a decrease in the rate of operative delivery and fetal macrosomia [31]. Currently, based on observational data suggesting an increased risk of small for gestational age, inadequate GWG is not encouraged. High-quality randomized controlled trials are also needed in this area.

Table 26.3 IOM guidelines for gestational weight gain [32]

Pregestational BMI category	BMI (kg/m²)	Recommended total weight gain (kg)	Recommended mean weight gain: trimesters 2 & 3 (kg/week)
Underweight	<18.5	12.5–18.0	0.51 (0.44–0.58)
Normal weight	18.5–24.9	11.5–16.0	0.42 (0.35–0.50)
Overweight	25.0–29.9	7.0–11.5	0.28 (0.23–0.33)
Obese	≥30.0	5.0–9.0	0.22 (0.17–0.27)

BMI: body mass index

26.4.2.3 Metabolic Disorders of Pregnancy

At risk women with obesity and metabolic syndrome should be screened for glucose intolerance and obstructive sleep apnoea at the first obstetric visit with history, physical examination and laboratory and clinical studies as needed [31]. Prompt treatment of obstructive sleep apnoea is required to reduce the risk of associated adverse outcomes including hypertensive pregnancy disorders and thromboembolism. Screening and care for women with diabetes in pregnancy are outlined in Chapter 27.

Blood pressure measurements should occur at each clinical encounter. An appropriate and consistent size of arm cuff is necessary to ensure reliable results. The Pre-eclampsia Community Guidelines (PRECOG) recommend that women with a booking BMI ≥35 kg/m^2 and any additional risk factor for pre-eclampsia (including first pregnancy, ≥10 years since last baby, family history of pre-eclampsia, underlying medical conditions such as hypertension or diabetes) should have early referral for early specialist care [36]. This encompasses all women with confirmed metabolic syndrome. Hypertensive disorders in pregnancy and eclampsia are discussed further in Chapter 25.

As previously described, it is anticipated that triglycerides will rise throughout pregnancy. Women with metabolic syndrome should be monitored throughout pregnancy, and if fasting triglyceride levels exceed 4 mmol/L pre-pregnancy or in early pregnancy, monthly assessment should occur. If the triglyceride levels rise to greater than 10 mmol/L despite a low-fat diet, specialist review will be necessary to escalate therapy. Options for therapy include nutritional supplements, fibrates, niacin-based preparations, heparin, insulin and therapeutic plasma exchange [18].

26.4.2.4 Fetal Monitoring

While obese women have an increased risk of fetal structural anomalies, detection using ultrasound is reduced as BMI increases. In addition, cell-free DNA screens, which have become increasingly popular in recent years, have an increased risk for inconclusive results among obese women [31]. Women should therefore be advised regarding the limitations of these common approaches to antenatal diagnosis of congenital anomalies. Fetal MRI is an option in certain situations but cost and availability limit its utility for routine practice.

There is no evidence that increased antepartum surveillance can reduce the elevated risks of early fetal loss and stillbirth in obese women [31].

26.4.2.5 Delivery Planning

Pregnant women with a BMI ≥40 kg/m^2 should have antenatal consultation with anaesthesiology to formulate a plan for labour and delivery. Epidural re-site rates have been reported to increase with increasing BMI and, combined with the elevated risk of caesarean delivery, an early epidural may be recommended [22]. Women considering a trial of labour after caesarean (TOLAC) should be informed that obesity reduces their risk of a successful VBAC. Home birth is not recommended due to the high risk of operative delivery and other complications.

26.4.3 Labour and Delivery

Obesity alone is not an indication for induction of labour, and although rates of abdominal delivery are increased, women should prepare for a normal vaginal delivery [31]. It is recommended that the anaesthetic team is aware of all obese patients in labour so abdominal delivery can be anticipated with availability of appropriate transfer equipment and senior personnel as necessary [22]. Venous access should be established early in labour.

There is considerable debate with regard to optimal antibiotic dosing in the setting of obesity. While broad-spectrum antimicrobial prophylaxis is recommended for all caesarean deliveries, there is no high-quality evidence addressing the question of weight-based dosage and so conclusive recommendations are not in place [31]. Finally, due to an increased risk of postpartum haemorrhage, obese women should have a managed third stage of labour [22].

26.4.4 Postpartum

26.4.4.1 Thromboprophylaxis

While thromboembolism in pregnancy is discussed in Chapter 30, it is important to note that in high-risk groups such as obese women with and without metabolic syndrome, thromboprophylaxis with low molecular weight heparin is commonly used in addition to pneumatic compression devices postpartum [31]. While enoxaparin 40 mg once daily is a commonly used dose, further studies are required to determine whether a weight-based dosing regimen would be superior. Early mobilization should be encouraged.

26.4.4.2 Infection

Surgical sites should be well maintained with early intervention if there are signs of infection. This may take the form of antibiotics, wound exploration and debridement. Options for managing the subsequent open wound include secondary closure or secondary intention using dressings or negative pressure wound therapy [31]. Postpartum glucose levels should be optimized to reduce infection risk and promote healing.

26.4.4.3 Breastfeeding

Obese mothers are less likely to breastfeed and less likely to seek support for breastfeeding in the first three months [37]. These women may benefit from extra education and support to ensure a successful lactation journey. In addition to the general benefits associated with breastfeeding, women with gestational diabetes who breastfeed experience significantly lower rates of abnormal glucose tolerance at the time of postpartum assessment (8.2 vs 18.4%) [38].

26.4.4.4 Weight Management

In a large cohort study of over 10 000 obese women; mild-to-moderate inter-pregnancy weight loss reduced the risk of subsequent large-for-gestational-age infants without increasing the risk of small-for-gestational-age infants [39]. The inter-pregnancy time period is therefore important for targeting weight loss. A Cochrane review evaluated the effect of diet, exercise or both for weight reduction in women after childbirth and included six trials involving 245 women in their analysis. They concluded that dieting and exercise together appear to be more effective than diet alone because the former improves cardiorespiratory fitness and preserves fat-free mass [40]. Ongoing investigation will clarify the effect of medications including glucagon-like-peptide (GLP-1) agonists on postpartum weight retention and development of type 2 diabetes in women with GDM.

26.5 Conclusions

A significant body of evidence links obesity and metabolic syndrome to multiple pregnancy complications. At risk women will ideally receive pre-pregnancy support and intervention to optimize their clinical status before embarking on pregnancy. Once pregnant, these women require management by a multidisciplinary team of specialists. Special attention should be given to gestational weight gain; nutritional supplementation; monitoring and treating metabolic complications; and delivery planning. Postpartum care includes provision of a diet and exercise programme with the aim of reducing inter-pregnancy weight gain.

References

1. World Health Organization. Obesity: preventing and managing the global epidemic. Report of a WHO consultation. 2000. www.who.int/nutrition/publications/obesity/WHO_TRS_894/en/Accessed

2. Hales CM, Carroll MD, Fryar CD, Ogden CL. Prevalence of obesity among adults and youth: United States, 2015–2016. *NCHS Data Brief.* 2017 (288):1–8.

3. Organization WH. Fact Sheet: Obesity and Overweight. www.who.int/newsroom/fact-sheets/detail/obesity-and-overweight. April 2020.

4. Dennedy MC, Avalos G, O'Reilly MW, et al. ATLANTIC-DIP: raised maternal body mass index (BMI) adversely affects maternal and fetal outcomes in glucose-tolerant women according to International Association of Diabetes and Pregnancy Study Groups (IADPSG) criteria. *J Clin Endocrinol Metab.* 2012;**97** (4):E608–12.

5. Owens LA, O'Sullivan EP, Kirwan B, et al. ATLANTIC DIP: the impact of obesity on pregnancy outcome in glucose-tolerant women. *Diabetes Care.* 2010;**33**(3):577–9.

6. Alberti KG, Eckel RH, Grundy SM, et al. Harmonizing the metabolic syndrome: a joint interim statement of the International Diabetes Federation Task Force on Epidemiology and Prevention; National Heart, Lung, and Blood Institute; American Heart Association; World Heart Federation; International Atherosclerosis Society; and International Association for the Study of Obesity. *Circulation.* 2009;**120** (16):1640–5.

7. Egan AM, Dennedy MC. Obesity and gestational outcomes. In Watson, RR, ed. *Handbook of Fertility: Nutrition, Diet, Lifestyle and Reproductive Health.* Elsevier; 2015.

8. Dağ Z, Dilbaz B. Impact of obesity on infertility in women. *J Turk Ger Gynecol Assoc.* 2015;**16**(2):111–17.

9. Boots C, Stephenson MD. Does obesity increase the risk of miscarriage in spontaneous conception: a systematic review. *Semin Reprod Med.* 2011;**29** (6):507–13.

10. Reddy UM, Branum AM, Klebanoff MA. Relationship of maternal body mass index and height to twinning. *Obstet Gynecol.* 2005;**105** (3):593–7.

11. Gaillard R, Steegers EA, Hofman A, Jaddoe VW. Associations of maternal obesity with blood pressure and the risks of gestational hypertensive disorders. The Generation R Study. *J Hypertens.* 2011;**29**(5):937–44.

12. Egan AM, Vellinga A, Harreiter J, et al. Epidemiology of gestational diabetes mellitus according to IADPSG/WHO 2013 criteria among obese pregnant women in Europe. *Diabetologia.* 2017;**60**(10):1913–21.

13. Pedersen J. *Diabetes and Pregnancy: Bloodsugar of Newborn Infants.* Copenhagen: Danish Science Press; 1952.

14. Metzger BE, Lowe LP, Dyer AR, et al. Hyperglycemia and adverse pregnancy outcomes. *N Engl J Med.* 2008;**358** (19):1991–2002.

15. Catalano PM, McIntyre HD, Cruickshank JK, et al. The hyperglycemia and adverse pregnancy outcome study: associations of GDM and obesity with pregnancy outcomes. *Diabetes Care.* 2012;**35**(4):780–6.

16. Catalano PM, Hauguel-De Mouzon S. Is it time to revisit the Pedersen hypothesis in the face of the obesity epidemic? *Am J Obstet Gynecol.* 2011;**204**(6):479–87.

17. Knopp RH, Warth MR, Charles D, et al. Lipoprotein metabolism in pregnancy, fat transport to the fetus, and the effects of diabetes. *Biol Neonate.* 1986;**50** (6):297–317.

18. Goldberg AS, Hegele RA. Severe hypertriglyceridemia in pregnancy. *J Clin Endocrinol Metab.* 2012;**97** (8):2589–96.

19. Ghaji N, Boulet SL, Tepper N, Hooper WC. Trends in venous thromboembolism among pregnancy-related hospitalizations, United States, 1994–2009. *Am J Obstet Gynecol.* 2013;**209**(5):433.e431–8.

20. Wolfe KB, Rossi RA, Warshak CR. The effect of maternal obesity on the rate of failed induction of labor. *Am J Obstet Gynecol.* 2011;**205**(2):128.e121–7.

21. Brost BC, Goldenberg RL, Mercer BM, et al. The Preterm Prediction Study: association of cesarean delivery with increases in maternal weight and body mass index. *Am J Obstet Gynecol.* 1997;**177** (2):333–7; discussion 337–41.

22. CMACE/RCOG Joint Guideline. *Management of Women with Obesity in Pregnancy* 2010. www.rcog.org.uk/globalassets/documents/guidelines/cmacercogjointguidelinemanagementwomenobesitypregnancya.pdf.

23. Sebire NJ, Jolly M, Harris JP, et al. Maternal obesity and pregnancy outcome: a study of 287,213 pregnancies in London. *Int J Obes Relat Metab Disord.* 2001;**25** (8):1175–82.

24. Stothard KJ, Tennant PW, Bell R, Rankin J. Maternal overweight and obesity and the risk of congenital anomalies: a systematic review and meta-analysis. *JAMA.* 2009;**301** (6):636–50.

25. Aune D, Saugstad OD, Henriksen T, Tonstad S. Maternal body mass index and the risk of fetal death, stillbirth, and infant death: a systematic review and

meta-analysis. *JAMA*. 2014;**311**(15):1536–46.

26. Edlow AG. Maternal obesity and neurodevelopmental and psychiatric disorders in offspring. *Prenat Diagn*. 2017;**37**(1):95–110.

27. Laitinen J, Power C, Järvelin MR. Family social class, maternal body mass index, childhood body mass index, and age at menarche as predictors of adult obesity. *Am J Clin Nutr*. 2001;**74**(3):287–94.

28. Furber CM, McGowan L, Bower P, et al. Antenatal interventions for reducing weight in obese women for improving pregnancy outcome. *Cochrane Database Syst Rev*. 2013(1):CD009334.

29. Maggard MA, Yermilov I, Li Z, et al. Pregnancy and fertility following bariatric surgery: a systematic review. *JAMA*. 2008;**300**(19):2286–96.

30. Shah M, Simha V, Garg A. Review: long-term impact of bariatric surgery on body weight, comorbidities, and nutritional status. *J Clin Endocrinol Metab*. 2006;**91**(11):4223–31.

31. ACOG Practice Bulletin No 156: Obesity in Pregnancy. *Obstet Gynecol*. 2015;**126**(6):e112–26.

32. Institute of Medicine (US) and National Research Council (US) Committee to Reexamine IOM Pregnancy Weight Guidelines. In Rasmussen KM, Yaktine AL, eds. *Weight Gain During Pregnancy: Reexamining the Guidelines*. Washington, DC: National Academies Press; 2009.

33. Egan AM, Dennedy MC, Al-Ramli W, et al. ATLANTIC-DIP: excessive gestational weight gain and pregnancy outcomes in women with gestational or pregestational diabetes mellitus. *J Clin Endocrinol Metab*. 2014;**99**(1):212–19.

34. Thangaratinam S, Rogozinska E, Jolly K, et al. Effects of interventions in pregnancy on maternal weight and obstetric outcomes: meta-analysis of randomised evidence. *BMJ*. 2012;**344**:e2088.

35. Egan AM, Simmons D. Lessons learned from lifestyle prevention trials in gestational diabetes mellitus. *Diabet Med*. 2019;**36**(2):142–50.

36. *PRECOG: The Pre-eclampsia Community Guideline*. 2004. https://action-on-pre-eclampsia.org.uk/wp-content/uploads/2012/07/PRECOG-Community-Guideline.pdf

37. Mok E, Multon C, Piguel L, et al. Decreased full breastfeeding, altered practices, perceptions, and infant weight change of prepregnant obese women: a need for extra support. *Pediatrics*. 2008;**121**(5):e1319–24.

38. O'Reilly MW, Avalos G, Dennedy MC, O'Sullivan EP, Dunne F. Atlantic DIP: high prevalence of abnormal glucose tolerance post partum is reduced by breast-feeding in women with prior gestational diabetes mellitus. *Eur J Endocrinol*. 2011;**165**(6):953–9.

39. Jain AP, Gavard JA, Rice JJ, et al. The impact of interpregnancy weight change on birthweight in obese women. *Am J Obstet Gynecol*. 2013;**208**(3):205.e201–7.

40. Amorim AR, Linne YM, Lourenco PM. Diet or exercise, or both, for weight reduction in women after childbirth. *Cochrane Database Syst Rev*. 2007(3):CD005627.

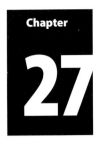

Chapter

27

Screening for Gestational Diabetes Mellitus and Care of Diabetes Mellitus in Pregnancy

Peter Hornnes & Jeannet Lauenborg

Diabetes in pregnancy can be classified as either pre-existing diabetes mellitus, if the diabetes is recognized before pregnancy, the most frequent forms being type 1 and type 2 diabetes, or as gestational diabetes mellitus (GDM), if diagnosed in pregnancy. The latter group may also cover women with undiagnosed pre-existing diabetes, as the definition of GDM is abnormal glucose tolerance or hyperglycaemia diagnosed for the first time in pregnancy [1]. GDM is one of the most frequent medical conditions complicating pregnancy, and affects up to almost 20% of the pregnancies in Europe depending on the population and criteria used (Table 27.1) [2].

Pregnancies in women with pre-existing diabetes are associated with increased risk of complications following higher glucose levels from early pregnancy, and co-morbidities such as hypertension and kidney disease, compared with women who develop diabetes during pregnancy. Women with pre-existing diabetes have a significantly higher risk of malformations due to poor glucose control at conception and in the first trimester, which is not the case with GDM. Due to this increased risk, they should be followed carefully before conception to obtain good glucose control [3].

In this chapter, we will discuss the screening for gestational diabetes and how to take care of women with gestational diabetes. We will briefly describe pregnancy care of women with pre-existing diabetes. Pre-conception care for women with pre-existing diabetes is beyond the scope of this chapter.

27.1 Gestational Diabetes Mellitus

Insulin resistance increases during pregnancy as a normal physiological trait of pregnancy [4]. Women developing GDM may be more insulin resistant already before pregnancy because of obesity or polycystic ovary syndrome, and they may not be capable of increasing insulin secretion sufficiently to maintain a normal glucose tolerance throughout pregnancy [5]. Among other pre-pregnancy risk factors are overweight/obesity before conception, a family history of diabetes (both first and second line relatives), a history of GDM or previous birth of a large-for-gestational-age infant [6]. Recent research may indicate that the microbiota could also play a role in the development of GDM [7]. Placental hormones have been related to the increasing insulin resistance during pregnancy, and possibly due to the larger placenta, multiple pregnancy is

Table 27.1 Screening method and criteria for GDM, and prevalence of GDM and type 2 diabetes in Europe

Country	Screening Criteria	Population	Prevalence (%) GDM	Type 2 DM 2017 [24]
Sweden	75 g 2 h OGTT, capillary BG ≥10 mmol/L		2012: 2.6 [25]	7.0
Denmark	Local, 75 g 2 h OGTT, 2 h plasma BG ≥9 mmol/L	Selective, risk based	2017: 4.1 [26]	9.3
Finland	IADPSG*	Selective, risk based	2017: 19 [27]	9.2
Belgium	2013 WHO, 75 g 2 h OGTT	Universal two step screening with GCT	2014–17: 9.1 [28]	6.1
France	IADPSG*	Selective, risk based	2016: 10.8§	7.3
UK	IADPSG*	Universal	12.1 [29]	5.1 [30]
Spain (Catalonia)			6.22§	10.4
Italy	Local, 75 g 2 h OGTT,	Selective, risk based	2015: 11.0 [31]	7.6
Malta	IADPSG*	Selective	2011: 19.7§	13.2

BG: blood glucose; DM: diabetes mellitus; GCT: glucose challenge test; IADPSG: International Association of the Diabetes and Pregnancy Study Groups; OGTT: oral glucose tolerance test; WHO: World Health Organization
* IADPSG criteria, venous plasma glucose measured at fasting >5.1 mmol/L, 1-hour >10.0 mmol/L, and 2-hour >8.5 mmol/L [17].
§ Personal communication

221

also a risk factor for developing GDM [8]. Besides glucosuria, women with GDM most often do not have any signs of the condition, unless there is excessive fetal growth, that influence the well-being of the woman. Rare symptoms are polydipsia or thirst [2]. An overview of risk factors where special focus in pregnancy care are warranted is given in Table 27.2.

Gestational diabetes mellitus is associated with increased morbidity for both mother and child, with both short- and long-term complications. These include hypertensive disorder, excessive fetal

growth, caesarean section and birth trauma and neonatal hypoglycaemia in the short run [9]. The risk of pregnancy and birth complications increase with increasing levels of glucose [10].

Being diagnosed with GDM or being born by a mother with GDM indicate a significantly increased risk of later metabolic disease [11, 12]. The risk may be reduced by proper lifestyle modification and weight loss, especially in people with impaired glucose tolerance (elevated 2-hour glucose level) after pregnancy [13]. Also, studies have shown a benefit of treating even milder degrees of hyperglycaemia during pregnancy for both mother and child [14]. Therefore, it is important to screen for and treat hyperglycaemia in pregnancy.

27.2 Diagnosing Gestational Diabetes

Most women developing GDM will be diagnosed after 24 weeks' gestation depending on screening strategy. Some countries screen all pregnant women for GDM (universal screening), others only screen based on risk factors (selective screening). The gold standard for diagnosing gestational diabetes is the oral glucose tolerance test (OGTT). The test is performed in the morning after an overnight fast, with an oral glucose load of either 75 g or 100 g, and by measuring glucose at either capillary or venous blood samples at different time intervals (fasting/1-hour/2-hour/3-hour). The cut-off differs between tests, as does the number of values that should be exceeded to fulfil the criteria for having GDM (Table 27.3) [15]. A glucose challenge test (GCT) is sometimes used for screening a large population to select those individuals with higher glucose levels who should be examined further with an OGTT. At a GCT, the glucose load is 50 g with measurement of 1-hour glucose. In case of a positive result, the woman is referred to an OGTT. In contrast to the OGTT, there is no restriction by time of day or relation to mealtime when performing a GCT, making this test more feasible to perform in a large-scale setting [16].

Several criteria have been published and used widely around the world. Some countries have universal screening with widely used tests, and some countries have their own criteria and screening strategy. The first set of criteria for diagnosing GDM was published in 1979 by the National Diabetes Data Group (NDDG) and the criteria were set to detect women at

Table 27.2 Risk factors for gestational diabetes

Pre-pregnancy	Pregnancy
Previous GDM ↑	Multiple pregnancy ↑
Previous birth of macrosomic or large-for-gestational-age child ↑	Glucosuria ↑
Previous shoulder dystocia ↑	Excessive gestational weight gain ↑
Previous stillbirth ↑	Excessive fetal growth ↑
Pregestational BMI ↑	Polyhydramnios ↑
Family history of diabetes ↑	(Polydipsia ↑)
Parity ↑	(Thirst ↑)
Age ↑	
Polycystic ovary syndrome ↑	
Ethnicity	
Microbiome	
Own birthweight	
Sucking ↓	

BMI: body mass index
Arrows indicate either a positive (↑) or a negative (↓) association

Table 27.3 Frequently used diagnostic tests for GDM

Test	Glucose load	Measure points	Cut-off (≥; mmol/L)	Values needed to meet criteria
O'Sullivan 1964	100 g	Fasting/1-h/2-h/3-h	5/9.2/8.1/6.9	≥2
NDDG 1979	100 g	Fasting/1-h/2-h/3-h	5.8/10.6/9.2/8.0	≥2
Carpenter and Coustan 1982	100 g	Fasting/1-h/2-h/3-h	5.3/10/8.6/7.8	≥2
WHO 1999	75 g	Fasting/2-h	7–0/7.8	≥1
IADPSG 2008	75 g	Fasting/1-h/2-h	5.1/10/8.5	≥1

IADPSG: International Association of Diabetes and Pregnancy Study Groups; NDDG: National Diabetes Data Group; WHO: World Health Organization

markedly increased risk of later type 2 diabetes. The most recent set of criteria for diagnosing GDM was published in 2008 by the International Association of the Diabetes and Pregnancy Study Groups (IADPSG) and was based on pregnancy and neonatal outcome [15]. The IADPSG criteria have now been accepted by several authorities across the world, including the World Health Organization (WHO) and the American Diabetes Association (ADA), and implemented in more or less modified versions all over the world. According to these criteria, all women should be screened at 24–28 weeks' gestation and blood samples drawn at fasting, 1 hour and 2 hours after ingestion of 75 g glucose. If one or more values exceed the cut-off of 5.1, 10 and 8.5 mmol/L at fasting, 1-hour and 2-hours, the woman has hyperglycaemia in pregnancy. In case of suspicion of diabetes in first trimester, the woman should be examined with glycated haemoglobin or fasting plasma glucose, and if haemoglobin A1c (HbA1c) is 48 mmol/molar higher, or plasma glucose 7 mmol/L or higher, the woman is classified as having pre-existing diabetes [17].

Haemoglobin A1c reflects the mean blood glucose level for the last 4 weeks and is used for evaluation of treatment effect during pregnancy. HbA1c is a screening tool for type 2 diabetes outside of pregnancy, and a high HbA1c in the first trimester may indicate a pre-gestational diabetes [1]. Several studies have evaluated the usefulness of measuring HbA1c in the beginning of pregnancy to define women at increased risk of GDM later in pregnancy but found that HbA1c is not a reliable tool for diagnosing GDM [16].

27.3 Treatment of Gestational Diabetes

High blood glucose levels increase risk of excessive fetal growth. Therefore, the goal in handling women with gestational diabetes is to prevent excessive fetal growth by lowering the glucose level. The glucose is often evaluated by self-monitoring or by continuous glucose measurement with a sensor. For women with diet-treated GDM, the glucose testing can be reduced to 2–3 meals a day, every second or third day. In cases on insulin therapy, the glucose should be measured before and after each main meal and at bedtime. Fasting or premeal blood glucose should not exceed 5.8 and 1-hour post-meal should not be higher than 7.8 [18]. Diet and physical activity are the cornerstones in the treatment of GDM. The intake of carbohydrates should be reduced. It is also advised to eat several times a day, with three main courses and two to three snacks [3]. Physical activity increases insulin sensitivity, and women with GDM should have at least 30 minutes of physical activity daily. The weight increase during pregnancy should follow the Institute of Medicine (IOM) guidelines for weight gain according to pre-pregnancy body mass index (BMI) [19]. If optimal glucose regulation cannot be obtained by diet alone, medication should be initiated. Insulin and metformin are the most widely used drugs in the medical treatment of GDM. The treatment for GDM may be initiated if two or more values exceed the pre- and post-meal threshold [3]. However, the indication for initiation of medical treatment is often based on an individual professional judgement.

As excessive fetal growth is more frequent in women with GDM, the women should be offered regular ultrasound examinations to evaluate fetal growth. Especially abdominal circumference is a marker for fetal growth. Evaluation of fetal growth should be

performed every 4–6 weeks from 28 weeks' gestation. At term (from week 38) fetal well-being can be further monitored by biophysical profile testing. In case of growth restriction or very poor glucose control, fetal surveillance may be intensified [3].

Women with GDM are not allowed to go post-term and are offered induction of labour at term even if glucose regulation and fetal growth are satisfactory on medical treatment. If glucose control is good and there is normal fetal growth on diet alone, the woman should await spontaneous labour until 40+6 weeks' gestation and then be induced. In case of very poor glucose regulation or excessive fetal growth, induction may be planned earlier than at term. During labour, blood glucose should be evaluated every hour or second hourly [3].

27.4 Postpartum Follow-Up after Gestational Diabetes

After delivery of the placenta, glucose tolerance will normalize within hours or days. The offspring is tested for hypoglycaemia around 2 hours after birth. If low, early feeding may be necessary. After birth, the women should be advised to attend a testing of the glucose tolerance about 2 months postpartum to exclude overt diabetes. Overweight women should be advised to lose weight by lifestyle modification. Lactation have also been shown to reduce risk for progression to overt diabetes and the women should be advised to lactate for at least three months [20]. It is well known that women with previous GDM have a very high risk of developing overt diabetes, especially type 2 diabetes, later in life [21]. Regular testing with 1–3 years' interval is therefore recommended.

Several intervention studies have examined the effect of lifestyle intervention for prevention of recurrence of GDM or progression to type 2 diabetes. Several studies show some effect of diet and physical intervention, but the intervention examined is often very intensive and showed only minor effect and is difficult and expensive to implement [13, 22].

27.5 Special Concerns Related to Pre-existing Diabetes

All risks for adverse pregnancy outcomes are increased in women with pre-existing diabetes, indicating that the care offered this group of women should be even more intense than for women with GDM [3]. They are often affiliated with a diabetes department/centre before pregnancy and will often continue care at their usual medical centre. Some women may have an insulin pump or wear a continuous glucose measurement device and receive treatment with insulin types not frequently used in pregnancy. Tight glucose control is even more crucial during pregnancy due to the increased risk of adverse pregnancy outcome. However, the more intensive and tight the glucose control, the higher the risk of hypoglycaemia, which can be dangerous, especially at nighttime [23]. Besides routine care and the additional care offered women with GDM, women with pre-existing diabetes should be offered assessment for diabetic retinopathy. At the ultrasound screening around 20 weeks' gestation, there should be special attention on structural abnormalities, including the fetal heart. Induction may be offered no later than 39 weeks' gestation [3].

References

1. 2. Classification and Diagnosis of Diabetes: *Standards of Medical Care in Diabetes-2018*. *Diabetes Care*. 2018;**41** (Suppl 1): S13–S27.

2. Tieu J, McPhee AJ, Crowther CA, Middleton P, Shepherd E. Screening for gestational diabetes mellitus based on different risk profiles and settings for improving maternal and infant health. *Cochrane Database Syst Rev*. 2017;(8): CD007222.

3. NICE. *Diabetes in Pregnancy: Management from Preconception to the Postnatal Period*. NICE Guideline NG3. 2015. www.nice.org.uk/gui dance/ng3.

4. Kuhl C. Etiology and pathogenesis of gestational diabetes. *Diabetes Care*. 1998;**21**(Suppl 2):B19–26.

5. Catalano PM, Kirwan JP, Haugel-de Mouzon S, King J. Gestational diabetes and insulin resistance: role in short- and long-term implications for mother and fetus. *J Nutr*. 2003;**133**(5 Suppl 2):1674s–83s.

6. Hartling L, Dryden DM, Guthrie A, et al. Screening and diagnosing gestational diabetes mellitus. *Evid Rep Technol Assess*. 2012(210):1–327.

7. Crusell MKW, Hansen TH, Nielsen T, et al. Gestational diabetes is associated with change in the gut microbiota composition in third trimester of pregnancy and postpartum. *Microbiome*. 2018;**6**(1):89.

8. Rauh-Hain JA, Rana S, Tamez H, et al. Risk for developing gestational diabetes in women with twin pregnancies. *J Matern Fetal Neonatal Med*. 2009;**22** (4):293–9.

9. Damm P, Houshmand-Oeregaard A, Kelstrup L, et al. Gestational diabetes mellitus and long-term consequences for mother and offspring: a view from Denmark. *Diabetologia*. 2016;**59** (7):1396–9.

10. Metzger BE, Lowe LP, Dyer AR, et al. Hyperglycemia and adverse pregnancy outcomes. *N Engl J Med*. 2008;**358** (19):1991–2002.

11. Clausen TD, Mathiesen ER, Hansen T, et al. High prevalence of type 2 diabetes and pre-diabetes in adult offspring of women with gestational diabetes mellitus or type 1 diabetes: the role of intrauterine hyperglycemia. *Diabetes Care*. 2008;**31**(2):340–6.

12. Lauenborg J, Mathiesen E, Hansen T, et al. The prevalence of the metabolic syndrome in a Danish population of women with previous gestational diabetes mellitus is three-fold higher than in the general population. *J Clin Endocrinol Metab*. 2005;**90**(7):4004–10.

13. Hemmingsen B, Gimenez-Perez G, Mauricio D, et al. Diet, physical activity or both for prevention or delay of type 2 diabetes mellitus and its associated complications in people at increased risk of developing type 2 diabetes mellitus. *Cochrane Database Syst Rev*. 2017;(12):Cd003054.

14. Han S, Crowther CA, Middleton P. Interventions for pregnant women with hyperglycaemia not meeting gestational diabetes and type 2 diabetes diagnostic criteria. *Cochrane Database Syst Rev*. 2012;(1):CD009037.

15. Noctor E, Dunne FP. Type 2 diabetes after gestational diabetes: The influence of changing diagnostic criteria. *World J Diabetes*. 2015;**6** (2):234–44.

16. Farrar D, Duley L, Dowswell T, Lawlor DA. Different strategies for diagnosing gestational diabetes to improve maternal and infant health. *Cochrane Database Syst Rev*. 2017;(8): CD007122.

17. Metzger BE, Gabbe SG, Persson B, et al. International association of diabetes and pregnancy study groups recommendations on the diagnosis and classification of hyperglycemia in pregnancy. *Diabetes Care*. 2010;**33** (3):676–82.

18. Martis R, Brown J, Alsweiler J, Crawford TJ, Crowther CA. Different intensities of glycaemic control for women with gestational diabetes mellitus. *Cochrane Database Syst Rev*. 2016;(4):CD011624.

19. ACOG Committee opinion no. 548: weight gain during pregnancy. *Obstet Gynecol*. 2013;**121**(1): 210–12.

20. Gunderson EP, Hurston SR, Ning X, et al. Lactation and progression to type 2 diabetes mellitus after gestational diabetes mellitus: a prospective cohort study. *Ann Intern Med*. 2015;**163** (12):889–98.

21. Kim C, Newton KM, Knopp RH. Gestational diabetes and the incidence of type 2 diabetes: a systematic review. *Diabetes Care*. 2002;**25**(10):1862–8.

22. Mijatovic-Vukas J, Capling L, Cheng S, et al. Associations of diet and physical activity with risk for gestational diabetes mellitus: a systematic review and meta-analysis. *Nutrients*. 2018;**10**(6).

23. Moy FM, Ray A, Buckley BS, West HM. Techniques of monitoring blood glucose during pregnancy for women with pre-existing diabetes. *Cochrane Database Syst Rev*. 2017;(6): CD009613.

24. IDF Europe Members. International Diabetes Federation; 2017. www.idf.org /our-network/regions-members/eur ope/members.html.

25. Ignell C, Claesson R, Anderberg E, Berntorp K. Trends in the prevalence of gestational diabetes mellitus in southern Sweden, 2003–2012. *Acta Obstet Gynecol Scand*. 2014;**93** (4):420–4.

26. Det Medicinske Fødselsregister (MFR). Sundhedsdatastyrelsen; 2018. www .esundhed.dk/sundhedsregistre/MFR/S ider/MFR06A.aspx.

27. Reports of Perinatal Statistics 2017 Finland. National Institute for Health and Welfare; 2018. https://thl.fi/tilasto liite/tilastoraportit/2018/Perinataalitila sto_ennakot_2017.pdf.

28. Benhalima K, Van Crombrugge P, Moyson C, et al. A modified two-step screening strategy for gestational diabetes mellitus based on the 2013 WHO criteria by combining the glucose challenge test and clinical risk factors. *J Clin Med*. 2018;7(10).

29. O'Sullivan EP, Avalos G, O'Reilly M, et al. Atlantic Diabetes in Pregnancy (DIP): the prevalence and outcomes of gestational diabetes mellitus using new diagnostic criteria. *Diabetologia*. 2011;**54**(7):1670–5.

30. Diabetes in the UK. 2010. Key statistics on diabetes 2010 25-01-2019. www .diabetes.org.uk/resources-s3/2017–11/ diabetes_in_the_uk_2010.pdf.

31. Di Cianni G, Gualdani E, Berni C, et al. Screening for gestational diabetes in Tuscany, Italy. A population study. *Diabetes Res Clin Pract*. 2017;**132**:149–56.

Cardiac Disease in Pregnancy

Sarah Vause, Anna Roberts & Bernard Clarke

28.1 Introduction

Major physiological changes occur in the maternal cardiovascular system during pregnancy. In women with pre-existing or previously undiagnosed cardiac disease, these changes may precipitate cardiac decompensation. The number of women with heart disease embarking on a pregnancy is increasing. Heart disease is the commonest cause of maternal death in the UK where all maternal deaths are critically reviewed. In approximately half of the women who died from cardiac disease in the UK, suboptimal care was identified. In the Netherlands, the maternal mortality rate from cardiac disease (2004–2006) was 3 per 100 000 maternities. Multidisciplinary teams working and co-location of clinical services are critically important to ensure the best care possible for pregnant women with cardiac conditions (Figure 28.1).

28.2 Epidemiology and Aetiology

The increase in the number of women with heart disease in pregnancy is due to both greater numbers of those with acquired heart disease (e.g. ischaemic and rheumatic heart disease), as well as an increase in women with inherited and congenital heart disease who are surviving to reproductive age and choosing to embark on pregnancy. Increasing maternal age, obesity and smoking result in more women with hypertension and these are all risk factors for the development of ischaemic heart disease. Immigration from developing countries means that an increased prevalence of rheumatic heart disease is now seen in Europe.

In the UK, cardiac disease remains the commonest cause of indirect maternal death. It is also the leading cause of maternal death overall, with deaths from acquired heart disease being significantly more frequent than those from congenital heart disease. Inherited cardiac conditions which may predispose to arrhythmias, cardiomyopathy or aortopathy are increasingly recognized (Figure 28.2).

28.3 Physiology

During pregnancy, oxygen consumption increases. This is in part because the fetus has its own increasing oxygen requirements and also because of the increasing size of the uterus and maternal metabolic rate. Cardiac output increases during pregnancy by at least 30%, with further significant elevation during labour and the immediate postpartum period.

The associated effects of pregnancy on the cardiovascular system are:

- Reduced systemic vascular resistance – decreased afterload

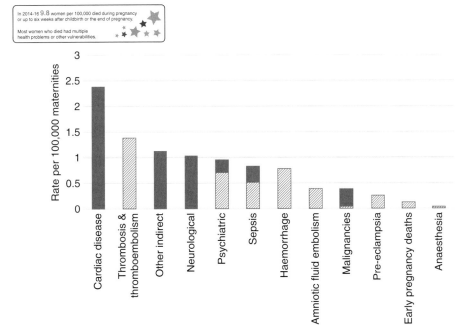

Causes of maternal death 2014–16

Figure 28.1 Causes of maternal mortality in the UK 2014–2016 (after MBRRACE-UK, 2016 [8])

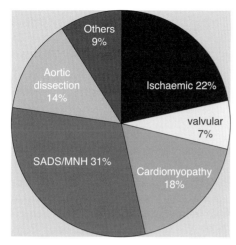

Figure 28.2 Type of cardiac disease for women who died (MBRRACE-UK, 2016 [8])

- Increased plasma volume – increased preload
- Increased stroke volume – occurs within the first trimester
- Increased heart rate by approximately 10 beats per minute (bpm) – mainly second and third trimesters
- Increased cardiac output by 30–50%; half of the total increase occurs by 8 weeks of gestation.

Whilst women with normal cardiac function tolerate these haemodynamic changes well, women with cardiac disease may decompensate during pregnancy. Women with heart disease are at greatest risk during periods when cardiac output is high or changing rapidly. Early pregnancy, the second stage of labour and immediately postpartum are times of greatest change, and therefore these periods carry the greatest risk of decompensation.

The ability of women with cardiac disease to tolerate pregnancy is mainly dictated by their functional status, rather than the underlying aetiology of their condition (Figure 28.3).

28.4 General Principles of Management

28.4.1 Pre-pregnancy

Women who are known to have heart disease should be offered pre-pregnancy counselling, ideally in a joint consultation with an obstetrician and cardiologist. This should include:

- A functional assessment
- Risk stratification (see below)
- A frank discussion of the risks involved for her and her baby to enable the woman to make an informed choice as to whether to embark on pregnancy or not
- Optimizing cardiac function (medically, e.g. control arrhythmias, or surgically, e.g. valvuloplasty)
- Review and adjust medication avoiding teratogens if possible
- Contraception advice if the woman decides against embarking on pregnancy
- Contact numbers to facilitate early referral once pregnant

Those undergoing assisted conception often have additional risk factors such as increased age, the risk of ovarian hyperstimulation and multiple pregnancy.

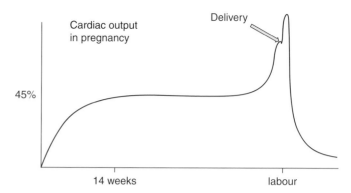

Figure 28.3 Cardiac output in pregnancy.

28.4.1.1 Risk Stratification

The level of risk associated with pregnancy is dependent on functional status, the underlying cardiac lesion and other co-morbidities. Information should be individualized for each woman.

Investigations which are helpful include echocardiography, electrocardiogram (ECG), formal cardiopulmonary exercise testing (CPET); and for some conditions advanced imaging techniques such as cardiac magnetic resonance (CMR) scanning or cardiac CT.

A modified World Health Organization (mWHO) classification can guide assessment of risk and planning of care during pregnancy (Table 28.1).

It is also important to discuss the risks to the fetus, including the risks of miscarriage, prematurity, growth restriction, risk of recurrence of the cardiac condition and any antenatal tests which may be offered.

28.4.2 Antenatal

Ideally, women with heart disease should be referred to a joint obstetric cardiac clinic as soon as they are pregnant. Services provided should include:

- Easy access to facilitate prompt referral
- A professional interpreter (if needed) to ensure that all relevant history is disclosed. Interpreters from within the family should not be used as in the family's desire to help the woman have a successful pregnancy, risks may not be accurately relayed to the patient.
- Easy access to termination of pregnancy services for those who choose not to continue with their pregnancy, in a hospital which can comprehensively care for a woman with heart disease.
- Fetal echocardiography if the mother has congenital heart disease
- Good communication between the clinicians involved in a woman's care, to facilitate rapid escalation of care should complications occur, is essential.

Antenatal care within a joint obstetric cardiology service should include:

- Risk stratification, following a detailed assessment of current condition and past medical history

Table 28.1 Modified WHO classification of maternal cardiovascular risk

	mWHO I	mWHO II	mWHO II–III	mWHO III	mWHO IV
Diagnosis (if otherwise well and uncomplicated)	Small or mild – pulmonary stenosis – patent ductus arteriosus – mitral valve prolapse Successfully repaired simple lesions (atrial or ventricular septal defect, patent ductus arteriosus, anomalous pulmonary venous drainage) Atrial or ventricular ectopic beats, isolated	Unoperated atrial or ventricular septal defect Repaired tetralogy of Fallot Most arrhythmias (supraventricular arrhythmias) Turner syndrome without aortic dilation	Mild left ventricular impairment (EF >45%) Hypertrophic cardiomyopathy Native or tissue valve disease not considered WHO I or IV (mild mitral stenosis, moderate aortic stenosis) Marfan or other HTAD syndrome without aortic dilation Aorta <45 mm in bicuspid aortic valve pathology Repaired coarctation Atrioventricular septal defect	Moderate left ventricular impairment (EF 30–45%) Previous peripartum cardiomyopathy without any residual left ventricular impairment Mechanical valve Systemic right ventricle with good or mildly decreased ventricular function Fontan circulation. If otherwise the patient is well and the cardiac condition uncomplicated Unrepaired cyanotic heart disease Other complex heart disease Moderate mitral stenosis Severe asymptomatic aortic stenosis Moderate aortic dilation (40–45 mm in Marfan syndrome or other HTAD; 45–50 mm in bicuspid aortic valve, Turner syndrome ASI 20–25 mm/m^2, tetralogy of Fallot <50 mm) Ventricular tachycardia	Pulmonary arterial hypertension Severe systemic ventricular dysfunction (EF <30% or NYHA class III–IV) Previous peripartum cardiomyopathy with any residual left ventricular impairment Severe mitral stenosis Severe symptomatic aortic stenosis Systemic right ventricle with moderate or severely decreased ventricular function Severe aortic dilation (>45 mm in Marfan syndrome or other HTAD, >50 mm in bicuspid aortic valve, Turner syndrome ASI >25 mm/m^2, tetralogy of Fallot >50 mm) Vascular Ehlers–Danlos Severe (re)coarctation Fontan with any complication
Risk	No detectable increased risk of maternal mortality and no/mild increased risk in morbidity	Small increased risk of maternal mortality or moderate increase in morbidity	Intermediate increased risk of maternal mortality or moderate to severe increase in morbidity	Significantly increased risk of maternal mortality or severe morbidity	Extremely high risk of maternal mortality or severe morbidity

Table 28.1 (cont.)

	mWHO I	mWHO II	mWHO II–III	mWHO III	mWHO IV
Maternal cardiac event rate	2.5–5%	5.7–10.5%	10–19%	19–27%	40–100%
Counselling	Yes	Yes	Yes	Yes: expert counselling required	Yes: pregnancy contraindicated: if pregnancy occurs, termination should be discussed
Care during pregnancy	Local hospital	Local hospital	Referral hospital	Expert centre for pregnancy and cardiac disease	Expert centre for pregnancy and cardiac disease
Minimal follow-up visits during pregnancy	Once or twice	Once per trimester	Bimonthly	Monthly or bimonthly	Monthly
Location of delivery	Local hospital	Local hospital	Referral hospital	Expert centre for pregnancy and cardiac disease	Expert centre for pregnancy and cardiac disease

ASI: aortic size index; EF: ejection fraction; HTAD: heritable thoracic aortic disease; mWHO: modified World Health Organization classification; NYHA: New York Heart Association; WHO: World Health Organization.

- Frank discussion of the risks involved to enable the woman to make an informed choice as to whether to continue with the pregnancy or not
- Review and adjustment of medication, for example, discontinuation of angiotensin-converting enzyme (ACE) inhibitors
- Anaesthetic review, usually in the second trimester, to discuss analgesia or anaesthesia for delivery
- A multidisciplinary care plan should be generated and circulated widely to everyone involved, including the woman

The number, timing and location of further appointments will be dependent on the nature and severity of cardiac disease. Women with low risk cardiac disease can be managed in their local hospital, but those with more severe cardiac disease will require specialist multidisciplinary care throughout in a tertiary centre.

28.4.2.1 Multidisciplinary Care Plan

This should include a plan for management during pregnancy, intrapartum and postpartum. Consideration should be given to what interventions and support may be needed around the time of delivery as this may affect the choice of hospital for delivery. The care plan should include contingency planning for such conditions as preterm labour and postpartum haemorrhage, and contact numbers for members of the multidisciplinary team. Anaesthetists, haematologists and neonatologists may all need to be involved in planning delivery. The woman's own views and wishes should be taken into account. The woman should be given a copy of her care plan to carry with her, in case she is admitted to a hospital where she has not previously been seen.

28.4.2.2 Cardiovascular Disease Presenting during Pregnancy

The majority of women who attend a joint obstetric cardiology clinic have congenital or inherited cardiac disease and were aware of it prior to pregnancy. However, many of the women who die from cardiac disease in pregnancy, have previously undiagnosed heart disease (acquired or inherited). It is therefore important for clinicians to be aware of relevant history, important signs and symptoms which may suggest a woman has cardiac disease; these should prompt timely referral to a cardiologist.

Examples include:

- New-onset breathlessness, particularly if associated with orthopnoea
- Severe chest pain not due to thromboembolism
- Interscapular pain
- Unexplained tachycardia
- Isolated systolic hypertension
- Unexplained polycythaemia

28.4.2.3 Appropriate Response to Cardiac Arrest in Pregnancy

When responding to a cardiac arrest in pregnancy, resuscitation should include:

- Manual displacement of the uterus to improve venous return by reducing compression of the inferior vena cava
- Early intubation with a cuffed endotracheal tube to protect the airway and prevent aspiration
- Perimortem caesarean section to facilitate resuscitation of the mother, should be performed as part of the resuscitation after 5 minutes. This is undertaken for maternal reasons, not to save the baby. It should be carried out if the woman is 'obviously pregnant' irrespective of whether the fetal heart is present or not.

28.4.3 Intrapartum

In most women with heart disease elective caesarean section carries no maternal benefit, and results in earlier delivery and lower birthweight of the baby. Vaginal delivery is associated with less blood loss, lower risk of infection and a lower chance of venous thromboembolism compared with caesarean section. It is therefore appropriate to aim for a vaginal delivery, unless a woman cannot safely raise her cardiac output sufficiently for labour or there is a high risk of aortic dissection. Caesarean section for cardiac indications may be appropriate in women with severely stenotic heart valves, poor ventricular function, ischaemia, cyanosis, pulmonary hypertension and those with a dilated aortic root.

Anaesthetic considerations, obstetric history, co-morbidities and the woman's preferences must also be taken into account when planning delivery.

An individualized, written, widely circulated, multidisciplinary care plan helps ensure consistent management.

As general principles, during labour in women with heart disease avoid hypotension or hypertension, provide good analgesia and ensure careful fluid balance. Allowing a longer passive second stage of labour can reduce the duration of the active second stage. Monitoring of progress and maternal condition in active second stage with timely intervention is necessary. Oxytocin 5 units in 20 mL saline given by an infusion over 10–20 minutes may be preferable to a bolus of syntometrine or bolus of syntocinon for management of the third stage, and this should be specified in the woman's care plan.

Given the lack of convincing evidence, antibiotic prophylaxis to prevent endocarditis is not routinely recommended for obstetric procedures and delivery [2, 3].

28.4.3.1 Contingency Plans

Preterm Labour

Atosiban is a specific oxytocin antagonist with no cardiac side effects and would be the tocolytic of choice in a woman with heart disease. Other tocolytics (e.g. ritodrine and nifedipine) have cardiovascular side effects.

Postpartum Haemorrhage

For postpartum haemorrhage mechanical methods (bimanual compression) and misoprostol are preferred for women with heart disease where sudden changes in haemodynamics may be detrimental. Although misoprostol has a longer time to onset of action than other uterotonic drugs it has less cardiac side effects. Oxytocin boluses can cause hypotension and tachycardia; ergometrine can cause a hypertensive surge, whilst carboprost (hemabate, prostaglandin F2α) may cause severe bronchoconstriction.

28.4.4 Postpartum Period

The majority of maternal deaths from cardiac causes occur postpartum. This is a time when increased vigilance is required, but when complacency often occurs. Maternal observations must be monitored regularly with an appropriate response if abnormal.

28.4.4.1 Breastfeeding

Women should be encouraged to breastfeed. Most medications required by postpartum women with heart disease are not contraindicated with breastfeeding. In particular, warfarin is not contraindicated. Enalapril can be used to treat breastfeeding women as they have no known adverse effects on babies receiving their breast milk.

28.4.5 Contraception

Appropriate contraceptive advice must be provided as soon as practicable, after any pregnancy. This allows time for reassessment of cardiac function and treatment if necessary, before another pregnancy ensues. One successful pregnancy must not engender complacency. Some conditions, such as peripartum cardiomyopathy, have a high recurrence risk and assessment and discussion should occur prior to embarking on a further pregnancy. Other conditions will naturally tend to worsen with age and in each subsequent pregnancy the risks will therefore increase. Contraceptive options should be discussed with women prior to discharge.

For some women with heart disease immediate postpartum contraception with either an intrauterine device (IUD) or long-acting reversible contraceptive (LARC) / progesterone implant is appropriate. These options should be discussed during pregnancy. The combined oral contraceptive pill should be avoided in women with heart disease who are at increased risk of thrombosis.

Guidance about contraception for women with heart disease is available on the Faculty of Sexual and Reproductive Health website – *Contraceptive Choices for Women with Cardiac Disease* 2014 [3].

28.5 Condition-Specific Management

28.5.1 Valvular Lesions

Heart valves can be regurgitant or stenotic. Although cardiac output increases in pregnancy, the reduction in systemic vascular resistance compensates in part for this, and pregnancy is generally well tolerated in women with regurgitant valves. Conversely, stenotic valves become more problematic in pregnancy as the increasing blood volume is forced through a fixed, narrowed valve.

28.5.1.1 Rheumatic Heart Disease and Mitral Stenosis

The most common cause of mitral stenosis is rheumatic endocarditis (75% of cases). Despite its decline in incidence, rheumatic heart disease is still an important problem in pregnancy, particularly if it is previously undiagnosed (as is often the case with recent immigrants from endemic areas).

The normal mitral valve surface area is 4 cm^2, but when the stenosis is severe (valve area $<1.5 \text{ cm}^2$) approximately two thirds of women will develop cardiac complications during pregnancy.

Pregnancy is associated with a 40% increase in preload. The combination of impaired diastolic flow through the stenotic valve, pregnancy-induced tachycardia and increased stroke volume causes increasing left atrial pressure and may result in pulmonary oedema and dyspnoea. The woman is then further compromised if atrial fibrillation supervenes and synchronized atrial transport is lost.

The cornerstones of treatment are diuretics, and meticulous rate control with β-blockade to allow increased left ventricular filling time. Anticoagulation (usually with low molecular weight heparin) should be used for women with atrial arrhythmia, a dilated left atrium, and during periods of reduced mobility.

The management plan for a woman with mitral stenosis should include:

Antenatal
- Treatment with beta blockade to slow the heart rate
- Vigilance regarding arrhythmias – treat and anticoagulate

Intrapartum
- Good analgesia in labour
- Careful fluid management: fluid overload must be avoided, and fluid restriction may be appropriate. Diuretics may be required. An abrupt increase of preload at delivery may lead to an increase in left atrial pressure and pulmonary oedema.
- May require a shortened active second stage or elective instrumental delivery
- Avoid syntometrine as this results in a rapid autotransfusion and can precipitate pulmonary oedema

28.5.1.2 Aortic Stenosis

The commonest causes of aortic stenosis are a congenital bicuspid valve or rheumatic heart disease. Symptoms occur late in the development of these conditions and include chest pain, syncope and heart failure. Sudden death may occur. On examination, a loud, greater than 3/6, harsh systolic murmur can be heard, but the bedside clinical signs are unreliable in critical aortic stenosis.

The woman's pre-conception functional class provides a good estimate of the woman's ability to tolerate pregnancy. Women asymptomatic before conception will, in general, tolerate pregnancy, while those with symptoms or severe stenosis (valve area $<1 \text{ cm}^2$) are at risk of sudden death or left ventricular failure. Those with severe aortic stenosis do not tolerate hypotension or tachycardia well. Adequate preload (volume of blood in the ventricle) is needed to generate sufficient pressure in the left ventricle to pump blood across the aortic valve. Blood loss, regional analgesia or vena caval compression can all compromise the woman's cardiac output.

The main objective is to avoid fluid depletion and hypotension. In labour, early placement of an arterial line, maintenance of left uterine displacement and aggressive treatment of blood loss are recommended. A bolus of intravenous oxytocin for third stage management can cause severe intractable hypotension, so an infusion of oxytocin (5 units over 20 minutes) reduces this risk. If postpartum haemorrhage occurs, there should be early recourse to mechanical methods (bimanual compression) and misoprostol. If there is significant haemorrhage, resulting in hypotension, syntometrine and other uterotonics can be used.

28.5.1.3 Valve Replacements

If a heart valve needs to be replaced either a mechanical prosthetic heart valve (MPHV) or a bioprosthetic (tissue) valve can be used.

Women with mechanical prosthetic heart valves require lifelong anticoagulation, usually with warfarin, to prevent valve thrombosis. During pregnancy, their thrombotic risk increases and the need for effective anticoagulation is greater. A recent UKOSS study has shown high rates of maternal and fetal morbidity and mortality [5]. There is no ideal anticoagulation regime. Warfarin treatment throughout pregnancy appears to have the lowest risk of maternal thrombotic complications but is associated with a higher fetal loss rate and can have damaging effects on the fetus (teratogenesis and fetotoxicity). Low molecular weight heparin is safe for the fetus, but doubts have been expressed about its efficacy in preventing maternal thrombotic complications. Factors such as the type and position of the mechanical valve, choice of anticoagulant regimen and patient compliance may all affect the rate of thrombosis.

Thrombotic complications, such as valve thrombosis, dysfunction or cerebrovascular accident (CVA), are the most common causes of maternal mortality and tend to occur antenatally. Serious haemorrhagic complications, such as intra-abdominal bleeding, secondary postpartum haemorrhage (PPH), wound haematoma and vaginal haematoma, are the most common cause of maternal morbidity occurring in the early postnatal period.

When bioprosthetic (tissue) valves are used for valve replacements, there is no need for long-term anticoagulation; however, the valve does deteriorate with time. Therefore, in a woman contemplating further pregnancies, a tissue valve is preferable to a mechanical prosthetic valve. Although it may subsequently need to be replaced, it will hopefully last until her family is complete. This should form part of any pre-pregnancy counselling.

28.5.1.4 Prophylaxis against Bacterial Endocarditis

National Institute for Health and Care Excellence (NICE) guidelines recommend that women at risk of infective endocarditis undergoing gynaecological and obstetric procedures do not require antibiotic prophylaxis regardless of the cardiac lesion. The strength of evidence on which this recommendation is based has been questioned [3].

28.5.2 Aortopathies

Aortopathy is a recognized feature of Marfan's syndrome, Ehlers–Danlos type IV, *ACTA2* mutation and Turner syndrome. Women with bicuspid aortic valves or those who have had a patent ductus arteriosus ligated are also at increased risk of aortic dissection.

Patients with Marfan's syndrome should have regular echocardiogram surveillance during pregnancy to detect any increase in the aortic root diameter.

In Marfan's syndrome the increased risk of aortic dissection associated with increasing aortic diameters in pregnancy has been well described. The risk of aortic dissection with an aortic root diameter less than 4 cm is 1%, whereas with a diameter of more than 4 cm the risk is 10%. The time of greatest risk is during labour and immediately postpartum when cardiac output is maximal. Hypertension increases the risk of dissection, thus the systolic blood pressure should be carefully monitored and controlled. Those with Ehlers–Danlos type IV are known to be at risk of aortic dissection even if the aortic root is of normal size. There is very little information on the risks associated with *ACTA2* mutation in pregnancy as this has only recently been described.

The diagnosis of aortic dissection should be considered in women with:

- Central chest pain, jaw pain or intrascapular pain – not all chest pain is due to pulmonary embolism
- Family history of aortic dissection (Marfan's and Ehlers–Danlos IV are autosomal dominant)
- Women with a known bicuspid aortic valve
- If there is uncontrolled hypertension or the blood pressure is significantly different in the two arms
- Women with unusual neurological symptoms, particularly in lower limbs or bowel

28.5.3 Cardiomyopathy

There are three different, principal types of cardiomyopathy seen in obstetric practice – peripartum, dilated and hypertrophic.

28.5.3.1 Peripartum Cardiomyopathy

Peripartum cardiomyopathy is a form of dilated cardiomyopathy and typically presents either as a woman approaches term or in the first few weeks after delivery, although it can occur up to five months postpartum. Whilst it is commoner in older, obese, black or hypertensive women, it can present in women with no risk factors who have previously been well. Unexplained breathlessness, tachycardia, gross oedema or supraventricular tachycardia should prompt a chest x-ray, ECG and echocardiography. Prior to delivery, peripartum cardiomyopathy can be treated with diuretics and beta blocking drugs, with ACE inhibitors being added after delivery. There is a high recurrence risk in future pregnancies, and women with cardiomyopathy should receive detailed preconceptual counselling prior to embarking on further pregnancies. Women whose ventricular function has returned to normal have approximately a 20% recurrence risk in future pregnancies, whilst those who do not achieve complete recovery of ventricular function have approximately a 50% recurrence risk in future pregnancies [6]. Serial echocardiography should therefore be performed to monitor ventricular function in women who have previously suffered from peripartum cardiomyopathy.

28.5.3.2 Dilated Cardiomyopathy

A dilated cardiomyopathy picture can be due to inherited, acquired (due to chemotherapy or ischaemia), peripartum or idiopathic causes. In pregnant women with a dilated cardiomyopathy, anticoagulation should be considered to prevent intracardiac thrombus formation. There should be a lower threshold for commencing anticoagulation during pregnancy, as pregnancy is a prothrombotic state. During pregnancy low molecular weight heparin should be used as warfarin is both teratogenic and fetotoxic. Beta-blockers and diuretics can be used, with the addition of ACE inhibitors or angiotensin receptor blockers (ARBs) in the postnatal period. Pro beta-natriuretic protein (proBNP) is a biomarker routinely used in the management of heart failure and can be measured serially to assess improvement or deterioration in heart function.

28.5.3.3 Hypertrophic Cardiomyopathy

Hypertrophic cardiomyopathy (HCM) is usually an autosomal dominant condition. There is thickening of the left ventricular wall, in particular the interventricular septum. Sometimes the thickening of the septum can cause obstruction to the left ventricular outflow tract, acting as a form of 'functional aortic stenosis' which worsens on exercise. Sometimes the ventricular hypertrophy results in a reduced ventricular volume, and hence a reduced stroke volume. Pregnancy outcome is usually good unless there is severe diastolic dysfunction, but cardiac output may be compromised by:

- Bleeding – therefore prevent/treat postpartum haemorrhage aggressively
- Tachycardia – therefore consider beta-blocking agents to prolong diastole and allow adequate ventricular filling, and ensure adequate analgesia in labour
- Vasodilation – therefore avoid nifedipine as a tocolytic
- Arrhythmias – therefore treat arrhythmia and consider anticoagulation
- Labour – if severe, caesarean section may be more appropriate

Women with inherited cardiomyopathy (dilated or hypertrophic) should be referred to a clinical geneticist to discuss the risks to the fetus, testing and follow-up.

28.5.4 Arrhythmias

Women are often more aware of ectopic beats in pregnancy, as well as a physiological increase in heart rate. Palpitations are

therefore a common symptom. Significant arrhythmias are rare, but can cause significant haemodynamic compromise.

28.5.4.1 History
Important features to ask about in the history are:
- Frequency of episodes
- Heart rhythm – is it regular or irregular?
- Length of time for which the palpitations occur – occasional extra beats or a sustained run?
- Associated syncope – requires referral for cardiology opinion
- Onset and offset – sudden onset and offset is more suggestive of arrhythmia
- Family history of sudden death
- Underlying medical problems (e.g. thyrotoxicosis or heart disease)

28.5.4.2 Investigations
- 12-lead ECG (ideally when an episode occurs)
- Thyroid function tests
- Haemoglobin
- 24-hour ECG (Holter monitoring) if palpitations are occurring sufficiently frequently to make this worthwhile
- Echocardiography and cardiology review for newly diagnosed arrhythmias in pregnancy to determine whether there is an underlying structural cardiac abnormality

28.5.4.3 Treatment
- Reassurance is sufficient for majority of women, where no significant arrhythmia is identified
- Pharmacological treatment
  o β-blockade
  o intravenous adenosine to terminate episodes of supraventricular tachycardia (this is safe for the fetus)
- Anticoagulation in women with atrial fibrillation
- DC cardioversion if unresponsive to medical therapy, or haemodynamic compromise

Women with pacemakers should be reviewed during pregnancy by a cardiologist, and have their pacemaker checked, but very few have problems in pregnancy. The main issue is battery longevity. Ideally, a generator change should be avoided in pregnancy, but sometimes this is unavoidable, and better performed if needed than the battery running out.

Intracardiac defibrillators can be deactivated by applying a magnet to the woman's chest, and reactivated by removing it. If women with intracardiac defibrillators have their device switched off around the time of delivery, it should be checked after it has been turned back on, prior to the woman's discharge from hospital.

Women with inherited arrhythmias (e.g. long QT syndrome) should be offered a consultation with a clinical geneticist to discuss follow-up and testing of the baby at an appropriate age.

28.5.4.4 Sudden Adult Death Syndrome (SADS) with a Morphologically Normal Heart (MNH)

This is increasingly being recognized as a cause of maternal death. The case definition for SADS is a sudden unexpected cardiac death (i.e. presumed fatal arrhythmia) where all other causes of sudden collapse are excluded, including a drug screen for stimulant drugs such as cocaine. Women with a family history of SADS, or relatives of a woman who had died suddenly should be screened for inherited cardiac conditions (e.g. long QT syndrome).

28.5.5 Ischaemic Heart Disease

The estimated incidence of non-fatal myocardial infarction in pregnancy has been estimated at 0.7 per 100 000 maternities [7], and 0.48 per 100 000 for maternal deaths from acute myocardial infarction or chronic ischaemic heart disease. The majority of women who suffer acute myocardial infarction or ischaemic heart disease have identifiable risk factors relating to lifestyle such as increased maternal age, obesity or smoking.

Failure to consider the diagnosis in women presenting with chest pain during pregnancy is common. Unlike some other cardiac enzymes (e.g. creatinine kinase-MB), troponin I remains within the normal range during labour and delivery. It can therefore be utilized in the diagnosis (or exclusion) of myocardial infarction during pregnancy and in the peripartum period. There should be a high index of suspicion for myocardial ischaemia or infarction, particularly if the woman is requiring opiate analgesia, and low threshold for further investigation including coronary angiography and percutaneous coronary intervention if appropriate. Although coronary artery dissection is rare in the non-pregnant population, it is a recognized complication of pregnancy and the puerperium. It can lead to coronary artery occlusion and myocardial infarction. The postpartum period is a time of particular risk.

28.5.6 Congenital Heart Disease

More women with congenital heart disease are now surviving until their childbearing years and are the group of women most commonly seen antenatally in a joint obstetric cardiac clinic. The biggest increase in survival has been seen in women with complex congenital heart disease. Since this group of women are known to healthcare services prior to pregnancy, there is an opportunity to offer preconceptual counselling for this group. Pre-pregnancy counselling should include a frank discussion of the risks involved in pregnancy to enable a woman to make an informed choice about whether to embark on pregnancy or not.

At the time of booking for antenatal care, it is important to define the lesion and determine what surgery has been done previously. Women with surgically corrected congenital heart disease are still at risk, as there may be residual uncorrected defects, or a predisposition to arrhythmias.

Those with complex congenital heart disease (e.g. pulmonary hypertension/Eisenmenger syndrome, cyanotic heart disease, Fontan circulation and transposition of the great arteries) are at highest risk of maternal and fetal complications [8].

There is still a significant risk of maternal mortality (approximately 25%) in women with pulmonary hypertension [9], and termination of pregnancy should be discussed and offered if women become unexpectedly pregnant [4].

Fetal echocardiography is indicated if either parent had congenital heart disease, as there is a 3–6% recurrence risk for the fetus.

Various scoring schemes have been used to try to predict the outcomes of pregnancy in women with congenital heart disease [10, 11]. Failure to increase heart rate during exercise testing appears to be associated with a poor fetal and maternal outcome [12].

28.5.6.1 Atrial Septal Defects and Patent Foramen Ovale

These are usually well tolerated. In view of the risk of paradoxical embolism to the systemic circulation, filters should be used on all intravenous infusions. Giving sets for electronic infusion pumps usually have filters built in.

28.5.6.2 Ventricular Septal Defects

Pregnancy is well tolerated in women with small or moderate ventricular septal defects (VSDs). Echocardiography should be performed to assess the load on the right side of the heart. A high-velocity jet across the ventricular septal defect shows that there is a significant pressure difference between the left and right sides of the heart, ruling out significant pulmonary hypertension.

If a large VSD, or right ventricular loading, is found prior to pregnancy, it is sensible to consider cardiac investigations with a view to closure (surgical or interventional) to prevent pulmonary hypertension developing.

Filters should be used on intravenous infusion lines to prevent paradoxical embolism.

28.5.6.3 Patent Ductus Arteriosus (PDA)

Pregnancy is well tolerated in women with a patent ductus arteriosus (PDA) and a left-to-right shunt. In women with a clinically evident PDA, this should be closed prior to pregnancy.

28.5.6.4 Tetralogy of Fallot

The four features which make up the tetralogy of Fallot are:

- Ventricular septal defect
- Pulmonary artery stenosis
- Overriding aorta
- Right ventricular hypertrophy.

Approximately 15% of women with tetralogy of Fallot have a deletion of chromosome 22q11. This increases the chance of the fetus also having congenital heart disease.

The most common situation encountered antenatally is where a woman has already had corrective surgery. Pregnancy is well tolerated in women who have had a repair of tetralogy of Fallot, as long as ventricular function is good and there is no significant right ventricular outflow tract obstruction. Many women have significant pulmonary regurgitation and may become more tired and breathless as pregnancy progresses, occasionally needing diuretic treatment or admission for observation.

28.5.6.5 Transposition of the Great Arteries (TGA)

Two different types of surgery have been used to correct congenital transposition of the great arteries (TGA). The operation which was developed first was an atrial switch procedure, and generally older women will have had this type of operation (Mustard or Senning procedure). Younger women may have had an arterial switch procedure. It is important to clarify which type of procedure the woman underwent, as they have different implications for the management during pregnancy.

Atrial Switch Procedures (Mustard or Senning procedure)

Following this operation, the right ventricle supplies the systemic circulation and the left ventricle supplies the lungs. With the increased cardiac output in pregnancy, right (systemic) ventricular function may decline. These women should be monitored for signs of ventricular failure and arrhythmias. Monitoring of heart function should continue into the postnatal period with close attention being paid to systemic (morphological right) ventricular function.

Arterial Switch Procedures

In this operation, the great arteries are switched round so that the left ventricle supplies the systemic circulation, and the right ventricle the pulmonary circulation as in the normal anatomical arrangement. This operation is a newer treatment; women tend to be younger, and there are fewer data about possible complications in pregnancy. Heart function is usually preserved as the left ventricle is the systemic ventricle.

28.5.6.6 Univentricular Heart – Fontan Circulation

A Fontan type procedure is a surgical operation that is required when the only way of correcting the heart is to change the circulation to a univentricular mode of circulation. Surgery is required in cases such as hypoplastic right heart or tricuspid atresia. The systemic venous return is diverted directly to the pulmonary arteries and it does not go through the right ventricle. From the lungs, the blood comes back to the left side of the heart and the left side of the heart pumps it around the body. One ventricle is doing all the work, pumping the blood around the systemic and pulmonary circulations. In pregnancy, the single ventricle has to cope with the increased volume load. Women with a Fontan circulation can, therefore, have problems with heart failure in pregnancy. Arrhythmias may also be problematic.

Since the blood is flowing slowly by the time it gets to the lungs, there is an increased thrombotic risk. Often, women with Fontan circulations are anticoagulated. If the woman becomes hypotensive, blood pressure may not be sufficient to maintain the circulation of blood through the body and then through the lungs. Cyanosis may develop quickly.

Women who themselves have had a Fontan repair have a 30% fetal loss rate in pregnancy. Many require premature delivery (Figure 28.4).

28.6 Key Messages

- Cardiac output increases significantly in pregnancy. Women with cardiac disease may be unable to tolerate this demand, and may decompensate.
- Cardiac disease is the commonest cause of maternal death with the majority of maternal deaths due to acquired heart disease, not congenital heart disease.

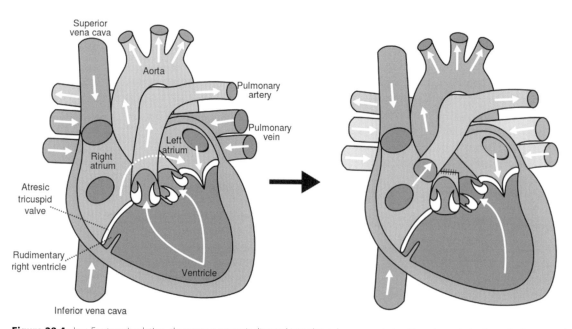

Figure 28.4 In a Fontan circulation, the venous return is directed into the pulmonary arteries. Flow through the lungs is slower, and systemic hypotension can compromise the venous return and therefore pulmonary blood flow.

- Pregnant women with known cardiac disease should be referred for consultant-led obstetric care with involvement of a cardiologist with expertise in the care of women with heart disease in pregnancy.
- There should be a low threshold for early referral to a cardiologist of women with symptoms which could represent cardiac disease.
- If an acute coronary syndrome is suspected in a pregnant woman, she should be investigated, managed and treated in the same way it would be if the woman were not pregnant. Investigations and treatment should not be withheld simply because the woman is pregnant.
- Resuscitation training should include training on how to modify resuscitation techniques for a pregnant woman.
- In pregnancy, stenotic valves are associated with a higher risk than regurgitant valves.
- Pregnant women with mechanical prosthetic valves are at very high risk during pregnancy.
- The number of women with congenital heart disease surviving to their childbearing years is increasing.
- All women with congenital heart disease should be offered preconceptual counselling.
- There is a wide spectrum of congenital heart disease, and therefore some women have minimal increase in risk, whereas others are at very high risk. All should be reassessed in a joint obstetric cardiology clinic.
- Increased vigilance is required in the postnatal period for women who have heart disease in pregnancy, as this is when deterioration can occur, and when the majority of deaths occur.

28.7 Key Guidelines Relevant to the Topic

The Task Force for the Management of Cardiovascular Diseases during Pregnancy of the European Society of Cardiology (ESC) 2018. ESC Guidelines for the management of cardiovascular diseases during pregnancy. *Eur Heart J.* 2018;**39**(34):3165–241. https://doi.org/10.1093/eurheartj/ehy340 [2]

National Institute for Health and Care Excellence. *Antimicrobial Prophylaxis Against Infective Endocarditis: In Adults and Children Undergoing Interventional Procedures.* Clinical Guideline 64. London: NICE; 2008. [2]

National Institute for Health and Care Excellence. *Hypertension in Pregnancy: Diagnosis and Management.* NICE Guideline CG107. London: NICE; 2010. [13]

Faculty of Sexual and Reproductive Healthcare. *Clinical Guideline: Contraceptive Choices for Women with Cardiac Disease.* London: FSRH; 2014. [3]

References

1. The Task Force for the Management of Cardiovascular Diseases during Pregnancy of the European Society of Cardiology (ESC). ESC Guidelines for the management of cardiovascular diseases during pregnancy. *Eur Heart J.* 2018;**39**(34):3165–241. https://doi.org/10.1093/eurheartj/ehy340

2. National Institute for Health and Care Excellence. *Antimicrobial Prophylaxis Against Infective Endocarditis: In Adults and Children Undergoing Interventional Procedures.* Clinical Guideline 64. London: NICE; 2008.

3. FSRH Clinical Effectiveness Unit (CEU). *FSRH Clinical Guideline: Contraceptive Choices for Women with Cardiac Disease.* London: FSRH; June 2014, www.fsrh.org/standards-and-guidance/documents/ceu-guidance-contraceptive-choices-for-women-with-cardiac/

4. Bedard E, Dimopoulos K, Gatzoulis MA. Has there been any progress made on pregnancy outcomes among women with pulmonary arterial hypertension? *Eur Heart J.* 2009;**30**:256–65.

5. Drenthen W, Boersma E, Balci A, on behalf of the ZAHARA Investigators. Predictors of pregnancy complications in women with congenital heart disease. *Eur Heart J.* 2007;**31**(17):2124–32.

6. Drenthen W, Pieper PG, Roos-Hesselink JW, on behalf of the ZAHARA Investigators. Outcome of pregnancy in women with congenital heart disease: A literature review. *J Am Coll Cardiol.* 2010;**49**:2303–11.

7. Elkayam U, Tummala PP, Rao K. Maternal and fetal outcomes of subsequent pregnancies in women with peripartum cardiomyopathy. *N Engl J Med.* 2001;**344**(21):1567–71.

8. Knight M, Nair M, Tuffnell D, et al. eds., on behalf of MBRRACE-UK. *Saving Lives, Improving Mothers' Care – Surveillance of Maternal Deaths in the UK 2012–14 and Lessons Learned to Inform Maternity Care from the UK and Ireland Confidential Enquiries into Maternal Deaths and Morbidity 2009–14.* Oxford: National Perinatal Epidemiology Unit, University of Oxford; 2016.

9. Knight M, Bunch K, Tuffnell D, et al. eds., on behalf of MBRRACE-UK. *Saving Lives, Improving Mothers' Care – Lessons Learned to Inform Maternity Care from the UK and Ireland Confidential Enquiries into Maternal Deaths and Morbidity 2014–16.* Oxford: National Perinatal Epidemiology Unit, University of Oxford; 2018.

10. Lui GK, Silversides CK, Khairy P, for the Alliance for Adult Research in Congenital Cardiology (AARCC). Heart rate response during exercise and pregnancy outcome in women with congenital heart disease. *Circulation.* 2011;**123**: 242–8.

11. Siu SC, Sermer M, Colman JM, et al. Prospective multicenter study of pregnancy outcomes in women with heart disease. *Circulation.* 2001;**104**:515–21.

12. Vause S, Clarke B, Tower CL, Hay C, Knight M. Pregnancy outcomes in women with mechanical prosthetic heart valves: a prospective population based study using the United Kingdom Obstetric Surveillance System (UKOSS) data collection system. *BJOG.* 2017;**124**:1411–19.

13. National Institute for Health and Care Excellence. *Hypertension in Pregnancy: Diagnosis and Management.* Clinical Guideline CG107. London: NICE; 2010.

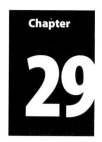

Respiratory Disease in Pregnancy

Katharine Rankin & Tahir A. Mahmood

29.1 Introduction

During the course of a normal pregnancy, the respiratory system undergoes both physiological and anatomical changes. These changes can predispose to the development of acute respiratory conditions; they can also affect the natural history of chronic pulmonary disease. Conversely, poorly controlled chronic pulmonary conditions can adversely affect the progress of pregnancy [1].

29.1.1 Anatomy

During pregnancy, progressive uterine distension causes lung volume and chest wall changes [2]. The function of the diaphragm and chest wall musculature appears to be unaffected in pregnancy [3]; however, the gravid uterus can cause the diaphragm to be elevated by up to 4 cm [2]. This results in a shorter chest height and a decrease in residual volume and expiratory reserve volume – thus resulting in a decreased functional residual capacity (FRC). By term, FRC can be reduced by up to 10–20% [3]. However, other thoracic dimensions increase in order to maintain constant total lung capacity [4, 5]: the subcostal angle widens as the transverse diameter of the thoracic cage increases by approximately 2 cm and thoracic circumference increases by around 6 cm [6].

Large airway function is unimpaired in normal pregnancy and therefore spirometry remains within normal limits: forced vital capacity (FVC), forced expiratory volume in 1 second (FEV1) and peak expiratory flow do not change significantly [2].

29.1.2 Physiology

Changes in respiratory physiology in pregnancy are due to an alteration in hormonal patterns and begin early in pregnancy. They are mainly mediated by oestrogen and progesterone, both of which gradually increase during pregnancy [2].

Increased levels of circulating oestrogen in pregnancy cause an increase in the number and sensitivity of progesterone receptors within the central neuronal respiratory-related areas in the hypothalamus and medulla [3].

Progesterone is thought to directly stimulate the primary respiratory centre and increase the sensitivity of the respiratory centre to carbon dioxide [3].This results in an increase in minute ventilation by 40–50% in pregnancy [7].This increase is mostly due to an increase in tidal volume, rather than in respiratory rate, which remains essentially unaffected [8]. Pregnant women therefore increase their ventilation by

breathing more deeply, rather than more quickly. Some women are aware of this physiological hyperventilation and this can lead to a subjective feeling of breathlessness. Up to three quarters of pregnant women are aware of this at some point during the course of their pregnancy [7]. It can occur even in early pregnancy [9].

This physiological hyperventilation results in a decrease in arterial and alveolar carbon dioxide pressure. This respiratory alkalosis is compensated by an increase in the renal excretion of bicarbonate. Thus arterial blood gases in normal women in pregnancy show a decreased partial pressure of carbon dioxide (PCO_2 26–30 mm Hg) and a slightly increased oxygen tension (PO_2 101–106 mm Hg) and a normal or slightly elevated pH (7.42–7.46) [8].

29.2 Asthma

Asthma is a common chronic inflammatory condition of the lung airways characterized by episodes of reversible bronchoconstriction [10]. It affects up to 8% of woman of childbearing age [11, 12] and is probably one of the most common chronic medical conditions encountered in pregnant women [13].

29.2.1 Diagnosis

Clinical diagnosis of asthma is based on the presence of symptoms and evidence of variable airflow obstruction [10]. Features of asthma include wheeze, breathlessness, chest tightness and cough. Symptoms are often worse at night and in the early morning; in response to exercise, cold air or allergen exposure; and after taking aspirin or beta-blockers. There is often an associated personal or family history of atopy. On examination, a widespread wheeze may be heard on chest auscultation. Investigation results which point to a diagnosis of asthma include an otherwise unexplained low FEV1 or peak expiratory flow (PEF) or an unexplained peripheral blood eosinophilia [14].

Diagnosis is confirmed by evidence of reversible airflow obstruction. Spirometry is preferable to measurement of PEF because it allows clearer identification of airflow obstruction and the results are less dependent on effort [14].

29.2.2 Effects of Asthma on Pregnancy

Maternal asthma has been associated with an increased risk of pregnancy complications. Rejno et al (2014) published a recent, large, prospective population-based study of pregnancy complications and adverse perinatal outcomes [15].

They found significant associations between maternal asthma and pre-eclampsia or eclampsia, haemorrhage and premature contractions and late preterm birth (32–36 weeks). They also found significant associations with emergency caesarean sections, low birthweight and small-for-gestational-age babies. Importantly, the relative risks of some adverse outcomes were reduced to non-significant by active asthma management (preterm labour and preterm delivery) [16].

29.2.3   Effects of Pregnancy on Asthma

In 1988, Schatz et al (1988) studied the clinical course of 366 pregnancies complicated by maternal asthma. They found that asthma improved in 28%, remained unchanged in 33% and worsened in 35% [17]. This seminal paper formed the basis of the widely quoted approximate rule of thirds and was subsequently supported by the conclusions of a meta-analysis including 14 studies [18]. However, a more recent cohort study by Grosso et al (2018) suggests that the percentage of women who have worsening asthma in pregnancy may have reduced [19], perhaps suggesting an important evolution in the understanding of asthma and important aspects of asthma care in pregnancy over the intervening 20 years.

While the mechanisms of the effects of pregnancy on asthma remain unclear, the effect of pregnancy tends to be consistent throughout successive gestations. This suggests that the changes observed are not solely due to fluctuations in the natural course of the disease [20].

If symptoms do worsen in pregnancy, this is most likely to be in the second and third trimesters [20]. Risk factors for exacerbation of asthma during pregnancy include difficult-to-control asthma pre-pregnancy and upper respiratory viral infections. Exacerbations are also noted to be more common and more severe in current smokers [13]. Other possible risk factors include obesity and African American ethnicity. Importantly, non-adherence with medication during pregnancy has also been demonstrated to be associated with an increased risk of acute exacerbations [13].

29.2.4   Management

29.2.4.1   Avoidance of Allergens/Triggers

Current emphasis in the management of asthma is on the prevention of, rather than the treatment of, acute attacks. Allergen and trigger avoidance should be discussed when atopy is also present [10]. Women who smoke should be offered appropriate support to stop.

29.2.4.2   Drug Therapy

Drug therapy in pregnancy is essentially the same as for the non-pregnant population. Globally, asthma guidelines strongly recommend that women continue their asthma medications during pregnancy. However, adherence to asthma medications during pregnancy can be a significant problem. Over one third of women have been shown to discontinue their asthma medications during pregnancy [21]. Women have also been shown to decrease their inhaled corticosteroid therapy

and are more reliant on their preventive therapy [22]. This highlights the imperative importance of clear communication between asthmatic women and the healthcare professionals looking after them in the perinatal period.

29.2.4.3   Chronic Asthma

Management of chronic asthma should follow the stepwise approach recommended by the British Thoracic Society guidelines on the management of asthma [14]. Mild intermittent asthma is managed with inhaled, short-acting β2-agonist medication as required. If usage of this exceeds more than once a day regular inhaled steroid should be commenced (200–800 micrograms/day). The next step is either the addition of a long-acting β2-agonist or an increase in the dose of inhaled steroid. Further steps involve a trial of additional therapies e.g. leukotriene receptor antagonists or slow release oral theophylline or an oral β2-agonist. If these measures fail to achieve adequate control, the continuous use of oral steroids may become necessary.

There is extensive evidence to show that steroid tablets are not teratogenic. Some studies have found an association between steroid use and pregnancy-induced hypertension, pre-eclampsia, preterm labour and intrauterine growth restriction. However, severe asthma is likely to confound these associations [23]. There has been a slight concern regarding an association with oral clefts; however, this association is by no means definite and the benefits of treatment to the mother and fetus in treating or preventing worsening asthma justify the use of oral steroids in pregnancy [20].

Drug safety evidence regarding leukotriene receptor antagonists is more limited. However, no evidence has been found of an increased risk of major malformations between women exposed to these drugs and women exposed to β2-agonists only [20].

29.2.4.4   Acute Asthma

Acute asthma attacks should be managed vigorously in pregnant women. They should be managed as per the non-pregnant population, with a low threshold for admission [10].

The features of acute severe asthma include: PEF rate (PEFR) 33–50% of best/predicted; respiratory rate >25/minute; heart rate >100 beats per minute (bpm); inability to complete sentences. Features of life-threatening asthma include PEFR <33% of best/predicted SpO$_2$ <92%, PaO$_2$ <8 kPa with normal PaCO$_2$, silent chest, cyanosis, feeble respiratory effort, hypotension and altered consciousness [14].

High flow oxygen should be given to maintain saturations of 94–98%. Intravenous (IV) rehydration should be commenced. High-dose inhaled β2-agonists should be given via oxygen-driven nebulizer. Nebulized ipratropium bromide (0.5 mg 4–6 hourly) should be added if there is a poor response or if there are any features of acute severe asthma. Systemic corticosteroids should be given in all cases for at least 5 days or until recovery (IV hydrocortisone 100 mg and/or oral prednisolone 40–50 mg daily). Other therapies which can be considered include intravenous magnesium sulphate, IV inhaled β2-agonist or IV aminophylline. Routine antibiotics are not recommended [14].

29.2.4.5 Labour and Delivery

Asthma exacerbations are uncommon in labour due to endogenous steroid production. Patients should continue their usual medical therapy during labour. If women do experience symptoms, these are usually controlled by inhaled β2-agonists. If they respond poorly, intravenous methylprednisolone should be administered [21].

In women receiving oral steroids, there is a theoretical risk of maternal hypothalamic-pituitary-adrenal (HPA) axis suppression: these women should therefore receive supplemental glucocorticoids during labour to cover for the stress of labour [21].

29.2.4.6 Drugs to Avoid

Many medications used for obstetric indications should be avoided in patients with asthma due to the risk of triggering bronchospasm. These include non-selective β-adrenergic blockers (e.g. labetalol), 15-methylprostaglandin F2α (e.g. carboprost) and nonsteroidal anti-inflammatory drugs (NSAIDs) in women with aspirin-sensitive asthma. Use of prostaglandin E2 gel or suppositories for cervical ripening or labour induction has not been reported to cause clinical exacerbations in asthmatic patients [10].

29.2.4.7 Breastfeeding

Women with asthma should be encouraged to breastfeed and to use their asthma medications as normal. None of the medicines used to treat asthma is contraindicated in breastfeeding [23].

29.3 Cystic Fibrosis

Cystic fibrosis (CF) is a common inherited autosomal recessive disorder resulting from mutations in the CF transmembrane conductance regulator (*CFTR*) gene on chromosome 7 [24]. This leads to abnormalities of the cystic fibrosis transmembrane chloride channel in epithelial cells [10], causing impaired movement of water and electrolytes across epithelial surfaces. This leads to thickened mucus and increased sweat sodium levels. In the lungs, the condition is characterized by viscous mucus that becomes chronically colonized with various organisms, leading to recurrent respiratory infections. Chronic inflammation leads to progressive bronchiectasis and declining respiratory function. Bowel, pancreatic and hepatobiliary organs are also affected, resulting in impaired digestion, reduced absorption, steatorrhoea and malnutrition, which may be further complicated by pancreatic insufficiency and biliary cirrhosis [25].

29.3.1 Effect on Fertility

There is little evidence that CF compromises female fertility. However, some literature hypothesizes that the composition of cervical mucus may be altered, and severely unwell women with a reduced body mass index may be anovulatory [26].

The first successful delivery of a baby in a woman with CF was reported in 1960 [27]. Advancements in the understanding and clinical management of CF have led to a progressive

increase in life expectancy – with a predicted survival of greater than 50 years in women born in the twenty-first century [28]. As a result, pregnancy in CF patients is becoming increasingly common [29]. Whilst pregnancy can be well-tolerated in patients with CF, the additional physiological demands of pregnancy can also lead to deterioration in maternal condition and detrimental effects of fetal health [30].

29.3.2 Genetic Counselling

If the carrier status of the father is unknown, the risk of a baby of a woman with CF being affected is 2–2.5%, based on a carrier frequency of 1 in 25 Caucasians. Screening panels need to include mutations common in people of the partner's ethnic background [24]. A negative result reduces the likelihood that the baby will have CF; however, CF does remain possible as screening is limited and the number of identified *CFTR* mutations now exceeds 1700 [31]. If the father is heterozygous for the gene, the risk of an affected child is 50%.

29.3.3 Effect of CF on Pregnancy

The most frequently encountered adverse fetal outcome is preterm delivery: 10–25% of babies are born before 37 weeks' gestation. Increased rates of low birthweight have been reported in some series, but not in all. Rates of congenital malformation do not appear to be increased and Apgar scores appear to be normal. Short-term neurological and cognitive development appears to be normal. However, subtle sequelae have not been thoroughly investigated [24]. In some reports, caesarean section is more common in women with an FEV1 less than 60% of predicted, although not in others.

29.3.4 Effect of Pregnancy on CF

Pregnancy does not appear to influence the long-term course of the disease. Maternal mortality is no greater than non-pregnant age-matched women with CF except in the presence of pulmonary hypertension, cyanosis, arterial hypoxaemia, moderate/severe lung disease (FEV1 <60% predicted) and/or malnutrition.

The main maternal morbidities in pregnancy include poor maternal weight gain; infective pulmonary exacerbations; congestive cardiac failure; and deterioration in lung function with worsening dyspnoea, exercise tolerance and oxygen saturation. Whilst there is often loss of lung function during pregnancy, this is regained following delivery.

29.3.5 Pregnancy in CF Post–Lung Transplantation

Survival rates following lung transplantation in patients with CF are progressively improving. The median survival rate is 7.5 years with 40% of patients surviving 10 years or more [24]. The long-term effect of pregnancy on lung allograft function has not been systematically explored. A case series published by Gyi et al in 2006 reported on 10 pregnancies in CF lung transplant recipients. They demonstrated the successful pregnancy post-transplant was feasible. There were nine livebirths and one therapeutic abortion. Five of the nine births were premature, three developed rejection during pregnancy and four women died within 38 months of delivery [32]. Pregnancy post–lung transplantation is therefore still considered high risk and requires detailed discussion between the obstetric, CF and transplant teams. Preparation is particularly important so that decisions regarding immunosuppressive medication can be considered.

29.3.6 Management

Women with mild disease may be reassured that pregnancy is usually safe. For more severe cases, liaison between a CF centre and obstetrician with a specialist interest should be planned. The presence of pulmonary hypertension, cor pulmonale or FEV1 <30–40% are contraindications to pregnancy. Colonization with *Burkholderia cepacia* may be associated with rapid deterioration in lung function. Recent acquisition or declining lung function in the presence of this organism may also be a contraindication to pregnancy – although no consensus exists [33].

29.3.6.1 Medication

Despite requirements for extensive drug therapy, excess fetal malformations have not been demonstrated. However, some commonly prescribed medications should be used with caution (e.g. ciprofloxacin, which has been associated with arthropathy in animal studies). Consensus guidelines outside pregnancy for patients chronically infected with *Pseudomonas* species include parenteral beta-lactam antibiotics in combination with an aminoglycoside. However, aminoglycosides have demonstrated selective uptake in fetal kidneys and have been associated with eighth cranial nerve damage after in utero exposure. Their use is often avoided; however, a risk/benefit analysis should be considered in a deteriorating mother. With tetracycline, there is a risk of discoloration of the child's teeth. Trimethoprim-sulfonamide combinations have been associated with several major malformations such as neural tube defects.

29.3.6.2 Nutrition

Impaired pre-pregnancy nutritional status is a significant risk factor for suboptimal maternal and fetal outcomes. In general, a pre-pregnancy BMI of $\geq$22 kg/m^2 is recommended [34] and pregnancy approached with caution if BMI is $\leq$18 kg/m^2 [24]. Pregnancy increases nutritional demands by approximately 300 kcal/day [35]. Many women with CF may struggle to meet this increased requirement and often struggle to gain weight. During pregnancy, the recommendation is for mothers to eat 120–150% of the non-CF age- and sex-matched patients [24]. They should aim for a weight gain of 11–12 kg [36]. Most patients with CF have pancreatic insufficiency, leading to malabsorption of fat-soluble vitamins A, D, E and K and require supplementation. Vitamin A supplementation is usually contraindicated in pregnancy due to concerns regarding teratogenicity; however, deficiency may be associated with increased risk of anaemia and infection [24]. If supplementation is required, a daily intake of less than 10 000 units is recommended [24]. Prothrombin time should also be checked regularly and parenteral vitamin K administered if prothrombin time is elevated [36].

29.3.6.3 Surveillance for Gestational Diabetes

A glucose tolerance test is recommended during each trimester in women with CF who do not have a diagnosis of CF-related diabetes (CFRD). In women who do have CFRD, insulin is the treatment of choice and is often required in women who develop CF-related gestational diabetes[34].

29.3.6.4 Labour and Delivery

In most cases, women with CF deliver vaginally at term [7]. However, optimal timing of delivery should be discussed in women with significant compromise of their respiratory function in the latter stages of pregnancy [33].

Caesarean section is necessary only for obstetric indications [7], and general anaesthesia should be avoided if possible to minimize the risk of atelectasis and retained secretions [33]. Low-dose epidural analgesia is recommended to provide high-quality pain relief and reduce cardiovascular and respiratory work in labour. Nitrous oxide may be complicated by gas trapping and barotrauma [34]. Patients with CF are particularly prone to pneumothoraces; this may be precipitated by repeated Valsalva manoeuvres. There may be a place for electing to shorten the second stage [34].

29.3.6.5 Breastfeeding

Breastfeeding should usually be encouraged although the mother may need to continue nutritional supplementation in the puerperium. However, exclusive breastfeeding may not be possible due the increased nutritional demand [37]. Analysis of breast milk of women with CF has shown a normal content of sodium and protein [38].

29.4 Sarcoidosis

Sarcoidosis is characterized by non-caseating epithelioid granulomas. These can affect any organ system and the clinical presentation is, therefore, variable. Most commonly, it involves granuloma formation in the lungs. The course of sarcoidosis can range from a self-limited acute disease to a chronic debilitating disease. Spontaneous remissions occur in nearly two thirds of patients; however, 10–30% of patients have a chronic progressive course [10]. Data on sarcoidosis in pregnancy are sparse and appear to be limited to case reports.

29.4.1 Effect of Sarcoidosis on Pregnancy

There is little evidence that sarcoidosis adversely affects pregnancy. However, in 2015 Hadid et al presented data on obstetric outcomes in a population-based cohort in the United States. They found that women with sarcoidosis were more likely to have pre-eclampsia, eclampsia, thromboembolism and premature delivery. There was also an increased risk of caesarean delivery and postpartum haemorrhage [39].

29.4.2 Effect of Pregnancy on Sarcoidosis

Sarcoidosis tends to improve or remain the same in pregnancy; however, there is a tendency to relapse in the puerperium. Factors indicating a poor prognosis include parenchymal lesions on chest x-ray, advanced radiographic staging, advanced maternal age, requirement for drugs other than steroids and presence of extra-pulmonary sarcoidosis [10].

29.4.3 Management

Ideally, patients should be evaluated pre-pregnancy to establish baseline pulmonary function, inflammatory activity, chronicity, staging and response to treatment. Systemic steroids should be continued during pregnancy; intravenous hydrocortisone should be administered in labour to women taking more than 7.5 mg of prednisolone daily. Angiotensin-converting enzyme levels are used as a marker of disease activity outside of pregnancy – however, these are unreliable in pregnancy. Hypercalciuria with or without hypercalcaemia is a well-known complication of sarcoidosis [40]. The pathogenesis of this is incompletely understood; however, pregnant women with sarcoidosis should be advised to avoid vitamin D because of the risk of hypercalcaemia [10].

29.5 Severe Restrictive Lung Disease

Restrictive ventilatory defects are characterized by a reduction in lung volumes and an increase in the ratio FEV1 to forced vital capacity (FVC). This occurs when lung expansion is limited and can be the result of abnormalities in the pleura (e.g. interstitial lung disease) or chest wall (e.g. kyphoscoliosis) or a neuromuscular abnormality [10]. Interstitial lung disease is a relatively uncommon cause of restrictive lung disease in pregnancy because most of these conditions have a point of onset after the reproductive years.

29.5.1 Effect of Pregnancy on Restrictive Lung Disease

The increased ventilatory requirement in pregnancy may be problematic in women with pre-existing restrictive pulmonary disease. Restrictive disease may limit the ability of pregnant women to increase her minute ventilation resulting in an increased risk of hypercapnic respiratory failure. The effects of mild to moderate hypercapnia in pregnancy are unclear; limited data from animal studies suggest that it may induce vigorous respiratory movements in the fetus thereby increasing their oxygen consumption [41].

29.5.2 Effect of Restrictive Lung Disease on Pregnancy

Interstitial lung disease may affect gas exchange and oxygenation – potentially putting the fetus at risk of hypoxia [42]. Kyphoscoliosis may be associated with pelvic abnormalities which impede normal delivery or predispose to malpresentation and significantly affect the ability to provide adequate epidural or spinal anaesthesia [10].

Some case series have reported on small numbers of women with restrictive lung disease with good outcomes [43]. However, some literature suggests that women with severe restrictive lung disease – defined as an FVC <1.0 litre – should be counselled to avoid pregnancy because of the increased maternal risk [44].

Recent data on this subject are sparse and generally limited to small case series. In 2014, Lapinsky et al published a retrospective review of 12 women with restrictive lung disease who undertook 15 pregnancies. They found that severe reduction in FVC may be tolerated in pregnancy. Three women went into spontaneous labour. The remaining 12 were induced or underwent elective caesarean section. The women with parenchymal lung disease underwent vaginal delivery with epidural anaesthesia – with the exception of one patient who required a caesarean section for pre-eclampsia. Among the women with chest wall or neuromuscular disease, all except one were delivered by caesarean section. In 50% of these deliveries, regional anaesthesia was not considered possible or failed, and these patients therefore required general anaesthesia.

Nine pregnancies were delivered preterm in the range of 31 to 36 weeks of gestation. Eleven of the 15 babies required high dependency support. However, there was no maternal or neonatal mortality – all survived to hospital discharge. Respiratory support was needed by five patients during labour and in the immediate postpartum period. Unfortunately, there was no comment on birthweight in this case series and no mention of other specific complications (e.g. postpartum haemorrhage) [42].

29.5.3 Management

A multidisciplinary approach is important to the management of these women – with shared care between obstetric and respiratory teams and involvement of anaesthetic colleagues [42]. Each case should be assessed and managed individually. Baseline lung function tests should be carried out as well as echocardiography to exclude pulmonary hypertension (mean pulmonary artery pressure of >25 mm Hg at rest). Lastly, it should be remembered that women with restrictive lung disease and associated polycythaemia are at an additional risk of thromboembolism [10] and consideration should be given to antenatal and postnatal prophylaxis.

29.6 Respiratory Infections

Pneumonia occurs in the pregnant population with the same frequency as in the general population. However, there is an increased risk of serious maternal complications, including respiratory failure and mortality. The spectrum of pathogens is similar in the pregnant population, and management is the same. Severe pneumonia can precipitate preterm delivery and also result in low birthweight infants [10].

29.6.1 Bacterial Pneumonia

Community-acquired pneumonia is most commonly caused by *Streptococcus pneumoniae*, *Haemophilus influenzae* and *Mycoplasma pneumoniae*. Women present with cough, fever, rigors, breathlessness and pleuritic pain. Signs include fever, purulent sputum, coarse crackles on auscultation and signs of lung consolidation. Diagnosis may be confirmed by chest x-ray; however, radiographic changes tend to lag behind the clinical signs. Bacterial pneumonia is associated with a rise in white cell count – although mycoplasma is not.

The mainstay of treatment is antibiotic therapy. Beta-lactam and macrolide antibiotics are safe in pregnancy, and amoxicillin and clarithromycin are current recommended treatment options for community-acquired pneumonia. Note that tetracyclines cause discolouration of the teeth of the fetus and should be avoided after 20 weeks of gestation. Supportive measures include oxygen therapy and intravenous rehydration. Chest physiotherapy will help clear secretions and aid oxygenation.

29.6.1.1 Pneumocystis Pneumonia (in association with HIV)

This is the most common opportunistic infection seen in patients progressing to acquired immune deficiency syndrome (AIDS). It should be suspected in the presence of profound hypoxia which is out of proportion to chest x-ray findings and bronchoscopy should be considered. Treatment is with high-dose cotrimoxazole – which is usually contraindicated in pregnancy because of the theoretical risks of neonatal kernicterus or haemolysis.

29.6.2 Influenza

Seasonal influenza epidemics and previous influenza pandemics have shown that pregnant women are generally at higher risk for influenza-associated morbidity and mortality. Influenza vaccinations can reduce the risk of hospitalization among pregnant women during influenza season and are not contraindicated in pregnancy. Oseltamivir should ideally be started within 48 hours of onset of symptoms.

29.6.2.1 Varicella Pneumonia

Varicella pneumonia can result in up to 10% of pregnant women with chickenpox. Severity of infection increases along with gestation. With antiviral therapy the mortality rates have fallen to 3–14%; however, it remains a very morbid infection. Between 1985 and 2005, there were nine indirect and one late maternal deaths reported in the UK as a result of maternal varicella pneumonia. Whilst the case fatality rate remains low, it is still five times that in the non-pregnant adult.

Women who develop chickenpox during pregnancy should be treated with aciclovir as per Royal College of Obstetricians and Gynaecologists guidelines. They should be referred immediately to hospital if they have signs of severity including chest or neurological symptoms; haemorrhagic rash or bleeding; and a dense rash or mucosal lesions. The use of IV aciclovir is felt to be justified due to the potential maternal and neonatal morbidity and mortality associated with chickenpox in pregnancy. Delivery during the viraemic period poses increased risk of bleeding, thrombocytopenia, disseminated intravascular coagulation, hepatitis and fetal varicella transmission and should be avoided if possible.

29.6.3 Tuberculosis (TB)

Globally, tuberculosis (TB) is one of the leading causes of death in women of reproductive age [45], and it is estimated that worldwide as many as 216 500 pregnant women have active TB [46]. *Mycobacterium tuberculosis* characteristically causes caseating granulomas [10]. Pulmonary TB is the most common manifestation of the disease and may present with cough, haemoptysis, weight loss and night sweats, although extrapulmonary manifestations also occur. Sputum microscopy for acid-fast bacilli (Ziehl–Neelsen stain), sputum (or tissue) culture and chest radiography are the mainstays of diagnosis. The minimum incidence estimate is 4.2 per 100 000 maternities in the UK – where the disease appears to be limited to ethnic minorities and is most common amongst recent immigrants [47].

Data regarding the relationship between active tuberculosis and pregnancy outcomes have been conflicting. In 2017, Sobhy et al published a rigorous systematic review and meta-analysis which found that maternal and perinatal outcomes were consistently poorer for women with active TB. There were increased odds of maternal morbidity, anaemia, perinatal death, preterm birth, low birthweight and fetal distress [48]. Better outcomes were found when treatment was initiated in the first trimester when compared to treatment initiated in the second or third trimester – thus highlighting the importance of having a high index of suspicion in women at risk of TB and rapid treatment.

Mother-to-child transmission of TB is rare; however, it may occur in utero through haematogenous spread via the umbilical vein or swallowing of infected amniotic fluid. Intrapartum, it can be transmitted via infected amniotic fluid or genital secretions, and postpartum infection may occur through aerosol spread. Symptoms of congenital TB are typically seen in the second and third weeks of life [48].

The World Health Organization recommends the treatment of TB in pregnant women should be the same as that in non-pregnant adults; the only notable exception to this is streptomycin, which should be avoided in pregnancy due to the risk of fetal ototoxicity [49]. The standard treatment is rifampicin, isoniazid, ethambutol and pyrazinamide for 2 months, followed by 4 months of isoniazid and rifampicin. The safety of these first line drugs has been established in pregnancy; second line drugs used in the setting of multi-drug-resistant TB have limited data [49].

After delivery, the neonate should be given prophylactic isoniazid if the mother is sputum positive and should be vaccinated as soon as possible. Breastfeeding is not contraindicated, as very little of the medications are excreted into breast milk. However, if a mother has newly diagnosed, active, untreated TB, she should be separated from her infant to reduce aerosol transmission [50].

References

1. Leighton B, Fish J. Pulmonary disease in pregnancy. In *The Global Library of Women's Medicine*. www.glowm.com/section_view/heading/Pulmonary%20Disease%20in%20Pregnancy/item/170

2. LoMauro A, Aliverti A. Respiratory physiology of pregnancy. *Breathe.* 2015;**11**:297–301.

3. Bhatia P, Bhatia K. Pregnancy and the lungs. *Postgrad Med J.* 2000 Nov 1;**76** (901):683.

4. Weinberger S, Weiss S, Cohen W, Weiss J, Johnson T. Pregnancy and the

lung. *Am Rev Respir Dis.*
1980;**121**:559–81.

5. Gilroy R, Mangura B, Lavietes M. Rib cage and abdominal volume displacements during breathing in pregnancy. *Am Rev Respir Dis.* 1988;**137**:668–72.

6. Cunningham F, Leveno K, Bloom S, eds. *Williams Obstetrics*, 22nd ed. New York: McGraw Hill; 2005.

7. Nelson-Piercy C. *Handbook of Obstetric Medicine*, 4th ed. London: Informa Healthcare; 2010.

8. Williams D, Kenyon A, Adamson D. Physiology. In Bennett P, Williamson C, eds. *Basic Science in Obstetrics and Gynaecology*, 4th ed. New York: Churchill Livingstone Elsevier; 2010. pp. 173–230.

9. Milne J, Howie A, Pack A. Dyspnoea during normal pregnancy. *Br J Obstet Gynecol.* 1978;**85**:260.

10. Stone S, Nelson-Piercy C. Respiratory disease in pregnancy. *Obstet Gynaecol Reprod Med.* 2012;**22**(10):290–8.

11. Skadhauge L, Baelum J, Siersted H. The occurrence of asthma among young adults. A population-based study in five west Danish countries. *Ugeskr Laeger.* 2005;**167**(6):648–51.

12. Kwon H, Triche E, Belanger K, Bracken M. The epidemiology of asthma during pregnancy: prevalence, diagnosis and symptoms. *Immunol Allergy Clin North Am.* 2006;**26**(1):29–62.

13. Ali Z, Suppli Urik C. Incidence and risk factors for exacerbations of asthma during pregnancy. *J Asthma Allergy.* 2013;**6**:53–60.

14. *British Guideline on the Management of Asthma*. London: British Thoracic Society; 2016 www.brit-thoracic.org.uk /document-library/clinical-information/asthma/btssign-asthma-guideline-quick-reference-guide-2016/

15. Rejno G, Lundholm C, Gong T, et al. Asthma during pregnancy in a population-based study – pregnancy complications and adverse perinatal outcomes. *PLoS ONE.* 2014;**9**(8): e104755.

16. Murphy V, Namazy J, Powell H, et al. A meta-analysis of adverse perinatal outcomes in women with asthma. *BJOG.* 2011;**118**:1314–23.

17. Schatz M, Harden K, Forsythe A. The course of asthma during pregnancy, post partum and with successive pregnancies: a prospective analysis.

J Allergy Clin Immunol. 1988;**81**:509–17.

18. Juniper E, Newhouse M. Effect of pregnancy on asthma: systematic review and meta-analysis. In Schatz M, Zeiger RS, Claman HN, eds. *Asthma and Immunological Diseases in Pregnancy and Early Infancy.* New York: Marcel Dekker; 1993. pp. 223–50.

19. Grosso A, Locatelli F, Gini E, et al. The course of asthma during pregnancy in a recent, multicase-control study on respiratory health. *Allergy Asthma Clin Immunol.* 2018 Apr 17;(14):16.

20. Wankhende U, Wadate A. Bronchial asthma in pregnancy. *Princ Crit Care Obstet.* 2016;**II**:3-n7.

21. Schatz M, Zeiger R, Falkoff R, Chambers C, Mellon M. Asthma and allergic diseases during pregnancy. In Burks AW, Holgate ST, O'Hehir RE, et al, eds. *Middleton's Allergy: Principles and Practice*, 9th ed. Edinburgh: Elsevier; 2019. pp. 951–69.

22. Sawicki E, Stewart K, Wong S, et al. Management of asthma by pregnant women attending an Australian maternity hospital. *Aust NZ J Obstet Gynaecol.* 2012;**52**(2):183–8.

23. Nelson-Piercy C. Asthma in pregnancy. *Thorax.* 2001;**56**:32.

24. Geake J, Tay G, Callaway L, Bell S. Pregnancy and cystic fibrosis: approach to contemporary management. *Obstet Med.* 2014;**7**(4):147–55.

25. Burden C, Ion R, Chung Y, Henry A, Downey D, Trinder J. Current pregnancy outcomes in women with cystic fibrosis. *Eur J Obstet Gynecol Reprod Biol.* 2012;**164**:142–5.

26. Thorpe-Beeston J, Madge S, Gyi K, Hodson M, Bilton D. The outcome of pregnancies in women with cystic fibrosis – single centre experience 1998–2011. *BJOG.* 2013;**120**:354–61.

27. Siegel B, Siegel S. Pregnancy and delivery in a patient with cystic fibrosis of the pancreas. *Obstet Gynecol.* 1960;**16**:438–40.

28. Dodge J, Lewis P, Stanton M, Wilsher J. Cystic fibrosis mortality and survival in the UK: 1947–2003. *Eur Respir J.* 2007;**29**:522–6.

29. Cystic Fibrosis in Pregnancy. UK Obstetric Surveillance System. www .npeu.ox.ac.uk/ukoss/current-surveillance/cfip

30. Renton M, Priestley L, Bennett L, Mackillop L, Chapman S. Pregnancy outcomes in cystic fibrosis: a 10-year experience from a UK centre. *Obstet Med.* 2015;**8**(2):99–101.

31. Cystic Fibrosis Foundation. About Cystic Fibrosis. www.cff.org/What-is-CF/About-Cystic-Fibrosis/

32. Gyi K, Hodson M, Yacoub M. Pregnancy in cystic fibrosis lung transplant recipients. Case series and review. *J Cyst Fibros.* 2006;**5**:171–5.

33. Lau E, Moriarty C, Ogle R, Bye P. Pregnancy and cystic fibrosis. *Paediatr Respir Rev.* 2010;**11**:90–4.

34. Edenborough FP, Borgo G, Knoop C, et al. Guidelines for the management of pregnancy in women with cystic fibrosis. *J Cyst Fibros.* 2008 Jan 1;7:S2–32.

35. Michel S, Mueller D. Nutrition for pregnant women who have cystic fibrosis. *J Acad Nutr Diet.* 2012;**112**(12):1943–8.

36. Whitty J. Cystic fibrosis in pregnancy. *Clin Obstet Gynecol.* 2010;**53**(2):369–76.

37. Goddard J, Bourke S. Cystic fibrosis and pregnancy. *TOG.* 2009;**11**:19–24.

38. Alpert S, Cormier A. Normal electrolyte and protein content in milk from mothers with cystic fibrosis: an explanation for the initial report of elevated milk sodium concentration. *J Pediatr.* 1983;**102**:77–80.

39. Hadid V, Patenaude V, Oddy L, Abenhaim H. Sarcoidosis and pregnancy: obstetric and neonatal outcomes in a population-based cohort of 7 million births. *J Perinat Med.* 2015;**43**(2):201–7.

40. Subramanian P, Chinthalapalli H, Krishnan M, et al. Pregnancy and sarcoidosis. An insight into the pathogenesis of hypercalciuria. *Chest.* 2004;**126**(3):995–8.

41. Rurak D, Cooper C, Taylor M. Fetal oxygen consumption and PO2 during hypercapnia in pregnant sheep. *J Dev Physiol.* 1986;**8**(6):447–59.

42. Lapinsky S, Tram C, Mehta S, Maxwell C. Restrictive lung disease in pregnancy. *Chest.* 2014;**145**(2):394–8.

43. Boggess K, Easterling T, Raghu G. Management and outcome of pregnant women with interstitial and restrictive lung disease. *Am J Obstet Gynecol.* 1995;**173**(4):1007–14.

44. King TJ. Restrictive lung disease in pregnancy. *Clin Chest Med.* 1992;**13**(4):607–22.

45. Say L, Chou D, Gemmill A, et al. Global causes of maternal death: a WHO systematic analysis. *Lancet Glob Health.* 2014 Jun 1;**2**(6): e323–33.

46. Sugarman J, Colvin C, Moran AC, Oxlade O. Tuberculosis in pregnancy: an estimate of the global burden of disease. *Lancet Glob Health.* 2014 Dec 1;2(12):e710–6.

47. Knight M, Kurinczuk J, Nelson-Piercy C, Spark P, Brocklehurst P. Tuberculosis in pregnancy in the UK. *BJOG Int J Obstet Gynaecol.* 2009 Mar 1;**116**(4):584–8.

48. Sobhy S, Babiker Z, Zamora J, Khan K, Kunst H. Maternal and perinatal mortality and morbidity associated with tuberculosis during pregnancy and the postpartum period: a systematic review and meta-analysis. *BJOG Int J Obstet Gynaecol.* 2017 Apr 1;**124**(5):727–33.

49. World Health Organization. *Treatment of Tuberculosis Guidelines.* World Health Organization; 2010.

50. Nhan-Chang C, Jones T. Tuberculosis in pregnancy. *Clin Obstet Gynecol.* 2010;**53**:311–21.

Thromboembolism in Pregnancy

Vrinda Arora & Sambit Mukhopadhyay

30.1 Introduction

Venous thromboembolism (VTE) is defined as a blood clot that forms in the veins and can migrate to other locations. It can be associated with a significant morbidity and mortality. The two most common types of VTE conditions are:

- Deep vein thrombosis (DVT): Blood clot (also known as thrombus) in the major deep veins of the leg (commonly) and/or pelvis.
- Pulmonary embolism (PE): Blood clot in the pulmonary circulation, when a part or whole clot of DVT migrates and lodges in the lung.

Thromboembolism (VTE) is the leading cause of direct maternal deaths in the UK. MBRRACE-UK 2018 [1] says, 'there has been no consistent decrease in mortality over the past 20 years, despite efforts from the colleges and national institutes as well as health professionals to provide preventive measures'. The MBRRACE-UK report also states that there were 39 deaths from VTE in the UK and Ireland between 2014 and 2016 (1.39 per 10 000 maternities), reflecting an increase from 1.01 per 10 000 maternities in 2011–2013 triennium [1].

30.2 Epidemiology

As compared to non-pregnant women, VTE risk is increased from 4- to 6-fold during pregnancy and there is a 60-fold increase during the first 3 months after birth [2, 3]. The absolute risk of VTE during pregnancy is 1–2 in 1000 pregnancies, even if the relative risk is high [3]. Within the UK, the incidence of antenatal PE is calculated as 1.3 per 10 000 maternities [4]. The Royal College of Obstetricians and Gynaecologists (RCOG) [3] cites absolute incidence of VTE in pregnancy and puerperium as 107 per 100 000 person years (95% confidence interval (CI) 93–122 per 1000 person years in the UK) and 107 per 10 000 pregnancy years during pregnancy compared with 175 per 100 000 puerperal years during puerperium reported from Denmark and 175 per 100 000 pregnancies from Canada.

30.3 Risk Factors

There are a number of risk factors that can exist either before pregnancy or can develop during pregnancy, during intrapartum or during postpartum period. It is important to be aware of these risks factors for woman who are planning to conceive and are attending for pre-pregnancy counselling. Furthermore, risk factor screening should be applied throughout pregnancy,

starting from the first antenatal booking appointment and continued at each antenatal visit during the intrapartum and the postpartum periods. The identification of risk factors would warrant either prophylactic or therapeutic treatment with low molecular weight heparin (LMWH) on their own, while some need to be present with other risk factors for intervention.

These risk factors can be divided into three categories, as shown in Table 30.1 [2], which provides a list of all the risk factors before pregnancy, during pregnancy and following birth which can lead to venous thrombosis in pregnant women [3].

30.4 Pathophysiology [4]

30.4.1 Pathophysiology of Deep Vein Thrombosis (DVT)

Venous valves are avascular, which in conjunction with reduced flow of oxygenated blood in veins predisposes the endothelium to be hypoxaemic. The endothelium around valves responds by expressing adhesion molecules that attract leukocytes. These cells transfer tissue factor to the endothelium, which can interact with activated factor VII to begin the coagulation cascade via the extrinsic pathway. The main component is fibrin (a product of coagulation cascade and red blood clots; platelets also contribute, but to a lesser extent). The skeletal muscle pump prevents DVT by moving blood past the valves which washes away activated clotting factors. If a clot (thrombus) is formed and does not resolve, it will extend along the popliteal and femoral veins. When plasminogen is converted into plasma (an enzyme that degrades fibrin into soluble peptides), it is known as a fibrinolysis. This natural process protects against formation of thrombi.

30.4.2 Pathophysiology of Pulmonary Embolism (PE)

In patients with DVT, the thrombus can dislodge, travel up the inferior vena cava to the right heart and lodge in the pulmonary vasculature. There are two types of presentations, depending on the size of the clot:

- Central PE – When a large clot blocks a large vessel, it causes haemodynamic instability due to mechanical occlusion of blood vessels.

Table 30.1 Risk factors for developing VTE in pregnancy

Pre-pregnancy

1. Thrombophilia

   a. Inherited

      i. Antithrombin deficiency
      ii. Protein C deficiency
      iii. Protein S deficiency
      iv. Factor V Leiden
      v. Prothrombin gene mutation

   b. Acquired

      i. Antiphospholipid antibodies
      (persistent lupus anticoagulant antibodies and/or persistent moderate / high titre cardiolipin antibodies and/or beta-2 glycoprotein 1 antibodies

2. Medical conditions

   a. Example: cardiac diseases, cancer, active systemic lupus erythematosus (SLE), inflammatory polyarthropathy or inflammatory bowel disease (IBD), nephrotic syndrome, type 1 diabetes mellitus with nephropathy, sickle cell disease, thalassaemia, current intravenous drug user.

3. Age >35 years
4. Obesity (body mass index (BMI) ≥30 kg/m^2)
5. Parity ≥3
6. Smoking
7. Gross varicose veins (symptomatic or above knee or with associated phlebitis, oedema/skin changes)
8. Paraplegia
9. Family history of VTE (unprovoked or oestrogen provoked in first degree relative)

Antenatal

1. In vitro fertilization (IVF) pregnancy / assisted reproduction
2. Multiple pregnancy
3. Hyperemesis / dehydration (admission only), unless other risk factors are present
4. Ovarian hyperstimulation syndrome (first trimester only)
5. Admission or immobility (≥3 days bed rest)
6. Current systemic infection (requiring admission or intravenous (IV) antibiotics)
7. Any surgical procedure in pregnancy or puerperium except immediate repair of the perineum (e.g. appendectomy, postpartum sterilization, bone fracture)
8. Pelvic girdle pain with restricted mobility
9. Long-distance travel (>4hours)
10. Current pre-eclampsia

Postpartum

1. Caesarean section
2. Prolonged labour (>24 hours)
3. Mid-cavity or rotational operative forceps
4. Stillbirth
5. Preterm birth
6. Postpartum haemorrhage (>1 litre /requiring transfusion)

- Peripheral PE – Small thrombi lodge in the peripheral vessels, thus causing pleural irritation (pleural chest pain), resulting in increased inflammation, and chemical mediators are released, leading to vasoconstriction and bronchoconstriction.

30.5 Prevention [3, 5, 6]

Venous thromboembolism can be prevented by assessing every woman during the pre-pregnancy period, during the antenatal period and postnatally, and by the timely institution of thrombo-prophylaxis with LMWH as the agent of choice, unless

245

contraindicated. If thromboprophylaxis is contraindicated (e.g. the woman is allergic to anticoagulation) and the woman is high risk for VTE, the haematologist should be involved for further advice. Compression stockings should be provided, and the woman should be counselled to keep hydrated and mobile. Depending on the need for thromboprophylaxis, there are four subgroups to which women at risk for VTE can be assigned:

30.5.1 Antenatal VTE Prophylaxis from the Start of Pregnancy with or without High Dose of LMWH (50%, 75% or full-treatment dose) and 6 Weeks Postpartum

a. Women with previous VTE associated with antithrombin deficiency (unprovoked or oestrogen related).
b. Women with previous VTE and antiphospholipid syndrome (APS).
c. Previous recurrent VTE (on long-term anticoagulation).
d. Those women who have four or more risk factors during risk assessment at the booking visit (they may not need a higher anticoagulation dose).
e. Those with asymptomatic inherited thrombophilia (antithrombin, protein C, protein S, homozygous prothrombin gene mutation and compound heterozygous) should be considered for antenatal LMWH from the start of pregnancy [7].
f. Those with the medical co-morbidities listed in Table 30.1.

These women should be managed by a multidisciplinary team comprising a haematologist who is an expert in thrombosis in pregnancy and an obstetrician who has special interest in high-risk pregnancy. Those on long-term anticoagulants such as warfarin need to be advised to stop warfarin and change to LMWH within 2 weeks of a missed period and before 6 weeks of pregnancy.

Warfarin can cross the placenta and lead to fetal complications.

30.5.2 Women Who Need LMWH Prophylaxis from 28 Weeks to 6 Weeks Postpartum (intermediate risk)

a. Women with previous VTE secondary to a major surgery and are currently not on long-term anticoagulant therapy.
b. Women with three risk factors for VTE (other than the high-risk factors).

30.5.3 Women Who Need LMWH Prophylaxis for 10 Days Postpartum

a. Those who have at least two risk factors for VTE.
This advice is only recommended by the RCOG, UK. The clinical practice guidelines for VTE in pregnancy by the Royal College of Physicians of Ireland and Institute of Obstetrics and Gynaecology [6] states that there appears to be different views in international guidelines and their recommendation is in line with the American College of Obstetricans and Gynecologists (ACOG) 'suggesting that if LMWH is indicated in postpartum, it should be given until the woman is fully ambulant.

Thromboprophylaxis beyond discharge from hospital need only to be offered to women at high risk of VTE' [5].

The RCOG [3] states that as the postpartum period has increased risk of VTE, especially if the age is above 35 years, the woman has high BMI and/or has had a caesarean section, VTE prophylaxis is advisable after discharge.

30.5.4 Women Who Require LMWH Only Short Term (hospital admission), When No Other Risk Factors Are Present

- Hyperemesis/dehydration (only during admission unless there are other risk factors present)
- Ovarian hyperstimulation (first trimester only)
- Surgery in pregnancy/postpartum
- Current systemic infection
- Long-distance travel / air travel

30.6 Family History and Testing for Thrombophilia [3]

The RCOG does not recommend testing for thrombophilia in pregnancy if a patient has risk factors that make her eligible for prophylactic LMWH. The following patients should be offered testing for thrombophilia after a discussion about the implications of the test results, whether positive or negative:

Family history of VTE and antithrombin deficiency.

Family history of VTE and specific thrombophilia has not been detected. These women should specifically be tested for antithrombin deficiency.

Women with history of unprovoked VTE. These women should specifically be tested for antiphospholipid antibodies, on two occasions 12 weeks apart.

The above thrombophilia risk categories are recommended for testing, as the dose of LMWH will need altering if they were reported to be positive. As the detection of other thrombophilia will not make any difference to the dose or anticoagulation agent, testing for them is not recommended. However, these patients should be tested for all thrombophilia 6 weeks after pregnancy. This is because, pregnancy alters proteins in pregnancy (e.g. protein S falls progressively in pregnancy and protein C increases marginally between 28 to 32 weeks of pregnancy) [8].

In 2010, Cochrane review [2] published a meta-analysis of 16 trials involving 2592 women and it stated that there is insufficient evidence to suggest that thromboprophylaxis in pregnancy, postnatal or after a caesarean section could prevent VTE. However, the RCOG [3] Green-top Guidelines are based on current thinking within the multiprofessional teams.

30.7 Choice of Anticoagulant Agent Medication

The Cochrane review [2] found no difference in using LMWH versus unfractionated heparin (UH). Both have their advantages and disadvantages.

30.7.1 Low Molecular Weight Heparin (LMWH)

The dose calculation is weight dependent. The booking weight is ideally used to calculate the dose, but most recent weight can be used as well. As LMWH has a renal clearance, a reduced dose should be used in women with renal impairment. It is safe in breastfeeding.

30.7.1.1 Advantages

- Low risk of heparin-induced thrombocytopenia (HIT)
- Does not require monitoring in women with normal weight, in an intermittent risk group or with no renal impairment
- Less risk of bleeding (<2%)

30.7.1.2 Disadvantages

- Long half-life. Twelve hours are needed before regional anaesthesia can be given for those on prophylaxis dose and 24 hours for those on therapeutic dose.
- Incomplete reversal of its activity by protamine sulphate.

30.7.2 Unfractionated Heparin (UFH)

30.7.2.1 Advantages

- Shorter half-life (6 hours with an intravenous dose)
- Complete reversal with protamine sulphate
- Can be used when there is an increased risk of haemorrhage in women with high risk of VTE (due to a shorter half-life)
- Can be given 6 hours before regional anaesthesia (if given as an intravenous dose)

30.7.2.2 Disadvantages

- High risk of HIT and need platelet monitoring
- Increased risk of bleeding
- Needs monitoring of activated partial thromboplastin time (APTT) if used for treatment

Contraindication to Anticoagulation

1. Women with risk of bleeding or active bleeding
2. Allergy to LMWH/UFH
3. Known bleeding disorders
4. Thrombocytopenia (platelet count <75 x 10^9/L)
5. Acute stroke in previous 4 weeks
6. Severe renal disease
7. Severe liver disease
8. Uncontrolled hypertension (systolic >200 mm Hg or diastolic 120 mm Hg)

On the basis of evidence above, the RCOG [3] suggests that LMWH may be used as the first line drug. The ACOG [5] suggests either LMWH or UFH can be used for prophylaxis or treatment.

30.8 Symptoms and Signs of Acute VTE in Pregnancy [9]

- Leg pain and swelling
- Lower abdomen pain (reflecting extension of thrombus into pelvic vessels and/or development of a collateral circulation)
- Dyspnoea
- Chest pain/pleuritic pain
- Haemoptysis
- Collapse
- Tachycardia
- Hypotension
- Increased respiratory rate and reduced saturation
- Rarely, low-grade pyrexia and leukocytosis.
- Iliac vein thrombosis can present as back and buttock pain and swelling of the entire limbs

30.9 Investigations and Diagnosis of Acute VTE (PE and/or DVT) [9]

It is important to suspect and assess for VTE in any pregnant woman presenting with the above said symptoms. The management starts with complete information gathering of the symptoms and assessment of the risk factors. A complete clinical examination is needed before starting investigations and treatment. There are no specific scores used in pregnancy to determine VTE.

The following steps should be taken to manage a pregnant mother with VTE. It is important to know that in such cases maternal treatment is of utmost importance.

- Bloods should be taken for full blood count, coagulation screen, urea and electrolytes and liver function test, as abnormal values in these tests could be a contraindication for anticoagulation therapy.
- Treatment dose of LMWH should be given after bloods come back as normal and if there are no contraindications.
- Multidisciplinary team involvement: senior obstetrician, radiologist and haematologist should be involved.
- If the symptoms suggest acute pulmonary embolism (PE), then an electrocardiogram (ECG) and chest x-ray should be performed.
- If symptoms are suggestive of DVT with or without PE, then compression duplex ultrasound should be performed. If DVT is confirmed, no further investigations is suggested as the treatment for DVT and PE is anticoagulation.
- If symptoms and signs suspect PE without DVT, a ventilation/perfusion (V/Q) lung scan or a computerized tomography pulmonary angiogram (CTPA) need to be performed.
- If the X-ray is normal, then a V/Q scan should be performed. The ventilation (V) component can be omitted to reduce the radiation exposure to the fetus.
- If the chest x-ray is abnormal, then it is suggested to perform a CTPA.
- In both the diagnostic investigations, the slight risk of childhood cancer following the exposure to V/Q scan and risk of breast cancer with exposure to CTPA should be discussed and consent should be obtained.
- If there is high suspicion of PE and V/Q scan or CTPA do not confirm the diagnosis of PE, then LMWH should be continued, and repeat testing should be done 3 to 4 days later.

- If there is a high suspicion of DVT and the ultrasound does not confirm DVT, then anticoagulant should be discontinued and ultrasound should be repeated on days 3 and 7. If repeat testing is negative, no further action is needed.

30.10 Management of a Life-Threatening PE in Pregnancy [9]

A collapsed or a shocked pregnant woman needs to be managed by a multidisciplinary team consisting of a consultant obstetrician, consultant haematologist, consultant in the resuscitation team and consultant anaesthetist, radiologist and physician.

- The basic life resuscitation needs to be carried out.
- Although the mode of treatment should be decided after assessment of the patient, intravenous unfractionated heparin is the preferred initial treatment.
- An urgent portable cardiogram or CTPA should be done in 1 hour. If massive PE is confirmed, immediate thrombolysis should be considered (with agents such as streptokinase, urokinase alteplase and telecteplase).
- In case of cardiac arrest, CPR (cardiopulmonary resuscitation) needs to be carried out and perimortem caesarean should be performed within 5 minutes if the pregnancy is 20 weeks or more.
- RCOG suggests a regime for UFH starting with a loading dose of 80 units/kg followed by a maintenance of 18 units/kg (if the patient was thrombolysed, omit the loading dose). Check APTT levels every 4–6 hours after loading dose and every 6 hours after any dose change. The therapeutic target for APTT ratio is usually 1.5–2.5 times the average laboratory control value. The above regime should be followed after discussion with a haematologist or according to local protocol.
- If a patient is not fit for thrombolysis, then discussion with the cardiothoracic surgeons should be done for an urgent thoracotomy.

The treatment dose of LMWH should be given for 6 weeks postnatally and should be continued until at least 3 months. These women should also have an outpatient follow-up with the haematologist and should have a plan for platelet or anti-Xa levels monitoring, if needed.

30.11 Anticoagulation Therapy or Prophylaxis during the Intrapartum Period [3, 8]

It is important to inform the woman who is on LMWH thrombophylaxis or treatment that once she thinks she is in labour or has symptoms suggesting that she is in labour, she should not self-administer any further LMWH/UFH.

The dosage of LMWH/UFH are weight dependent. Table 30.2 provides comparative dosage for three commonly used anticoagulant preparations. LMWH are commonly used and dosages have been summarized in Table 30.3.

Women should be advised to present to the hospital for assessment and for advice on taking further doses. If a delivery is planned (by elective caesarean section or induction of labour), LMWH should be discontinued 12 hours before planned delivery if the patient is on prophylactic dose and 24 hours before if she is on the therapeutic dose. Regional anaesthesia should not be given until at least 12 hours after previous prophylactic LMWH and 24 hours if a therapeutic dose has been given. This precaution will reduce the risk of epidural haematoma. The highest risk for formation of epidural haematoma is around the time for epidural catheter removal, therefore it is important that this procedure is carried out by an obstetric anaesthetist [10]. It is recommended that the prophylaxis dose of LMWH should be withheld for at least 4 hours after the use of spinal anaesthesia or the epidural catheter has been removed. If a woman is taking the prophylaxis dose of LMWH, then the epidural catheter should not be removed within 12 hours of the most recent injection. If she is on the therapeutic dose of LMWH, then the risk of epidural bleeding should be assessed before removing the catheter [11].

o Normal risk – catheter should be removed more than 24 hours after therapeutic dose of LMWH

o Increased risk – removal between 12 and 24 hours

o High risk – removal between 6 and 12 hours

The RCOG [8] recommends that in women on a therapeutic dose of LMWH, the risk of wound haematoma post-caesarean section is 9%. Hence it is recommended that wound drains and interrupted skin sutures should be considered to allow drainage of any subcutaneous haematoma.

Table 30.2 Drug and dose for thromboprophylaxis in pregnancy as per weight [3]

Weight	Enoxaparin	Dalteparin	Tinzaparin (75 U/kg/day)
<50 kg	20 mg daily	2 500 units daily	3 500 units daily
50–90 kg	40 mg daily	5 000 units daily	4 500 units daily
91–130 kg	60 mg daily	7 500 units daily	7 000 units daily
131–170 kg	80 mg daily	10 000 units daily	9 000 units daily
>170 kg	0.6 mg/kg/day	75 U/kg/day	75 U/kg/day
High prophylactic dose for women weighing 50–90 kg	40 mg 12 hourly	5 000 units 12 hourly	4 500 units 12 hourly

Table 30.3 Therapeutic drugs and dose for LMWH [4]

Booking or early pregnancy weight	Initial dose of enoxaparin
<50 kg	40 mg twice daily or 60 mg once daily
50–69 kg	60 mg twice daily or 90 mg once daily
70–89 kg	80 mg twice daily or 120 mg once daily
90–109 kg	100 mg twice daily or 150 mg once daily
110–125 kg	120 mg twice daily or 180 mg once daily
>125 kg	Discuss with haematologist
Booking or early pregnancy weight	**Initial dose of dalteparin**
<50 kg	5 000 IU twice daily or 10 000 IU once daily
50–69 kg	6 000 IU twice daily or 12 000 IU once daily
70–89 kg	8 000 IU twice daily or 16 000 IU once daily
90–109	10 000 IU twice daily or 20 000 IU once daily
110–125 kg	12 000 IU twice daily or 24 000 IU daily
>125 kg	Discuss with haematologist

Initial dose of tinzaparin (based on booking or early pregnancy weight)

175 units/kg once daily

30.12 Choice of Heparin Agents and Treatment in Case of High Risk of Haemorrhage

Women who are at an increased risk for haemorrhage (e.g. placenta praevia), as well as requiring continuance of their heparin treatment, should be managed after a discussion with the haematologist. If a woman requires a caesarean section, a general anaesthesia may be considered [12]. In case of antepartum or postpartum haemorrhage, or a wound haematoma not needing surgical intervention, unfractionated heparin should be considered. This is because UFH can be completely reversed by protamine sulphate, as its half-life is 6 hours if given intravenously (12 hours for subcutaneous administration). Unfortunately, protamine sulphate reverses the anti-IIa fraction of LMWH, but does not fully reverse the anti-Xa effect.

30.13 Anti-Xa Monitoring

Both the RCOG [3] and the Irish guidelines for thromboembolism in pregnancy [6] suggest that anti-Xa monitoring is routinely not indicated for all women on treatment with LMWH .This is because weight-based LMWH helps maintain 3 hours post-injection peak anti-Xa activity of 0.5–1.2 U/mL. This may not be the case in some women with complicating factors and thus the need for therapeutic LMWH. Anti-Xa monitoring is recommended for the following groups of women:

o Extremes of body weight (<50 kg and ≥90 kg)
o Renal impairment (LMWH is cleared via the renal route)
o Pre-eclampsia (as the kidneys can be affected)
o Recurrent VTE (to check that anti-Xa levels are maintained)
o Those on treatment dose for prophylaxis with previous history of VTE and antithrombin deficiency.

30.14 Warfarin

Warfarin is a vitamin K antagonist. Unlike heparin (LMWH and UFH), it is known to readily cross the placenta. It affects the fetus and is associated with increased risk of miscarriage, warfarin embryopathy (hypoplasia of nasal bridge, congenital heart defects, ventriculomegaly, agenesis of corpus collosum, stippled epiphyses), prematurity, low birthweight, neurodevelopment issues and fetal and neonatal bleeding, stillbirth or neonatal death [12]. Hence the use of warfarin is not recommended to be used in pregnancy, where it is classed as a category X drug, except in women with mechanical heart valves, where it is classified a category D drug.

The above fetal complications usually occur if there is fetal exposure of >5 mg of warfarin per day. Those women on long-term anticoagulants such as warfarin need to be advised to stop warfarin and change to LMWH within 2 weeks of a missed period. These women can be switched back to warfarin from LMWH 5–7 days after delivery. It is safe to use during breastfeeding.

30.15 Other Anticoagulants [3, 8]

30.15.1 Dextran

Dextran is a complex branch glucan that is used as an anticoagulant in non-pregnant patients due to its antiplatelet activities. As it has a high risk of anaphylactic reactions, it should be avoided both antenatally and in the intrapartum period.

30.15.2 Non-Vitamin K Antagonist Oral Anticoagulants (NOACs)

Drugs such as dabigatran, rivaroxaban and apixaban work through direct inhibition of thrombin or factor Xa. It is not licensed or recommended for use in pregnancy and breastfeeding. No data are currently available for the use of NOACs in pregnancy, breastfeeding, or children [13]. They are likely to cross the placenta.

30.15.3 Argatroban and r-Hirudin

Argatroban and r-hirudin are direct thrombin inhibitors. They are not licensed for use in pregnancy but some evidence of safety and efficacy in pregnancy has been reported.

30.16 Alternative Anticoagulants for Women Who Are Intolerant to Heparin [3, 8]

30.16.1 Danaparoid

Danaparoid is a heparinoid that is used in patients who do not tolerate or are allergic to heparin. It has a half-life of 24 hours and regional anaesthesia should be avoided within that time. It is safe in pregnancy and breastfeeding.

30.16.2 Fondaparinux

Fondaparinux is a synthetic pentasaccharide that acts through inhibition of factor Xa via antithrombin. It is another alternative agent used in patients who cannot tolerate heparin. It has been used in pregnancy without any adverse effects on the mother or fetus being reported. Its half-life is 18 hours, and 36–42 hours should pass following the previous dose before regional anaesthesia can be considered.

Both danaparoid and fondaparinux should be used only after discussion with a consultant haematologist.

30.17 Anti-embolism (mechanical methods of prophylaxis and therapeutics) [3, 8]

The anti-embolism stockings are recommended for prophylaxis as well as for therapeutic use.

30.17.1 For Prophylaxis Use

- Appropriate size should be used.
- Should provide graduated compression with calf pressure of 14–15 mm Hg.
- Recommended for all women who are pregnant and admitted to the hospital, where there is a contraindication to the administration of LMWH, those who are at high risk and those who plan to travel long distances >4 hours.

30.17.2 For Therapeutic Use

- Should be used as a part of the initial management with LMWH and elevation of legs.
- The graduated elastic stockings should be worn to reduce oedema.
- The size should be measured to fit accurately.
- The current national guidance in the UK recommends that with proximal DVT, below-knee compression stockings with ankle pressure >23 mm Hg needs to be fitted.
- The unaffected leg does not need to be fitted with the stocking.
- If the hosiery does not fit (e.g. in those with a very high BMI), then intermittent pneumatic compression devises or foot impulse devices can be used while the patient is in the hospital. The mechanism of action of all the above mechanical devices is to keep the blood flowing and prevent or manage VTE.

30.18 Inferior Vena Cava Filters (IVCFs) [8, 14]

There have been reports of IVCF placement in pregnant women who have been assessed as being at high risk of VTE and where heparin therapy is either contraindicated or has failed. The ideal candidates are those who are at term, near labour, high risk of preterm delivery or who need high-dose heparin due to thromboembolic complications. It is also used to prevent PE in cases of pregnant women with thrombophilia and severe heparin-induced thrombocytopenia. This needs to be done with a multidisciplinary team of medical professionals.

The complications associated with IVCF are:

- Fetal radiation exposure, which is around 7 mcg (minimal)
- Migration of the filter

30.19 Post-thrombotic Syndrome (PTS) [8]

Post-thrombotic syndrome (PTS) is characterized by chronic persistent leg swelling, pain and feeling of heaviness, dependent cyanosis, telangiectasia, chronic pigmentation, eczema, associated varicose veins and, in the most severe cases, venous ulceration. Although the role of compression stockings has been questioned to prevent PTS, the national guideline recommends its use for at least 2 years.

References

1. Knight M, Bunch K, Tuffnell D, et al, eds., on behalf of MBRRACE-UK. *Saving Lives, Improving Mothers' Care: Lessons Learned to Inform Maternity Care from the UK and Ireland Confidential Enquiries into Maternal Deaths and Morbidity 2014–16*. Oxford: National Perinatal Epidemiology Unit, University of Oxford; 2018.

2. Bain E, Wilson A, Tooher R, et al. Prophylaxis for venous thromboembolic disease in pregnancy and the early postnatal period. *Cochrane Database Syst Rev*. 2014 Feb **11**;(2):CD001689.

3. *Reducing the Risk of Venous Thromboembolism during Pregnancy and the Puerperium*, Green-top Guideline No 37a. London: RCOG, 2015.

4. Wong, E, Chaudhry S. Venous thromboembolism (VTE). *McMaster Pathophysiology Review*. Ontario, Canada: McMaster University; 2012–2018. www.pathophys.org/vte/

5. American College of Obstetricians and Gynecologists practice bulletin no. 196: thromboembolism in pregnancy. *Obstet Gynecol*. 2018;**132**(1):243–8. doi: 10.1097/aog.0000000000002707

6. Institute of Obstetricians & Gynaecologists. *Venous Thromboprophylaxis in Pregnancy*. Clinical Practice Guideline. RCPI, 2013.

7. Croles FN, Nasserinejad K, Duvekot JJ, et al. Pregnancy, thrombophilia, and the risk of a first venous thrombosis:

systematic review and bayesian meta-analysis. *BMJ.* 2017;**359**:j4452. Review.

8. Warwick R, Hutton RA, Goff L, Letsky E, Heard M. Changes in protein C and free protein S during pregnancy and following hysterectomy. *J R Soc Med.* 1989 Oct;**82**(10):591–4.

9. *The Acute Management of Thrombosis and Embolism during Pregnancy and Puerperium*, Green-top Guideline No 37b. London: RCOG, 2015.

10. Nelson-Piercy C. *Handbook of Obstetric Medicine*, chapter 3. New York: Informa Healthcare; 2010.

11. Association of Anaesthetists of Great Britain & Ireland, Obstetric Anaesthetists' Association and Regional Anaesthesia UK. Regional anesthesia and patients with abnormalities of coagulation. *Anaesthesia.* 2013;**68**:966–72.

12. Alshawabkeh L, Economy KE, Valente AM. Anticoagulation during pregnancy: evolving strategies with a focus on mechanical valves. *J Am Coll Cardiol.* 2016;**68** (16):18041813. doi: 10.1016/j.jacc.2016.06.076

13. González-Mesa E, Azumendi P, Marsac A, et al. Use of a temporary inferior vena cava filter during pregnancy in patients with thromboembolic events. *J Obst Gynaecol.* 2015;**35**:8, 771–6, doi: 10.3109/01443615.2015.1007928

Chapter 31

Haemoglobinopathies in Pregnancy

Panos Antsaklis, Maria Papamichail, George J. Daskalakis & Aris J. Antsaklis

31.1 Introduction

Haemoglobinopathies constitute a heterogeneous group of autosomal recessive inherited disorders, affecting either haemoglobin synthesis (i.e. thalassaemia) or structure (i.e. sickle cell disease) [1], and they represent the most common single-gene disorder in humans [2]. According to the World Health Organization (WHO), about 5% of the world's population are carriers of a potentially pathological haemoglobin gene. Annually, about 300 000 infants are born all around the world with a dominant haemoglobinopathy, with 30% of them suffering from thalassaemia syndromes and the remaining 70% from sickle cell anaemia [3]. Sickle cell disease appears to be more prevalent in Africa, α-thalassaemia in South East Asia and β-thalassaemia in the Mediterranean, Middle East and Asia. This geographic allocation is due to the fact that individuals carrying one pathological and one normal gene (heterozygous carriers trait) were protected from malaria, and these regions had the highest prevalence of this fatal disease.

A few decades ago, pregnancy in women with α- or β-thalassaemia was almost impossible, as women with transfusion-dependent thalassaemia had hypogonadism and ovulation abnormalities [4]. In addition, as a pregnancy in women with a haemoglobinopathy is considered high risk, getting pregnant was discouraged. Nowadays, due to the improvement in treatment options, such as recurrent blood transfusions and chelation agents, organ disorders and malfunctions have been eliminated, leading to a higher life expectancy and greater possibility of pregnancy.

As haemoglobinopathies are inherited disorders, they can affect the fetuses of ostensibly healthy parents. Therefore, screening and timely diagnosis of the couple's haemoglobin status have an extremely high significance, especially in couples who originated from areas with a high prevalence of haemoglobinopathies. When genetic counselling can be given, couples can be armed with the information to help them make decisions about pregnancy in their particular situations [5].

In this chapter, an overview of the synthesis and structure of the haemoglobin molecule will be discussed, haemoglobinopathies will be briefly presented and the most common and serious consequences that may affect a pregnancy of a woman with a haemoglobinopathy will be reviewed. Finally, the algorithm of screening and management will be presented.

31.2 Haemoglobin Synthesis and Structure

Haemoglobin (Hb) is a protein found in the red blood cells and it is responsible for the oxygen transfer to the body's tissues [2].

It is a tetrameric protein, composed of four interlocking polypeptide chains. Each chain has attached a haem molecule, resulting in each haemoglobin molecule carrying four haem molecules [5]. These polypeptide chains are named after the first six letters of the Greek alphabet: α-alpha, β-beta, γ-gamma, δ-delta, ε-epsilon or the ζ-zeta. The genes responsible for the expression of these proteins are located on chromosome 16 (chains α and ζ) and on chromosome 11 (chains β, γ, δ and ε). For a deeper understanding of α-thalassaemia, it is important to know that the production of the α-chain is controlled by four genes (two genes from the maternal chromosome 16 and two from the paternal chromosome 16) [1].

In humans, six different combinations of the polypeptide chains have been detected. Three of them are present only during embryonic development and they will not be mentioned further here. The other three are presented in variable proportions during fetal and adult life [2]. The fetal haemoglobin (HbF) is composed of two α- and two γ-chains and it is present in fetal blood starting in the 12th week of gestation [5]. In the third trimester, the expression of the β-gene begins, leading to the first appearance of the HbA – the adult haemoglobin. HbA is composed of two α- and two β-chains. The third clinically significant haemoglobin molecule is HbA_2, consisting of two α- and two δ-chains [6]. Normally, when a baby is born, its red blood cells carry 70% HbF and 30% HbA. The percentage of the HbF drops significantly in the 4th–6th months of extrauterine life, making the baby now dependent on HbA synthesis. This leads to α-disorders being presented in utero or at birth, while the symptoms of β-disorders start to become apparent after the 4th month of life [2]. In healthy adults, HbA constitutes 98% of haemoglobin molecules, while the remaining 2% are HbA_2 [6].

31.3 A Brief Overview of Haemoglobinopathies

As mentioned above, haemoglobinopathies can be divided into two subgroups. The first includes the production of an abnormal haemoglobin molecule, the most common of which is sickle cell disease. The second group constitutes a quantitative defect represented by the thalassaemias (quantitative haemoglobinopathies). Thalassaemias are inherited disorders where a reduction in the synthesis of the globin chains results in instability of the haemoglobin molecule. Microcytic anaemia is the outcome upon blood examination and is due to ineffective red blood cell production [1, 5].

31.3.1 The Sickle Cell Disorders

The sickle cell disorders are a group of autosomal inherited disorders causing production of abnormal haemoglobin molecules. The defect on the DNA material involves a single nucleotide substitution of thymine for adenine in the β-chain gene. This has been translated into a substitution in the number six position of the β-polypeptide chain of HbA. Valine takes the place of glutamine acid, resulting in an abnormal haemoglobin molecule which is insoluble in decreased oxygen situations [1]. When only the one gene of the β-chain is affected (heterozygous), individuals are asymptomatic and they are said to be carriers or to have the sickle cell trait. The most severe clinical status occurs when both the genes are affected, resulting in sickle cell anaemia. Africans seem to have the highest prevalence rate of the sickle cell trait, as 1 in 12 African Americans is a carrier, while 1 in 300 is homozygous for HbS [7]. HbS is also found in Greek, Italian, Turk, Arab, Iranian and Asian Indian populations.

When a person is homozygous for HbS, in low-oxygen tension situations, the red blood cells take a sickle shape and they are removed from the circulation, causing haemolytic anaemia. Additionally, when this alteration of the red blood cells' shape takes place in the minor blood vessels, vaso-occlusive crisis occurs, causing microvascular obstruction in several organs including the spleen, heart, lungs, kidneys and brain [5]. It is important to mention that due to the recurrent microvascular obstructions in the spleen, homozygous adults for the HbS gene are functionally asplenic, making them vulnerable to serious infections from bacteria such as *Streptococcus pneumoniae*. The most severe expression of sickle cell disease is acute chest syndrome, with the patient experiencing extreme chest pain, dyspnoea, fever and cough. The optimal treatment of this condition is hydration and high dosages of opioids [8].

The group of sickle cell disorders includes doubly heterozygous states of HbS and either α- or β-thalassaemia. The different combinations lead to variable clinical phenotypes [9].

The diagnosis of sickle cell disease is made by haemoglobin electrophoresis. In the homozygous HbSS, HbS is found at levels greater than 90%, with the remaining 10% consisting of HbF and small amounts of HbA$_2$. Heterozygous HbAS has larger amounts of HbA [5].

31.3.2 The Thalassaemias Group

α-Thalassaemia is the most common single-gene disorder and it has a higher frequency in Asia and in the Mediterranean region. In most of the cases, it is caused by a deletion of one or more of the four genes responsible for the production of the α-chain [9]. If one of the four genes is deleted (heterozygous α-thalassaemia, -α/αα), the only expression is a mild microcytosis. A mild hypochromic microcytic anaemia is the result of the loss of two genes, either on the same chromosome 16 (–/αα) or on the opposite chromosomes 16 (-α/-α). Loss of three genes (–/-α) causes the HbH disease, resulting in mild or moderate haemolyticanaemia, requiring frequent blood transfusions. When none of the four genes is present (–/–) the disorder is called Bart's hydrops and it

is incompatible with life, with the affected fetus dying in utero or shortly after birth. An interesting fact is that HbH disease and Bart's hydrops can only occur when at least one of the parents carries the *cis* mutation (–/αα), which is found only in South East Asia and the Mediterranean basin. The *trans* mutation (-α/-α) is found globally and couples who are both carriers are not at high risk of having a fetus with Bart's hydrops [2].

β-Thalassaemia is the most common quantitative haemoglobinopathy. The higher prevalence is found in the Mediterranean basin, Asia, Middle East, West India and in the Hispanic population [5]. It is caused by either a point mutation, a small deletion or an insertion mutation in the β-globin genes [10], with more than 200 different DNA detected around the world. More interestingly, these defects are highly associated with geographic allocation [2]. Due to these DNA defects, the production of the β-chain is either absent or reduced, resulting in an α-β chain imbalance and, therefore, in the absence of the HbA. When one gene is affected, individuals have β-thalassaemia minor and they present with microcytic anaemia. When both the genes are affected, individuals have β-thalassaemia major – or Cooley's anaemia. β-Thalassaemia minor is a severe disorder, with severe anaemia, causing extramedullary erythropoiesis, delayed sexual development and poor growth. Those with clinical manifestations between these two are said to have a manifestation called β-thalassaemia intermedia [5].

In haemoglobin electrophoresis, HbA2 levels are elevated (>3.5%) and HbF exceeds frequently 7% [9].

31.4 Screening

31.4.1 Parental Screening

As haemoglobinopathies are inherited disorders with an autosomal recessive pattern, carrier screening is the key for prevention, and for correct and timely management of the couples that are at high risk for having an affected baby. Screening programmes have improved significantly over the few last decades, especially in populations where haemoglobinopathies are highly prevalent. Often, the carrier of sickle cell disease or thalassaemia is living a normal life, unaware of their haemoglobinopathy status, but their babies are at a high risk of having a severe disease or even in utero death [2]. Therefore, genetic testing is offered to asymptomatic individuals at a high risk for being carriers, while prenatal diagnosis is offered to couples with a known haemoglobinopathy trait.

Ideally, screening should be performed before pregnancy, so that the correct diagnostic tools are in place and genetic counselling can be scheduled. The main aim of antenatal screening is first to detect those women with a clinically significant trait who are in danger of having an affected fetus when the father is also a carrier. Second, women with a severe, although unknown, haemoglobinopathy can be identified. Therefore, extra care can be offered to these pregnant women, in order to eliminate the possibility of unpleasant outcomes, as maternal or perinatal mortality and morbidity [1]. As a result, couples have the opportunity to decide on partner screening, prenatal diagnosis or even termination of the pregnancy.

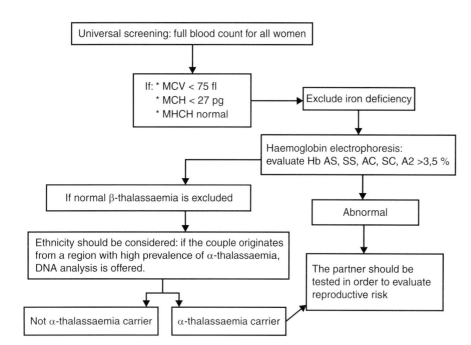

Figure 31.1 The recommended algorithm for screening of haemoglobinopathies

An algorithm of the recommended screening [5] is represented in Figure 31.1. Generally, all pregnant women should have a full blood count at their first antenatal care, as a universal screening for thalassaemia, with mean cell haemoglobin (MCH) to be the most sensitive marker for identifying thalassaemia traits [1]. α-Thalassaemia can only be detected through molecular genetic testing.

The solubility test is the primary screening for HbS in the general population. The solubility test is used when rapid results are required, but it fails to identify other haemoglobin variants that play a significant role for the fetal outcomes. Isoelectric focusing and the high-performance liquid chromatography (HPLC) test also help in making a diagnosis [2].

31.4.2 Ultrasound Assessment

In addition to screening the parents, if the algorithm in Figure 31.1 cannot reach a conclusive result, ultrasound assessments of the fetus at high risk are important. Anaemia or hydrops will be presented only by fetuses with α-thalassaemia major or Bart's hydrops, as the HbF is β-chain independent. The classic sign of Bart's hydrops, the hydrops fetalis, is not present until the 20th week of gestation [2]. However, there are some ultrasound findings which can detect fetal anaemia in the early second trimester such as the increased peak systolic velocity (PSV) in the middle cerebral artery, increased cardiac output, increased forward velocities in the ductus venosus and cardiomegaly. Interestingly, 90% of the affected fetuses have an increased placental thickness between the 14th and the 23th week of gestation, and much earlier than the appearance of hydrops fetalis [11].

31.4.3 Prenatal Diagnosis

When both the parents are carriers or they are in any kind of an increased risk for having an affected fetus, invasive prenatal tests are available in order to evaluate the fetal DNA and therefore to detect fetuses with haemoglobinopathies. The knowledge of the

baby's haemoglobinopathy status gives the parents the opportunity to know what is occurring in the pregnancy. Genetic counselling is needed to review the natural history of these disorders and the possible treatment and clinical status of the baby. Finally, the decision to terminate may be made at this point [5].

In the late first trimester (11th–15th week of gestation), chorionic villus sampling (CVS) can be performed in order to obtain fetal DNA. Amniocentesis is the alternative choice which is performed after the 16th week of gestation. CVS is the optimal method because it is performed earlier, giving the parents the choice of an earlier and therefore a less painful termination. In addition, CVS has the advantage of quicker results, as amniocentesis requires more than 10–14 days to culture the fetal cells [12]. One other choice, especially for couples ambivalent about terminating a pregnancy, is the pre-implantation genetic diagnosis, where the major disadvantage is the need for the in vitro fertilization (IVF) procedure [13].

31.5 Fertility and Pre-conception Evaluation

In the past, despite the small possibility of a spontaneous pregnancy, women with haemoglobinopathies were always recommended not to become pregnant, as they were considered as high-risk.

Although women with sickle cell disease do not have infertility problems, pregnancy is not very common, as females usually do not survive until the reproductive age, due to the high mortality associated with this disorder. However, significant improvements of both the treatment and management of women with sickle cell disease have led to improved pregnancy outcomes [2].

Concerning the women with homozygous β-thalassaemia, the vast majority (40–90%) [4] of them have associated hormonal insufficiencies, mainly due to the iron overload [14]. The most frequently encountered endocrinological disorders are hypopituitarism and hypogonadotrophic hypogonadism [2].

Therefore, women with transfusion-dependent thalassaemia have to use ovulation induction or assisted reproduction techniques in order to achieve pregnancy [2]. As ovulation induction can be used, there exists a variety of regimens and monitoring parameters including the evaluation of anti-Müllerian hormone (AMH) and oestradiol levels and transvaginal ultrasound (US) to evaluate the size of the follicles [22].

In all women with haemoglobinopathies, a multispecialty assessment, including reproductive medicine specialists, obstetricians, endocrinologists, haematologists and psychologists, should be performed prior to conception. Besides the determination of the fetal risk of having a haemoglobinopathy, the maternal transfusion and chelation therapy needs, in addition to the iron-overload status, end-organ dysfunction, liver and cardiac function, glucose tolerance, red blood cell antibodies and thrombotic risk, have to be evaluated. It is very important to evaluate for red blood cell antibodies, as these can cause severe morbidity of the newborn, due to the haemolytic disease [1]. Moreover, the exposure of chronic infections such as hepatitis B and C and HIV should be detected. Additionally, it is important to confirm that vaccines for hepatitis B and *S. pneumoniae* have been given. In this way, both the fetal and maternal outcomes are optimized, resulting in higher survival rates for both the mother and fetus [4]. Finally, especially in women with transfusion-dependent thalassaemia (TDT), assessment of bone mineral density with dual-energy x-ray absorptiometry (DEXA) should be performed prior to conception, in addition with an evaluation of the vitamin D levels.

Pregnancy should be avoided in women with unacceptable iron levels and end-organ damage. An MRI scan of the heart is recommended, and if in the T2 analysis, significant iron overload and cardiac dysfunction are identified, pregnancy should be planned when the maternal condition is optimized [2].

31.5.1 Pre-conception Treatment

The need of aggressive chelation and the reassurance that iron levels are as low as possible should be assessed prior to pregnancy, as chelation agents are contraindicated throughout pregnancy [1], because they have been blamed for embryotoxicity and teratogenicity [9]. Although the usage of oral hypoglycaemic agents in pregnancy is controversial, insulin transition is recommended. In addition, folic acid in higher dosages of 5 mg per day is recommended, and calcium and vitamin D supplements periconceptionally are highly recommended [2]. Vitamin C and calcium supplementation does not only optimize the bone health for both the mother and fetus, they can also reduce the risk for gestational diabetes [21]. Vitamin D and calcium should be continued throughout the entire pregnancy and breastfeeding period [19]. Iron supplementation should be given only to women who have documented iron deficiency.

31.6 Pregnancy Complications in Women with Haemoglobinopathies

It is well established that pregnancy affects every system of the mother's body, causing significant changes in her physiology [2]. Frequently, normal alterations due to pregnancy must be distinguished from pathological disorders, as maternal adaptations to pregnancy might exacerbate an underlying disorder. In women with haemoglobinopathies, physiological changes in the cardiovascular, haematological and respiratory systems are significant [2].

During pregnancy, blood volume increases significantly, by about 1.5 litres. However, this increase is not proportional – as plasma increases by 1.2 L while red blood cells only by 300 mL– resulting in a mild dilutional anaemia. Although in healthy pregnant women this alteration does not lead the haemoglobin levels to drop beyond 11 mg/dL, women with haemoglobinopathies often experience a higher haemoglobin level reduction, leading to a suboptimal oxygenation of fetal and maternal tissues. In extremely severe situations, maternal haemoglobin might be less than 6 mg/dL requiring supportive blood transfusions [2].

31.6.1 Maternal Complications

31.6.1.1 Complications in the Thalassaemias Group

The cardiovascular system in pregnancy has to be adjusted to the increased blood volume and metabolic demands. Therefore, the myocardium undergoes hypertrophy and the chambers enlarge, causing mild multivalvular regurgitation [4]. These alterations are finely managed in healthy pregnant women. In women with transfusion-dependent anaemia, where myocytes have exceeded iron deposition and cardiac reserve is decreased, cellular destruction is the result [15]. Moreover, left ventricular dysfunction or right-sided strain might be also present due to pulmonary hypertension, in addition to the chronic anaemia and increased vascular resistance. Women with haemoglobinopathies have to be closely monitored for these disorders, in addition to dysrhythmias and cardiac failure, as cardiac complications are the primary cause of death in individuals with TDT [16]. This makes the evaluation of the iron levels prior to conception an essential requisite.

Thrombotic risk is also increased in women with thalassaemia. In pregnancy, fibrin and coagulation factors increase, while fibrinolytic activity, protein S levels and venous flow velocity decrease. In thalassaemia, additional hypercoagulable factors are present, especially in patients who are non-transfused and splenectomized, involving interactions of the disrupted thalassaemic red blood cell membranes with the platelets, and endothelium [17-18].

Pregnant women with thalassaemia are vulnerable to infections, because of the elevated oestrogen levels of pregnancy, the variable state of iron overload and, in some cases, the absence of the spleen [19]. More specifically, pregnant women with HbH disease are at risk of having a haemolytic crisis in response to infections, fever or drugs usage. Moreover, osteopaenia and osteoporosis are also common in TDT [20].

Severe pregnancy and intrapartum complications for the mother can be present when the fetus has Hb Bart's hydrops. These include early-onset severe pre-eclampsia and primary postpartum haemorrhage. The latter is due to the delivery of a grossly hydropic fetus and placenta [1].

Severe early-onset pre-eclampsia is also very likely to be presented by women having either α- or β-thalassaemia [1]. In women with β-thalassaemia, the enlargement of the spleen is found to be associated with dystocia and hypersplenism [23]. Other common obstetric complications are placental ischaemic disease, placental abruption, polyhydramnios, gestational hypertension, gestational diabetes, renal and gallbladder stones and urinary tract infections [19].

31.6.1.2 Complications in the Sickle Cell Disorders

Due to improvements in transfusion medicine and neonatology and timely and evidence-based prenatal care, pregnancy complications in women with sickle cell disease have significantly decreased. However, they do exist and they occur with a higher frequency in them compared to healthy women.

Women carrying the HbS trait are not at an increased risk for adverse fetal or maternal outcomes. However, they are at risk of presenting with urinary tract infection, such as pyelonephritis or bacteriuria [24]. Therefore, they have to be monitored closely, and if any suspicion of an infection is present, treatment should be given immediately. Haematuria is also common in HbS trait, with no need for a specific medication, besides hydration and rest.

Women with sickle cell disease are at high risk for presenting with a sickle cell crisis, as pregnancy, labour and delivery are situations where infections, decreased oxygen tension status and dehydration are met frequently, predisposing the red blood cells to sickle [1]. Forty-eight per cent of women with sickle cell disease experience a crisis during pregnancy [25]. In this group, urinary tract infections are represented and managed in the same way as the trait's group. Additionally, pneumonia and puerperal sepsis are also common [19]. A clinical study which took place in Atlanta in 2001 [28] concluded that pregnant women with sickle cell anaemia are more likely to be admitted to hospital, with the main reasons being sickle pain crisis, pyelonephritis and anaemia. In addition, postpartum infections, mainly endometritis and pyelonephritis, were found in a higher prevalence compared to healthy women. These complications were found to be more frequent during the third trimester and puerperium [19].

Parvovirus B19 is also a threat for pregnant women with sickle cell disease. Besides the known complications of this infection for the fetus [29] (fetal anaemia, non-immune hydrops, fetal death and congenital anomalies affecting the eyes, the central nervous system and cranium), the parvovirus can also cause an aplastic crisis in the mother resulting in an extreme anaemia and worsening the symptoms of a possible respiratory or gastrointestinal infection [1].

Like women with thalassaemia, women with sickle cell disease are also at a higher risk for presenting with severe pre-eclampsia [2].

Resende Cardoso et al [26] studied the factors predisposing to severe or even fatal complications in pregnant women with sickle cell disease. They found that multiparity, baseline red blood macrocytosis evaluated by the mean corpuscular volume (MCV), and baseline hypoxia were significantly associated with high mortality in this group of patients. Furthermore,

the highest morbidity was due to pulmonary complications, such as severe acute chest syndrome leading to acute respiratory distress syndrome (ARDS), acute respiratory failure and need for mechanical ventilation.

31.6.2 Fetal Complications

Complications for fetuses whose mother suffers from both groups of haemoglobinopathies include intrauterine growth restriction (IUGR), premature rapture of the membranes and preterm birth [1, 2]. As a result, low-birthweight newborns are very likely to be delivered [26]. There is a theory, claiming that IUGR in sickle cell disease is due to vascular stasis in the uteroplacental unit [27]. Additionally, miscarriage and stillbirth occur with a high frequency in women with sickle cell disease, with a significant increase in perinatal mortality.

31.7 Management and Treatment in Women with Haemoglobinopathies

Correct and timely management of women with haemoglobinopathies is the key for the optimization of both the fetal and maternal outcomes, since the anaemia and the multi-organ dysfunction associated with these disorders have the potential to elevate maternal and perinatal mortality. The knowledge that every person is unique is important, as it offers the opportunity of the individualized management and therapy [1].

As fetal complications are common in women suffering from both groups of haemoglobinopathies, fetal surveillance has high significance. In this way, both the obstetrician and the mother can be reassured of fetal well-being, and if any indication of fetal distress is present, timely and correct management must be instituted [5]. Fetal biometry evaluation should be performed every 4 weeks, after the 24th week of gestation, in order to detect fetuses with IUGR. Specifically in women with thalassaemias, where multiple pregnancies are more common than the general population, the initial ultrasound scan should be performed carefully at the 7th–9th week of gestation [19]. Women with haemoglobinopathies should be screened for gestational diabetes at the 16th week of gestation, and if the result is negative, a repetitive test should be performed at the 28th week.

Generally, haemoglobin levels in pregnant women with haemoglobinopathies should be at least 10 mg/dL. However, a disagreement among the medical community is present concerning blood transfusions. Prophylactic blood transfusions in women with sickle cell disease throughout pregnancy are not globally accepted. The main reason for this disagreement is that blood transfusions increase the risk of transmission of blood-borne viral infections, promote isoimmunization, iron overload and increased rates of admissions to hospitals, despite the decrease of painful crises and severe anaemia [2, 5, 30]. Pregnancy outcomes are not different in women in whom blood transfusions were prophylactically used, compared to those in whom transfusions were used only as a corrective measure [31]. Additionally, alloantibodies added to the maternal system via the transfusions can cross the placenta, causing haemolytic neonatal anaemia. Therefore, extended genotype and antibody screening is required before any transfusion is undertaken.

31.7.1 Management in the Thalassaemias Group

When managing women with thalassaemias, the clinician should be continuously on the alert for any possible condition predisposing to complications, such as hypersplenism. Oxidative agents, infections, alcohol and smoking must be avoided while lifestyle and diet should be also modified to the 'pregnancy status' [2, 19].

Regular blood transfusions in women with thalassaemias are used as a corrective measure if the anaemia is worsening and if the fetus is not growing as expected. In women who are not on a regular blood transfusion schedule, and whose haemoglobin levels drop beyond 8 mg/dL before the 36th week of gestation, an alternative to the transfusions is erythropoietin administration [19].

Although chelation agents are contraindicated throughout pregnancy, use of desferioxamine (DFO) should be an option if the benefits of treatment are greater than the potential risks concerning both the maternal and fetal outcomes. The most representative example of a situation where DFO is beneficial is when the mother develops left-ventricular dysfunction and the organogenesis of the fetus has already taken place [19]. Additionally, DFO can be used safely during labour, as iron overload might lead to fatal cardiac dysrhythmias.

Thromboprophylaxis is relevant in the management of women with thalassaemias. Low molecular weight heparin should be offered to splenectomized women with a platelet count greater than 600 000, if they had history of recurrent abortions, or they are not receiving transfusions [32]. Thromboprophylaxis should continue for 7 days after vaginal delivery or 6 weeks after a caesarean section [33].

Delivery mode in women with thalassaemias should be individualized. Caesarean sections should be performed only for obstetric indications. Routine caesarean section is a choice for women with cardiac dysfunction. The main reasons for delivering via an emergency caesarean section are maternal short structure, skeletal deformities and cephalopelvic disproportion [19]. Nevertheless, epidural analgesia is preferred over general analgesia.

31.7.2 Management in Sickle Cell Disorders

31.7.2.1 General Management

Hydroxyurea is the drug which is the most used in sickle cell anaemia, as it can correct the globin chain imbalance, resulting in an increase in haemoglobin levels and therefore making sickling less possible [9]. The mechanism of action is said to be the rapid erythroid progenitor regeneration. However, hydroxyurea has been found to be teratogenic and therefore its use is contraindicated throughout pregnancy [5].

Preventing sickling can be achieved by avoiding a cold environment, heavy physical exercise, dehydration and stress. Correct nutrition is also equally significant. Prophylactic usage of penicillin due to the hypersplenism is another issue that must be considered.

31.7.2.2 Management of Acute Pain Syndrome

In pregnancy, acute pain syndrome has to be treated in the same way as in the non-pregnant state – with hydration and analgesia [1]. However, analgesia throughout pregnancy presents a challenge. Chronic nonsteroidal anti-inflammatory agents are contraindicated in gestations beyond the 32nd week, as they can be responsible for premature closure of the ductus arteriosus and oligohydramnios [1, 2]. On the other hand, chronic opiate use might lead to neonatal withdrawal syndrome. The solution is to adopt scheduled usage of morphine, with bolus dosage if required.

31.7.2.3 The Role of Transfusion

The controversial theories about prophylactic transfusion have been discussed above. Curative blood transfusion can be the treatment of choice for women with aplastic crisis due to parvovirus B19 infection, acute pain syndrome or where haemoglobin levels drop by more than 5 mg/dL [1]. Exchange transfusion might be an alternative treatment to acute pain syndrome [5].

31.7.2.4 Mode of Delivery

Although spontaneous labour is preferred in women with sickle cell disease, as the medication used for labour induction has the potential of causing sickling of the red blood cells [2], these women are more likely to deliver with caesarean section [28]. Generally, though, caesarean section should be reserved only for obstetric indications. If a caesarean section is unavoidable, epidural analgesia is preferred, as general anaesthesia might cause hypotension and hypoxaemia, predisposing to sickle crisis [5]. Regardless the mode of delivery, intravenous fluids and oxygen must be given the whole time, in order to prevent dehydration and hypoxia, respectively [1].

31.8 Haemoglobinopathies Prevention Programme in Greece

There is a need for universally agreed protocols for the prevention of thalassaemias in future generations. Here we share our dilemma and approach in Greece as we have a high endemicity of β-thalassaemia, with a frequency of 8%. The population of Greece is about 11 million and the number of marriages per year are around 58 000. The distribution of β-thalassaemia carriers is quite heterogeneous and varies from 5% to 20% within the country. There are also several foci of sickle cell syndromes, a mean frequency of haemoglobin 'S' carriers in the order of 1%. α-Thalassaemia also occurs in Greece, but these cases rarely result in severe Hb 'H' disease and hydrops fetalis, which have been reported in very few cases. National prevention and prenatal diagnosis programmes allow individuals and couples at risk to choose from the fullest range of available options. The best time for carrier screening is probably around the end of high school education. Approximately 70 000 persons are examined every year in Greece, and pre-conceptional carrier screening is mandatory. The couples at risk thus identified have enough time to choose from the fullest range of available options. Experience with adolescent screening in the schools suggests that acceptance rates are high, and the information is

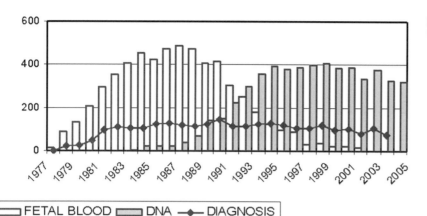

Fig 31.2 Prenatal diagnosis of β-thalassaemia and haemoglobinopathies in Greece (1977–2005)

well understood. There has been a significant drop in birth rates in Greece since 1977 (144 000 births (15.4%) down to 103 500 births (9.43) in 2003). The successful implementation of this programme is shown in Figure 31.2. These data demonstrate the efficacy of newer diagnostic tools.

The Prevention Programme for Thalassaemia and Haemoglobinopathies in Greece include:

1. Sensitization of the public,
2. Screening test for the identification of carriers,
3. Genetic counselling and
4. Prenatal diagnosis.

In Greece, Target Health Education Programmes for immigrants involve screening for haemoglobinopathies, genetic counselling and prenatal diagnosis. Carrier identification is carried out in all units following a standard approach:

• Complete blood tests (by electronic measurement: Hb, RBC, MCH, red cell distribution width (RDW), red blood cell morphology)
• Electrophoresis

• Measurement of haemoglobin fractions (HbA2, HbF)

The presence of α-thalassaemia sometimes makes screening more complicated as precise diagnosis of α-thalassaemia requires the demonstration of inclusion bodies in the red cells and is suggested by the study of DNA or a high β/α globin chain synthetic ratio. In these subjects, the parents and other family members are studied for the globin chain synthetic ratios and DNA for specific mutations or a combination of β- and δ-thalassaemias.

31.9 Conclusion

It is important to appreciate that haemoglobinopathies can have many different clinical presentations, challenging diagnosis and management. The key to having the optimal fetal and maternal outcomes is a clear appreciation and understanding of the risk the couple present, leading to correct screening. After detection of the affected individuals, management from a multispecialty team is essential to reduce the morbidity and mortality of both women and fetuses with haemoglobinopathies.

References

1. Johnston TA. Haemoglobinopathies in pregnancy. *Obstet Gynaecol.* 2005;7:149–57.

2. Rappaport VJ, Valazquez M, Williams K. Haemoglobinopathies in pregnancy. *Obstet Gynecol Clin N Am.* 2004;**31**:287–317.

3. Executive Board, 118. Thalassaemia and other haemoglobinopathies: report by the Secretariat. World Health Organization. 2006.

4. Carlberg KT, Singer ST, Vichinsky EP. Fertility and pregnancy in women with transfusion-dependent thalassaemia. *Hematol Oncol Clin North Am.* 2018 Apr;**32**(2):297–315.

5. ACOG Committee on Obstetrics. ACOG Practice Bulletin No. 78:

hemoglobinopathies in pregnancy. *Obstet Gynecol.* 2007;**109**(1):229–37.

6. Huntsman RG. Haemoglobinopathies in pregnancy. *J Clin Path (R Coll Pathol).* 1976;**10**:42–53.

7. Davies SC, Cronin E, Gill M, et al. Screening for sickle cell disease and thalassemia: a systematic review with supplementary research. *Health Technol Assess.* 2000;**4**:i–v,1–99. (Level III)

8. Yaster M, Kost-Byerly S, Maxwell LG. The management of pain in sickle cell disease. *Pediatr Clin North Am.* 2000;**47**:699–710.

9. Krafft A, Breymann C. Haemoglobinopathies in pregnancy.

Diagnosis and treatment, *Curr Clin Med.* 2004;**11**:2903–9.

10. Bergstrome JA, Poon A. Evaluation of a single-tube multiplex polymerase chain reaction screen for detection of common alpha-thalassemia genotypes in a clinical laboratory. *Am J Clin Pathol.* 2002;**118**: 18–24.

11. Ko TM, Tseng LH, Hsu PM, et al. Ultrasonographic scanning of placental thickness and the prenatal diagnosis of homozygous alpha-thalassaemia 1 in the second trimester. *Prenat Diagn.* 1995;**15**:7–11.

12. Wang X, Seaman C, Paik M, et al. Experience with 500 prenatal diagnoses of sickle cell diseases: the effect of

gestational age on affected pregnancy outcome. *Prenat Diagn.* 1994;**14**:851–7.

13. Xu K, Shi ZM, Veeck LL, Hughes MR, Rosenwaks Z. First unaffected pregnancy using preimplantation genetic diagnosis for sickle cell anemia. *JAMA.* 1999;**281**:1701–6.

14. Skordis N, Christou S, Koliou M, et al. Fertility in female patients with thalassemia. *J Pediatr Endocrinol Metab.* 1998;**11**(Suppl 3):935–43.

15. Tsironi M, Karagiorga M, Aessopos A. Iron overload, cardiac and other factors affecting pregnancy in thalassemia major. *Hemoglobin.* 2010;**34**(3):240–50.

16. Lao TT. Obstetric care for women with thalassemia. *Best Pract Res Clin Obstet Gynaecol.* 2017;**39**:89–100.

17. Leung TY, Lao TT. Thalassaemia in pregnancy. *Best Pract Res Clin Obstet Gynaecol.* 2012;**26**(1):37–51.

18. Ambroggio S, Peris C, Picardo E, et al. beta-thalassemia patients and gynecological approach: review and clinical experience. *Gynecol Endocrinol.* 2016;**32**(3):171–6.

19. Petrakos G, Andriopoulos P, Tsironi M. Pregnancy in women with thalassemia: challenges and solutions. *Int J Womens Health.* 2016;**8**:441–51.

20. Vogiatzi MG, Macklin EA, Fung EB, et al. Bone disease in thalassemia: a frequent and still unresolved problem. *J Bone Miner Res.* 2009;**24**(3):543–57.

21. Triunfo S, Lanzone A, Lindqvist PG. Low maternal circulating levels of vitamin D as potential determinant in the development of gestational diabetes mellitus. *J Endocrinol Invest.* 2017;**40**:1049–59.

22. Cassinerio E, Baldini IM, Alameddine RS, et al. Pregnancy in patients with thalassemia major: a cohort study and conclusions for an adequate care management approach. *Ann Hematol.* 2017;**96**(6):1015–21.

23. Aessopos A, Karabatsos F, Farmakis D, et al. Pregnancy in patients with well-treated b-thalassemia: outcome for mothers and newborn infants. *Am J Obstet Gynecol.* 1999;**180**:360–5.

24. Dale DC. Hematopoiesis. In Dale DC, ed. *Scientific American Medicine.* Seattle: University of Washington Medical Center; 1995.

25. Ismai KMK, Kilby MD. Human parvovirus B19 infection and pregnancy. *Obstet Gynecol.* 2003;**5**:4–9.

26. Resende Cardoso PS, Pessoa de Aguiar AL, Viana MB. Clinical complications in pregnant women with sickle cell disease: prospective study of factors predicting maternal death or near miss. *Rev Bras Hematol Hemoter.* 2014;**36**(4):256–63.

27. Pantanowitz L, Schwartz R, Balogh K. The placenta in sickle cell disease. *Arch Pathol Lab Med.* 2000;**124**:1565.

28. Sun PM, Wilburn W, Raynor BD, Jamieson D. Sickle cell disease in pregnancy: twenty years of experience at Grady Memorial Hospital, Atlanta, Georgia. *Am J Obstet Gynecol.* 2001 May;**184**(6):1127–30.

29. Giorgio E, De Oronzo MA, Iozza E, et al. Parvovirus B19 during pregnancy: a review. *J Prenat Med.* 2010 Oct-Dec; **4**(4):63–6.

30. Koshy M, Burd L, Wallace D, et al. Prophylactic red-cell transfusions in pregnant patients with sickle cell disease: a randomized cooperative study. *N Engl J Med.* 1988;**319**:1447–52.

31. Morrison JC, Schneider JM, Whybrew WD, Bucovaz ET, Menzel DM. Prophylactic transfusions in pregnant patients with sickle cell hemoglobinopathies: benefit versus risk. *Obstet Gynecol.* 1980;**56**:274–80.

32. Origa R, Piga A, Quarta G, et al. Pregnancy and β-thalassemia: an Italian multicenter experience. *Haematologica.* 2010;**95**:376–81.

33. Lekawanvijit S, Chattipakorn N. Iron overload thalassemic cardiomyopathy: iron status assessment and mechanisms of mechanical and electrical disturbance due to iron toxicity. *Can J Cardiol.* 2009;**25**:213–18.

Kidney Diseases in Pregnancy

Giorgina Barbara Piccoli, Rossella Attini & Gianfranca Cabiddu

32.1 Introduction: Riding Out the Storm

The link between kidney diseases and adverse pregnancy outcomes has been acknowledged since the birth of nephrology as a discipline. At the beginning of the twentieth century, a clinical paper in *The Lancet* listed the situations in which pregnancy was affected by a kidney disease, and some of these findings hold true today: the differential diagnosis between pre-existing kidney disease and pre-eclampsia may be difficult if not impossible to make and the two conditions frequently merge [1].

About 70 years later, another editorial in *The Lancet*, entitled 'Pregnancy and Renal Disease', started with the following sentence: *'Children of women with renal disease used to be born dangerously or not at all – not at all if their doctors had their way.'* The paper reflected the then current opinion on the grim prognosis of a 'CKD pregnancy'. However, the final advice deserves being cited: *'The woman should be told that there is a considerable risk to her infant and a small risk to herself, but dogmatic prohibitions do not seem justified today. Instead, obstetrician and physician must batten down the hatches and prepare to ride out the storm together with those determined to set sail'* [2].

What has changed in recent decades to make pregnancy in chronic kidney disease (CKD) more common?

The advances made in maternal-fetal medicine, with a progressive expansion of the fetal viability zone to 22–24 weeks, and improvements in the care of the 'small' and 'very small' babies have made possible a more tolerant attitude towards high-risk pregnancies. The definition of CKD has also changed, from the identification with renal insufficiency, to the acknowledgement of the importance of the early stages in which some kind of damage is already present, but where kidney function is still normal [3]. This is of relevance for pregnancy, where even initial kidney damage increases the risk of adverse pregnancy outcomes (Table 32.1). In the last decade, 'intensive dialysis protocols' have significantly improved the prognosis of pregnancy on dialysis, highlighting new frontiers for dialysis efficiency [4].

From the social perspective, the changes in the patient–physician relationship, shifting from a paternalistic view focused on the ethical imperative to 'do no harm' to awareness of patients' autonomy, have modified attitudes towards high-risk pregnancies so they are no longer routinely banned [5]. Furthermore, the results reported from countries where having a large family is a deeply rooted social value have led to reconsideration of the minimalist style of counselling usually employed in Western countries. In a wider perspective, acknowledging the differences in the care of kidney diseases in pregnancy supports global initiatives to reduce mortality and morbidity in 'CKD pregnancy', which are higher in low- and middle-income countries [6, 7].

32.2 Epidemiology and Aetiology: Chronic Kidney Disease (CKD)

Many initial forms of CKD are not symptomatic and are not recognized unless searched for as described in Table 32.1. For this reason, the actual prevalence of CKD in pregnancy is not known and the figures that are most frequently reported derive from interpolations of data obtained in the overall population, based on the assumption that fertility is not reduced in the initial CKD stages, and may be progressively reduced in further stages. The figures most often cited are a prevalence of about 3% in the early CKD stages (1–3a) and of between 1:150 to 1:750 pregnancies in the later ones (3b–5) [8].

'Chronic kidney disease' is an umbrella term for several diseases that may differently affect pregnancy. Immunological nephropathies are at risk of flare-ups during and after pregnancy. Pyelonephritis and renal malformations share a risk of urinary tract infections. Polycystic kidney disease presents complex ethical problems for prenatal counselling. Diabetic nephropathy is the only disease associated with a higher risk for non-renal malformations, mainly due to the presence of diabetes itself.

As will be further discussed, beside the aetiology of kidney disease, prognosis is modulated by degree of kidney impairment, the presence and severity of hypertension and proteinuria. Their interactions are complex, and so far have not been completely elucidated.

32.3 Epidemiology and Aetiology: Acute Kidney Injury (AKI)

Pregnancy-related AKI (p-AKI) has not disappeared in high-income countries and is the leading cause of AKI in women in the developing world [7]. The epidemiology is not completely known, since its definition ranges from an increase in serum creatinine by 0.5 mg/dL to need for

Table 32.1 Chronic kidney disease (CKD) classification based upon e-GFR and examples for pregnancy

CKD stage	definition	Example	Notes for pregnancy
1	**e-GFR >90 mL/min:** normal kidney function, associated with persistent signs of kidney damage.	Initial phases of glomerulonephritis; kidney scars due to reflux nephropathy or pyelonephritis; recurrent lithiasis and previous AKI; kidney donors are frequently in this group.	Risk of preterm delivery is about twice that of the overall population in many studies; proteinuria and hypertension before pregnancy or at referral increase risk. Small but overall significant increase in risk of PE.
2	**e-GFR 60–90 mL/min:** a slight reduction in kidney function does not classify a patient as CKD unless other persistent signs of kidney damage are present.	**As stage 1;** in both cases hyperfiltration in pregnancy may mask a more severe kidney disease.	Risks increase with respect to stage 1 CKD, suggesting a direct relationship between reduced kidney function and outcomes.
3a	**e-GFR 45–60 mL/min** the old definition of renal insufficiency starts from this phase.	Chronic glomerulonephritis, reflux nephropathy, diabetic nephropathy or ADPKD may fall in this category at childbearing age.	Risk of preterm delivery is further increased; proteinuria and hypertension before pregnancy or at referral increase the risk. Risk of developing PE, worsening hypertension or proteinuria is greater. Risk of delivering small-for-gestational-age babies may increase, in particular in immunological diseases.
3b	**e-GFR 30–45 mL/min**		
4	**e-GFR 15–30 mL/min**	**As above.** Due to the frequent slow progression of many forms of CKD, these last stages mainly comprise severe immunological diseases, diabetic nephropathy in a context of poor metabolic control, or severe malformations, with or without superimposed infection.	Risks are further increased, including PE, worsening hypertension or proteinuria. Overall risk of delivering small-for-gestational-age babies increases, and is modulated by obstetric policy.
5	**e-GFR <15 mL/min or on renal replacement therapy**	**Last 'pre-dialysis stage' (see above).** Patients without contraindications should be waitlisted for transplantation (but off waitlist when pregnant). An AV fistula can be proposed, given potential advantage compared to a tunnelled catheter on haemodialysis	**As above.** In stage 5, dialysis start may be needed. Indications and advantages with respect to 'conservative' treatment are not clear. Case by case decisions, based on the experiences of each group, are needed.

AKI: acute kidney injury; AV: arterio-venous fistula for dialysis; e-GFR: estimated glomerular filtration rate; PE: pre-eclampsia.

dialysis, and even then the need for dialysis may be underestimated due to the lack of availability of this treatment in low-income settings. Even though AKI was considered to be an all-or-nothing condition, in which complete reversal was the rule in surviving patients, it is now known to be associated with future risk for CKD, hypertension and cardiovascular diseases. The epidemiology of p-AKI varies widely from country to country and closely follows the epidemiology of death in pregnancy: according to WomenAid International, the probability that an African woman will die from pregnancy-related complications is 100 times higher than for women in high-income settings. The main causes are haemorrhage, sepsis, pre-eclampsia-eclampsia and septic abortion, all of which also cause AKI. According to the World Health Organization, the Maternal Mortality Ratio is 12:100 000 in high-income regions and 239:100 000 in low-income ones.

The causes of p-AKI vary: septic abortion is the leading cause of early p-AKI in countries where legal abortions are not available, while PE after assisted fertilization (egg donation in particular) is becoming a cause of p-AKI in high-income countries. Furthermore, CKD may present as p-AKI and p-AKI increases in the hypertensive disorders of pregnancy, which increase in CKD. Table 32.2 provides an extensive, albeit non-exhaustive, classification of the most common causes of p-AKI (modified from [7]).

32.4 Physiopathology of CKD in Pregnancy: Measuring Kidney Function in Pregnancy

In physiological conditions, the indexes of kidney function increase in pregnancy: renal plasma flow, fractional filtration, glomerular filtration rate (GFR) increase, with a consequent reduction of serum creatinine and an increase in proteinuria. The excretory system increases its compliance, which is one of the elements favouring urinary tract infections [9]. As a consequence, the normality ranges of serum creatinine are not applicable in pregnancy and none of the formulae on which the usual estimation of GFR (e-GFR) is based are validated in pregnancy. The hyperfiltration response is frequently preserved in a diseased kidney, and this may alter CKD staging, or, more importantly, make it more difficult to diagnose CKD. The problem is even more relevant if we consider that many kidney diseases are asymptomatic, and that pregnancy is a precious occasion for diagnosing CKD.

When pre-conception serum creatinine is known, the fact that there is no decrease suggests the presence of a kidney disease; however, this is often not the case, since kidney function evaluation is not included in the usual pre-pregnancy workup, and attention to the kidney in pregnancy is still mainly focused on proteinuria, both as a sign of kidney disease (if detected before 20 gestational weeks) or as a marker of pre-eclampsia (PE).

Otherwise, a correction in the usual creatinine range has recently been suggested and may represent a way to account at least in part for pregnancy-related hyperfiltration [10].

32.5 Pathogenesis of Adverse Pregnancy Outcomes in CKD Pregnancies

All the main complications of pregnancy increase in CKD; this starts from the early stages and rises in parallel with the reduction in kidney function, being negatively modulated by the presence of hypertension and proteinuria (see Table 32.1). The reasons why adverse pregnancy outcomes are more common in pregnancy in patients with CKD is

not known. In the presence of severe kidney disease, a pathogenic role for the 'uraemic toxins' can be postulated and is in keeping with the observation that intensive dialysis extends the duration of pregnancy and makes possible better fetal growth [4].

In patients with hypertension, immunological diseases, diabetes or severe proteinuria, endothelial damage is common. However, the reasons for increases in adverse pregnancy outcomes in patients with normal kidney function, normotension and without proteinuria remain obscure. This increase is consistently described in kidney donors, the best example of a 'healthy' reduction in kidney tissue, in patients with kidney stones or other interstitial kidney diseases, in the pre-clinical phase of polycystic kidney disease, or following an episode of AKI, even when the kidney function has normalized.

On these bases, some groups hold that all patients with CKD should be managed as 'high-risk pregnancies' and closely monitored by both a nephrologist and obstetrician whenever possible (see Section 32.14 on guidelines).

32.6 Clinical Features and Clinical Management in the Different Phases of CKD

Schematically, CKD in pregnancy can be divided into three main phases:

- Early CKD (stages 1–2), in which prognosis and clinical management deal with the underlying disease or its complications (hypertension and proteinuria);
- Advanced CKD (stages 3–5), in which the picture is increasingly dominated by the reduction in kidney function;
- Renal replacement therapy, which is in turn divided into dialysis and kidney transplantation.

32.7 Early Disease: CKD Stages 1–2

The current definition of CKD, which includes all patients with signs of kidney disease regardless of their kidney function, dates to the beginning of the new millennium. Consequently, most of the older studies concern advanced CKD and most of the studies on early kidney disease in pregnancy are recent [11]. Table 32.3 summarizes the adverse maternal-fetal outcomes observed in CKD patients, including pre-eclampsia, pregnancy-induced hypertension and preterm delivery.

In the early-CKD cohort, the risks of maternal death are very low, especially in high-income countries, and are almost entirely limited to active immunological diseases. The risk of death is higher in poorly resourced countries; p-AKI and PE are closely associated with a risk of death in disfavoured settings, where underlying CKD may be particularly difficult to diagnose [12].

The risks of worsening of the kidney function, developing hypertension and developing or increasing proteinuria increase along with CKD stage; in the early stages, they are higher in diseases with glomerular involvement, but not specific to them. While the presence of proteinuria before the 20th

Table 32.2 A general, but non-exhaustive, classification of the main causes of pregnancy-related acute kidney injury (p-AKI)

PRERENAL			
Type of damage	**Phase**	**Condition**	**Main clinical features**
Hypovolaemic	Early	Hyperemesis gravidarum	May be severe, associated with nutritional deficits, and is more common in patients with a nutritional disorder or malnutrition; may reflect psychological problems. More commonly diagnosed in developed countries, it is probably underestimated in developing ones.
	Any time	Other causes of vomiting	Infectious diseases, nutritional disorders; acute fatty liver of pregnancy; metabolic acidosis, uraemia.
Haemorrhagic	Early	Abortion	Early fetal loss can cause severe haemorrhaging, but unsafe, illegal abortions are the most common cause of massive bleeding, usually associated with sepsis. More common in low- and middle-income countries, and where abortion is illegal.
	Late	Placental abruption	Can cause massive bleeding, as well as fetal loss; usually occurs in late pregnancy.
Hypotensive	Any time	Hypovolaemia, cardiopathy, sepsis	Hypotension is usually a concomitant cause and a marker of severity of the above. The rare, but sometimes severe, cardiomyopathy of pregnancy can lead to severe hypotension and AKI. Sepsis (any cause, any phase) is often associated with hypotension up to hypotensive shock, and associated with tubular necrosis (see below).
Combined pathogenesis	Any time	Septic abortion, placental abruption, sepsis, puerperal sepsis	Severe bleeding is associated with hypovolaemia and hypotension. While the 'usual' classification of AKI may be of help, focusing on one element only may avert attention from treating all associated factors.

PARENCHYMAL (except pre-eclampsia)			
Structure primarily involved	**Phase**	**Condition**	**Clinical features**
Glomerular	Any time	CKD (known or undiagnosed)	The presence of CKD is associated with adverse pregnancy outcomes starting from the early stages. Immunological diseases may relapse or appear in pregnancy. CKD worsening is described in 20–80% of patients.
	Usually late	Microangiopathies	Haemolytic uraemic syndrome and related diseases are an emerging concern, particularly in developed countries, perhaps because they fail to be diagnosed in low-income settings.
Interstitial	Any time	Iatrogenic, associated with other causes of AKI	The causes are the same encountered outside of pregnancy but the consequences may be more severe. Whether the 'pregnant kidney' is associated with increased risk is a matter of debate.
	Any time	Pyelonephritis and upper urinary tract infections	These infections seldom cause AKI, although they can be severe and life threatening. In this context, AKI is usually linked to sepsis or is iatrogenic.
Combined	Any time	Tubular necrosis- cortical necrosis	Tubular necrosis may result from any severe AKI, and may be multifactorial.

(continued)

Table 32.2 (cont.)

POSTRENAL–OBSTRUCTIVE			
Pathogenesis	**Phase**	**Condition**	**Clinical features**
Mechanical	Any time	Stone disease	Hypercalciuria can occur in pregnancy. Pain due to the passage of a stone may be misinterpreted, especially at term; infection and undiagnosed obstruction may be life- and function-threatening.
	Postpartum	Iatrogenic	Ligature of the ureters is a rare but serious iatrogenic complication of caesarean section or other surgery.
	Any time	Neoplasia	Kidney and urinary tract neoplasia are rare but occasionally encountered in young women. Diagnosis should be considered in macroscopic haematuria, in particular if there are clots.
	Usually late	ADPKD and other cystic diseases of the kidney	Cystic diseases of the kidney may go unrecognized in younger women. Large non-symptomatic cysts may become symptomatic, cause pain or obstruction, or become infected in pregnancy.
Functional	Usually late	Functional obstruction and hydronephrosis	Mild urinary tract dilation (usually on the right side) is common, and usually without consequences; pyelo-ureteral junction anomaly, may decompensate in pregnancy leading to giant hydronephrosis. Severe urinary tract dilation is occasionally described in patients with reflux nephropathy.
Combined	Any time	Infection, bleeding in obstructed kidney	All the above causes are associated with infection, sepsis (mainly Gram negative), merging intrarenal, prerenal and obstructive pathogenesis.

e-GFR: estimated glomerular filtration rate; AKI: acute kidney injury; PE: pre-eclampsia; ADPKD: autosomal dominant polycystic kidney disease (modified from [7]).

Table 32.3 Adverse pregnancy outcomes in CKD patients and main risks in their offspring

Term	Definition	Main issues in CKD
Maternal death	Death in pregnancy or within 1 week – 1 month postpartum	Too rare to be quantified, at least in highly resourced settings, where cases are in the setting of severe flares of immunological diseases (SLE *in primis*).
CKD progression	Decrease in GFR, rise in sCr, shift to a higher CKD stage	Differently estimated; may be linked to obstetric policy (anticipating delivery in the case of worsening of the kidney function); 20% to 80% in advanced CKD. Probably no increase in early CKD (stages 1–3a).
Immunological flares and neonatal SLE	Flares of immunological diseases in pregnancy	Once thought to increase in pregnancy, in particular in SLE, probably a risk in patients who start pregnancy with an active disease, or recent flare. Definition of a 'safe' zone not uniformly agreed; in quiescent, well-controlled SLE, flares do not appear to increase compared to non-pregnant, carefully matched controls.
Transplant rejection	Acute rejection in pregnancy	Similar to SLE, rejection episodes are not higher compared to matched controls; may be an issue in unplanned pregnancies, in unstable patients.
Abortion	Fetal loss, before 21–24 gestational weeks	May increase in CKD, but data are scant. An issue in immunological diseases (eventually, but not exclusively linked to the presence of LLAC) and in diabetic nephropathy.
Stillbirth	Delivery of a non-viable infant, after 21–24 gestational weeks	Probably no increase in early CKD, too few data in late CKD; may be an issue in dialysis patients; when not linked to extreme prematurity, may specifically be linked to SLE, immunological diseases and diabetic nephropathy.

Table 32.3 (cont.)

Term	Definition	Main issues in CKD
Neonatal death	Death within 1 week – 1 month from delivery	Usually a result of extreme prematurity, which bears a risk of respiratory distress, neonatal sepsis, cerebral haemorrhage.
Small, very small baby	A baby weighting <2500–1500 g at birth	The weight has to be analyzed considering gestational age; however, very low birthweight bears important risks for future health, even when growth is adequate for gestational age. Different cut-points are used, the most common are 1500 for very small and 2500 for small baby.
Preterm, early preterm, extremely preterm	Delivery before 37; 32 or 34; 28 completed gestational weeks	Increase in risk of preterm and early preterm delivery across CKD stages; extremely preterm may be an important issue in undiagnosed or late-referral CKD and PE-AKI. The definition of preterm is agreed at <37 weeks; two cut-points, at 32 and 34 weeks are used for dividing late from early preterm, while 28 weeks is agreed for extremely preterm delivery.
SGA: Small for gestational age	<5th or <10th centile for gestational age	SGA and IUGR may be associated, but IUGR is also a dynamic event, characterized by flattening of the growth curve. Both are better defined when ample data on pregnancy are available.
IUGR: Intrauterine growth restriction	<5th centile or flattening of the growth curve	Small, SGA and IUGR babies are at higher risk of developing hypertension, metabolic syndrome and CKD in adulthood.
Malformations	Any kind of malformations	Malformations are not more common in CKD patients not treated with teratogen drugs (MMF, mTor inhibitors, ACEi, ARBS), with the following exceptions: diabetic nephropathy (attributed to diabetes); hereditary diseases, such as PKD, reflux nephropathy, CAKUT may be evident at birth.
Hereditary kidney diseases	Any kind of CKD	In several forms of CKD there is a recognizable hereditary pattern or predisposition; besides PKD, reflux and CAKUT, Alport's disease, IgA, kidney tubular disorders and mitochondrial diseases have a genetic background, usually evident in adulthood, but not always elucidated.
CKD – hypertension	Higher risk of hypertension and CKD in adulthood	Late maturation of nephrons results in a lower nephron number in preterm babies; the risks are probably higher in SGA-IUGR babies than in preterm babies adequate for gestational age.
Other long-term issues	Developmental disorders	Mainly due to prematurity. Cerebral haemorrhage or neonatal sepsis, are not specific to CKD, but are a threat in all preterm babies.

ACEi: angiotensin-converting enzyme inhibitor; ADPKD: autosomal dominant polycystic kidney disease; AKI: acute kidney injury; ARBS: angiotensin II receptor blockers; CAKUT: congenital anomalies of the kidney and urinary tract; e-GFR: estimated glomerular filtration rate; IgA: immunoglobulin A; IUGR: intrauterine growth restriction; LLAC: lupus-like anticoagulant; MMF: mycophenolate mofetil; mTor: mechanistic target of rapamycin; PE: pre-eclampsia; PE-AKI: pre-eclampsia acute kidney injury; PKD: polycystic kidney disease; sCR: serum creatinine; SGA: small for gestational age; SLE: systemic lupus erythematosus (modified from [6]).

gestational week, in a singleton pregnancy, is highly suggestive of a pre-existing glomerular disease, pregnancy-induced proteinuria and PE can occur in any kind of kidney disease; however, since proteinuria post-delivery is the most common disease marker employed, and kidney ultrasounds are not a part of the usual post-PE workup, the role of interstitial and malformative diseases is not yet fully understood.

The short- and long-term fetal risks are mainly related to prematurity. Small or premature children have an increased probability of having a low nephron number and of developing

CKD later in life, along with the panoply of metabolic diseases described in preterm babies [13–14]. This risk may be further increased in the children of CKD mothers, due to the multifactorial genetic background of CKD.

Perinatal death increases in lupus nephropathy, diabetic nephropathy, and other immunological systemic diseases, even in the early CKD stages. The reasons are not completely understood, and absence of specific antibodies in lupus nephropathy or presence of good metabolic control in diabetic nephropathy does not completely rule out these risks.

Conversely, malformations not linked to hereditary kidney diseases do not increase. Although data were not confirmed in later studies, one report found only a two- to threefold increase in different types of malformations in diabetic nephropathy.

Regardless of kidney function, risks for adverse maternal-fetal outcomes increase in multiple pregnancies, in particular if they are the result of assisted fertilization techniques. Conversely, the risk for worsening of the kidney function is considered minimal in the early CKD stages and increased, albeit differently quantified, in advanced CKD [11].

32.7.1 Specific Diseases and Specific Signs: Glomerulonephritis

Since many forms of CKD are fully asymptomatic, pregnancy is often the moment when 'isolated' urinary anomalies are discovered; in pregnancy, attention is often focused on proteinuria, and haematuria is often overlooked. Microscopic haematuria is very common during pregnancy, detected in up to 20% of women, limiting the value of this semeiotic element; however, micro-haematuria persists after delivery in up to 25% of these women, who should undergo an extensive nephrology workup [15].

The most common potentially progressive glomerulonephritis which presents with isolated haematuria in pregnancy is immunoglobulin A (IgA) nephropathy (the most common glomerulonephritis worldwide), but haematuria may be the initial presentation of complex immunological diseases including lupus, or a sign of 'benign' familial haematuria or Alport syndrome, which usually has an attenuated presentation in females.

When proteinuria during pregnancy is not associated with PE, it may reflect a primary glomerulonephritis. Interestingly, when not associated with pregnancy, the most common presentation of IgA nephropathy is haematuria; in pregnancy, nephrotic syndrome is common, and may completely or partially remit after delivery. Other causes of intense proteinuria, besides diabetic nephropathy, which is usually self-evident, are focal segmental glomerulosclerosis, minimal change nephropathy and membranous nephropathy. Minimal change nephropathy may be suggested by the presence of proteinuria almost exclusively constituted by albumin, with a decrease in serum albumin that is out of proportion with total proteins. However, all types of glomerulonephritis may present with intense proteinuria in pregnancy and occasionally have a rapidly progressive course [16].

The indications for renal biopsy are limited: the risk of bleeding increases in pregnancy, in keeping with increased renal blood flow; secondly, many immune-depressive drugs, including mycophenolate mofetil, rapamycin and cyclophosphamide, are not prescribed, thus limiting the subsequent therapeutic options (Table 32.4). Renal biopsy may be considered in early pregnancy, in the presence of rapidly progressive kidney function impairment or severe nephrotic syndrome; in the third trimester of pregnancy, the risks of bleeding and the delay between the kidney biopsy and its results need to be balanced against the risks linked with inducing premature delivery.

Table 32.4a Main immunosuppressive drugs for chronic treatment in pregnant CKD patients

DRUG	MAIN FEATURES	FDA
	Usually considered as RELATIVELY SAFE, WHEN ABSOLUTELY NEEDED	
Azathioprine	This is the most widely used immunosuppressive drug. It is teratogenic in animal models, but not in humans, possibly because the fetal liver is not able to activate the drug. KDIGO and European Best Practice Guidelines suggest switching from mycophenolate to azathioprine before pregnancy.	D
Cyclosporine A	This calcineurin inhibitor has not been associated with increased teratogenicity; however, small-for-gestational-age babies and preterm delivery have been reported, possibly due to maternal disease rather than the drug; levels may vary in pregnancy and the hypertensive, hyperglycaemic and nephrotoxic effects should be mentioned	C
Tacrolimus	The drug has similar effects and side effects as cyclosporine A; since it is a relatively new drug, experience is more limited than with the previous drug.	C
Steroids	Together with azathioprine these are the most often employed and best-known drugs. The most frequently used short-acting corticosteroids include prednisone, methylprednisolone and prednisolone, while betamethasone and dexamethasone are among the long-acting drugs. No major malformations have been reported, and the issue of labiopalatoschisis is debated. A higher risk of premature rupture of membranes has been reported. Other relevant side effects include infectious risk, and an increased risk of gestational diabetes.	C
Hydroxychloroquine	This synthetic anti-malaric agent crosses the placenta but has not been found to be associated with fetal toxicity.	B

Table 32.4a (cont.)

DRUG	MAIN FEATURES	FDA
	TO BE AVOIDED	
Cyclophosphamide	This alkylating agent is contraindicated in pregnancy; a few reports suggest that pregnancy termination is common in cases of inadvertent use or the need for lifesaving therapy. A few positive reports, mainly in women with SLE are available.	D
Mycophenolate	Severe fetal malformations are reported, mainly involving cardiovascular and cranial malformations. Discontinuation for at least 6 months, to stabilize kidney function, is usually indicated after kidney transplantation.	D
Rituximab	There are no data on whether rituximab can cause fetal harm. Rituximab was detected postnatally in the serum of infants exposed in-utero: B-cell lymphocytopenia generally lasting less than six months can occur in infants. The manufacturer recommends contraception for up to 12 months following therapy.	C
m-Tor inhibitors	Very few studies consider their use in pregnancy. They are teratogenic in animals and discontinuation in humans is a matter of debate; KDIGO guidelines suggest discontinuation in anticipation of pregnancy	C

Table 32.4b Main anti-hypertensive drugs in pregnant patients with CKD

DRUG	MAIN FEATURES	FDA	SOGC
	Usually considered FIRST CHOICE drugs		
Alpha-methyldopa	Widely used in pregnancy, with no reported negative effects on the fetus or on its subsequent development. May not be able to correct severe hypertension in CKD.	B	1-A
Nifedipine	The long-acting drug most commonly used in hypertension in pregnancy. The increase in peripheral oedema may be a relevant side effect in CKD patients.	C	1-A
Labetalol	Usually well tolerated, should be avoided in subjects with asthma. In one RCT it was shown to be comparable to alpha-methyldopa.	C	1-A
	Usually considered SECOND CHOICE drugs		
Beta blockers	The main drawback in older studies was fetal growth restriction, possibly as an effect of overzealous correction. Beta1 selective beta blockers (atenolol) are more often involved. Beta blockers may be more effective than alpha-methyldopa in severe hypertension, alone or in a combined therapy. At delivery they may induce hypoglycaemia, hypotension and bradycardia (usually mild and transient)	D atenolol B pindolol C metoprolol	1-B
Clonidine	The effect is similar to alpha-methyldopa; side effects may be more common and hypertensive rebounds at discontinuation are common; slowed fetal growth is occasionally reported	C	
Alpha blockers	Other drugs should be preferred as there are no controlled studies.	C	
Diuretics	They are usually avoided in pregnancy except for nephrological or cardiological indications. Thiazides may be continued in patients previously on treatment. In selected cases with Gitelman syndrome, amiloride may be employed.	B hydrochlorothiazide amiloride	
	TO BE AVOIDED		
Short-acting nifedipine	Contraindicated by the FDA, RCOG and AIPE due to the risk of severe sudden hypotension with detrimental effects on placental flows.	D	
ACEi ARB and related drugs	Both drugs are contraindicated in all phases of pregnancy because of the risk of major malformations, including cardiovascular, central nervous system, renal and bone malformations.	C 1st D 2nd 3rd trimester	II 2E

Table 32.4c Other drugs for pregnant CKD women

Drug	Characteristics	FDA
	Usually considered as safe, when needed	
Acetyl salicylate	Low doses during pregnancy needed for the treatment of diverse medical conditions have not been shown to cause fetal harm; may protect against pre-eclampsia, favouring placentation; discontinuation before delivery is recommended.	NC
LMWH	Low molecular weight heparin (LMWH) does not cross the placenta and is safe for the fetus, although bleeding at the uteroplacental junction cannot be ruled out. Individualized doses of LMWH are well tolerated and safe for prophylaxis and treatment of thromboembolic complications during pregnancy, and postpartum. Twice-daily heparin should be discontinued prior to induction of labour or planned caesarean delivery and can be resumed after delivery.	C
ESAs	In vitro studies suggest that recombinant erythropoietin does not cross the human placenta; higher doses may be needed in dialysis.	C
Allopurinol	Adverse events were observed in animal studies. Allopurinol crosses the placenta. An increased risk of malformations has not been observed in humans (limited data).	C
Vitamin D	The role for vitamin D supplementation in pregnancy is controversial, but there is no evidence of a reduction in adverse pregnancy outcomes (e.g. pre-eclampsia, stillbirth, neonatal death) or improvement in bone mineral content in children in studies in which supplementation was given independently from blood levels. *Cholecalciferol (vitamin D3)* crosses the placenta but the transfer to the fetus from the mother is low. Maternal supplementation has not been shown to affect pregnancy outcomes. *Ergocalciferol.* Adverse events have been observed in animal studies. The ergocalciferol (vitamin D_2) metabolite, 25(OH)D, crosses the placenta; maternal serum concentrations correlate with fetal concentrations at birth. *Calcitriol.* Teratogenic effects have been observed in animal studies. Adverse effects on fetal development were not observed in women with pseudo vitamin D-dependent rickets. *Paricalcitol.* Adverse events have been observed in some animal reproduction studies. Vitamin D deficiency in a pregnant woman can lead to deficiency in the neonate. Serum 25(OH)D concentrations should be measured in pregnant women at increased risk of deficiency. Current guidelines recommend an intake of 1000 to 2000 units/per day until more safety data are available. Vitamin D and calcium levels should be monitored and kept in the low normal range.	C

AIPE: Italian Association on Pre-eclampsia; ESA: erythropoiesis-stimulating agent; FDA: US Food and Drug Administration; RCOG: Royal College of Obstetricians and Gynaecologists; RCT: randomized controlled trial; SOGC: Society of Obstetricians and Gynaecologists of Canada:
FDA Classification: A Controlled human studies show no risk; B No evidence of risk in studies; C Risk cannot be ruled out; D Positive evidence of risk; X Contraindicated in pregnancy. NC not classified
Modified from guidelines on best-practices on kidney diseases in pregnancy of the Italian Society of Nephrology

Since pulse steroids are a part of the treatment of most of primary nephropathies, some authors suggest that empiric steroid treatment, eventually combined with anticalcineurin inhibitors in the case of severe proteinuria, can help postpone the kidney biopsy to the puerperium. Since the enzyme 11b-hydroxysteroid dehydrogenase 2, present in the placenta, sharply reduces the transplacental passage of prednisolone, this drug should be preferred to betamethasone or dexamethasone; treatment should however be discussed with an experienced nephrologist.

While many glomerulonephritis do not have specific biomarkers, presence of antibodies directed against the phospholipase A2 receptor 1 (PLA2R) is a highly specific indication of primary membranous nephropathy; they are easily detectable using commercial kits, allowing diagnosis without the need for a kidney biopsy, which can be postponed until after pregnancy to allow for staging of the disease.

Since hypercoagulability is one of the main risks of the nephrotic syndrome, treatment with aspirin or low molecular weight heparin should be considered. Early prophylactic treatment with aspirin is usually suggested in patients with known IgA nephropathy, on the basis of positive results obtained in relatively small series, and, in the absence of specific evidence, it is often used in other glomerular diseases. While the effect on prevention of PE is probably limited to the start of treatment in the first trimester of pregnancy, the target of reducing systemic thrombotic risk and possibly secondary placental damage should be pursued in all phases (Table 32.5).

32.7.2 Specific Diseases and Specific Signs: Lupus Nephropathy

Pregnancy in women with lupus nephritis is the paradigm of pregnancy in the course of autoimmune diseases with renal involvement (for pregnancy in systemic lupus erythaematosus (SLE), see Chapter 34). The 'ideal' situation is a planned pregnancy in an informed woman with stable and prolonged remission of SLE, normal renal function, normal blood pressure and negative antiphospholipid antibodies. This is not always the case and the management of lupus nephropathy is often quite challenging. An extensive clinical, biochemical and immunological evaluation, in particular to determine an extractable nuclear antigen antibodies (ENA) profile and the presence of antiphospholipid antibodies, is advised before pregnancy, and, when this is not possible, at referral; ideally, cyclophosphamide should be withdrawn at least 3 months before pregnancy and mycophenolate replaced by azathioprine at least 6 weeks prior to pregnancy in order to minimize the risk of SLE flares.

The risk of a renal flare of lupus nephritis during pregnancy ranges from 15% to 30%; severe flares probably account for about 1:10 of all flares. In the case of renal flares, pulse steroids and high-dose immunoglobulins are reported as safe and effective. Low molecular weight heparin (LMWH) should be added to low-dose aspirin, if not already prescribed, in case of intense proteinuria.

The definition of superimposed PE may be difficult; however, all the hypertensive disorders of pregnancy increase fetal loss, stillbirth and neonatal death increase more compared to the overall population; active lupus nephritis at conception, hypertension, reduced kidney function and proteinuria specifically increase the risk. While even severe kidney function impairment is not an absolute contraindication to pregnancy, this may increase the risk of needing dialysis in pregnancy. Severe pulmonary hypertension, restrictive lung disease and heart failure are associated with an increased risk of maternal death.

Multidisciplinary follow-up of lupus nephropathy should not end at delivery, since renal flares may be more frequent in the first 6–12 months after birth ([17] and guidelines).

32.7.3 Specific Diseases and Specific Signs: Other Vasculitis

Most types of vasculitis are rare diseases that, except for Takayasu disease, peak at an age typically over 40; multiorgan involvement often discourages the few patients of childbearing age to plan a pregnancy, and frequently used immunosuppressive drugs, such as cyclophosphamide, may induce premature menopause and sterility [18].

As in lupus nephropathy, the presence of kidney involvement is associated with a higher risk of adverse pregnancy outcomes, and with life-threatening complications, including pulmonary haemorrhage, polyneuritis and myocarditis. Rapidly progressive glomerulonephritis, whose occurrence may increase up to 1 year after delivery, is the most feared kidney complication. Because of their rarity, follow-up should be planned in tertiary care centres and therapeutic strategies need to be individualized. As in lupus nephropathy, low-dose acetyl salicylic acid can be used for preventing PE. Pulse steroids, plasma-exchange, high-dose immunoglobulin, azathioprine and, according to a few reports, rituximab may make continuation of pregnancy possible in an attempt to balance maternal and fetal risks [18].

32.7.4 Specific Diseases and Specific Signs: Diabetic Nephropathy

The prevalence of diabetic nephropathy, broadly defined as the presence of any sign of renal disease including microalbuminuria, ranges from 5% to over 25% in type 1 diabetic pregnant women; the prevalence of nephropathy in the context of type 2 diabetes in pregnancy is less known [19]. In pregnancy, a sharp increase in proteinuria, not necessarily in the context of PE, is probably more common than in other kidney diseases; therefore, critical decisions on pregnancy management in patients with diabetic nephropathy should not rely on this isolated issue.

Besides the general risks of prematurity or intrauterine growth restriction (IUGR), risk of stillbirth or fetal death is specific of diabetic nephropathy and of lupus nephropathy. Furthermore, there may be a higher incidence of malformations in diabetic nephropathy as compared to diabetes without kidney involvement, not offset by an optimized metabolic balance (see also best practice on CKD).

32.7.5 Specific Diseases and Specific Signs: Autosomal Dominant Polycystic Kidney Disease (ADPKD)

Autosomal dominant polycystic kidney disease (ADPKD) is one of the most common monogenic diseases and an example of epigenetic variability. While the prevalence of a mutation in the *ADPKD1* or *ADPKD2* gene is estimated to occur in 1:500 to 1:1000 individuals, ADPKD accounts for only 5–10% of the patients on renal replacement therapy (representing about 1:1000 individuals in settings where dialysis and transplantation are available without restriction). Due to the fact that the disease is frequently non-symptomatic until the third to fifth decade, it may escape diagnosis before pregnancy, and reports in pregnancy are limited. Within these limits, it is thought that hypertensive disorders of pregnancy, urinary tract infections and preterm delivery are more frequent in ADPKD patients [20]. The old tenet that women with ADPKD should deliver by caesarean section because the peaks in abdominal pressure at parturition increase the risk of intracystic bleeding is not supported by the current evidence; caesarean section should be reserved for cases with very large cysts or a history of recurrent bleeding.

Pre-conception and pre-implantation diagnosis is now possible in cases in which the disease is linked to a mutation in the major genes (PKD1 and PKD2, which account for about 90% of cases); this possibility gives rise to ethical issues, both with respect to pregnancy interruption for a condition which may be asymptomatic throughout life or only become evident 30–50 years later and given the increased rate of complications caused by assisted fertilization procedures.

32.7.6 Specific Diseases and Specific Signs: Chronic Pyelonephritis, Kidney Scars and Kidney Stones

Chronic pyelonephritis is an umbrella diagnosis encompassing many causes in which a mechanic (including high pressure vesico-ureteral reflux, obstruction secondary to kidney stones) or infectious disease produce damage resulting in kidney scars. Kidney scars may involve one or both kidneys, be minimal or numerous enough to distort the renal architecture; imaging techniques are obviously required for diagnosis [21].

Since many of these diseases do not lead to end-stage kidney disease, and are frequently overlooked in the asymptomatic phases, the actual prevalence in different age groups is not known.

Conversely, asymptomatic bacteriuria is the most common infectious problem encountered during gestation, found in 2–7% of pregnancies, when specifically searched for (since urinary tract infections are usually asymptomatic during pregnancy). Pregnancy predisposes to urinary tract infections as a result of urinary stasis, associated with physiological hypotonia and decreased ureteral peristaltic activity induced by progesterone and by the compression of the gravid uterus; furthermore, pregnancy-induced glycosuria and aminoaciduria often facilitate bacterial colonization.

A history of urinary tract infections, diabetes, obesity, low socio-economic status, older maternal age and urological abnormalities are associated with an increased risk of bacteriuria and upper urinary tract infections. Even when asymptomatic, bacteriuria has been associated with an increased risk of miscarriage, preterm birth, low birthweight and perinatal mortality, thus leading to the current practice of performing one urinary culture in early pregnancy even in low-risk pregnancies.

Since even high-grade bacteriuria in pregnancy may be fully asymptomatic or present with frequency and urgency only, the classic signs and symptoms (dysuria, suprapubic pain and haematuria) are not required for starting treatment, which should wait for the antibiogram in the absence of upper urinary tract involvement (flank pain, fever usually with chills, abdominal or pelvic pain, up to full-blown sepsis). Upper urinary tract infections are reported in 1–3% of all pregnancies and, besides sepsis, may be complicated by p-AKI in 2–25% of cases.

In cases of recurrent lower urinary tract infections, in particular in cases at risk for upper urinary infections, including ADPKD reflux nephropathy or kidney scars, 'suppressive'

therapy should be considered, usually consisting of low-dose nitrofurantoin or cephalexin at bedtime, up to 2–4 weeks before the date of expected delivery.

Kidney stones are rare in pregnancy but are associated with PE and preterm delivery; renal colic is more frequent in the second and third trimesters, and besides the classic hallmark of flank pain, it may cause gross, sometimes painless haematuria. In most cases, the dilation of the urinary tract favours stone emission and only symptomatic therapy is needed. Albeit rarely, surgical management may be required, and when it is, must be performed by experienced hands.

Upper urinary tract infection is one of the most feared complications of all these diseases. Due to the fact that lower urinary tract infections are often asymptomatic, severe acute urinary tract infections may develop abruptly, and the information on how to minimize their risks is scant. On the basis of one rather old survey, considering the time needed by the most frequent urinary pathogens, Escherichia coli, to colonize the urinary tract to the kidney (1–2 weeks), some authors suggest that for patients at high risk of urinary tract infections (reflux nephropathy, history of acute pyelonephritis with kidney scars, ADPKD, kidney stones and complex renal malformations), urinalysis and urinary culture should be performed every 1 to 2 weeks, and those with positive urinary cultures should be systematically treated (see best practices).

32.8 Advanced CKD (stages 3–5 not on dialysis)

Although the specific challenges linked to different diseases are not offset by severe CKD, and, for example, patients with an immunological disease remain at high risk of flares, or the risk of further infections does not decrease in patients with chronic pyelonephritis, the clinical picture is increasingly dominated by a reduction in kidney function which is increasingly, albeit non-invariably, accompanied by hypertension and proteinuria [3, 11, 22].

32.8.1 Reduction in Kidney Function and Indications for Dialysis Start

The reason why a reduction in kidney function is accompanied by an increased risk of adverse pregnancy outcomes is not fully understood, even if the presence of uraemic toxins, whose role is indirectly demonstrated by an improvement in pregnancy results in patients on intensive dialysis versus patients treated using conventional schedules, are thought to be important [4].

The indications on when to start dialysis in pregnancy are not established. Some authors retain that dialysis should be started at the same levels of blood urea that guide dialysis treatment in patients already on chronic dialysis (urea of about 100 mg/dL or blood urea nitrogen of about 50 mg/dL), while others hold that initiation of dialysis should be guided in pregnancy by the same indications established for the overall population, in which early dialysis start is associated with excess morbidity. Following this line, dialysis should be started when a good metabolic and fluid balance cannot be achieved by conservative treatment, rather than on blood urea-based thresholds. The phase of pregnancy should be taken into account, balancing the risks and benefit of starting dialysis versus inducing delivery.

The main benefits of dialysis for metabolic control and volume and blood pressure management should be weighed on an individual basis versus the potentially negative effects of catheter-related complications. When dialysis is started with a central venous access, these include the need for surgical intervention and the stress related to fistula placement, as well as an increased risk of haemorrhage from dialysis anti-coagulation and the risk of dialysis-related hypotension, that may precipitate fetal-placental hypoperfusion [23, 24].

32.8.2 CKD in Pregnancy

Target blood pressure values are periodically reviewed in the hypertensive disorders of pregnancy, a setting in which a shared recommendation is to avoid overcorrection of hypertension, which can negatively affect fetal growth. However, blood pressure targets in hypertensive CKD pregnancies are less well established; out of pregnancy, a 'low normal' target level of 110–120 systolic and 70–80 mm Hg diastolic blood pressure is common for young patients, with the aim of reducing the progression of kidney disease. In pregnancy, while avoiding overcorrection is obviously wise, most authors consider that the same low blood pressure targets should be pursued, under strict medical control and with self-monitoring of blood pressure [25].

The main list of anti-hypertensive drugs that can be used is shown in Table 32.6. None is fully safe, and the issue of teratogenicity of ACEi and ARBs is still a matter of debate. While some authors suggest discontinuing these drugs before pregnancy, others support discontinuation at the first positive pregnancy test to maximize the benefits of control of protei-nuria, at least in compliant patients [24].

32.8.3 Specific Issues: Proteinuria

An increase in proteinuria is frequent in CKD pregnancy. There are two elements that may induce it: the need for dis-continuation of ACEi and ARBs, and hyperfiltration linked to pregnancy. These two elements combine with PE, or flares of immunological disease; furthermore, isolated proteinuria may appear in pregnancy, even without hypertension.

Since the entity of proteinuria in pregnancy is not closely correlated to the severity of kidney disease, monitoring should focus on albumin levels (effective volaemia), and consider coagulation (and antithrombin III levels), and immunoglobulin levels, to establish a comprehensive evaluation of the severity of protein loss. Anticoagulation should be added in the absence of contraindications. No benefit from albumin infusion in increasing albumin levels and reducing the risk of placental hypoperfusion is reported and albumin infusion should be avoided, considering the risk of adverse reactions, and of further increasing proteinuria by enhancing hyperfiltration.

In the absence of specific anti-proteinuric treatment in pregnancy, small studies suggest that a plant-based diet, with a controlled protein intake (0.6–0.8 g/kg/day) may at least partly counteract hyperfiltration without a negative effect

(and possibly with a small advantage) on fetal growth [26]. The effect may be due to a combination of reduction of the workload for the intact nephrons, in keeping with what is observed out of pregnancy, and the antioxidant power of plant-based diets. The safety data are in keeping with the position of the American Dietary Association, provided that B12, iron and vitamin D are controlled and supplied when needed.

32.9 Renal Replacement Therapy

32.9.1 Dialysis

The first report, in the early 1970s, of a successful pregnancy on dialysis was met with fascination and disbelief, and since then pregnancy on dialysis has been alternatively regarded as a miracle or as an event to discourage [23].

There are many reasons why this attitude is changing, even though pregnancy is still very rare in dialysis patients, who have roughly 1:100 probability of a live-born baby compared to the overall population. The reasons for this reduced fertility are both physical and psychological: derangements of the hypothalamus-hypophysis-ovarian axis are common in advanced CKD, driven by hyperprolactinemia, anaemia, stress and phar-macological interferences [8]. The stigmatization of dialysis patients as 'too ill to lead a normal life', and the widespread opinion that for them successful pregnancy was impossible constituted important psychological barriers. In fact, in many series, most pregnancies on dialysis were unplanned [5]. The diffusion of dialysis in settings with a strong cultural drive towards large families and less attention to 'invisible diseases', such as end-stage kidney disease, has made it possible to gather large series of pregnancies on dialysis from emerging countries. Patients' empowerment may have contributed to increasing pregnancy on dialysis in the Western world.

Dialysis patients should not be considered as infertile; the increase in dialysis efficiency, the correction of anaemia, attention to a more comprehensive metabolic balance now mean that the hormonal milieu can be restored, at least in some cases. Once pregnancy has started, the impressive advances in dialy-sis efficiency allowed by 'intensive' non-conventional sche-dules (the reference schedules is 8 hours of overnight dialysis 6 days per week, which represent a fourfold increase in dialysis duration compared to 'conventional' schedules of 4 hours 3 days per week) now allow most pregnancies to go to term or near term, with good results for fetal growth [4].

32.9.2 Peritoneal Dialysis or Haemodialysis in Pregnancy

There is still no randomized study comparing peritoneal dialysis (PD) and extracorporeal dialysis (HD) in pregnancy. There are reports of pregnancies on both dialysis modalities, and the lower number of cases on PD is at least in part a reflection of the less widespread use of this technique. Overall, the best data are those reported on daily long-hour haemodialysis and some authors therefore suggest switching from PD to HD in pregnant patients, while others suggest that this policy should be reserved to patients who have a low efficiency of PD, without residual diuresis or with PD-related problems [24].

The disadvantages of each therapy, namely, the risk of peritonitis and the lower efficiency of PD, and the risk of too rapid fluid and electrolyte shifts, of anticoagulation and the higher intrusiveness in daily life of HD need to be explained in counselling.

Whatever the choice, dialysis intensity (frequency and duration) should be increased in pregnancy; on haemodialysis, quotidian or nightly sessions (6–7 days per week) should be the standard at least for patients without residual renal clearances (with 36 hours of haemodialysis per week the probability of a successful pregnancy reaches 85%). Other prescriptions should be individualized, and bicarbonate, potassium, sodium, calcium and vitamins should be controlled (folic acid is usually supplemented in pregnancy, intensive dialysis is associated with loss of hydro-soluble vitamins, in particular vitamin C; iron, vitamin B12 and vitamin D, which also need to be monitored and supplemented when needed). The loss of small-size proteins, in particular albumin, via highly permeable dialysis membranes, should also be kept in mind in planning dietary interventions [27].

32.10 Kidney Transplantation

The history of pregnancy after kidney transplantation starts with a kidney donation from one young woman to her identical twin in 1956. After restoration of good health, the patient recovered her menstrual cycles and soon afterwards became pregnant, giving birth to a healthy baby. The donor and recipient were enthusiastic enough to give birth to a total of 5 babies, all in good health. Their case was reported in *The New England Journal of Medicine* [28].

Since then, kidney transplantation has come to be recognized as the best method for restoring fertility in a woman with advanced CKD or on dialysis; while higher compared to women on dialysis, the probability of having a child after kidney transplantation is however reduced: about 1:10 with respect to the overall population. Even if the outcomes are better than on dialysis, pregnancies after kidney transplantation are not devoid of risks, which encompass prematurity, small-for-gestational-age babies and the hypertensive disorders of pregnancy [29]. Overall, if teratogen drugs are avoided (Table 32.4), the risks are similar to those observed in patients with CKD, for the same level of kidney function. No difference between the 'allowed' immunosuppressive drugs is evident, although calcineurin inhibitors have been occasionally associated with fetal growth restriction. As in the settings of other kidney diseases, PE is differently defined, and this impairs calculating its real incidence. The clinical choices in cases at high risk for malformations or kidney function impairment require merging clinical and ethical approaches in which, besides the mother and child dyad, the grafted kidney is a crucial 'third element', since pregnancy may precipitate kidney loss in the case of impaired kidney function at baseline.

32.10.1 The 'Ideal and Non-ideal' Profile of a Kidney Transplant Patient Who Wants to Start a Pregnancy

An ideal pre-pregnancy profile after kidney transplantation includes normal kidney function, scant or no proteinuria, normotension, no recent acute rejection, good compliance and low-dose immunosuppression, without potentially dangerous drugs (mycophenolic acid and mTor inhibitors), at least 1 to 2 years after transplantation [30].

In such a setting, the risks of worsening of the kidney function are minor, and the outcomes are overall reported as good, even if the incidence of preterm delivery, small babies and the hypertensive disorders of pregnancy is 2 to 10 times higher than in the overall population.

Less is known about how to manage 'non-ideal' situations, such as pregnancy shortly after transplantation, in the context of proteinuria and/or hypertension or with a failing kidney. While our experience in such cases is limited, and the risks of worsening the renal function are differently reported, the risks are probably higher in the presence of reduced kidney function and proteinuria, while well-controlled hypertension alone seems less relevant for outcomes.

32.11 Differential Diagnosis between CKD, Pre-eclampsia and Superimposed Pre-eclampsia

The definition of CKD (any alteration in the kidney morphology or function lasting for at least 3 months, or e-GFR lower than 60 mL/min (see Table 32.1)) has several points in common with that of pre-eclampsia (PE), classically defined as a reversible condition characterized by the association of hypertension and proteinuria (above 300 mg/day), occurring after the 20th week of pregnancy in previously normotensive, non-proteinuric women. According to the American College of Obstetricians and Gynecologists' guidelines, demonstration of proteinuria is no longer needed for diagnosis, and serum creatinine increase is mentioned among the alternative criteria.

In any case, proteinuria, hypertension or kidney function impairment should disappear within 1–3 months after delivery. In fact, PE has been defined as a transitory and reversible kidney disease, ultimately cured by delivery.

Pre-eclampsia and CKD are closely related: both are characterized by micro-vascular involvement, and sometimes by combinations of hypertension and proteinuria, and are related in pregnancy, where one condition may favour the development of the other [31].

There is no fully agreed on definition of 'superimposed' PE. The condition encompasses worsening of hypertension or an increase in proteinuria in a setting in which they are already present, and grading this 'worsening' may be difficult, in particular when measures for improving blood pressure control or reducing proteinuria have already been undertaken.

Independently from the definition, there are three conditions in which making a differential diagnosis between PE and CKD is almost impossible: when no data before 20 gestational weeks is available; when CKD flares in pregnancy; when kidney disease develops in pregnancy. In the few studies addressed to this issue, the main suggestions for differential diagnosis are based upon the degree of placental involvement. In this regard, 'early' or 'placental' PE is characterized by a deficit in placentation, leading to an early impairment of uteroplacental flows, and ischaemia, reflected by an unbalance in angiogenic and anti-angiogenic biomarkers. So far only soluble Fms-like tyrosine kinase 1 (sFlt1), placental growth factor (PlGF) and their ratio have been integrated in the clinical practice [32]. Figure 32.1 reports the scheme developed by the Italian Society of Nephrology's study group on kidney diseases and pregnancy, as a pragmatic support for differential diagnosis and further follow-up (see best practices on pre-eclampsia).

While an extensive discussion of this subject is beyond the scope of this chapter, it should be mentioned that PE represents a risk factor for the development of CKD; the question is whether PE is an epiphenomenon of a pre-existent kidney disease, or a pathogenic agent [33]. In the absence of specific indications, some authors suggest following all PE patients for at least 6 months, and prescribing yearly controls of blood pressure, kidney function and proteinuria. Children born to PE mothers should be considered as at risk for developing cardiovascular diseases, including CKD, and followed accordingly, with attention paid to preventing obesity, and carefully monitoring other predisposing factors [14].

32.12 The Treatment and Planning of Follow-Up

There is no specific treatment for CKD pregnancies; however, several therapies that are used in CKD are contraindicated and should be discontinued or replaced in pregnancy (Table 32.4).

The main goals of a joint nephrology and obstetric follow-up are early identification and treatment of potential complications, including hypertension, proteinuria, anaemia, coagulation disorders and flares of immunological diseases.

A logical suggestion is to intensify follow-up in CKD patients in comparison with normal pregnancies, increasing the frequency of visits in line with the increase in CKD stages and according to the presence of hypertension, proteinuria and systemic diseases. However, no fixed rule exists. Figure 32.2 reports a proposed frequency of controls in various situations.

Due to the lack of agreed formulae for establishing kidney function in pregnancy, assessment of creatinine clearance on 24-hour urine collection is probably the best option, allowing for precise quantification of proteinuria.

Patients at risk of recurrent urinary tract infections or immunological flares or those with glomerulonephritis in remission should have urinalysis for proteinuria and/or urinary cultures every 1–2 weeks, so that urinary tract infections and immunological flares can be promptly identified. The drugs most commonly used in CKD and limitations on their used in pregnancy are reported in Table 32.4.

32.13 Key Messages

1. CKD is increasingly encountered in pregnancy, and patients with chronic diseases, including CKD, are increasingly deciding to become pregnant. The prevalence of CKD in pregnancy has reached 3%, considering the early CKD stages.
2. The adverse pregnancy outcomes encountered in CKD patients are preterm delivery, small-for-gestational-age babies and the development of hypertension and proteinuria, with or without a picture of pre-eclampsia.
3. The risks start increasing from the first CKD stage, in which signs of kidney damage (including kidney scars or solitary kidney) are present, but kidney function

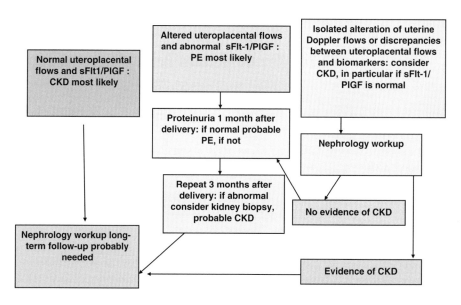

Figure 32.1 A proposed flow chart for the differential diagnosis between CKD and PE (modified from the best-practices on kidney diseases in pregnancy of the Italian Society of Nephrology)

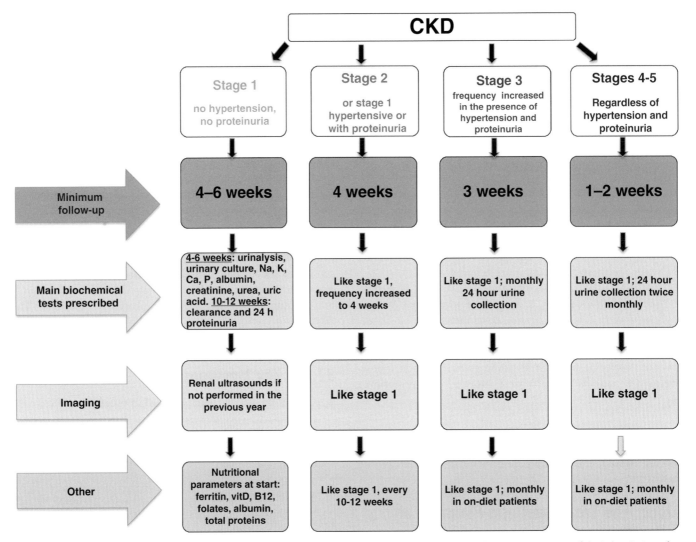

Figure 32.2 A proposed flow chart of controls in CKD pregnancy (modified from the best-practices on kidney diseases in pregnancy of the Italian Society of Nephrology)

may still be normal, and increase along with kidney function reduction.

4. The presence of hypertension and proteinuria increase the risks mentioned above.

5. Malformations are not increased in CKD pregnancy, in the absence of teratogen drugs or genetic diseases. A possible exception is diabetic nephropathy.

6. There is no fixed threshold for dialysis start in pregnancy; however, when dialysis is started, intensive schedules yield the best results.

7. Follow-up of CKD in pregnancy should be intensive and multidisciplinary, and should continue after pregnancy, at least for patients with immunological diseases, in which flares may also increase in puerperium.

8. There have been significant changes in therapies, attitudes to the patient's right to self-determination and the definitions of CKD and PE. The evidence on what constitute the best counselling and follow-up procedures is scattered and fragmentary. This lack of certitudes should be

mentioned during counselling, and strongly supports shared choices in the context of multidisciplinary care.

32.14 Key Guidelines Relevant to the Topic

There is a lack of guidelines on pregnancy in kidney diseases, with the partial exception of kidney transplantation.

The Italian Study Group on Kidney and Pregnancy compiled a series of 'best practices':

1. Cabiddu G, Castellino S, Gernone G, et al. Best practices on pregnancy on dialysis: the Italian Study Group on Kidney and Pregnancy. *J Nephrol.* 2015 Jun;28(3):279–88.

2. Cabiddu G, Castellino S, Gernone G, et al. A best practice position statement on pregnancy in chronic kidney disease: the Italian Study Group on Kidney and Pregnancy. *J Nephrol.* 2016 Jun;29(3):277–303.

3. Piccoli GB, Cabiddu G, Castellino S, et al. A best practice position statement on the role of the nephrologist in the prevention and follow-up of preeclampsia: the Italian Study

Group on Kidney and Pregnancy. *J Nephrol.* 2017 Jun;**30**(3):307–317.

4. Cabiddu G, Spotti D, Gernone G, et al. A best-practice position statement on pregnancy after kidney transplantation: focusing on the unsolved questions. The Italian Society of Nephrology's Study Group on Disease and Pregnancy. *J Nephrol.* 2018 Oct;**31**(5):665–81.

Management of lupus nephritis during pregnancy is discussed in:

Wilhelmus S, Bajema IM, Bertsias GK, et al. Lupus nephritis management guidelines compared. *Nephrol Dial Transplant.* 2016 Jun;**31**(6):904–13.

The recent EULAR guidelines are available at:

Andreoli L, Bertsias GK, Agmon-Levin N, et al. EULAR recommendations for women's health and the management of family planning, assisted reproduction, pregnancy and menopause in patients with systemic lupus erythematosus and/or antiphospholipid syndrome. *Ann Rheum Dis.* 2017 Mar;**76**(3):476–85.

For further information on lupus nephropathy or on diabetic nephropathy, see the specific chapters on these topics in this book.

The suggestions of an international panel of experts on glomerular diseases in pregnancy, based upon a systematic review, are also available: Blom K, Odutayo A, Bramham K, Hladunewich MA. Pregnancy and glomerular disease: a systematic review of the literature with management guidelines. *Clin J Am Soc Nephrol.* 2017 Nov 7;**12**(11):1862–72.

Kidney transplantation guidelines are available at:

European best practice guidelines for renal transplantation. Section IV: Long-term management of the transplant recipient. IV.10. Pregnancy in renal transplant recipients. EBPG Expert Group on Renal Transplantation. *Nephrol Dial Transplant.* 2002; **17** Suppl 4:50–5.

And at https://uroweb.org/wp-content/uploads/EAU-Guidelines-Renal-Transplantation-2009.pdf

References

1. A Lecture ON THE ALBUMINURIA OF PREGNANCY AND THE KIDNEY OF PREGNANCY. Delivered at University College Hospital on Nov. 8th, 1905, BY G. F. BLACKER, M.D. LOND., F.R.C.P. LOND, F.R.C.S. ENG., OBSTETRIC PHYSICIAN TO THE HOSPITAL AND TO THE GREAT NORTHERN HOSPITAL. *Lancet.* 1905;**166**(4295):1819–22.

2. [No authors listed] Pregnancy and renal disease. *Lancet.* 1975 Oct 25;**2**(7939):801–2.

3. Piccoli GB, Attini R, Vasario E, et al. Pregnancy and chronic kidney disease: a challenge in all CKD stages. *Clin J Am Soc Nephrol.* 2010 May;**5**(5):844–55.

4. Hladunewich MA, Hou S, Odutayo A, et al. Intensive hemodialysis associates with improved pregnancy outcomes: a Canadian and United States cohort comparison. *J Am Soc Nephrol.* 2014 May;**25**(5):1103–9.

5. Tong A, Jesudason S, Craig JC, Winkelmayer WC. Perspectives on pregnancy in women with chronic kidney disease: systematic review of qualitative studies. *Nephrol Dial Transplant.* 2015 Apr;**30**(4):652–61.

6. Piccoli GB, Zakharova E, Attini R, et al. Pregnancy in chronic kidney disease: need for higher awareness. a pragmatic review focused on what could be improved in the different CKD stages and phases. *J Clin Med.* 2018 Nov 5;**7**(11).pii: E415.

7. Piccoli GB, Zakharova E, Attini R, et al. Acute kidney injury in pregnancy: the need for higher awareness. A pragmatic review focused on what could be improved in the prevention and care of pregnancy-related AKI, in the year dedicated to women and kidney diseases. *J Clin Med.* 2018 Oct 1;**7**(10).

8. Williams D, Davison J. Chronic kidney disease in pregnancy. *BMJ.* 2008 Jan 26;**336**(7637):211–15.

9. August P. Obstetric nephrology: pregnancy and the kidney–inextricably linked. *Clin J Am Soc Nephrol.* 2012 Dec;**7**(12):2071–2.

10. Wiles K, Bramham K, Seed PT, Nelson-Piercy C, Lightstone L, Chappell LC. Serum creatinine in pregnancy: a systematic review. *Kidney Int Reports.* 2019;**4**;408–19

11. Zhang JJ, Ma XX, Hao L, et al. A systematic review and meta-analysis of outcomes of pregnancy in CKD and CKD outcomes in pregnancy. *Clin J Am Soc Nephrol.* 2015 Nov 6;**10**(11):1964–78.

12. Ibarra-Hernández M, Orozco-Guillén OA, de la Alcantar-Vallín ML, et al. Acute kidney injury in pregnancy and the role of underlying CKD: a point of view from México. *J Nephrol.* 2017 Dec;**30**(6):773–80.

13. Chehade H, Simeoni U, Guignard JP, Boubred F. Preterm birth: long term cardiovascular and renal consequences. *Curr Pediatr Rev.* 2018;**14**(4):219–26.

14. Luyckx VA. Preterm birth and its impact on renal health. *Semin Nephrol.* 2017 Jul;**37**(4):311–19.

15. Brown MA, Holt JL, Mangos GJ, et al. Microscopic hematuria in pregnancy: relevance to pregnancy outcome. *Am J Kidney Dis.* 2005 Apr;**45**(4):667–73.

16. Blom K, Odutayo A, Bramham K, Hladunewich MA. Pregnancy and glomerular disease: a systematic review of the literature with management guidelines. *Clin J Am Soc Nephrol.* 2017 Nov 7;**12**(11):1862–72.

17. Sammaritano LR. Management of systemic lupus erythematosus during pregnancy. *Ann Rev Med.* 2017 Jan 14;**68**:271–85.

18. Machen L, Clowse ME. Vasculitis and pregnancy. *Rheum Dis Clin North Am.* 2017 May;**43**(2):239–47.

19. Spotti D. Pregnancy in women with diabetic nephropathy. *J Nephrol.* 2018 Nov 15;**32**(3):379–88. doi: 10.1007/s40620-018-0553-8. [Epub ahead of print]

20. Wu M, Wang D, Zand L, et al. Pregnancy outcomes in autosomal dominant polycystic kidney disease: a case-control study. *J Matern Fetal Neonatal Med.* 2016 Mar;**29**(5):807–12.

21. Attini R, Kooij I, Montersino B, et al. Reflux nephropathy and the risk of preeclampsia and of other adverse pregnancy-related outcomes: a systematic review and meta-analysis of case series and reports in the new millennium. *J Nephrol.* 2018 Dec;**31**(6):833–46.

22. Imbasciati E, Gregorini G, Cabiddu G, et al. Pregnancy in CKD stages 3 to 5:

fetal and maternal outcomes. *Am J Kidney Dis.* 2007 Jun;**49**(6):753–62.

23. Cabiddu G, Castellino S, Gernone G, et al. Best practices on pregnancy on dialysis: the Italian Study Group on Kidney and Pregnancy. *J Nephrol.* 2015 Jun;**28**(3):279–88.

24. Cabiddu G, Castellino S, Gernone G, et al. A best practice position statement on pregnancy in chronic kidney disease: the Italian Study Group on Kidney and Pregnancy. *J Nephrol.* 2016 Jun;**29**(3):277–303.

25. Piccoli GB, Cabiddu G, Attini R, et al. Hypertension in CKD pregnancy: a question of cause and effect (cause or effect? this is the question). *Curr Hypertens Rep.* 2016 Apr;**18**(5):35.

26. Attini R, Leone F, Parisi S, et al. Vegan-vegetarian low-protein supplemented diets in pregnant CKD patients: fifteen years of experience. *BMC Nephrol.* 2016 Sep 20;**17**(1):132.

27. Tangren J, Nadel M, Hladunewich MA. Pregnancy and end-stage renal disease. *Blood Purif.* 2018;**45**(1–3):194–200. doi: 10.1159/000485157. Epub 2018 Jan 26.

28. Murray JE, Reid DE, Harrison JH, Merrill JP. Successful pregnancies after human renal transplantation. *N Engl J Med.* 1963 Aug **15**;269:341–3.

29. Deshpande NA, James NT, Kucirka LM, et al. Pregnancy outcomes in kidney transplant recipients: a systematic review and meta-analysis. *Am J Transplant.* 2011 Nov;**11**(11):2388–404.

30. https://uroweb.org/wp-content/uploads/EAU-Guidelines-Renal-Transplantation-2009.pdf

31. Rolfo A, Attini R, Nuzzo AM, et al. Chronic kidney disease may be differentially diagnosed from preeclampsia by serum biomarkers. *Kidney Int.* 2013 Jan;**83**(1):177–81.

32. Zeisler H, Llurba E, Chantraine F, et al. Predictive value of the sFlt-1: PlGF ratio in women with suspected preeclampsia. *N Engl J Med.* 2016 Jan 7;**374**(1):13–22.

33. Vikse BE, Irgens LM, Leivestad T, Skjaerven R, Iversen BM. Preeclampsia and the risk of end-stage renal disease. *N Engl J Med.* 2008 Aug 21;**359**(8):800–9.

Chapter 33

Gastrointestinal Disorders in Pregnancy

Laura Kitto & Hasnain M. Jafferbhoy

Gastrointestinal (GI) conditions are common in women of childbearing age. The physiological changes that occur during pregnancy can influence differential diagnosis, affect the interpretation of diagnostic tests and prevent the use of diagnostic or therapeutic procedures [1]. This chapter will summarize the clinical features, pathophysiology, diagnosis and management of common hepatology and luminal GI conditions occurring in pregnancy.

33.1 Hepatology

33.1.1 Physiological Changes in Pregnancy

The incidence of abnormal liver function tests (LFTs) in pregnancy is approximately 3–5% [2]. The majority of LFTs remain in the normal range, except those produced by the placenta (alkaline phosphatase (ALP), alpha-fetoprotein (AFP)) or those affected by haemodilution (albumin). Any abnormality in bilirubin or transaminases requires investigation (Table 33.1).

33.1.2 Pathological Changes in Pregnancy

Liver disease occurring in pregnancy can be classified as shown in Table 33.2.

33.1.2.1 Liver Disease Unique to Pregnancy

33.1.2.1.1 Intrahepatic Cholestasis of Pregnancy (ICP)

Intrahepatic cholestasis of pregnancy (ICP) is the most common liver disease unique to pregnancy. It is a reversible form of cholestasis, characterized by pruritis, elevated serum bile acids and abnormal LFTs, which resolve within 6 weeks of delivery [3]. ICP typically presents in the third trimester but can occur as early as 20 weeks' gestation. Whilst pruritis in pregnancy is common (23% of pregnancies), only a small proportion of women have ICP [4] (Table 33.2).

33.1.2.1.1.1 Pathogenesis -- The aetiology of ICP is not completely understood but involves an interplay between genetic susceptibility, hormonal (increased circulating oestrogen and

Table 33.1 Physiological changes in haematological and biochemical parameters during pregnancy

Increased	Decreased	Unchanged
Alkaline phosphatase (ALP)	Haemoglobin	Aminotransferases (ALT/AST)
Cholesterol/triglycerides	Albumin	Gamma-glutamyltransferase (GGT)
White blood count	Urea	Bilirubin
Alpha-fetoprotein		Lactate dehydrogenase (LDH)
Caeruloplasmin		Prothrombin time (PT)

Table 33.2 Classification of liver diseases occurring in pregnancy and timing of presentation

	Liver disease	Trimester of presentation
1. Liver disease unique to pregnancy	Intrahepatic cholestasis of pregnancy	Second/third
	Acute fatty liver of pregnancy	Third
	Hypertension-related liver diseases:	
	• Pre-eclampsia and eclampsia	Second/third/postpartum
	• HELLP syndrome	Third/postpartum
	Hyperemesis gravidarum	First (but can present second/third)
2. Liver disease coincidental to pregnancy	Gallstones	Second/third
	Viral hepatitis	Any
3. Pre-existing liver disease	Chronic viral hepatitis	
	Cirrhosis from any cause	

progesterone) and environmental (seasonal and geographic) factors. There is a greater incidence of ICP in women with a past medical history of chronic hepatitis C or a family or personal history of ICP. More than 50% of women are >35 years old [5].

33.1.2.1.1.2 Clinical Features --
- Intrahepatic cholestasis of pregnancy typically presents with pruritis, which is generalized but starts on the palms and soles. This is often worse overnight.
- Right upper quadrant pain, nausea, poor appetite and steatorrhoea may occur.
- Jaundice occurs in less than 25% of patients [2], with onset after the development of pruritis. Jaundice without pruritis is rare and should prompt full investigation.
- Physical examination is normal, aside from excoriations.

33.1.2.1.1.3 Diagnosis -- Intrahepatic cholestasis of pregnancy is a clinical diagnosis, requiring a typical history of pruritis, abnormal liver function tests, elevated serum bile acids and exclusion of other causes. Pruritis can precede LFT abnormalities and serial measurements are therefore required.

- An increase in serum total bile acid concentration is the key finding and may be the first and only biochemical abnormality.
- Weekly monitoring of LFTs is recommended. Abnormalities may include:
  - Mildly elevated transaminases (less than 2x the upper limit of normal)
  - Raised ALP and GGT (20% of cases)
  - Mild hyperbilirubinaemia
- A full liver screen (including viral serology and autoantibodies) should be obtained and hepatitis C infection should be excluded.
- Abdominal ultrasound is normal in ICP but is recommended to exclude other pathology.

33.1.2.1.1.4 Pregnancy Considerations -- Although pruritis is unpleasant, ICP is not usually associated with serious maternal consequences. Vitamin K deficiency may occur due to fat malabsorption or cholestyramine treatment and this may be reflected by a prolonged PT. In this setting vitamin K replacement may reduce the risk of maternal and fetal bleeding.

The clinical significance of ICP lies in the potential fetal risk. Maternal bile acids can cross the placenta and accumulate in amniotic fluid, posing a significant risk to the fetus. Most fetal complications occur when serum bile acids exceed 40 µmol/L [2, 6]. Complications include intrauterine demise, meconium-stained amniotic fluid, preterm delivery and neonatal respiratory distress syndrome. The incidence of stillbirth after 37 weeks of gestation is reported at 1.2% and increases with higher bile acid levels and gestational age. There is no evidence that fetal monitoring with cardiotocography (CTG) or ultrasound (fetal growth, fluid volume or umbilical artery Doppler) predicts fetal compromise or improves outcome.

33.1.2.1.1.5 Management -- The management of ICP focuses on:

1. Reduction of maternal pruritis
2. Reduction of perinatal morbidity and mortality
3. Optimal timing of delivery

In mild disease (bile acids <40 µmol/L), expectant management is appropriate [3]. First line therapy for ICP is ursodeoxoycholic acid (UDCA), which increases the expression of bile salt export pumps and placental bile transporters. UDCA improves maternal pruritis and biochemistry in approximately 75% of cases. However, there is a lack of robust data to support improved fetal outcomes [2, 4]. Antihistamines and anion exchange resins, such as cholestyramine (often poorly tolerated) can be used for symptomatic relief but are less effective than UDCA.

The timing and risks of delivery should be discussed on an individual basis. The Royal College of Obstetricians and Gynaecologists UK recommend that induction of labour should be discussed after 37 weeks of gestation. The case for early induction may be stronger in those with more severe biochemical abnormality [4].

Postnatal resolution of symptoms and biochemistry is required to secure the diagnosis. Pruritis usually disappears in the first few days following delivery, followed by normalization of biochemical parameters by 10 days. ICP has a high recurrence rate in subsequent pregnancies and oestrogen containing oral contraceptives should be avoided.

33.1.2.1.2 Acute Fatty Liver of Pregnancy (AFLP)

Acute fatty liver of pregnancy (AFLP) is a rare obstetric emergency, characterized by fatty infiltration of the liver, which can result in hepatic failure. Early recognition, prompt delivery and supportive care are vital, as the interval between symptom onset and termination of pregnancy has a significant impact on maternal and fetal morbidity and mortality [2] (see Table 33.2).

33.1.2.1.2.1 Pathogenesis -- The pathogenesis of AFLP is not well understood but defects in fatty acid metabolism appear to be important; fatty acids normally increase in pregnancy to support fetoplacental growth but in AFLP, impaired maternal fatty acid metabolism leads to accumulation in hepatocytes. Risk factors include previous AFLP, multiple pregnancy (20% of cases), male fetal sex (ratio 3:1), low maternal body mass index (BMI) (<20 kg/m^2) and fetal longchain 3-hydroxyacyl CoA dehydrogenase (LCHAD) deficiency. Given the link between LCHAD deficiency and AFLP, babies born to mothers with AFLP should undergo molecular testing for this, as early diagnosis of LCHAD can be lifesaving.

33.1.2.1.2.2 Clinical Features --
- Presenting features are often non-specific and may include nausea, vomiting and abdominal pain (Table 33.3).
- Pre-eclampsia is present in 50% of cases and mothers may have hypertension, with or without proteinuria [2].

- Signs of acute liver failure (including jaundice, encephalopathy, coagulopathy, hypoglycaemia and ascites) develop rapidly.
- Most patients develop acute kidney injury and may progress to multi-organ failure.

33.1.2.1.2.3 Diagnosis – – Acute fatty liver of pregnancy is a clinical diagnosis based on the presence of characteristic symptoms in a woman in the second half of pregnancy (median gestation 36 weeks) with significant hepatic dysfunction, after other causes have been excluded. The differential diagnosis includes HELLP (haemolysis, elevated liver enzymes, low platelet count) and pre-eclampsia with severe features. There is significant clinical overlap between these entities, and it can be impossible to differentiate amongst them. The 'Swansea Criteria' (Table 33.3) are a diagnostic model, which have been validated in a large cohort in the UK.

Markers of severity of AFLP include prolonged prothrombin time, hypoglycaemia, encephalopathy, acidosis and elevated lactate.

33.1.2.1.2.4 Pregnancy Considerations – – Acute fatty liver of pregnancy is an obstetric emergency, associated with significant maternal and fetal morbidity and mortality. Women with AFLP develop varying degrees of hepatic impairment, which

Table 33.3 Swansea Criteria for the diagnosis of acute fatty liver of pregnancy

Six or more criteria required without evidence of another cause		
Clinical Features	Vomiting Abdominal Pain Polydipsia/Polyuria Encephalopathy	
Biochemical Features Hepatic	Hyperbilirubinaemia	>14 μmol
	Elevated transaminases (usually 5–10x the upper limit of normal)	>42 IU/L
	Elevated ammonia	>47 μmol/L
Renal	Elevated uric acid	>340 μmol/L
	Elevated creatinine	>150 μmol/L
Endocrine	Hypoglycaemia	<4 mmol/L
Haematological	Leukocytosis	>11 x 10^9/L
	Coagulopathy – increased prothrombin time	>14 sec
Radiological Features	Abdominal ultrasound scan	Fatty liver or ascites
Histological Features	Liver biopsy (rarely required for diagnosis)	Microvascular steatosis

can rapidly progress to fulminant hepatic failure. Adverse fetal outcomes usually occur secondary to maternal decompensation or preterm birth.

33.1.2.1.2.5 Management – – The management of AFLP focuses on:
1. Expedient delivery of the fetus
2. Support of maternal recovery

Initial management of AFLP includes prompt delivery of the fetus, regardless of gestational age. Coagulopathy and hypoglycaemia should be treated aggressively prior to this. Whilst it may not be possible to distinguish between AFPL, HELLP syndrome and pre-eclampsia with severe features, the management is the same and delivery should not be delayed whilst attempting to ascertain a diagnosis. Early recognition and rapid delivery of the fetus vastly improves prognosis for both mother and baby.

Following delivery, women may require organ support in an intensive care environment. Those with fulminant hepatic failure should be urgently discussed with a specialist liver transplant unit. Coagulopathy increases the risk of postpartum haemorrhage.

Acute fatty liver of pregnancy usually resolves completely after delivery, with return of normal liver function within a week, without long-term hepatic damage. If maternal hepatic function does not rapidly improve, evaluation for liver transplant offers the best chance of survival. AFLP has been reported in subsequent pregnancies, even in the absence of LCHAD deficiency but the exact risk of recurrence is unknown.

33.1.2.1.3 HELLP Syndrome

HELLP syndrome is characterized by haemolysis, elevated liver enzymes and low platelets. It is thought to be a variant of severe pre-eclampsia, though not all patients with HELLP have preceding hypertension or proteinuria. Both entities, however, are associated with serious hepatic manifestations and maternal and fetal consequences (see Table 33.2).

33.1.2.1.3.1 Pathogenesis – – The pathogenesis of HELLP syndrome is unclear, although it is thought to occur secondary to abnormal placentation. Risk factors include white ethnicity, advanced maternal age, previous pre-eclampsia (with or without HELLP), obesity, chronic hypertension, diabetes and multiparity.

33.1.2.1.3.2 Clinical Features – – HELLP syndrome typically presents between 28 and 36 weeks of gestation, though 30% of patients manifest symptoms postpartum [7].

- Patients with HELLP may be asymptomatic or present with non-specific symptoms such as epigastric pain, nausea, vomiting, malaise, headache and oedema.
- Hypertension (>140/90 mm Hg) and proteinuria occur in 85% of patients [2] but either, or both may be absent in severe HELLP syndrome.
- Jaundice is uncommon (less than 5% of cases) [2].
- Brisk tendon reflexes may be elicited on clinical examination.

33.1.2.1.3.3 Diagnosis --
- The diagnosis of HELLP is made through typical laboratory results, including:
  - Microangiopathic haemolytic anaemia with characteristic schistocytes on blood smear. Anaemia is rarely severe. Lactate dehydrogenase is elevated but this is non-specific and can also occur secondary to hepatic impairment.
  - Thrombocytopenia (usually <100 x 10^9/L)
  - Transaminitis with serum AST/ALT >2x the upper limit of normal
  - Unconjugated hyperbilirubinaemia >20.5 µmol/L
  - A small proportion of women may develop disseminated intravascular coagulation (DIC), with PT prolongation and reduced fibrinogen.
  - Elevated protein creatinine ratio
- Abdominal ultrasound scan may be helpful to exclude hepatic complications. However, when transaminases are greater than 1000 U/L or abdominal pain radiates to the right shoulder, cross-sectional imaging is recommended to exclude hepatic complications with more accuracy than ultrasound.

Differential diagnosis includes AFLP, haemolytic uraemic syndrome (HUS) and thrombocytopenic purpura (TTP). These conditions (AFLP, HUS, TTP, pre-eclampsia) represent a spectrum of endothelial disease and differentiation may be difficult.

33.1.2.1.3.4 Pregnancy Considerations -- HELLP syndrome is a serious condition associated with progressive and sometimes rapid maternal and fetal deterioration [8]. The risk of maternal morbidity correlates with increasingly severe symptoms and biochemical abnormalities. Serious maternal illness may be present at initial presentation or rapidly develop.

Major maternal morbidity may include (Table 33.4):
- ***Hepatic Complications:*** Hepatic infarction should be suspected when right upper quadrant pain and fever occur in this clinical setting. Hepatic rupture can result in abdominal swelling from haemoperitoneum and hypovolaemic shock. Subcapsular hepatic haematoma and intraparenchymal haemorrhage are also possible.
- ***Cardiopulmonary Complications:*** Congestive heart failure, pulmonary oedema and pleural or pericardial effusion.

- ***Haematological Complications:*** DIC
- ***Central Nervous System Complications:*** Stroke, cerebral oedema, hypertensive encephalopathy and posterior reversible encephalopathy syndrome (PRES)
- ***Renal Complications:*** Acute tubular necrosis and acute renal failure

The Martin/Mississippi Classification can be used to estimate maternal risk [8, 9].

Fetal prognosis is most strongly associated with gestational age at delivery and birthweight.

33.1.2.1.3.5 Management – – The management of HELLP focuses on:
1. Stabilizing maternal condition
2. Assessing fetal condition and minimizing perinatal morbidity and mortality
3. Optimal timing of delivery

All women with HELLP should be admitted to a high dependency unit with frequent monitoring of blood pressure and observations. Blood pressure should be reduced to a level that prevents end-organ damage, with a goal systolic blood pressure of <160 mm Hg. Intravenous infusion of antihypertensives may be required. Magnesium sulphate should be considered as seizure prophylaxis for any woman with severe hypertension or pre-eclampsia with a history of previous eclamptic fits, or when birth is planned within 24 hours. Following delivery, the infusion should continue for 24 hours.

Having ensured adequate blood pressure control, seizure prophylaxis and correction of coagulopathy, the optimal treatment of HELLP syndrome is delivery of the baby. The American College of Obstetricians and Gynecologists recommend [10]:
- Prompt delivery if HELLP syndrome develops beyond 34 weeks, or earlier if evidence of major maternal morbidity or non-reassuring fetal status.
- Before the gestational age of fetal viability delivery should occur rapidly, after maternal stabilization.
- Between the age of fetal viability and 34 weeks' gestation, delivery should be delayed for 24 to 48 hours if maternal and fetal condition are stable, to allow corticosteroid administration for fetal benefit.

Thrombocytopenia can be marked and there is no contraindication to platelet transfusion, especially where procedures are planned. Although delivery is the only cure, serious

Table 33.4 Martin/Mississippi Classification for estimation of major maternal morbidity

	Platelets	LDH	ALT and/or AST	Risk of major maternal morbidity (see complications above)
Class 1	0 to ≤ 50 x 10^9/L	≥ 600 IU/L	≥ 70 IU/L	40 to 60%
Class 2	>50 to ≤ 100 x 10^9/L	≥ 600 IU/L	≥ 70 IU/L	20 to 40%
Class 3	>100 to ≤ 150 x 10^9/L	≥ 600 IU/L	≥ 40 IU/L	20%

manifestations of the disease continue into the immediate postpartum period and 30% of cases of HELLP arise postpartum. Laboratory parameters may initially deteriorate after delivery but usually begin to normalise by 48 hours postpartum. The majority of women recover completely with no long-term hepatic sequelae. In future pregnancies, these women are more likely to develop pre-eclampsia.

33.1.2.1.4   Hyperemesis Gravidarum (see also Chapter 9)

Hyperemesis gravidarum (HG) presents in the first trimester and is diagnosed in the setting of protracted vomiting, dehydration, ketosis and weight loss of greater than 5%. It may be associated with abnormal LFTs in up to 50% of cases [6], including:

- Transaminitis (ALT usually <200 U/L)
- Mild elevation in bilirubin (jaundice is not common)

The degree of abnormality correlates with the severity of vomiting. As hyperemesis improves, these abnormalities in liver function tests also resolve, with no long-term hepatic damage. If LFTs fail to resolve on cessation of vomiting, other diagnoses should be considered [6].

33.1.2.2   Liver Disease Coincidental to Pregnancy

33.1.2.2.1   Gallbladder Disease

Asymptomatic gallstones are present in approximately 10% of pregnant women and cholecystitis occurs in 0.1% of pregnancies [11].

33.1.2.2.1.1 Pathogenesis – – Cholelithiasis is common in pregnancy due to an increase in bile lithogenicity caused by cholesterol supersaturation of bile (secondary to increased oestrogen), impaired gallbladder contractility and gallbladder stasis. Multiparity, elevated BMI and increasing age are risk factors for gallstone development.

33.1.2.2.1.2 Clinical Features ––

Clinical features are similar to non-pregnant women:

- Typical pain occurs in the right upper quadrant or epigastrium and may radiate to the back. Acute cholecystitis can occur at any time during pregnancy and causes severe pain, fever and features of sepsis.
- Nausea, vomiting and dyspepsia are common.
- Jaundice or pancreatitis may occur in the setting of impacted ductal stones.

33.1.2.2.1.3 Diagnosis ––

- Typical laboratory results may be suggestive, including:
  - Cholestatic LFTs
  - Hyperbilirubinaemia
  - Elevated leukocytes in the case of cholecystitis
  - A mildly raised amylase (twofold) – greater rises should raise suspicion of pancreatitis.
- Abdominal ultrasound is safe in pregnancy and accurate in the diagnosis of gallstones. It can differentiate between

choledocholithiasis and cholecystitis (thickening of gallbladder wall, pericholecystic fluid).

33.1.2.2.1.4 Management ––

Management is the same as in the non-pregnant patient with intravenous fluids, antibiotics and analgesia. Cholecystitis had previously been managed conservatively but this was associated with high rates of recurrent symptoms, preterm labour and spontaneous abortions [2]. Therefore, early surgical intervention with laparoscopic cholecystectomy, on its own or after endoscopic retrograde cholangiopancreatography (ERCP), is preferred. ERCP is indicated in the case of biliary disease strongly necessitating intervention (pancreatitis, cholangitis, symptomatic choledocholithiasis) and should be performed with minimal radiation.

33.1.2.2.2   Acute Viral Hepatitis (HAV, HEV, HSV, HBV)

Acute viral hepatitis is the most common cause of jaundice occurring in pregnancy. All pregnant women presenting with acute hepatitis should be tested for common aetiologies of acute liver injury including hepatitis A (HAV), hepatitis E (HEV), herpes simplex (HSV) and hepatitis B (HBV).

HAV: HAV is transmitted by the faecal-oral route and causes an acute, self-limiting illness, which does not result in chronic infection. Pregnancy does not alter the course of acute HAV infection. Acute HAV during the third trimester has been associated with preterm labour and premature rupture of membranes but without a significant impact on maternal or fetal outcomes [2]. Vertical transmission of HAV has been reported. In addition to careful infection control precautions, the American College of Gastroenterology guidelines recommend administration of HAV immune globulin to the neonate if HAV infection occurs within 2 weeks of delivery [2]. Treatment is otherwise supportive.

HEV: HEV is transmitted by the faecal-oral route, and in non-pregnant women causes a mild, self-limiting disease. However, there is a significant increase in morbidity and mortality in pregnancy, with increased risk of fulminant hepatic failure (15–20% risk), particularly when occurring in the third trimester [2]. Women with HEV infection also have a higher risk of obstetric complications, including antepartum haemorrhage, intrauterine fetal death, prematurity and stillbirth [6]. Treatment is supportive but may require specialist hepatology input as patients with fulminant hepatic failure may require liver transplant evaluation.

HSV: HSV hepatitis is rare but can result in fulminant hepatic failure in pregnant women. Clinical features include fever, upper respiratory tract symptoms and anicteric hepatitis. Mucocutaneous lesions are present in <50% of patients. Diagnosis is challenging due to limited sensitivity and specificity of HSV-IgM testing and HSV PCR should be requested when HSV hepatitis is suspected. Maternal mortality is high, and acyclovir should be started as soon as the diagnosis is suspected.

HBV: HBV is a blood-borne virus and transmission is sexual, vertical or via blood. Acute HBV or reactivation of chronic HBV can occur during pregnancy and these entities can be difficult to differentiate. All pregnant women should be tested for hepatitis B surface antigen (HBsAg) [12]. HBsAg positivity may indicate acute or chronic infection and HBV core IgM may be required to distinguish. Acute HBV is not associated with increased maternal or fetal mortality.

33.1.2.3   Pre-existing Liver Disease

33.1.2.3.1   Chronic HBV

Women with chronic HBV should be monitored closely in pregnancy and the postpartum period for disease flares. The risk of perinatal infection is high and is greatest from mothers who are both HbSAg positive and HBV e-antigen (HBsAg) positive. Viral load is also important, and risk of transmission increases with maternal viraemia [2]. Transmission usually occurs at the time of delivery but can be transplacental (5% of cases). The risk of developing chronic HBV is strongly related to age of exposure and is particularly high in infants (up to 90%) [2], with the associated risks of cirrhosis and hepatocellular carcinoma in later life.

Women with chronic HBV and high viral load should be offered antiviral therapy in the third trimester to reduce peri-natal transmission. Active-passive immunoprophylaxis with Hep B immune globulin and the HBV vaccination series should be administered to all infants born to HBsAg positive mothers (within 12 hours of delivery) to prevent perinatal transmission [2]. Immunization is 85–95% effective at preventing HBV infection and chronic carrier state. Caesarean section should not be performed electively in HBV-positive mothers, in order to prevent fetal infection. Breastfeeding is safe for babies who have been vaccinated.

33.1.2.3.2   Hepatitis C

Hepatitis C (HCV) is a blood-borne virus, although transmission can occur less commonly via sexual or vertical routes. The most common risk factor for HCV infection in the UK is current or past intravenous drug use. All pregnant women with risk factors for HCV should be screened for infection with anti-HCV antibody. There is a significant risk of chronic infection (80%), with development of cirrhosis over time.

Hepatitis C has little impact during pregnancy, with minimal risk to mother or fetus. However, there may be a higher risk of ICP, premature rupture of membranes or gestational diabetes [13]. Viral load and ALT fluctuate, but these changes are not usually of clinical significance [2].

Vertical transmission occurs in 3–5% of cases and is higher with higher maternal viraemia and HIV co-infection. There is no specific perinatal management strategy to decrease the risk of transmission, but invasive procedures such as amniocentesis and invasive fetal monitoring should be avoided. Treatment is not recommended during pregnancy due to lack of safety and efficacy data [14]. Caesarean section should not be performed electively to prevent fetal infection. Breastfeeding is safe but should be avoided in the case of skin breakdown.

33.1.2.3.3   Cirrhosis and Portal Hypertension

Pregnancy in women with cirrhosis has been associated with prematurity, spontaneous abortions and maternal-fetal mortality. There is very little evidence to guide the management of cirrhotic patients during pregnancy – largely due to its low prevalence in women of reproductive age and reduced fertility in this patient cohort.

Outcomes of pregnancy are related to the severity of maternal liver disease rather than underlying aetiology. Use of prognostic scoring systems (UKELD, MELD) can be used to predict risk of maternal decompensation and to guide pre-conception counselling of women with cirrhosis [15].

Pregnancy has a variable effect in women with cirrhosis and in some cases can precipitate decompensation, including encephalopathy, ascites and variceal haemorrhage [15, 16]. Variceal haemorrhage is the most frequent complication (30% of cirrhotic pregnant women), owing to increased intravascular volume and IVC compression from the gravid uterus. Maternal and fetal mortality rates are significant. Pregnant women with suspected portal hypertension (PHT) should undergo variceal screening with upper GI endoscopy in the second trimester [16] and those with varices should be treated with beta blockers or band ligation.

There are no recommendations as to the preferred mode of delivery in patients with PHT, though a shortened second stage of labour is recommended to avoid excessive straining.

33.1.2.3.4   Liver Disease of Other Aetiologies

The presentation of these rare conditions and the effects of pregnancy have been summarized in Table 33.5. Patients with chronic liver disease are managed by a multidisciplinary team comprising an obstetrician, hepatalogist and laboratory medicine specialist.

33.2   Luminal Gastroenterology

33.2.1   Physiological Changes in Pregnancy

Gastrointestinal symptoms are very common during pregnancy. Elevated levels of oestrogen and progesterone mediate changes in GI motility, causing smooth muscle relaxation and resulting in:

- Decreased lower oesophageal sphincter pressure
- Decreased gastric peristalsis and delayed gastric emptying
- Increased small and large bowel transit times

These changes contribute to the common pregnancy symptoms of constipation, nausea and vomiting.

33.2.2   Pathological Changes in Pregnancy

The spectrum of GI disease in pregnancy can range from conditions that are specific to the pregnancy state to previously existing conditions. The physiological changes attending the pregnancy state may further promote or alter GI symptomatology.

Table 33.5 Management of liver disease in pregnancy

Aetiology	Advice
Autoimmune hepatitis	- Mild disease is unlikely to cause problems in pregnancy. - Immunosuppression should be continued to prevent relapse.
Primary biliary cholangitis	- Stable disease is unlikely to cause problems and UDCA should be continued. - Pruritis may worsen and women may develop ICP.
Primary sclerosing cholangitis	- Pregnancy outcomes are usually good but worsening pruritis may develop.
Liver transplant	- Pregnancy should be delayed for up to 12 months after transplant to allow stabilization of graft function and immunosuppressive therapy [15]. - Immunosuppression must be continued and closely monitored during pregnancy. - Tacrolimus, prednisolone and azathioprine are not associated with teratogenesis. - There is an increased risk of preterm delivery and maternal and fetal complications, but outcome is usually good.

Table 33.6 Classification of luminal gastroenterological diseases occurring in pregnancy and timing of presentation

	Condition	Trimester of presentation
1. GI disease unique to pregnancy	Hyperemesis gravidarum	First
2. Common GI complaints during pregnancy	Gastro-oesophageal reflux disease Constipation and bloating	Any trimester but may be exacerbated later in pregnancy
3. Pre-existing luminal GI disease	Inflammatory bowel disease Coeliac disease	

33.2.2.1 GI Disease Unique to Pregnancy

33.2.2.1.1 Hyperemesis Gravidarum (HG) (see Chapter 9 as well)

Nausea and vomiting are common in pregnancy and are usually self-limiting. Approximately 80% of women experience nausea and at least 50% have one episode of vomiting [11, 17]. This is more common in the first trimester. Hyperemesis gravidarum (HG) is the term used to describe severe nausea and vomiting (including loss of more than 5% pre-pregnancy body weight) and is much less common, occurring in only 0.1–1% of pregnancies (Table 33.6). Hyperemesis gravidarum is a clinical diagnosis and other causes of nausea and vomiting should be excluded, particularly where vomiting occurs for the first time after 10 weeks' gestation. Vomiting occurring later in pregnancy is abnormal and may be a sign of acute liver failure. The diagnosis and management of HG has been covered in detail in a previous chapter.

33.2.2.2 Common GI Complaints during Pregnancy

33.2.2.2.1 Gastro-oesophageal Reflux Disease (GORD)

Heartburn is common, with up to 80% of women experiencing dyspepsia at some point during pregnancy, most commonly in the third trimester [17].

33.2.2.2.1.1 Pathogenesis –– Reflux of acidic gastric contents into the oesophagus causes inflammation of the oesophageal mucosa. Functional and structural alterations of the gastro-oesophageal junction are responsible for the high prevalence of reflux occurring in pregnancy. Reduced lower oesophageal sphincter pressures, an increase in gastric pressure secondary to enlarging uterus, decreased gastric peristalsis and delayed gastric emptying all contribute.

33.2.2.2.1.2 Clinical Features –– Clinical features are similar to those experienced in the general population:

- Heartburn and regurgitation are the most predominant symptoms and are exacerbated by lying in a recumbent position and after meals.
- Nausea, vomiting or nocturnal cough may occur in some cases.

33.2.2.2.1.3 Diagnosis –– Serious complications of GORD are rare during pregnancy and diagnostic tests (such as endoscopy) are rarely required.

33.2.2.2.1.4 Management –– Reflux symptoms during pregnancy should be treated according to a step-up algorithm (Figure 33.1).

33.2.2.2.2 Constipation

Constipation and abdominal bloating are common in pregnancy (25–40% of cases) [17]. Women who are predisposed to constipation prior to pregnancy often experience a worsening of symptoms.

33.2.2.2.2.1 Pathogenesis –– There are a number of aetiological factors which contribute to constipation and bloating,

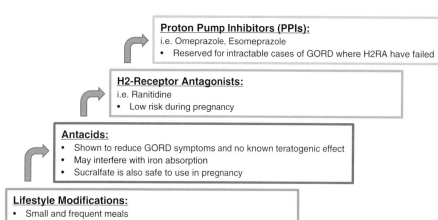

Figure 33.1 Algorithm approach for the management of GORD during pregnancy

including changes in water absorption, mechanical factors (pressure on rectum by gravid uterus), dietary factors (reduced oral intake in the context of nausea and vomiting), reduced physical activity and hormonal effects on gastrointestinal motility [18]. Gastrointestinal transit time is prolonged during the second and third trimesters and contributes to constipation. Oral iron supplements may contribute, causing either constipation or diarrhoea.

33.2.2.2.2.2 Clinical Features --
- Decreased frequency of defecation and increased difficulty passing stool
- Bloating, lower abdominal discomfort and flatus
- Constipation may exacerbate or cause haemorrhoids and anal fissures, which typically present with bleeding, itching and pain on defecation.

33.2.2.2.2.3 Management -- Women should be reassured that constipation is a normal feature of pregnancy. They should be initially recommended to increase their water and dietary fibre intake. Light physical exercise can improve gastrointestinal transit. Temporary cessation of iron tablets may also be beneficial. Laxatives should only be used in severe cases, when lifestyle measures fail to alleviate symptoms. The American Gastroenterological Association guidelines recommend a faecal softener, followed by an osmotic laxative [17].

Therapeutic options include the following:
- Faecal softeners (sodium docusate) are safe for use in pregnancy and act as a stimulant as well as a softening agent.
- Osmotic laxatives (i.e. lactulose) are regarded as low risk.
- Bulk-forming laxatives (i.e. ispaghula husk) have been shown to increase the frequency of defecation and soften stool in pregnant women [17]. However, may exacerbate bloating and abdominal pain.
- Stimulant laxatives (i.e. senna, glycerol suppositories) are safe for use in pregnancy. Danthron should be avoided.

33.2.2.3 Pre-existing luminal GI disease

33.2.2.3.1 Inflammatory Bowel Disease (IBD)
Inflammatory bowel disease (IBD) comprises the chronic inflammatory disorders, Crohn's disease (CD) and ulcerative colitis (UC). IBD is most commonly diagnosed in the third and fourth decades and is often encountered in pregnancy. Maintaining disease control is vital for maternal and fetal health.

33.2.2.3.1.1 Pathogenesis -- The aetiology of IBD is incompletely understood but it arises from a complex interplay between the immune system and environmental factors, in genetically susceptible individuals.

33.2.2.3.1.2 Clinical Features -- Inflammatory bowel disease follows an unpredictable pattern of relapse and remission with significant variation in symptoms between different patients. Ulcerative colitis is characterized by relapsing and remitting episodes of inflammation that are limited to the mucosal layer of the colon, almost invariably involving the rectum and extending proximally in a continuous fashion. Crohn's disease is characterized by non-continuous, transmural inflammation that can involve any part of the GI tract but most commonly affects the distal small intestine.

Symptom onset tends to be insidious but may also present acutely, mimicking infective aetiology. Inflammatory bowel disease has a varied phenotype and clinical features depend on anatomical distribution and severity but may include:
- UC: bloody diarrhoea, urgency and colicky abdominal pain.
- CD: diarrhoea (with or without blood and mucus), abdominal pain and weight loss.
- Systemic manifestations such as malaise, anorexia or fever (more common in CD).
- Extra-intestinal manifestations (particularly CD), including gallstones, axial and peripheral arthritis, acute ocular inflammation, erythema nodosum and pyoderma gangrenosum.

33.2.2.3.1.3 Diagnosis – – Diagnosis encompasses clinical, laboratory, radiological, endoscopic and histological findings in order to establish the disease type, extent and severity. Flexible sigmoidoscopy is safe in pregnancy and allows histological examination to differentiate between UC and CD.

33.2.2.3.1.4 Pregnancy Considerations – – Infertility is more likely in patients with active disease [19]. Pre-conception planning is important to minimize disease activity and ensure the best possible pregnancy outcomes [20].

Pregnancy has little effect on the course of IBD and the risk of flares is similar to that in non-pregnant women. Disease activity at conception influences disease course during pregnancy [19]. Exacerbations of IBD tend to be mild and occur during the first two trimesters. Many of the adverse outcomes in pregnancy are related to active disease, rather than medications given to treat this. Women with IBD are more likely to experience preterm labour and low birthweight babies, especially in the context of active disease [19].

In women with quiescent disease at the time of conception, the rates of miscarriage, stillbirth and fetal abnormalities are no different to the general population. Neonates born to mothers receiving immunosuppressive and anti-TNF (tumour necrosis factor) drugs are considered to be immunosuppressed and should not receive live vaccines for at least 6 months after birth [21].

33.2.2.3.1.5 Management – – Management of remission and disease flares is not significantly altered by pregnancy. Patients with acute severe colitis should be managed as the non-pregnant patient, including abdominal radiograph and treatment with steroids where indicated [19]. Patients hospitalized with acute, severe IBD should receive thromboprophylaxis. Combined care between gastroenterologists and obstetricians is mandatory. Table 33.7 summarizes medical management options for patients with IBD during pregnancy.

Caesarean section is usually only required for obstetric indications. However, in cases of severe perianal CD, vaginal delivery should be avoided due to perineal inelasticity and reduced healing ability of episiotomy scars [22]. In some cases, women with ileal pouch anal anastomosis should also avoid vaginal delivery.

33.2.2.3.2 Coeliac Disease

Coeliac disease is an autoimmune disorder primarily affecting the small intestine. It occurs in the setting of an inflammatory reaction to gluten in those who are genetically predisposed. Upon exposure to gluten-containing foods, inflammation within the small intestine (predominantly duodenum) results in villous atrophy and nutrient malabsorption.

Coeliac disease can present in many different ways or may even be asymptomatic. The diagnosis should be considered in those with anaemia (B12, folate or iron deficiency), fat-soluble vitamin deficiency, weight loss or unexplained infertility. It is

Table 33.7 Therapeutic options for IBD in pregnancy

Medication	Indication	Role in pregnancy
Aminosalicylates (sulfasalazine, mesalazine)	Maintaining and inducing remission in UC	- Safe in pregnancy and breastfeeding up to 3 g/day. - Sulfasalazine is a dihydrofolate reductase inhibitor that blocks the conversion of folate to its more active metabolites. Folic acid 5 mg/day pre-conception and in pregnancy is important to prevent increased risk of neural tube defects and cleft palate.
Antibiotics (i.e. metronidazole)	Perianal CD	- Metronidazole is safe for use in pregnancy.
Corticosteroids, budesonide	Acute flares of UC and CD to induce remission	- Risk to pregnancy from active disease is greater than risk of steroid use. - Both oral and rectal preparations can be used.
Thiopurines (azathioprine, 6-mercaptopurine)	Maintaining remission in UC and CD	- Thought to be safe in pregnancy and should be continued to maintain remission in these patients.
Cyclosporin	Induction of remission in UC	- Higher rate of prematurity and low birthweight but a high survival rate. - Not thought to be related to congenital abnormalities and probably safe in pregnancy.
Methotrexate	Maintaining remission in UC and CD	- Absolutely contraindicated in pregnancy. - Should be stopped 3 months prior to conception.
Anti-TNF (i.e. infliximab, adalimumab)	Induction and maintenance of remission in UC and CD	- Safety data is accumulating, though longer-term data are lacking. - Should be used cautiously, though in patients who are already established on treatment, they can probably be continued safely [22]. - If considering starting in pregnancy, women require full risk counselling vs. risk of active disease [19]. - Should be discontinued by 30–32 weeks to allow time for the fetus to clear the drug prior to delivery.

diagnosed through a combination of blood tests (detection of IgA anti-endomysial antibodies or anti-transglutaminase antibodies) and pathognomonic changes on duodenal biopsies. Diagnostic serological testing and oesophago-gastro-duodenoscopy (OGD) can be performed as normal in pregnancy.

Uncontrolled disease in pregnancy is associated with miscarriage, low birthweight babies and intrauterine growth retardation [1]. Management is the same as in the non-pregnant population, with strict compliance to a gluten-free diet.

References

1. Frise C, Williamson C. Gastrointestinal and liver disease in pregnancy. *Clin. Med.* 2013;**13**:269–74.

2. Tran TT, Ahn J, Reau NS. ACG clinical guideline: Liver disease and pregnancy. *Am. J. Gastroenterol.* 2016;**111**:176–94.

3. EASL Clinical Practice. Guidelines: Management of cholestatic liver diseases. *J Hepatol.* 2009;**51**:237–67.

4. *Obstetric Cholestasis*, Green-top Guideline No 43. London: Royal College of Obstetricians and Gynaecologists, 2011.

5. Debbs RH. Cholestasis of pregnancy. *BMJ Best Pract.* 2017. Available online.

6. Westbrook RH, Dusheiko G, Williamson C. Pregnancy and liver disease. *J. Hepatol.* 2016;**64**:933–45.

7. Sibai B. Diagnosis, controversies and management of the syndrome of haemolysis, elevated liver enzymes and low platelet count. *Obs. Gynaecol.* 2014;**123**:618–27.

8. Martin JN Jr, Brewer JM, Wallace K, et al. HELLP syndrome and composite major maternal morbidity: importance of Mississippi Classification system. *J Matern Fetal Neonatal Med.* 2013 Aug;**26**(12):1201–6. doi: 10.3109/14767058.2013.773308

9. Haram K, Svendsen E, Abildgaard U. The HELLP syndrome: clinical issues and management. A review. *BMC Pregnancy Childbirth.* 2009;**9**:1–15.

10. Hypertension in pregnancy. Report of the American College of Obstetricians and Gynecologists' Task Force on Hypertension in Pregnancy. *Obstet Gynaecol.* 2013;**122**:1122–31.

11. Boregowda G, Shehata HA. Gastrointestinal and liver disease in pregnancy. *Best Pract Res Clin Obstet Gynaecol.* 2013;**27**:835–53.

12. Society for Maternal-Fetal Medicine (SMFM), Dionne-Odom J, Tita A, Silverman NS. #38: Hepatitis B in pregnancy-screening, treatment and prevention of vertical transmission. *Am J Obstet Gynecol.* 2016;**214**:6–14.

13. Redddik K, Jhaveri R, Gandhi M et al. Pregnancy outcomes associated with viral hepatitis. *J Viral Hepat.* 2011;**18**:e394–8.

14. American Association for the Study of Liver Diseases. AASLD-IDSA recommendations for testing, managing and treating adults infected with hepatitis C virus. *Hepatology.* 2015;**62**:932–54.

15. Esposti S. Pregnancy in patients with advanced chronic liver disease. *Clin. Liver Dis.* 2014;**4**:62–8.

16. Garcia-Tsao G, Sanyal A, Grace N et al. Prevention and management of gastroesophageal varices and variceal hemorrhage in cirrhosis. *Hepatology.* 2007;**46**:922–38.

17. Keller J, Frederking D, Layer P. The spectrum and treatment of gastrointestinal disorders during pregnancy. *Nat Clin Pract Gastroenterol Hepatol.* 2008;**5**:430–43.

18. Cullen G, O'Donoghue D. Constipation and pregnancy. *Best Pr Res Clin Gastroenterol.* 2007;**21**:807–18.

19. Mowat C, Cole A, Windsor A, et al. Guidelines for the management of inflammatory bowel disease in adults. *Gut.* 2011;**60**:571–607.

20. Vermeire S Carbonnel F, Coulie PG, et al. Management of inflammatory bowel disease in pregnancy. *J Crohns Colitis.* 2012;**6**:811–23.

21. Kalla R, Ventham N, Satsangi J et al. Crohn's disease. *BMJ.* 2014;**349**:g6670.

22. Nguyen G, Seow C, Maxwell C. The Toronto consensus statements for the management of inflammatory bowel disease in pregnancy. *Gastroenterology.* 2016;**150**:734–57.

Chapter 34

Systemic Lupus Erythematosus and Pregnancy

Sarah McRobbie & Katrina Shearer

Systemic lupus erythematosus (SLE) is a chronic multi-organ inflammatory disease which can involve any organ or system. It is an autoimmune condition with an overproduction of autoantibodies directed against various nuclear components and cell-surface antigens. The underlying cause of the condition is unknown, but it is likely multifactorial with genetic and environmental factors having a role. The incidence is higher in women than in men; some sources quote this as high as 9:1, and is even higher during the reproductive years [1, 2].

The course of the condition is very variable, and episodes of quiescence will be experienced with intermittent episodes of active disease. Sometimes these flare-ups can result in permanent organ damage and disease progression.

Systemic lupus erythematosus affects approximately 1:500 women of reproductive age [1]. During pregnancy, flare-ups are more common particularly in later pregnancy and postnatally [1, 2]; however, pregnancy does not affect the long-term course of SLE itself. This highlights the importance of multidisciplinary team (MDT) care to identify and therefore treat flare-ups early.

34.1 Pre-pregnancy Counselling

As with pregnancy in any woman with a pre-existing medical condition, women with SLE should be considered high risk. Pre-pregnancy counselling for optimization of disease and review of medication and planning for careful monitoring by an MDT during pregnancy allow for the best outcomes for both mother and baby. A summary of recommended pre-conception care and advice is listed at the end of this section.

Pre-conceptually, previous pregnancies should be discussed including a history of pre-eclampsia and pregnancy-induced hypertension.

Women should be advised to avoid pregnancy within 6–12 months of a flare-up [2]. Pregnancy within this time frame increases the risk of flare-up both during the pregnancy and postnatally. Flare-ups will usually be typical of those experienced by the woman outside of pregnancy. In addition, lupus nephritis flare-ups can cause a particular diagnostic problem during pregnancy because of its superficial similarity to pre-eclampsia (PE). It is important to counsel a woman that pregnancy in some situations is not safe – including active lupus nephritis, severe renal impairment, significant pulmonary hypertension, advanced heart failure and stroke within the last 6 months. Deferring pregnancy (or complete avoidance in certain severe cases) until clinically more stable may be advisable [1, 2, 3].

Hypertension, pre-eclampsia, preterm delivery and poorer outcomes for the fetus including intrauterine growth restriction (IUGR) are all more likely where pregnancy occurs within 6 months of a flare-up.

Drug history must be elicited and rationalized. Angiotensin-converting enzyme (ACE) inhibitors, angiotensin receptor blockers (ARBs), mycophenolate mofetil, methotrexate and cyclophosphamide are all used in the treatment of SLE and are teratogenic and should be stopped [2, 3]. It is vital that after any change in medication, time is allowed to ensure that the disease remains in remission and blood pressure remains well controlled.

Hydroxychloroquine, sulfasalazine, azathioprine, cyclosporine, tacrolimus and biologic agents are all considered safe in pregnancy and should be continued [1, 2].

Antiphospholipid antibodies (aPL; lupus anticoagulant and anticardiolipin antibodies) should be checked. If positive, the pregnancy should be considered higher risk [1].

Anti-Ro and anti-La antibodies are present in some women with SLE and are associated with neonatal heart block, which is permanent and may be present from early second trimester as well as the transient neonatal cutaneous lupus syndrome that may also result due to their presence (see neonatal section later in this chapter) [1, 2].

Renal function and proteinuria should be quantified. The presence of either predicts poorer outcomes [3].

The usual healthy living advice about smoking, diet, alcohol and drugs should also be given.

34.1.1 Summary of Pre-conception Care in SLE [1, 2, 3, 4]

1. **Counselling** – MDT involvement, current medication, disease activity, previous obstetric history, renal function, presence of aPL and anti-Ro/La antibodies.
2. **Advise against pregnancy** if active lupus nephritis, severe renal impairment, significant pulmonary hypertension, advanced heart failure and stroke within the last 6 months.
3. **Defer pregnancy until disease in remission for 6–12 months.**
4. **Baseline investigations**– full blood count, thyroid function tests, blood pressure, renal function, autoantibody profile (including anti-Ro, anti-La, anti-dsDNA, aPL), C3/4 levels, quantification of proteinuria and haematuria.
   Echocardiogram or chest x-ray if respiratory involvement/pulmonary hypertension or cardiomyopathy.

5. **Contraception** –especially during (and immediately in the 6 months after) flare-ups and/or if on potentially teratogenic medication.
6. **Treat hypertension** – review of medications to ensure safe in pregnancy.
7. **Review and adjust medications**– risk/benefit to mother and fetus.
8. **Thrombosis risk assessment** – review need for anticoagulation.
9. **Individualized care plan**

A management plan for pregnancy including early booking with consultant-led care and close involvement of the MDT should be made. With advances in medical knowledge and pharmacological treatments, women who previously may have been advised to avoid pregnancy can potentially have successful pregnancies with tailored, individualized care. Additionally, a clear plan of care postnatally including advice on contraception is equally important, as SLE can flare up during this period [1].

34.2 Diagnosis of SLE

Systemic lupus erythematosus is a multisystem disease and, hence, diagnosis can be difficult due to the diverse presentation and on occasion may be confused with pregnancy symptoms such as fatigue, skin changes and joint pain [2, 3]. Figure 34.1 highlights where diagnosis should be considered if two or more features are identified and demonstrates the heterogeneous presentation. Most commonly encountered features are musculoskeletal and skin complaints [5].

Renal involvement is the main prognostic factor in pregnancy with poorer outcomes clearly evidenced in these women [2].

The American College of Rheumatology [6] has a classification system for diagnosing SLE (Table 34.1). If

a patient at any time in their medical history exhibits 4 of the 11 criteria documented, a diagnosis of SLE can be made with 95% specificity and 85% sensitivity. However, in the presence of specific antibodies, a diagnosis can be made where fewer criteria are met.

Table 34.1 American College of Rheumatology SLE diagnostic criteria [6]

Finding	Description
Malar rash	Fixed erythema over malar eminences in shape of butterfly
Discoid rash	Erythematous raised patches with scaling and scarring may occur in older lesions
Photosensitivity	Skin rash following exposure to sunlight
Oral ulceration	Oral or nasopharyngeal ulcers
Arthritis	Nonerosive arthritis (tenderness, swelling or effusion) involving two or more peripheral joints
Serositis	Pleuritis or pericarditis
Renal disorder	Persistent proteinuria (>0.5 g/day) or cellular casts
Neurological disorder	Seizures or psychosis without other cause including drug or metabolic condition
Haematological disorder	Haemolytic anaemia, leukopenia, lymphopenia, or thrombocytopenia
Immunological disorder	Anti-DNA, anti-Sm, or antiphospholipid antibodies
Antinuclear antibody	Antinuclear antibody (ANA) detected in the absence of any drug that can cause this

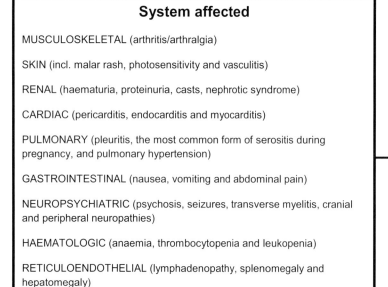
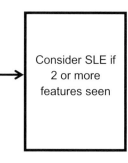

Figure 34.1 Symptomatology of SLE.
Adapted from [5]

34.3 Antibodies

Autoimmune antibodies are common in connective tissue disorders. Antinuclear antibodies (ANA) bind to various proteins or protein complexes within the cell nucleus (Box 34.1).

Antinuclear antibodies can be detected in up to 99% of patients with SLE but are also found in other conditions including infection and cancer. Importantly, evidence shows they are found in up to 25% of the general population, and in only 2.5% are they found to be significantly elevated. Thus, for the majority their presence has no obvious immediate significance, but a small percentage may be diagnosed with an autoimmune condition later in life. Overall, autoimmune disease is found in 5–7% of the population and SLE is diagnosed in 0.1% [7].

There are many subtypes of ANAs including anti-Ro/SS-A antibodies, anti La/SS-B antibodies, anti-Smith (Sm) antibodies and anti-double-stranded (dsDNA) antibodies [2].

Anti-dsDNA is most specific to SLE and found in around 75% of patients. Titres often correspond to disease activity, and along with low complement levels can be a useful tool to recognize a flare-up. Anti-Sm antibodies are found in 20% of individuals with SLE; lupus nephritis occurs more commonly in the presence of this antibody [2].

Anti-Ro and anti-La antibodies are noted in around 30% of individuals with SLE and antiphospholipid antibodies in about 40%; their presence is important in determining potential risks to the fetus and secondary antiphospholipid syndrome, amongst other concerns [2].

34.4 Management of SLE

In non-pregnant women, the management and treatment of SLE depends on the system affected and the aims are for the acute treatment of symptoms as well as the prevention of disease progression. Treatment may include topical sunscreens to prevent cutaneous flare-ups from exposure to ultraviolet (UV) light, antimalarial agents such as hydroxychloroquine (especially where there is skin and joint involvement) for preventing flare-ups and topical or oral glucocorticoids which may also be needed to improve quality of life [8]. A number of medications that may be used in SLE are outlined in brief in Table 34.2 with reference to their safety in pregnancy [1, 2, 3].

34.4.1 Severe Disease Management

Life-threatening lupus may be secondary to various causes including deteriorating lupus nephritis resulting in rapidly progressive renal failure. Cardiac failure, severe anaemia and thrombocytopenia also contribute to significant morbidity and mortality.

High-dose glucocorticoids may be needed, as well as immunosuppressive and potentially cytotoxic agents which can pose significant risks to the fetus in pregnancy. The exact choice of drug will depend on the nature and severity of the condition. Intravenous gamma globulin and splenectomy are also treatment options for thrombocytopenia.

Despite treatment, deterioration can occur, and end-stage renal disease may require dialysis and/or renal transplantation [8.]

Table 34.2 highlights a number of immunosuppressants and whether they are safe to use in pregnancy and breastfeeding.

34.5 Pregnancy and SLE

Flare-up is more common during pregnancy, the highest risk time being postnatally. Studies have shown that a flare-up in the 6 months prior to pregnancy or in previous pregnancies is a good indicator of potential flare-up and type in future pregnancy. Outcome in pregnancy is very much driven by the presence of renal disease. Table 34.3 outlines the increased potential risks to mother and baby and the factors that influence this [1, 2, 3, 4].

34.6 Antenatal Care in SLE

Table 34.4 summarizes the antenatal care instituted in the management of a pregnant woman with SLE. Care must encompass and consider the potential risks to mother and baby as already described above, in addition to instituting measures for prevention including aspirin usually from 12 weeks to delivery to reduce risk of pre-eclampsia [9], and commencing thromboprophylaxis in women with antiphospholipid antibodies or active disease to reduce risk of venous thromboembolism. Maternal and fetal health should be monitored by regular blood pressure (BP) checks and urine assessment, bloods (to monitor renal, liver and haematological systems, as well as monitoring disease stability with antibody/complement levels). Fetal growth should be monitored at least 4 weekly [1], with additional fetal heart auscultation weekly from 16 weeks [4] if the fetus is at risk of heart block (positive maternal antibodies for anti-Ro and/or anti-La). Management should be delivered by the MDT and very much patient centred with an individualized care plan.

34.7 Lupus Flare-Ups in Pregnancy

It is generally unpredictable who will encounter a flare-up in pregnancy but potential factors influencing this include active disease within the last 6 months prior to pregnancy or a history of flare-up during a previous pregnancy. It can on occasion be difficult to distinguish physiological pregnancy symptoms from a flare-up, as many of the signs and symptoms are

Table 34.2 Medications used in autoimmune conditions and in pregnancy

Medication	Action	Safe to continue/ commence in pregnancy	Contraindicated	Safe to breastfeed
Methotrexate	Folic antagonist	No Discontinue 3 months prior to pregnancy	Yes – teratogenic	No
Corticosteroids – e.g. prednisolone	Act on steroid receptors – suppress inflammation and immunity	Can be used and relatively safe in low doses Preferable to NSAIDs Various routes depending on clinical need – oral, IM, IV or intra-articular If on long-term/high dose steroids (e.g. >7.5 mg prednisolone daily) for >2 weeks, then may need to consider parenteral steroids to cover the 'stress' of labour	No Increased risk preterm labour and gestational diabetes with steroids in pregnancy	Yes
Leflunomide	Pyrimidine synthesis inhibitor	No Delay conception for 2 years – long half-life, unless eliminated with cholestyramine or active charcoal	Yes – teratogenic	No
Sulfasalazine	Dihydrofolate reductase inhibitor	Yes (+ give with folic acid 5 mg/day)	No	Yes
Azathioprine	Antiproliferative immunosuppressive	Yes Fetal liver lacks enzyme that converts azathioprine to its active metabolites Useful as steroid sparing agent	No	Yes (theoretical risk)
TNFα antagonists – Etanercept	Suppress response to TNF, hence, suppressing inflammatory response	Not enough evidence with these new agents to fully advise – risk / benefit should be discussed and where possible discontinue by 30–32 weeks	No	Yes
Antimalarials – Hydroxychloroquine	Decrease formation of protein complexes required to stimulate CD4+ T cells	Yes	No	Yes
Cyclophosphamide	Alkylating agent	No Discontinue 3 months prior to pregnancy May need in late pregnancy for life-threatening disease	Yes	No

Table 34.2 (cont.)

Medication	Action	Safe to continue/commence in pregnancy	Contraindicated	Safe to breastfeed
Mycophenolate mofetil (MMF)	Antiproliferative immunosuppressive	No Stop 3 months prior to conception	Yes	No
Rituximab	Monoclonal antibody	No Stop 1 year prior to conception	Yes	No

Table 34.3 Potential risks to mother and baby secondary to SLE [1,2,3,4]

Effects on mother	Increased risk of pre-eclampsia (PE), risk of deep vein thrombosis (DVT) (in the presence of secondary antiphospholipid syndrome) or active disease and infection Long-term course of SLE unaffected by pregnancy	Adverse outcomes are significantly related to the presence of various factors including: 1. Anticardiolipin antibodies 2. Lupus anticoagulant 3. History of lupus nephritis 4. Active disease at time of conception/flare-up in pregnancy 5. Hypertension 6. Proteinuria 7. Thrombocytopenia
Effects on baby	Increased risk of miscarriage, IUGR (10–30% affected), premature rupture of membranes (PROM), abruption, preterm delivery, intrauterine death (IUD), neonatal lupus syndromes	

Table 34.4 Antenatal care in SLE

Antenatal care for women with SLE in pregnancy [1,2,3,4]

Multidisciplinary care with early booking

- Review pre-conception plan of care.

- Review of previous obstetric history and plan for current care based around this.

- MDT involvement – monitoring disease activity and placental insufficiency.

- Baseline bloods with minimum of 4 weekly repeat including: renal function, liver function, full blood count, urate, urine protein creatinine (PCR), anti-dsDNA antibody and serum complement titres (C3/C4).

- Close monitoring of BP – at least monthly monitoring aiming for BP <140/90 [1].

- Control hypertension with anti-hypertensives which are considered safe for use in pregnancy including methyldopa, labetalol and nifedipine.

- Advise low-dose aspirin 75 mg (or 150 mg) daily from 12 weeks until delivery as per NICE Hypertension guidance [9] for patients with autoimmune disease. May commence pre-conception if APS.

- If antiphospholipid antibodies present (and/or active disease) – will require low-dose aspirin and prophylactic low molecular weight heparin (LMWH) from as early as 6 weeks. LMWH should be continued for 6 weeks after end of pregnancy.

- If anti-Ro or anti-La antibody positive, fetal heart should be listened to and noted every visit from as early as 16 weeks. Heart block necessitates referral to tertiary fetal medicine unit [3].

- Serial growth measurements of baby (and umbilical artery Doppler at 24 weeks).

- Identify and manage flare-up.

- Supplementation with calcium, vitamin D and folic acid.

- Screening for gestational diabetes if on moderate/high-dose steroids.

analogous to the changes that occur in 'normal' pregnancy including oedema, fatigue, anaemia, thrombocytopenia and joint and muscle aches and pains [2, 3].

34.7.1 Blood Results Suggestive of Flare-Up

- Increasing anti-dsDNA titres
- Decreasing complement C3/4 level (even with normal limits) [4]

Managing a lupus flare-up during pregnancy must involve the wider MDT and depends on the severity and the system(s) affected. Treatment is usually limited to medications considered safe in pregnancy. It may be simply symptomatic relief such as analgesics (NSAIDs) for controlling mild arthritic symptoms and mild serositis. Hydroxychloroquine (a randomized, placebo-controlled study supports its use [10]), oral steroids and azathioprine can be safely used in pregnancy. In moderate to severe cases, IV steroids or immunoglobulins and plasmapheresis can be used. If severe, delivery may be required so that specific medications unsafe for use in pregnancy can be given [4]. With the agreement of the mother, the maternal condition should always be given priority.

34.8 Lupus Nephritis versus Pre-eclampsia (PE)

Renal activity is a predictor of adverse pregnancy outcome and should be closely monitored by measuring and quantifying proteinuria, urine sediment analysis (for presence of glomerular haematuria or red cell casts) and serum creatinine / glomerular filtration rate [1].

It can be difficult to determine if lupus nephritis or PE or both is the cause of hypertension and proteinuria in pregnancy. The diagnosis can be critical particularly if the presentation is around extremely premature gestations.

There are a few factors that can help predict which is more likely (see Table 34.5) but the only way to be diagnostically certain is renal biopsy. This is very rarely undertaken during pregnancy but may be necessary at the extremes of fetal viability if the alternative is termination of the pregnancy to allow for treatment of the mother. However, at later gestations, often when faced with this diagnostic dilemma it may be more appropriate to deliver; PE will resolve following delivery but lupus nephritis persists and delivery allows treatments such as cyclophosphamide or mycophenolate mofetil which may be

lifesaving to be administered without associated fetal risks [1, 2, 3, 4] but all undertaken with specialist/MDT discussion.

34.9 Heavy Proteinuria in Pregnancy

Proteinuria is often encountered in the antenatal setting, sometimes intermittently and sometimes related to urinary tract infection, but in the setting of persistent heavy proteinuria without a recognizable cause this needs to be investigated to exclude PE or underlying renal disease secondary to a number of conditions including diabetes, reflux nephropathy, glomerulonephritis and SLE [11].

Initial investigations should at least include:

- Formal quantification of proteinuria – urinary protein: creatinine ratio (uPCR), an abnormal result is > 30 mg/ mmol
- Serum creatinine (should be interpreted using pregnancy values)

34.10 Timing of Delivery

Umbilical and uterine artery Doppler at 20–24 weeks has good negative predictive value but modest positive predictive value for placental-associated problems [4] including PE and IUGR, so regular 4 weekly fetal scan assessment for growth with increased surveillance where needed is essential [1]. The mode and timing of delivery will depend on both maternal and fetal factors, but delivery by term at the latest should be considered in all women with SLE. If antiphospholipid antibodies are also present, delivery could be considered from 37 weeks.

34.11 Neonatal Lupus Syndromes

Lupus syndromes in the fetus and neonate are the consequence of passively acquired autoimmunity from transplacental anti-Ro and anti-La antibodies from an ANA-positive mother [2].

All women with SLE should be screened for anti-Ro and anti-La antibodies both pre-conceptually and in early pregnancy.

Anti-Ro and anti-La antibodies can be found in entirely asymptomatic women who have never had a diagnosis of SLE. Their babies are at a similar risk of fetal/neonatal lupus syndromes as are those women with SLE who are antibody positive [2, 12].

Table 34.5 Differences in distinguishing lupus nephritis from PE

Lupus nephritis	Encountered with both Lupus nephritis and PE	PE
Reduced complement (C3)	Hypertension	Raised urate
Raised anti-dsDNA antibody	(prior to 20 weeks may be more suggestive	Raised liver transaminases
May respond to steroids	of lupus)	No response to steroids
May have cutaneous/joint manifestations	Proteinuria	Past history
	(prior to 20 weeks more suggestive of lupus)	Abnormal liver function tests (LFTs)
	Thrombocytopenia	

Anti-Ro antibody is most commonly associated with fetal and neonatal sequelae (90%), although in 50–70% of cases anti-La is also present [2].

The two main presentations are:

1. **Cutaneous (5% risk)** [2]
2. **Cardiac (2% risk)** [2]

Other presentations, including haematological and hepatic, are rare [3].

34.12 Cutaneous Neonatal Lupus

This presents with erythematous lesions usually affecting the scalp, face and neck at birth or within the first 2 weeks of life after exposure to sun/UV light. It is a photosensitive condition, and avoidance of sunlight/phototherapy is recommended. It can last weeks or months and resolves once maternal antibodies are cleared, usually by around 6–8 months [1, 2, 3].

34.13 Cardiac Neonatal Lupus

Antibodies cause an inflammatory response affecting calcium channels in the conducting system of the heart, resulting in permanent damage due to scarring and fibrosis and consequent congenital heart block (CHB) with resultant impaired cardiac output and congestive cardiac failure in complete block. Congenital heart block affects 2% of children born to primiparous women with anti-Ro antibodies. Other factors that may increase risk include high antibody levels and maternal hypothyroidism [3]. Evidence suggests a 16% recurrence rate with a previous child affected [1, 2, 3]. The first finding may be detection of bradycardia and atrioventricular (AV) dissociation on scan. There may also be myocarditis and pericardial effusion present [2].

Complete heart block is associated with neonatal mortality (30%). Cardiac failure leading to hydrops can be present before the fetus is viable, usually presenting between 18 and 28 weeks [1]. Input from a fetal medicine unit and neonatologists should be sought.

A pacemaker may be needed immediately in the neonatal period and consideration will need to be given to place of delivery. Approximately 50–60% of those who survive require a pacemaker in early infancy and due to the risk of sudden death [1]. It is recommended that all these children are fitted with a pacemaker by their early teenage years [2].

34.14 Antiphospholipid Syndrome (APS) Is Not a Subgroup of SLE

It is important to make a distinction between SLE and antiphospholipid syndrome (APS) (diagnosed by 2 or more positive readings for lupus anticoagulant and/or anticardiolipin antibodies at least 12 weeks apart in addition to one clinical criteria – history of thrombosis (venous, arterial or small vessel) or poor pregnancy morbidity ($\geq$3 consecutive miscarriages at <10 weeks' gestation, $\geq$1 fetal death at >10 weeks' gestations with normal morphology or $\geq$1 premature birth <34 weeks' gestation)) [2]. Women who have SLE do not necessarily have APS and vice versa. Equally, positive antibodies alone do not equate to a diagnosis of APS. This can cause confusion in antenatal care and it is important to recognize they are two different conditions with consequent differing management approaches. Antiphospholipid syndrome is not discussed in detail in this chapter.

34.15 Summary Key Points – SLE in Pregnancy

Systemic lupus erythematosus should be considered a high-risk condition and hence involvement of an MDT is important to manage obstetric care for women appropriately. Regular review is needed antenatally to monitor mother and baby.

Pre-conception review is paramount to achieving the best outcome in terms of both maternal and fetal morbidity.

Obstetricians (and the MDT) should strongly recommend (and have a duty of care to prevent harm) to women to avoid pregnancy until disease stability is achieved or complete avoidance if risk to maternal health is significant in women with current/recent flare-up or severe disease.

Suggested Reading

Cauldwell M, Nelson-Piercy C. Maternal and fetal complications of systemic lupus erythematosus. *Obstet Gynaecol.* 2012;**14**:167–74.

LUPUS UK. www.lupusuk.org.uk/lupus-and-pregnancy/ Recommended for patient information. [accessed online 6th December 2019]

RCOG online StratOG learning resource: Connective tissue, bone and joint disorders tutorial.

Lateef A, Petri M. Managing lupus patients during pregnancy. *Best Pract Res Clin Rheumatol.* 2013;

27(3):435–47. doi: 10.1016/j.berh.2013.07.005

References

1. Cauldwell M, Nelson-Piercy C. Maternal and fetal complications of systemic lupus erythematosus. *Obstet Gynaecol.*2012;**14**:167–74.

2. Nelson-Piercy C, ed. Chapter 8. In *Handbook of Obstetric Medicine*, 4th ed. London: Informa Healthcare;2010.

3. Lateef A, Petri M. Managing lupus patients during pregnancy. *Best Pract Res Clin Rheumatol.*2013;27(3):435–47. doi: 10.1016/j.berh.2013.07.0057

4. Andreoli L, Bertsias GK, Agmon-Levin N, et al. EULAR recommendations for women's health and the management of family planning, assisted reproduction, pregnancy and menopause in patients with systemic lupus erythematosus and/or antiphospholipid syndrome. *Ann Rheum Dis.* 2017;**76**:476–85.

5. Gladman, DD, Urowitz, MB, Esdaile, et al. Guidelines for referral and management of systemic lupus erythematosus in adults. *Arthritis Rheum.* 1999;**42**(9): 1785–96.

6. American College of Rheumatology. ACR-endorsed criteria for rheumatic diseases. www.rheumatology.org/Practice-Quality/

Clinical-Support/Criteria/ACR-Endorsed-Criteria [accessed online 11th Dec 2019]

7. Grygiel-Górniak B, Rogacka N, Puszczewicz M. Antinuclear antibodies in healthy people and non-rheumatic diseases – diagnostic and clinical implications. *Reumatologia.*2018;**56** (4),243–8. doi: 10.5114/reum.2018.77976

8. Gordon C, Amissah-Arthur MB, Gayed M, et al., for the British Society for Rheumatology Standards, Audit and Guidelines Working Group. The British Society for Rheumatology guideline for the management of systemic lupus erythematosus in adults. *Rheumatology.* 2018;**57**(1):e1–e45, https://doi.org/10 .1093/rheumatology/kex286

9. National Institute for Health and Care Excellence. (2019) Hypertension in pregnancy: diagnosis and management (NICE Guideline 133).

10. Levy RA, Vilela VS, Cataldo MJ, et al. Hydroxychloroquine (HCQ) in lupus pregnancy: double-blind and placebo-controlled study. *Lupus.* 2001;**10**:401–4.

11. Nelson-Piercy C, ed. Section B, Differential diagnosis of medical problems in pregnancy – Proteinuria. In *Handbook of Obstetric Medicine*, 4th ed. London: Informa Healthcare; 2010. p. 294.

12. Kapur A, Dey M, Tangri M, Bandhu HC. Maternal anti-Ro/SSA and anti-La/SSB antibodies and fetal congenital heart block. *J Obstet Gynaecol India.*2015;**65**(3): 193–95. doi: 10.1007/s13224-014-0608-2

Autoimmune Rheumatic Disorders in Pregnancy

Laura Andreoli, Maria Chiara Gerardi & Angela Tincani

35.1 Introduction

Autoimmune rheumatic diseases (ARDs) are chronic inflammatory systemic conditions which mainly affect women and whose onset is often during childbearing age. These diseases can be characterized by either a predominant articular involvement (chronic forms of arthritis) or by a multisystemic impairment (connective tissue diseases (CTDs)). Reproductive issues such as fertility, contraception and family planning are topics of crucial interest for women with ARDs [1]. For a long time, pregnancy has been discouraged in patients with ARDs because of the concerns about poor maternal and fetal prognosis. In the last decades, the increasing knowledge about the use of antirheumatic drugs during pregnancy and lactation has paved the way to a more effective maternal disease control, leading to the improvement of pregnancy outcomes. Preconception risk stratification is the key point and should be part of the physician–patient communication [2]. However, this task may be overlooked by either the rheumatologist or by the gynaecologist, yielding to an unmet need in the care of women with ARDs of childbearing age [3, 4].

35.2 Pre-conception Counselling

35.2.1 Fertility and Assisted Reproductive Techniques (ARTs)

Patients of childbearing age should be aware that the disease itself is not a cause of infertility; the majority of women with ARDs is indeed fertile [5]. They should be counselled for general risk factors of infertility (increasing age, cigarette smoking, alcohol consumption, etc.) and referred for fertility assessment with their partners after 12 months of unprotected intercourses (6 months if the patient is over 35 years of age) [1]. Women with ARDs can have transiently or permanently reduced fertility due to disease-related factors in the case of high disease activity, chronic renal insufficiency, use of alkylating drugs such as cyclophosphamide, and the 'unruptured follicle syndrome' because of chronic use of nonsteroidal anti-inflammatory drugs (NSAIDs) [1].

Women with ARDs can be candidates for assisted reproductive techniques (ARTs) [6]. If the type of ARTs suggested to the patient includes ovarian stimulation with hormones, it is appropriate to assess the individual risk for thrombosis (general and disease-specific risk factors, such as antiphospholipid antibodies (aPL)). The patients at higher risk of thrombosis can be counselled to use low-dose aspirin (LDA) and/or heparin (at prophylactic or anticoagulant dosage, based on individual risk stratification) during the period of ovarian stimulation. The rate of live births induced by ARTs in patients with ARDs has not been extensively investigated; a recent case-control study showed that patients with rheumatoid arthritis (RA) seem to have fewer live births because of an increased rate of implantation failures after ARTs [7]. Regarding maternal risks for disease flare-up and thrombosis, it was shown in a multicentre cohort of patients with systemic lupus erythematosus (SLE) and/or the antiphospholipid syndrome (APS) that risks are negligible if the patients are treated during ARTs procedures and pregnancy [8].

35.2.2 Risk of Maternal Complications

The disease course during pregnancy may vary upon different ARDs (Table 35.1), mainly depending on the characteristics of the disease (articular involvement vs. systemic involvement). Rheumatoid arthritis and juvenile idiopathic arthritis seem less likely to flare up during pregnancy, although more recent prospective studies indicate that only 50–60% of women with RA may experience disease remission in pregnancy rather than the higher rates reported by retrospective studies in the past [9]. Different study design, improved treatment and the possibility to get pregnant also for women with more severe disease could account for this difference. Spondylarthritis tends to be stable or to get worse during pregnancy, even though the available literature is scarce [2]. In SLE, the reported rate of flare-ups during pregnancy may be different from study to study, this reflecting the severity of different disease subsets (e.g. renal vs. non-renal SLE) and different management during pregnancy (e.g. withdrawal of treatment prior to pregnancy is a risk factor for flare-up) [10]. The effect of other CTDs on pregnancy or vice versa has been less investigated. Systemic sclerosis generally remains stable in most pregnancies, but patients with severe pulmonary hypertension or severe interstitial lung disease should avoid pregnancy on account of the high maternal mortality risk [11]. A special consideration should be given to APS because obstetric complications are hallmarks of the disease [2]. Pregnancy does not seem to worsen the activity of systemic vasculitis, but a disease flare-up during pregnancy can lead to severe complications [12].

In general, high disease activity is associated with maternal complications such as hypertensive disorders (pre-eclampsia, HELLP syndrome) and with fetal complications (intrauterine death (IUD); intrauterine growth restriction (IUGR)). Active disease during pregnancy can lead to preterm birth (mainly

Table 35.1 Maternal and fetal risks in autoimmune rheumatic diseases during pregnancy

	Disease	Maternal risks	Fetal risks	Counselling
Prevalent joint involvement	RA	Active disease in 10–40% of pregnancies	Prematurity and SGA with active maternal diseases	Low to moderate risk if maternal disease in remission. Continue immunosuppressive therapy compatible with pregnancy.
	ax-SpA	Active disease in approximately 50% of pregnancies	Prematurity and SGA with active maternal diseases	Low to moderate risk. Control maternal diseases with immunosuppressive therapy compatible with pregnancy.
	PsA	Active disease in approximately 40% of pregnancies	Prematurity and SGA with active maternal diseases	Low to moderate risk. Control maternal diseases with immunosuppressive therapy compatible with pregnancy.
	JIA	Active disease in 30–40% of pregnancies	Prematurity and SGA with active maternal diseases	Low to moderate risk. Control maternal diseases with immunosuppressive therapy compatible with pregnancy.
Systemic involvement	SLE	Flare in 35–70% of patients; Hypertension and PE/E	Fetal loss, IUGR, prematurity, SGA, anti-Ro/SSA-associated neonatal lupus	High-risk pregnancy. Continue immunosuppressive therapy compatible with pregnancy; consider LDA±heparin if increased risk for PE (e.g. lupus nephritis, positive aPL).
	APS	Thrombosis, PE/E, HELLP syndrome	Fetal loss, IUGR, prematurity, SGA	High-risk pregnancy. Start conventional treatment of LDA±heparin at positive pregnancy index and continue throughout pregnancy; consider additional immunomodulatory treatments if history of refractory obstetric APS.
	SSc	Majority of women, no disease worsening	IUGR, prematurity, SGA	High risk, especially if moderate to severe vital organ involvement
	Systemic vasculitis	If in remission, low-moderate risk for flare. Hypertension, PE	Fetal loss, IUGR, prematurity, SGA	High risk, especially if moderate to severe vital organ involvement

Source: Modified from Østensen M. Preconception counselling. *Rheum Dis Clin North Am.* 2017; 43:189–99.

aPL: antiphospholipid antibodies; APS: antiphospholipid syndrome; ax-SpA: axial spondyloarthritis; CTDs: connective tissue diseases; E: eclampsia; HELLP syndrome: haemolysis, elevated liver enzyme levels, low platelet count syndrome; IUGR: intrauterine growth restriction; JIA: juvenile idiopathic arthritis; LDA: low-dose of aspirin; PE: pre-eclampsia; PsA: psoriatic arthritis; RA: rheumatoid arthritis; SLE: systemic lupus erythematosus; SSc: systemic sclerosis; SGA: small-for-gestational-age.

due to preterm prelabour rupture of membranes (PPROM) and small-for-gestational-age (SGA) neonates). Therefore, it is currently stressed that stable disease remission prior to conception and during pregnancy is the key point for minimizing the risk of maternal and fetal complications. In addition, women who carry aPL should be monitored for and offered prophylaxis against thrombotic events, with particular attention to those with a 'high-risk aPL profile' (see Section 35.2.4). Women with ARDs should be encouraged to plan the pregnancy and discuss with their doctors the best timing for embarking on a pregnancy [2].

35.2.3 Risk of Fetal Complications

Fetal complications can be caused by maternal active disease and/or maternal disease factors such as autoantibodies that can have a negative impact on pregnancy outcome and fetal well-being. Complications can occur during any trimester of gestation and include pregnancy loss (miscarriage, IUD), IUGR, preterm birth, SGA infants. Certain maternal autoantibodies can have a negative impact on fetal development: aPL; anti-Ro/SSA ± anti-La/SSB. aPL can impair placentation through multiple mechanisms (pro-thrombotic and pro-inflammatory) and lead to placental insufficiency, whose consequences can be IUD, IUGR, preterm birth (±pre-eclampsia), SGA infants [2]. Anti-Ro/SSA ± anti-La/SSB can be responsible for the so-called neonatal lupus syndrome, a rare condition which is a model of secondary autoimmunity due to the transplacental passage of maternal autoantibodies [2]. The less severe form consists of erythematosus skin lesions, cytopenia, elevated liver enzymes during the first months of life, with spontaneous resolution within the first year of age. Anti-Ro/SSA ± anti-La/SSB can also exert proinflammatory actions at the level of fetal heart. Atrioventricular block (AVB) can develop (incomplete vs. complete), possibly in association with dilative cardiomyopathy and endocardial fibroelastosis. Complete AVB (grade III) requires in 50–80% of the cases the implantation of a cardiac pacemaker soon after birth. Incomplete AVB (grade II) has been managed with different treatments (dexamethasone, intravenous immunoglobulins, plasma exchange), although it was not possible to show a clear advantage in the prevention of progression towards complete AVB. Fetal cardiac involvement is the most severe and life-threatening manifestation of the neonatal lupus syndrome, but it is estimated to be quite rare (1–2% of pregnancies with anti-Ro/SSA ± anti-La/SSB) [10, 13, 14].

35.2.4 Risk Stratification

Individual risk stratification is the main objective of pre-conception counselling and should include both disease-specific and general risk factors (Figure 35.1), assessed by different specialists. A multidisciplinary approach for the care of a pregnant woman is indicated. The joined assessment of disease-specific and general obstetric risk factors will yield an individual risk profile for tailoring a treatment plan.

Rheumatologists will assess disease activity and modify the treatment if necessary for reaching a stable disease remission

prior to conception (ideally 6–12 months), using drugs that are compatible with pregnancy. In addition, autoantibodies with a potential negative impact such as aPL and anti-Ro/SSA ± anti-La/SSB should be searched. Although the frequency of positivity for these autoantibodies is variable upon different ARDs (more common in patients with connective tissue disorders (CTDs) as compared to women with chronic arthritis), it may be considered to check any women with ARDs prior to pregnancy in order to broaden the spectrum of risk stratification.

Regarding aPL, the three 'criteria' tests should be available (lupus anticoagulant, anticardiolipin antibodies, anti-beta2glycoprotein I antibodies) to define the so-called aPL profile.

It is accepted by consensus that a 'high-risk' aPL profile (risk of thrombosis and pregnancy morbidity) is identified as the presence of:

1. positive lupus anticoagulant;
2. triple aPL positivity (all three tests positive);
3. the presence of medium-high titres of IgG anticardiolipin and anti-beta2glycoprotein I;
4. persistence of positive aPL overtime (transient aPL are more likely to be non-autoimmune, non-pathogenic aPL) [14].

Obstetricians will focus on maternal co-morbidities (e.g. arterial hypertension, obesity), harmful lifestyle habits (e.g. cigarette smoking) and previous pregnancy complications.

35.2.5 Contraindications to Pregnancy

It can be wise to suggest postponing pregnancy in patients with either new-onset ARDs, or active disease (especially if renal involvement) or recent arterial thrombosis (stroke, myocardial infarction).

Patients with ARDs should be discouraged from pregnancy in the case of severe organ involvement (e.g. pulmonary hypertension, cardiomyopathy) or previous pre-eclampsia with HELLP syndrome while on treatment [2]. Contraindicating a pregnancy is no easy task; therefore, it is important that the reasons are explained from the point of view of both the rheumatologist and the obstetrician.

35.3 Management of Pregnancy

35.3.1 Maternal Assessment

Pregnant patients with ARDs should be closely monitored for clinical and laboratory signs of disease activity. Evaluations can be performed every 4–6 weeks, depending on the type of disease and individual situation (Figure 35.2). For instance, patients with lupus nephritis should be regularly checked for renal parameters (urine analysis, 24 hours' proteinuria) and for C3/C4 levels and anti-dsDNA titres).

35.3.2 Fetal Assessment

Besides the routine ultrasound examinations performed during pregnancy in healthy women, patients with ARDs should undergo additional obstetric ultrasound (see Figure 35.2), with

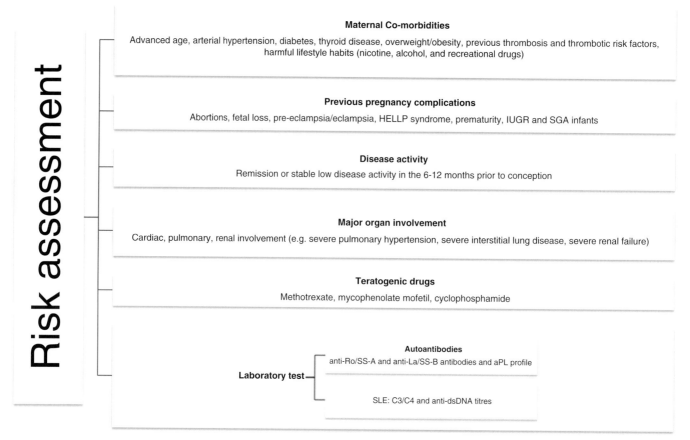

Figure 35.1 Pre-conception risk assessment
aPL: antiphospholipid antibodies; aPL profile: Lupus Anticoagulanti, anticardiolipin antibodies, anti-beta2glycoprotein I antibodies; HELLP syndrome: haemolysis, elevated liver enzyme levels, low platelet count syndrome; IUGR: intrauterine growth restriction; SGA: small-for-gestational-age.

the main purpose of detecting early or late IUGR and establishing the correct timing for delivery.

In women with positive anti-Ro/SSA ± anti-La/SSB, fetal echocardiography is usually performed during 16 and 26 weeks of gestation with a weekly or biweekly schedule. It is currently debated whether it is cost-effective to perform such a highly intensive surveillance for AVB, as there is no effective treatment. In any case, the timely diagnosis of this rare condition can be useful to plan a highly specialized follow-up of the pregnancy, which is usually available only in a few referral centres [10].

35.3.3 Delivery

Patients with ARDs do not have any contraindication to vaginal delivery, with a few exceptions for those patients who have problems at the hips as a consequence of their inflammatory disease [16]. Epidural anaesthesia can be performed in accordance with the practice scheduled by the obstetrician and the anaesthetist.

Several patients do believe that having ARDs is an indication for caesarean section and that this mode of delivery is safer. Obstetric counselling should reassure the patients and their families about the indications towards a specific mode of delivery, explaining advantages and drawbacks.

35.4 Postpartum Care

35.4.1 Maternal Assessment

Maternal disease can flare up in the period after delivery; therefore, patients with ARDs should be followed up 40–50 days after delivery and in the following 6 months. In the case of a disease flare-up, the treatment should be discussed according to the patient's preference regarding breastfeeding.

Patients who carry positive aPL should receive antithrombotic treatment with heparin at prophylactic dosage for 4–6 weeks after delivery. Women who were anticoagulated with vitamin K antagonists prior to pregnancy, can resume the treatment after delivery as it is compatible with breastfeeding.

Systemic vasculitis seems to be at higher risk of ischaemic events in the postpartum period; hence, antithrombotic treatment with heparin at prophylactic dosage for 4–6 weeks after delivery should be used also in these women, especially after caesarean section [17].

35.4.2 Methods of Contraception

Women with ARDs may need contraception for several reasons: 1) family planning; 2) to avoid pregnancy while on teratogenic drugs; 3) to avoid pregnancy during disease

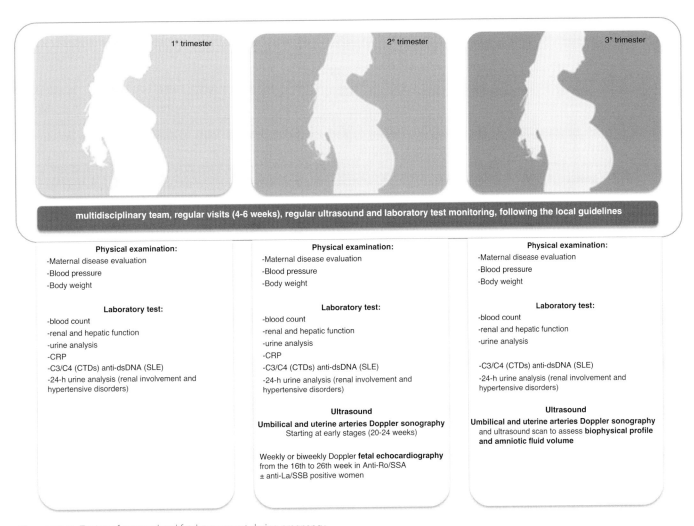

1° trimester	2° trimester	3° trimester

multidisciplinary team, regular visits (4-6 weeks), regular ultrasound and laboratory test monitoring, following the local guidelines

Physical examination:
- Maternal disease evaluation
- Blood pressure
- Body weight

Laboratory test:
- blood count
- renal and hepatic function
- urine analysis
- CRP
- C3/C4 (CTDs) anti-dsDNA (SLE)
- 24-h urine analysis (renal involvement and hypertensive disorders)

Physical examination:
- Maternal disease evaluation
- Blood pressure
- Body weight

Laboratory test:
- blood count
- renal and hepatic function
- urine analysis
- CRP
- C3/C4 (CTDs) anti-dsDNA (SLE)
- 24-h urine analysis (renal involvement and hypertensive disorders)

Ultrasound
Umbilical and uterine arteries Doppler sonography
Starting at early stages (20-24 weeks)

Weekly or biweekly Doppler **fetal echocardiography** from the 16th to 26th week in Anti-Ro/SSA ± anti-La/SSB positive women

Physical examination:
- Maternal disease evaluation
- Blood pressure
- Body weight

Laboratory test:
- blood count
- renal and hepatic function
- urine analysis

- C3/C4 (CTDs) anti-dsDNA (SLE)
- 24-h urine analysis (renal involvement and hypertensive disorders)

Ultrasound
Umbilical and uterine arteries Doppler sonography
and ultrasound scan to assess **biophysical profile and amniotic fluid volume**

Figure 35.2 Timing of maternal and fetal assessment during pregnancy.

flare-ups or situations that transiently/permanently contra-indicate pregnancy [18]. In addition, they may need hormonal treatments for the management of gynaecological conditions [19].

In order to select the best female contraceptive method for a woman with ARDs, two major disease-related factors should be taken into account: 1) type of ARDs; 2) aPL profile. These factors should be combined with individual risk factors (obesity, cigarette smoking, etc.), preference of the patient and gynaecological contraindications [19].

Oestrogen–progesterone-containing compounds are not contraindicated in women with chronic arthritis (they even seem to be protective against severe evolution of disease), while they should be limited to patients with connective tissue disorders (especially SLE) who have inactive or stable active disease [20].

The presence of aPL, especially if high-risk profile, is a contraindication to the use of oestrogen-containing compounds, regardless of the disease of the patient. Patients with aPL can use progesterone compounds (first or second

generations progestins are preferred for lower thrombotic risk as compared to ultimate generation progestin). The levonorgestrel-releasing intrauterine device can be useful to manage metrorrhagia in patients who take oral anticoagulation, particularly patients with APS [21].

Nulliparity and chronic use of immunosuppressive drugs are no longer considered contraindications to the use of the intrauterine device (as long as the patient is compliant with the gynaecological follow-up) [20].

Emergency contraception is suitable in patients with ARDs [20].

35.5 Treatment during Pregnancy and Lactation

35.5.1 Conventional Disease-modifying Antirheumatic Drugs (DMARDs)

While counselling women with ARDs, it should be stressed that maternal active disease during pregnancy can negatively impact on fetal development and pregnancy outcome [22, 23]. Active disease is deleterious; therefore, it is convenient to keep the disease under control by using drugs that are not harmful to the fetus.

The large majority of conventional disease-modifying anti-rheumatic drugs (DMARDs) can be used during pregnancy and lactation (see Figure 35.3) [24–26]. Very few are known teratogens (methotrexate, cyclophosphamide, mycophenolate mofetil) and need to be withdrawn prior to conceptions (allowing a period of wash-out: 6 weeks for mycophenolate, 3 months for methotrexate and 6 months for cyclophosphamide). It is wise to wait for longer periods after the withdrawal of these drugs (and switch to others) to ascertain that the disease is well controlled.

Particular attention should be given to hydroxychloroquine (HCQ). Older and recent studies have shown multiple beneficial properties of HCQ in SLE pregnancy [27]. HCQ is able to prevent SLE flare-up during pregnancy, while HCQ discontinuation at positive pregnancy test is associated with increased risk for flare-ups. HCQ was able to reduce by 85% the rate of SGA neonates in women with lupus nephritis. Novel properties of HCQ include the chance for reducing the risk of recurrence of AVB in anti-Ro-positive women who already had a baby with AVB, reducing the risk for skin manifestations of neonatal lupus in anti-Ro-positive women, and improving pregnancy outcome in women with primary obstetric APS refractory to conventional treatment. These findings highlight the importance of maintaining HCQ throughout pregnancy if already on treatment or to consider starting it when pregnancy is planned.

Some drugs are currently not recommended during pregnancy and lactation (Figure 35.3). This is not because of proof of harm, but rather because data are lacking. In the case in which the drug is the only available choice, the benefit/risk ratio should be discussed with the patient. It is important to share with the patient what is known and what is not about the use of a drug during pregnancy and lactation, to let her and her family make an informed decision.

The new Pregnancy Labelling System released by the Food and Drug Administration (FDA) will help physicians to have a clear picture of the data available for each drug (www.fda.gov /drugs/developmentapprovalprocess/developmentresources/l abeling/ucm093307.htm).

35.5.2 Biologic Disease-Modifying Antirheumatic Drugs (bDMARDs)

As a consequence of the 'revolution' in rheumatology due to the introduction of bDMARDs nearly 20 years ago, there is an increasing need for data about the use of these drugs during pregnancy and lactation.

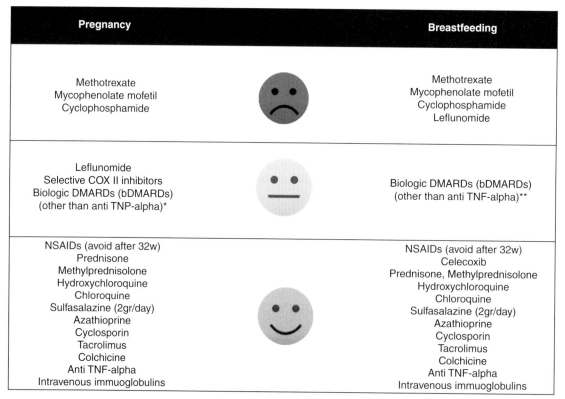

Figure 35.3 Antirheumatic drugs compatible with pregnancy and breastfeeding.
*The molecular structure of many of these drugs (monoclonal antibodies) suggests that their transplacental passage may be virtually absent until the second trimester due to the 'immaturity' of the placenta. In theory, receiving these drugs during the first trimester should not cause effects on the fetus. Their use can be prescribed if there is no other therapeutic option.
**These drugs are large protein molecules having little chance of passing into breast milk. Even if it was present in the breast milk, the drug would degrade in the digestive system of the newborn being impossible of absorption. The possibility of breastfeeding during therapy should be discussed.

Biologic disease-modifying antirheumatic drugs can differ in molecular structure; however, they are all big size proteins which cannot passively diffuse and reach the fetus during the first trimester of gestation. Based on this assumption, unintended pregnancies exposed to these drugs are not a problem. Moreover, it is currently suggested to maintain the treatment during pregnancy, as the discontinuation of TNF inhibitors (TNFi) (the biological agents with more published evidence) at positive pregnancy index has been associated with maternal disease flare-ups during pregnancy (and poorer pregnancy outcomes as a consequence) [28].

As the active transport of IgG immunoglobulins across the placenta becomes significant after week 16 of gestation, it is understood that those bDMARDs which are IgG monoclonal antibodies will be transferred to the fetus. It was demonstrated that the drug concentration of monoclonal antibodies was higher in the newborn as compared to the mother, as expected for any IgG. Therefore, it is recommended to stop bDMARDs (with different timing according to their structure) in the second trimester–early third trimester in order to minimize the exposure to the drug and avoid that the newborn will be immunosuppressed because of the drug received from the mother [29].

Among TNFi, certolizumab pegol (CTZ) does not have the Fc portion needed for transplacental passage. Based on this peculiarity, the CRIB study demonstrated that no to minimal drug was detectable in the blood of neonates whose mothers received the drug until delivery; these children did not have any particular adverse event in the first two months of life [30]. The CRADLE study was a milk-specific study showing the absence of the drug in breast milk and the absence of adverse events in children who were breastfed while their mothers were taking CTZ [31].

Regarding breastfeeding, it is possible to consider bDMARDs as a homogeneous class. They are all large proteins, which are unlikely excreted in breast milk due to their high molecular weight. But even if they were present in breast milk, bDMARDs will be degraded in the newborn's digestive tract with no chance for absorption (consider that bDMARDs are administered intravenously or subcutaneously, not orally) [29].

The exposure to immunosuppressive drugs, especially to bDMARDs, during late pregnancy poses the question about the immune competence of the neonate and the approach towards vaccinations. Data from large administrative US databases showed that children exposed during the third trimester to TNFi did not have an increased risk for serious infections during the first year of life [32]. The only concern about vaccinations is about live vaccines; it is recommended to postpone these vaccinations after 4–6 months after the last administration of drug during pregnancy.

35.5.3 Prophylactic Treatment with Low-Dose Aspirin (LDA) and Heparin

In patients with definite criteria for obstetric APS, combination treatment with LDA and heparin (at prophylactic or therapeutic dosage, based on individual risk stratification) is recommended to decrease the risk of adverse pregnancy outcomes [15] (see Figure 35.4). In refractory obstetric APS, data are few and not sufficient to show superiority of a therapeutic regimen over another one. Hydroxychloroquine, prednisolone 10 mg/day in the first trimester, intravenous immunoglobulin or plasma-exchange can be currently considered for refractory obstetric APS [15]. Strong evidence is also lacking for the management of asymptomatic women positive for aPL or in women not fulfilling clinical or laboratory criteria for APS; however, it is reasonable to assume that they will benefit from combination therapy if they have a high-risk profile. Women with a low-risk profile could be treated during pregnancy only with LDA (see Figure 35.4). In APS patients with previous thrombosis, vitamin K antagonist should be stopped before week 6 of gestation and therapeutic heparin should be started [15]. The management of these women during puerperium has been discussed above (see Section 35.4.1).

Patients with other ARDs at higher risk of pre-eclampsia (e.g. SLE with lupus nephritis) will benefit from LDA, preferably given pre-conceptionally or no later than week 16 of gestation [21].

35.6 Key Messages

- Reproductive issues are important topics in women with ARDs.
- Multidisciplinary pre-conception counselling, individual risk stratification and assessment are of fundamental importance to reduce pregnancy adverse outcomes in ARDs.
- It is crucial to maintain disease remission or treat disease flare-ups with drugs which are not harmful during pregnancy and lactation to pursue good pregnancy outcomes and well-being of the mother–child dyad.

  - Reproductive issues such as fertility, contraception, and family planning should be addressed in all women of childbearing age with ARDs.
  - Fertility in women with ARDs can be reduced as compared with healthy women of a similar age, but the causes are usually multifactorial. Women with ARDs can be candidate to ARTs, given individual risk stratification.
  - Risk assessment for maternal and/or fetal complications during pregnancy is essential for counselling each patient and tailor treatment.
  - Monitoring women with ARDs before, during and after pregnancy should be performed by a multidisciplinary team (rheumatologist, gynaecologist/obstetrician and neonatologist).
  - Treatment of patients with rheumatic disease before/during pregnancy and lactation should aim at preventing or suppressing maternal disease activity with drugs which are not harmful to the fetus/breastfed newborn.

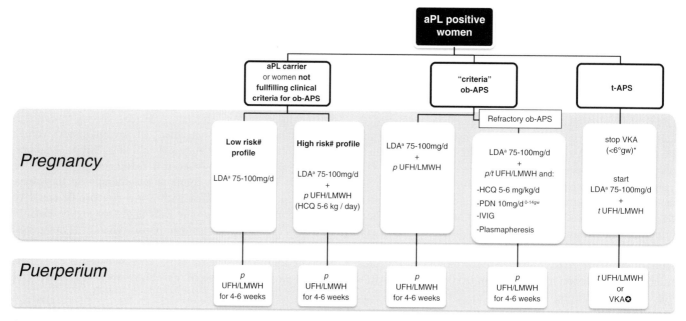

Figure 35.4 Proposed maternal management of antiphospholipid syndrome

aPL: antiphospholipid antibodies; APS: antiphospholipid syndrome; CAPS: catastrophic antiphospholipid syndrome; d: day; gw: gestational week; IVIG: intravenous immunoglobulins; ob-APS: obstetric-antiphospholipid syndrome; LDA: low-dose aspirin; LMWH: low molecular weight heparin; kg: kilogram; hr: hour; mg: milligram; p: prophylactic; PDN: prednisone; t: therapeutic; RTX: rituximab; t-APS: thrombotic APS; UFH: unfractionated heparin; U: units; VKA: vitamin K antagonists.

#'low-risk' profile (patients with isolated, intermittently positive aCLor aβ2GPI at low-medium titres); 'high-risk' aPLprofile: LA positivity, or 'triple positivity' – LA + aCL + aβ2GPI – or medium-high titres of IgG aCLor IgG aβ2GPI.

*Warfarin: teratogenic, specially between the 6th and 10th week of gestation; risk of fetal bleeding specially after the 12th week of gestation. During puerperium, it can be restarted after bridging therapy with heparin

a Depending on formulations of the drug available in different countries.

Note: LDA should be started prior to conception and stopped before delivery depending on the local protocol. Heparin should be started when pregnancy is confirmed (at positive pregnancy test or after ultrasound confirmation, depending on local protocols) and stopped before delivery depending on the type of heparin and delivery.

✪In pregnant women with APS and thrombocytopenia, a frequent APS non-criteria manifestation, the use of heparin, LDA, and VKA should be carefully evaluated due to the increased risk of bleeding. If thrombocytopenia is mild, above 50 x 10⁹/L, and no signs of bleeding, antithrombotic treatment can be continued. If platelet count is below 50 x 10⁹/L, the use of antithrombotic drugs should be weighed against the risk of clotting.

References

1. Østensen M. Sexual and reproductive health in rheumatic disease. *Nat Rev Rheumatol.* 2017;**13**:485–93.

2. Østensen M. Preconception counseling. *Rheum Dis Clin North Am.* 2017;**43**:189–99.

3. Andreoli L, Lazzaroni MG, Carini C, et al. 'Disease knowledge index' and perspectives on reproductive issues: a nationwide study on 398 women with autoimmune rheumatic diseases. *Joint Bone Spine.* 2019 Jul;**86**(4):475–81.

4. Clowse MEB, Eudy AM, Revels J, Neil L, Sanders GD. Provider perceptions on the management of lupus during pregnancy: barriers to improved care. *Lupus.* 2019 Jan;**28**(1):86–98. doi: 10.1177/0961203318815594

5. Eudy AM, McDaniel G, Hurd WW, Clowse MEB. Fertility and ovarian reserve among women with rheumatoid arthritis. *J Rheumatol.* 2019 May;**46**(5):455–9.

6. Reggia R, Andreoli L, Sebbar H, et al. An observational multicentre study on the efficacy and safety of assisted reproductive technologies in women with rheumatic diseases. *Rheumatol Adv Pract.* 2019;**3**(1):rkz005.

7. Nørgård BM, Larsen MD, Friedman S, Knudsen T, Fedder J. Decreased chance of a live born child in women with rheumatoid arthritis after assisted reproduction treatment: a nationwide cohort study. *Ann Rheum Dis.* 2019 Mar;**78**(3):328–34. doi: 10.1136/annrheumdis-2018-214619

8. Orquevaux P, Masseau A, Le Guern V, et al. In vitro fertilization in 37 women with systemic lupus erythematosus or antiphospholipid syndrome: a series of 97 procedures. *J Rheumatol.* 2017;**44**:613–18.

9. Jethwa H, Lam S, Smith C, Giles I. Does rheumatoid arthritis really improve during pregnancy? a systematic review and metaanalysis. *J Rheumatol.* 2019 Mar;**46**(3):245–50. doi: 10.3899/jrheum.180226

10. Lateef A, Petri M. Systemic lupus erythematosus and pregnancy. *Rheum Dis Clin North Am.* 2017; **43**:215–226.

11. Betelli M, Breda S, Ramoni V, et al. Pregnancy in systemic sclerosis. *J Scleroderma Relat Disord.* 2018;**3**:21–9.

12. Machen L, Clowse MEB. Vasculitis and pregnancy. *Rheum Dis Clin N Am.* 2017;**43**:239–47.

13. Clowse MEB, Eudy AM, Kiernan E, et al. The prevention, screening and treatment of congenital heart block from neonatal lupus: a survey of provider practices. *Rheumatology (Oxford).* 2018;**57**:v9-v17.

14. Brucato A, Tincani A, Fredi M, et al. Should we treat congenital heart block with fluorinated corticosteroids? *Autoimmun Rev.* 2017;**16**:1115–18.

15. Chighizola CB, Andreoli L, Gerosa M, et al. The treatment of anti-phospolipid syndrome; a comprehensive clinical approach. *J Autoimmun.* 2018; **90**:1–27.

16. Eudy AM, Jayasundara M, Haroun T, et al. Reasons for cesarean and medically indicated deliveries in pregnancies in women with systemic lupus erythematosus. *Lupus.* 2018;**27**:351–6.

17. Fredi M, Lazzaroni MG, Tani C, et al. Systemic vasculitis and pregnancy: a multicenter study on maternal and neonatal outcome of 65 prospectively followed pregnancies. *Autoimmun Rev.* 2015;**14**:686–91.

18. Clowse ME, Eudy AM, Revels J, Sanders GD, Criscione-Schreiber L. Rheumatologists' knowledge of contraception, teratogens, and pregnancy risks. *Obstet Med.* 2018;**11**:182–5.

19. Birru Talabi M, Clowse MEB, Blalock SJ, et al. Contraception use among reproductive-age women with rheumatic diseases. *Arthritis Care Res (Hoboken).* 2019 Aug;**71**(8):1132–40. 14. doi: 10.1002/acr.23724.

20. Sammaritano LR. Contraception in patients with rheumatic disease. *Rheum Dis Clin North Am.* 2017;**43**:173–88.

21. Andreoli L, Bertsias GK, Agmon-Levin N, et al. EULAR recommendations for women's health and the management of family planning, assisted reproduction, pregnancy and menopause in patients with systemic lupus erythematosus and/or antiphospholipid syndrome. *Ann Rheum Dis.* 2017;**76**:476–85.

22. Zbinden A, van den Brandt S, Østensen M, Villiger PM, Förger F. Risk for adverse pregnancy outcome in axial spondyloarthritis and rheumatoid arthritis: disease activity matters. *Rheumatology (Oxford).* 2018 Jul1;**57** (7):1235–42. doi: 10.1093/ rheumatology/key053

23. Smith CJF, Förger F, Bandoli G, Chambers CD. Factors associated with preterm delivery among women with rheumatoid arthritis and juvenile idiopathic arthritis. *Arthritis Care Res (Hoboken).* 2019 Aug;**71**(8):1019–27. doi: 10.1002/acr.23730.

24. Flint J, Panchal S, Hurrell A, et al. BSR and BHPR guideline on prescribing drugs in pregnancy and breastfeeding – Part I: standard and biologic disease modifying anti-rheumatic drugs and corticosteroids. *Rheumatology (Oxford).* 2016;**55**:1693–702.

25. Flint J, Panchal S, Hurrell A, et al. BSR and BHPR guideline on prescribing drugs in pregnancy and breastfeeding – Part II: analgesics and other drugs used in rheumatology practice. *Rheumatology (Oxford).* 2016;**55**:1698–702.

26. Skorpen CG, Hoeltzenbein M, Tincani A, et al. The EULAR points to consider for use of antirheumatic drugs before pregnancy, and during pregnancy and lactation. *Ann Rheum Dis.* 2016;**75**:795–810.

27. Andreoli L, Crisafulli F, Tincani A. Pregnancy and reproductive aspects of systemic lupus erythematosus. *Curr Opin Rheumatol.* 2017;**29**:473–9.

28. van den Brandt S, Zbinden A, Baeten D, et al. Risk factors for flare and treatment of disease flares during pregnancy in rheumatoid arthritis and axial spondyloarthritis patients. *Arthritis Res Ther.* 2017;**19**:64.

29. Østensen M. The use of biologics in pregnant patients with rheumatic disease. *Expert Rev Clin Pharmacol.* 2017;**10**:661–9.

30. Mariette X, Förger F, Abraham B, et al. Lack of placental transfer of certolizumab pegol during pregnancy: results from CRIB, a prospective, postmarketing, pharmacokinetic study. *Ann Rheum Dis.* 2018;**77**: 228–33.

31. Clowse ME, Förger F, Hwang C, et al. Minimal to no transfer of certolizumab pegol into breast milk: results from CRADLE, a prospective, postmarketing, multicentre, pharmacokinetic study. *Ann Rheum Dis.* 2017;**76**:1890–6.

32. Vinet É, De Moura C, Pineau CA, et al. Serious infections in rheumatoid arthritis offspring exposed to tumor necrosis factor inhibitors: a cohort study. *Arthritis Rheumatol.* 2018;**70**:1565–71.

Chapter 36

Thyroid Disease in Pregnancy

Anastasios Malakasis & Francoise H. Harlow

36.1 Introduction

Thyroid disease is a common finding in the female population. The prevalence of hypothyroidism is 1–2 per 100 women and the prevalence of hyperthyroidism is between 5 and 20 per 1000 women in iodine-replete communities [1]. These numbers may be higher in areas with iodine insufficiency. Thyroid disease is 10-fold higher in the female population in comparison to the male [1]. Considering the high prevalence in the female population, we understand that thyroid disease is very common in pregnant women, with the overall rate of overt thyroid dysfunction being as high as 1% of all pregnancies [2]. In this chapter, we will review the physiology in pregnancy, the normal adaptations of the thyroid gland and hormones and will mention the challenges in thyroid function tests in pregnancy. Furthermore, we will also concentrate on the impact of hypothyroidism and hyperthyroidism on pregnancy, and the diagnosis and management of both. We will also briefly overview postpartum thyroiditis and thyroid cancer in pregnancy.

36.2 Thyroid Physiology in Pregnancy

36.2.1 Brief Overview of Normal Thyroid Physiology

The iodination of tyrosine residues in thyroglobulin that takes place in the thyroid gland results in the formation of mono-iodotyrosine and di-iodotyrosine. These molecules are coupled to form thyroid hormones T3 and T4. The majority of released hormone from the thyroid gland is T4, which then is converted to T3 in peripheral tissues. Both T4 and T3 are bound to carrier proteins in the serum, predominantly the serum thyroxine-binding globulin (TBG). Other carrier proteins are thyroxine-binding pre-albumin or transthyretin and albumin [3]. The unbound component of thyroid hormones, FT3 (free T3) and FT4 (free T4), is the physiologically active element that can be transported to the target cells and exert the hormonal activity. The unbound FT4 represents only 0.04% of the total T4.

The main regulator of thyroid stimulation is the thyroid-stimulating hormone (TSH). TSH is produced in the anterior pituitary gland and its synthesis is influenced by thyrotropin-releasing hormone (TRH), which is produced in the hypothalamus and also by the circulating thyroid hormone via a negative feedback mechanism [4].

Low levels of serum thyroid hormone stimulate the synthesis of TRH in the hypothalamus, which, in turn, stimulates TSH production, resulting in increased levels of serum thyroid hormones. Conversely, high levels of serum hormones suppress the axis with the aim of decreasing the levels.

Thyroid hormones target every organ in the human body, leading to an increase in basal metabolic rate. They bind to intracellular receptors in mitochondria causing an increase in adenosine triphosphate (ATP) production, leading to temperature increase. In the heart, they cause an increase in heart rate, and in the gastrointestinal tract, they cause increase in motility. In addition, thyroid hormones are important for neurological development and also increase the sympathetic tone in the body [5].

36.2.2 Changes of Thyroid Physiology in Pregnancy

Pregnancy is associated with significant reversible changes that affect thyroid physiology. The most important changes and their effects are the following:

a) Elevation of beta-hCG in the first trimester, which results in an increase in FT3 and FT4 and a subsequent decrease in TSH. This happens because TSH and beta-hCG have structural homology and the latter has weak thyroid-stimulating activity [6].

b) Increase in serum TBG because of high oestrogen levels in pregnancy, which provokes an increase in serum T3 and T4. TBG increases rapidly at the beginning of pregnancy, and by 20 weeks it has doubled. As a consequence, and in order to maintain the pool of unbound free thyroid hormones, serum T3 and T4 are rapidly increased.

c) Increased plasma volume results in increasing T4 and T3 pool size so that FT3 and FT4 are maintained unchanged.

d) Increased renal clearance results in increased iodine clearance. That makes necessary the adequate iodine supplementation and, if iodine is insufficient, poses the risk of maternal hypothyroidism and goitre [7].

e) Transfer of iodine to the fetus, also makes necessary the sufficient storage of iodine in maternal body.

f) Placental de-iodination of T4 and T3 increases the metabolism rate of T4 and T3 and increases the need of their production [8] (Table 36.1).

36.2.3 Iodine Intake and Supplementation in Pregnancy

Iodine is an important component, essential for the production of thyroid hormones. As already mentioned, the increase in

Table 36.1 Physiological changes and thyroid consequences in pregnancy

Physiological change	Thyroid-related result
hCG increases	FT3 and FT4 increases – TSH decreases
TBG increases	Total T3 and T4 increase
Plasma volume increases	T3 and T4 pool size increases
Renal clearance increases	Increased iodine clearance – Need for adequate iodine intake in pregnancy
Fetal need for iodine	Need for adequate iodine intake in pregnancy
Placental de-iodination of T3 and T4	Increased need for T3 and T4

renal glomerular filtration rate, the fetal needs for iodine and the increased thyroid hormones production in pregnancy make adequate iodine intake paramount. In iodine-replete communities, women with adequate intake have no problem in adapting to pregnancy changes. In those women, total iodine levels remain stable throughout pregnancy [9]. Conversely, in areas of iodine deficiency the thyroid iodine stores are decreased in pregnancy. The consequences of iodine deprivation in pregnancy are very serious. Severe iodine deficiency is associated with increased pregnancy loss, stillbirth and increased perinatal mortality [10]. It is also related to adverse effects on the cognitive function of the offspring due to lack of thyroid hormones. The use of iodized salt has significantly reduced iodine deficiency, but there are still 30 countries which are considered iodine-deficient areas. In addition, many countries that are considered iodine-replete have recorded iodine deficiency in pregnant women. The World Health Organization (WHO) recommends that daily intake of iodine should be 250 μg for a pregnant or breastfeeding woman [11], achieved by either diet or supplementation or both. It is also very difficult to identify the iodine status of a pregnant woman. Considering that iodine supplementation improves outcome in mild, moderate and severe iodine deficiency, recent guidelines recommend that women who are planning pregnancy or are pregnant should supplement their diet with a daily oral supplement that contains 150 μg of iodine in the form of potassium iodide [12]. Conversely, daily intake greater than 500 μg should be avoided in pregnancy, but this is highly unlikely with a controlled diet and supplementation.

36.2.4 Thyroid Function Testing in Pregnancy

Thyroid function test (TFT) levels change in pregnancy because of the changes in a woman's physiology. Therefore, TFT levels in a healthy pregnancy are significantly different from those in a non-pregnant woman. During pregnancy, TSH levels shift downwards, with the largest decrease happening in

the first trimester due to an increase in serum hCG. At second and third trimester, the decrease is smaller but TSH is still below the reference range of a non-pregnant woman. Older studies first led to recommendations for a TSH upper reference limit of 2.5 mU/L in the first trimester and 3.0 mU/L in the second and third trimesters [13]. However, more recent studies in pregnant women have demonstrated only a modest reduction in the upper reference limit. Considering this, it is important when possible to use population-based trimester-specific reference ranges for serum TSH.

In addition, FT4 measurement in pregnancy is difficult due to technical problems with the methods in current use, mainly due to the increase of TBG in pregnancy. These challenges in measurement of FT4 make it important to use method- and trimester-specific reference ranges when measured.

An alternative and more reliable test of thyroid hormones is the measurement of total T4 (TT4), but this test is more valid in the second half of pregnancy and does not provide accuracy at early gestation.

Another reliable test in pregnancy is the FT4 index, which takes into consideration the changes in TBG. We understand that there are specific challenges with TFTs in pregnancy, so we should be very careful in how we interpret these tests in pregnancy.

36.3 Thyroid Dysfunction and Pregnancy

36.3.1 Hypothyroidism in Pregnancy

36.3.1.1 Overt Hypothyroidism

Overt hypothyroidism is defined by elevated TSH and decreased FT4, both outside the reference range or TSH above 10 mIU/L. The most common causes of overt hypothyroidism are Hashimoto's thyroiditis and iatrogenic intervention (surgery, radioactive treatment) for treatment of hyperthyroidism, goitre or cancer [14]. Overt hypothyroidism is associated with significant adverse outcomes in pregnancy. The most serious risks are premature birth, low birthweight, pregnancy loss and lower offspring IQ [15]. Women who are planning pregnancy should optimize TSH before conception due to the risks already mentioned. Pregnant women with overt hypothyroidism should be treated [16]. Treatment is in the form of oral levothyroxine (LT4). Women who are already on treatment for hypothyroidism should adjust their dose of LT4. After conception, an adjustment to the dose is recommended as soon as possible. The dose should be increased by 20–30%, and an easy approach is to increase the previously taken 7 tablets a week to 9 tablets. The monitoring of TSH should be every 4 weeks until mid-gestation and then at least once near 30 weeks or every 6–8 weeks after mid-gestation [17]. The goal of treatment is to maintain TSH in the lower half of the trimester's specific range. If there is no trimester-specific range, then a goal of TSH below 2.5 mU/L is optimal. Every time the dose is adjusted, TSH should be measured 4 weeks after adjustment. After delivery, the LT4 dose should return to the pre-conception dose, as the needs of pregnancy cease and thyroid function should be checked 4–6 weeks postpartum

Table 36.2 Differences in guidance for treatment of hypothyroidism between ATA and ETA

	ATA (American Thyroid Association)	ETA (European Thyroid Association)
Overt hypothyroidism	Treatment	Treatment
Subclinical hypothyroidism	1. TSH above 10 – treatment 2. TSH > reference range and TPO-Ab positive – treatment 3. TSH >2.5 and <reference range (or 4) and TPO-Ab positive – consider treatment 4. TSH > reference range (or 4) and <10 – consider treatment 5. TSH <4 and TPO-Ab negative – No treatment	Treatment
Isolated hypothyroxinemia	No treatment	Treatment in first trimester

[18]. In pregnant women with adequate treatment, there is no need for extra fetal monitoring with serial scans.

36.3.1.2 Subclinical Hypothyroidism

Subclinical hypothyroidism (SCH) is defined by elevated levels of TSH – between 2.5 and 10 mU/L – with normal levels of thyroxine. It is a condition that it is associated with adverse outcomes in pregnancy as pregnancy loss, preterm delivery, pre-eclampsia and placental abruption [19]. The association of subclinical hypothyroidism with cognitive problems of the offspring still remains controversial.

Treatment of SCH still remains debatable, and so we will analyze the two main schools of management.

According to the recent guidelines by the American Thyroid Association (ATA, 2017) women with SCH should also be checked for thyroid peroxidase antibodies (TPO-Ab), as many studies have found that the risk is higher in TPO-Ab-positive women [20]. After this test, the treatment should be as follows:

a) LT4 should be started in all women with TSH above 10mU/L.

b) LT4 should be started in TPO-Ab-positive women with TSH above the pregnancy-specific reference range.

c) LT4 should be considered in TPO-Ab-positive women with TSH between 2.5 mU/L and below the upper limit of the pregnancy-specific reference range (if unavailable, use TSH of 4 mU/L)

d) LT4 should be considered in all woman irrespective of the antibodies status with TSH above the pregnancy-specific reference range and below 10 mU/L.

e) LT4 is not recommended in women who are TPO-Ab negative and have TSH within the pregnancy reference range or TSH below 4 mU/L.

Conversely, the European Thyroid Association (ETA) recommends that all women with subclinical hypothyroidism should be treated with oral levothyroxine.

The starting dose in newly diagnosed SCH in pregnancy should be 1.2 mcg/kg/day and the goal should be a TSH level below 2.5 mU/L. Thyroid function should be checked every 4 weeks in the first trimester and then once in the second and third trimesters. Following delivery, the levothyroxine dose should be reduced to the pre-conception dose. Women diagnosed with SCH during pregnancy with TSH less than 5 mU/L and negative TPO-Ab could stop levothyroxine after delivery and have their thyroid function checked 6 weeks after delivery. Women diagnosed with SCH during pregnancy should be re-evaluated 6 months and 1 year after delivery to ascertain the continuing requirement for levothyroxine. Subclinical hypothyroidism in pregnancy when appropriately managed is not an indication for additional obstetric surveillance.

36.3.1.3 Isolated Hypothyroxinaemia

Isolated hypothyroxinaemia (IH) is characterized by normal TSH but low FT4 levels (either below the reference range or between the 2.5th and 10th centile of the normal pregnant population) [21]. The studies so far give conflicting results in terms of the association of IH and adverse pregnancy outcomes. Overall, available evidence appears to show an association between hypothyroxinaemia and effects on cognitive development of the offspring, with uncertain effects on prematurity and low birthweight. At the moment, there is no study to show that treatment of IH with oral levothyroxine prevents any of these adverse outcomes. That is why there are conflicting recommendations between different associations. The ATA recommends no treatment of IH in pregnancy; the ETA recommends treatment in the first trimester but not in the second and third trimesters (Table 36.2).

36.4 Hyperthyroidism in Pregnancy

36.4.1 Introduction

Overt thyrotoxicosis in pregnancy occurs in 0.2–0.4% of population. It is characterized by suppressed TSH levels and elevated FT4, both outside the pregnancy reference range. Causes of thyrotoxicosis include common ones that are found in the general population and some pregnancy-specific causes [22]. The commonest cause is Graves' disease (GD) with a prevalence of 0.2% during pregnancy. Less common, non-pregnancy-specific causes include toxic adenoma and toxic multinodular goitre, as well as rarer conditions such as pituitary adenoma, struma ovarii and thyroid cancer metastases. Conversely, the most common pregnancy-specific cause of thyrotoxicosis is gestational transient thyrotoxicosis, which is diagnosed in about 1–3% of pregnancies. Other conditions associated with hCG-induced thyrotoxicosis include multiple gestation, hydatidiform mole and choriocarcinoma [23].

36.4.2 Graves' Disease

36.4.2.1 Pre-pregnancy Counselling

Several studies have shown that maternal hyperthyroidism is associated with adverse outcomes in pregnancy, such as pregnancy loss, pregnancy-induced hypertension, prematurity, low birthweight, intrauterine growth restriction, stillbirth, thyroid storm and maternal congestive heart failure [24]. It is very important that women with Graves' disease who are thinking of becoming pregnant be informed appropriately about the risks of hyperthyroidism in pregnancy and the options of treatment before pregnancy. It is paramount to become euthyroid before pregnancy; this means having two sets of normal TFTs 1 month apart without a change in the treatment. Until this euthyroid state is achieved, the pregnancy should be postponed, and contraception is highly recommended. The treatment options include the following and the advantages and disadvantages for the future pregnancy are highlighted:

a) Surgical management (thyroidectomy). This is a definite treatment and the euthyroid state can be easily achieved with oral levothyroxine soon after the operation. On the other hand, surgical complications can occur and need for lifelong levothyroxine is mandatory.

b) Radioactive iodine. It is relatively easy, as oral administration is used and future relapse is rare. In terms of future pregnancy, there are some disadvantages. After treatment, TSH receptor antibody (TRAb) levels are increased, so pregnancy should be avoided for at least 6 months after treatment even if euthyroid status is achieved. In addition, some patients who undergo ablative treatment do not become euthyroid for almost a year, which delays the pregnancy even longer. It is also a treatment that is not allowed in pregnancy. In addition, the use of levothyroxine will be needed for the rest of the woman's life.

c) Antithyroid drugs (ATD). These include propylthiouracil (PTU) and carbimazole (CBZ), which is a prodrug of methimazole (MMI). It is an easy and inexpensive treatment, and euthyroid status is easily achieved in 1–2 months. Women who opt for ATD should be informed of its disadvantages. Both drugs are associated with birth defects. Specifically, MMI is associated with aplasia cutis and other defects such as choanal or oesophageal atresia, various types of abdominal wall defects and ventricular septal defects [25]. On the other hand, PTU was previously considered a safe medication but a recent study from Denmark showed that 2–3% of children exposed to PTU developed birth defects (face and neck cysts) associated with this therapy [26]. These are considered less severe than those associated with MMI exposure. In addition, one of

the major risks of treatment with PTU is hepatotoxicity and it is considered the third most frequent cause of drug-induced liver transplantation in the USA.

A woman who has hyperthyroidism and wants to become pregnant should have appropriate counselling by a doctor with expertise in management of this condition in pregnancy.

36.4.2.2 Management of Graves' Disease in Pregnancy

The management of GD in pregnancy is complicated and very important for the mother and the fetus.

In pregnant women who are euthyroid and are on low doses of ATD, that is, MMI <5–10 mg/d or PTU <100–200 mg/d, discontinuation of treatment may be considered in pregnancy in view of teratogenic effects. Of note, this is not an easy decision and should take into account the disease history, goitre size, duration of therapy, results of recent thyroid function tests and TRAb measurement. If discontinuation is decided, then TFTs should be done every 1–2 weeks in the beginning, and if mother remains euthyroid and clinically stable, then every 2–4 weeks.

In pregnant women with a high risk of thyrotoxicosis (e.g. women who are hyperthyroid or receive high doses of ATDs), then PTU is recommended until 16 weeks, so if she is receiving MMI this should be changed to PTU. After the first trimester, it is still controversial to switch to MMI, again due to PTU hepatotoxicity, as recent studies have shown no advantage for that change. Pregnant women should have their TFTs checked regularly about every 3–4 weeks whilst on PTU treatment [27].

It is very important in pregnant women with overt hyperthyroidism or history of hyperthyroidism to appropriately measure TRAb. TRAb is known to cross the placenta and can stimulate fetal thyroid when present in high concentrations. Features suggestive of fetal thyroid dysfunction include goitre, growth restriction, hydrops, tachycardia and heart failure [28]. If the patient has a history of previously treated GD (radioactive ablation or surgery) but currently is not on treatment, an early pregnancy serum TRAb concentration should be checked. If it is low or undetectable, no further testing is needed. If it is elevated, TRAb should be checked at each trimester. If a mother is on treatment in pregnancy, then TRAb should be checked in each trimester. A value of >5 IU/L or 3 times the upper limit of normal in the mother indicates that the fetal thyroid may be strongly stimulated by TRAb passing through the placenta and that triggers the need for neonatal monitoring. If fetal hyperthyroidism is present and is thought to endanger the pregnancy, ATD should be given to the mother to suppress the fetal thyroid. This represents the only potential indication for concomitant use of ATD and levothyroxine ('block and replace' regime) in pregnancy.

Serial ultrasound scans should be performed in women with hyperthyroidism and high levels of TRAb in pregnancy to assess the growth, the fetal heart rate, the anatomy and the presence of goitre (rare finding).

36.4.3 Gestational Transient Hyperthyroidism and Subclinical Hyperthyroidism

36.4.3.1 Gestational Transient Hyperthyroidism

Gestational transient hyperthyroidism (GTH) is defined by suppressed TSH and elevated FT4 in the first half of pregnancy but without any clinical or antibody evidence of thyroid autoimmunity. A TRAb check that is negative in gestational transient thyrotoxicosis is helpful to clarify the cause of thyrotoxicosis. In addition, FT3 is rarely elevated. It complicates 0.5–10 per 1000 pregnancies. It is commonly associated with hyperemesis gravidarum and high levels of hCG. The majority of patients with GTH do not require any antithyroid treatment. In women with hyperemesis gravidarum, symptomatic treatment is required with intravenous fluid and control of vomiting. In some cases, hospitalization is required. In patients with GTH, thyroid function normalizes by the second trimester when hCG levels stabilize. Obstetric outcome is not improved by the use of ATD [29]. In rare cases in which the woman is clinically symptomatic of hyperthyroidism, small amounts of beta-blockers for a short period of time may be considered.

36.4.3.2 Subclinical Hyperthyroidism

Subclinical hyperthyroidism is defined by suppressed levels of TSH but normal FT4 and FT3. It is not associated with any pregnancy or neonatal adverse outcome. Most often, it is considered a normal variant (due to high hCG levels) or it is attributed to non-thyroidal illness. Treatment should be definitely avoided [30].

36.5 Postpartum Thyroiditis

Postpartum thyroiditis (PPT) is a condition related to the changes in the immune system of the woman that take place after delivery. The Th2 (T-helper 2) immune status that is dominant in pregnancy and is characterized by cytokines such as IL4 abruptly reverts back to the non-pregnant Th1 (T-helper 1) status. The consequences of that shift are that antithyroid peroxidase antibodies (anti-TPO-Ab), which are found in 10% of pregnant women and are decreased at second and third trimester, rebound after delivery and reach a maximum between 3 and 6 months postpartum ('immune rebound phenomenon').The prevalence of postpartum thyroiditis varies from 1% to 17% and is more common in women with type 1 diabetes, a family history of hypothyroidism and in euthyroid pregnant women with TPO-Ab positivity. The classical pattern of postpartum thyroiditis is characterized by transient thyrotoxicosis followed by transient or, in 5% of cases, permanent hypothyroidism, before a return to a euthyroid state, usually within the 12-month postpartum period [31]. Permanent hypothyroidism is reported in as many as 30% of these cases after 3 years, and in 50% at 7–10 years .

The diagnosis of PPT is clinical and biochemical. The hyperthyroid phase most of the time passes undetected but occasionally the symptoms can be severe enough to interfere with the mother's functioning due to sleep deprivation, nervousness and irritability or palpitations. The biochemical findings are suppressed TSH together with an elevated FT4 or FT3. The hyperthyroid phase of PPT should be distinguished by postpartum Graves' disease where TRAb levels are high and the clinical symptoms more profound. The hypothyroid phase in the postpartum period is diagnosed when either TSH is >3.6 mU/L together with FT4 <8 pmol/L or FT3 <4.2 pmol/L or TSH higher than 10mU/L on one or more occasions. The most frequent symptoms have been found to be lack of energy, aches and pains, poor memory, dry skin and cold intolerance. There are some studies that show association of PPT with postpartum depression, so all patients with postpartum depression should be checked for thyroid dysfunction.

In regards to the management of PPT, if there are severe symptoms during the hyperthyroid phase, propranolol should be considered but antithyroid drugs are not indicated as the condition is a destructive thyroiditis.

In terms of the hypothyroid phase, close monitoring of TFTs is really important for patient management. If hypothyroidism develops, then treatment with levothyroxine is only indicated if this is persistent or symptomatic or the woman plans a pregnancy in the near future. If the FT4 is low but slowly rising and the patient is asymptomatic, then no treatment is required. It is recommended that women with postpartum thyroiditis be monitored with annual TSH and FT4 measurements, as 50% will develop permanent hypothyroidism in the first 7 years. In addition, TFTs should be checked in the postpartum period of future pregnancies, given the high risk of recurrence which is up to 70% [32].

36.6 Thyroid Nodules and Thyroid Cancer and Pregnancy

The management of thyroid nodules and thyroid cancer in pregnancy is challenging for clinicians. There are limited studies regarding the prevalence of thyroid nodules in pregnancy and the effect of pregnancy on them. According to these, the prevalence varies between 3% and 21% and there is an increase in nodular volume during pregnancy [33]. In addition, the prevalence of thyroid cancer in pregnancy is 14.4 per 100 000 pregnancies [34].

The investigation of thyroid nodules in pregnancy should comprise a detailed medical history and clinical examination, as well as TSH measurement and ultrasound imaging. Fine needle aspiration (FNA) of the nodule can be performed in every trimester without any adverse outcome in pregnancy and should be decided according to the nodules' characteristics and based on the established guidelines for non-pregnant patients. Radionuclide scan is contraindicated in pregnancy. All cytologically benign nodules should be monitored as in non-pregnant patients. The cytologically indeterminate nodules without any signs of metastatic disease can also be monitored and operated on after pregnancy.

All studies agree that pregnancy does not alter the prognosis of women diagnosed with differentiated thyroid cancer

Table 36.3 A summary of thyroid disorders and their management during pregnancy

Hypothyroidism	• Overt hypothyroidism needs treatment with LT4 • Some clinicians increase LT4 during pregnancy routinely • Treatment of subclinical hypothyroidism is controversial in view of TSH limits • TSH monitoring on treatment
Hyperthyroidism	• Pre-pregnancy counselling for Graves' disease is crucial and euthyroid status is paramount • Teratogenicity of antithyroid drugs – propylthiouracil is preferred in 1st trimester • TRAB or thyroid-stimulating antibodies (TSA) check and TFTs monitoring • Gestational hyperthyroidism is related to hyperemesis gravidarum and no treatment is needed
Postpartum thyroiditis	• Transient hyperthyroidism followed by transient hypothyroidism • Risk of permanent hypothyroidism • Annual TFTs
Thyroid nodules and cancer	• FNA is safe in all trimesters • If surgery is needed better to be done at 2nd trimester • Pregnancy does not alter the prognosis of DTC • TSH suppression is required (<0.1 in high-risk patients) • Ultrasound and Tg monitoring should be performed during pregnancy in women diagnosed with well-differentiated thyroid cancer and a biochemically or structurally incomplete response to therapy, or in patients known to have active recurrent or residual disease

(DTC). In addition, the timing of surgery, either during pregnancy or after delivery, does not change the survival prognosis. The impact of pregnancy on women with medullary or anaplastic carcinoma is unknown.

Surgery is the treatment of choice for DTC and can safely be deferred until the postpartum period if it is not at advanced stage. If surgery is to be done during pregnancy, the second trimester is the optimal period for the operation. However, delaying operating on medullary or anaplastic carcinoma probably has adverse outcome, so surgery should be strongly considered during pregnancy.

Pregnant women with previous diagnosis and treatment for DTC should maintain pre-conception established TSH suppression. For high-risk patients, the limit of TSH suppression is 0.1 and below and in low-risk patients it should be at the lower half of the reference range. TSH should be monitored approximately every 4 weeks until 16–20 weeks of gestation, and at least once between 26 and 32 weeks of gestation. In addition, women with incomplete response to therapy or active recurrent or residual disease should have ultrasound and thyroglobulin (Tg) monitoring during pregnancy. In previously treated DTC and in the absence of Tg antibodies, there is no need for ultrasound and Tg monitoring in pregnancy. Table 36.3 provides a summary of thyroid disorders and their management during pregnancy.

References

1. Vanderpump MPJ. The epidemiology of thyroid disease. *Br Med Bull.* 2011;**99**:39–51.

2. Klein RZ, Haddow JE, Faix JD, et al. Prevalence of thyroid deficiency in pregnant women. *Clin Endocrinol (Oxford).* 1991;**35**:41–6.

3. Schussler GC. The thyroxine-binding proteins. *Thyroid.* 2000;**10**(2):141–9.

4. Stathatos N. Thyroid physiology. *Med Clin North Am.* 2012 Mar;**96**(2):165–73.

5. Shahid MA, Sharma S. Physiology, thyroid hormone. In StatPearls Internet. Treasure Island, FL: StatPearls Publishing; 2018 Jan–. Updated 2018 Oct 27.

6. Hershman JM. Physiological and pathological aspects of the effect of human chorionic gonadotropin on the thyroid. *Best Pract Res Clin Endocrinol Metab.* 2004;**18**:249-65.

7. Powrie RO, Greene MF, Camman W. *De Swiet's Medical Disorders in Obstetric Practice,* 5th ed. London: Wiley-Blackwell; 2010. pp. 322–34

8. Lazarus J. Thyroid regulation and dysfunction in the pregnant patient. In De Groot LJ, Chrousos G, Dungan K, et al., eds. *Endotext Internet.* South Dartmouth, MA: MDText.com, Inc.; 2000–. Updated 2016 Jul 21.

9. Liberman CS, Pino SC, Fang SL, Braverman LE, Emerson CH. Circulating iodide concentrations during and after pregnancy. *J Clin Endocrinol Metab.* 1998;**83**:3545–9.

10. Delange FM, Dunn JT. Iodine deficiency. In Braverman LE, Utiger RD, eds. *Werner and Ingbar's The Thyroid: A Fundamental and Clinical Text,* 9th ed. Philadelphia: Lippincott, Williams and Wilkins; 2005. pp 264–88.

11. World Health Organization/International Council for the Control of the Iodine Deficiency Disorders/United Nations Children's Fund (WHO/ICCIDD/UNICEF) *Assessment of the Iodine Deficiency Disorders and Monitoring Their Elimination.* Geneva: World Health Organization;2007.

12. Alexander EK, Pearce EN, Brent GA, et al. Guidelines of the American Thyroid Association for the diagnosis and management of thyroid disease during pregnancy and the postpartum. *Thyroid.* 2017 Mar;**27**(3):315–89.

13. Stagnaro-Green A, Abalovich M, Alexander E, et al., American Thyroid Association Taskforce on Thyroid

Disease During Pregnancy and Postpartum. Guidelines of the American Thyroid Association for the diagnosis and management of thyroid disease during pregnancy and postpartum. *Thyroid.* 2011;**21**:1081–1125.

14. Tingi E, Syed AA, Kyriacou A, Mastorakos G, Kyriacou A. Benign thyroid disease in pregnancy: a state of the art review. *J Clin Transl Endocrinol.* 2016;**6**:37–49.

15. van den Boogaard E, Vissenberg R, Land JA, et al. Significance of (sub) clinical thyroid dysfunction and thyroid autoimmunity before conception and in early pregnancy: a systematic review. *Hum Reprod Update.*2011;**17**:605–19.

16. Smith A, Eccles-Smith J, D'Emden M, Lust K. Thyroid disorders in pregnancy and postpartum. *Aust Prescr.* 2017;**40** (6):214–19.

17. Lazarus J, Brown RS, Daumerie C, et al. European Thyroid Association guidelines for the management of subclinical hypothyroidism in pregnancy and in children. *Eur Thyroid J.* 2014;**3**:76–94.

18. Yassa L, Marqusee E, Fawcett R, Alexander EK. Thyroid hormone early adjustment in pregnancy (the THERAPY) trial. *J Clin Endocrinol Metab.* 2010;**95**:3234–41.

19. Chan S, Boelaert K. Optimal management of hypothyroidism, hypothyroxinaemia and euthyroid TPO antibody positivity preconception and in pregnancy. *Clin. Endocrinol (Oxford).* 2015;**82**:313–26.

20. Liu H, Shan Z, Li C, et al. Maternal subclinical hypothyroidism, thyroid autoimmunity, and the risk of miscarriage: a prospective cohort study. *Thyroid.* 2014;**24**:1642–9.

21. Moleti M, Trimarchi F, Vermiglio F. Doubts and concerns about isolated maternal hypothyroxinemia. *J Thyroid Res.* 2011;**2011**:463029.

22. Marx H, Amin P, Lazarus JH. Hyperthyroidism and pregnancy. *Brit Med J.* 2008;**336**:663–7.

23. Hershman JM. Human chorionic gonadotropin and the thyroid: hyperemesis gravidarum and trophoblastic tumors. *Thyroid.* 1999;**9**:653–7.

24. Davis LE, Lucas MJ, Hankins GD, Roark ML, Cunningham FG. Thyrotoxicosis complicating pregnancy. *Am J Obstet Gynecol.* 1989;**160**:63–70.

25. Yoshihara A, Noh J, Yamaguchi T, et al. Treatment of Graves' disease with antithyroid drugs in the first trimester of pregnancy and the prevalence of congenital malformation. *J Clin Endocrinol Metab.* 2012;**97**: 2396–2403.

26. Andersen SL, Olsen J, Wu CS, Laurberg P. Birth defects after early pregnancy use of antithyroid drugs: a Danish nationwide study. *J Clin Endocrinol Metab.* 2013;**98**:4373–81.

27. Patil-Sisodia K, Mestman JH. Graves hyperthyroidism and pregnancy: a clinical update. *Endocr Pract.* 2010;**16**:118–29.

28. Alamdari S, Azizi F, Delshad H, et al. Management of hyperthyroidism in pregnancy: comparison of recommendations of american thyroid association and endocrine society. *J Thyroid Res.* 2013;**2013**:878467.

29. Bouillon R, Naesens M, Van Assche FA, et al. Thyroid function in patients with hyperemesis gravidarum. *Am J Obstet Gynecol.* 1982;**143**:922–6.

30. Ross DS, Burch HB, Cooper DS, et al. American Thyroid Association guidelines for diagnosis and management of hyperthyroidism and other causes of thyrotoxicosis. *Thyroid.* 2016;**26**:1343–421.

31. Muller AF, Drexhage HA, Berghout A. Postpartum thyroiditis and autoimmune thyroiditis in women of childbearing age: recent insights and consequences for antenatal and postnatal care. *Endocr Rev.* 2001;**22**:605–30.

32. Nicholson WK, Robinson KA, Smallridge RC, Ladenson PW, Powe NR. Prevalence of postpartum thyroid dysfunction: a quantitative review. *Thyroid.* 2006;**16**:573–82.

33. Kung AW, Chau MT, Lao TT, Tam SC, Low LC. The effect of pregnancy on thyroid nodule formation. *J Clin Endocrinol Metab.* 2002;**87**:1010–14.

34. Smith LH, Danielsen B, Allen ME, Cress R. Cancer associated with obstetric delivery: results of linkage with the California cancer registry. *Am J Obstet Gynecol.* 2003;**189**:1128–35.

Chapter 37

Infections in Pregnancy

Sarah McRobbie

37.1 Introduction

It is important to recognize and treat infection appropriately, as sepsis is a leading cause of maternal mortality and still features highly in reports [1]. Consideration should be given to recent suggested measures that may have significant positive impact including early recognition of an unwell woman's clinical condition regardless of her vital signs to instigate timely treatment. Additionally, all pregnant women should be offered the influenza immunization as part of antenatal care [1].

37.2 Sepsis Six

Sepsis is 'a life-threatening condition defined as organ dysfunction resulting from infection during pregnancy, childbirth, post-abortion, or postpartum period' [2]. One of the major recent impacts on improvement in maternal morbidity and mortality is the introduction of 'Sepsis Six' [3]. The key features of this campaign include consideration, early recognition and management of likely sepsis, treating with the most appropriate antibiotics and giving intravenous (IV) fluids within 1 hour of recognition, ensuring bloods including lactate and blood cultures are taken, arterial blood gases (ABG) +/– oxygen and hourly urine output monitoring. In addition to the 'Sepsis Six', other factors that need to be considered include early senior input/expert help [1] and early involvement and discussion with Microbiology, especially where a woman fails to respond to initial management. Regular review is vital to assess whether there has been improvement or deterioration.

37.3 Overview of Infection in Pregnancy

It is important to remember that many infections encountered in pregnancy often have little effect on maternal health and may result in minimal or no maternal symptoms unless the mother is immunocompromised. Moreover, incidental findings may be seen at ultrasound including echogenic bowel, intracranial calcification or intrauterine growth restriction (IUGR); infection will be in the differential diagnosis. In addition, following an intrauterine death (IUD), women are screened for infections including toxoplasmosis, parvovirus and cytomegalovirus (CMV) as a cause [4]. What is more, timing of infection in relation to the pregnancy gestation may determine the potential effect(s) on the fetus. Infections such as HIV are important to be aware of and treat both in relation to promoting maternal health and reducing the risk of mother-to-child transmission (MTCT) [5].

37.4 Routine Antenatal Infection Screening

The recommended routine antenatal screening by the National Institute for Health and Care Excellence (NICE) [6] is outlined below:

1. UTI + treatment of asymptomatic bacteriuria
2. Hepatitis B
3. Syphilis
4. HIV

Chlamydia – women under age 25 advised of local national screening programme.
  NOT part of routine screening –
  Toxoplasmosis, CMV, hepatitis C, varicella zoster
  Rubella screening is no longer recommended.

37.4.1 TORCH Screen

The acronym TORCH (*Toxoplasma gondii*, **O**ther, **R**ubella, **C**ytomegalovirus, **H**erpes simplex) highlights the various infections that could be vertically transmitted to the fetus and cause morbidity. However, it is outdated as not all infections will be tested for and will depend on clinical indication.

TORCH [2] when first introduced stood for *TOxoplasma gondii*, **R**ubella, **C**ytomegalovirus, **H**erpes, after which variations have been used, including TORCHES, for **TO**xoplasmosis, **R**ubella, **C**ytomegalovirus, **HE**rpes simplex, and **S**yphilis, and also O became 'Other' to include infections such as varicella-zoster, syphilis, listeriosis, chlamydia, parvovirus B19, coxsackievirus.

Perinatal infections are reported to account for 2–3% of all congenital anomalies [4].

37.4.2 Antibodies in Infection

The summary below is a basic overview of antibodies in relation to current/recent infection. However, it is important to seek appropriate advice if there is concern.

- IgG and IgM negative = absence of infection or extremely recent acute infection
- IgG positive, IgM negative = indicative of previous infection
- IgM (+/– IgG) positive = indicative of current infection (though not in all cases)
- IgM and IgG positive = indicative of recent infection or a false-positive test result.

In testing for many infections, paired (acute and convalescent) serological testing is often advised to obtain a baseline.

A repeat test may be done 2–3 weeks later and a 4-fold rise in IgG antibody titre indicates recent infection. IgG antibodies can cross the placenta [7].

37.5 Urinary Tract Infection (UTI)

Urinary tract infections (UTIs) are commonly encountered in pregnancy. Treatment for asymptomatic bacteriuria is advised, as the risk of ascending infection and consequent risk of pyelonephritis is significant (up to 40%) [8] as a consequence of pregnancy-related physiological and anatomical changes in the renal tract including dilation in up to 80% of women which may or may not occur with coexisting hydronephrosis. *Escherichia coli* is thought to be the most common organism as a bowel commensal. UTIs need treatment to reduce maternal morbidity but also to reduce fetal risks including prematurity; infection can be a trigger for labour at any gestation [9].

Women reporting symptoms and diagnosed with symptomatic bacteriuria in pregnancy are reported to be around 17–20%. From 2–9% of pregnant women are bacteriuric in the first trimester and 10 to 30% go on to develop ascending infection in the second or third trimester; hence, treatment for asymptomatic bacteriuria is vital with regular urine screening antenatally [10].

A 7-day course of antibiotics is generally recommended, with treatment according to urine sensitivities and local antibiotic prescribing guidance. It is important to ensure test for cure and repeat urine culture 7 days after completion of treatment, especially in women with symptomatic bacteriuria [10]. Nitrofurantoin is generally avoided in the third trimester due to haemolytic anaemia; trimethoprim is avoided in the first trimester due to antifolate teratogenicity [11].

37.6 Group B Streptococcus (*Streptococcus agalactiae*) (GBS)

Group B streptococcus (GBS) in relation to the urinary tract is the commonest cause of severe early-onset infection in the newborn. Intrapartum antibiotics reduced the incidence of early-onset GBS, but have no impact on late onset (after 7 days), which is not associated with maternal GBS [12].

37.6.1 GBS Screening – the Argument against Screening

Testing assesses the women's GBS status at that specific point in time and, if negative, there is a possibility she may test positive at a later date. Thus, the appropriate timing of screening and other factors such as cost, potential risks posed by exposing the mother and child to antibiotics (including anaphylaxis) and unnecessary medicalization and management of labour if she tests positive need to be given due consideration; equally, she may clear the GBS and subsequently test negative [12].

37.6.2 Management of Positive GBS Result

If a GBS UTI is identified in pregnancy, this should be treated antenatally, as well as offering intrapartum antibiotics.

Intrapartum antibiotics should be given to women found to have GBS bacteriuria or GBS identified on low vaginal and/or anorectal swab during current pregnancy or who had a previous baby affected by GBS [12].

Any woman with ruptured membranes at term with GBS should be advised regarding expediting delivery. In preterm rupture, management with GBS depends on factors such as gestation and maternal and fetal condition. Generally, the risks of delivery prior to 34 weeks are likely to be greater than infection risk; beyond 34 weeks expedited delivery should be considered [12].

37.7 Mastitis

Mastitis tends to affect women postnatally, and most commonly in the first few months postpartum and may result secondary to infection. Inflammation is caused by an obstructed milk duct, resulting in the breast or a 'wedge' area becoming swollen, painful, erythematous and firm. It is important to encourage continued breastfeeding to try and unblock the duct. Milk stasis as a result of duct blockage provides the ideal medium for culture of microorganisms and resultant infection. Flu-like symptoms are common. It is important to include breast examination in the assessment of an unwell pregnant/postnatal woman.

NICE recommends that antibiotic therapy should be commenced if there is an infected nipple fissure, no improvement and/or worsening symptoms after 12–24 hours or if milk culture is positive (*Streptococcus* or *Staphylococcus* are often isolated) [13].

Empirical treatment is usually with flucloxacillin for 14 days, unless penicillin allergic where erythromycin may be an alternative. In most cases the newborn is unaffected and NICE recommends observation only if there is positive milk culture [13].

If there is no improvement and ongoing concerns, seek expert opinion including the advice of the breast team, as imaging may be required to ensure there is not an underlying breast abscess requiring surgical intervention.

37.8 Genital Herpes

Genital herpes is a sexually transmitted infection caused by herpes simplex virus 1 or 2 (HSV1 or HSV2) and is usually the first chronic/reactivating condition that many individuals encounter in their lifetime [14].

When a mother presents with likely HSV infection in pregnancy, it is important to ascertain whether this is likely to be primary or secondary. Most important, if primary confirmed, is the timing of the episode in relation to gestation, as this will impact on potential risks to the baby and advice on delivery mode.

37.8.1 Presentation of Infection

Primary HSV infection tends to be the most severe episode.

The classical features and presentation include:

- small vulval vesicles that ulcerate (a virology swab should be taken)
- significant pain

Urinary problems can result including dysuria and autonomic neuropathy leading to retention. There may also be painful inguinal lymphadenopathy and flu-like symptoms. More severe complications include encephalitis, hepatitis and transverse myelitis but usually seen if the patient is immunocompromised. In contrast, some women have few symptoms or may actually have secondary/recurrent HSV but not attributed previous minimal symptoms to HSV, hence the importance of determining primary/secondary to guide management.

Specific recognized potential pregnancy risks include links to miscarriage or preterm labour but there is no evidence suggesting correlation with congenital defects. Intrauterine (congenital) infection is rare.

Neonatal infection (1–2 per 100 000) as outlined in Royal College of Obstetricians and Gynaecologists (RCOG) Green-top guidance can present in three ways and preventing neonatal infection is the main outcome of deciding on mode of delivery [14]:

1. **Localized herpes** – localized to skin, eyes and mouth
2. **CNS herpes** (e.g. encephalitis)
3. **Disseminated herpes** – widespread involvement of multiple organs – significant mortality (up to 70%) and survivors are at risk of long-term sequelae including mental retardation.

37.8.2 Reducing Risk – the Role of Aciclovir and Transplacental Antibodies

The risk is dependent on timing and whether maternal infection is primary or secondary. The greatest risk to the baby is primary maternal infection in the third trimester within 6 weeks of delivery, as the baby will not have had the chance to gain protection from transplacental antibodies. If there is ongoing viral shedding, exposure increases.

37.8.3 Management

See Table 37.1. Of note, in all cases if there is concern or uncertainty about results, liaison with genitourinary medicine (GUM) is vital. Referral to GUM is indicated with a positive primary diagnosis for a full sexual health screen, partner notification and appropriate counselling. Generally antiviral treatment with aciclovir (usually oral but IV for disseminated herpes) is recommended at onset to try and reduce the duration and severity of symptoms and decrease the period of viral shedding. Although not licensed for use in pregnancy, inform women aciclovir is considered safe.

37.8.4 Type-specific Antibody Testing

This is particularly important to ascertain, especially when women present with a suspected first episode in the third trimester. Thus, type-specific antibody (IgG antibodies to HSV1 and HSV2) testing should be undertaken and compared to HSV isolated from the viral PCR swab. The presence of antibodies that match the same type as that isolated from the swab suggest recurrence and vaginal delivery possible unless not advisable otherwise.

If the woman wishes vaginal delivery despite counselling around risks, specific consideration is given to minimizing transmission to baby including avoidance of procedures that may increase risk (fetal blood sampling, fetal scalp electrodes, artificial rupture of membranes and instrumental deliveries) especially if active primary HSV lesions, in addition to considering intrapartum IV aciclovir.

37.8.5 Recurrent HSV Infection in HIV-Positive Women

There is some evidence, albeit inconsistent, that women who are HIV positive and have active HSV lesions are more likely to transmit HIV infection. These women should be offered daily oral aciclovir from 32 weeks (increased risk of preterm labour if HIV positive) to reduce risk of transmission, especially where vaginal delivery is planned. However, mode will depend on various factors, including viral load and other obstetric considerations [14].

37.8.6 Neonatal Surveillance

Monitoring the neonate and informing the neonatal team of exposure to HSV antenatally or intrapartum, along with monitoring and assessment at 24 hours of age, are usually enough [14].

37.9 Chlamydia

All pregnant women under 25 years should be advised of the high incidence of chlamydia in this age group and given advice and details on their local national screening programme [6].

Any woman who has symptoms of infection and/or has a positive chlamydia result should be treated. Azithromycin is recommended first line treatment [15, 16]. Given the potential associations with preterm rupture of membranes and premature delivery as well as risks to the baby such as neonatal conjunctivitis and neonatal pneumonia, it is important to ensure cure, and BASHH advises test of cure at 6 weeks [16].

As with all other sexually transmitted infections (STIs), referral to GUM for appropriate counselling, partner notification and full sexual health screen is recommended.

37.10 Chicken Pox (varicella-zoster virus (VZV))

At booking, enquire about a women's previous history of chicken pox (varicella-zoster virus (VZV)) or shingles. It is thought that approximately 90% of women are immune and the incidence of primary infection in pregnancy is around 3 in 1000 [17]. Avoidance in pregnancy is advised if no previous history.

With regard to exposure, the history must determine the significance of contact and the woman's susceptibility to infection. Consider the type, timing and closeness of exposure. For instance, significant is face-to-face (direct) contact for 15 minutes with a child with exposed lesions. The incubation period is 14–21 days and the period of infectivity is from 1–2 days prior to rash appearing until all lesions have crusted over [17].

313

Table 37.1 Summary of RCOG guidance on management of herpes in pregnancy [14]

	Management	Intrapartum care	Neonatal risk
Primary herpes Onset up to 27+6 weeks	Refer to GUM Viral PCR swab to confirm this is herpes Commence aciclovir at onset for 5 days Consider aciclovir from 36 weeks	Aim for vaginal delivery unless otherwise indicated	Risk of affecting baby low due to development of transplacental antibodies
Primary herpes Onset beyond 28 weeks	Refer to GUM Viral polymerase chain reaction (PCR) swab HSV IgG antibody assessment to HSV 1 and 2 – to determine whether primary or secondary infection Commence aciclovir and continue until delivery	Advise delivery by caesarean section especially if infection within 6 weeks of delivery If declines/wishes vaginal delivery – consider intravenous (IV) aciclovir in labour and avoid invasive procedures such as fetal blood sampling (FBS) and fetal scalp electrodes (FSE)	Risk of affecting baby significant as not long enough for transplacental antibodies to provide protection – risk of transmission can be as high as 41%
Secondary herpes	Liaise with GUM HSV IgG antibody assessment as above Viral PCR swab Above tests to confirm secondary and not primary infection Consider starting aciclovir at 36 weeks especially if frequent flare-ups, unless HIV positive where recommended to start at 32 weeks	Aim for vaginal delivery unless otherwise indicated Can use invasive procedures as advice suggests that any increase in risk associated with invasive procedures is unlikely to be significant	Risk of affecting baby low – small risk of localized disease if affected

37.10.1 Role of VZIG Immunoglobulin

If there is no previous exposure/history of infection, a blood test is required to assess if there is VZV immunity. IgG suggests immunity requiring no further action, whilst IgM suggests acute infection. If there is no immunity, then varicella-zoster immunoglobulin (VZIG) should be offered (where available) as soon as possible; this is effective if given up to 10 days after contact. These women should be treated as potentially infectious from 8–28 days after exposure if they receive VZIG and 8–21 if they do not. Occasionally, a second dose may be needed if subsequent exposure occurs and more than 3 weeks since the last dose.

37.10.2 Chicken Pox in Adulthood

Chicken pox occurring in adulthood is often associated with increased morbidity compared to childhood. It can result in potentially life-threatening hepatitis, pneumonitis and encephalitis. Pregnant women are amongst those more susceptible.

37.10.3 Treatment for Chicken Pox in Pregnancy

Guidance advises that in any pregnancy over 20 weeks oral aciclovir should be offered within 24 hours of rash appearing due to increased risk of pneumonitis in later pregnancy, but before 20 weeks weigh up and discuss the risks and benefits with the mother. Treatment via IV is recommended if the woman is unwell. Hospitalization requires isolation and close liaison with at least obstetric, microbiology (virologist), infectious disease and neonatal teams [17].

37.10.4 Risks to the Fetus

The most significant risk is in early pregnancy; the risk of fetal varicella syndrome (FVS) is greatest in the first 16 weeks and occurs in about 2% [17].

The features of FVS include skin scarring in dermatomal distribution, eye lesions (microphthalmia, chorioretinitis or cataracts), hypoplasia of the ipsilateral limb as well as neurological abnormalities. Fetal varicella syndrome is a result of subsequent herpes zoster reactivation in utero and not an occurrence at the time of acute infection. It may be suspected at ultrasound if limb deformity, microcephaly, hydrocephalus, soft tissue calcification and fetal growth restriction are noted.

If maternal infection is confirmed, refer to a fetal medicine specialist after 5 weeks (or at 16–20 weeks) for ultrasound assessment [17].

37.10.5 Delivery

Ideally, delivery should be avoided before 7 days of onset to try and ensure some passive transfer of antibodies. Infection acquired in the last 4 weeks of pregnancy poses a significant risk of infection (neonatal varicella) at around 20% [17].

37.10.6 Postnatal

Varicella-zoster immunoglobulin may be given to newborns at significant risk of VZV infection such as maternal rash/infection within days of delivery. As with any infection, inform neonatal colleagues of exposure antenatally who can assess the need for neonatal ophthalmic examination or otherwise.

37.11 Parvovirus B19 'Slapped Cheek'/ Erythema Infectosium/Fifth Disease

Parvovirus is spread by respiratory droplets with an incubation period of 4–20 days and often occurs in epidemic waves every 2–3 years in primary-aged children [18]. It is thought that about 50% of women are immune in the UK. Primary infection is not often encountered in pregnancy.

As with many infections, the mother is often relatively asymptomatic but may have a malar rash: 'slapped cheek'. It is difficult to differentiate between rubella and parvovirus B19 on clinical grounds, as both present with a similar rash, fever and arthralgia and both should be considered if a woman is not known to be immune unless definite parvovirus exposure.

NICE [18] clinical guidance advises that anyone thought to have parvovirus should be referred to the Health Protection Unit (HPU). Determination of significant contact is as per VZV, 15-minute face-to-face contact and, in the case of parvovirus, in the last 3 weeks. The infectious phase of parvovirus is prior to the rash; once the rash appears, the individual is no longer infectious. Immediate serological screening is indicated if significant contact.

37.11.1 Diagnosis

The diagnosis is confirmed by checking paired serological samples >10 days apart, IgM antibodies present and IgG increasing.

37.11.2 Risks to Mother and Fetus

Most women are relatively unaffected, but if a patient is immunocompromised, haemolysis and aplastic anaemia pose risks. Furthermore, 'mirror syndrome' is rare and presents with significant fetal compromise (hydrops) and maternal presentation 'mirroring' this with swollen legs, hypertension, proteinuria and anaemia [19].

Fetal infection is thought to occur in around 25–30% of cases and the consequence of the infection to the baby is as a result of suppression of erythropoiesis (+/– thrombocytopenia) and resultant anaemia and cardiotoxicity, which can lead to cardiac failure and hydrops. Amniocentesis may be indicated to confirm infection.

37.11.3 Fetal Assessment

Refer to a fetal medicine specialist for review 4 weeks after infection. Ultrasound may show evidence of pleural and pericardial effusions, ascites, skin oedema and cardiomegaly with infection. Repeated scanning 1–2 weekly until 30 weeks is recommended. If hydrops is evident, serial ultrasound scans measuring middle cerebral artery peak systolic velocity to assess need for tertiary referral for intrauterine fetal blood transfusion are required.

Depending on gestation, delivery may be indicated in some affected cases.

37.12 Cytomegalovirus (CMV)

Cytomegalovirus (CMV) is a herpes virus and incidence of primary infection in pregnancy is around 1 in 100. As in various other infections, women are generally asymptomatic but may also present with non-specific symptoms such as fever, malaise and lymphadenopathy [22]. There is no routine screening in the UK but strategies to prevent transmission exist including education and hygiene.

Infection is usually confirmed by paired maternal serological samples. Evidence of maternal seroconversion (negative to positive IgM or a 4-fold increase in IgG antibody titre over a 4- to 6-week period) confirms primary infection. However, unlike many other infections, isolated positive IgM does not confirm primary infection, as IgM antibodies can persist for months or years.

37.12.1 CMV MTCT

Primary CMV infection results in around 30–40% risk of vertical transmission. However, only 10–20% will be symptomatic and have evidence of infection at birth. Unfortunately, a third of those who become infected will die and two thirds will have long-term effects.

Infection in the fetus may lead to IUGR, microcephaly, hepatosplenomegaly, chorioretinitis, psychomotor retardation and sensorineural hearing loss (the leading cause of non-genetic hearing loss) [20].

Ultrasound features of CMV include intracranial calcifications, echogenic bowel, hepatosplenomegaly, IUGR, microcephaly and evidence of hydrops [16]. A number of the features are not specific to CMV and not every CMV-infected fetus (around 15%) will have ultrasound changes. Ultrasound abnormalities alongside serological evidence of primary infection are strongly suggestive of fetal infection. Amniocentesis may be advised to confirm infection after 20 weeks. False negative results are possible prior to this, as the virus is slow growing and may not be excreted by the fetal kidney in high enough quantities.

If viral culture and PCR for CMV are positive, suggesting infection, the consequent fetal effects are unknown. Follow-up scanning is indicated antenatally, and infection should be confirmed by isolating CMV in fetal urine and/or saliva postnatally.

37.13 Rubella

The significant effects of rubella on the fetus were first described by Gregg in 1941 [21], but since the introduction of a vaccination programme rubella is not often encountered in the UK. Women are no longer routinely screened at booking [6].

Rubella is caused by an RNA togavirus and is spread by respiratory droplets with an incubation of 14–21 days. The individual is infectious for 7 days before and after the appearance of the rash [21].

Importantly, as NICE clinical advice states, parvovirus and rubella in symptomatic women are very similar and, as already discussed, unless there is definite known contact with parvovirus, the woman should be tested for both.

Confirmation requires paired samples in the acute and convalescent phase 21–28 days later. Recent infection is suggested by the presence of IgM antibodies and at least 4-fold increase in IgG antibodies on repeat testing.

37.13.1 Fetal Effects

The fetal effects of rubella are secondary to the disruption it causes to mitosis. The earlier the onset of infection, the more significant consequences will be. Thus, infection before 13 weeks results in almost all fetuses being affected, leading to microcephaly and mental retardation, eye lesions (microphthalmia and congenital cataracts), cardiac and sensorineural deafness, to name but a few. In this situation, if there is confirmed maternal infection, termination may be offered without invasive prenatal diagnosis. At between 13 and 16 weeks, around 35% of fetuses will be affected and primarily by deafness. Beyond 16 weeks reassurance should be given, as it is rare for there to be fetal infection [21, 22].

37.14 Toxoplasmosis

Toxoplasmosis due to *Toxoplasma gondii* (protozoan parasite) causing congenital toxoplasmosis is rare but includes severe neurological or ocular disease as well as cerebral and cardiac abnormalities [23]. This affects around 1 in 500 pregnancies.

The classical spread of the infection is by contact with oocyte-infected cat faeces and by eating undercooked meat. The incubation period is <2 days and it is estimated that approximately 20% of women are immune [23].

37.14.1 Risk Prevention

Many women are aware of the potential routes of contracting toxoplasmosis and it is important to re-emphasize these at booking. NICE guidance advises that pregnant women are educated about these measures including washing hands before handling food, ensuring meat is thoroughly cooked, washing fruit and vegetables and avoiding contact with cat faeces [6].

37.14.2 Maternal Infection

In general, like many infections already described most individuals are asymptomatic, with few experiencing vague symptoms including fever, myalgia and lymphadenopathy and, rarely, visual disturbance. However, the immunocompromised can have significant morbidity including encephalitis, myocarditis, pneumonitis and hepatitis. The diagnosis is based on serological testing with paired samples 28 days apart.

Screening is not routinely recommended but may be recommended if high risk (HIV positive) or ultrasound findings show features that indicate possible infection including hydrocephalus, intracranial calcifications, microcephaly/ventriculomegaly, IUGR, ascites and hepatosplenomegaly. Toxoplasmosis has been associated with an increased risk of first trimester miscarriage and as a cause of intrauterine death (IUD) [23]. Of note, most affected fetuses will have a normal scan and are unaffected at delivery [23].

37.14.3 Treatment

There is some evidence to suggest that maternal infection in the first trimester likely results in fetal infection in around 15% of cases and is more likely to be severe than in later gestations.

However, infection later in pregnancy is associated with increased risk of vertical transmission but usually less severe. Spiramycin is given to the mother to try to prevent MTCT; however, if fetal infection is suspected or confirmed (positive PCR – amniotic fluid), combination treatment is recommended as spiramycin doesn't cross the placenta.

Amniocentesis should not be undertaken prior to 18–20 weeks' gestation and not before 4 weeks after suspected infection. IgM antibodies in amniotic fluid is diagnostic.

37.15 Malaria

Malaria is the most common tropical parasitic infection seen in the UK with potential for significant associated morbidity and mortality [24]. Malaria results from the bite of a female *Anopheles* mosquito. The majority of infections are caused by *Plasmodium falciparum* (75%) but others are caused by *P. vivax*, *P. malariae* and *P. ovale* (and rarely *P. knowlesi*) [24, 25]. Falciparum is mainly seen in Africa, but in Asia infection is usually secondary to *P. vivax* and *P. ovale* [25]. The relatively unique hallmark of falciparum is sequestration in the placenta and this facilitates evasion of splenic processing and filtration [24], but unique to *P. vivax* and *P. ovale* is the ability for dormant sporozoites to persist in the liver, which can result in relapses months or years later. Rarely, infection is a consequence of blood transfusion or vertical transmission [26].

It has been suggested that about 1 in 4 women in sub-Saharan Africa will have had malaria at the time of birth in pregnancy [24], and hence this is a significant threat to global health, with 40% of the world's pregnant population thought to be at risk [26]. Moreover, decreased immunity in pregnancy makes women more susceptible, and some evidence suggests that the physiological changes in pregnancy, including increased skin blood flow, also increase infection risk [26].

37.15.1 Prevention

Prevention of malaria is a key focus; avoidance and/or postponing travel in pregnancy to areas where malaria is known to be endemic is the ideal unless it is absolutely unavoidable to travel [25]. If travel is necessary, expert advice should be sought. However, for many women of reproductive age worldwide, avoidance is not an option if they live within an endemic area and preventive measures and compliance with these become essential if they can be accessed.

The RCOG suggests an **ABCD** approach to prevention – **A**wareness, **B**ite prevention, **C**hemoprophylaxis and prompt **D**iagnosis and treatment.

Anti-mosquito measures include skin repellents such as 50% DEET, knock-down room sprays containing permethrin and pyrethroid, insecticide-treated bed nets (pyrethroid impregnated) and clothing that covers as much of the body as possible to reduce risk of bites that typically occur from dusk until dawn [25].

Chemoprophylaxis in pregnancy does not completely remove the risk of malaria; therefore, if the woman is symptomatic including fever and flu-like illness, medical review is essential.

It is vital to discuss risks and benefits of chemoprophylaxis versus the potential risk of malaria. It is vital that up-to-date details by country are reviewed and advice sought. Chemoprophylaxis can be causal (directed against the liver schizont stage and medication would need to continue for 7 days after leaving a malaria endemic area) or suppressive (directed against the erythrocyte stage and need to continue for 4 weeks after leaving a malaria area). Mefloquine (contraindications include current or pervious history of depression, neuropsychiatric disorder, epilepsy) is often suggested for chemoprophylaxis in the second and third trimesters and it may be used in the first trimester for high-risk areas of falciparum, but discussion including expert advice is essential [25].

37.15.2 Presentation

Malarial presentation may be non-specific. It is vital to take a full history including recent travel and consider the diagnosis in any presentation of pyrexia of unknown origin (PUO). Symptoms include fevers/sweats, headache, myalgia, cough, general malaise and gastrointestinal (GI) upset, including abdominal pain, nausea and vomiting and diarrhoea. Signs include pyrexia (fever pattern varies for each species), jaundice, sweating, pallor, splenomegaly, tender hepatomegaly and respiratory distress [24, 26]. Markers of severe disease included impaired consciousness, hypoglycaemia, respiratory distress, convulsions, pulmonary oedema, circulatory collapse, abnormal bleeding and disseminated intravascular coagulation (DIC), jaundice, haemoglobinuria and acute renal failure [24, 26].

After a bite, asexual multiplication of the virus occurs in the liver, and subsequently this occurs in erythrocytes and results in various problems including consumption of haemoglobin and jaundice due to haemolysis and damage to the red cell membrane, with consequent adherence to blood vessels and end-organ damage [24, 26].

37.15.3 Diagnosis

The gold standard for diagnosis is a blood film – a thick film allows diagnosis and a thin film identifies the species [24, 26]. Of note, high parasitaemia usually occurs several hours after rupture of liver schizonts and there is a resultant temperature spike. Serial samples may be needed to confirm a diagnosis [26], and repeat samples may also be needed in confirmed cases where there is clinical deterioration.

37.15.4 Treatment

Treatment involves supportive measures, antimalarial measures and treatment of complications. In pregnancy, urgent treatment is vital and admission to hospital for monitoring is recommended to monitor for side effects of treatment; deterioration can occur quickly. In severe malaria, admission to the intensive treatment unit (ITU) and involvement of the multidisciplinary team (MDT) are essential [24, 26].

Antimalarial treatment should include discussion with Infectious Diseases department, as drugs used will depend on pattern of resistance, disease severity, drug safety and in some countries drug availability. For *P. vivax* and *P. ovale*, treatment

includes eradicative cure due to the infection's ability to lie dormant in the liver [26]. Artesunate IV may be recommended for severe falciparum malaria (or quinine IV); quinine and clindamycin may be used to treat uncomplicated falciparum. Chloroquine may be used to treat *P. vivax*, *P. ovale* or *P. malariae* [24].

Supportive measures include antipyretics for fever and anaemia, which may range from oral iron and folic acid to blood transfusion with furosemide in more severe anaemia and blood products in DIC patients [24]. Hypoglycaemia may also occur directly as a result of maternal infection or quinine-induced hyperinsulinism. It may co-exist with raised lactate, which can impact significantly on morbidity and mortality of both mother and baby [26]. Furthermore, sepsis needs to be treated in the presence of hypotension due to secondary bacterial infection and endotoxic shock. Pulmonary oedema is a very poor prognostic marker and associated with 50% mortality [24].

Alongside maternal management, where appropriate fetal monitoring and monitoring for preterm labour are vital and use of steroids may need to be considered for lung maturity [26].

37.15.5 Risks to Pregnancy

Maternal and fetal risks resulting from infection are:

1. Systemic infection – maternal and fetal mortality, miscarriage, stillbirth and preterm labour
2. Parasitization itself – fetal growth restriction and low birthweight, maternal and fetal anaemia, susceptibility of infant to malaria

Following recovery from acute infection, regular follow-up is vital, regular maternal monitoring of various parameters including haemoglobin, platelets and glucose is needed as well as fetal growth scans. In an endemic country, ongoing protective measures are essential [24].

37.15.6 Postnatal Care of Baby

All babies of affected women should be screened with thick and thin blood film at birth and weekly until 28 days [24]. There is some evidence that maternal infection can affect an infant's health postnatally and result in reduced response to vaccination in infancy [27].

Current ongoing research includes looking at a vaccine based on VAR2CSA (falciparum-derived protein that mediates sequestration and is found on the surface of infected erythrocytes). This has started phase 1 clinical trials to address the question, 'Can a vaccine based on VAR2CSA or other antigens prevent malaria in pregnancy and its adverse consequences for offspring?' [27].

37.16 Zika Virus

Zika virus infection and potential association with risks to the unborn baby first arose in 2015 in Brazil; few outbreaks were reported until this time [28, 29] and this outbreak led to an International Public Health concern by the World Health Organization (WHO) in February 2016 [32].

Zika virus is a flavivirus [28] and was first found in a rhesus monkey in Uganda in 1947 [29] and then subsequently found in humans in 1952 [28]. It is transmitted predominantly by an infected female *Aedes* mosquito, but occasional cases of blood transfusion and sexual transmission have been reported. This mosquito is known to transmit other viruses, including yellow fever and dengue, and may need to be excluded in symptomatic women [28, 29]. Various countries are considered endemic, including the Americas and the Caribbean as well as much of Africa and Asia [31].

Symptoms may be seen from day 3 to day 12, but this is not absolute and can vary [31] and about 1 in 5 of those infected develop symptoms. Usually infected individuals are asymptomatic or have minimal symptoms, but if more symptomatic it tends to be short-lived (2 to 7 days)and self-limiting [28]. Signs and symptoms include macular or maculopapular rash, pruritus, fever, arthralgia/arthritis and conjunctivitis, as well as myalgia, headache, oedema, vomiting and lower back pain [28, 31]. Symptoms can mirror other infections including dengue fever [31]. Pregnant women (unlike with malaria) do not appear to be more susceptible or experience more severe infection [28, 31].

The WHO stated that infection during pregnancy is a cause of congenital brain abnormalities including microcephaly (this is undoubtedly the focus of the worldwide media reports and the significant heightened concern) but it is also known that Zika can be a trigger for Guillain-Barré syndrome [31], neuropathy and myelitis [32].Increasing evidence since the outbreaks arose suggest that maternal-fetal transmission can occur throughout pregnancy but it is not entirely clear the significance of this [28]. It is estimated that 5–15% of infants in women with confirmed Zika virus during pregnancy have evidence of Zika-related complications [32]. Interestingly, UKOSS report that the risk of congenital Zika virus infection for travellers returning from Zika-affected countries is small [30]. However, what may be more important is the gestation at which infection occurred, and if it is in early pregnancy, fetal infection may be more likely [31].

37.17 Congenital Zika Virus Syndrome

This syndrome includes a plethora of cranial (including microcephaly, ventriculomegaly, microphthalmia, choroid plexus cyst, periventricular cysts and cerebellar abnormalities) and extra-cranial abnormalities (including intrauterine fetal growth restriction, oligohydramnios, intrauterine fetal death and talipes) [28,31].

The potential for a false positive test for microcephaly is very high and true microcephaly is rare. There is no universally accepted definition of congenital Zika virus syndrome, but it should be considered where a head measurement is more than 2 or 3 standard deviations (SDs) below the mean for gestational age [29]. However, the higher the SD below the mean, the higher the correlation will be with microcephaly [28]. Based on other infections such as CMV, the presence of microcephaly and/or central nervous system (CNS) involvement is usually always associated with poorer prognosis including neurodevelopmental delay, intellectual disability, visual disturbance and neurosensory hearing loss [28]. If there is an ultrasound abnormality, counselling for amniocentesis should be offered. If amniocentesis is PCR positive, this confirms likely infection and the woman needs to be counselled on all options including termination where appropriate. With ongoing pregnancy, liaison with paediatrics is essential [31].

37.17.1 Prevention

Akin to malaria, pregnant women should be advised to postpone travel to endemic areas [29], but if travel is is unavoidable personal protection as already described for malaria is recommended. Slightly different to malaria, though, the involved mosquito is primarily active during daylight hours [31]. There is currently no vaccine or drug available to prevent Zika infection, but other measures to prevent transmission include abstaining from intercourse or using condoms for the duration of pregnancy if a male partner resides in or travelled to an endemic area [28].

If a pregnant woman has recently been in an endemic area for Zika virus transmission, she should advise the healthcare team so appropriate monitoring and/or testing can be instigated [31]. Box 37.1 provides advice regarding travel and Zika virus avoidance from the Royal College of Obstetricians and Gynaecologists.

37.17.2 Diagnosis

Infection should be considered and tested for in any women who experiences symptoms suggestive of Zika within 2 weeks of leaving an endemic area or within 2 weeks of sexual contact

---

Box 37.1 RCOG Advice [31]

Avoid becoming pregnant while travelling in a country or area with risk of Zika virus transmission.

If the couple is considering pregnancy, consistent use of effective contraception and barrier methods (e.g. condoms) is advised and should be started prior to travel and followed for:

- 3 months after return from an area with risk of Zika transmission or last possible Zika exposure, if both partners travelled.
- 3 months after return from an area with risk for Zika transmission or last possible Zika exposure, if just the male partner travelled.
- 2 months after return from an area with risk for Zika transmission or last possible Zika exposure, if just female partner travelled.

with a male sexual partner who has recently travelled to an endemic area [28,31]. It is a notifiable disease.

Detection of the virus in serum using reverse transcription-polymerase chain reaction (RT-PCR) within 1 week of symptoms is advised, but viral clearance can occur within 1 week and a negative result 5–7 days after symptom onset may therefore not totally exclude infection due to viral clearance [28, 29]. It is possible to test other fluids including urine, saliva, semen (often found after no longer detected in blood or urine) and amniotic fluid, but serum is the recommended standard for testing [28]. Of note, if Zika virus antibodies are not detected in serum 4 or more weeks after the last possible exposure, infection can be excluded and in pregnancy no additional scans are needed unless new concerns arise [31].

Amniocentesis is invasive and should only be undertaken by fetal medicine specialists. It is primarily considered when a woman tests negative but brain abnormality is seen on ultrasound, and it is used for screening both genetic abnormalities and congenital infections, ideally done after 15 weeks' gestation [28].

37.17.3 Treatment

There is no specific treatment. Supportive treatment, including rest, personal protection and topical emollients, is usually all that is required if the woman is symptomatic [28].

If there is a positive diagnosis in symptomatic women, a baseline fetal ultrasound and referral to a fetal medicine service for further assessment and ongoing care are indicated.

In women who have been to an endemic area but are asymptomatic, routine testing in pregnancy is not done but baseline fetal ultrasound is advised and repeated at 18–20 weeks and then consideration of repeat at 28–30 weeks in line with WHO guidance [31].

37.18 Group A Streptococcus (GAS) – Notifiable to Public Health

Group A streptococcus (GAS) can result in significant invasive infection in pregnancy and postpartum, including endometritis and toxic shock syndrome, and is associated with mortality rates around 30–50%. Symptoms can be atypical and vague; despite being uncommonly encountered in day-to-day clinical practice, it needs to be considered in the differential due to potentially significant and catastrophic outcomes [33, 34]. In the last MBRRACE-UK report, 7 women died from genital tract sepsis; in 2 of the women, puerperal sepsis secondary to GAS after normal delivery was the cause [1]. A cross-sectional study by Leonard et al [33] showed that often the genital tract is the source of infection, but sometimes it can be acquired from another route/external source, including respiratory, and usually women have had contact with young children. Moreover, the study also showed two clusters and raised concerns that a healthcare worker colonized could inadvertently infect a patient by touch [34, 35]. This ties in with evidence by Ignaz Semmelweis in 1847 whose work showed that hand

washing in Austria in 1847 reduced maternal mortality secondary to puerperal sepsis significantly [36].

37.19 Key Messages

1. Infection has various presentations in pregnancy from acute maternal infection with potential significant morbidity with infection (such as pyelonephritis) to infection with minimal/no maternal symptoms.
2. The timing of infection in relation to gestation has significant impact on the timing of the mode of delivery and thus the potential impact and consequences of the infection on the fetus.
3. ALWAYS liaise with the MDT including microbiologists, infectious disease specialists, virologists, fetal medicine specialists and paediatricians to ensure the best clinical care is in place for mother and child.
4. Reducing morbidity and risk of infection is of utmost importance from encouraging immunization programme uptake prenatally and postnatally, to preventive measures including hygiene, personal protection and chemoprophylaxis, early identification and treatment of asymptomatic bacteriuria, to implementing current best practice when infection occurs and following local guidance on prescribing.
5. Antibodies in paired samples can be extremely useful to help determine the nature of an infection; however, results can be difficult to understand and are not always clear cut. Thus, the importance of liaising with colleagues in Infectious Disease/GUM/Immunology cannot be emphasized enough.

37.20 Key Guidelines

- Rhodes A, Evans LE, Alhazzani W, et al (2016) Surviving Sepsis Campaign: international guidelines for management of sepsis and septic shock. *Crit Care Med.* 2017;45(3):486–552.
- *Bacterial Sepsis in Pregnancy*, Green-top Guideline No 64a. London: Royal College of Obstetricians and Gynaecologists, 2012.
- Scottish Intercollegiate Guidelines Network (SIGN). *SIGN 88 – Management of Suspected Bacterial Urinary Tract Infection in Adults: A National Clinical Guideline.* Edinburgh: SIGN; 2012.
- RCOG/RCM/PHE/HPS Clinical guidelines. *Zika Virus Infection and Pregnancy: Information for Healthcare Professionals.* 17 June 2016, updated 27 February 2019. www.rcog.org.uk/globalassets/documents/guidelines/zika-virus-rcog-feb-2019.pdf

37.21 Summary

Table 37.2 summarizes a number of infections that may be encountered in pregnancy, but it is not an exhaustive list.

Table 37.2 Infections in pregnancy

Infection	Common organism(s) encountered	Treatment	Treatment cautions/ avoidance/notes	Follow-up	Special features
UTI	E. coli Klebsiella	As per local guidance	Trimethoprim – avoid in 1st trimester Nitrofurantoin – avoid in 3rd trimester	MSSU after 7 days of completion of treatment – to ensure cure	Grp B Strep found in urine – antibiotics in labour advised
Mastitis	Staphylococcus aureus Streptococcus	Penicillin – usually Flucloxacillin Erythromycin if penicillin allergic	Usually 14 days	Consider breast abscess if not responding to treatment	Encourage to continue breastfeeding
Herpes – Primary Secondary	Herpes simplex virus 1 or 2 (HSV1 or HSV2)	Antiviral – usually Aciclovir	Aciclovir	May wish to consider Aciclovir from 36 weeks (32 weeks if HIV positive) Liaise with GUM	If primary and within 6 weeks of delivery – recommend caesarean section as delivery mode
STIs – Chlamydia (Commonest STI encountered in UK)	Chlamydia trachomatis	First line treatment – Azithromycin (other treatment options: Erythromycin or Amoxicillin)		Test of cure vital in all pregnant women – NAAT testing undertaken for this at 6 weeks following Azithromycin Liaise with GUM	Partner notification and testing Ensure safe sex advice given
Toxoplasmosis	Toxoplasmosis gondii parasite	Spiramycin (if fetal infection confirmed – combination treatment recommended) e.g. pyrimethamine-sulfadoxine)	Spiramycin does not cross placenta	Follow-up ultrasounds and may consider amniocentesis after 20 weeks	Primary prevention advice paramount to reducing infection risk – e.g. cooking raw meat thoroughly, avoid contact with cat faeces in soil or cat litter
CMV	Cytomegalovirus Herpes virus	No specific treatment – symptomatic		Scanning	Immunocompromised most susceptible to infection or its reactivation
Chicken pox	Varicella-zoster virus – DNA virus	Aciclovir especially if present within 24 hours of rash and >20 weeks' gestation	Could consider Aciclovir if under 20 weeks' gestation	Occurrence as an adult has greater morbidity than childhood – risk of hepatitis, encephalitis and pneumonitis and further increased risk in immunocompromised	If significant exposure and not immune – VZIG could be considered if within 10 days of exposure Risk of FVS in first 16 weeks of pregnancy

Zika	Flavivirus usually transmitted by female *Aedes* mosquito	No specific treatment – supportive measures	Personal protection vital for prevention in endemic areas	If symptomatic – testing within 2 weeks Fetal scans if exposure risk	Condoms if male partner symptomatic or in endemic area for duration of pregnancy
Parvovirus B19 'Slapped cheek'	Parvovirus B19 – DNA virus	No specific maternal treatment	Immunocompromised may be significantly affected and require transfusion if aplastic anaemia results	If confirmed fetal infection – monitor middle cerebral artery peak systolic velocity and monitor for evidence of hydrops	If peak systolic velocity increased, referral to tertiary centre with a view to intrauterine transfusion indicated
Chorioamnionitis	Various infections including *E. coli*	Follow local antibiotic guidance – potentially co-amoxiclav	If concerns – delivery recommended ASAP	Maternal pyrexia, offensive vaginal discharge and fetal tachycardia indicate clinical chorioamnionitis	10 days erythromycin recommended for PPROM
Rubella	Rubella- RNA togavirus	No specific treatment		Routine screening at booking to determine immunity no longer undertaken TOP may be discussed if infection confirmed <13 weeks' gestation as most fetuses infected if maternal infection in first trimester	Live vaccine (MMR) given postnatally and hence advised avoidance of pregnancy and hence to use contraception for 10–12 weeks
Malaria	Parasite – commonest *P. falciparum*	Antimalarial – commonest IV artesunate or quinine especially severe infection	Liaise with Infectious Disease Consultant for advice, treatment options and chemoprophylaxis as significant resistance	Growth scans	

References

1. Knight M, Nair M, Tuffnell D, et al., eds. *Saving Lives, Improving Mothers' Care: Surveillance of Maternal Deaths in the UK 2012–14 and Lessons Learned to Inform Maternity Care from the UK and Ireland Confidential Enquiries into Maternal Deaths and Morbidity 2009–14*. Oxford: National Perinatal Epidemiology Unit, University of Oxford; 2016.

2. World Health Organization. Statement on Maternal Sepsis. 2017. https://apps.who.int/iris/bitstream/handle/10665/254608/WHO-RHR-17.02-eng.pdf?sequence=1[accessed online 30Nov 2019]

3. Rhodes A, Evans LE, Alhazzani W, et al. Surviving Sepsis Campaign: international guidelines for management of sepsis and septic shock. *Crit Care Med.*2017;**45**(3):486–552.

4. Stegman BJ, Carey, JC. TORCH Infections. Toxoplasmosis, other (syphilis, varicella-zoster, parvovirus B19), rubella, cytomegalovirus (CMV), and herpes infections. *Curr Womens Health Rep.*2002;**2**(4):253–83.

5. British HIV Association guidelines for the management of HIV infection in pregnant women. *HIV Medicine.* 2012;**13**(2):87–157.

6. NICE. *Antenatal Care for Uncomplicated Pregnancies*. Clinical Guideline 62. Guidance issued March 2008; last modified December 2014.

7. Palmeira P, Quinello C, LuciaSilveira-Lessa A, AugustaZago C, Carneiro-Sampaio M. IgG placental transfer in healthy and pathological pregnancies. *J Immun Res.* 2012;**2012**, Article ID 985646. doi: 10.1155/2012/985646

8. Schnarr J, Smaill F. Asymptomatic bacteriuria and symptomatic urinary tract infection in pregnancy. *Eur J Clin Invest.* 2008;**38**(2):50–7.

9. Vazquez JC, Abalos E. Treatments for symptomatic urinary tract infections during pregnancy. *Cochrane Database Syst Rev.* 2011 Jan 19;**2011**(1): CD002256.

10. Scottish Intercollegiate Guidelines Network (SIGN). *SIGN 88 – Management of Suspected Bacterial Urinary Tract Infection in Adults: A National Clinical Guideline*. Edinburgh: SIGN; 2012.

11. Lee M, Bozzo P, Einarson A, Koren G. Urinary tract infections in pregnancy. *Can Fam Physician.* 2008;**54**(6),853–84.

12. *The Prevention of Early-onset Neonatal Group B Streptococcal Disease*, Green-top Guideline No 36. London: Royal College of Obstetricians and Gynaecologists, 2017.

13. NICE. *Mastitis and Breast Abscess*. Clinical Knowledge Summaries. 2015. http://cks.nice.org.uk/mastitis-and-breast-abscess

14. BASHH and Royal College of Obstetricians and Gynaecologists (RCOG). *Management of Genital Herpes in pregnancy*, London: RCOG; 2014.

15. Scottish Intercollegiate Guidelines Network (SIGN). *SIGN 109 – Management of Genital Chlamydia Trachomatis Infection: A National Clinical Guideline*. Edinburgh: SIGN; 2012.

16. *Chlamydia Diagnosis and Management*. BASHH Guidelines. www.bashhguidelines.org/current-guidelines/urethritis-and-cervicitis/chlamydia-2015/.

17. *Chicken Pox in Pregnancy*, Green-top Guideline No 13. London: Royal College of Obstetricians and Gynaecologists, 2015.

18. NICE. *Parvovirus B19 Infection Scenario: Suspected Parvovirus B19 or Possible Exposure – Pregnant Women*. Clinical Knowledge Summaries. 2010. http://cks.nice.org.uk/parvovirus-b19-infection#!scenario:2

19. Brochot C, Collinet P, Provost N, Subtil D. Mirror syndrome due to parvovirus B19 hydrops complicated by severe maternal pulmonary effusion. *Prenat Diagn.* 2006;**26**:179–80. doi: 10.1002/pd.1342.

20. Carlson A, Norwitz ER, Stiller RJ. Cytomegalovirus infection in pregnancy: should all women be screened? *Rev Obstet Gynecol.* 2010;**3**(4):172–9.

21. Puder KS, Treadwell MC, Gonik B. Ultrasound characteristics of in utero infection. *Infect Dis Obstet Gynecol.* 1997;**5**:262–70.

22. Nelson-Piercy, C. ed. Chapter 15. In *Handbook of Obstetric Medicine*, 4th ed. London: Informa Healthcare;2010.

23. Paquet C, Yudin MH. Toxoplasmosis in pregnancy: prevention, screening, and treatment. *J Obstet Gynaecol Can.* 2013 Jan;**35**(1):78–81.

24. *The Diagnosis and Treatment of Malaria in Pregnancy*, Green-top Guideline No 54b. London: Royal College of Obstetricians and Gynaecologists, 2010.

25. *The Prevention of Malaria in Pregnancy*, Green-top Guideline 54a. London: Royal College of Obstetricians and Gynaecologists, 2010.

26. Gitau G, Eldred J. Malaria in pregnancy: clinical, therapeutic and prophylactic considerations. *Obstet Gynaecol.* 2005;**7**:5–11

27. Rogerson S, Desai M, Mayor A, et al. Burden, pathology and costs of malaria in pregnancy: new developments for an old problem. *Lancet Infect Dis.* 2018;**18**: e107–e118.

28. *Pregnancy Management in the Context of Zika Virus Infection*. World Health Organisation Interim Guidance Update. 13 May 2016. https://apps.who.int/iris/bitstream/handle/10665/204520/WHO_ZIKV_MOC_16.2_eng.pdf;jsessionid=B3164F862927FBB741B7F84B4E5DC74 C?sequence=1

29. Meaney-Delman D, Rasmussen S, Staples J, et al. Zika virus and pregnancy. What obstetric healthcare providers need to know. *Obstet Gynaecol.* 2016;**127**(4):642–8. https//doi: 10.1097/AOG.0000000000001378

30. Oeser C, Aarons E, Heath PT, et al. Surveillance of congenital Zika syndrome in England and Wales: methods and results of laboratory, obstetric and paediatric surveillance. *Epidemiol Infect.* 2019;**147**:e262.

31. RCOG/RCM/PHE/HPS Clinical Guidelines. *Zika Virus Infection and Pregnancy: Information for Healthcare Professionals*. 17 June 2016, updated 27 February 2019. www.rcog.org.uk/globalassets/documents/guidelines/zika-virus-rcog-feb-2019.pdf

32. World Health Organization. *Zika Virus.* 20 July 2018. www.who.int/en/news-room/fact-sheets/detail/zika-virus

33. Leonard A, Wright A, Saavedra-Campos M, et al. Severe group A streptococcal infections in mothers and their newborns in London and the South East, 2010–2016: assessment of risk and audit of public health

management. *BJOG*. 2018;**126**(1):44–53 https://doi.org/10.1111/1471–0528 .15415

34. Hughes BL. Group A streptococcus puerperal sepsis: an emerging obstetric infection? *BJOG*.2018;**126**(1).

https://doi.org/10.1111/1471–0528 .15485

35. *Bacterial Sepsis in Pregnancy*, Green-top Guideline No 64a. London: Royal College of Obstetricians and Gynaecologists, 2012.

36. Semmelweis I. (1861) *Die Aetiologie, der Begriff und die Prophylaxis des Kindbettfiebers.* [The etiology, concept and prophylaxis of childbed fever]. Pest, Wien und Leipzig: Hartleben's Verlag–Expedition.

38 HIV Infection in Pregnancy

Christine M. Bates

38.1 Introduction

Human immunodeficiency virus (HIV) is a retrovirus which causes depletion of CD4 lymphocytes, leading to susceptibility to opportunistic infections and certain cancers.

It is transmitted through sexual activity, sharing needles, blood and blood products and mother-to-child transfer (MTCT) during pregnancy and breastfeeding. Management of HIV infection pre-conception and during antenatal and postnatal phases of pregnancy aims to reduce the risk of MTCT to the minimum.

38.2 Epidemiology and Aetiology

In the early 1980s there were reports of men who have sex with men in the USA presenting with what is now recognized as acquired immunodeficiency syndrome (AIDS). The causative agent was identified in 1983 as the human immunodeficiency virus (HIV) [1].

Subsequent studies show that HIV had been present in Central Africa since the early twentieth century. The theory that there has been zoonotic transmission of simian immunodeficiency virus (SIV) from monkeys and chimpanzees to humans is supported by molecular phylogenetic studies [2].

Since 1981 infection with HIV has developed into a global pandemic: 36.9 million people were living with HIV/AIDS worldwide in 2017. It is estimated that just over half of these are women, with the highest prevalence of people living with HIV (PLWHIV] in the World Health Organziation (WHO) African region where nearly 1 in 25 adults are HIV positive [3].

The infection is spread through sexual activity, contaminated hypodermic needles, blood and blood products and mother-to-child transmission during pregnancy and breastfeeding.

HIV is divided into 2 types:

1. HIV-1, which is the commonest, is thought to have originated from an SIV in apes. Within this type there are four groups: N, O, P and M; the latter is the pandemic strain and is further divided into nine clades or subtypes (A–D, F–H, J–K). Subtype C is found in about half of all HIV-1 infections globally and is found mainly in southern Africa and India; while subtype B is principally found in the Americas, Western and Central Europe and the Caribbean.
2. HIV-2 accounts for about 5% of global infections and is thought to have originated from an SIV in monkeys. This type was endemic in Western Africa but is now found globally. Compared with HIV-1 it has a longer incubation period, a more indolent course and an innate resistance to some antiretrovirals.

38.3 Pathogenesis/Pathophysiology

HIV is a retrovirus from the family of lentiviruses containing only RNA. It replicates by using reverse transcriptase enzyme to transcribe its RNA to host cell proviral DNA. Once the virus enters the body, HIV reproduces using the DNA of CD4 lymphocytes rapidly resulting in an acute viraemia reaching levels of HIV up to millions of virus copies/mL and a reduction on CD4 lymphocytes as they are lysed during the process. The life cycle of HIV has seven stages: binding, fusion, reverse transcription, integration, replication, assembly and budding.

HIV-1 binds to CD4 lymphocytes that express CCR5; these are mainly found in the mucosal surfaces including the intestine. During the acute phase, CD8 lymphocytes are activated and kill the infected cells contributing to the fall in CD4 cells. The immune response brings the infection under control, which then enters a latent or chronic phase; this may last many years during which the CD4 cell count gradually declines, resulting in increased susceptibility to opportunistic infections and some cancers.

HIV can be transmitted during pregnancy, labour, delivery and breastfeeding. Without intervention, the rate of transmission is between 15% and 45% [4]. Factors that increase the likelihood of vertical transmission are a high maternal viral load, prolonged rupture of membranes and the presence of other sexually transmitted infections (STIs). In utero transmission tends to occur towards the end of pregnancy and may be related to factors such as high maternal viral load, chorioamnionitis and low birthweight [5].

During delivery, the infant may be infected directly by maternal-fetal transfusion or by the infant ingesting HIV-infected genital tract fluid [6]. MTCT may occur through breastfeeding; a high viral load and breast problems such as mastitis or cracked/bleeding nipples increase the risk of transmission.

38.4 Clinical Features

In 80% of cases, a seroconversion illness occurs in 1–3 weeks following exposure to HIV with symptoms of fever, sore throat, myalgia, headache, rash and lymphadenopathy. This coincides with the acute viraemia phase, with levels of HIV up to millions of virus copies/mL and a reduction on CD4 lymphocytes.

The patient may be asymptomatic for several years during the chronic phase until the CD4 count drops to a point where there is increasing risk of opportunistic infections.

Table 38.1 Diagnostic paradigm for blood testing following risk exposure

Test	Days from exposure to positive result	
	Earliest	Average
HIV RNA or DNA	3	7–14
HIV p24 antigen	7	16
HIV antibodies	14	28

38.4.1 HIV Testing

Screening for HIV is by an immunoassay which tests for HIV-1 and HIV-2 antibodies and HIV-1 p24 antigen (an antigen/antibody combination immunoassay).

A fourth generation assay will typically be positive in 95% within 4 weeks and >99.9% within 3 months after infection. A reactive test should be confirmed by HIV-1/HIV-2 antibody differentiation assay (e.g. Western blot). If acute infection, i.e. seroconversion, is suspected, HIV RNA testing may be positive before the presence of antibodies (Table 38.1).

38.4.2 Differential Diagnosis of Acute HIV Infection

HIV seroconversion illness may be mistaken for other infections such as Epstein–Barr virus infection, influenza, viral gastroenteritis, viral hepatitis, upper respiratory tract infection or drug reaction.

38.5 Clinical Management

38.5.1 Pre-conception

38.5.1.1 General Advice

HIV-positive women on treatment intending to conceive should have their combination antiretroviral treatment (cART) reviewed in light of current knowledge regarding efficacy and possible association with birth defects.

Screening for and treatment of other sexually transmitted infections is advised as is the optimization of cART to attain virological suppression. Where viral suppression is achieved, condomless sexual intercourse should be limited to 2–3 days before and at ovulation, i.e. the time of peak fertility. There is no evidence currently to support the addition of pre-exposure prophylaxis (PrEP), consisting of daily tenofovir/emtricitabine, for the HIV-negative partner.

If the one of the partners living with HIV has detectable virus or the viral load is unknown, then the HIV-negative partner may take PrEP to protect against transmission of the virus. Other options include assisted insemination with sperm from the HIV-negative male where the woman has a detectable viral load; the use of donor semen from a male without HIV; or sperm washing where the male partner has a detectable viral load. Where both partners are living with HIV, they should be on cART and have attained viral suppression before trying to conceive.

38.5.2 Antenatal Care

HIV-positive pregnant women should be managed by a multidisciplinary team (MDT) consisting of HIV physicians, obstetricians, neonatologists, paediatricians and midwives. Universal HIV testing is recommended early in pregnancy to identify patients not already known to have the infection. Repeat testing later in pregnancy is indicated if risk factors are present such as a history of intravenous (IV) drug misuse or multiple sexual partners including those with HIV.

If the woman presents for the first time in labour without having been previously screened, a rapid HIV test, where results are available within an hour, should be undertaken. If this test is positive, treatment with antiretroviral medication should be started intrapartum and the baby given ART prophylaxis once born, rather than waiting for confirmatory HIV blood tests.

38.5.2.1 Medical History Should Include

- STIs
- Medication (including if already on antiretrovirals)
- Vaccinations
- Opportunistic infections which might indicate advanced HIV infection (AIDS)
- Mental health

38.5.2.2 New Diagnosis of HIV during Pregnancy

The pregnant woman diagnosed for the first time as HIV positive at antenatal testing should have the following tests:

- CD4 count early in the pregnancy and at delivery – this becomes less reliable later in pregnancy due to the haemodilution effect
- HIV RNA viral load
- HIV resistance test to guide choice of antiretroviral medication
- HLA B5701
- Renal and liver function tests
- Hepatitis B and C status
- Toxoplasma titres
- Screening tests for other STIs

The woman will further require social and psychological support following a diagnosis of HIV and it is recommended that she should start antiretroviral treatment as soon as possible to reduce the viral load quickly to undetectable. The viral load should be closely monitored to ensure full suppression of the virus throughout the pregnancy.

38.5.2.3 Antiretroviral Treatment

HIV-positive women not already on treatment should be started on an appropriate combination of antiretrovirals as soon as possible. The regimen choice should follow current standard antiretroviral (ARV) recommendations guided by resistance and HLA B5701 testing and will usually consist of a three-drug combination regimen. Other factors that need to be taken into account when deciding upon the medication regimen include maternal co-morbidities (e.g. co-infection

Table 38.2 Mode of action of drugs used in the treatment of HIV patients

Stage of HIV life cycle	Class of drug	Examples of drugs
Binding	CCR5 antagonist	maraviroc
Fusion	Fusion inhibitor	enfuvirtide
Reverse transcription	Nucleoside reverse transcription inhibitors (NRTIs)	zidovudine lamivudine abacavir tenofovir (alafenamide or disoproxil fumarate) emtricitabine
	Non-nucleoside transcription inhibitors (NNRTIs)	nevirapine efavirenz rilpivirine doravirine etravirine
Integration	Integrase inhibitors	dolutegravir raltegravir bictegravir elvitegravir
Budding	Protease inhibitors [PIs] [boosted with ritonavir or cobicistat]	darunavir atazanavir lopinavir nelfinavir saquinavir fosamprenavir tipranavir

with hepatitis B), drug–drug interactions, adverse side effects, as well as the woman's preferences (Table 38.2). Antiretroviral medications interfere at different stages of the HIV life cycle.

The UK, European and US guidelines for commencing cART in pregnancy where the woman is ARV naïve all recommend combinations of two NRTIs together with either a boosted protease inhibitor (PI) or integrase inhibitor as the third agent. The UK BHIVA and European guidelines also recommend an NNRTI as the third agent.

Table 38.3 is a summary of preferred combinations.

Antiretrovirals and the Placenta

Most NRTIs cross the placenta barrier, although currently there is insufficient evidence regarding tenofovir alafenamide. Nevirapine, an NNRTI, if taken at least an hour before delivery, results in a high serum concentration in the fetus. This applies also to the integrase inhibitor, raltegravir; however, protease inhibitors cross the placenta less well [7].

Women who conceive while already on cART should in principle continue on their regimen; however, switching or dosing adjustments may need to be considered in certain circumstances, as some antiretrovirals are not recommended in pregnancy or may have lower plasma concentrations in the second and third trimesters.

Pregnant women presenting in the first trimester should be counselled regarding the risks and benefits of cART. Most commonly used antiretrovirals are not associated with birth

Table 38.3 Mode of action of third agent drugs in HIV patients

ARV class		Antiretroviral
NRTI		tenofovir/emtricitabine or abacavir/lamivudine
3rd agent	PI	atazanavir/ritonavir or darunavir/ritonavir
	NNRTI	efavirenz or rilpivirine
	Integrase inhibitor	raltegravir or dolutegravir [after 1st trimester]

defects; however, knowledge is limited for the newer medications.

Information regarding birth defects and antiretrovirals is collected by the Antenatal Pregnancy Registry [8].

38.5.2.4 Screening for Fetal Abnormality

Screening should follow guidelines common to all pregnant women i.e. ultrasound scanning, combined screening test for trisomies 13, 18 and 21 and non-invasive prenatal testing. Where invasive testing is necessary, e.g. amniocentesis, it is recommended that this be delayed until the HIV viral load is <50 copies/mL.

38.5.2.5 Screening for Sexually Transmitted Infections

Screening begun early in pregnancy and repeated at 28 weeks is recommended in women with HIV. *Chlamydia trachomatis*, *Neisseria gonorrhoeae*, and bacterial vaginitis are associated with chorioamnionitis, which, together with prolonged rupture of membranes and premature birth, increases the risk of vertical HIV transmission [9].

38.6 Intrapartum

38.6.1 Mode of Delivery

The mode of delivery chosen is dependent on the maternal HIV viral load at 36 weeks. Where this is <50 copies/mL in women taking cART, the vertical transmission rate has been shown to be <0.5% whatever the mode of delivery [10, 11]. However, in situations where the virus is not suppressed, the risk of vertical transmission is increased. The following advice regarding choice of mode of delivery can be considered:

o <50 copies/mL – vaginal delivery
o 51–399 copies/mL – consider elective caesarean section (CS)
o >400 copies/mL – elective CS at 38 weeks

An elective CS for obstetric reasons with a viral load <50 copies/mL should be performed as a normal procedure after 39 weeks.

38.6.2 Instrumentation and Fetal Monitoring

In a planned vaginal delivery, the artificial rupture of membranes, application of fetal scalp electrodes, instrumental delivery and episiotomy have generally been avoided in the past due to concerns of increasing mother-to-child transmission; however, most studies suggesting increased risk of vertical transmission were carried out in the pre-cART era.

38.6.3 Management of Spontaneous Rupture of Membranes (SROM)

Prolonged rupture of membranes (>4 hours) is associated with increased risk of MTCT. In the presence of rupture of membranes before onset of established labour, induction or augmentation is recommended with a view to delivery within 24 hours. If SROM occurs and the viral load is >400 copies/mL, immediate CS should be performed. Chorioamnionitis increases the risk of MTCT, so pyrexia during labour should be actively treated as per guideline protocols.

38.6.4 Intrapartum Antiretroviral Treatment

Antiretroviral medication should be continued during labour and the postpartum period. Intravenous zidovudine, started 3 hours before delivery, is recommended where the HIV viral load >1000 copies /mL or unknown in untreated HIV-positive

women and may be further considered where the HIV viral load is between 50 and 1000 copies/mL.

Where a woman with undetermined HIV status presents in labour or with SROM, it is recommended that she should have an urgent point-of-care HIV test. If this is reactive, then immediate treatment should be given to prevent MTCT with the following regimen:

nevirapine 200 mg orally stat dose

zidovudine 300 mg orally twice a day

lamivudine 150 mg orally twice a day

raltegravir 400 mg orally twice a day

zidovudine IV during labour and delivery plus a double dose of tenofovir if premature

The neonate in this situation is managed as high risk and given three-drug post-exposure prophylaxis (PEP).

38.7 Postnatal Care

38.7.1 Mother

Women established on cART should continue their treatment in the postpartum period with a review by the HIV physician at 6 weeks post-delivery. Their mental health should be assessed and appropriate support given. Additionally, contraception choices should be addressed, as menstruation may resume quickly after birth when not breastfeeding. Contraception should be initiated by day 21 after childbirth and may be started sooner depending on patient choice and eligibility.

38.7.2 Infant

It is recommended that all infants born to HIV mothers should receive antiretroviral treatment following delivery (within 6–12 hours). Infants with a very low risk of transmission are those who are born after 34 weeks of gestation and whose maternal viral load was <50 copies/mL at 36 weeks, or whose mother was on cART for >10 weeks with 2 viral loads <50 copies/mL documented 4 weeks apart. These should receive zidovudine for 2 weeks. Infants at low risk should receive zidovudine for 4 weeks. Those born to mothers whose viral load is >50 copies/mL at delivery should have combination drug therapy consisting of zidovudine, lamivudine and nevirapine for 4 weeks.

38.7.3 Testing for HIV in the Neonate

Tests for HIV DNA or, if not available, RNA are recommended as follows:

Non-breastfed
- Within 48 hours of birth and before discharge from hospital
- 2 weeks of age if high risk
- 6 weeks (or 2 weeks after PEP completed)
- 12 weeks (or 8 weeks after PEP completed)

Breastfed
- Within 48 hours of birth and before discharge from hospital

- 2 weeks of age if high risk
- Monthly for the duration of breastfeeding
- 4 and 8 weeks after stopping breastfeeding

All infants should have an HIV antibody test performed at 18–24 months to confirm loss of maternal antibodies.

38.7.4 Breastfeeding

HIV can be transmitted via breast milk and the risk increases the longer the infant is breastfed. Maternal factors that increase the risk are an unsuppressed virus, mastitis, nipple cracks/inflammation. Infant factors include oral or intestinal infection or inflammation. Additionally, early weaning to solid food increases the risk of MTCT.

The risk of transmission via breast milk is reduced but not eliminated if the viral load is <50 copies/mL. Therefore, in high resource settings such as Europe and the USA, it is recommended that infants of HIV-positive women receive formula milk.

The option of not breastfeeding should be discussed with women during pregnancy so they are aware of the rationale and support arranged to implement this, including psychological and financial help. Lactation suppression therapy, e.g. cabergoline, should be offered to women not intending to breastfeed.

Women with a viral load <50 copies/mL and a good history of adherence to cART who decide to breastfeed should have monthly viral load checks on both themselves and their infant while breastfeeding and for 2 months after stopping.

In resource-poor settings where formula feeding may not be an option (e.g. lack of access to clean water, high infant morbidity/mortality due to gastrointestinal infection), the WHO advises women to exclusively breastfeed for 6 months in addition to taking cART themselves.

38.8 Key Messages

- Universal HIV screening in early pregnancy repeated later if at high risk of infection
- Treatment to attain virological suppression during pregnancy/labour and postpartum
- Planned caesarean section where viral load is >400 copies/mL
- Baby to be formula fed where possible

38.9 Key Guidelines

www.eacsociety.org/files/guidelines_9.0-english.pdf

www.bhiva.org/file/5bfd30be95deb/BHIVA-guidelines-for-the-management-of-HIV-in-pregnancy.pdf

https://aidsinfo.nih.gov/

www.acog.org/-/media/Committee-Opinions/Committee-on-Obstetric-Practice/co751.pdf?dmc=1&ts=20190124T1038488881

References

1. Barre-Sinoussi F, Chermann JC, Rey F, et al. Isolation of a T-lymphotropic retrovirus from a patient at risk for acquired immune deficiency syndrome (AIDS). *Science.* 1983;**220**:868–71.

2. Hahn BH, Shaw GM, De Cock KM, Sharp PM. AIDS as a zoonosis: scientific and public health implications. *Science.* 2000;**287**(5453):607–14.

3. www.unaids.org/sites/default/files/media_asset/UNAIDS_FactSheet_en.pdf

4. www.who.int/hiv/topics/mtct/about/en/

5. Magder LS, Mofenson L, Paul ME. Risk factors for in utero and intrapartum transmission of HIV. *J Acquir Immune Defic Syndr.* 2005;**38**:87–95.

6. Cavarelli M., Scarlatti G. Human immunodeficiency virus type 1 mother-to-child transmission and prevention: successes and controversies (Symposium). *J Intern Med.* 2011;**270**: 561–79.

7. Navér L, Albert J, Carlander C, et al. Prophylaxis and treatment of HIV-1 infection in pregnancy – Swedish Recommendations 2017. *Infect Dis.* 2018;**50**(7):495–506.

8. www.apregistry.com/

9. Czikk MJ, McCarthy FP, Murphy KE. Chorioamnionitis: from pathogenesis to treatment. *Clin Microbiol Infect.* 2011;**17**(9):1304–11.

10. Aho I, Kaijomaa M, Kivelä P, et al. Most women living with HIV can deliver vaginally – national data from Finland 1993–2013. *PLoS ONE.* 2018;**13**(3): e0194370.

11. Townsend, CL, Cortina-Borja, M, Peckham, CS, et al. Low rates of mother-to-child transmission of HIV following effective pregnancy interventions in the United Kingdom and Ireland, 2000–2006. *AIDS.* 2008;**22**:973–81.

Chapter 39

Acute Management of Sepsis in Pregnancy

Lucy Maudlin & Francoise H. Harlow

39.1 Introduction

Sepsis is the body's life-threatening response to severe infection. Classification of sepsis is currently based on mortality and amount of organ dysfunction as defined by the Third International Consensus Definitions for Sepsis and Septic Shock (Sepsis-3) [1]. The World Health Organization (WHO) has added to these to incorporate the definition of maternal sepsis [2] as described in Table 39.1.

The SOFA scoring system was identified by the same Sepsis-3 consensus group. It assumes that a baseline of between 0 and ≥2 points is associated with increased mortality of about 10% in adult general hospital patients who have an infection. Septic shock is the most severe end of the spectrum of an infection and has the highest mortality risk with a hospital mortality of ≥40%. Septic shock is ongoing hypotension which needs vasopressors to keep the mean arterial pressure (MAP) ≥65 mm Hg and serum lactate level ≥2 mmol/L despite adequate volume resuscitation.

Identifying maternal sepsis can be difficult and should be considered when a woman has a confirmed or suspected infection and the following other signs of organ dysfunction: tachycardia, hypotension, tachypnoea, altered mental status and reduced urine output.

Table 39.1 International Definitions

Sepsis	Life-threatening organ dysfunction caused by dysregulated host response to infection
Maternal sepsis	Life-threatening organ dysfunction resulting from infection during pregnancy, childbirth, post-abortion or postpartum period
Organ dysfunction	Acute change in identified physiological parameters known as Sequential Organ Failure Assessment (SOFA)
Septic shock	Sepsis with underlying circulatory and cellular/metabolic abnormalities severe enough to substantially increase mortality. Clinically – hypotension requiring vasopressors and raised serum lactate ≥2 mmol/L despite fluid resuscitation

39.2 Epidemiology and Aetiology

The UK publishes regular reports into maternal deaths known as MBRRACE-UK (Mothers and Babies: Reducing Risk through Audit and Confidential Enquiries in the UK) [3]. These data reveal that sepsis was the cause of death of 24 women in the UK and Ireland between 2014 and 2016. Overall, the report states that 225 women died in pregnancy or within 6 weeks of having a baby, which is an incidence of 9.8 per 100 000. This means that sepsis represents about 10% of UK maternal deaths. However, only 7 of these women died from lower genital tract sepsis. The others died from a wide variety of different infections. The Centers for Disease Control and Prevention in the USA gives sepsis as cause of death in 12.7% of maternal deaths during 2011–2013.

Major themes to emerge from the UK report include delayed recognition of sepsis, the failure to initiate treatment in a timely fashion and communication problems between staff members.

39.3 Pathophysiology

The initial infective pathogen stimulates the host defence cells. This leads to activation of the inflammatory cascade, causing systemic inflammation with resulting end tissue damage. There are increased cortisol levels and decreased corticotropin levels.

The exact pathogenesis of the excess inflammatory reaction is still not well understood [4]. Several factors involved include:

- Sudden increase in pro-inflammatory mediators such as tumour necrosis factor-alpha (TNF-α), interleukins and macrophage migration inhibitory factor (MIF), leukotrienes and tissue factor
- Apoptosis of total numbers of lymphocytes
- Delayed neutrophil apoptosis
- Coagulation cascade abnormalities, including fibrin (which is deposited intra-vascularly), accelerated production of platelet-activating factor and abnormal thromboxane production

Risk factors for a patient developing sepsis are mostly associated with immunocompromise. Pregnancy by itself is an immunocompromised physiological state, but this can be made more risky with superimposed co-morbidities.

Maternal factors which increase risk of developing sepsis include impaired glucose tolerance and diabetes, obesity, HIV, anaemia, a history of recent or current vaginal discharge, previous splenectomy, corticosteroid use (chronic or high dose), immune-modifying drugs (for autoimmune disease or transplant) and rarer diseases such as active malignancy in pregnancy. Pregnancy factors include prolonged rupture of membranes, infection in a previous pregnancy and cervical cerclage (to reduce risk of preterm birth). There are thought to be genetic links to susceptibility to sepsis; however, these are still being investigated [5].

39.4 Pathology

The pathogenesis behind sepsis can be bacterial, fungal, viral or parasitic in nature. The majority of adult sepsis cases are gram-positive and gram-negative bacteria in origin. Common source organs during pregnancy are the urinary tract, lungs and genital tract. Almost all of these infections can be transferred to the fetus or the baby during delivery or postnatally, many babies affected require special care from the neonatologists.

39.4.1 Chorioamnionitis

Chorioamnionitis is a general term for inflammation of the fetal membranes, cord and amniotic fluid leading to illness in the baby and mother. The usual cause is vertical transmission of infection from the genital tract of the mother. The chorion is infiltrated by neutrophils and can eventually lead to necrosis and abscess in the membranes and fluid. There can also be vasculitis seen in the umbilical vessels in response to the fetal inflammatory system activation. Common bacterial causes are group B streptococcus, *Escherichia coli* (*E. coli*), anerobic bacteria, chlamydia and bacterial vaginosis, and less common pathogens include HIV, gonorrhoea and syphilis.

The most common cause of chorioamnionitis is group B streptococcus, which can be identified on genital swabs, or in serum or urine of the mother antenatally. Group B streptococcus is a common commensal carried by 20% of the female population in their digestive and genital tracts. It is usually asymptomatic for these women, but it can cause preterm birth. It also increases risk of cerebral palsy and peri-ventricular leukomalacia in the baby. Women carrying these bacteria have a 1 in 1750 chance of transferring the infection to their baby. Some countries routinely screen for group B streptococcus from 32 weeks' gestation. In the UK a risk-stratifying system is used to determine which patients to test and treat. Those affected in a previous pregnancy would automatically be offered prophylactic antibiotics in labour, as their risk of continued carriage is 50%. Those found to have the infection incidentally or through intentional testing outside of the national programme are offered prophylaxis. Women with known group B streptococcus or those with unknown status are offered induction of labour at 24 hours post spontaneous rupture of membranes to try and reduce the risk of transmission to the baby [6].

39.4.2 Urinary Tract Infection

Urinary tract infection affects up to 5% of pregnant women. There is ureteric dilation and physiological hydronephrosis in pregnancy starting at around 22 weeks' gestation combined with progesterone and oestrogen hormone levels rising leading to decreased ureteric and bladder tone. These lead to urinary stasis and ureto-vesical reflux both predisposing to infection. Usually caused by *E. coli* in 90% of cases, there are other bacteria such as *Proteus mirabilis*, *Klebsiella pneumonia*, *Gardnerella vaginalis* and *Ureaplasma ureolyticum* which can cause infections. Rarely, group B streptococcus and *Staphylococcus haemolyticus* can also cause urinary infections. If left untreated, these infections lead to acute cystitis, pyelonephritis and sepsis. These all increase risk of preterm birth and low birthweight.

39.4.3 Surgical Site Infection

Surgical site infection (caesarean section) is increasing in incidence as we deliver more babies this way and with medical co-morbidities such as diabetes and obesity. International data show up to 15% of caesarean surgeries can be complicated by infection primarily with *Staphylococcus aureus*. Other organisms include gram-negative bacilli, coagulase negative staphylococci and *E. coli*. However, amongst surgical site infections, post-caesarean section infections are often polymicrobial and have aerobic and anaerobic components making it potentially difficult to treat. This mix of pathogens makes it important to introduce risk-reducing strategies such as good preoperative preparation of the skin with chlorhexidine solution, not using shaving at the time of surgery (introduces micro-cuts into the skin), antibiotic prophylaxis at induction of anaesthesia or after regional anaesthesia is sited and maternal factors such as good long-term glycaemic control. There are also some surgical techniques such as using a Joel-Cohen entry and closure of the subcutaneous tissue layer [7].

39.4.4 Puerperal Mastitis

Lactation or puerperal mastitis is common and usually caused by milk stasis from problems with incorrect attachment of the baby when feeding, sucking problems with the baby and irregular or missed feedings. Staphylococci and streptococci are common pathogens and cause rapid-onset symptoms and can lead to abscess formation.

39.4.5 Group A Streptococcal Infection

Group A streptococcus can cause severe infection leading to sepsis. It may initially present with the usual throat infection but can cause sepsis, including when it is spread to the genital tract after a vaginal birth.

39.4.6 Influenza

Influenza has an extremely high mortality rate amongst pregnant women. The H1N1 influenza A outbreak amongst other strains caused 1 in 11 maternal deaths in the UK in 2009–2012. Public Health England has recommended all pregnant women should be vaccinated against seasonal and pandemic influenza strains with inactivated vaccine; however, uptake continues to be challenging.

39.4.7 Other Infections

More unusual but serious infections include endocarditis, atypical pneumonias and pneumococcal or meningococcal meningitis.

39.5 Clinical Features

Early identification of sepsis is crucial to changing the outcome for these patients. All hospitals in the UK use a form of 'early warning system' with adapted parameters to suit the physiological changes that occur in pregnancy, often termed MEOWS (modified early obstetric warning system) – see below for further detail.

MBRRACE-UK reminds all caregivers to 'think sepsis' in any unwell pregnant patient and recommends that where sepsis is identified a 'care bundle' be instigated to ensure timely and appropriate treatment and management of the pregnant or postnatal patient. This will be discussed further in Section 39.8 on clinical management.

Clinical presentation, deterioration of clinical signs and features and regular observations are the key to identifying sepsis early. Any patient with a suspected infection (from whatever source) whose condition deteriorates should prompt the clinical team to consider a diagnosis of sepsis. The patient may look clammy, pale, be in respiratory distress, appear confused or be in significant pain. However, the patient may also look well, and only the physiological parameters measured at the bedside may lead to a diagnosis. Pregnant women are able to physiologically compensate extremely well and so by the time they appear very unwell they may be at an advanced stage of illness.

The modified early obstetric warning system (MEOWS) is calculated using known physiological changes that occur in pregnancy. There is an increased minute ventilation, tidal volume and oxygen requirement, combined with diaphragmatic splinting to give a raised respiratory rate. Tachypnoea is an early and sensitive sign of deterioration in pregnant women. The pH is slightly more alkalotic in pregnancy

(7.40–7.46) compared to non-pregnant adults (7.34–7.44). There is a raised heart rate and increased circulating volume and cardiac output, so loss of blood volume is less easily recognized, meaning that hypotension is a late sign. Table 39.2 shows a MEOWS scoring system suggested by the Royal College of Obstetricians and Gynaecologists [3, 8]. The sum of scores for respirations, temperature, systolic blood pressure (BP) and diastolic BP and heart rate is calculated and then a specific escalation policy is used to summon the correct staff members to review the patient and act on their findings. This escalation policy should be determined by each individual maternity unit according to their staffing capabilities and services available, such as whether intensive care is on or off site. As an example, a low score of 2–4 would mean four-hourly observations. A medium score of 4–5 would prompt an urgent response from the obstetric registrar within an hour and observations would be re-checked. A high score of ≥6 would warrant an immediate response from the registrar including initiation of treatment of suspected sepsis.

In combination with this MEOWS chart, a standard way of communicating the deterioration of the patient with the clinical team requested can be used, such as the SBAR (Situation Background Assessment Response) tool. These words allow a simple framework to assist any level of caregiver to provide succinct information and to convey level of seriousness to the next clinical team member.

Worrying features, or 'red flags', in a pregnant or postnatal patient may include abnormal observations as described above but may also include abdominal pain (multiple causes include appendicitis, infective flare of inflammatory bowel disease, post-caesarean infection, pancreatitis), renal angle tenderness (pyelonephritis), sudden onset breathlessness, orthopnoea, new wheeze (cardiac or respiratory causes), headache and neck stiffness or any new neurological sign (meningitis, encephalitis), diarrhoea and vomiting (intra-abdominal sepsis, gastroenteritis), fainting or dizziness. Other significant points in the history could include spontaneous rupture of membranes

Table 39.2 MEOWS

Score	2	1	0	1	2
Central nervous system	-	-	Awake	Only responds to verbal commands	Only responds to pain or unresponsive
Oxygen saturation%	<95	95–96	97–100	-	-
Respiratory rate	<10	-	10–20	-	>20
Heart rate	<40	41–50	51–89	90–100	>100
Systolic blood pressure (mm Hg)	<90	90–100	101–149	150–159	≥160
Diastolic blood pressure (mm Hg)	<50	-	50–79	80–89	≥90
Temperature °C	<36	-	36.1–37	37.1–37.9	≥38
Urine output	<20	20–40	>40	-	-

or vaginal discharge (rising infection and chorioamnionitis), uterine tenderness and reduced or absent fetal movements (or absent fetal heart rate indicating fetal demise).

Sequential Organ Failure Assessment (SOFA) can be used to identify patients with suspected infections who have an increased risk of a prolonged admission to intensive care and increased risk of death. The Sepsis 3 Consensus uses a quick SOFA for adults which incorporates respiratory rate ≥22 - per minute, altered mental state and systolic blood pressure ≤100 mm Hg. It goes on to identify septic shock as sepsis with abnormalities severe enough to increase mortality (circulatory and cellular or metabolic abnormalities). Septic shock is defined in this way as persistent hypotension requiring vaso-pressors to maintain mean arterial pressure (MAP) ≥65 mm Hg and serum lactate level ≥2 mmol/L (18 mg/dL) despite adequate volume resuscitation. In adults it is associated with hospital mortality ≥40%.

39.6 Investigations

When the patient is identified as being at risk of sepsis or it is clinically suspected, there are many tests which aid the clinician to confirm the diagnosis and assess the significance of the disease process, and there are some which enable planning of management beyond the initial empirical stage.

39.6.1 Standard Blood Serum Tests

Standard blood serum tests include a full blood count (also known as complete blood count), urea and electrolytes screen, liver function tests, test of clotting and inflammatory markers. The full blood count would reveal any anaemia, neutrophilia (associated mostly with bacterial infection), lymphocytosis (often seen in viral infection), monocytosis (raised in bacterial infection, tuberculosis and ulcerative colitis) or eosinophilia (found with parasitic infections although also raised in allergic reactions and patients with asthma). Normal adult values are as follows:

Haemoglobin 115–155 g/L

Platelets 150–450 x 10^9/L

Total white cell count 4–11 x 10^9/L

Neutrophils 2–7 x 10^9/L

Lymphocytes 1–3.5 x 10^9/L

Monocytes 0.2–1.0 x 10^9/L

Eosinophils 0–0.5 x 10^9/L

The total white cell count rises when an infection starts but does not fall immediately on recovery. Red blood cells become deformed and damaged in sepsis; examination of a blood film under a microscope can show these cells experience shearing forces which lead to haemolysis. Haemolysis can be caused by disseminated intravascular coagulation, haemolytic pathogens, abnormal capillary blood flow and red cell apoptosis as well as red cell membrane abnormalities. Clotting abnormalities are a fairly late sign for patients with sepsis. Abnormal clotting values

should also prompt a discussion about mode of delivery and which type of anaesthesia would be most suitable.

Renal function tests may become abnormal if the kidneys become hypoperfused (acute kidney injury, AKI). There may be oliguria in septic patients, and regular renal function tests may become necessary during a hospital admission. There would be raised creatinine and reduced urine output if the kidneys were involved in sepsis. This acute insult to the kidneys may leave the patient with a chronic kidney injury. Liver function tests can show evidence of hepatitis or an obstructive type picture. Alkaline phosphatase (ALP) increases in pregnancy from the placenta and can reach three times the normal adult values, making differentiation from obstruction difficult. Transaminases can be raised with systemic inflammation and sepsis. A serum amylase can be useful to diagnose acute pancreatitis. Another metabolic dysfunction in sepsis is hyperglycaemia, and so it is important to measure and control glycaemic levels in unwell septic patients.

39.6.2 Inflammatory Markers

C-reactive protein (CRP) is an acute-phase protein found in blood plasma and forms part of our innate immunity. It is independent of pregnancy and gestation. It rises in response to infection and inflammation. The complement system is activated when it binds to phosphocholine on the surface of dead or dying cells and also on some bacteria and other foreign bodies. This causes phagocytosis by macrophages to aid removal of cells undergoing apoptosis and also foreign bacteria. This rise occurs in inflammatory processes both acute and chronic: infections, autoimmune diseases, trauma (including surgery), allergic reaction and malignancy. Normal levels are usually ≤10 mg/L. CRP rises within 4 to 6 hours of the inflammation and doubles every 8 hours until it reaches a peak between 36 and 50 hours after the initial insult. When the inflammation or infection starts to resolve, the levels fall swiftly as CRP has a short half-life of only 19 hours.

39.6.3 Arterial Blood Gases

An arterial blood gas sample is useful in an acute setting, as this will provide information on any acid-base balance disturbances and oxygen levels. Septic patients will often display a metabolic acidosis and have decreased oxygen levels according to the source of their infection and whether complications such as acute respiratory distress syndrome (ARDS) have occurred. Most modern blood gas analyzers will also return several other values such as a rapid haemoglobin estimate, glucose and lactate (from a venous or arterial sample).

39.6.4 Lactate Levels

Lactate is an important source of energy for the body formed from the reduction of pyruvate generated (mostly) by anaerobic glycolysis. When there is lack of oxygen in the tissues, there is increased production of lactate and so increased lactate can reflect septic shock. Lactate is eliminated mostly by the liver but also by kidneys and, less significantly, by the heart and skeletal muscle. When there is tissue hypoxia, lactate clearance is overwhelmed by lactate production and so there is overall acidosis seen by its conversion to lactic acid. This is then worsened if there is any renal or hepatic dysfunction. Physiological shock from sepsis causes raised lactate levels. Raised lactate levels can cause depression of cardiac function and decrease the response of vasopressors. Normal venous lactate levels are <2 mmol/L. Adult patients with sepsis who have hypotension and lactate ≥4 mmol/L have a mortality of more than 30%. Those with lactate ≥4 mmol/L after good initial resuscitation should be considered for intensive care unit (ICU) treatment. Decreasing or normalizing lactate levels can be seen as a sign that the patient is improving. Normalization of lactate levels occurs prior to CRP levels reducing to baseline.

39.6.5 Procalcitonin Levels

Procalcitonin (PCT) is another test usually only found in the critical care setting and is currently not recommended by national guidelines outside intensive care in the UK. Procalcitonin is produced by several cell types when inflammation occurs in response to significant bacterial infection. It has several roles in sepsis, including altering induction of pro-inflammatory cytokines, changing cell migration to areas of inflammation and also affecting contraction of blood vessels through nitrogen-oxide synthase. Procalcitonin rises rapidly with onset of infection and falls swiftly as the patient improves and also enables clinicians to stop antimicrobial drugs if a non-bacterial source is more likely.

39.6.6 Blood Cultures

Blood cultures are a crucial investigative tool in the diagnosis and treatment for a septic patient. Ideally, the sample should be taken before any antimicrobial therapy is administered. The skin must be appropriately cleaned (e.g. using chlorhexidine single-use wipes) and two venous samples collected for aerobic and anaerobic growth patterns. Urine infections are extremely common and can cause sepsis from rising infection to the kidneys and beyond; therefore, initially a bedside dip is useful followed by a mid-stream sample to send for microbiological culture. Urine output is measured using a urinary catheter, in which case a catheter-tubing sample should be obtained. Microbiological charcoal swabs should be used to collect samples from the throat, skin, wounds, vagina or breast milk. Any pus seen can be collected in a sterile empty container to be sent for analysis. Specialized methicillin-resistant *Staphylococcus aureus* (MRSA) swabs are used to test for nasal and skin carriage. Influenza outbreaks often are tested with throat or nasal viral culture swabs.

In cases of suspected meningitis, the cerebral spinal fluids removed during a lumbar puncture procedure can also be analyzed for culture and sensitivities. Bacterial meningitis lumbar puncture results show an elevated opening pressure, high white cell count and decreased serum-to-glucose ratio. A viral meningitis may show a low white cell count and a normal serum-to-glucose ratio.

39.6.7 Imaging

Imaging the patient can aid diagnosis and enable treatment to be more focused and effective. Any exposure to ionizing radiation must be carefully considered in a risk-benefit way to ensure a pregnant woman is not needlessly exposed. Plain-film x-rays can be particularly useful for chest infections, and some screening of the fetus can be achieved with lead panels placed over the abdomen. Computed tomography (CT) scans involve much larger amounts of radiation; therefore, their use in the postpartum patient in whom breast tissue is hormonally very active should be carefully weighed, as CT scans can lead to an increased risk of breast cancer in these patients [9]. This type of scan can give detailed images of the location of a source of infection such as meningitis or any chest or intra-abdominal focus. It can also be used postoperatively to investigate whether a cause of abdominal pain and infection is related to the recent surgery. A magnetic resonance imaging (MRI) scan does not use ionizing radiation and can be used in place of a CT scan if required during pregnancy. Ultrasound also uses non-ionizing radiation to image soft tissues with good results particularly for ovaries, fallopian tubes, uterus, appendix, gallbladder, pancreas and pelvic spaces such as the pouch of Douglas. The radiologist can use ultrasound-guided drainage to remove a focus of infection in a relatively low-risk procedure compared to major surgery required for usual drainage.

39.7 Differential Diagnosis

Consideration should be given to alternative diagnoses, which may also have a systemic inflammatory response such as severe trauma, significant burns and drug reactions. Other causes of persistent low blood pressure include bleeding (hypovolaemic shock), neurogenic shock, adrenocortical insufficiency, cardiogenic shock (including cardiac tamponade) and anaphylactic shock.

39.8 Clinical Management

Early intervention after early identification of sepsis can make a difference in outcomes for mother and baby. See Section 39.11 for a summary overview of management.

Immediate resuscitation (medical management) should start with the application of high-flow oxygen at the bedside through a facemask allowing maximum flow. Oxygen saturations and arterial blood gas samples will show whether there is any hypoxia and, if so, whether it is improving. Any sepsis-related hypotension should be managed with a bolus of crystalloid intravenous (IV) fluid such as Hartmann's solution (Ringer's lactate) ≥30 mL/kg in the first 3 hours; this choice of fluid can be altered according to individual electrolyte balance as more information is gathered. Observations of blood pressure, respiratory rate, heart rate and urine output provide bedside information about the status of fluid responsiveness. There are methods of measuring response in more invasive ways such as using an arterial line to detect central venous pressure, the arterial waveform, pulse pressure variations and stroke volume variation. If the blood pressure responds well initially to the intravenous fluid bolus but falls again or the venous lactate level is raised, then a further bolus of crystalloid should be administered [10].

High-dose intravenous antibiotics should be administered within ONE HOUR of a suspected case of sepsis being diagnosed to change the course and severity of the illness. If delivered within this hour, especially as soon as any hypotension is recognized, there is reduced mortality in those patients with severe sepsis and septic shock.

Empirical treatment of suitable broad-spectrum antibiotics should be used according to the presumed source, local resistance patterns and any personal history of antibiotic use or allergies the patient may have. Antibiotics with gram-negative cover should be given first. The choice should have action against gram-negative bacteria, and against toxins produced from gram-positive bacteria. The choice should be refined once more information is available from microbiological examination.

Common antibiotics are provided in Table 39.3.

There should be consideration of anti-fungal agents if there is strong suspicion as many of this class of drugs are toxic to the fetus. Anti-viral agents (e.g. aciclovir) should also be considered where there is strong suspicion of a viral source such as influenza and these have been used extensively in pregnancy without problems with either the patient or fetus. Influenza can be identified with a rapid test in under an hour and treated with an anti-viral such as oseltamivir (Tamiflu*), reducing the duration and severity of influenza.

Surgical management is important in intra-abdominal sepsis (especially with postoperative infection), as the patient will not improve even with antibiotics if there is a large internal reservoir of infection. A laparoscopy or laparotomy and wash-out can be lifesaving and should not be delayed with a deteriorating patient where the source is known from imaging.

Delivery management should be focused on after initial care of the unwell woman has been instigated. The timing and mode of birth will be a risk-benefit scenario dependent on many factors and should be made with a senior obstetrician and the woman if she is well enough. An anaesthetist may also

take part in this decision-making process to include care of the woman during delivery and postnatal place of care such as high dependency or intensive care requirements.

Corticosteroids for fetal lung maturation should be considered if a preterm birth becomes likely or necessary. Magnesium sulphate can also be given to protect the fetal brain in cases of preterm birth [11]. If there is confirmed or suspected intrapartum sepsis, then continuous electronic fetal monitoring should be used in labour. Electronic fetal monitoring may show changes including a raised baseline, and new decelerations (which indicate that the fetus is also being affected by sepsis) should prompt the birth to be expedited. Ideally, the woman should be stabilized before attempting delivery of the baby as this can increase maternal and neonatal mortality rates. However, when the woman is critically unwell, a prompt delivery may reduce the physiological strain on her body and may be required to save her life.

Adjuncts to management of sepsis should always include risk assessment and prophylaxis for venous thromboembolism. This should include measured graduated compression stockings plus administration of subcutaneous low molecular weight heparin if required.

39.8.1 Special Case of Early-Pregnancy-Related Sepsis

Sepsis can cause the body to spontaneously miscarry if the patient is unwell enough, specifically if there is a prolonged high temperature. Infections associated with causing miscarriage include bacterial vaginosis. An infection after miscarriage, abortion (medical or surgical) or retained products of conception are relatively common; however, it is rare in the UK for this to lead to sepsis. Infection after miscarriage is rarely due to sexually transmitted infections (*Chlamydia trachomatis* is routinely tested for in the UK); these infections are more often caused by group B streptococcus and *Staphylococcus aureus*. Surgical removal of pregnancy tissue (whether early pregnancy or retained products after delivery) removes the source of infection and can help the

Table 39.3 Empirical antibiotic choices

Antibiotic	Cover and limitations
Co-amoxiclav (Clavulanic acid + amoxicillin)	Good broad-spectrum cover; however, no MRSA or *Pseudomonas* cover Some concern about risk of necrotizing enterocolitis in the neonate when exposed during pregnancy; however, it is commonly used
Metronidazole	Anaerobes covered only
Clindamycin	Streptococci and staphylococci mostly covered including MRSA Stops exotoxin production Not nephrotoxic
Tazocin (piperacillin + tazobactam)	Excellent broad-spectrum cover excluding MRSA
Carbapenems, e.g meropenem	Excellent broad-spectrum cover excluding MRSA
Aminoglycosides, e.g. gentamicin	Can be nephrotoxic. Usually safe as single daily dose gentamicin with normal renal function.

patient to recover faster. However, suction evacuation in the presence of infection is a more difficult procedure, with increased risk of uterine perforation and complications such as bleeding [12].

39.9 Prevention

Consideration for prevention of spread of any kind of infection should be in line with national and local guidelines.

Confirmed group A streptococcus in the peripartum period requires the neonatology team to be informed. They will take blood cultures and swabs and start prophylactic antibiotics for the baby. Any healthcare worker exposed to respiratory secretions or those in the same household would be encouraged to attend for immediate antibiotic prophylaxis. In the UK, the Health Protection Agency produces guidelines about managing communicable diseases [13].

Any woman with group B streptococcus should have been given antibiotics in labour or delivery to prevent transmission. A baby born to a mother with a positive result but who is apparently not clinically unwell would be observed for at least 24 hours after birth, including temperature observations.

Vaccination plays an important part in preventing infection and therefore sepsis in pregnant women. All pregnant women and healthcare workers are offered influenza vaccination in the UK. All young adults aged 18–20 are now routinely offered vaccination for meningitis types A, C, W and Y.

Premature rupture of membranes is an obvious source of infection for both mother and fetus and so a 10-day prophylactic antibiotic course of erythromycin is offered to these women in the UK after the outcomes of a large trial published in the *Lancet* [14, 15]. Those women who also experience threatened preterm labour with intact membranes may be offered antibiotics if the source of infection is identified. Those women who do not start labour within 24 hours of the rupture of membranes after 37 weeks' gestation would routinely be offered induction of labour as per NICE guidelines to reduce risk of maternal and fetal infection and compromise [16].

Simple health measures such as good hand hygiene in any clinical area and between patients are important at reducing spread of infection in the healthcare setting. According to the suspected source and type of infection, there may be a need for increased infection control procedures. These may include isolation nursing (moving the patient to an individual or side room) and personal protective equipment for staff such as gloves, gowns and masks. Contact tracing may also be required to ensure that the infection does not become a problem outside of the healthcare setting; this is guided by Public Health England in the UK, who also provide a list of communicable diseases that need to be reported to them [17].

39.10 Complications and Sequelae and Prognosis

Indications for consideration of transfer to the ICU include ongoing hypotension despite adequate fluid resuscitation or rising lactate requiring inotropic support, pulmonary oedema requiring mechanical ventilation or airway protection, renal dialysis, decreased conscious levels, worsening acidosis, hypothermia or evidence of multi-organ failure.

Vasopressor treatment is administered via central access and the first line drug used is noradrenaline (norepinephrine), followed by vasopressin if required.

Adjuncts to care used in the intensive care setting include transfusion, glucose control using an insulin infusion and stress-ulcer prophylaxis with histamine-2 receptor antagonist of proton pump inhibitor drugs. Nutrition support should also be considered. Extra-corporeal membrane oxygenation (ECMO) is a technology used at tertiary intensive care settings when adequate oxygenation to end-organs is not being achieved by conventional means. It supports the failing lungs by allowing gas exchange to the patient using a device that removes carbon dioxide then re-oxygenates the blood outside of the body.

A very rare and dangerous complication of any wound is necrotizing fasciitis. These difficult to manage polymicrobial infections often end up with multiple surgical procedures to try and stop the spread of infection and require complex skin grafts and intensive care support for a considerable time. There is some evidence that using nonsteroidal anti-inflammatory drugs (NSAIDs) can increase the risk of this complication occurring.

Rare complications include necrosis leading to loss of digits and limbs, and end-organ damage requiring organ transplant.

39.11 Key Messages

Sepsis in an important cause of morbidity and mortality in pregnant and postnatal women in the UK. There are excellent bundles of care used throughout the UK. Multiple studies have shown that recognizing an unwell patient who is deteriorating to become septic and then supplying appropriate care immediately can save lives [18, 19]. Table 39.4 is a short summary of tasks required to improve outcomes for pregnant women and their babies.

Finally, human interaction can cause delays with septic patients; however, working as cohesive teams who communicate well will enable us to '**Spot it, Treat it, Beat it**', as described by the Sepsis Trust [20].

Table 39.4 Six tasks to manage sepsis

	Primary task	Related tasks
1	Give oxygen	
2	Take blood cultures	Identify source
3	Give antibiotics	
4	Consider IV fluids	
5	Take blood (full blood count, CRP lactate)	Arterial blood gas
6	Monitor urine output	Insert catheter

References

1. Singer M, Deutschman CS, Seymour CW, et al. The Third International Consensus Definitions for Sepsis and Septic Shock (Sepsis-3). *JAMA*. 2016 Feb 23;**315**(8):801–10

2. World Health Organization (WHO). Statement of Maternal Sepsis. 2017. WHO/RHR/17.02

3. Knight M, Bunch K, Tuffnell D, et al, eds., on behalf of MBRRACE-UK. *Saving Lives, Improving Mothers' Care: Lessons Learned to Inform Maternity Care from the UK and Ireland Confidential Enquiries into Maternal Deaths and Morbidity 2014–16*. Oxford: National Perinatal Epidemiology Unit, University of Oxford; 2018.

4. Stearns-Kurosawa D, Osuchowski M, Valentine C, Kurosawa S, Remick DG. The pathogenesis of sepsis. *Annu Rev Pathol*. 2011;**6**(1):19–48.

5. *Bacterial Sepsis in Pregnancy* and *Bacterial Sepsis Following Pregnancy*, Green-top Guidelines Nos 64a and 64b. London: Royal College of Obstetricians and Gynaecologists, April 2012.

6. *Prevention of Early-onset Neonatal Group B Streptococcal Disease*, Green-top Guideline No 36. London: Royal College of Obstetricians and Gynaecologists, September 2017.

7. Zuarez-Easton S, Zafran N, Garmi G, Salim R. Postcesarean wound infection: prevalence, impact, prevention, and management challenges. *Int J Womens Health*. 2017;**9**:81–8.

8. Royal College of Physicians. *National Early Warning Score (NEWS): Standardising the Assessment of Acute-Illness Severity in the NHS*. London: RCP; 2012

9. Protection of Pregnant Patients during Diagnostic Medical Exposures to Ionising Radiation. Health Protection Agency and Royal College of Radiologists; 2009. www.rcr.ac.uk/publication/protection-pregnant-patients-during-diagnostic-medical-exposures-ionising-radiation

10. *The Sepsis Manual*. 4th ed. 2017–2018 https://sepsistrust.org/wp-content/uploads/2018/06/Sepsis_Manual_2017_web_download.pdf

11. Doyle L, Crowther CA, Middleton P, Marret S. Magnesium sulphate for women at risk of preterm birth for neuroprotection of the fetus. *Cochrane Database Syst Rev*. 2009;(1):CD004661

12. NICE. *Ectopic Pregnancy and Miscarriage: Diagnosis and Initial Management*. Clinical Guideline 154. 2012. www.nice.org.uk/guidance/CG154

13. Public Health England. *Hand Hygiene Audit Tool for Care Homes*. www.infectionpreventioncontrol.co.uk/resources/hand-hygiene/

14. Kenyon, S, Pike K, Jones DR. Childhood outcomes following prescription of antibiotics to pregnant women with preterm rupture of the membranes: 7-year follow-up of the Oracle I trial. *Lancet*. 2008;**372**:1310–18.

15. Kenyon, S, Pike K, Jones DR. Childhood outcomes following prescription of antibiotics to pregnant women with spontaneous preterm labour: 7-year follow-up of the Oracle II trial. *Lancet*. 2008;**372**:1319–27.

16. NICE. *Inducing Labour*. Clinical Guideline 70. 2008. www.nice.org.uk/guidance/cg70/chapter/1-guidance

17. Public Health England. www.england.nhs.uk/south/wp-content/uploads/sites/6/2017/09/spotty-book-2018.pdf

18. Royal College of Emergency Medicine and the UK Sepsis Trust. Sepsis: A Toolkit for Emergency Departments. 2014. www.rcem.ac.uk/docs/Sepsis/Sepsis%20Toolkit.pdf

19. Dellinger RP, Levy MM, Rhodes A, et al; Surviving Sepsis Campaign Guidelines Committee Including the Pediatric Subgroup. Surviving Sepsis Campaign: international guidelines for management of severe sepsis and septic shock: 2012. *Crit Care Med*. 2013;**41**(2):580–637.

20. Sepsis Trust. *The Sepsis Manual*. 2017. https://sepsistrust.org/wp-content/uploads/2018/06/Sepsis_Manual_2017_web_download.pdf

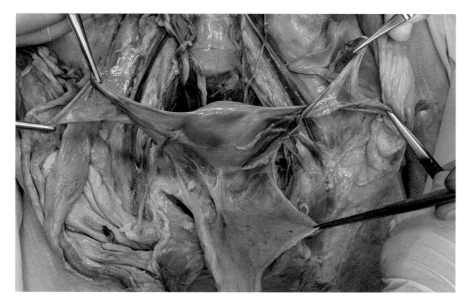

Figure 1.3 Dissection of the female pelvis (carried out on a Thiel embalmed cadaver at the Department of Anatomy, University of Malta). A black and white version of this figure will appear in some formats.

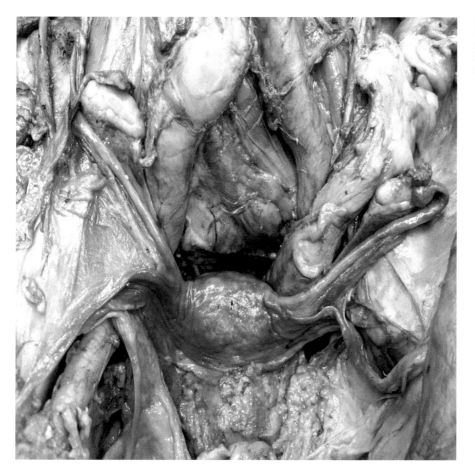

Figure 1.4 Dissection of the uterus, tubes and ovaries (carried out on a Thiel embalmed cadaver at the Department of Anatomy, University of Malta). A black and white version of this figure will appear in some formats.

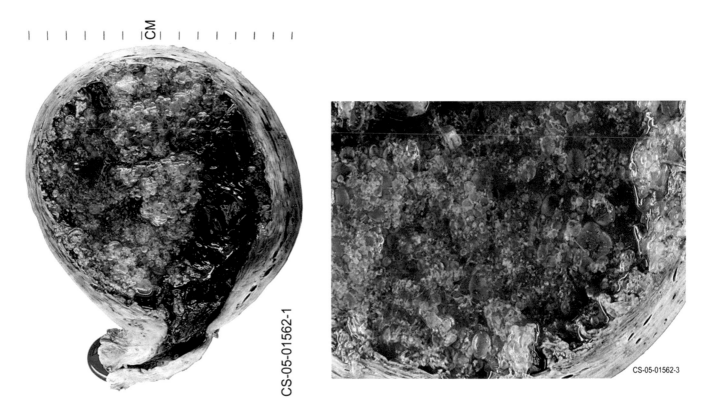

Figure 8.4 Macroscopic appearance of complete hydatidiform mole. A black and white version of this figure will appear in some formats.

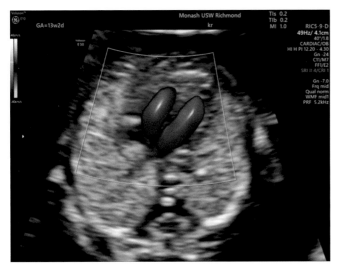

Figure 11.9 Fetal cardiac 4-chamber view at 13 weeks of gestation. Fetal spine posterior. Colour Doppler demonstrating blood flow from the left atrium into the left ventricle and from the right atrium into the right ventricle. Red = blood flow towards the ultrasound transducer. A black and white version of this figure will appear in some formats.

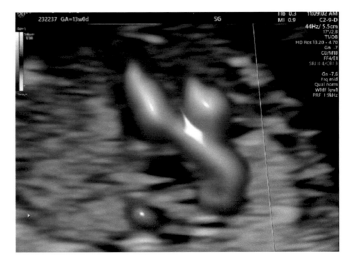

Figure 11.10 Normal crossing of the cardiac arterial outflow representing the ascending aorta and pulmonary artery at 13 weeks of gestation. Blue = blood flow away from the ultrasound transducer. A black and white version of this figure will appear in some formats.

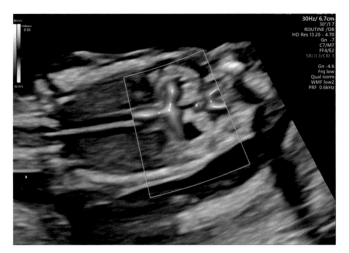

Figure 11.11 Fetal kidneys at 12 weeks of gestation. Note the colour Doppler images of the fetal descending aorta and branching of the renal arteries and common iliac arteries. A black and white version of this figure will appear in some formats.

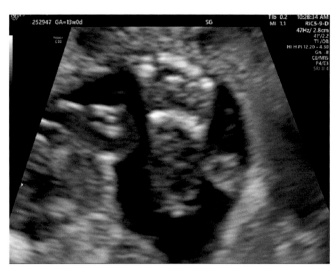

Figure 11.12 Fetal footprints displaying all five toes at 13 weeks of gestation. A black and white version of this figure will appear in some formats.

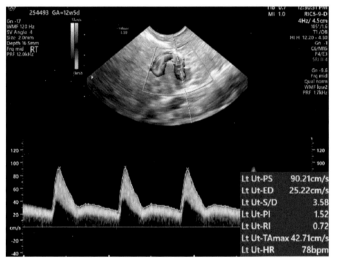

Figure 11.19 Maternal uterine artery waveform recording using colour Doppler ultrasound at 12+ weeks of gestation. A black and white version of this figure will appear in some formats.

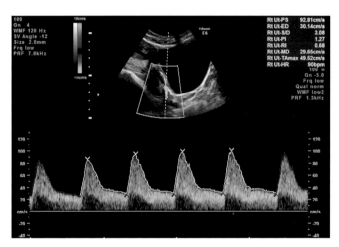

Figure 17.1 Transabdominal Doppler ultrasound examination of uterine artery in the first trimester. The peak systolic velocity should be >60 cm/s (here 92.81 cm/s) to verify that the uterine artery is being examined.. A black and white version of this figure will appear in some formats.

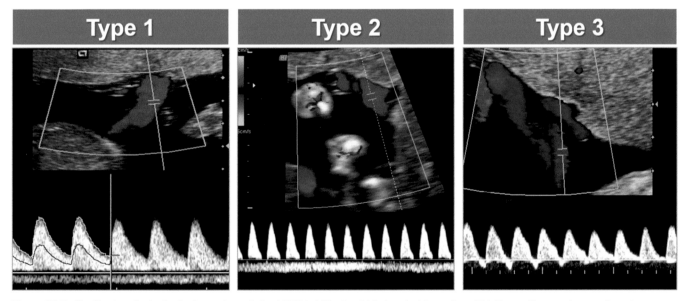

Figure 18.5 Classification of selective fetal growth restriction (sFGR) in MC twins. A black and white version of this figure will appear in some formats.

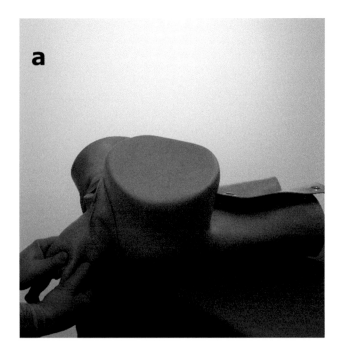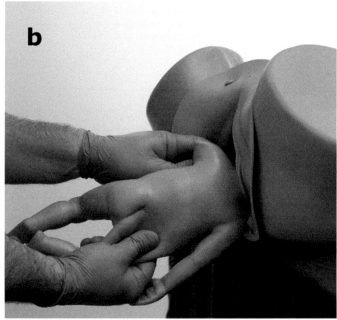

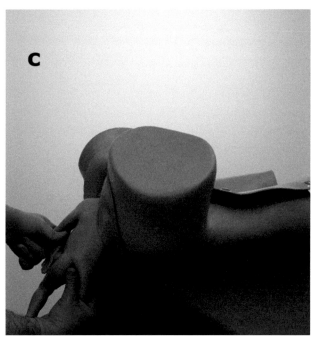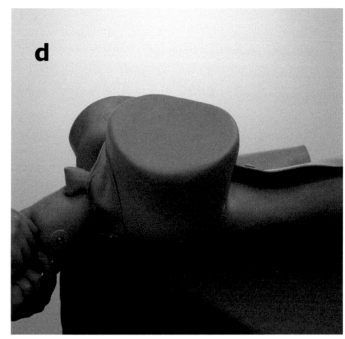

Figure 51.1 Demonstration of Lovset's manoeuvre for delivery of twin 2 (breech). (a) The obstetrician's thumbs are placed on the infant's sacrum and the other fingers hold the hips and the pelvis. (b) Turn the infant 90° so as to bring the anterior shoulder under the symphysis pubis; (c) engage the anterior arm and deliver it. (d) Then, continue with 180° counter rotation, and the posterior arm that is now moved under the symphysis pubis is delivered. A black and white version of this figure will appear in some formats.

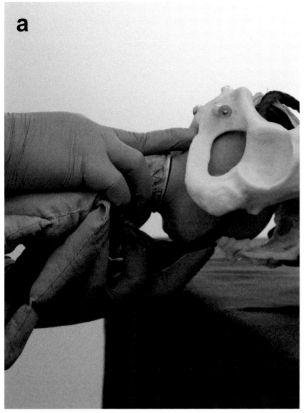 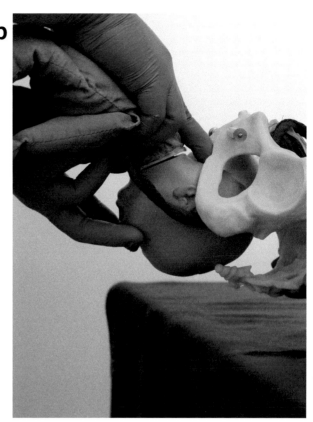

Figure 51.2 Mauriceau–Smellie–Veit manoeuvre for delivery of twin 2 (breech). (a) The obstetrician inserts the non-dominant hand into the vagina: he or she palpates the fetal maxilla with the index and middle fingers and places these fingers on the neonate's cheekbone. The index and ring fingers of other hand are used to hook the baby's shoulders, while the middle finger presses the occiput in order to flex the head. (b) The head is flexed gently towards the chest until the hairline is visible. Then the obstetrician continues to raise the baby, holding in place the non-dominant hand until the head is free. A black and white version of this figure will appear in some formats.

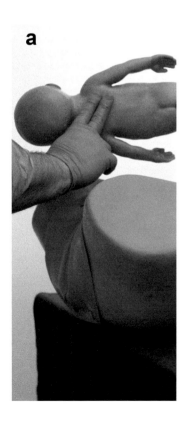 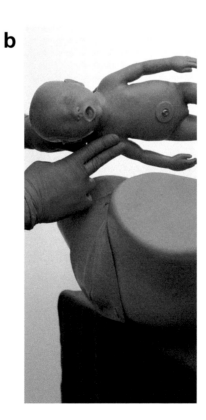

Figure 53.1 Woods screw manoeuvre for disengagement of the anterior shoulder. (a) Using the fingers of the right hand for the right fetal shoulder (and vice versa for the left) placed posteriorly and applying gentle pressure. (b) Assisting the back pressure using the fingers of the opposite hand on the front side of the shoulder to apply pressure. A black and white version of this figure will appear in some formats.

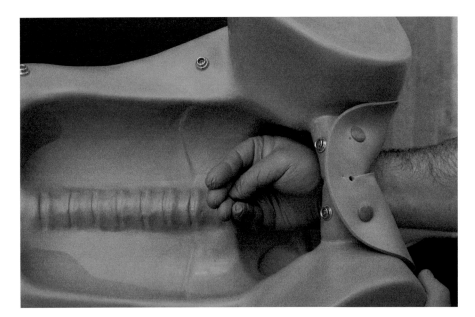

Figure 53.2 Proper placement of two thirds of the hand and the forearm in the vagina to perform elevation of the inverted uterine fundus towards the abdominal cavity. Keeping fingers as shown at the level of the uterine isthmus, proceed to lift the fundus of the uterus above the umbilicus. A black and white version of this figure will appear in some formats.

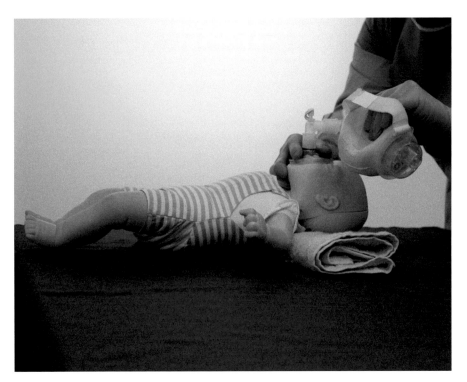

Figure 53.3 Proper neonatal ventilation requires adequate support of the mandible to ensure an open upper airway. A black and white version of this figure will appear in some formats.

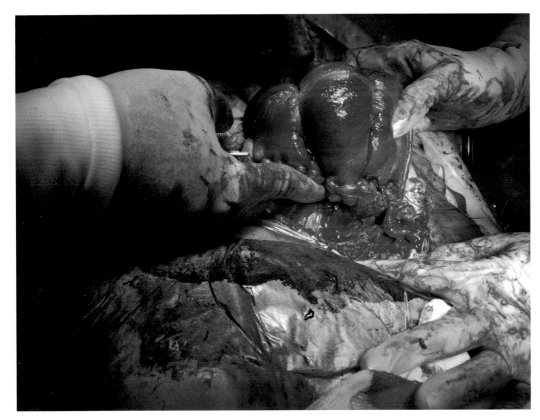

Figure 57.1 Vertical compression sutures. A black and white version of this figure will appear in some formats.

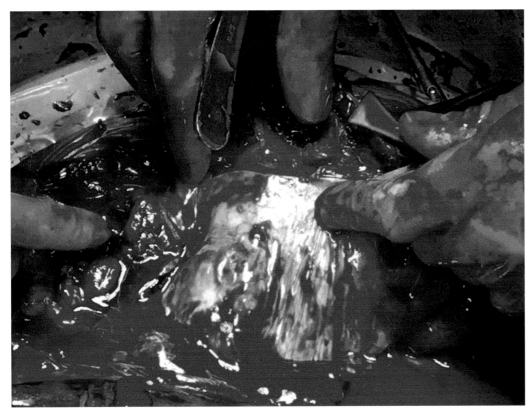

Figure 57.2 Placenta percreta. A black and white version of this figure will appear in some formats.

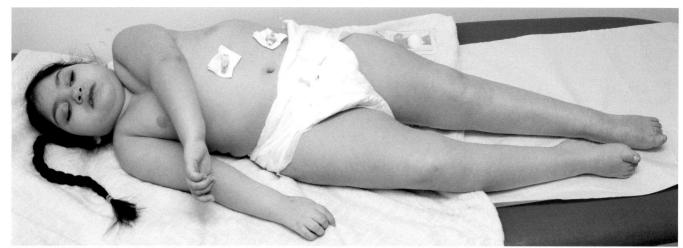

Figure 60.4 School-age child with post-HIE severe spastic tetraplegia.

A 10-year old with post-HIE spastic cerebral palsy, who is failing to grow appropriately, had recurrent chest infections, feeding difficulties (has a gastrostomy tube to clear secretions in view of severe oesophageal reflux and an ileostomy for feeds) and seizures. She also has limited awareness, communication and cognition, and global developmental delay (e.g. still requires nappies), generalized spasticity, muscle atrophy, contractures and immobility (hence, she is lying on a soft fleece rug to prevent pressure sores). A black and white version of this figure will appear in some formats.

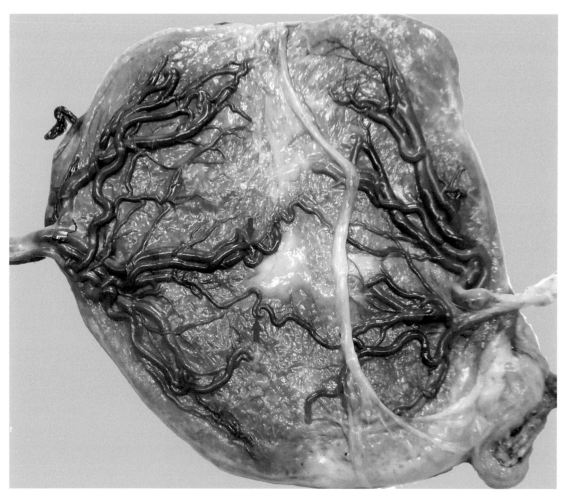

Figure 62.3 Monochorionic twin placenta with vascular anastomosis. A black and white version of this figure will appear in some formats.

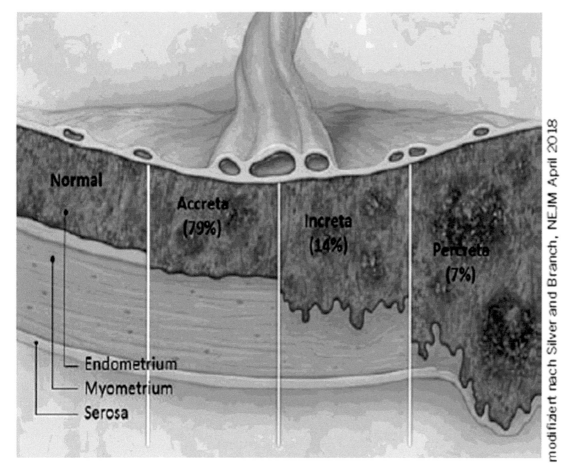

Figure 63.1 Schematic presentation of abnormally invasive placenta with its incidence. A black and white version of this figure will appear in some formats. Source: according to Hürter et al 2017 [7]

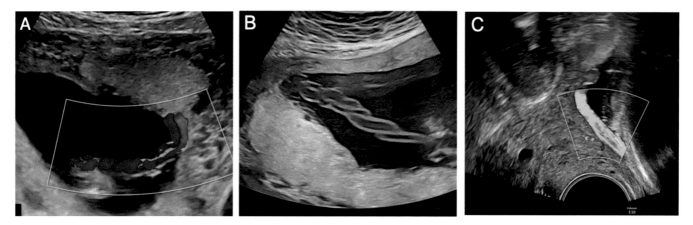

Figure 63.3 Umbilical cord abnormalities and vasa praevia – A: marginal cord insertion; B: velamentous cord insertion; C: vasa praevia. A black and white version of this figure will appear in some formats.

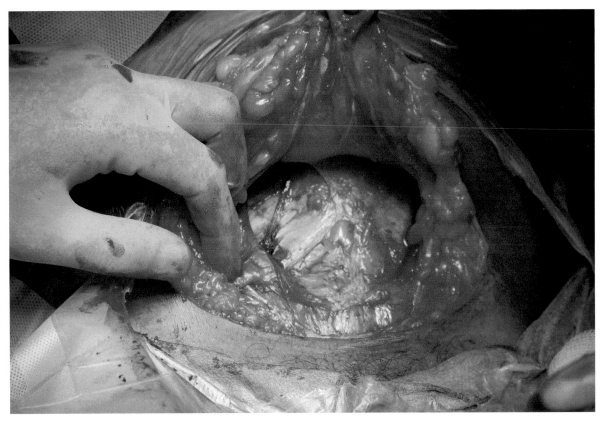

Figure 64.5 The rectus sheath is incised like a 'boat' so that the base of the incision is at a higher level. A black and white version of this figure will appear in some formats.

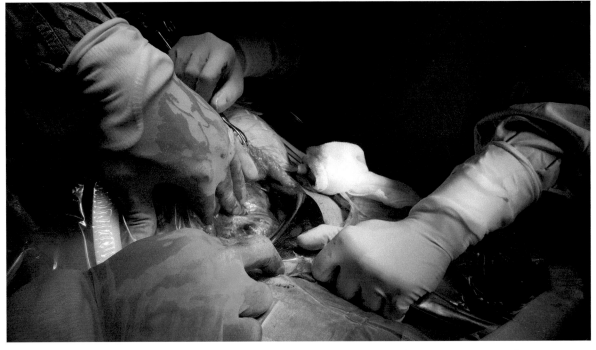

Figure 64.6 Access above the upper border of the placenta. A black and white version of this figure will appear in some formats.

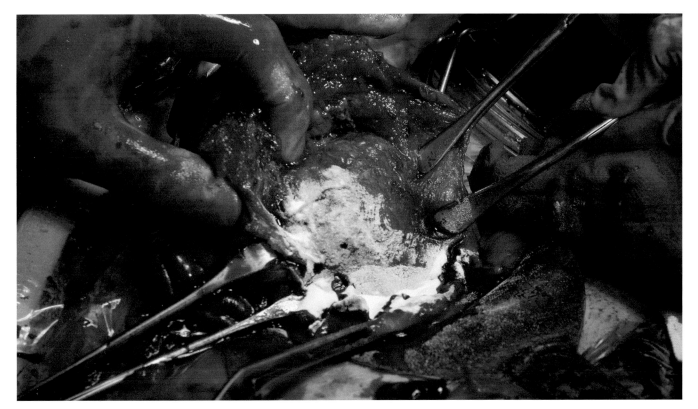

Figure 64.7 Copious amount of local haemostat (PerClot) is applied to the bleeding placental venous sinuses at the area of invasion of the urinary bladder. A black and white version of this figure will appear in some formats.

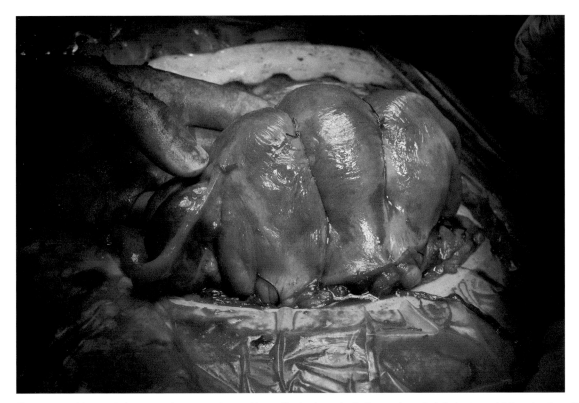

Figure 64.8 Two vertical compression sutures inserted immediately above the balloon, prior to its inflation to avoid the migration of the uterine tamponade balloon into the upper segment. A black and white version of this figure will appear in some formats.

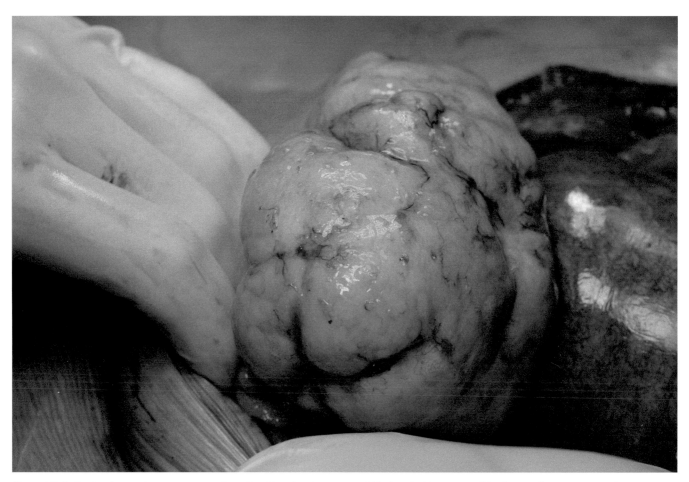

Figure 74.4 Ovarian dysgerminoma, surgery performed at 14 weeks of pregnancy. A black and white version of this figure will appear in some formats.

Psychological Disorders in Pregnancy

Sibil Tschudin

40.1 Introduction

Psychological disorders always have an impact not only on the individual, but also on all family members, especially partners and children. In the case of a pregnancy, the situation becomes even more complex, as the psychological problem and its treatment might in addition have an impact on the unborn child. Furthermore, psychological problems may compromise fertility and the course of pregnancy, as well as the peri- and postnatal period, and they might be aggravated due to pregnancy and the challenges of motherhood. Pregnancy implies emotional, physical and social changes for the mother, her partner and the rest of the family, but while many mothers greatly enjoy these changes and adapt well to them, others – and especially women at risk for or with pre-existing psychological disorders –may react with severe distress. Women´s socio-economic and cultural context features are modulators of the adaptive responses to the pregnancy, and unfavourable economic conditions or specific social circumstances make it harder to cope. In order to prevent negative long-term effects on the newborn, the mother and the entire family, early detection and adequate care of all pregnant women at risk for psychological maladjustment is of utmost importance and has an impact on mental health and well-being. This chapter describes psychological disorders pregnant women may suffer from, discusses diagnostic procedures as well as treatment options and explains preventive strategies.

40.2 Epidemiology

Psychological morbidity is in general considerably high in women of reproductive age. A systematic review and meta-analysis covering findings pooled across all studies of the period (1980–2013) indicated that on average 1 in 5 adults (17.6%) experienced a common mental disorder within the past 12 months and 29.2% across their lifetime. In high- as well as low- and middle-income countries, females were more likely to experience a mood or anxiety disorder, and males were more likely to experience an alcohol or other substance use disorder. The lifetime prevalence for women was 14.0% for mood disorders, 18.2% for anxiety disorders and 5.0% for substance use disorders, respectively [1]. These findings concur broadly with the estimates of depression and anxiety disorder prevalence produced by the Global Burden of Disease 2010 review as well as with another major source of global information on the prevalence of mood disorder, the 2002–03 *WHO World Mental Health Survey* [2, 3].

In the perinatal period particularly, mood and anxiety disorders are a common, even if often not recognized, but still taboo problem and at least as frequent during pregnancy as in the postpartum period [4, 5]. According to a large-scale retrospective observational database study conducted in Germany and including 38 000 pregnancies, the prevalence of the four distinguished categories of depression, anxiety disorders, somatoform disorders and acute stress reactions was 9.3%, 16.9%, 24.2% and 11.7%, respectively [6]. Furthermore, the prevalence of mental disorders is increasing throughout pregnancy [7, 8].

40.3 Aetiology

The variation in the presentation, course and outcomes of mental health problems in pregnancy and the postnatal period is reflected in the breadth of theoretical explanations for their aetiology, including genetic, biochemical, endocrine, psychological and social factors. Mental health problems are not unique to pregnancy and the postnatal period. Thus, the aetiological factors involved are the same as for mental health problems at other times in women's lives and include a history of psychopathology, psychosocial adversity, childhood and adulthood abuse, and lack of social support. There is evidence for heredity tendency for the trigger of postpartum psychosis and for a 'subtype' of depression characterized by a particular sensitivity to changes in reproductive hormones. Specific traumata including stillbirth, infant complications and other forms of traumatic childbirth experiences are associated with mental health problems, particularly post-traumatic stress disorder (PTSD) (Table 40.1). There is emerging evidence, as well, that refugees, asylum seekers and trafficked pregnant women are at increased risk of mental health problems [9].

40.4 Clinical Features

40.4.1 Perinatal Depression

Although research and clinical care has generally placed the greatest emphasis on the postnatal period, depression in pregnancy is also of considerable importance. According to Heron et al, the prevalence of depression during pregnancy is even higher than in the postpartum period: 11.4%, 13.1%, 8.9% and 7.9% at 18 weeks of gestation, 32 weeks of gestation, 8 weeks postpartum and 8 months postpartum, respectively [10]. Nevertheless, depression during pregnancy is a risk factor for

Table 40.1 Risk factors for perinatal depression

Affective disorders in patient history
- Number of preceding episodes
- Early onset of depression (adolescence)
- Last episode ≤6 months
- Short interval to discontinuation of antidepressants

Childhood abuse
Positive family history

Young age

Low education
Multiparity

Partnership conflicts

Socio-economic problems
Housing problems
Lack of social support

Table 40.2 Effects and consequences of perinatal depression

Pregnancy and delivery	Mother and child
Loss of appetite and weight	High risk of postpartum depression
Nicotine/ drug/alcohol consumption	Dysfunction in mother–child relationship
Malcompliance/non-adherence concerning antenatal care	Impairment of the child's neurobehavioural development
Low birthweight	Long-term effect on the child
Risk of prematurity	
Higher rate of caesarean sections	
Complications during labour	

postpartum depression. Table 40.1 gives an overview on the various risk factors of perinatal depression that have been identified [11].

During pregnancy, depression manifests itself often by atypical symptoms, such as changes in appetite and weight, anxiety and somatic complaints. Alder et al could identify nausea, premature contractions and frequent use of analgesics as indirect signs for depression [12]. Furthermore, the stress associated with pregnancy can also exacerbate the symptoms.

Depression has an impact on pregnancy and the postpartum period, on both the woman and the child (Table 40.2). Depressed pregnant women may experience loss of appetite and weight, they are more prone to nicotine/drug/alcohol consumption and they are often insufficiently compliant with regard to antenatal care. Low birthweight is more prevalent in children of depressed women. There is a higher risk for prematurity and for complications during delivery as well as for caesarean sections [7, 13–15].

Untreated depression may result in dysfunction in the mother–child relationship, in impairment of the child's neurobehavioural development and in negative long-term effects on the child [16].

40.4.2 Anxiety Disorders

A large US-population-based study found a 13% past-year prevalence of any anxiety disorder in currently pregnant or postnatal women, which was comparable to non-pregnant women [17]. Anxiety symptoms seem to be present even more frequently during pregnancy than postpartum, and there is a high level of co-morbidity with depression [10, 18, 19]. That pregnant women experience childbirth anxieties is very common, but these anxieties do generally not reach pathological levels. Precise data on

the prevalence of true fear of childbirth, be they primary, possibly pre-dating pregnancy, or secondary due to a traumatic birth experience, are lacking. Secondary fear of childbirth, however, may more helpfully be conceptualized as a trauma symptom or as part of a presentation of PTSD. A recent systematic review and meta-analysis across community samples in studies considering rates 1–18 months postnatally reported rates of 3.1% for PTSD with symptoms related specifically to childbirth [20]. Stillbirth has also been identified as a stressor for PTSD symptoms during a subsequent pregnancy [21].

40.4.3 Eating Disorders

Eating disorders (EDs), such as anorexia nervosa (AN), bulimia nervosa (BN), binge eating disorder and other specified feeding and eating disorders, are common among women of reproductive age (5–10%) and among pregnant women (5–8%). In a longitudinal population-based cohort study including 83 826 from the Danish National Birth Cohort, lifetime anorexia nervosa and lifetime anorexia and bulimia nervosa were prospectively associated with restricted fetal growth and higher odds of small-for-gestational-age (SGA) newborns compared with unexposed women. There was evidence of worse outcomes in women with active disorder [22]. Furthermore, eating disorders were also associated with an increased risk of depression and anxiety in pregnancy and the postnatal period [23].

40.4.4. Psychotic Disorders (schizophrenia, bipolar disorder and postpartum psychosis)

There are limited data on the prevalence and incidence of psychotic disorders in pregnancy. However, in women with high levels of depressive symptoms in pregnancy and in the postnatal period, Lydsdottir et al and Wisner et al reported bipolar disorders rates of 13% and 22%, respectively [18, 19]. Prospective cohort studies suggest an increased risk of relapse of psychotic disorders in pregnancy in women with bipolar disorder who discontinue prophylactic medication such as mood stabilizers [24]. There is little evidence on the course of schizophrenia in pregnancy. For women with bipolar disorders, both retrospective and population registry studies suggest at least a 1 in 5 risk of having a severe recurrence following childbirth [24]. This increased risk of relapse occurs in the first few months after childbirth for women with bipolar disorder and for women with schizophrenia throughout the first postnatal year [25]. It remains an issue of controversy whether the so-called postpartum psychosis is a distinct diagnosis. Commonly it takes the form of mania, severe depression or a mixed episode. It is characterized by early onset in the postpartum period up to 3 months after childbirth and has an incidence rate of about 1 in 1000 deliveries.

40.4.5 Drug and Alcohol Use Disorders

Drug and alcohol misuse in pregnancy are markers of complex pregnancies, multiple co-morbidities and adverse obstetric outcomes, and are often associated with limited access to healthcare during pregnancy. Obviously, the exact number of drug-dependent women is unknown because epidemiological data rely almost exclusively on voluntary patient reports. Substance abuse not only harms the patient herself but also the unborn child. Table 40.3 shows a summary of the effects of different substances on mother and child. Problems include preterm labour and low birthweight in general as well as teratogenic effects in the case of alcohol and specific complications such as myocardial infarction, cerebrovascular accidents and placental abruption in cocaine-using women, owing to the vasoconstrictive effects of the drug. Examining direct effects of specific drugs, however, is challenging since most of the women are poly-drug users. The fact that the effects on mother and child are likely to be multifactorial complicates care even more. Factors such as smoking, poor diet, stress and chaotic lifestyle appear to be the most important contributing factors. Furthermore, there is a paucity of research regarding newer drugs such as Ecstasy, bath salts or synthetic cannabinoids [26].

40.5 Investigations

Considering the impact and unfavourable long-term effects on mother and child of psychological disorders during pregnancy and postpartum – especially if undetected and untreated – early detection is of utmost importance. Perinatal care varies from country to country, and consequently it might be predominantly in the hands of obstetricians, midwives or general practitioners. All health professionals in charge of perinatal care should be familiar with the symptomatology of psychological disorders in pregnancy and with diagnostic and screening procedures. Aside from anxiety disorders, depression is the most prevalent psychological problem in the perinatal period and fortunately, with the depression-screening (Whooley) questions in combination with the Edinburgh Postnatal Depression Scale (EPDS), there exists a valid strategy to screen for this condition [27, 28]. Considering the risk factors for depression, attention should also be paid to experience of (partnership) violence and symptoms of PTSD . Pregnancy is in fact a period of high risk for domestic violence (DV) occurring for the first time or escalating during this period [29]. This speaks for a systematic or at least opportunistic screening for DV during pregnancy, which seems generally well received and accepted by pregnant women, provided that health professionals carefully choose adequate wording and the right moment to ask questions and can give advice, in case the patient discloses recent or current experiences of DV (Table 40.4).

To date no well-established screening tools for other than depressive disorders exist. Therefore, history taking that includes questions about previous psychological problems of the pregnant woman and her family as well as current symptoms of anxiety, eating habits and alcohol and illicit drug use are crucial. For a woman with history of a past or current psychiatric condition, counselling should ideally start before conception. The severity of the mental health problem can then be assessed in time; psychotropic medication can be checked for compatibility with pregnancy and lactation and be adapted if necessary. Many women are reluctant to disclose psychological distress to others, including caregivers, because of the stigma of mental illness. Furthermore, a woman might be hesitant to disclose her mental health problems due to fears about loss of custody of her newborn or other children. Attention should therefore be paid to providing a safe environment and access to non-stigmatizing support that is regarded by women as appropriate to their needs.

40.6 Clinical Management

Considering the consequences of untreated mental health problems during pregnancy, routine antenatal care should include mental health aspects and should include optimization of the woman's psychological well-being and the provision of psychosocial support. This is best assured when health professionals consider the biopsychosocial model of care and chose an interdisciplinary approach, in all cases where basic psychosocial support turns out to be insufficiently effective. When a woman is not pregnant or caring for her baby, she is the sole focus of care and treatment. In pregnancy and the postnatal period, however, the emphasis shifts to a concern for the fetus and baby as well as the woman, which can contribute to different and difficult experiences of care, particularly where the needs of the mother and fetus or baby conflict. Even if the use of any medication during pregnancy has to be considered carefully, discontinuation of a treatment is discouraged, in case of a pre-existing, psychiatric disorder requiring psychotropic medication. Ideally, a necessary adaptation of the dosage or a change to another preparation occurs in close collaboration with the attending psychiatrist.

40.6.1 Treatment of Perinatal Depression

First line treatment for clinically relevant depressive symptoms during pregnancy or in the postpartum period is psychosocial support and/or psychotherapy. There is evidence that especially cognitive behavioural therapy (CBT) has a beneficial effect on depressive symptoms during pregnancy. If this approach is not sufficiently efficient and the severity of the symptoms affords it, adequate medication with antidepressants should be started. No consistent association between use of antidepressant medication during pregnancy and negative long-term effects on the child has been demonstrated, and the potential impact of maternal psychiatric illness on the child should be taken into account when considering drug use during pregnancy [30]. Dosage of selective serotonin reuptake inhibitors (SSRIs) should be as low as possible, but as high as

Table 40.3 Drug effects on mother and child

Drug/Substance	Effects on mother	Effects on fetus
Opiates (heroine, methadone, morphine)	- Constipation - Vasodilation - Drug interactions (pulmonary oedema, β2-sympathomimetics) - Premature contractions - Protracted delivery	- SGA - Prematurity - IUGR - Intrauterine demise - Withdrawal symptoms - SIDS - Impaired intellectual development
Cocaine	- Loss of appetite, sleep - Increased sympathetic activity - Reduced placental perfusion - Placental abruption - Premature contractions - Hypertension - Cerebrovascular events - Myocardial infarction	- SGA - IUGR - Prematurity - Intrauterine demise - Malformations (heart and musculoskeletal, urogenital tract) - Microcephalus - Perinatal cerebral infarction
Cannabis resp. THC	- Increased sympathetic activity - (General vasoconstriction) - Placental abruption - Formation of ketone bodies (*cave* gestational diabetes!) - Convulsions (*cave* pre-eclampsia, premature contractions)	- SGA - IUGR - Prematurity - Impaired postnatal intellectual development
Amphetamines/ Ecstasy	- Increased sympathetic activity - Mental hyperactivity - Compulsive chewing - Dysfunctional thermoregulation - Constriction of placental vessels - Placental abruption	- Fetal distress - IUGR - Malformations (heart, skeleton)
LSD	- Increased sympathetic activity - Visual hallucination - Panic attacks	- Chromosomal aberrations - Skeletal dysplasias (hands, feet) - Ocular dysplasia (suspected)
Alcohol	- Gastric hyperacidity - Sedation - Tocolytic effect	- FASD / FAS facial dysmorphogenesis, cardiac septal effects, joint abnormalities

SGA: small for gestational age; IUGR: intrauterine growth restriction; SIDS: sudden infant death syndrome; FASD / FAS: fetal alcohol spectrum disorder / fetal alcohol syndrome

needed. Sertraline or citalopram are the preferred SSRI, above all during the third trimester. Antenatal medication can be reduced as much as possible to prevent neonatal behavioural syndrome, but the perinatal risk of relapse has to be considered.

40.6.2 Management of Drug and Alcohol Use Disorders during Pregnancy

Pregnancies of drug-using women should be considered as potential high-risk pregnancies. Aspects that might be neglected when assessing drug-using women are concomitant factors such as cigarette smoking, alcohol use and poor social circumstances, which are all common in women using illicit drugs. Institutionalized toxicology screenings are recommended since they are more easily accepted. This can be in the form of questionnaires or urine drug tests. Most importantly, the screening tools have to be consistent and easy to use, and the care team should approach the patient in a non-judgemental way.

Nowadays, there is consensus that drug-using pregnant women are in need of multidisciplinary prenatal care with medical, social and psychological support. Research suggests that comprehensive, interdisciplinary treatment programmes have a positive impact on outcomes. Depending on the individual situation and needs for care, disciplines such as drug

Table 40.4 Screening for depression

Step 1:
Ask 2 screening questions according to Whooley:
1) During the past month, have you often been bothered by feeling down, depressed or hopeless?
2) During the past month, have you often been bothered by little interest or pleasure in doing things?
Interpretation: If both questions are answered with yes, there is need for further investigation with regard to a depressive disorder
→ step 2

Step 2:
Edinburgh Postnatal Depression Scale (EPDS):
10 items; scoring range 0–3 each; maximum score 30
Interpretation: cut-off >10 affords further clinical investigations for a depressive disorder

substitution centres, social workers, neonatologists, psychiatrists, paediatric psychiatrists and child welfare authorities have to be involved [26].

40.6.3 Management during Delivery and Postpartum

Giving birth is a unique experience for every woman, and individual reactions may sometimes be unpredictable, especially in women with a psychosocial disorder. Thus, assisting at the birth of a woman with a personality, psychotic or anxiety disorder can be particularly challenging for the obstetrician and midwife in charge. A timely discussion and decision making with regard to the mode of delivery are highly recommended.

Special attention should be paid to the care of women with a drug disorder. At presentation in the delivery ward, midwives and obstetricians need to be aware of unusual behaviour or agitation. They have to pay attention to physiological signs of drug abuse, such as dilated or constricted pupils, increased or decreased respirations, bradycardia or tachycardia, hypotension or hypertension, all depending on the substance used. These can be both signs of intoxication and of withdrawal and should prompt further testing to confirm drug use and rule out pre-eclampsia. As substance use and smoking are associated with an increased risk of placental insufficiency, growth restriction and possible fetal distress, monitoring has to be especially thorough. Neonatal care should be readily available in the maternity ward. Postnatal care needs to be adjusted to the needs (e.g. withdrawal signs) of the newborn.

Breastfeeding is beneficial in a number of ways and facilitates bonding. As women with psychosocial disorders often have difficulties in building a relationship with the child, breastfeeding might be particularly advisable. Drug-using women should be encouraged to breastfeed, depending on the substitution and parallel consumption of other drugs; breastfeeding might even reduce the severity of neonatal

withdrawal symptoms. For women under psychotropic medication, the decision for or against breastfeeding depends on the available evidence concerning effects on the neonate of the substances concerned.

Support and counselling by a paediatric psychiatrist with respect to all questions around bonding may reasonably complement psychiatric and/or psychosocial care of the mother. Furthermore, including the partner and other family members at all stages of care is crucial as well.

40.7 Key Messages

- Psychological morbidity is in general considerably high in women of reproductive age.
- In the perinatal period, particularly mood and anxiety disorders are a common, even if often not recognized, and still a taboo problem in pregnant women.
- Mood and anxiety disorders are at least as frequent during pregnancy as in the postpartum period.
- Psychological problems during pregnancy have an impact not only on the woman herself, but also on the unborn.
- In women with known psychological disorders or at risk for developing perinatal depression, care should start when a pregnancy is intended, be maintained throughout pregnancy and extend beyond delivery.
- Continuity of care and support is crucial and should be warranted even beyond the early postpartum.

40.8 Key Guidelines

The NICE guideline *Antenatal and Postnatal Mental Health: Clinical Management and Service Guidance* provides excellent pathways and defined quality standards for the care of women with mental health problems from pre-conception counselling throughout pregnancy to the postpartum period (www.nice.org.uk/guidance/cg192).

References

1. Steel Z, Marnane C, Iranpour C, et al. The global prevalence of common mental disorders: a systematic review and meta-analysis 1980–2013. *Int J Epidemiol.* 2014;**43**(2):476–93.

2. Kessler RC, Ustun TB, eds. *The WHO World Mental Health Surveys. Global Perspectives on the Epidemiology of Mental Disorders.* Cambridge: Cambridge University Press; 2010.

3. Murray CJL, Vos T, Lozano R, et al. Disability-adjusted life years (DALYs) for 291 diseases and injuries in 21 regions, 1990–2010: a systematic analysis for the Global Burden of Disease Study 2010. *Lancet.* 2012;**380**(9859):2197–223.

4. O'Hara M. Postpartum depression: what we know. *J Clin Psychol.* 2009;**65** (12):1258–69.

5. O'Hara MW, Wisner KL. Perinatal mental illness: definition, description and aetiology. *Best Pract Res Clin Obstet Gynaecol.* 2014;**28**(1):3–12.

6. Wallwiener S, Goetz M, Lanfer A, et al. Epidemiology of mental disorders during pregnancy and link to birth outcome: a large-scale retrospective observational database study including 38,000 pregnancies. *Arch Gynecol Obstet.* 2019;**299**(3):755–63.

7. Bennett HA, Einarson A, Taddio A, et al. Prevalence of depression during pregnancy: systematic review. *Obstet Gynecol.* 2004;**103**(4):698–709.

8. Gaynes BN, Gavin N, Meltzer-Brody S, et al. Perinatal depression: prevalence, screening accuracy, and screening outcomes. *AHRQ Evidence Report Summary,* 2005(119):1–8.

9. NICE. *Antenatal and Postnatal Mental Health: Management and Service Guidance,* Clinical Guideline 192. 17 December 2014. Updated 11 February 2020.

10. Heron J, O'Connor TG, Evans J, et al. The course of anxiety and depression through pregnancy and the postpartum in a community sample. *J Affect Disord.* 2004;**80**(1):65–73.

11. Yonkers KA, Vigod S, Ross LE. Diagnosis, pathophysiology, and management of mood disorders in pregnant and postpartum women. *Obstet Gynecol.* 2011;**117**(4):961–77.

12. Alder J, Fink N, Urech C, et al. Identification of antenatal depression in obstetric care. *Arch Gynecol Obstet.* 2011;**284**(6):1403–9.

13. Evans J, Heron J, Patel R, et al. Depressive symptoms during pregnancy and low birth weight at term: longitudinal study. *Br J Psychiatry.* 2007;**191**:84–5.

14. Grigoriadis, S., VonderPorten EH, Mamisashvili L, et al. The impact of maternal depression during pregnancy on perinatal outcomes: a systematic review and meta-analysis. *J Clin Psychiatry.* 2013;**74**(4):e321–41.

15. Kelly RH, Russo J, Katon W. Somatic complaints among pregnant women cared for in obstetrics: normal pregnancy or depressive and anxiety symptom amplification revisited? *Gen Hosp Psychiatry.* 2001;**23**(3):107–13.

16. Field T. Prenatal depression effects on early development: a review. *Infant Behav Dev.* 2011;**34**(1):1–14.

17. Vesga-Lopez O, Blanco C, Keyes K, et al. Psychiatric disorders in pregnant and postpartum women in the United States. *Arch Gen Psychiatry.* 2008;**65** (7):805–15.

18. Lydsdottir LB, Howard LM, Olafsdottir H, et al. The mental health characteristics of pregnant women with depressive symptoms identified by the Edinburgh Postnatal Depression Scale. *J Clin Psychiatry.* 2014;**75**(4):393–8.

19. Wisner KL, Sit DKY, McShea MC, et al. Onset timing, thoughts of self-harm, and diagnoses in postpartum women with screen-positive depression findings. *JAMA Psychiatry.* 2013;**70** (5):490–8.

20. Grekin R, O'Hara MW. Prevalence and risk factors of postpartum posttraumatic stress disorder: a meta-analysis. *Clin Psychology Rev.* 2014;**34**(5):389–401.

21. Turton, P, Hughes P, Evans CD, Fainman D. Incidence, correlates and predictors of post-traumatic stress disorder in the pregnancy after stillbirth. *Br J Psychiatry.* 2001;**178**: 556–60.

22. Micali, N. Size at birth and preterm birth in women with lifetime eating disorders: a prospective population-based study. *BJOG.* 2016;**123**(8):1301–10.

23. Micali, N., Simonoff E, Treasure J. Pregnancy and post-partum depression and anxiety in a longitudinal general population cohort: the effect of eating disorders and past depression. *J Affect Disord.* 2011;**131**(1–3):150–7.

24. Viguera AC. Risk of recurrence in women with bipolar disorder during pregnancy: prospective study of mood stabilizer discontinuation. *Am J Psychiatry.* 2007;**164**(12):1817–24; quiz 1923.

25. Munk-Olsen T. Risks and predictors of readmission for a mental disorder during the postpartum period. *Arch Gen Psychiatry.* 2009;**66**(2):189–95.

26. Goettler SM, Tschudin S. Care of drug-addicted pregnant women: current concepts and future strategies – an overview. *Womens Health (Lond).* 2014;**10**(2):167–77.

27. Cox JL, Holden JM, Sagovsky R. Detection of postnatal depression. Development of the 10-item Edinburgh Postnatal Depression Scale. *Br J Psychiatry.* 1987;**150**:782–6.

28. Gibson J, McKenzie-McHarg K, Shakespeare J, Price J, Gray R. A systematic review of studies validating the Edinburgh Postnatal Depression Scale in antepartum and postpartum women. *Acta Psychiatr Scand.* 2009;**119**(5):350–64.

29. James L, Brody D, Hamilton Z. Risk factors for domestic violence during pregnancy: a meta-analytic review. *Violence Victims.* 2013;**28**(3):359–80.

30. Chisolm MS, Payne JL. Management of psychotropic drugs during pregnancy. *BMJ.* 2016;**532**:h5918.

Chapter 41

Pregnancy after Solid Organ Transplantation

Giuseppe Benagiano, Patrick Puttemans & Ivo Brosens

41.1 Introduction

Over the past 50 years, thousands of young women have attempted pregnancy after solid vital organ transplantation, often with full success. In theory, since pregnancy induces a state of immunotolerance, gestation should not pose any specific threat [1]. Unfortunately, data available from the Transplantation Pregnancy Registry tell a different story: gestation following a solid organ transplant is associated with an increased risk of major obstetric syndromes, including preterm birth and fetal growth restriction, pre-eclampsia and pregnancy-induced hypertension. Collectively these complications are known as the 'Great Obstetric Syndromes' (GOS) [2]. Given this reality, close follow-up must not end at delivery, and specific care must become part of the woman's reproductive healthcare needs.

Professional information must be provided on all aspects of pre- and post-conceptional care for these women, as well as on the type of post-pregnancy healthcare most beneficial to them. Detailed information must include: (a) the incidence of major obstetric syndromes following different solid organ transplantation; (b) the unique risks associated with uterus transplantation; (c) a description of the critical uterine functions affected by solid organ transplantation; (d) the kind of post-delivery care to be given to these women and their babies, including guidelines for breastfeeding.

This group of women requires a multidisciplinary team (MDT) approach for continuous management to monitor not only the woman's care, but also that of the fetus in what should always be considered a high-risk pregnancy.

Finding the most efficient way to deliver appropriate care to the population of transplanted individuals can be usefully employed in improving pregnancy outcomes in women with a solid organ transplant.

41.2 Historical Overview

In 1960, Murray et al [3] published an evaluation of 6 patients who had received bone marrow, kidney or skin homotransplantation, followed by total body irradiation. Of these, the only long-term success was obtained in the case in which the donor was the biovular twin; she conceived within 2 years of the transplantation, without any immunosuppressive treatment, and delivered twice by caesarean section two healthy babies at term [4].

Then, in 1986, the first case was published of a successful pregnancy following kidney–pancreas transplantation. This woman had been diabetic for 24 years and became pregnant at age 33. She received immunosuppression with cyclosporine throughout gestation and she was delivered by caesarean section at 35 weeks, soon after becoming hypertensive [5].

Almost 30 years later, the first successful pregnancy and delivery occurred in a woman with a transplanted heart, who was treated throughout pregnancy with cyclosporine and prednisone and delivered vaginally with a satisfactory outcome for both the mother and the newborn [6]. A full review of 29 pregnancies in allograft heart recipients and 3 in women with a heart–lung graft reported that two thirds of the women delivered vaginally, and common complications were hypertension in 44%, premature labour in 30% and pre-eclampsia in 22% [7]. The first case of pregnancy after bilateral lung transplantation was reported in 1996, complicated by acute and chronic allograft rejection, resulting in irreversible loss of lung function [8].

The first live birth from a transplanted uterus occurred at 32 weeks, following the development of pre-eclampsia in 2015 [9]. A 33-year-old woman with Mayer–Rokitansky–Küster–Hauser syndrome delivered at 36 weeks a live infant following donor uterus transplantation in 2017 [10].

It seems therefore that pregnancy has become an integral part of the expectations of women to whom a vital organ had been grafted, and successful pregnancy is today included among the benefits granted to these women. In spite of thousands of successful pregnancies in transplant recipients, full information on the expected course, the likelihood of pregnancy and the anticipated fetal outcomes in these patients, up to some 10 years ago, information on the subject was considered unsatisfactory even for the most frequent type of graft, the kidney [11]. It is for this reason that in 2014 a full issue of the journal *Best Practice & Research: Clinical Obstetrics and Gynaecology* was dedicated to the subject [12].

41.3 Fertility in Transplanted Women

The effect of a solid organ transplantation on fertility was reviewed a little over 10 years ago [13]. With regard to kidney disease, although treatment of end-stage renal failure with repeated peritoneal dialysis and haemodialysis improves the patient's general health, reduced fertility persists. Grafting results in a major improvement, although it seems that restoration of normal function of the hypothalamic-pituitary-ovarian (HPO) axis after renal transplantation is primarily influenced by graft efficiency. Poor contraceptive practices seemed to be responsible for a high frequency of unintended pregnancy, reaching in one study 48.5% [14]. In the case of liver grafts, it seems that in young patients who underwent transplantation early in adolescence, mean age at menarche was statistically significantly delayed [15].

Several surveys have been carried out on fertility, contraception and pre-conception counselling in women who had received a solid organ graft [16–18]; one study reported that before transplantations, 44% of the women were not aware that they could become pregnant. Another study showed that, in general, transplant patients were being counselled against attempting pregnancy, in spite of acceptable risks of complications and no specific effects on long-term graft function. A third study indicated that the most common contraceptive method used in both the year preceding transplant and the year after transplant was condoms, concluding that recipients of solid organ transplants need better counselling on highly effective methods.

It has been known that women with chronic renal failure suffer from hyperprolactinaemia with an increased luteinizing hormone to follicle-stimulating hormone (LH-to-FSH) ratio [19], leading to gonadal dysfunction of mainly hypothalamic origin [20, 21]. As the condition progresses, menstrual patterns become unpredictable, leading in a majority of cases to oligomenorrhoea and amenorrhoea [22]. Menstrual irregularities persist in the vast majority of these women while undergoing dialysis, but following transplantation and in the presence of a stable kidney function, most women resume normal menstrual cycles [23] and premature ovarian failure seems to be a rare event.

Women with severe liver disfunction may be also be affected by disturbances of the hypothalamic-pituitary-ovarian axis and suffer from menstrual abnormalities, possibly related in part to the consequences of metabolic abnormalities and substance abuse (i.e. alcoholism) [24]. Amenorrhoea is common also in women with non-alcoholic chronic liver disease, and there is a great variance in serum concentrations of testosterone, oestradiol, prolactin, FSH and LH, leading to the conclusion that amenorrhoea in these subjects arises from hypothalamic-pituitary dysfunction and can occur at any stage of the disease. Findings, however, are not uniform: in some cases, amenorrhoea is associated to hypo-oestrogenism and related to undernutrition, whereas in others LH and oestrogen are normal or even high. When oestradiol levels are elevated, this may be due, at least in part, to a portosystemic shunting of less potent androgens and to peripheral oestrogen conversion [25]. In this case too, liver transplant improves the situation and restores a normal menstrual pattern, although it has been estimated that up to 50% of women of reproductive age with end-stage liver disease will remain subfertile after receiving a grafted liver [26].

Women receiving a heart transplant may be fertile, although they would have been discouraged from becoming pregnant in view of the inherent risks that gestation may induce in these subjects. In particular, if heart transplantation had been performed because of a congenital condition, such as mitochondrial myopathies, dilated cardiomyopathy, etc., offspring are at risk of similar anomalies and a pre-conception genetic counselling is warranted [24].

41.4 Outcome of Pregnancy in Solid Organ Recipients

Data on the outcome of pregnancies, as well as the risk of major obstetric syndromes after solid organ transplantation, are available through various registries: the National Transplantation Pregnancy Registry (NTPR) [27] in the USA, now renamed the Transplantation Pregnancy Registry International (TPR) [28] (Table 41.1); the United Kingdom Transplant Pregnancy Registry [29]; the Australia and New Zealand Dialysis and Transplant Registry (ANZDATA) and the Australian National Perinatal Epidemiology and Statistics Unit (NPESU) [30, 31]; the Italian Registry of Dialysis and Transplantation [32], the French Organ Transplant Data System [33] and the German data collection system [34]. Information has also been published about a number of other countries (e.g. Hungary [35], Sweden [36], Spain [37]).

The comparison of pregnancy outcomes after kidney and liver transplantation shows a significant increase in the risk of major obstetric complications, including pre-eclampsia (PE), preterm birth (PTB) and low birthweight (LBW) [28].

41.4.1 Kidney

Pregnancy outcomes in recipients of kidney transplants have been evaluated through systematic reviews and meta-analyses. A study in the *American Journal of Transplantation* [38] reported on 4706 pregnancies in 3570 recipients, with an overall live birth and miscarriage rates higher than the general US population (73.5% vs. 66.7% and 14.0% vs. 17.1%, respectively). Conversely, pregnancy complications, such as PE (27.0%), gestational diabetes (8.0%) and PTB (45.6%) were significantly higher than the general US population (3.8%, 3.9% and 12.5%, respectively).

Another large study, based on data from the ANZDATA and the NPESU, reported on 695 pregnancies in 447 kidney transplant recipients [39]. The mean gestational age at birth was 35±5 weeks in transplant recipients, significantly shorter than the national average of 39 weeks (P<0.0001). The mean

Table 41.1 Transplant pregnancy registry topics

- Pregnancy Registry Annual and Overall Statistical Reports
- Contraception for Transplant Recipients
- Kidney Transplantation and Pregnancy
- Liver Transplantation and Pregnancy
- Kidney/Pancreas Transplantation and Pregnancy
- Heart Transplantation and Pregnancy
- Lung Transplantation and Pregnancy
- Immunosuppressive Medications during Pregnancy
- Teratology and Immunosuppressive Medications
- Pregnancy after Paediatric Transplantation
- Obstetric Management of Transplant Recipients
- Breastfeeding while on Immunosuppression
- Fatherhood after Transplantation
- Follow-up Reports on the Offspring of Transplant Recipient

From [28]

live birthweight for transplant recipients was lower than the national average (2485±783 vs. 3358±2 g), a difference that remained significant after controlling for gestational age.

In Sweden, the outcome of pregnancy in women recipients of a renal graft who conceived spontaneously has been compared to that in women submitted to in vitro fertilization and embryo transfer (IVF-ET) [40]. There were 199 single births after a renal graft in subjects who conceived spontaneously. The rates of PE (23.6%), PTB (48.5%), LBW (43.7%) and small for gestational age (SGA) (21.2%) were significantly higher than in pregnancies with no transplantation. Follow-up for a mean of 14.7 years of the children of grafted mothers indicated that acute bronchitis, systemic lupus erythematosus and hyperactivity disorders were more common. The study reported on 7 singletons and one set of twins. Two of the single pregnancies ended in PTB, one had a very LBW neonate (672 g) and one was SGA. Two infants had minor birth defects. One woman developed PE.

A long-term retrospective study evaluated maternal and fetal outcomes and the evolution of graft function in 22 pregnancies in young subjects (mean age 22.32; range, 19.45–33.1 years) post-kidney and kidney–pancreas transplantation and there was an increased frequency of PE, PTB and LBW. Graft failure was higher (although non-significantly) among subjects who had become pregnant [41].

Pregnancy after kidney transplantation seems to produce a significant increase of mean serum creatinine from baseline to the third trimester of pregnancy, and this negative effect was maintained at follow-up (Table 41.2).

Guidelines aimed at optimizing pregnancy outcomes after kidney transplantation have now been proposed [42]. An ideal profile of the potential mother includes normal kidney function (e.g. a glomerular filtration rate (GFR) ≥60 mL/min), scant or no proteinuria, normal or well-controlled blood pressure, no recent acute rejection, good compliance and low-dose immunosuppression).

It can be concluded that pregnancies after kidney transplantation are generally successful but can be associated with serious maternal and fetal complications.

41.4.2 Kidney–Pancreas Transplants

The International Pancreas Transplant Registry (IPTR) provides data on a total of 9012 pancreatic transplants [43]. Nineteen pregnancies were recorded in 17 female recipients of simultaneous pancreas–kidney transplants and resulted in 19 live births. Metabolic control during pregnancy was satisfactory in all cases. Mean duration of gestation was 35.2 ± 2.2

weeks. Mean birthweight was 2150 ± 680 g. One pancreas and one kidney graft were lost in two different recipients.

Subsequently, single successful cases have been reported: in one instance [44], the baby was delivered at 35 weeks because of maternal hypertension; in another case [45], delivery was anticipated at 30 weeks because of deterioration in renal indices; the infant weighed 1.18 kg, appropriate for the gestational age. In a third instance, an unplanned and unexpected pregnancy was incidentally discovered at around 18 weeks' gestation in a woman recipient of an intestine–pancreas transplant. She had chronic graft dysfunction and needed immunosuppression and parenteral nutrition at the time of conception. Yet, a healthy infant was delivered vaginally at term [46]. Finally, a small series reported on 6 gestations all delivered by caesarean section at a mean gestational age of 32.8 weeks with an LBW [47].

Unusual but serious complications have been reported in one case where a dilated right fallopian tube strongly suggested an ectopic pregnancy and salpingectomy was performed. No pancreatic dysfunction occurred subsequently [48]. Another serious problem related to pregnancy, but observed in non-pregnant recipients, consisted in the transmission of an undiagnosed choriocarcinoma in a pregnant multiple organ donor [40]. Interestingly, the recipient of the combined pancreas–kidney remained in complete remission 2 years after the beginning of chemotherapy without removal of the grafted organs, which showed optimal function. The second kidney was quickly removed from a second recipient, who is also in remission, whereas the recipient of the liver showed intestinal metastases and died from digestive haemorrhage; diffuse metastases were found also in the heart of the recipient [49].

41.4.3 Liver Transplants

A systematic review and meta-analysis of articles published between 2000 and 2011 provided information on outcomes of pregnancies in liver transplant recipients [50]. It included data from 8 studies for a total of 450 pregnancies in 306 recipient women. The review found that live birth rates for women with a liver graft were higher and miscarriage rates were lower than rates for the US general population (76.9% vs. 66.7% and 15.6% vs. 17.1%, respectively). However, complications rates were higher than in the general population: for PE they were 21.9% vs. 3.8%; and for PTB 39.4% vs. 12.5%. Interestingly, these rates were lower than the post-kidney transplant rates. Mean gestational age and mean birthweight were highly significantly greater for liver vs. kidney recipients.

Table 41.2 Pregnancy after kidney transplantation

Variable	Baseline	1 Trimester	2 Trimester	3 Trimester	Follow-up	p
Serum creatinine, mg/dL	1.19±0.07	1.08±0.07	1.17±0.10	1.47±0.15	1.59±0.20	<0.001
Estimated GFR, mL/ min/1.73m^2	72.23±26.77	81.10±27.01	80.98±34.66	60.75±23.42	62.04±25.90	<0.001
Proteinuria, g/L	08±0.2	0.12±0.03	0.18±0.05	0.40±0.08	0.28±0.06	<0.001

From [111]

In Japan, a national survey following living donor grafts collected information on 38 pregnancies in 30 recipients with 31 live births, 3 induced first trimester abortions, 1 miscarriage and 3 fetal deaths. Complications included PTB (<37 weeks), pregnancy-induced hypertension, and fetal growth restriction (FGR). Acute rejection developed during 2 pregnancies [51]. Biopsy-proven acute cellular rejection occurred in 15% of another series from Japan [52].

Recently published series confirmed both the success and complications in pregnancies after liver transplantation [53, 54]. In 2018 a publication detailed the outcomes of 41 pregnancies in 28 transplanted women, 6 of whom conceived following a second liver transplant after the first was rejected [55]. Maternal complications included pregnancy-induced hypertension (n = 10), deterioration in renal function (n = 6), gestational diabetes (n = 4) and graft deterioration (n = 2). There were 2 miscarriages, 3 stillbirths, 1 neonatal death and 5 small-for-gestational-age infants. Mean gestational age at delivery was 36.7±4.2 weeks, with 14 (38.9%) PTBs. They concluded that immunosuppressants and high-dose glucocorticoids can be safely used for maintenance of graft function and management of graft deterioration during gestation. Finally, also in 2018, using the liver transplant database of Birmingham (UK), morbidities and outcomes of 139 pregnancies occurring between August 1986 and May 2016 were evaluated in 83 women. Overall, 69% of the pregnancies resulted in live births, 19% in miscarriages or stillbirths and 9% were terminated. Tacrolimus exposure was associated with a higher risk of premature delivery and caesarean section than cyclosporine exposure [56].

An attempt has been made at identifying factors predictive of adverse pregnancy outcomes in liver transplant recipients using clinical information of 162 conceptions in 93 women with a live birth rate of 75% and a prematurity rate of 35%. Preconception creatinine levels were higher in patients who had a preterm birth (P = 0.008); pre-conception glomerular filtration rate (GFR) <90 mL/minute was significantly associated with preterm delivery (P = 0.04); gestational length declined with increasing chronic kidney disease; risk of PTB was greatest in women with a GFR <60 mL/minute (P = 0.004) [57].

Finally, there have been a few cases of liver transplant during pregnancy for acute liver failure; one in particular had a successful outcome [58].

41.4.4 Heart Transplantation

In order to minimize risks for both the mother and the fetus, pregnancy after heart grafting requires adequate preconception counselling aimed at identifying optimal timing and modifying immunosuppressive therapy [59].

Following the first successful pregnancy after heart transplantation in 1988 [6], the 2010 NTPR report [27] indicated an incidence of PE for cardiac recipients of 18%, lower than that seen in kidney transplant recipients, but higher than the 2.7% in healthy nulliparous women [60]. A comprehensive review in 2012 [61] included 103 pregnancies in 58 recipients, reporting that the risk of PE increases after this type of grafting. Management of a gestation in women with a heart graft was reviewed in 2015 [62] and concluded that with careful planning, monitoring and

appropriate therapies, pregnancy is a viable option in select patients. Recently, a report of 12 pregnancies in 11 women showed that gestation was basically uneventful, without severe complications or rejections. As invariably reported in these cases, birthweight rates were in the lower range in most of the newborns; this was attributed to in utero cyclosporine exposure, although haemodynamic problems cannot be excluded [59].

Pregnancy in heart transplant recipients is possible, often successful and reasonably safe, but specific cautionary considerations must be considered and discussed [63].

41.4.5 Lung Transplantation

Pregnancy after lung transplant had been considered more problematic than in the case of other solid organ drafts [8 , 64].

A study published in *Progress in Transplantation* [65] analyzed 30 pregnancies with 32 outcomes (one triplet) in 21 lung transplant recipients, in a majority affected by cystic fibrosis, and reported 12 outcomes (7 live births, 3 spontaneous and 2 therapeutic abortions).

Another early review [66] reporting the outcome of pregnancies after thoracic organ transplantation mentioned that the risk of rejection during and after pregnancy remains significant, especially for lung transplants which have a high rate of rejection requiring long-term immunosuppression. A 5-year mortality rate of 50% was mentioned, stressing the ethical need for proper counselling.

41.4.6 Heart–Lung Transplantation

A report from Scandinavia in 2011 provided information on 25 women with 42 pregnancies following heart and heart–lung transplantation [67]. All women survived the pregnancy, and in a number of them complications were relatively minor (proteinuria, hypertension and diabetes). However, major problems were also encountered: there were two rejections in early postpartum, two had severe renal failures and seven developed PE. Five patients died after 2 to 12 years following delivery. There were also problems with the newborn: one was born with cancer and one died early after inheriting the mother's cardiomyopathy.

Several comprehensive reports appeared during 2014 [68–70] emphasizing the existence of problems with these pregnancies, first and foremost that particularly lung transplant recipients are at increased risk for maternal and neonatal pregnancy-related complications, postpartum graft loss, long-term morbidity and mortality compared to other solid organ recipients. Unplanned pregnancies are common and therefore women awaiting transplantation should be encouraged to use effective contraception. Pregnancy should be avoided for a minimum of 1 to 2 years post-allograft and a series of complications are likely to appear: increased risk of miscarriage; hypertension, gestational diabetes, PE, PTB, FGR. Problems appeared also in the postpartum period, such as pneumonia and obliterative bronchiolitis. Monitoring during labour is mandatory and epidural anaesthesia recommended. Finally, vaginal delivery should be the standard modality and caesarean sections should be performed for obstetric reasons.

41.4.7 Pregnancy Complications Common to All Solid Organ Recipients

Common factors influencing the outcome of a pregnancy in all recipients of a grafted organ include age, parity, time from transplantation, chronic hypertension, diabetes and renal disease. Specifically, pre-gestational chronic hypertension can unfavourably influence gestations in all recipients and is associated with early-onset PE, FGR and fetal death. The high frequency of chronic hypertension in kidney recipients may explain the excess of severe obstetric disorders in this population [71]. A comparison of infant outcomes in women who delivered before and also after organ transplantation is presented in Table 41.3 and Figure 41.1.

Table 41.3 Preterm birth (<37 weeks), low birthweight (<2500 g) and small for date (≤2 SD) among singleton infants born before and after maternal organ transplantation

Preterm birth		
All	202/965 = 21%	60/139 = 43%
Only kidney	154/637 = 24%	58/126 = 46%
Only liver	26/214 = 12%	4/10 = 40%
Low birthweight		
All	182/965 = 19%	58/143 = 41%
Only kidney	150/635 = 24%	52/126 = 41%
Only liver	14/215 = 6.5%	2/12 = 17%
Small for date		
All	90/982 = 9.2%	24/143 = 17%
Only kidney	73/634 = 11.5%	23/126 = 18%
Only liver	9/214 = 4.2%	0/12 = 0.0%

From [36]

41.4.8 Uterus Transplantation

Ethical issues around uterine transplant in women born without a uterus, such as in cases of Mayer–Rokitansky–Küster–Hauser (MRKH) syndrome, had been discussed by two expert groups [72, 73]. The first successful pregnancy following transplantation from a cadaver [10] has totally changed the perspective in these women.

The first, partially successful, uterus transplantation from a living donor was carried out in 2000 in a 26-year-old and the donor was a 46-year-old woman who had to undergo surgery for 'multiloculated ovarian cysts'. Three months after surgery, the recipient developed acute vascular thrombosis and hysterectomy became necessary [74, 75]. Following several attempts [76, 77], a successful first live birth occurred [9] in 2015. The following year, the same group reported the birth (at 35 weeks) of a second live infant following uterus transplantation from a living donor who was the mother of the recipient; she was hysterectomized with vascular pedicles of uterine vessels and proximal vessels up to and including parts of the internal iliac arteries. Surgery in the recipient, a woman with MRKH syndrome, included bilateral vascular connections to external iliac arteries, vaginal-vaginal anastomosis and uterine fixation. Some 100 days after delivery the recipient was hysterectomized to prevent complications [78]. Finally, as mentioned above, in 2017 a group in São Paulo (Brazil) reported the first successful pregnancy in a uterus donated postmortem [10].

The situation in this fast-moving area has now been summarized [79], indicating the existence of several yet unpublished cases. As of 2018 approximately 40 procedures have been carried out, mostly with live donors. Following the attempt in Saudi Arabia, a group in Gothenburg (Sweden) initiated a systematic research approach [80]. Eventually they moved to the clinical part with nine cases (eight subjects with MRKH and one with cervical cancer and radical hysterectomy) [81] with the first live birth [9]. More recently, some 30 live donor procedures have been performed in China, Germany and the USA. So far, only one case with a successful pregnancy

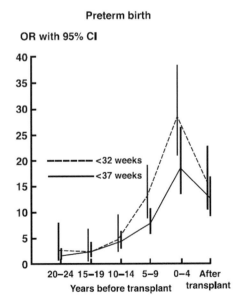

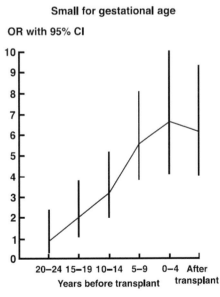

Figure 41.1 Odds ratios (OR) with 95% confidence intervals (95% CI) for preterm birth (<32 weeks, <37 weeks) or small for gestational age (SGA). ORs are adjusted for year of birth, maternal age, parity and (after 1982) maternal smoking habits. *From* [36]

has been reported [82]; the Chinese report is of interest because of the innovative and simplified procedure utilized [83].

The first attempt at a transplantation from a deceased donor occurred in Turkey in 2011 [84]; the second and the third procedures were performed in 2016 in the USA [85] and in Brazil [10], and the latter produced a live baby.

Grafting a uterus poses unique biological problems since the uterus is not a 'steady-state' organ and requires great plasticity of the anastomosed vessels to accommodate the increase of blood flow during the second half of pregnancy. Indeed, it was questionable whether the extensive vascular adaptations associated with human deep placentation could be tolerated after uterine artery anastomotic surgery, with its inevitable scar formation, particularly after a prolonged interval between surgery and pregnancy [73]. This is because deep placentation in humans involves the transformation of arterioles with a diameter of 50 mm into large amorphic channels capable of accommodating 90% of the uterine blood supply to the intervillous space. In this respect, there is increasing evidence that cyclic waves of spontaneous decidualization, menstruation and endometrial regeneration play an important role in embryo selection at implantation and in the preconditioning of the vasculature prior to deep trophoblast invasion [80].

41.5 Pathophysiology of Pregnancies in Organ Transplant Recipients

An important research field has dealt with how the presence of a 'foreign organ' can affect physiological mechanisms active in pregnancy.

41.5.1 Defective Deep Placentation in Solid Organ Recipient Pregnancies

During pregnancy, there is a critical interface coined 'the placental bed' [86]. This term identifies the basal plate of the placenta, the underlying decidua and the inner myometrium (the so-called myometrial junctional zone, or JZ) (Figure 41.2), encompassing the spiral arteries supplying maternal blood to the placenta. Changes in this critical area may jeopardize an adequate maternal blood supply to the intervillous space of the placenta [87]. Indeed, the process of deep haemochorial placentation typical of *Homo sapiens* females requires not only decidualization of the endometrium, but also substantial changes in the spiral arteries in the JZ, characterized by their intravascular invasion by cytotrophoblasts. If decidualization is impaired, the physiological intravascular trophoblast invasion may be compromised. Because the decidual process in the human is controlled by crosstalk between sex steroid hormones and locally released cytokines during the luteal phase of the cycle, the failure of subsequent deep placentation may already have been determined in the conception cycle [88].

As mentioned, pregnant women with a transplanted solid organ are at an increased risk of pregnancy complications and therefore it can be hypothesized that in these subjects the

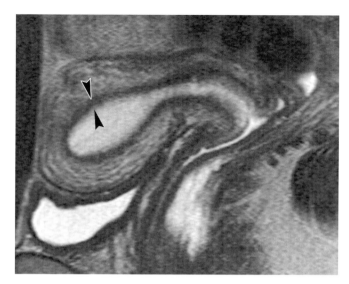

Figure 41.2 Myometrial junctional zone as seen on MRI (normal JZ: see arrow heads)

frequency of defective deep placentation may be a more common eventuality. Unfortunately, no systematic research of the endometrium and the placental bed has been performed to explain this high risk of obstetric complications.

41.5.2 Other Critical Uterine Functions

Besides decidualization, several uterine functions may be impaired in women with a grafted organ, among them the ability of decidualized stromal cells to respond to individual embryos in a manner that either promotes implantation and further development or facilitates early rejection [89–92]. Early and late fetal development occurs in very different environments [93], but the end result is that for proper fetal growth and well-being, in the third trimester uterine and placental perfusion rate should be respectively on the order of 750 and 600 mL per minute [94].

41.5.3 Complex Chimerism

A unique immunological situation characterizes pregnancies in women who have received a transplanted organ because of the presence in these subjects of multiple allogeneic or semi-allogeneic cell populations originating from the donated organ, the fetus and the mother of the pregnant woman. This situation has been labelled multiple or complex *microchimerism*. Possible short- or long-term consequences of this unique situation have yet to be evaluated, but the problem exists and may influence pregnancy outcome. In connection to this, several questions have been posed, such as a possible role of the mechanisms responsible for organ allograft rejection during pregnancy and during the postpartum period. The latter is of specific relevance since it is characterized by an increased T cell auto-reactivity, and complex microchimeras may be at higher risk [95].

41.6 Management of Major Obstetric Syndromes in Solid Organ Recipients

41.6.1 A Multidisciplinary Approach

Before conception, during the whole pregnancy and following delivery, the recipient needs to be monitored very closely through a multidisciplinary approach involving obstetricians, paediatricians and the transplant team. Such a coordinated action is of the utmost importance for an optimal graft and pregnancy outcome [96].

Following transplantation surgery, conception should be delayed at least a year, individualized according to the general health of the patient, her fertility potential and a stable, immunosuppressed graft function [27].

Major considerations in the management of pregnancy in subjects with a grafted organ are summarized in Table 41.4.

41.6.2 Pre-conception Counselling

In 2003 a consensus conference organized by the Women's Health Committee of the American Society of Transplantation issued guidelines for the transplant and obstetric teams [97]. They pointed out that it is still uncertain how pregnancy precisely influences the graft and the patient herself, and the long-term risks to the fetus are not known. A premature delivery, especially before 34 weeks of pregnancy, may lead to neonatal death or may be followed by long-term morbidities such as cerebral palsy, blindness, deafness, learning disorders and low IQ. In addition to these immediate consequences, low birthweight is associated with an increased risk of diabetes, hypertension and coronary artery disease later on (i.e. in adulthood) [98].

41.6.3 Immunosuppression in Pregnancy

Deep placentation and spiral artery remodelling implicate the influx and presence of immune cells, such as the uterine natural killer (uNK) cells and the T lymphocytes, in the uteroplacental interface (i.e. the decidua and the myometrial JZ). Immunosuppression may affect the functions of these cells.

Data from the literature and the NTPR support the notion that, to minimize the possibility of rejection, during pregnancy immunosuppressive therapy should be maintained at a sufficient level [99]. Today the majority of maintenance regimens combine the use of different immunosuppressive agents, usually based on cyclosporine or tacrolimus. This maintenance treatment is prescribed to most female graft recipients before, during and after pregnancy.

For some treatments (e.g. monoclonal antibodies and mycophenolate mofetil) there is either specific concern or lack of safety data, and therefore these drugs should not be used during pregnancy [99].

Meanwhile, ample experimental data have demonstrated that changes in the immune cell population or function at the level of the maternal-fetal interface contribute to the pathological pathways that induce obstetric disorders.

A few years ago, a nested case-control study [100] examined whether early- and late-onset PE have different pathophysiologies. The study showed that the more childbirth was premature, the higher was the frequency of placental lesions consistent with maternal underperfusion. This indicated that the so-called early- and late-onset variants of PE rather follows a continuum, with no precise and unambiguous gestational age at which lesions consistent with underperfusion develop. This state of underperfusion causing placental lesions has been linked to an imbalance in circulating concentrations of angiogenic versus anti-angiogenic factors [101].

41.6.4 First Trimester Diagnosis of Major Obstetric Disorders

There has been a considerable interest in the first trimester screening of women at risk for severe adverse pregnancy outcomes, using both risk assessments and biological assays. Several promising biomarkers have been proposed in the literature to identify women with an increased risk of PE, PTB and FGR [102].

41.6.4.1 Pre-eclampsia

The placental vascular bed is more prone to developing obstructive atherosclerotic lesions in the presence of subclinical hypertensive disorders when compared to other vascular beds. For this reason, in kidney transplant recipients, the increased risk of placental disease in the event of a pregnancy is often present many years prior to transplantation. In these women, alterations in the endothelial cell morphology of glomerular capillaries, termed glomerular endotheliosis, also occur in unmodified spiral arteries and are characterized by endothelial cell swelling and lipid accumulation [103, 104].

In this respect, there is prospective evidence that impaired placental development may be associated with subsequent development of severe pre-eclampsia, and levels of βhCG are

Table 41.4 Important considerations in pregnancy after transplant

- *The Mother*: Potential for risks to her long-term health, survival, and ability to be a parent.
- *The Graft*: Potential for risks of dysfunction and/or loss related to the pregnancy itself and the potential for changes in drug metabolism during pregnancy that could increase the susceptibility to rejection.
- *The Fetus/Neonate*: High incidences of prematurity and low birthweight. Potential for teratogenic risks associated with immunosuppression and other medications. Some birth defects may comprise subtle developmental changes, which might not become apparent until later in life.
- *Family and Social Issues*: The ability of a parent with a transplant to cope with unexpected illnesses and/or graft dysfunction while child rearing and the impact on the child if the transplanted parent is ill or dies.

From [112]

significantly lower in pregnancies that subsequently developed pre-eclampsia [105, 106].

41.6.4.2 Fetal Growth Restriction

In 2014, a population-based prospective cohort study [107] showed that early fetal life might be a critical period for cardiovascular health in later life. In 1184 children, first trimester fetal crown to rump length measurements were taken. Their mothers had a reliable first day of their last menstrual period and a regular menstrual cycle. Subsequently, at the median age of 6.0 (90% range 5.7–6.8) years the children's body mass index, total and abdominal fat distribution, blood pressure and blood concentrations of cholesterol, triglycerides, insulin and C peptide were measured. The childhood body mass index fully explained the associations of first trimester fetal crown to rump length with childhood total fat mass. Investigators concluded that impaired first trimester fetal growth is associated with an adverse cardiovascular risk profile in school-age children.

Therefore, early fetal life might be a critical period for cardiovascular health in later life.

41.6.4.3 Preterm Birth

Assessing the risk for preterm birth using maternal characteristics or a woman's previous obstetric history is known to have a poor predictive value [108, 109]. Biochemical assays reliably predicting subsequent preterm birth are also lacking. Measuring the cervical length with transvaginal ultrasound is the mainstay of mid-trimester screening of women at risk. A short cervix before 12 weeks alone, however, does not predict a subsequent premature labour before 34 weeks [110].

41.7 Conclusions

The experience of several thousand cases (particularly in kidney and liver transplants) has now properly established that pregnancy following all types of solid organ grafting, when compared to the general population, is invariably associated with an increased frequency in the occurrence of all major obstetric syndromes.

It seems that pregnancy complications, including hypertension, PE, PTB, FGR, occur more frequently in kidney than in liver or other solid organ transplantations. However, the most problematic is gestation following the grafting of a lung (alone or in associations with a heart).

Over recent years, several important insights have emerged to elucidate the causes of this phenomenon, indicating the existence of a complex interplay of different pathophysiological modifications. Among them, the fact that solid organ transplantation likely increases the risk of defective deep placentation in a subsequent pregnancy. Kidney transplant recipients have the highest risk, presumably reflecting the presence of pre-existing hypertensive and vascular diseases. Indeed, it has been shown that in women with renal disease a similar increased risk of complications was already present in pregnancies during the years before the transplantation.

It must be borne in mind that, in contrast to other vascular beds, uterine arteries in the event of a pregnancy must quickly undergo substantial changes to accommodate a major increase in blood supply. Even a minor impairment in this mechanism, such as the presence of subclinical hypertensive disease, will increase the risk of developing obstructive, atherosclerotic lesions and complications such as pre-eclampsia.

A definite role is probably played by immunosuppression in perturbing vascular remodelling in pregnancy; these drugs may affect key immune cells, such as uNK cells, present at the fetomaternal interface. Unfortunately, no attempts have been made to obtain placental bed biopsies and study the vascular changes after organ transplantation. Finally, the long-term consequences of the singular phenomenon of multiple microchimerism in these women will have to be investigated.

Uterus transplantation presents unique problems and, from the very limited experience gathered so far, it seems that establishing proper vascular connections plays a pivotal role in this type of grafting.

In terms of prevention of complications, the best avenue is provided by the early detection of any underlying maternal hypertensive or vascular disorder. This must include a strict antihypertensive treatment from the earliest stage of pregnancy. Multidisciplinary care before and throughout pregnancy, as well as in the critical postpartum period, is required, as signs of fetal growth restriction can be detected from the early stage of pregnancy.

References

1. Schjenken JE, Zhang B, Chan HY, et al. miRNA regulation of immune tolerance in early pregnancy. *Am J Reprod Immunol*. 2016;**75**:272–80.

2. Brosens I, Pijnenborg R, Vercruysse L, Romero R. The 'Great Obstetrical Syndromes' are associated with disorders of deep placentation. *Am J Obstet Gynecol*. 2011;**204**:193–201.

3. Murray JE, Merrill JP, Dammin GJ, et al. Study of transplantation immunity after total body irradiation: clinical and experimental investigation. *Surgery*. 1960;**48**:272–84.

4. Murray JE, Reid DE, Harrison JH, Merrill JP. Successful pregnancies after human renal transplantation. *New Engl J Med*. 1963;**269**:341e3.

5. Castro LA, Baltzer U, Hillebrand G, et al. Pregnancy in juvenile diabetes mellitus under cyclosporine treatment after combined kidney and pancreas transplantation. *Transplant Proc*. 1986;**18**:1780–1.

6. Löwenstein BR, Vain NW, Perrone SV, et al. Successful pregnancy and vaginal delivery after heart transplantation. *Am J Obstet Gynecol*. 1988;**158**:589–90.

7. Wagoner LE, Taylor DO, Olsen SL, et al. Immunosuppressive therapy, management, and outcome of heart transplant recipients during pregnancy. *J Heart Lung Transplant*. 1993;**12**:993–9.

8. Donaldson S, Novotny D, Paradowski L, Aris R. Acute and chronic lung allograft rejection during pregnancy. *Chest*. 1996;**110**:293–6.

9. Brännström M, Johannesson L, Bokström H, et al. Livebirth after uterus transplantation. *Lancet*. 2015;**385** (9968):607–16.

10. Ejzenberg D, Andraus W, Baratelli Carelli Mendes LR, et al. Livebirth after uterus transplantation from a deceased donor in a recipient with uterine infertility. *Lancet.* 2018;**392** (10165):2697–704.

11. McKay DB, Josephson MA. Pregnancy after kidney transplantation. *Clin J Am Soc Nephrol.* 2008;**3**(Suppl. 2):S117e25.

12. Brosens I, Benagiano G. Pregnancy and reproductive health after solid organ transplantation. *Best Pract Res Clin Obstet Gynaecol.* 2014;**28**:1113.

13. Shah M, Sauer MV. Fertility and reproductive disorders in female solid organ transplant recipients.*Semin Perinatol.* 2007;**31**:332–8.

14. Lessan-Pezeshki M, Ghazizadeh S, Khatami MR, et al. Fertility and contraceptive issues after kidney transplantation in women. *Transplant Proc.* 2004;**36**:1405–6.

15. Viner RM, Forton JT, Cole TJ, et al. Growth of long-term survivors of liver transplantation. *Arch Dis Child.* 1999;**80**:235–40.

16. French VA, Davis JS, Sayles HS, Wu SS. Contraception and fertility awareness among women with solid organ transplants. *Obstet Gynecol.* 2013;**122**:809–14.

17. Rupley DM, Janda AM, Kapeles SR, et al. Preconception counseling, fertility, and pregnancy complications after abdominal organ transplantation: a survey and cohort study of 532 recipients. *Clin Transplant.* 2014;**28**:937–45.

18. Rafie S, Lai S, Garcia JE, Mody SK. Contraceptive use in female recipients of a solid-organ transplant. *Prog Transplant.* 2014;**24**:344–8.

19. Gomez F de la Cueva R, Wauters JP, Lemarchand-Béraud T. Endocrine abnormalities in patients undergoing long-term hemodialysis. The role of prolactin. *Am J Med.* 1980;**68**: 522–30.

20. Lim VS, Henriquez C, Sievertsen G, Frohman LA. Ovarian function in chronic renal failure: evidence suggesting hypothalamic anovulation. *Ann Intern Med.* 1980;**93**:21–7.

21. Zingraff J, Jungers P, Pélissier C, et al. Pituitary and ovarian dysfunctions in women on haemodialysis. *Nephron.* 1982;**30**:149–53.

22. Handelsman DJ, Dong Q. Hypothalamo-pituitary gonadal axis in chronic renal failure. *Endocrinol Metab Clin North Am.* 1993;**22**:145–61.

23. Kim JH Chun CJ, Kang CM, Kwak JY. Kidney transplantation and menstrual changes. *Transplant Proc.* 1998;**30**:3057–9.

24. De Pinho JC, Sauer MV. Infertility and ART after transplantation. *Best Pract Res Clin Obstet Gynaecol.* 2014;**28**:1235–50.

25. Cundy TF, Butler J, Pope RM, et al. Amenorrhoea in women with non-alcoholic chronic liver disease. *Gut.* 1991;**32**:202–6.

26. Christopher V, Al-Chalabi T, Richardson PD, et al. Pregnancy outcome after liver transplantation: A single-center experience of 71 pregnancies in 45 recipients. *Liver Transplant.* 2006;**12**:1138–43.

27. Coscia LA, Constantinescu S, Moritz MJ, et al. Report from the National Transplantation Pregnancy Registry (NTPR): outcomes of pregnancy after transplantation. *Clin Transplant.* 2010:65e85.

28. The Gift of Life Institute. The Transplant Pregnancy Registry International. www .transplantpregnancyregistry.org/

29. Sibanda N, Briggs JD, Davison JM, Johnson RJ, Rudge CJ. Pregnancy after organ transplantation: a report from the UK Transplant Pregnancy Registry. *Transplantation* 2007;**83**:1301e7.

30. Shahir AK, Briggs N, Katsoulis J, Levidiotis V. An observational outcomes study from 1966–2008, examining pregnancy and neonatal outcomes from dialysed women using data from the ANZDATA Registry. *Nephrology (Carlton, Vic).* 2013;**18**:276e84.

31. McDonald SP, Russ GR. Australian registries-ANZDATA and ANZOD. *Transpl Rev (Orlando, Fla).* 2013;**27**:46e9.

32. Nordio M, Limido A, Conte F, et al. Il Registro Italiano Dialisi e trapianti 2011–2013 [Italian Registry Dialysis and Transplant 2011–2013]. *G Ital Nefrol.* 2016;33.

33. Strang WN, Tuppin P, Atinault A, Jacquelinet C. The French organ transplant data system. *Stud Health Technol Inform.* 2005;**116**:77–82.

34. Nashan B, Hugo C, Strassburg CP, et al. Transplantation in Germany. *Transplantation.* 2017;**101**:213–18.

35. Gerlei Z, Wettstein D, Rigó J, Asztalos L, Langer RM. Childbirth after organ transplantation in Hungary. *Transplant Proc.* 2011;**43**:1223–4.

36. Källén B, Westgren M, Åberg A, Otterblad Olausson P. Pregnancy outcome after maternal organ transplantation in Sweden. *Br J Obstet Gynaecol.* 2005; **112**:904–9.

37. López V, Martínez D, Viñolo C, et al. Pregnancy in kidney transplant recipients: effects on mother and newborn. *Transplant Proc.* 2011;**43**:2177–8.

38. Deshpande NA, James NT, Kucirka LM, et al. Pregnancy outcomes in kidney transplant recipients: a systematic review and meta-analysis. *Am J Transplant.* 2011;**11**:2388e404.

39. Wyld ML, Clayton PA, Jesudason S, Chadban SJ, Alexander SI. Pregnancy outcomes for kidney transplant recipients. *Am J Transplant.* 2013;**13**:3173e82.

40. Norrman E, Bergh C, Wennerholm UB. Pregnancy outcome and long-term follow-up after in vitro fertilization in women with renal transplantation. *Hum Reprod.* 2015;**30**:205–13.

41. Svetitsky S, Baruch R, Schwartz IF, et al. Long-term effects of pregnancy on renal graft function in women after kidney transplantation compared with matched controls. *Transplant Proc.* 2018;**50**:1461–5.

42. Cabiddu G, Spotti D, Gernone G, et al.; The Kidney and Pregnancy Study Group of the Italian Society of Nephrology.A best-practice position statement on pregnancy after kidney transplantation: focusing on the unsolved questions. The Kidney and Pregnancy Study Group of the Italian Society of Nephrology. *J Nephrol.* 2018;**31**:665–681.

43. Barrou BM, Gruessner AC, Sutherland DE, Gruessner RW. Pregnancy after pancreas transplantation in the cyclosporine era: report from the International Pancreas Transplant Registry. *Transplantation.* 1998;**65**:524–7.

44. Van Winter JT, Ogburn PL Jr, Ramin KD, Evans MP, Velosa JA. Pregnancy after pancreatic-renal transplantation because of diabetes. *Mayo Clin Proc.* 1997;**72**:1044–7.

45. Smyth A, Gaffney G, Hickey D, et al. Successful pregnancy after simultaneous pancreas-kidney

transplantation. *Case Rep Obstet Gynecol.* 2011;**2011**:983592.

46. Marcus EA, Wozniak LJ, Venick RS, et al. Successful term pregnancy in an intestine-pancreas transplant recipient with chronic graft dysfunction and parenteral nutrition dependence: a case report. *Transplant Proc.* 2015;**47**:863–7.

47. Yamamoto S, Nelander M. Ectopic pregnancy in simultaneous pancreas-kidney transplantation: A case report. *Int J Surg Case Rep.* 2016;**28**:152–4.

48. Bösmüller C, Pratschke J, Ollinger R. Successful management of six pregnancies resulting in live births after simultaneous pancreas kidney transplantation: a single-center experience. *Transplant Int.* 2014;**27**: e129-31.

49. Braun-Parvez L, Charlin E, Caillard S, et al. Gestational choriocarcinoma transmission following multiorgan donation. *Am J Transpl.* 2010;**10**:2541–6.

50. Deshpande NA, James NT, Kucirka LM, et al. Pregnancy outcomes of liver transplant recipients: a systematic review and meta-analysis. *Liver Transpl.* 2012;**18**:621e9.

51. Kubo S, Uemoto S, Furukawa H, Umeshita K, Tachibana D; Japanese Liver Transplantation Society. Pregnancy outcomes after living donor liver transplantation: results from a Japanese survey. *Liver Transpl.* 2014;**20**:576–83.

52. Kanzaki Y, Kondoh E, Kawasaki K, et al. Pregnancy outcomes in liver transplant recipients: a 15-year single-center experience. *J Obstet Gynaecol Res.* 2016;**42**:1476–82.

53. Akarsu M, Unek T, Avcu A, et al. Evaluation of pregnancy outcomes after liver transplantation. *Transplant Proc.* 2016;**48**:3373–7.

54. Mattila M, Kemppainen H, Isoniemi H, Polo-Kantola P. Pregnancy outcomes after liver transplantation in Finland. *Acta Obstet Gynecol Scand.* 2017;**96**:1106–11.

55. Zaffar N, Soete E, Gandhi S, et al. Pregnancy outcomes following single and repeat liver transplantation: An international 2-center cohort. *Liver Transpl.* 2018;**24**:769–78.

56. Kamarajah SK, Arntdz K, Bundred J, et al. Outcomes of pregnancy in recipients of liver transplants. *Clin Gastroenterol Hepatol.* 2019;**27** (7):1398–1404.e1.

57. Lim TY, Gonsalkorala E, Cannon MD, et al. Successful pregnancy outcomes following liver transplantation is predicted by renal function. *Liver Transpl.* 2018;**24**:606–15.

58. Kimmich N, Dutkowski P, Krähenmann F, et al. Liver transplantation during pregnancy for acute liver failure due to HBV infection: a case report. *Case Rep Obstet Gynecol.* 2013;**2013**:356560

59. Macera F, Occhi L, Masciocco G, Varrenti M, Frigerio M. A new life: motherhood after heart transplantation. A single center experience and review of literature. *Transplantation.* 2018;**102**:1538–44.

60. Lisonkova S, Joseph KS. Incidence of preeclampsia: risk factors and outcomes associated with early- versus late-onset disease. *Am J Obstet Gynecol* 2013;**209**:544.e1e544.e12.

61. Cowan SW, Davison JM, Doria C, et al. Pregnancy after cardiac transplantation. *Cardiol Clin.* 2012;**30**:441e52.

62. Tran DD, Kobashigawa J. A review of the management of pregnancy after cardiac transplantation. *Clin Transpl.* 2015;**31**:151–61.

63. Potena L, Moriconi V, Presta E. Pregnancy and heart transplantation: giving birth after a new life. *Transplantation.* 2018;**102**:1411–12.

64. Parry D, Hextall A, Robinson VP, Banner NR, Yacoub MH. Pregnancy following a single lung transplant. *Thorax.* 1996;**51**:1162–4.

65. Shaner J, Coscia LA, Constantinescu S, et al. Pregnancy after lung transplant. *Prog Transplant.* 2012;**22**:134e40.

66. Wu DW, Wilt J, Restaino S. Pregnancy after thoracic organ transplantation. *Sem Perinatol.* 2007;**31**:354e62.

67. Estensen M, Gude E, Ekmehag B, et al. Pregnancy in heart- and heart/lung recipients can be problematic. *Scand Cardiovasc J.* 2011;**45**:349–53.

68. Lund LH, Edwards LB, Kucheryavaya AY, et al. The registry of the International Society for Heart and Lung Transplantation: thirty-first official adult heart transplant report – 2014; focus theme: retransplantation. *J Heart Lung Transplant.* 2014;**33**:996–1008.

69. Vos R, Ruttens D, Verleden SE, et al. Pregnancy after heart and lung transplantation. *Best Pract Res Clin Obstet Gynaecol.* 2014;**28**:1146–62.

70. Thakrar MV, Morley K, Lordan JL, et al. Pregnancy after lung and heart-lung transplantation. *J Heart Lung Transplant.* 2014;**33**:593–8.

71. Wielgos M, Szpotanska-Sikorska M, Mazanowska N, et al. Pregnancy risk in female kidney and liver recipients: a retrospective comparative study. *J Matern Fetal Neonatal Med.* 2012;**25**:1090e5.

72. Milliez J. Uterine transplantation FIGO Committee for the Ethical Aspects of Human Reproduction and Women's Health. *Int J Gynecol Obstet.* 2009;**106**:270.

73. Benagiano G, Landeweerd L, Brosens I. Medical and ethical considerations in uterus transplantation. *Int J Obstet Gynecol.* 2013;**123**:173–7.

74. Fageeh W, Raffa H, Jabbad H, Marzouki A. Transplantation of the human uterus. *Int J Gynecol Obstet.* 2002;**76**:245–51.

75. Kandela P. Uterine transplantation failure causes Saudi Arabian government clampdown. *Lancet.* 2000;**356**(9232):838.

76. Hansen A. Swedish surgeons report world's first uterus transplantations from mother to daughter. *BMJ.* 2012;**345**:e6357.

77. Ozkan O, Akar ME, Ozkan O, et al. Preliminary results of the first human uterus transplantation from a multiorgan donor. *Fertil Steril.* 2013;**99**:470–6.

78. Brännström M, Bokström H, Dahm-Kähler P, et al. One uterus bridging three generations: first live birth after mother-to-daughter uterus transplantation. *Fertil Steril.* 2016;**106**:261–6.

79. Brännström M. Current status and future direction of uterus transplantation. *Curr Opin Organ Transplant.* 2018;**23**:592–7.

80. Brännström M, Diaz-Garcia C, Olausson M, Tzakis A. Uterus transplantation: animal research and human possibilities. *Fertil Steril.* 2012;**97**:1269–6.

81. Brännström M, Johannesson L, Dahm-Kähler P, et al. The first clinical uterus transplantation trial: a six months report. *Fertil Steril.* 2014;**101**: 1228–36.

82. Testa G, McKenna GJ, Gunby RT Jr, et al. First live birth after uterus transplantation in the United States. *Am J Transplant.* 2018;**18**:1270–4.

83. Wei L, Xue T, Tao KS, et al. Modified human uterus transplantation using ovarian veins for venous drainage: the first report of surgically successful robotic-assisted uterus procurement and follow-up for 12 months. *Fertil Steril.* 2017;**108**:346–56.

84. Ozkan O, Erman Akar M, Ozkan O, et al. Preliminary results of the first human uterus transplantation from multiorgan donor. *Fertil Steril.* 2013;**99**:470–6.

85. Flyckt RL, Farrell RM, Perni UC, Tzakis AG, Falcone T. Deceased donor uterine transplantation: innovation and adaptation. *Obstet Gynecol.* 2016;**128**:837–42.

86. Dixon HG, Robertson WB. A study of the vessels of the placental bed in normotensive and hypertensive women. *J Obstet Gynaecol Br Emp.* 1958;**65**:803e9.

87. Brosens I, Robertson WB, Dixon HG. The physiological response of the vessels of the placental bed to normal pregnancy. *J Pathol Bacteriol.* 1967;**93**:569e79.

88. Brosens JJ, Pijnenborg R, Brosens IA. The myometrial junctional zone spiral arteries in normal and abnormal pregnancies. *Am J Obstet Gynecol.* 2002;**187**:1416e23.

89. Brosens JJ, Salker MS, Teklenburg G, et al. Uterine selection of human embryos at implantation. *Sci Rep.* 2014;**6**:3894.

90. Salker M, Teklenburg G, Molokhia M, et al. Natural selection of human embryos: impaired decidualization of endometrium disables embryo-maternal interactions and causes recurrent pregnancy loss. *PLoS ONE.* 2010;**5**:e10287.

91. Salker MS, Christian M, Steel JH, et al. Deregulation of the serum- and glucocorticoid-inducible kinase SGK1 in the endometrium causes reproductive failure. *Nat Med.* 2011;**17**:1509e13.

92. Salker MS, Nautiyal J, Steel JH, et al. Disordered IL-33/ST2 activation in decidualizing stromal cells prolongs uterine receptivity in women with recurrent pregnancy loss. *PLoS ONE.* 2012;**7**:e52252.

93. Burton GJ, Jaunaiux E. Maternal vascularisation of the human placenta: does the embryo develop in a hypoxic environment? *Gynecol Obstet Fertil.* 2003;**29**:503e8.

94. Browne JC, Veall N. The maternal placental blood flow in normotensive and hypertensive women. *J Obstet Gynaecol Br Emp.* 1953;**60**:141e7.

95. Ma KK, Petroff MG, Coscia LA, Armenti VT, Adams Waldorf KM. Complex chimerism: pregnancy after solid organ transplantation. *Chimerism.* 2013;**4**:71–7.

96. Benagiano G., Brosens I. The multidisciplinary approach. *Best Pract Res Clin Obstet Gynaecol.* 2014;**28**:1114–22.

97. McKay DB, Josephson MA. Reproduction and transplantation: report on the AST consensus conference on reproductive issues and transplantation. *Am J Transplant.* 2005;**5**:1592e9.

98. Robinson R. The fetal origins of adult disease: no longer just a hypothesis and may be critically important in south Asia. *BMJ.* 2001;**322** (7283):375e6.

99. Armenti VT, Daller JA, Constantinescu S, et al. Report from the National Transplantation Pregnancy Registry: outcomes of pregnancy after transplantation. *Clin Transplants.* 2006:57e70.

100. Ogge G, Chaiworapongsa T, Romero R, et al. Placental lesions associated with maternal underperfusion are more frequent in early-onset than in late-onset preeclampsia. *J Perinat Med.* 2011;**39**:641e52.

101. Soto E, Romero R, Kusanovic JP, et al. Late-onset preeclampsia is associated with an imbalance of angiogenic and antiangiogenic factors in patients with and without placental lesions consistent with maternal underperfusion. *J Matern Fetal Neonatal Med.* 2012;**25**:498e507.

102. Sharp AN, Alfirevic Z. First trimester screening can predict adverse pregnancy outcomes. *Prenat Diagn.* 2014;**34**:660e7.

103. Khong TY, Sawyer IH, Heryet AR. An immunohistologic study of endothelialization of uteroplacental vessels in human pregnancy - evidence that endothelium is focally disrupted by trophoblast in preeclampsia. *Am J Obstet Gynecol.* 1992;**167**:751e6.

104. Ferris TF. Preeclampsia and postpartum renal failure: examples of pregnancy-induced microangiopathy. *Am J Med.* 1995;**99**:343e7.

105. Karahasanovic A, Sørensen S, Nilas L. First trimester pregnancy-associated plasma protein a and human chorionic gonadotropin-beta in early and late pre-eclampsia. *Clin Chem Lab Med.* 2014;**52**:521e5.

106. Åsvold BO, Vatten LJ, Tanbo TG, et al. Concentrations of human chorionic gonadotrophin in very early pregnancy and subsequent pre-eclampsia: a cohort study. *Hum Reprod.* 2014;**29**:1153e60.

107. Jaddoe VWV, De Jonge LL, Hofman A, et al. First trimester fetal growth restriction and cardiovascular risk factors in school age children: population based cohort study. *BMJ (Online).* 2014;**348**:g14.

108. Sananes N, Meyer N, Gaudineau A, et al. Prediction of spontaneous preterm delivery in the first trimester of pregnancy. *Eur J Obstet Gynecol Reprod Biol.* 2013;**171**:18e22.

109. Beta J, Akolekar R, Ventura W. Prediction of spontaneous preterm delivery form maternal factors, obstetric history and placental perfusion and function at 11–13 weeks. *Prenat Diagn.* 2011;**31**:75e83.

110. Parra-Cordero M, Sepulveda-Martinez A, Rencoret G, et al. Is there a role for cervical assessment and uterine artery Doppler in the first trimester of pregnancy as a screening test for spontaneous preterm delivery? *Ultrasound Obstet Gynecol.* 2014;**43**:291e6.

111. Candido C, Cristelli MP, Fernandes AR, et al. Pregnancy after kidney transplantation: high rates of maternal complications. *J Bras Nefrol.* 2016;**38**:421–6.

112. Rao S, Ghanta M, Moritz MJ, Constantinescu S. Long-term functional recovery, quality of life, and pregnancy after solid organ transplantation. *Med Clin North Am.* 2016;**100**:613–29.

Oral Health and Periodontal Diseases in Pregnancy

Hans Ulrich Brauer, Irene Hösli & Gwendolin Manegold-Brauer

42.1 Introduction

Diseases in the oral cavity affecting the periodontal connective tissue are summarized under the term *periodontal diseases*. Periodontitis, the most relevant periodontal disease, is caused by a bacterial inflammation of the tissues supporting the teeth. Periodontal diseases are highly prevalent. Relevant risk factors are diabetes, smoking and stress.

Gingivitis, the mildest and reversible form of periodontal disease, affects up to 50–90% of the worldwide population [1]. Gingivitis during pregnancy is called pregnancy gingivitis and is known to be the basis for the development of oral pregnancy tumours, which are rare, but can cause clinical symptoms. Gingivitis can be a precursor of periodontitis. Periodontitis is clinically relevant and can be an underlying factor causing adverse pregnancy outcomes (Figure 42.1). Treatment options include optimization of oral hygiene by proper instruction, professional cleaning, antibiotic treatment and surgical treatment [1].

42.1.1 Structure of the Healthy Periodontium

The periodontium functionally anchors the teeth in the bone and protects the germ-free ecosystem of the internal tissues from the bacterially colonized oral cavity. The periodontium consists of gingiva (gums), cement, alveolar bone and periodontal ligaments. The healthy periodontium shows the gums with a mostly pale pink, slightly dipped oral surface. Healthy gums do not bleed when touched, the interdental spaces are completely filled by the interdental papilla and the teeth are free of dental plaque [1, 2].

42.1.2 Gingivitis and Periodontitis

The common signs of periodontal diseases are loss of attachment and alveolar bone loss. The loss of connective tissue and alveolar bone may lead to the loss of teeth. While gingivitis is a plaque-induced inflammation of the gingiva and is a reversible form of periodontal disease (Figure 42.2), the periodontium is irreversibly destroyed in chronic or aggressive periodontitis [1].

Periodontitis results in the formation of soft tissue pockets or recessed gaps between the gingiva and the root surface. Reasons for the formation of the pockets are accumulations of bacteria in the form of plaque (biofilm). As a result, the body's defence system is activated and initiates the destruction of the periodontium. *Porphyromonas gingivalis*, *Tannerella forsythensis*, *Treponema denticola* and *Aggregatibacter actinomycetemcomitans* are typical organisms causing the disease [1]. Recently a new, complex periodontitis classification system was proposed [3]. This classification scheme includes a multidimensional staging and grading system that might be relevant in future literature. Traditionally, chronic periodontitis progresses slowly and is classified according to its distribution pattern (localized/

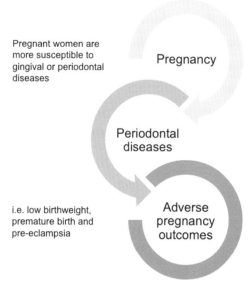

Figure 42.1 Potential association between diseases in the oral cavity and pregnancy.

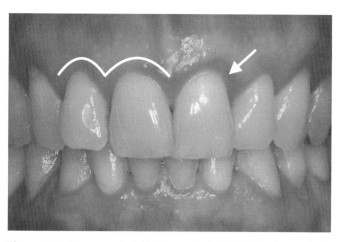

Figure 42.2 Pregnancy gingivitis. The marginal gingiva (white line marks the border to the gingiva propria) is reddened and slightly thickened (white arrow). Frequently, the gingiva bleeds when touched. Bone destruction is not present in gingivitis.

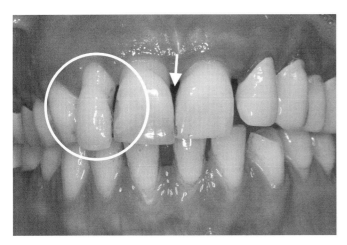

Figure 42.3 Advanced stage periodontitis. Severe form of regression of the gingiva and advanced bone resorption. As a result, 'black triangles' have developed between individual teeth (white arrow). The teeth seem to be longer. Late features include the elongated, slightly rotated, right lateral maxillary anterior tooth (white circle).

generalized) and severity (mild/moderate/severe). Clinical signs of advanced stages are tooth mobility and tooth migration. In the majority of cases, the patients do not report pain as a leading symptom. For aggressive periodontitis familial clustering is typical. The patient is clinically healthy except for periodontitis, even though there is a rapidly progressive tissue destruction. Both chronic and aggressive periodontitis show a significant association with adverse pregnancy outcome. In periodontitis, the teeth seem to be longer due to the reduction of the periodontium. In advanced stages, the interdental papilla, which normally fill the space between two adjacent teeth, diminish (Figure 42.3).

42.2 Gingival and Periodontal Diseases in Pregnancy

Due to hormonal changes during pregnancy, pregnant women are generally more susceptible to developing gingival or periodontal diseases.

42.2.1 Pregnancy Gingivitis

Gingivitis in pregnancy is usually referred to as pregnancy gingivitis. Several studies have shown that pregnant women are more often affected by gingivitis than women who are not pregnant [4].

42.2.1.1 Clinical Features

Gingivitis is characterized by bleeding gums and thickened papillae without degradation of the alveolar bone. Some clinical features of gingivitis may be more pronounced in pregnancy (see Figure 42.2). Due to the increased vascularity and extravasation of red blood cells, the gingiva is dark red and bleeds easily [4]. Other clinical features are the oedema-related smooth appearance of the gingiva, thickening of the gingival margin and hyperplastic interdental papillae [1, 4].

42.2.1.2 Aetiology

In the case of pregnancy gingivitis, it is assumed that initially a plaque-induced gingivitis is present, which is intensified by

the hormonal changes [4]. One explanation for pregnancy-related gingival changes is the increased tissue vascularity and vascular flow [4]. Other proposed mechanisms include changes in the immune system and the changes in connective tissue metabolism [4].

42.2.1.3 Dental Treatment

The intervention to treat gingivitis in pregnancy should have the goal of reducing the bacterial load and the signs of inflammation. This goal is reached with professional cleaning, cleaning instruction and mouth rinse, hereby aiming at an improvement of dental hygiene. A plaque-free tooth surface with a healthy gingiva at the onset of the pregnancy and maintenance of good oral hygiene prevent clinical signs of gingival inflammation in pregnancy [4].

42.2.2 Oral Pregnancy Tumour

Oral pregnancy tumour (OPT), also known as pyogenic granuloma, epulis gravidarum or granuloma gravidarum, is a benign, rare, hyperplastic oral mucosal lesion in pregnancy [5, 6]. Certain individual cases of OPT can cause significant impairment and bleeding [7].

42.2.2.1 Clinical Features

Oral pregnancy tumour is known to involve the gingiva most commonly and usually remains under 1 cm in diameter [8]. OPT is a smooth or lobulated exophytic lesion manifesting as small, red erythematous papule appearing in the second and third trimesters of pregnancy [9, 10].

42.2.2.2 Aetiology and Histopathology

The aetiology of OPT is still unclear. Hormonal changes, including increased oestrogen and progesterone levels, are thought to affect the periodontal tissues, immunity and/or the composition of the oral microflora [5, 6]. Oral pregnancy tumour can arise in response to various stimuli such as low-grade local irritation, traumatic injury or hormonal factors. OPT is histologically identical to the pyogenic granuloma, but has unique biological behaviour such as spontaneous remission after pregnancy [10]. A biopsy is needed to exclude malignancy. Microscopic examination of OPT shows a highly vascular proliferation that resembles granulation tissue and is partly or completely covered by parakeratotic or non-keratinized stratified squamous epithelium [6].

42.2.2.3 Treatment and Management Strategies

Surgical excision is the treatment of choice, but OPT has a high recurrence rate of 3–23% [6]. Lesions that do not cause significant functional or aesthetic problems should not be excised during pregnancy, because they may recur and ultimately can resolve spontaneously after delivery [10].

42.2.3 Clinical Recommendations for Oral Health

- During pregnancy, careful oral hygiene, removal of dental plaque and use of soft toothbrushes are very important to avoid occurrence and recurrence of a gingivitis or an oral pyogenic granuloma [10].

- Oral pregnancy tumour is an intraoral lesion during pregnancy that is histologically identical to the pyogenic granuloma but has unique biological features [10].
- Obstetricians should be able to recognize periodontal disease and pyogenic granuloma in a routine follow-up to ensure referral to a dentist for appropriate treatment [9].
- Ideally, any existing gingival inflammation should be treated before conception. For this reason, advising women to seek appropriate dental care might be worthwhile to integrate into pre-conception counselling and the topic of dental hygiene should not be neglected during pregnancy care [9].

42.3 Maternal Periodontal Disease and Adverse Pregnancy Outcomes

The relationship between maternal periodontitis and adverse pregnancy outcomes (APO) such as premature delivery has been controversial for more than 20 years. Numerous epidemiological studies and intervention trials have attempted to prove the relationships between maternal periodontal diseases and APO. The first study was published by Offenbacher et al in 1996 [11]. Adverse pregnancy outcomes discussed in the context of periodontal diseases are low birthweight (<2500 g), very low birthweight (<1500 g), premature delivery (<37 weeks), very early premature delivery (<32 weeks), pre-eclampsia, miscarriage, stillbirth and gestational diabetes [12–14].

42.3.1 Scientific Data

The increased risk for preterm low birthweight in pregnant women with periodontitis with an odds ratio of 7.9 found by Offenbacher et al (1996) could not be consistently confirmed in subsequent studies. After evaluation of the literature, there are a series of high-quality studies that find an association, but also numerous studies with the same level of quality that did not establish a connection. The differing study results are explained by differences in the definition of periodontitis and unequal study populations [13]. Therefore, several researchers have attempted to reveal the relationship between periodontal diseases and APO in systematic reviews and meta-analyses [15, 16]. It should be noted that low birthweight, premature birth and pre-eclampsia may be associated with maternal periodontitis, according to current data. The connection seems to be moderate [4, 16].

The efficacy of periodontal treatment (nonsurgical periodontal therapy) during pregnancy to reduce the incidence of adverse pregnancy outcomes is also controversial [17]. Though some reports found efficacy of periodontal treatment during pregnancy in high-risk mothers, most of the studies concluded that the treatment of periodontal diseases could not reduce the incidence of adverse pregnancy outcomes [17]. Periodontal disorders are an independent risk factor for APO, according to epidemiological and experimental studies [17].

42.3.2 Biological Mechanism

There are two pathways triggering an inflammatory/immune response and/or suppression of local growth factors (such as IGF-2) in the fetoplacental unit [16, 18].

There is a direct pathway where oral microorganisms and/or their components reach the fetoplacental unit via haematogenous dissemination from the oral cavity [18].

It is also postulated that periodontal disease has an indirect association to APO, the link possibly being the fact that poor oral hygiene is commoner in low socio-economic status patients who are prone to APO.

The other concept suggests that inflammatory mediators locally produced in periodontal tissues, for example, PGE-2, TNF-alpha, circulate in maternal blood and impact the fetoplacental unit indirectly (indirect pathway). Another indirect pathway is that inflammatory mediators and/or microbial components circulate to the maternal liver, enhancing cytokine production (e.g. IL-6) and acute phase protein responses (e.g. C-reactive protein (CRP)), which then impacts the fetoplacental unit [18].

Periodontal bacteria, especially *Porphyromonas gingivalis*, and their components can injure the trophoblast morphologically and functionally [16]. Moreover, inflammatory mediators from periodontal pockets might elicit an inflammatory immune response at the fetoplacental unit. However, periodontal treatment during pregnancy seems to have little effect on the prevention of APO incidence [17, 19]. Although dental care is effective in curing periodontal diseases, dissemination of the bacteria into the maternal blood has already occurred and therefore one can speculate that dental care during pregnancy may occur too late to significantly reduce pregnancy complications [17, 19].

42.3.3 Clinical Recommendations

- During pregnancy, a consistent and thorough oral hygiene is important to reduce the amount of plaque at the gingival margin and thus prevent the development of any periodontal disease [4].
- It is recommended to include dental care as an integral part of pre-conception counselling [2]. Any existing periodontal inflammation should be treated before conception. Treatment of periodontitis in pregnancy with the aim to reduce adverse pregnancy outcomes might be too late [17].

42.4 Conclusion

There are a number of interactions between diseases in the oral cavity and pregnancy. Every periodontal inflammation should ideally be treated before conception. During pregnancy, a consistent and thorough oral hygiene is important to reduce the amount of plaque at the gingival margin and thus prevent the development of any periodontal disease.

For pre-conception health counselling and antepartum pregnancy counselling, information on periodontal disease should be regularly updated and prepared according to what is most current practice.

References

1. Pihlstrom BL, Michalowicz BS, Johnson NW. Periodontal diseases. *Lancet.* 2005;**366**:1809–20.

2. Manegold-Brauer G, Hoesli I, Brauer HU, Beikler T. Periodontal diseases – a review on the association between maternal periodontitis and adverse pregnancy outcome. *Z Geburtshilfe Neonatol.* 2014;**218**:248–53.

3. Papapanou P, Sanz M, Buduneli N, et.al Periodontitis: consensus report of workgroup 2 of the 2017 World Workshop on the Classification of Periodontal and Peri-Implant Diseases and Conditions. *J Periodontol.* 2018;**89** (Suppl 1):S173–182.

4. Laine MA. Effect of pregnancy on periodontal and dental health. *Acta Odontol Scand.* 2002;**60**: 257–64.

5. Kamal R, Dahiya P, Puri A. Oral pyogenic granuloma: Various concepts of etiopathogenesis. *J Oral Maxillofac Pathol.* 2012;**16**:79–82.

6. Sills ES, Zegarelli DJ, Hoschander MM, Strider WE. Clinical diagnosis and management of hormonally responsive oral pregnancy tumor (pyogenic granuloma). *J Reprod Med.* 1996;**41**:467–70.

7. Durairaj J, Balasubramanian K, Rani PR, Sagili, Pramya N. Giant lingual granuloma gravidarum. *J Obstet Gynaeco.l* 2011;**31**:769–70.

8. Manegold-Brauer G, Brauer HU. Oral pregnancy tumour: an update. *J Obstet Gynaecol.* 2014;**34**:187–8.

9. Wang PH, Chao HT, Lee Wl, Yuan CC, Ng HT. Severe bleeding from a pregnancy tumor. A case report. *J Reprod Med.* 1997;**42**:359–62.

10. Daley TD, Nartey NO, Wysocki GP. Pregnancy tumor: an analysis. *Oral Surg Oral Med Oral Pathol.* 1991;**72**:196–9.

11. Offenbacher S, Katz V, Fertik G, et al. Periodontal infection as a possible risk factor for preterm low birth weight. *J Periodontol.* 1996;**67**:1103–13.

12. Brauer HU, Manegold-Brauer G, Hoesli I, Beikler T. Parodontitis und negative Schwangerschaftsoutcomes. *ZWR.* 2015;**124**:160–1.

13. Ide M, Papapanou PN. Epidemiology of association between maternal periodontal disease and adverse pregnancy outcomes – systematic review. *J Periodontol.* 2013;**84**:S181–94.

14. Gogeneni H, Buduneli N, Ceyhan-Öztürk B, et al. Increased infection with key periodontal pathogens during gestational diabetes mellitus. *J Clin Periodontol.* 2015;**42**(6): 506–12.

15. Daalderop LA, Wieland BV, Tomsin K, et al. Periodontal disease and pregnancy outcomes: overview of systematic reviews. *JDR Clin Trans Res.* 2018;**3**:10–27.

16. Komine-Aizawa S, Aizawa S, Hayakawa S. Periodontal diseases and adverse pregnancy outcomes. *J Obstet Gynaecol Res.* 2019;**45**:5–12.

17. Michalowicz BS, Gustafsson A, Thumbigere-Math V, Buhlin K. The effects of periodontal treatment on pregnancy outcomes. *J Periodontol.* 2013;**84**:S195–208.

18. Sanz M, Kornman K; Working Group 3 of the Joint EFP/AAP Workshop. Periodontitis and adverse pregnancy outcomes: consensus report of the joint EFP/AAP workshop on periodontitis and systemic diseases. *J Periodontol.* 2013;**84**:S164–9.

19. Iheozor-Ejiofor Z, Middleton P, Esposito M, Glenny AM. Treating periodontal disease for preventing adverse birth outcomes in pregnant women. *Cochrane Database Syst Rev.* 2017 Jun 12;6:CD005297.

43

Normal Labour

Silvia Serrano & Diogo Ayres-de-Campos

43.1 Introduction

Labour is defined as a series of physiological phenomena whereby the fetus, membranes and placenta are expelled from the uterus at a period in pregnancy where extrauterine survival is possible. The onset of labour implies the occurrence of rhythmic and effective uterine contractions that lead to progressive effacement and dilation of the cervix. This process is required before the fetus can progress through the birth canal.

The physiological processes behind the onset of labour are incompletely understood, as the mechanisms of labour in humans are unique, and cannot be extrapolated from other species. It is useful to consider the periods just before the beginning of labour. Quiescence corresponds to the time in which the uterine muscle ceases to suffer the inhibitory effects of progesterone, PGI2 (prostacyclin), nitric oxide and other metabolites that prevent contractility. During the activation phase, oestrogen facilitates the expression and opening of myometrial receptors for prostaglandins and oxytocin, increasing the permeability of gap junctions between myometrial cells, and consequently the initiation of contractions. The process may be prolonged in humans, occurring for days or weeks [1–3].

The influence of the human fetus on the initiation of parturition is largely unknown, unlike what happens in other mammals where it plays an important role in the course of labour. A decrease in progesterone levels is not necessary for the initiation of uterine contractions in humans, although there is some evidence suggesting a decrease in functional progesterone, consisting in a reduction in progesterone receptors and a change in their isoforms [4].

Oxytocin is a peptide hormone, synthesized in the hypothalamus and secreted in a pulsatile form by the posterior lobe of the pituitary gland. It has a biological half-life of 3–6 minutes and is degraded by placental oxytocinase, mainly in the liver and kidneys. Oxytocin concentration in maternal circulation remains stable during pregnancy and increases significantly during the active phase of labour [5]. After the onset of spontaneous labour, the fetus also synthesizes oxytocin, releasing it in increasing concentrations. Oxytocin stimulates uterine contractility, and myometrial receptors are found predominantly in the uterine fundus, becoming scarcer in the lower uterine segment and cervix. During gestation, the number of receptors progressively increase, reaching a maximum concentration in the beginning of labour. Oxytocin also stimulates the amnion and decidua to produce prostaglandins, which are additional promoters of uterine contractions [6].

43.2 Uterine Activity

Rhythmic uterine contractions are essential for the progression of labour, promoting cervical effacement, dilation and fetal descent. At the end of pregnancy, contractions usually become more frequent, stronger and perceptible. They may also become painful. Irregular contractions (Braxton Hicks contractions) are frequent at term, being usually shorter and less intense than those of true labour, and are not associated with cervical changes. Changing position and analgesia will often reduce the discomfort caused by these contractions. Particularly in first-time mothers, the fetal head may descend into the pelvis before labour. This may lead to an increasing urge to urinate because of urinary bladder compression. Passage of the mucus plug occupying the cervical canal, sometimes accompanied by a small amount of bleeding from the cervix, may also occur before the onset of labour.

True labour is defined by the occurrence of rhythmic contractions of progressive frequency and intensity. Physiologically, these contractions are also more coordinated than those arising before labour: contractile waves start in the uterine fundus and propagate to the cervix. The upper part of the uterus is where most muscle fibres concentrate, and during delivery this segment contracts actively. The lower portion, formed by the lower uterine segment and the cervix, has a more passive role, and becomes thinner with labour progression. Abdominal palpation during labour allows a clear distinction between the two segments. The transition zone between them is marked by a discrete prominence in the inner surface of the uterus called the physiological retraction ring. During prolonged labour, this ring may become prominent, and in these situations, it is called a pathological retraction ring or Bandl ring.

43.3 Fetal Position

The anatomical relation between the fetal body and the birth canal is described by various terms: fetal **attitude** refers to how the main fetal body parts are positioned inside the uterus, which is usually characterized by generalized flexion of all joints. Occasionally, one or both of the upper/lower extremities may not be fully flexed.

Fetal **lie** is the relationship between the major axes of the maternal and fetal body. Longitudinal lie is by far the most frequent and refers to the situation whereby these axes are parallel, so that the presenting part is cephalic or breech. Transverse lie refers to the situation of crossing axes, whereby the presenting part is usually the shoulder. Oblique lies are transitory and during labour rotate to longitudinal or transverse lies.

The **presenting part** is the fetal structure that first descends through the birth canal. It can be cephalic (which is further subdivided in vertex, face or brow), breech or shoulder. Vertex presentations occur in circa 96% of all labours, while breech presentations occur in circa 4%. Face, brow and shoulder presentations are very rare.

Fetal **position** describes the relationship between a given reference point of the presenting part and the maternal birth canal. In vertex presentations, the reference point is the occiput, in face presentations it is the mentum and in breech presentations it is the sacrum. In vertex presentations, when the occiput faces the anterior and left part of the birth canal, it is referred to as left anterior occiput (LOA), and likewise for other positions (Figure 43.1). Occiput transverse (OT) and occiput posterior (OP) positions are less frequent and usually associated with more prolonged labours.

Fetal **station** describes the level of descent of the lowest portion of the presenting part in relation to the plane of the maternal ischial spines. It is quantified on a scale ranging from −5 to +5, according to the level of descent (in centimetres) above or below the spines. When the presenting part reaches the level of the ischial spines, it is at 0 station. Above the ischial spines, the presenting part descends through −5, −4, −3, −2 and −1 stations. Below the ischial spines, it descends through +1, +2, +3, +4 and +5 stations, towards the pelvic outlet. When the fetal head reaches the introitus, it is considered to be at +5 station (Figure 43.2).

43.4 Maternal Pelvis

The maternal bony pelvis consists of the sacro-coccygeal part of the spine, the innominate bones formed by the ileum, ischium and pubis that join through the pubic symphysis. Three sections of the bony pelvis are usually considered:

The **pelvic inlet** is demarcated posteriorly by the promontory and anterior ala of the sacrum, laterally by the arcuate line of the ilium and anteriorly by the pectineal line of the pubis and the pubic symphysis. The anteroposterior diameter of this plane is the only one that can be estimated clinically on vaginal examination: It corresponds to the shorter distance between the sacral promontory and the pubic symphysis (obstetric conjugate).

The **pelvic midcavity** is formed by the posterior aspect of the pubis and the sacral concavity. The interspinous diameter is measured between the protrusion of the sciatic spines.

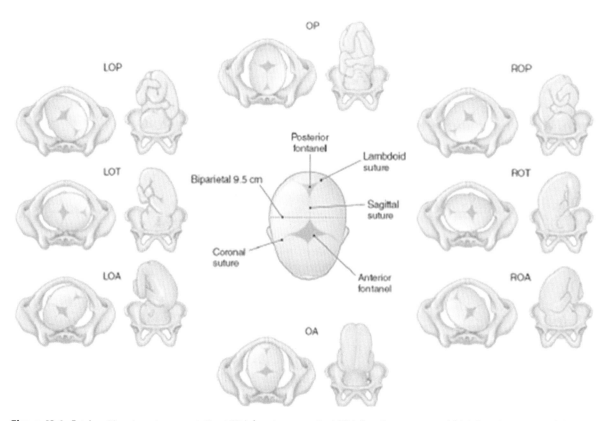

Figure 43.1 Fetal positions in vertex presentation. LOP, left occiput posterior; LOT, left occiput transverse; LOA, left occiput anterior; OA, occiput anterior; ROA, right occiput anterior; ROT, right occiput transverse; ROP; right occiput posterior; OP, occiput posterior;

The **pelvic outlet** is constituted anteriorly by the lower portion of the pubic symphysis, posteriorly by the coccyx and laterally by the sciatic and lower branches of the pubis.

The global shape of the maternal pelvis is classically classified into gynecoid, anthropoid, android and platypelloid forms. However, it is well recognized that clinical evaluation of these characteristics is imprecise, and most women do not fall into a typical pattern. Therefore, this subdivision is usually of reduced clinical value except in extreme cases.

43.5 Cardinal Movements of Labour

The cardinal movements of labour describe the actions undergone by the fetus when passing through the birth canal, and usually refer to vertex presentations in anterior positions. They are the following: engagement, flexion, descent, internal rotation, extension, external rotation and expulsion. Although described independently, in reality the mechanics of labour condition an overlap in these movements (Figure 43.3).

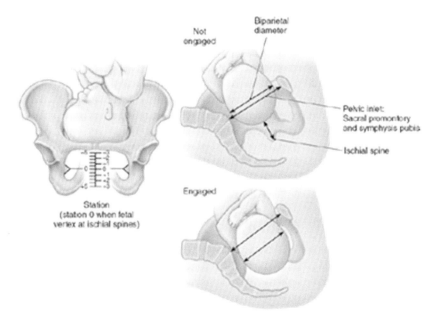

Figure 43.2 Fetal station and engagement of the fetal head.

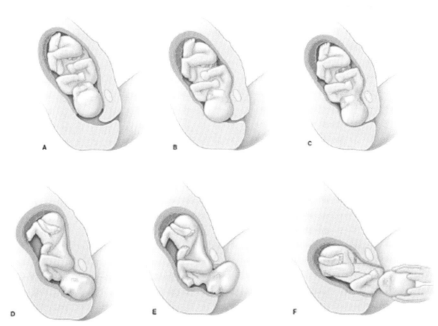

Figure 43.3 The cardinal movements of labour: engagement (**A**), flexion (**B**), descent (**C**), internal rotation (**D**), extension (**E**), and external rotation (**F**).

Engagement corresponds to the passage of the largest transverse diameter of the fetal head (the biparietal diameter) through the pelvic inlet. On vaginal examination, engagement occurs when the presenting part is at the level of the ischial spines. It may occur in the last weeks of pregnancy, particularly in white nulliparous women, or during labour. When the fetal head encounters resistance from the birth canal, **flexion** of the neck usually follows, as this results in the presentation of smaller diameters. **Descent** of the presenting part through the birth canal occurs by the action of uterine contractions arising in the fundus, together with reduced resistance from the lower uterine segment and cervix. **Internal rotation** of the occiput towards the pubic symphysis (from LOA or ROA to OA) usually occurs after the head has reached the ischial spines. When the lowest part of the head reaches the introitus and the base of the occiput comes into direct contact with the lower margin of the pubic symphysis, **extension** of the head occurs, due to increased resistance from the posterior structures of the birth canal (coccyx and perineum). Thus, the head is progressively exteriorized starting with the occiput, bregma, forehead, nose, mouth and finally the mentum. After delivery of the fetal head, the latter usually rotates to the position in which it became engaged, a movement called **external rotation**. For **expulsion** of the fetal body, the biacromial diameter of the shoulders usually rotates to the antero-posterior diameter of the pelvic outlet. The anterior shoulder appears under the pubic symphysis and the posterior shoulder distends the posterior perineum.

43.6 Stages of Labour

Labour is usually divided into three stages. The **first stage** corresponds to the period between the onset of regular uterine contractions (beginning of labour) and complete cervical dilation (10 cm). It is subdivided into two phases: classically, the **latent phase** occurs from the beginning of labour until the cervix is 4 cm dilated and almost completely effaced [7]. Recent data has challenged this definition and proposed that it should last until the cervix is 5 or 6 cm dilated [8]. The latent phase has variable duration, with progress of cervical dilation being usually slow, and it can be influenced by external factors such as sedation and oxytocin augmentation. It may last up to 20 hours, during which the cervix progressively softens, becomes effaced, and dilates. Uterine contractions are usually of moderate intensity, relatively short duration and variable frequency. During the **active phase** the cervix dilates at a relatively fixed rate, until it reaches full dilation (conventionally described as 10 cm). At this point the cervix is no longer palpable between the vaginal walls and the fetal presenting part. Dilation rates during this phase are more constant than in the latent phase [9], although wide variations still occur [10].

The **second stage** of labour begins with complete cervical dilation and ends with the full delivery of the fetus. This stage can also be subdivided into two phases: the **latent phase**, between the moment when complete cervical dilation occurs and the onset of pushing and the **active phase**, between the onset of pushing and full delivery of the fetus. Naturally, the moment of complete cervical dilation is rarely diagnosed with

precision, as vaginal examinations cannot and should not be performed too frequently. Therefore, the total duration of the second stage and that of its latent phase are usually imprecise measurements. With use of regional analgesia in labour, the natural occurrence of the urge to push is usually delayed, and some women may need to be encouraged to start pushing without feeling this urge, when the latent phase of the second stage becomes prolonged.

The **third stage** of labour is the period between full delivery of the fetus and delivery of the placenta. After the fetus is born, the uterus continues to contract intermittently. The decrease in uterine dimensions leads to a reduction in the area of placental implantation, with subsequent placental detachment. After detachment has occurred, further maternal pushing or controlled cord traction will usually exteriorize the placenta.

Some authors also describe a fourth stage of labour, corresponding to 2 hours that follow placental delivery. After the placenta is exteriorized, the uterus usually contracts in a sustained fashion, thereby collapsing the vessels that formerly irrigated the placental bed. With an average blood perfusion of 600 mL/minute at term, sustained uterine contraction is essential to control blood loss. The uterus usually remains contracted for about 1–2 hours, and close observation is recommended during this period.

43.7 Diagnosis of Labour

Women are usually advised in prenatal visits to seek professional care if one of the following symptoms appear: **rhythmic uterine contractions**, approximately one every 5–10 minutes, that do not subside with movement or oral analgesia, and usually become longer (lasting up to 90 seconds) and more painful, typically in the hypogastric area and irradiating to the back; a **sudden gush or constant flow of fluid** from the vagina, usually corresponding to amniotic fluid when the membranes rupture. In these situations, a short **clinical history** should be taken, including gestational age, complications occurring during the present and previous pregnancies, past medical and surgical history, medication and allergies. Labour is mainly a clinical diagnosis, so it is important to characterize the location, frequency, intensity, duration and irradiation of pain, as well as possible alleviating factors. Other important information relates to the loss of liquid or blood, fetal movements and other symptoms. The results of ultrasound and blood tests performed during pregnancy should be reviewed.

Abdominal examination is useful to identify fetal lie, presentation and engagement, using Leopold manoeuvres. Contractions may also be identified during these manoeuvres, and their duration and frequency evaluated. Rarely, **transabdominal ultrasound** may be indicated, if palpation was inconclusive, or if there are uncertainties regarding placental location, etc.

When rupture of membranes is suspected, a sterile **speculum examination** should be performed before vaginal examination, to document the presence and characteristics of amniotic fluid flowing from the cervical canal.

Digital **vaginal examination** is an essential part of the diagnosis of labour. At term, the only situation when it should be avoided is when there is a suspected placenta praevia. Vaginal examination allows identification of the following four characteristics of the cervix: **consistency**, which can be soft (similar to the consistency of the lip) or firm (similar to the consistency of the nose); **position**, which can be posterior (behind the main axis of the fetus), intermediate (along the main axis of the fetus) or anterior (in front of the main axis of the fetus); **effacement** (evaluating the percentage of cervical canal length that has disappeared – outside labour it is usually 3–4 cm long); and **dilation**, which varies from 0 (closed) to 10 cm (fully dilated). Sometimes the cervix is permeable to one or two fingers, but it closes when these are removed. In these situations, there is no cervical dilation. Vaginal examination also allows the identification of the following three fetal characteristics: **presenting part**, **position** (see above) and **level of descent**. It may only be possible to evaluate fetal position later on in labour, depending on whether the reference points are or not accessible through the cervical canal. Evaluation of the integrity of the amniotic membranes also forms part of routine evaluation.

43.8 Management of the First Stage of Labour

Labour and delivery can occur in different settings, ranging from classical labour wards to midwife-led birthing units, and even to home births. The pros and cons of these options fall outside the scope of this chapter. The management considered below forms part of routine care in most modern-day European labour wards.

Current expectations regarding intrapartum care in Europe are for a positive outcome for all mothers and babies arriving in hospital with term pregnancies and a non-malformed well-oxygenated fetus, while at the same time avoiding unnecessary obstetric interventions. Additionally, there is a strong focus on providing women with a positive birth experience, as this is one of the most important days for them and their families. Careful monitoring of labour progress and fetal oxygenation, as well as strong empathy and support are all required for this.

Stratification of patients into **high-risk** and **low-risk** is common in pregnancy and during labour, but not all high-risk pregnancies condition a high-risk labour, and vice versa. Among the most important risk factors for labour are **previous caesarean section, suspected fetal macrosomia, fetal growth restriction, antepartum haemorrhage** and **previous cardiotocographic (CTG) abnormalities**. However, the vast majority of labour complications occur in patients with no identified risk factors, so careful monitoring is required in all women.

Monitoring of fetal oxygenation in labour is discussed in a separate chapter. Regarding monitoring of labour progress, **vaginal examinations** are usually repeated circa every 4 hours. These intervals may be shortened, particularly during the active phase of labour, in women with induced or accelerated labours, in those with a previous caesarean section, or when there is no labour progress. The temporal evolution of cervical dilation and effacement, together with fetal position and

descent, are registered in a **partograph**. Maternal vital signs, fetal monitoring records and medications are also regularly recorded. While the rate of cervical dilation is known to vary immensely in the latent phase, it is more consistent during the active phase. Average rates of 1.2 cm/hour in nulliparous women and 1.5 cm/hour in multiparous women were described in the 1950s by Friedman [9]. More recently, wide variations have also been documented in the active phase [8]. Together with a well-documented interobserver variability in evaluation of cervical characteristics [11], these findings have led to a more conservative approach towards monitoring of labour progress. Frequent vaginal examinations should be discouraged, as they are not useful and predispose to infection [12]. More conservative definitions of protracted and arrested labour should also be used (described in a separate chapter).

There is no evidence of benefit from performing **routine amniotomy** in women with spontaneous labour and normal progress. Amniotomy is associated with risks, including fetal heart rate changes, umbilical cord prolapse and increased incidence of infections when labour becomes prolonged. Labour duration is not significantly reduced with routine amniotomy [13].

During the latent phase of labour, women usually find walking more comfortable than lying down. They should **remain fully mobile**, and be encouraged to walk, as this has been shown to reduce the duration of the latent phase [14]. They should be allowed to adopt the position they find most comfortable and not remain restricted to bed, even after the membranes have ruptured, as long as the cervix is well adapted to the presenting part, thus precluding cord prolapse. Sitting on a birthing ball and using rocking movements is an alternative to walking and can be adopted intermittently. If a woman decides to lie down, she should preferably adopt a lateral decubitus position, as this avoids compression of the aorta and inferior vena cava by the pregnant uterus, which can affect cardiac output and uteroplacental flow [15].

Unless there is a specific medical contraindication, women should be allowed **to drink moderate quantities of clear liquids** (water, juices with no pulp, coffee, tea with and without sugar) and eat gelatine [16]. Ingestion of solid foods in labour is more controversial, although regularly used in some settings [17]. **Intravenous fluids** are indicated when oral intake is insufficient. Their routine use is controversial, although they have been associated with shorter durations of labour [18]. **Pain control** in labour is considered in a separate chapter.

43.9 Management of the Second Stage of Labour

With vaginal examinations being carried out intermittently, determining the start of the second stage of labour is naturally somewhat inaccurate. More objective is the moment when the woman starts to feel the urge to push during contractions (start of the active second stage of labour). But with increasing use of epidural analgesia, even this moment can become uncertain, as the urge to push may disappear after an epidural bolus. More importantly, it is normal for some time to elapse between full dilation and the urge to push, and artificially reducing this period usually results in increased intervention rates. On the one hand, a more expectant attitude towards the **latent phase** of the second stage of labour has been shown to result in decreased intervention rates, but on the other hand excessive duration results in increased perinatal infection [19].

In many hospitals, a 2- to 3-hour maximum duration of the latent phase is established, with action required when these limits are exceeded. Evaluation of fetal position becomes particularly important at this stage. With persistent posterior positions, manual rotation of the fetal head may be attempted, and has been associated with reduced intervention rates [20]. The clinician's hand is inserted into the vagina, the fetal parietal bones are grasped with the tips of the fingers and in between contractions the head is slightly elevated and rotated slowly to an anterior position. The procedure may be painful without epidural analgesia and should be stopped on the woman's request or after 2–3 unsuccessful attempts. High success rates have been reported [20], but this is naturally dependent on the clinician's experience.

Moulding of the fetal head (overlapping of the cranial bones), persistent transverse positions and extensive caput succedaneum (fetal scalp oedema) suggest the presence of relative cephalopelvic disproportion, but on their own they are not sufficiently specific to affect management. Prolonged latent phases of the second stage of labour should lead to a trial of pushing, even if there is no spontaneous urge to do this. This is particularly frequent in women with epidural analgesia, which can block the urge to push. Women may remain fully mobile during this stage, although many will prefer to sit or lie down.

The **active phase of the second stage** starts with maternal pushing. Although adaptations may be acceptable, based on the frequency of contractions and maternal physical condition, pushing should usually not exceed 1 hour. When this occurs, instrumental vaginal delivery or caesarean section need to be considered, as described in a separate chapter.

There is no strong evidence that a given position for delivery is better than the others. Vertical positions seem to condition shorter durations of the second stage and reduced instrumental vaginal deliveries. On the other hand, horizontal positions condition are associated with less haemorrhage [21]. In women with epidural analgesia, horizontal positions leads to condition more normal deliveries [22].

Women may prefer to push according to their own instinct or may benefit from some guidance. Directed pushing encourages the mother to perform forced inspiration at the start of a contraction, and while holding her breath, exert downward force with her diaphragm (corresponding to a high-intensity Valsalva manoeuvre). There is no strong evidence that directed pushing is superior to other forms of pushing, although it is widely applied [23].

The moment the fetal head starts to extend the vaginal outlet is called **crowning**. Disinfection of the vulva and perineal region may be performed around this moment, and sterile protections placed around the lower limbs and below the perineum. **Perineal massage** in between contractions is recommended, as it has been associated with a large reduction in third- and fourth-degree perineal lacerations [24]. Descent of the fetal head is usually slow and, unless there is concern regarding fetal oxygenation, does not need to be rushed. Slow distention of the maternal soft tissues is required to avoid lacerations. **Protection of the perineum** is performed by placing a stretched hand just below the introitus and exerting inward pressure on the perineum during contractions. It aims to avoid over distention of the perineum and to help the extension of the fetal head. Importantly, the perineum should be continuously observed for signs of imminent laceration during pushing – extreme thinning, whitening and cracking of the skin and mucosa. If this occurs, an episiotomy should be performed (see below). Very slow distention of the vulva is required to avoid lacerations and to achieve an intact perineum. This can be accomplished by carefully controlling the descent of the fetal head with the hand that is not protecting the perineum, and is particularly important when the largest diameters are passing the introitus, and when the fetal nose and brows are exteriorizing.

Episiotomy consists of an incision to the outer part of the vaginal wall and perineal body, aimed at avoiding uncontrolled lacerations that may reach the anal sphincter. Routine episiotomy has not been shown to be effective in preventing severe lacerations [25], and can cause pain, infection, bleeding and dyspareunia. Conversely, selective episiotomy (i.e. when there are signs of imminent laceration – see above) is recommended, resulting in fewer severe lacerations than routine episiotomy. A mediolateral episiotomy is usually performed, as medial episiotomy increases the risk of third-degree perineal injury [26]. For mediolateral episiotomy, a 60° angle to the perineal body should be respected, as vulvar distention affects local anatomy, and this converts into a 30° angle after birth [27].

Downward pressure on the uterine fundus during contractions (the Kristeller manoeuvre) is not recommended, as it does not result in a quicker second stage of labour, and causes more cervical lacerations and increased pain in the early postpartum period [28]. There are also anecdotic reports of maternal liver and spleen lacerations with this technique [29].

After delivery of the fetal head, the region of the neck should be inspected to identify nuchal cords (umbilical cord wrapped around the neck). When these occur, they can almost invariably be freed by passing the cord around the fetal head, or freeing a small loop of cord that allows it pass around the shoulders as the fetal body is exteriorized. Very rarely, when the cord is tightly wrapped around the neck and no freeing of a loop is possible, double clamping and cutting are necessary. This usually results in a more anaemic newborn.

Given time, the head will rotate to the position in which it became engaged (external rotation), and the shoulders will rotate to the anteroposterior diameter of the pelvic outlet. Aided delivery of the shoulders may be useful to decrease perineal lacerations, but there is insufficient evidence to evaluate this. When aided delivery of the shoulders is performed, continuous traction on the head along the largest fetal axis is performed to release the anterior shoulder. When this has occurred, the posterior shoulder is delivered with slow and gentle upward traction on the fetal head, with direct visualization and protection of the perineum using the opposite hand. Very slow release of the posterior shoulder is another essential manoeuvre to achieve an intact perineum. The remaining fetal body is easily removed by gentle traction.

43.10 Management of the Third Stage of Labour

After birth, the newborn may be placed directly on the mother's abdomen or in her arms, if the length of the umbilical cord allows. After a few seconds it will usually become clear whether the newborn is vigorous (with good tonus, movements and normal collar). With vigorous newborns, the mouth and nose usually do not require aspiration, except when there is thick meconium or exaggerated secretions, or further support [30]. Early skin-to-skin contact and breastfeeding (except when contraindicated, such as in HIV-positive mothers) has been shown to increase the overall duration of breastfeeding [31]. A detailed description of neonatal support is outside the scope of this chapter.

To decrease the duration of the third stage and reduce haemorrhage associated with uterine atony, **prophylactic oxytocin** is recommended in all labours [32]. This can be given intravenously (usually in perfusion) or intramuscularly at a dose of 10 IU.

When **umbilical blood sampling** for blood gas analysis is needed, it should be performed as soon as possible after birth, and previous cord clamping is not required for this [33]. Umbilical cord blood for other purposes should preferably be collected after the cord is clamped, to avoid reducing the newborn circulation. Late cord clamping (at least 2 minutes after birth) is associated with several benefits such as increased haemoglobin levels and reduced iron deficiency, but also with increased needs for phototherapy [34]. In preterm newborns, it is associated with less neurodevelopmental complications [35]. A plastic clamp is placed circa 3 cm from the umbilical stump, a Kelly forceps is placed a further 2 cm away from this and the cord is cut between the two.

Frequent evaluation of genital haemorrhage and maternal vital signs is necessary during this period. With the continuation of uterine contractions, the placenta becomes separated from the uterine wall and comes to lie in the uterine cavity and upper part of the vagina – the process usually takes less than 15 minutes. Usual signs of placental detachment are sustained contraction of the uterus, further exteriorization of the cord and a gush of blood from the vagina. Traction on the umbilical cord should be avoided before placental detachment. To confirm that this has occurred, the uterus is pushed upwards through the abdominal wall, and the umbilical cord observed. If it retracts into the vagina, the placenta remains attached to the uterus; if no retraction occurs, detachment has occurred. Gentle and continued cord traction together with further maternal pushing or gentle external uterine massage will usually cause **placental exteriorization**. Once at the level of the vulva, the placenta can be exteriorized with the help of gravity or by twisting it several times around its main axis. This usually avoids the retention of fragmented membranes inside the uterus.

Macroscopic **examination of the placenta** involves inspecting the maternal side to evaluate whether there are any missing cotyledons, and the fetal side to evaluate whether there are sectioned vessels on the placental margin, suggesting a succenturiate or bilobed placenta. Ultrasound is indicated in the latter cases.

After the placenta is exteriorized, the uterus will usually contract in a sustained fashion to prevent bleeding from the vessels irrigating the placental bed. A contracted uterus can be palpated as a firm round mass, with the fundus circa halfway between the umbilical stump and the pubic symphysis.

The birth canal should be examined for lacerations, namely, evaluating vulvar, perineal and anal sphincter integrity. Anal sphincter lacerations and those that are actively bleeding or cause a relevant distortion in vaginal or vulvar anatomy should be surgically corrected.

Continued vigilance of vital signs, contracted uterus and genital bleeding is necessary during the first 2 hours after birth, as this is the period with the highest risk of uterine atony and vaginal haemorrhage. Ingestion of solid foods is usually deferred until the end of this 2-hour period.

References

1. Liao J, Buhimschi C, Norwitz E. Normal labour: mechanism and duration. *Obstet Gynecol Clin North Am.* 2005;**32**:14564.

2. Garfield R, Blennerhassett M, Miller S. Control of myometrial contractility: role and regulation of gap junctions. *Oxford Rev Reprod Biol.* 1988;**10**:43690.

3. Nathanielsz P. Comparative studies on the initiation of labour. *Eur J Obstet Gynecol Reprod Biol.*1998;**78**:12732.

4. Oh S, Kim C, Park I, et al. Progesterone receptor isoform (A/B) ratio of human fetal membranes increases during term parturition. *Am J Obstet Gynecol.* 2005;**193**:115660.

5. Dawood M, Wang C, Gupta R, et al. Foetal contribution to oxytocin in human labour. *Obstet Gynecol.* 1978;**52**:2059.

6. Zeeman G, Khan-Dawood F, Dawood M. Oxytocin and its receptor in pregnancy and parturition: current concepts and clinical implications. *Obstet Gynecol.* 1997;**89**:87383.

7. Albers LL, Schiff M, Gorwoda JG. The length of active labour in normal pregnancies. *Obstet Gynecol.* 1996 Mar;**87**(3):355–9.

8. Zhang J, Duan T. The physiologic pattern of normal labour progression. *BJOG.* 2018;**125**:944–54.

9. Friedman EA. Primigravid labour; a graphicostatistical analysis. *Obstet Gynecol.* 1955;**6**:56789.

10. Friedman EA. *Labour: Clinical Evaluation and Management*, 2nd ed. New York: Appleton-Century-Crofts; 1978.

11. Nizard J, Haberman S, Paltieli Y, et al. How reliable is the determination of cervical dilation? Comparison of vaginal examination with spatial position-tracking ruler. *Am J Obstet Gynecol.* 2009;**200**:402.e14.

12. Downe S, Gyte GML, Dahlen HG, Singata M. Routine vaginal examinations for assessing progress of labour to improve outcomes for women

and babies at term. *Cochrane Database Syst Rev.* 2013 Jul 15;(7):CD010088.

13. Smyth RMD, Markham C, Dowswell T. Amniotomy for shortening spontaneous labour. *Cochrane Database Syst Rev.* 2013 Jun 18;(6):CD006167.

14. Lawrence A, Lewis L, Hofmeyr GJ, Styles C. Maternal positions and mobility during first stage labour. *Cochrane Database Syst Rev.* 2013 Oct 9;(10):CD003934.

15. Roberts J, Mendez-Bauer C. A perspective of maternal position during labour. *J Perinat Med.* 1980;**8**(6):255–64.

16. American Society of Anesthesiologists. Press release. Most healthy women would benefit from light meal during labour. www.asahq.org/about-asa/newsroom/news-releases/2015/10/eating-a-light-meal-during-labour. Published November 6, 2015. Accessed February 9, 2019.

17. Singata M, Tranmer J, Gyte GMI. Restricting oral fluid and food intake during labour. *Cochrane Database Syst Rev.* 2010 Jan 20;(1):CD003930.

18. Ciardulli A, Saccone G, Anastasio H, Berghella V. Less-restrictive food intake during labour in low-risk singleton pregnancies: asystematic review and meta-analysis. *Obstet Gynecol.* 2017 Mar;**129**(3):473–80.

19. Janni W, Schiessl B, Peschers U, et al. The prognostic impact of a prolonged second stage of labour on maternal and foetal outcome. *Acta Obstet Gynecol Scand.* 2002 Mar. **81**(3):214–21.

20. Shaffer BL, Cheng YW, Vargas JE, Laros RK Jr, Caughey AB. Manual rotation of the foetal occiput: predictors of success and delivery. *Am J Obstet Gynecol.* 2006;**194**(5):e7–9.

21. Gupta JK, Sood A, Hofmeyr GJ, Vogel JP. Position in the second stage of labour for women without epidural anaesthesia. *Cochrane Database Syst Rev.* 2017 May 25(5):CD002006.

22. The Epidural and Position Trial Collaborative Group. Upright versus lying down position in second stage of labour in nulliparous women with low dose epidural: BUMPES randomised controlled trial. *BMJ.* 2017;**359**:j4471.

23. Lemos A, Amorim MMR, Dornelas de Andrade A, et al. Pushing/bearing down methods for the second stage of labour. *Cochrane Database of Systematic Rev.* 2015 Oct 9;(10):CD009124.

24. Aasheim V, Nilsen ABV, Reinar LM, Lukasse M, Reinar LM. Perineal techniques during the second stage of labour for reducing perineal trauma. *Cochrane Database Syst Rev.* 2011 Dec 7;(12):CD006672.

25. Jiang H, Qian X, Carroli G, Garner P. Selective versus routine use of episiotomy for vaginal birth. *Cochrane Database Syst Rev.* 2017 Feb 8;(2):CD000081.

26. Van Bavel J, Hukkelhoven CWPM, de Vries C, et al. The effectiveness of mediolateral episiotomy in preventing obstetric anal sphincter injuries during operative vaginal delivery: a ten-year analysis of a national registry. *Int Urogynecol J.* 2018;**29**:407413.

27. Eogan M, Daly L, O'Connell PR, O'Herlihy C. Does the angle of episiotomy affect the incidence of anal sphincter injury? *BJOG.* 2006;**113**:1904.

28. Hofmeyr GJ, Vogel JP, Cuthbert A, Singata M. Fundal pressure during the second stage of labour. *Cochrane Database Syst Rev.* 2017 Mar 7(3):CD006067.

29. Simpson KR, Knox GE. Fundal pressure during the second stage of labour. *MCN Am J Matern Child Nurs.* 2001;**26**(2):64–70.

30. Wyllie J, Bruinenberg J, Roehr CC, et al. European Resuscitation Council guidelines for resuscitation 2015: Section 7. Resuscitation and support of transition of babies at birth. *Resuscitation.* 2015;**95**:249–63.

31. Moore ER, Bergman N, Anderson GC, Medley N. Early skin-to-skin contact for mothers and their healthy newborn infants. *Cochrane Database Syst Rev.* 2016 Nov;(11):CD003519.

32. Westhoff G, Cotter AM, Tolosa JE. Prophylactic oxytocin for the third stage of labour to prevent postpartum haemorrhage. *Cochrane Database Syst Rev.* 2013 Oct 30;(10):CD001808.

33. Ayres-de-Campos D, Arulkumaran S; FIGO Intrapartum Foetal Monitoring Expert Consensus Panel. FIGO consensus guidelines on intrapartum foetal monitoring: Physiology of foetal oxygenation and the main goals of intrapartum foetal monitoring. *Int J Gynaecol Obstet.* 2015;**131**(1):5–8.

34. McDonald SJ, Middleton P, Dowswell T, Morris PS. Effect of timing of umbilical cord clamping of term infants on maternal and neonatal outcomes. *Cochrane Database Syst Rev.* 2013 Jul(7):CD004074.

35. Andersson O, Lindquist B, Lindgren M, et al. Effect of delayed cord clamping on neurodevelopment at 4 years of age: a randomized clinical trial. *JAMA Pediatr.* 2015;**169**:6318.

Chapter

44

Issues during Labour for Migrant Populations

Apostolos M. Mamopoulos, Ioannis Tsakiridis & Apostolos P. Athanasiadis

44.1 Introduction – Epidemiology

According to the United Nation's definition, an international migrant is "a person who is living in a country other than his or her country of birth". By mid-2015, the UN reported that the number of new refugees and asylum seekers was about 15.1 million, and 1.6 million applications for asylum or refugee status were filed in 2014 alone. The hardship associated with the refugee experience can be especially pronounced for women who face the risk of discrimination and of physical and/or sexual violence. Past traumas that occurred in the country of origin can aggravate that feeling.

During pregnancy, labour and the postpartum period, research has found that, especially for migrant women, inadequate access and utilization of prenatal care, lack of interpretation services, incongruent cultural understanding and postpartum depression are significant risks. In such circumstances, medical care should be adapted to the specific requirements of migrants, as they represent a population with increased rates of total morbidity and mortality. The majority of migrants have late or no access to appropriate antenatal care, which is also highly correlated with adverse perinatal outcomes.

44.2 Ethnicity-related Issues

44.2.1 The 'Healthy Migrant Effect'

The 'healthy migrant effect', according to which migrants are healthier than people of similar ethnic backgrounds who were born in the host country, is paradoxical because many migrants have low socio-economic status, which should logically lead to less healthy lifestyles, fewer health-promoting behaviours and less access to primary healthcare in the high-income host countries [1]. The literature suggests that the healthy migrant effect on perinatal outcomes often varies, depending on country of origin and type of birth outcome, as well as healthcare and integration policies of the receiving countries [2]. When talking about the healthy migrant effect, selective migration should also be mentioned. Selective migration suggests that healthier individuals are more likely to migrate to a new country than their less healthy counterparts [3]. According to Norman et al [4], migrants are generally healthier than non-migrants when moving from more to less economically deprived locations, whereas migrants who relocate to more economically deprived areas tend to be less healthy than non-migrants.

44.2.2 Maternal and Child Health

Contradictory evidence exists for maternal and child health since a systematic review states that, although perinatal health outcomes were not consistently poorer among migrant women in general, geographic origin was important, with Asian and African migrants being at increased risk of fetal-neonatal mortality and preterm birth than the majority of migrant populations in Western industrialized countries [2]. Up to 15% of pregnant women experience life-threatening obstetric complications after leaving their homeland [5]. Moreover, Simsek et al reported a frequency of 47.7% of pregnancy losses among Syrian refugee women in Turkey [6]. The risk for an adverse perinatal outcome including stillbirth [7, 8], perinatal mortality [2, 9], caesarean section [9, 10], preterm birth [2, 10] and low birthweight [9, 10] appears to be increased among migrant women compared to women born in resettlement countries. Evaluating pregnancy outcomes for a heterogeneous migrant population may be limited by possible bias due to differences between women that are often undetectable in routine clinical datasets (e.g. cultural beliefs, dietary habits or genetic background). For example, female genital mutilation is a risk factor for adverse pregnancy outcomes that varies in prevalence and severity between African regions [11]. A recently published systematic review of systematic reviews [12] found that perinatal health outcomes were worse for migrant women than women in the host country, including mental health disorders, maternal mortality, preterm birth and congenital anomalies of the newborn.

44.2.3 Healthcare Providers' Gender Issues

Gender of the provider has been a contentious issue in obstetrics since the medicalization of childbirth, while the term *midwife* literally means 'with woman'. Overall, male obstetricians-gynaecologists are clearly a barrier for many migrant women accessing obstetric healthcare, mainly due to religious influences but also due to feeling more comfortable with female healthcare providers. It was only after 1700 that a male in the medical profession got involved in childbirth, but since then the male's presence at childbirth remains contested; the majority of women worldwide show a preference for a female obstetrician-gynaecologist. Especially for women originating from specific religious or cultural environments where separation of genders is the societal norm, preference for female healthcare providers is of even greater importance. On the other hand, a patient's refusal of care in terms of gender could be defined as gender discrimination. The Society of

Obstetricians and Gynaecologists of Canada (SOGC) states that, in order to provide the best care for all women, 'provision of (time sensitive or urgent) services cannot and should not ever be based on gender, race, sexual orientation, age, practice patterns or religious connections of either the patient or the provider' [13]. A systematic review found that there is a high preference for female obstetricians among migrant women, especially for Muslims [14]. Similarly, a qualitative study of African refugees in the USA found that even in an emergency, only 5 of 18 women would accept care from a male physician [15]. On the contrary, other qualitative studies have shown that women would consequently accept care from male providers [16] despite the significant preference for female providers; women themselves valued competency and respect over any concern regarding gender of their provider. Enhanced communication in the antenatal period between the healthcare provider and the female patient is most likely the key component in addressing such concerns.

44.3 Delivery Issues

44.3.1 Caesarean Section

Several studies have reported mixed results regarding the frequency of caesarean and operative vaginal delivery in the migrant population, and those results varied according to the country of origin and the host country [2]. Increased odds of caesarean section were reported for migrants from Caribbean states, South Asia, the Philippines and Somalia. In addition, a recently published study (2016) [17] found that migrant women from sub-Saharan Africa had high caesarean section rates, while migrants from Eastern Europe had lower rates. Higher rates of emergency caesarean deliveries were also reported for women who had migrated from Latin America, North Africa and the Middle East. A study that investigated migration status found no differences in the incidence of caesarean section between African women of refugee and non-refugee background [18]. On the other hand, a significantly higher prevalence of caesarean sections has been observed in refugee women than in a local population in Canada [19]. Those findings are similar to those of Gagnon et al who found a higher risk of caesarean sections among newly arrived migrants [20]. Consequently, certain groups of international migrants have different rates of caesarean sections than do local women. There is still insufficient evidence to explain these differences.

Similar to non-migrant women, it appears that all efforts should predominantly focus on aiming to reduce the primary caesarean rate, particularly the need for emergency caesareans due to more 'obscure' indications, such as abnormal fetal heart rate, and to increase the rates of vaginal births after a caesarean [21]. Statements in high-income countries, directed towards reducing the need for a caesarean section [22–24] recommend the following: easy access to prenatal care and education, continuous support during labour, no interventions during labour unless medically indicated, options for pharmacological as well as non-pharmacological pain management, more patience for labour to progress and allowing women to push longer. Women should be properly informed and participate in every

decision, while respect and consideration should be paid for the psychological and social aspects of labour and birth when providing care.

There are many risk factors that possibly affect the risk of caesarean section in migrants. First, a greater prevalence of excess weight and obesity among certain groups of women, including women from sub-Saharan Africa and North Africa, as well as migrant women arriving from 'humanitarian' source countries, has been shown. Research suggests that excess weight may be a causal factor in high caesarean section rates for some migrants. Adoption of more 'Western' dietary habits and sedentary lifestyles has been cited as one of the possible causes of migrants gaining excess weight. Two systematic reviews have indicated the association of increased body mass index and excessive gestational weight gain with an increased risk of fetal macrosomia and caesarean delivery [25, 26]. Human immunodeficiency virus (HIV), a known indication for a caesarean, is also known to be more prevalent in migrants. Insensitivity and improper care of women with genital cutting are probably the explanation for high caesarean section rates among these women rather than the scar itself. Genital cutting should not be considered an indication for caesarean.

44.3.2 Barriers

44.3.2.1 Cultural

It seems that culture and women's experiences before migration affect expectations of maternity care. Some women migrate from countries such as Brazil, which is known to have a very high caesarean rate and where it appears to be culturally preferred to have a caesarean. Conversely, consistently lower rates of caesarean sections among migrants from Eastern Europe have been suggested to be due to their cultural preference for less interventional care during labour. A large Norwegian study including women from 133 countries found evidence that the caesarean rate of a migrant's country of origin is associated with her likelihood to have a caesarean section [27]. Greater acculturation is also associated with higher caesarean rates for some migrants. *Acculturation* refers to the extent to which women have adopted the attitudes, behaviours and traditions of the receiving country.

44.3.2.2 Language

Language barriers have also been frequently suggested to play a role in migrant women's risk for a caesarean section. In the intrapartum period, documentation of assessments should be detailed in the relevant partograms to avoid repeat examinations. During labour, women may not understand what is happening and may be unable to effectively communicate about their preferences and support needs, including pain management. Explaining the normal labour stages dispels fear and helps the normal process. In the migrant population, however, such communication is quite difficult or even impossible because of the aforementioned barrier. Difficulties in communication often prevent obstetricians or midwives from providing the proper care that would lead to vaginal labour, such as adoption of alternative postures or pain-relief methods. Lack of communication enhances fear and may lead to unnecessary interventions. Migrant women often report problems with communication and caregivers' attitudes; they are made to feel anxious and not welcomed when they arrive at the hospital in labour.

Finally, barriers including limited or no health insurance and impediments to access to prenatal care need to be addressed to ensure all migrant women receive prenatal care; interpreters and translated materials should be used to ensure effective screening, treatment, education and health promotion of all migrant women.

44.3.3 Group B Streptococcus

Group B streptococcus (GBS, *Streptococcus agalactiae*) is a leading cause of neonatal sepsis in the developed world. According to National Institute for Health and Care Excellence (NICE) [28], pregnant women should not be offered routine antenatal screening for group B streptococcus because evidence of its clinical and cost-effectiveness remains uncertain. Historically, infection with GBS has been reported to be rare in the developing world. Intrapartum antibiotics given to women colonized with GBS have been shown to reduce the incidence of early-onset GBS neonatal sepsis. A cross-sectional study [29] in a refugee pregnant population in South East Asia found that the GBS carriage rate was 12%; all GBS isolates were susceptible to penicillin, ceftriaxone and vancomycin and 91.5% were susceptible to erythromycin and clindamycin. The prevalence of GBS colonization in this population was lower than that reported in developed countries (20–30%).

44.3.4 Pain Management

Healthcare professionals should think about how their own values and beliefs form their attitude to coping with pain in labour and ensure their care supports the woman's choice [23]. If a woman chooses to use breathing and relaxation techniques in labour, her choices should be supported. If a woman chooses to use massage techniques in labour that have been taught to birth companions, her choice should also be supported. The woman should be offered the opportunity to labour in water for pain relief. Acupuncture, acupressure or hypnosis should not be offered, but women who wish to use these techniques should not be prevented from doing so. If a woman is contemplating regional analgesia, she should be informed about the risks and benefits and the implications for her labour. If a woman in labour asks for regional analgesia, the healthcare provider should comply with her request. This includes women in severe pain in the latent first stage of labour. Any woman with infibulated genital mutilation should also be informed of the risks of difficulty with vaginal examination, catheterization and application of fetal scalp electrodes. She should be informed of the risks of delay in the second stage and spontaneous laceration together with the need for an anterior episiotomy and the possible need for defibulation in labour. African migrant women have previously been reported to be less likely to use analgesia during labour.

44.3.5 Episiotomy

The use of episiotomy during labour, especially in cases of female genital mutilation, is often used in order to reduce severe perineal trauma. The American College of Obstetricians and Gynecologists and the Society of Obstetricians and Gynaecologists of Canada recommend a restrictive episiotomy over a routine episiotomy, while the Royal College of Obstetricians and Gynaecologists states that clinicians should explain to women that there is conflicting evidence for the protective effect of episiotomy [30]. A systematic review showed that routine episiotomy offered no maternal benefit regarding the severity of perineal laceration, pelvic floor dysfunction or pelvic organ prolapse over the restrictive use of episiotomy [31]. In general, refugee women tend to have significantly fewer episiotomies and less severe perineal traumas.

44.4 Complications

44.4.1 Preterm Labour

Several studies have examined the risk of preterm birth in migrant women. A meta-review of 65 European studies [32] reported that migrant women tend to have significantly worse birth outcomes than women from the host country, including greater prevalence of low birthweight (43%), preterm birth (24%), perinatal mortality (50%) and congenital malformations (61%). Another meta-analysis [2] found also higher odds of preterm birth (<37 gestational weeks) among migrant women. On the other hand, the healthy migrant effect may have an impact on the prevalence of preterm birth: length of residence seems to affect the prevalence of preterm birth in migrants, since those with less than 5 years of residence had a lower prevalence of preterm birth compared with women in the host countries [33]. Previous studies have demonstrated that the incidence of preterm birth among migrant women may vary based on geographic region of origin: migrants from sub-Saharan Africa and Asia tend to have higher likelihood of preterm birth than native-born populations in developed countries [34]. A systematic review, published in 2009 [2], compared birth outcomes between migrants and native residents of Western industrialized countries. Preterm birth outcomes of migrant women, compared to native women, were worse in 36.4%, better in 45.5% and no different in 18.2% of examined reports. Another study examined how the combination of migrancy and mother's education influences the birth outcome [35]. Hence, it was proven that foreign-born status was associated with an increased risk for preterm birth in university-educated mothers only. Collectively, the above-mentioned contrasting findings may be explained by several factors such as differences in the countries of origin, the percentages of refugees, selective migration, access to care compared to previous studies and inaccurate pregnancy dating.

44.4.2 Low Birthweight

In a comparison, Shah et al found that foreign-born women had a greater risk of having low birthweight infants and deliveries by caesarean sections [36]. The evidence related to birthweight is still not clear. A meta-analysis [32] found that low birthweight (<2500 g) was increased in migrant women residing in Europe, while another meta-analysis showed a reduced prevalence of low birthweight infants among migrants [2]. Studies have proposed that the healthy migrant effect, as already mentioned above, may have an impact on the birthweight of the neonate [33]. Indeed, the results of a Portuguese study [37] showed that migrants were reported with a lower risk of low birthweight and small-for-gestational-age fetus, even after adjustment for important co-variates. Moreover, it is observed that migrants with low levels of education have better outcomes regarding birthweight of the neonate, when compared with non-migrant populations [33]. Another systematic review [38] examined how the apparent healthy migrant effect in the USA (where migrant populations often have improved outcomes compared with non-migrant populations) is contrasted by the health inequalities in Europe, where the associations are reversed and an increased risk of low birthweight neonates is observed, showing that the healthy migrant effect might disappear under certain circumstances. Evidence from a study in Turkey [39] showed that compared to Turkish pregnant women, Syrian refugees had a significantly lower gestational age at delivery, lower rates of caesarean sections and shorter length of hospitalization, but no significant differences in birthweight of the newborns were identified. In addition, maternal (e.g. postpartum haemorrhage) and fetal complications (e.g. admission to neonatal intensive care unit) and fetal anomaly rates were similar for both groups. Hence, there are inconsistent findings regarding the prevalence of low birthweight neonates among migrants. The lack of individua-lized methods of assessment of the estimated fetal weight or the birthweight might be one of the causes. The development of international estimated fetal weight standards, such as those proposed by the INTERGROWTH-21st study, has become, nowadays, almost imperative [40]. As a result, low birthweight neonates should be identified with caution when analyzing different populations. Finally, an increased risk of congenital anomalies and admission to the neonatal intensive care unit have been reported for migrants [32].

44.5 Conclusions

According to NICE, maternity services should provide a model of care that supports one-to-one care in labour for all women [23].

All parturients should be treated with respect and they should be in control of and involved in all decisions about their care in labour. To facilitate this, a rapport should be established with all women, and their expectations regarding labour should, ideally, be discussed beforehand and documented in the pregnancy notes. Both physicians and midwives involved in the intrapartum care of migrants should be aware of the importance of tone and demeanor and of the actual words used. In addition, all women should receive information during the antenatal period about what to expect in each stage of labour. Each woman in established labour should be provided with supportive one-to-one care.

Healthcare providers should be particularly aware of the requirements of pregnant migrants and should adapt primary healthcare strategies accordingly. They should always explain to those pregnant women who are at low risk of complications that giving birth is generally very safe for both the woman and her baby [23]. Clinical care should not deviate from the host country's recommendations, but extra caution and sensitivity are needed in order to make sure that they are adapted to the special needs of each woman from different minority groups. Optimized maternal healthcare may be an effective method to improve pregnancy outcomes, as well as long-term maternal and offspring outcomes.

44.6 Key Messages

- Migrants should have 24-hour access to host countries' health systems in order to give birth.
- A professional interpreter, preferably a non-relative, should be provided during labour, preferably via face-to-face contact.
- Healthcare providers' gender should be taken into consideration according to women's preferences, if possible.
- Continuous emotional support to the women and appropriate training to all staff working with migrant pregnant women should be provided, in order to successfully overcome the language, cultural and financial barriers during the intrapartum period.
- Labour and delivery issues should be based on local guidelines, despite the 'healthy migrant effect'.
- Bearing in mind that accurate pregnancy dating is not always available, there is an urgent need for an adoption of estimated fetal weight charts in order to avoid false diagnosis of macrosomia or fetal growth restriction.

References

1. Gould JB, Madan A, Qin C, Chavez G. Perinatal outcomes in two dissimilar immigrant populations in the United States: a dual epidemiologic paradox. *Pediatrics.* 2003 Jun; **111**(6 Pt 1): e676–82.

2. Gagnon AJ, Zimbeck M, Zeitlin J, et al. Migration to Western industrialised countries and perinatal health: a systematic review. *Soc Sci Med.* 2009 Sep;**69**(6):934–46.

3. Crimmins EM, Kim JK, Alley DE, Karlamangla A, Seeman T. Hispanic paradox in biological risk profiles. *Am J Public Health.* 2007 Jul;**97** (7):1305–10.

4. Norman P, Boyle P, Rees P. Selective migration, health and deprivation: a longitudinal analysis. *Soc Sci Med.* 2005 Jun;**60**(12):2755–71.

5. Women's Refugee Commission. Available online: www.womensrefugee commission.org/empower/resources/ practitioners-forum/facts-and-figures (accessed on 17 October 2018).

6. Simsek Z, Yentur Doni N, Gul Hilali N, Yildirimkaya G. A community-based survey on Syrian refugee women's health and its predictors in Sanliurfa, Turkey. *Women Health.* 2018 Jul;**58** (6):617–31.

7. Ravelli AC, Tromp M, Eskes M, et al. Ethnic differences in stillbirth and early neonatal mortality in The Netherlands. *J Epidemiol Community He*alth. 2011 Aug;**65**(8):696–701.

8. Ekeus C, Cnattingius S, Essen B, Hjern A. Stillbirth among foreign-born women in Sweden. *Eur J Public Health.* 2011 Dec;**21**(6):788–92.

9. Malin M, Gissler M. Maternal care and birth outcomes among ethnic minority women in Finland. *BMC Public Health.* 2009 Mar **20**;9:84.

10. Zanconato G, Iacovella C, Parazzini F, Bergamini V, Franchi M. Pregnancy outcome of migrant women delivering in a public institution in northern Italy. *Gynecol Obstet Invest.* 2011;**72** (3):157–62.

11. Banks E, Meirik O, Farley T, Akande O, Bathija H, Ali M. Female genital mutilation and obstetric outcome: WHO collaborative prospective study in six African countries. *Lancet.* 2006 Jun 3;**367**(9525):1835–41.

12. Heslehurst N, Brown H, Pemu A, Coleman H, Rankin J. Perinatal health outcomes and care among asylum seekers and refugees: a systematic review of systematic reviews. *BMC Med.* 2018 Jun 12;**16**(1):89.

13. Society of Obstetricians and Gynaecologists of Canada. *SOGC Position Statement: When a Patient Asks for Another Physician on Cultural or Religious Grounds.* Ottawa: Society of Obstetricians and Gynaecologists of Canada; 2013.

14. Small R, Roth C, Raval M, et al. Immigrant and non-immigrant women's experiences of maternity care: a systematic and comparative review of studies in five countries. *BMC Pregnancy Childbirth.* 2014 Apr **29**;14:152.

15. Carroll J, Epstein R, Fiscella K, et al. Caring for Somali women: implications for clinician-patient communication. *Patient Educ Couns.* 2007 Jun;**66** (3):337–45.

16. Murray L, Windsor C, Parker E, Tewfik O. The experiences of African women giving birth in Brisbane, Australia. *Health Care Women Int.* 2010 May;**31**(5):458–72.

17. Merry L, Vangen S, Small R. Caesarean births among migrant women in high-income countries. *Best Pract Res Clin Obstet Gynaecol.* 2016 Apr;**32**:88–99.

18. Gagnon AJ, Van Hulst A, Merry L, et al. Cesarean section rate differences by migration indicators. *Arch Gynecol Obstet.* 2013 Apr;**287**(4):633–9.

19. Kandasamy T, Cherniak R, Shah R, Yudin MH, Spitzer R. Obstetric risks and outcomes of refugee women at a single centre in Toronto. *J Obstet Gynaecol Can.* 2014 Apr;**36** (4):296–302.

20. Gagnon AJ, Dougherty G, Platt RW, et al. Refugee and refugee-claimant women and infants post-birth: migration histories as a predictor of Canadian health system response to needs. *Can J Public Health.* 2007 Jul–Aug;**98**(4):287–91.

21. Tsakiridis I, Mamopoulos A, Athanasiadis A, Dagklis T. Vaginal birth after previous cesarean birth: a comparison of 3 national guidelines. *Obstet Gynecol Surv.* 2018 Sep;**73** (9):537–43.

22. American College of Obstetricians and Gynecologists, Society for Maternal-Fetal M, Caughey AB, Cahill AG, Guise JM, et al. Safe prevention of the primary cesarean delivery. *Am J Obstet Gynecol.* 2014 Mar;**210**(3):179–93.

23. NICE. *Intrapartum Care for Healthy Women and Babies.* Clinical Guideline. 3 December 2014.

24. Executive and Council of the Society of Obstetricians and Gynaecologists of Canada (SOGC), The Association of Women's Health Obstetric and Neonatal Nurses of Canada (AWHONN Canada), The Canadian Association of Midwives (CAM), The College of Family Physicians of Canada (CFPC), and the Society of Rural Physicians of Canada (SRPC). SOGC Joint Policy Statement on Normal Childbirth. *J Obstet Gynaecol Can.* 2008;**30**:1163e5.

25. Goldstein RF, Abell SK, Ranasinha S, et al. Association of gestational weight gain with maternal and infant outcomes: a systematic review and meta-analysis. *JAMA.* 2017 Jun 6;**317** (21):2207–25.

26. Poobalan AS, Aucott LS, Gurung T, Smith WC, Bhattacharya S. Obesity as an independent risk factor for elective and emergency caesarean delivery in nulliparous women–systematic review and meta-analysis of cohort studies. *Obes Rev.* 2009 Jan;**10**(1):28–35.

27. Grytten J, Skau I, Sørensen R. Do mothers decide? The impact of preferences in healthcare. *J Hum Resour* 2013;**48**: 142e68.

28. NICE. *Antenatal Care for Uncomplicated Pregnancies.* Clinical Guideline. 26 March 2008.

29. Turner C, Turner P, Po L, et al. Group B streptococcal carriage, serotype distribution and antibiotic susceptibilities in pregnant women at the time of delivery in a refugee population on the Thai-Myanmar border. *BMC Infect Dis.* 2012 Feb 8;12:34.

30. Tsakiridis I, Mamopoulos A, Athanasiadis A, Dagklis T. Obstetric anal sphincter injuries at vaginal delivery: a review of recently published national guidelines. *Obstet Gynecol Surv.* 2018 Dec;**73** (12):695–702.

31. Hartmann K, Viswanathan M, Palmieri R, et al. Outcomes of routine episiotomy: a systematic review. *JAMA.* 2005 May 4;**293**(17):2141–8.

32. Bollini P, Pampallona S, Wanner P, Kupelnick B. Pregnancy outcome of migrant women and integration policy: a systematic review of the international literature. *Soc Sci Med.* 2009 Feb;**68** (3):452–61.

33. De Maio FG. Immigration as pathogenic: a systematic review of the health of immigrants to Canada. *Int J Equity Health.* 2010 Nov **24**;(9): 27.

34. Zeitlin J, Blondel B, Ananth CV. Characteristics of childbearing women, obstetrical interventions and preterm delivery: a comparison of the US and France. *Matern Child Health J.* 2015 May;**19**(5):1107–14.

35. Auger N, Luo ZC, Platt RW, Daniel M. Do mother's education and foreign born status interact to influence birth outcomes? Clarifying the epidemiological paradox and the healthy migrant effect. *J Epidemiol Community Health.* 2008 May;**62** (5):402–9.

36. Shah RR, Ray JG, Taback N, Meffe F, Glazier RH. Adverse pregnancy outcomes among foreign-born

371

Canadians. *J Obstet Gynaecol Can.* 2011 Mar;**33**(3):207–15.

37. Kana MA, Correia S, Barros H. Adverse pregnancy outcomes: a comparison of risk factors and prevalence in native and migrant mothers of Portuguese generation XXI birth cohort. *J Immigr Minor Health.* 2019 Apr;**21**(2): 307–14.

38. Villalonga-Olives E, Kawachi I, von Steinbuchel N. Pregnancy and birth outcomes among immigrant women in the US and Europe: a systematic review. *J Immigr Minor Health.* 2017 Dec;**19** (6):1469–87.

39. Gungor ES, Seval O, Ilhan G, Verit FF. Do Syrian refugees have increased risk for worser pregnancy outcomes?

Results of a tertiary center in Istanbul. *Turk J Obstet Gynecol.* 2018 Mar;**15** (1):23–7.

40. Stirnemann J, Villar J, Salomon LJ, et al. International estimated fetal weight standards of the INTERGROWTH-21(st) Project. *Ultrasound Obstet Gynecol.* 2017 Apr;**49** (4):478–86.

Chapter 45

Prolonged Pregnancy

Christina I. Messini & Alexandros Daponte

45.1 Introduction

Prolongation of pregnancy was described for the first time in the nineteenth century as case reports. The fact that a fetus remaining longer than what is considered normal in the uterine environment can have harmful effects on the fetus was first reported in 1911 by Adam Wright, who recommended 'induction of labour' as a routine procedure within two or three days after due date [1].

Prolongation of gestation is defined as the increase in the duration of pregnancy beyond 42+0 weeks of gestation, measured from the first day of the last menstrual period, in women with a menstrual cycle of 28 days' duration. Although the aetiopathogenetic mechanism remains largely unknown, it is believed that most prolonged pregnancies are due to an incorrect estimation of the last menstrual period or ovulation. Therefore, the main reason for diagnosing prolongation of pregnancy is the inaccurate determination of the age of pregnancy. Nevertheless, with the established use of ultrasound for dating, prolonged pregnancies nowadays are less common.

It has become clear, therefore, that the precise determination of the age of pregnancy is necessary, because prolonged pregnancies are considered high-risk pregnancies with increased rates of perinatal morbidity and mortality. This is due to many factors, such as the increased birthweight of the fetus, the decreased volume of amniotic fluid and the aging of the placenta.

In general, prolongation of pregnancy occurs mostly in primigravida women, in women with previous prolongation of pregnancy or in pregnancies with congenital abnormalities of the fetus. Proper dating for diagnosis as well as recognition and confirmation of possible complications are very important.

There are no ways to prevent prolonged pregnancy apart possibly from stripping or sweeping the membranes near term. Therefore, the management of a prolonged pregnancy depends on possible fetal distress and/or on the presence of various risk factors for mother and fetus with the aim of reducing perinatal mortality.

45.2 Definition

According to the World Health Organization (WHO) and the American College of Obstetricians and Gynecologists (ACOG), prolongation of pregnancy or post-term pregnancy is defined as a pregnancy lasting more than 294 days or 42+0 gestational weeks (Table 45.1) (Figure 45.1) [2]. Measurement of the duration is calculated from the first day of the last

Table 45.1 Definition of term pregnancy – ACOG

Definition	Weeks of gestation
Full-term pregnancy	From 39+0 to 40+6
Late-term pregnancy	From 41+0 to 41+6
Post-term / prolonged pregnancy	From 42+0 and more (≥294 days)

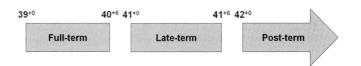

Figure 45.1 Prolonged pregnancy definition according to ACOG

menstrual period in women with a fixed menstrual cycle of 28 days. In these women, ovulation is estimated to occur around the 14th day of the menstrual cycle. Mean duration of a pregnancy is 280 days or 40+0 weeks of gestation. Full-term pregnancy occurs between 39+0 and 40+6 gestational weeks and late-term pregnancy is referred to as the period between 41+0 and 41+6 gestational weeks. However, it is worth noting that there is no consensus regarding the definition of this condition, as, for example, based on the French College of Gynecologists and Obstetricians (CNGOF), the pregnancy is considered prolonged when the duration is from 41+0 up to 41+6 gestational weeks and post-term when the duration is 42+0 gestational weeks and more (Table 45.2) [3].

Although the last menstrual period is the usual parameter on which the definition of prolongation of pregnancy is based, the widespread use of ultrasound has provided significant help in defining prolonged pregnancy more accurately. In a recent large cohort study from Denmark, in which 8551 singleton pregnancies delivered spontaneously were included and different dating methods were compared, it was shown that with first versus second trimester dating by ultrasound, the post-term delivery rate was lower [4]. The dating methods in that study included the last menstrual period, crown–rump length, biparietal diameter and head circumference. Ultrasound, when used by experienced staff, is a reliable method and is recommended routinely in the first trimester. However, dating can be affected by many other factors, such as maternal age, parity, gender of

Table 45.2 Definition of term pregnancy – CNGOF

Definition	Weeks of gestation
Term pregnancy	From 37+0 to 40+6
Prolonged pregnancy	From 41+0 to 41+6
Post-term / prolonged pregnancy	From 42+0 and more

the fetus, smoking, etc. It has been also shown that, in nulliparous women, increased length of the cervix in the second trimester noted by ultrasound is associated with increased possibility of prolonged pregnancy.

45.3 Epidemiology and Aetiology

Due to the lack of consensus regarding the definition of prolonged pregnancy, in the literature, there are significant variations of the incidence of this condition. In the UK and USA, an incidence has been reported ranging from 4.4 to 5.3%. In Sweden, the incidence reaches 6.5%, while in France the incidence of prolonged pregnancy is about 15–20% and that of post-term pregnancy only 1% [3, 5]. It is necessary, therefore, to distinguish between true and false prolongation of pregnancy. In an earlier study, when the menstrual dating was used, an incidence of 7.5% was found, while the incidence was decreased to 2.6% when it was based on ultrasound examination and to 1.1% when the two methods were used together [6]. The prevalence of post-date pregnancy is affected not only by the accuracy of gestational age estimation but also by the time that elective induction of labour is decided [7].

The aetiology of true prolonged pregnancy is not well known. Observational studies have shown potential predisposing factors for post-term pregnancy. These factors, some of which will be explained below, include null parity, prior post-term pregnancy, genes-related post-term pregnancy, a male fetus, congenital fetal abnormalities and increased maternal body mass index (BMI) [8]. The importance of various biological mechanisms has not been delineated. Normally, the spontaneous onset of labour involves many interactions between a variety of mechanisms, in which hormonal factors play a pivotal role. In this process, the role of corticotropin-releasing hormone (CRH) is central, which is produced by the placenta. Expression of this substance in the placenta has been found to increase over the last weeks of pregnancy both in term and preterm labour. In spontaneous onset of labour, CRH and oestriol are correlated and the levels of both increase at term. This together with progesterone withdrawal may participate in the initiation of labour. Possible failed interactions between the key factors towards the end of pregnancy, also including a slower increase in placental CRH expression, may contribute to the occurrence of prolonged pregnancy.

45.3.1 Parity and Prolonged Pregnancy

An association between parity and prolongation of pregnancy has been reported in many studies [9]. There seems to be a greater probability of post-term pregnancy in primipara women when compared to multipara.

45.3.2 Recurrence and Prolonged Pregnancy

Studies have shown that a previous post-term pregnancy increases the risk of pregnancy prolongation in a subsequent birth. Women who had their first delivery after 42+0 gestational weeks have a higher risk of repeated post-term delivery in the next gestation. There seems to be a relation between gestational age at delivery during the first pregnancy and gestational age at delivery in the second pregnancy. The recurrence of post-term pregnancy suggests that genetic factors may influence this increased risk [10].

45.3.3 Genetic Factors and Prolonged Pregnancy

The tendency of repeated post-term pregnancies in the same woman suggests that prolongation of pregnancy is not only related to environmental causes, but that it may be also biologically determined. Heredity may play a role, while possible genetic and epigenetic factors may interact with environmental factors contributing to pregnancy prolongation [11]. Studies show that family history of post-term pregnancy is related to the appearance of a prolongation in another pregnancy. More specifically, women's sisters with prolongation of pregnancy are more likely to experience post-term pregnancy, while there is no significant difference in brothers' partners, suggesting that maternal but not paternal genes influence post-term pregnancy [12]. Meanwhile, other studies have found a relation between paternal genes and prolongation of pregnancy, suggesting that it is important to consider the woman's personal history and the possible change of partner [13]. In a Danish study of 2588 same-sex twin pairs, it was observed that the rate of correlation of genetic factors with post-term pregnancy reached 30% [14]. Carrying of a male fetus appears to predispose significantly to prolongation of pregnancy after 43 weeks of gestation [15].

45.3.4 Body Mass Index (BMI) and Prolonged Pregnancy

The mechanism by which the mother's weight affects the duration of pregnancy and the delivery time is not known. However, it seems that women who are obese have a statistically higher incidence of prolonged pregnancy. This is particularly evident for women giving birth after 42+0 weeks if they belong to class III obesity (BMI ≥40) [16].

45.3.5 Antioxidant Status and Prolonged Pregnancy

During normal pregnancy, there seems to be a balance between antioxidants and oxidative concentrations. As pregnancy progresses and gets closer to due date, an increase in the oxidation process has been reported. A disturbance in this balance has been implicated in the aetiopathogenesis of various obstetric complications. It is likely that reduced oxidative stress is associated with the occurrence of prolonged gestation [17].

45.3.6 Oestrogens and Prolonged Pregnancy

Oestrogens play an important role in the regulation of many functions during pregnancy. In particular, oestriol (E3) and oestradiol (E2) have a key role in labour control. Reduced production of oestradiol appears to be related to prolongation of pregnancy. Rare fetal-placental factors related to this reduction that predispose to post-term pregnancy are fetal anencephaly, absence of fetal pituitary gland, abnormal functioning of fetal adrenal gland and deficiency of placental sulphatase [18, 19].

45.4 Pathogenesis/Pathophysiology

It has become clear that the potential risks of prolonged pregnancy derive from postmature placenta and oligohydramnios [20]. Although placental pathophysiology in post-term pregnancies is not well understood, it is known that as pregnancy progresses, the placenta ages with consequent formation of infarcts due to an increased amount of calcium deposition on blood vessels. Additionally, the aging placenta diminishes in diameter, while the length of chorionic villi decreases. This results in placental dysfunction and decreased oxygen transportation to the fetus. Infarcts are found in about 10–25% of term and 60–80% of post-term placentas. These changes in the morphology of the placenta can be detected by ultrasound classified into grades, which correspond to changes in placental functionality. On the other hand, if the placenta continues to function normally in post-term pregnancies, this will lead to an increase in the fetal weight. That is the reason why 20–25% of neonates delivered after 42 gestational weeks have a birthweight of 4000 g and more as compared to newborns delivered at 40±0 gestational weeks. Overweight fetuses may be the cause of obstetric complications related to the mother and/ or the fetus itself. Additionally, a continuous reduction of amniotic fluid contributes to the increased risk of perinatal morbidity and mortality [5].

45.5 Complications

Several studies have demonstrated that pregnancies beyond 42+0 weeks of gestation are associated with a number of complications, such as increased risk of stillbirth, increased perinatal mortality and morbidity and increased risk of caesarean delivery (Table 45.3).

45.5.1 Postmaturity Syndrome

In 1954, Stewart H. Clifford was the first to describe a clinical syndrome that often occurred in prolonged pregnancies characterized by intrauterine fetal growth restriction, coloured amniotic fluid and signs of fetal distress during labour, now known as postmaturity syndrome [21]. This syndrome was associated with increased fetal morbidity and mortality.

The incidence of postmaturity syndrome has not been determined. An incidence of about 10% has been reported in prolonged pregnancies, but depending on the presence of other factors, such as oligohydramnios or the suboptimal nonstress test (NST), the incidence can be higher [22]. Postmature

Table 45.3 Complications of prolonged pregnancies

Fetal–neonatal	Maternal
Postmaturity syndrome	Prolonged labour (dystocia)
Oligohydramnios	Increased rate of instrumental vaginal delivery
Meconium aspiration syndrome	Injuries of birth canal
Macrosomia	Increased caesarean section rate
Stillbirth	Chorioamnionitis
Shoulder dystocia	Puerperal endometritis
Increased perinatal morbidity	Postpartum haemorrhage
Increased perinatal mortality	

neonates usually have a typical appearance: loss of subcutaneous fat with minimal fat deposition; overgrown nails covered with meconium; abundant scalp hair; dry, peeling skin with either brown, green or yellow discoloration due to meconium; and wrinkled palms and soles of the feet. The term *dysmaturity* has been also used.

Postmaturity syndrome is associated with other complications, such as oligohydramnios, meconium aspiration and macrosomia. An increased risk of stillbirth is particularly evident when gestational age is 43+0 weeks or more [23].

45.5.2 Oligohydramnios

In normal pregnancy, amniotic fluid volume reaches a peak of 1000 mL at 38 weeks, decreasing thereafter, so that fluid volume is less than 500 mL at 42 weeks and less than 200 mL at 44 weeks [24]. Diminished amniotic fluid can be determined by ultrasound by measuring either amniotic fluid index (AFI) or the deepest vertical amniotic fluid pocket (Figure 45.2). To define oligohydramnios, AFI must be lower than 5 cm or the deepest vertical pocket less than 1–2 cm. The smaller the amniotic fluid pocket, the greater will be the likelihood of a clinically significant oligohydramnios.

The incidence of oligohydramnios is higher in post-term pregnancies than in pregnancies less than 42+0 gestational weeks. The mechanism via which oligohydramnios is developed has not been fully explained. The process resembles a vicious circle since it cannot be determined whether the fetus, due to the already decreasing amniotic fluid, swallows less fluid and therefore produces less urine, which is incapable of refilling the amniotic cavity [25]. When oligohydramnios occurs, there is an increased risk of fetal malformations, umbilical cord compression and thick meconium aspiration. Normally, changes occur not only in the quantity but also in the quality of the amniotic fluid. Especially with the progress of pregnancy, there is an increase in the amount of lipids related to fetal lung maturity, while after 40 weeks the amniotic fluid becomes cloudy due to the presence of flakes of vernix caseosa. The colour of the fluid becomes yellow or green if the fetus passes meconium, a finding that is not uncommon in post-term pregnancy.

45.5.3 Meconium Aspiration Syndrome

An important complication of prolonged pregnancy is meconium aspiration. When oligohydramnios coexists and the meconium is thick, there is an increased likelihood of bad perinatal outcome and intense fetal distress. It should be noted that thin meconium at the onset of labour does not mean that the meconium will not become thick by the time of birth. Meconium aspiration syndrome is statistically higher when delivery occurs after 42+0 weeks of gestation [26] and is more frequent when there is also fetal tachycardia with no fetal accelerations [27].

45.5.4 Macrosomia

Fetal macrosomia has been defined by birthweight greater than 4000–4500 g or greater than the 90th percentile for a given gestational age [28]. Fetuses in prolonged pregnancy continue to gain weight, although growth velocity slows down at that time. Studies have shown that post-term pregnancies have a twofold increased risk of macrosomia and higher risk of cephalopelvic disproportion (CPD) or shoulder dystocia during labour [26, 29]. The latter can be a very serious event resulting in fetal damage that includes brachial plexus injury, fracture of the humerus or clavicle and severe asphyxia leading to neurological manifestations. Additionally, due to macrosomia, cephalohaematoma or fractures of the fetal skull may occur. Instrumental vaginal delivery may increase the risk for these complications.

45.5.5 Perinatal Morbidity and Mortality

As normal pregnancy progresses, placental function displays a gradual reduction that usually does not affect oxygenation and adequate supply of components to the fetus. However, in some cases this deterioration of placental function (placental 'aging') is such that the placenta cannot meet the needs of the fetus, resulting either in increased risk of endometrial death or fetal distress and birth of a neonate with varying degrees of perinatal asphyxia (Table 45.4).

Perinatal morbidity appears to increase in neonates born after 42+0 weeks of gestation who receive treatment in a neonatal intensive care unit (NICU). Increased perinatal mortality of post-term pregnancies has been associated mainly with small-for-gestational-age (SGA) neonates when compared to the appropriate-for-gestational-age (AGA) neonates [30].

Table 45.4 Perinatal outcome in prolonged pregnancy in relation to placental and fetal risk factors

Risk factors	Perinatal outcome
Placental aging	Severe perinatal asphyxia Endometrial death
Macrosomia	Dysfunctional labour Shoulder dystocia Severe perineal injury
Oligohydramnios	Meconium aspiration syndrome Fetal malformations Umbilical cord compression

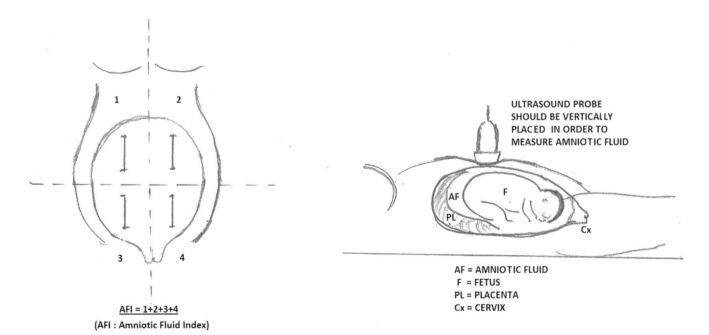

AFI = 1+2+3+4
(AFI : Amniotic Fluid Index)

ULTRASOUND PROBE SHOULD BE VERTICALLY PLACED IN ORDER TO MEASURE AMNIOTIC FLUID

AF = AMNIOTIC FLUID
F = FETUS
PL = PLACENTA
Cx = CERVIX

Figure 45.2 Measurement of amniotic fluid

45.5.6 Stillbirth

The risk of stillbirth in post-term pregnancies is considered to be low. Nevertheless, as weeks of gestation advance beyond 42+0, the risk of neonatal mortality and stillbirth is higher. The incidence of stillbirth is increased after 42 weeks in both primipara and multipara women [31].

45.5.7 Maternal Risks

Because of fetal macrosomia in post-term pregnancies, the likelihood of prolonged labour and operative vaginal delivery is increasing as well as severe perineal injury and postpartum haemorrhage. Routine induction of labour or secondary arrest due to macrosomia may increase the rates of a caesarean delivery. As pregnancy progresses, the incidence of chorioamnionitis and endometritis is also increased [32].

45.6 Antepartum Management

Due to the increased perinatal morbidity and mortality in post-term pregnancies, early induction of labour might be an option. Nevertheless, there is still debate as to whether induction of labour should be offered to these women and when would be the optimal time of delivery.

The primary concern is to have correctly identified the due dates for the proper management of post-term pregnancy. As discussed above, the expected date of delivery (EDD) calculated by last menstrual period has flaws because of possible irregular menstrual cycles or vaginal bleeding in early pregnancy.

Nevertheless, an antenatal surveillance process may be organized and offered to every woman with prolonged pregnancy in order to ensure fetal well-being and normal function of the fetoplacental unit and to minimize perinatal morbidity and mortality. Management of women with post-term pregnancy should be individualized, taking into consideration any findings from monitoring them.

45.6.1 Monitoring and Expectant Management

When dealing with post-term pregnancies, expectant management is an option. Women, after being given a complete explanation of what to expect and consensus has been achieved, may choose expectant management, which is waiting for spontaneous onset of labour. Most systematic reviews conclude that expectant management has a lower risk of an emergency caesarean delivery than induction of labour and no statistically different risk for an operative vaginal delivery. Nevertheless, it seems that with induction of labour, the rate of complications is significantly reduced.

To ensure a good perinatal outcome, a series of tests are currently being used such as a non-stress test (NST), biophysical profile and ultrasound assessment of amniotic fluid. There does not seem to be a statistical difference in the outcome with the use of NST alone versus a biophysical profile, although the latter may increase the rate of caesarean delivery. In an NST, monitoring of fetal heart rate, fetal movements and uterine contractions should be performed for at least 20 minutes. The biophysical profile has some parameters (Table 45.5) that also

Table 45.5 Biophysical profile

Parameters	Normal – 2	Abnormal – 0
NST	≥2 accelerations in 20 min	<2 accelerations in 20 min
Ultrasound (US) of fetal breathing movements	≥1 movement of 20 sec or 30 sec in 30 min	No movements of less than 20 sec or 30 sec
US fetal body movements	≥3 movements of body or limbs in 30 min	<3 movements of body or limbs
US fetal muscle tone	≥1 episode of active bending and straightening of the limb	None
US amniotic fluid	≥1 vertical pocket of >2 cm or AFI >5 cm	Largest vertical pocket ≤2 cm or AFI ≤5 cm

include an NST and the measurement of amniotic fluid. The total score is the sum of points, with the highest score at 10 and the lowest at 0. Measurement of the deepest vertical amniotic pocket is important for early detection of oligohydramnios.

The ACOG supports that surveillance of pregnancies of more than 41+0 weeks twice a week is almost the same as once a week, but no firm recommendation has been made. After 42 weeks, either antenatal surveillance or induction of labour is recommended [33], despite there being less evidence that antepartum fetal surveillance in prolonged pregnancies decreases perinatal morbidity and mortality.

45.6.2 Induction of Labour

The opinion of preventing prolongation of pregnancies by induction of labour has been considered by some studies as the best way of management in order to reduce perinatal morbidity, although no significant differences in the rate of neonates admitted in NICU have been reported. The WHO recommends induction of labour for women who have completed 41 gestational weeks [34], relying on systematic reviews that show a reduction in perinatal deaths, caesarean deliveries as well as less operative vaginal births when induction of labour is performed after 41+0 weeks. It should be also noted that the absolute risk of perinatal mortality in post-term pregnancies is rather small [35]. Elective caesarean delivery is not recommended by WHO because of a significant increase risk of NICU admission [36] when compared either with induction of labour or with expectant management.

On the other hand, inducing labour may increase the risk not only of operative vaginal delivery but also caesarean delivery rate. Thus, women should be appropriately informed in order to be aware of the options and the risks of either induction of labour or surveillance.

In order to make a decision on the management of post-term pregnancy, it is important to assess the state of the cervix and the station of the vertex in the pelvis. For this, the Bishop score (Table 45.6) is calculated (highest score is 13, lowest is 0), using five parameters: consistency of the cervix, dilation of the cervix, position of the cervix, effacement of the cervix and station of the presenting part of the fetus within the pelvis. It has been reported that when the Bishop score is ≥8, the possibility of vaginal delivery is greater than when it is below 8. Apart from the Bishop score, cervical ripening has been suggested.

45.6.2.1 Cervical Ripening

For cervical ripening (Figure 45.3), the effort is to increase prostaglandin levels locally. This can be achieved either by inserting dinoprostone or misoprostol in the vagina or by sweeping the membranes. A Foley catheter can be inserted in the cervix, which also increases prostaglandin levels.

In a systematic review and meta-analysis of 2252 participants, it was shown that membrane sweeping can facilitate initiation of spontaneous labour in post-term pregnancies and reduce the induction of labour rate [37]. When stripping is performed around 38 to 40 gestational weeks, the number of pregnancies

that extend beyond 41+0 weeks decreases. It should be noted that membrane stripping is contraindicated when placenta position is unknown or in placenta praevia or vasa praevia and in previous caesarean delivery. Whether this can be performed when there is a vaginal culture positive for group B streptococcus (GBS) is not yet clear, because there is not adequate evidence to support that the risk of GBS for neonates is increased [38].

As far as the use of a Foley catheter is concerned versus dinoprostone or misoprostol, all systematic reviews conclude that the catheter is as efficient as the use of a medication for cervical ripening without affecting perinatal outcome [39].

45.7 Intrapartum Management

Due to the increased perinatal morbidity and mortality in prolonged pregnancy, women should be advised that labour should be performed in a hospital under close surveillance of uterine contractions and fetal heart rate in order to avoid an adverse outcome.

If labour does not start spontaneously or if induction of labour has been decided upon, the use of prostaglandins or performing amniotomy and administering oxytocin will depend on the degree of maturity of the cervix according to

Table 45.6 Bishop score

Parameters	Score			
	0	1	2	3
Cervical position	Posterior	Middle	Anterior	-
Cervical effacement	0–30%	40–50%	60–70%	≥80%
Cervical consistency	Firm	Medium	Soft	-
Cervical dilation	0	1–2 cm	3–4 cm	≥5 cm
Station of vertex	−3	−2	−1, 0	+1, +2

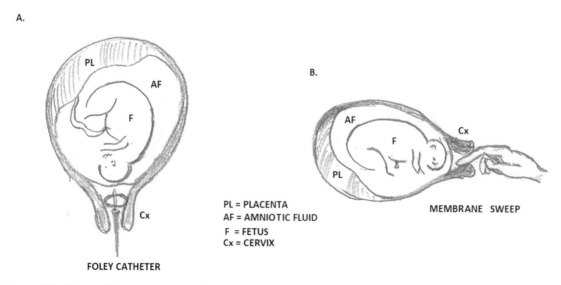

PL = PLACENTA
AF = AMNIOTIC FLUID
F = FETUS
Cx = CERVIX

Figure 45.3 A. Cervical ripening. B. Fetal membrane sweep.

the Bishop score, on the presence of uterine contractions and on the presence/absence of fetal distress.

Cervical maturation, which usually leads to a progression of labour, is a normal process. In a mature cervix with a Bishop score ≥7, only rupture of fetal membranes with or without intravenous administration of oxytocin is recommended. In prolonged pregnancies, if oligohydramnios occurs, amniotomy should be very carefully performed due to possible umbilical cord compression. This procedure is very helpful in detecting thick meconium in order to decide if caesarean delivery is the most appropriate method, especially if the woman with prolonged pregnancy is a primipara. In case of a Bishop score less than 7, maturation of the cervix is the better way to proceed, performed with one of the methods mentioned above.

In case of suspected cephalopelvic disproportion, fetal distress, thick meconium or dysfunctional labour, caesarean delivery should be considered. In this process, it is very important to detect any changes in fetal heart rate due to bradycardia and loss of beat-to-beat variability. There are two main reasons for fetal decelerations: the compression of the umbilical cord because of the oligohydramnios and insufficiency of the placenta.

45.8 Previous Caesarean Section

In women who have had a previous caesarean section, vaginal delivery can be attempted in order to avoid a repeat section. This procedure of vaginal birth after caesarean delivery (VBAC) is applicable in cases of uncomplicated pregnancies, since the rate of uterine rupture in well-organized obstetric centres is relatively small [40]. Nevertheless, in the case of prolonged pregnancies, there are insufficient data to justify such a procedure.

45.9 Conclusions

Prolonged or post-term pregnancy even today is poorly defined. In most studies, such a pregnancy is considered to be one of over 42+0 weeks of gestation, but there is variability in the incidence of this condition. The main reason for the discrepancy is inaccurate dating. The use of ultrasound for dating in the first trimester shows advantages over second trimester measurements or when considering the last menstrual period. With ultrasonography, a lower incidence of post-term delivery has been reported and consequently this method is recommended routinely in the first trimester. Fetal, neonatal and maternal complications can occur after 40+0 weeks of gestation and the incidence increases further after 42+0 gestational weeks. Antepartum management involving surveillance of the fetus with the use of biophysical methods is very important in order to find the optimal time for the safest intervention. Additionally, estimation of fetal weight before the onset of labour will reduce the risk of birth trauma and will ensure the delivery of a healthy newborn. Intrapartum fetal distress should be diagnosed as early as possible in order to avoid harmful consequences for the neonate. With regard to prevention of post-term delivery, there are no specific measures. Although stripping of the membranes and early induction of labour have been suggested, such an action does not seem to have any advantages over waiting for the spontaneous onset of labour and may increase the number of caesarean deliveries. Nevertheless, caesarean section may be a safe mode of delivery for many post-term babies, taking into account possible risk factors and their consequences.

References

1. Wright AH. Prolonged pregnancy. *Can Med Assoc J.* 1911 Oct;**1**(10):944–7.

2. The American College of Obstetricians and Gynecologists Committee on Obstetric Practice Society for Maternal-Fetal Medicine, Committee Opinion, Definition of Term Pregnancy, Number 579, November 2013 (Reaffirmed 2017).

3. Vayssière C, Haumonte JB, Chantry A, et al; French College of Gynecologists and Obstetricians (CNGOF). Prolonged and post-term pregnancies: guidelines for clinical practice from the French College of Gynecologists and Obstetricians (CNGOF). *Eur J Obstet Gynecol Reprod Biol.* 2013 Jul;**169**(1):10–16.

4. Näslund Thagaard I, Krebs L, Lausten-Thomsen U, et al. Dating of pregnancy in first versus second trimester in relation to post-term birth rate: a cohort study. *PLoS One.* 2016 Jan 13;**11**(1):e0147109.

5. Weiss E, Abele H, Bartz C, et al. S1-guideline: management of late-term and post-term pregnancy* short version –

AWMF Registry Number: 015/065. *Geburtshilfe Frauenheilkd.* 2014 Dec;**74**(12):1099–1103.

6. Boyd ME, Usher RH, McLean FH, Kramer MS Obstetric consequences of postmaturity. *Am J Obstet Gynecol.* 1988 Feb;**158**(2):334–8.

7. Caughey AB, Snegovskikh VV, Norwitz ER. Postterm pregnancy: how can we improve outcomes? *Obstet Gynecol Surv.* 2008 Nov;**63**(11):715–24.

8. American College of Obstetricians and Gynecologists. Practice Bulletin No. 146: management of late-term and postterm pregnancies. *Obstet Gynecol.* 2014 Aug;**124**(2 Pt 1):390–6.

9. Nadhifa Anwar M, Tutik R. Hubungan Usia, Paritas Ibu Bersalin Dengan Kejadian Persalinan Postterm [The Relationship between Age and Maternity Parity with Postterm Birth]. *Jurnal Berkala Epidemiologi.* 2018;**6**(1):27–34.

10. Kortekaas JC, Kazemier BM, Ravelli AC, et al. Recurrence rate and outcome of postterm pregnancy,

a national cohort study. *Eur J Obstet Gynecol Reprod Biol.* 2015 Oct;**193**:70–4.

11. Schierding W, O'Sullivan JM, Derraik JG, Cutfield WS. Genes and post-term birth: late for delivery. *BMC Res Notes.* 2014 Oct 14;**7**:720.

12. Oberg AS, Frisell T, Svensson AC, Iliadou AN. Maternal and fetal genetic contributions to postterm birth: familial clustering in a population-based sample of 475,429 Swedish births. *Am J Epidemiol.* 2013 Mar 15;**177**(6):531–7.

13. Olesen AW, Basso O, Olsen J. Risk of recurrence of prolonged pregnancy *BMJ.* 2003 Mar 1;**326**(7387):476.

14. Divon MY, Haglund B, Nisell H, Otterblad PO, Westgren M. Fetal and neonatal mortality in the postterm pregnancy: the impact of gestational age and fetal growth restriction. *Am J Obstet Gynecol.* 1998 Apr;**178**(4):726–31.

15. Divon MY, Ferber A, Nisell H, Westgren M. Male gender predisposes

to prolongation of pregnancy. *Am J Obstet Gynecol.* 2002 Oct;**187**(4):1081–3.

16. Heslehurst N, Vieira R, Hayes L, et al. Maternal body mass index and post-term birth: a systematic review and meta-analysis. *Obes Rev.* 2017 Mar; **18**(3): 293–308.

17. Kaya S, Keskin HL, Kaya B, Ustuner I, Avsar AF. Reduced total antioxidant status in postterm pregnancies. *Hippokratia.* 2013 Jan–Mar;**17**(1): 55–9.

18. Mannino F. Neonatal complications of postterm gestation. *J Reprod Med.* 1988 Mar;**33**(3):271–6.

19. Reynolds JW, Burry K, Carlson CV. Fetoplacental steroid metabolism in prolonged pregnancies. *Am J Obstet Gynecol.* 1986 Jan;**154**(1):74–9.

20. Vorherr H. Placental insufficiency in relation to postterm pregnancy and fetal postmaturity. Evaluation of fetoplacental function; management of the postterm gravida. *Am J Obstet Gynecol.* 1975 Sep 1;**123**(1):67–103.

21. Clifford SH. Postmaturity, with placental dysfunction; clinical syndrome and pathologic findings. *J Pediatr.* 1954 Jan;**44**(1):1–13.

22. Shime J, Gare DJ, Andrews J, et al. Prolonged pregnancy: surveillance of the fetus and the neonate and the course of labor and delivery. *Am J Obstet Gynecol.* 1984 Mar 1;**148**(5):547–52.

23. Campbell MK, Ostbye T, Irgens LM. Post-term birth: risk factors and outcomes in a 10-year cohort of Norwegian births. *Obstet Gynecol.* 1997 Apr;**89**(4):543–8.

24. Ounpraseuth ST, Magann EF, Spencer HJ, Rabie NZ, Sandlin AT. Normal amniotic fluid volume across gestation: Comparison of statistical approaches in 1190 normal amniotic fluid volumes. *J Obstet Gynaecol Res.* 2017 Jul;**43**(7):1122–31.

25. Trimmer KJ, Leveno KJ, Peters MT, Kelly MA. Observations on the cause of oligohydramnios in prolonged pregnancy. *Am J Obstet Gynecol.* 1990 Dec;**163**(6 Pt 1):1900–3.

26. Cheng YW, Nicholson JM, Nakagawa S, et al. Perinatal outcomes in low-risk term pregnancies: do they differ by week of gestation? *Am J Obstet Gynecol.* 2008 Oct;**199**(4):370.e1–7.

27. Rossi EM, Philipson EH, Williams TG, Kalhan SC. Meconium aspiration syndrome: intrapartum and neonatal attributes. *Am J Obstet Gynecol.* 1989 Nov;**161**(5):1106–10.

28. American College of Obstetricians and Gynecologists' Committee on Practice Bulletins – Obstetrics. Practice Bulletin No. 173: Fetal Macrosomia. *Obstet Gynecol.* 2016 Nov;**128**(5):e195–e209.

29. Maoz O, Wainstock T, Sheiner E, Walfisch A. Immediate perinatal outcomes of postterm deliveries. *J Matern Fetal Neonatal Med.* 2018 Jan 4:1–6.

30. Nakling J, Backe B. Pregnancy risk increases from 41 weeks of gestation. *Acta Obstet Gynecol Scand.* 2006;**85**(6):663–8.

31. Ingemarsson I, Källén K. Stillbirths and rate of neonatal deaths in 76,761 post-term pregnancies in Sweden, 1982–1991: a register study. *Acta Obstet Gynecol Scand.* 1997 Aug;**76**(7):658–62.

32. Caughey AB, Musci TJ. Complications of term pregnancies beyond 37 weeks of gestation. *Obstet Gynecol.* 2004 Jan;**103**(1):57–62.

33. ACOG Practice Bulletin Number 146: Management of Late-Term and Postterm Pregnancies, August 2014. *Obstet Gynecol.* 2014;**124**:390–6.

34. WHO. *World Health Organization Recommendations for Induction of Labour.* 2011. http://apps.who.int//iris/handle/10665/44531.

35. Middleton P, Shepherd E, Crowther CA. Induction of labour for improving birth outcomes for women at or beyond term. *Cochrane Database Syst Rev.* 2018 May 9;(5):CD004945.

36. Mya KS, Laopaiboon M, Vogel JP, et al.; WHO Multi-Country Survey on Maternal and Newborn Health Research Network. Management of pregnancy at and beyond 41 completed weeks of gestation in low-risk women: a secondary analysis of two WHO multi-country surveys on maternal and newborn health. *Reprod Health.* 2017 Oct 30;**14**(1):141.

37. Avdiyovski H, Haith-Cooper M, Scally A. Membrane sweeping at term to promote spontaneous labour and reduce the likelihood of a formal induction of labour for postmaturity: a systematic review and meta-analysis *J Obstet Gynaecol.* 2019 Jan;**39**(1):54–62.

38. Heilman E, Sushereba E. Amniotic membrane sweeping. *Semin Perinatol.* 2015 Oct;**39**(6):466–70.

39. Chen W, Xue J, Peprah MK, et al. A systematic review and network meta-analysis comparing the use of Foley catheters, misoprostol, and dinoprostone for cervical ripening in the induction of labour. *BJOG.* 2016 Feb;**123**(3):346–54.

40. Yeh S, Huang X, Phelan JP. Postterm pregnancy after previous cesarean section. *J Reprod Med.* 1984 Jan;**29**(1):41–4.

Chapter 46

Induction of Labour

Yves Muscat Baron & Martina Schembri

46.1 Introduction

Medical interest in labour induction has existed since the time of Hippocrates. This interest may have originated from both scientific curiosity and the innate fear of every obstetrician of experiencing a term stillbirth. The utilization of oxytocics was initiated in obstetric practice with its treatment for postpartum haemorrhage but later was employed for labour induction. In many countries the frequency of labour induction has doubled over the past three decades. Post-dates pregnancies are the commonest reason for induction of labour. Accordingly, a dating scan is crucial for high-quality antenatal care to assess growth and establish an accurate expected date of delivery. Advanced maternal age is increasingly becoming another common indication for induction of labour (IOL). Besides post-dates pregnancy and advanced maternal age, there are other valid reasons for IOL; however, obstetricians need to apply judicious clinical judgement and evidence-based medicine to justify intervention by IOL as the preferred option to the continuation of pregnancy and allowing spontaneous onset of labour to occur. Antenatal surveillance has expanded significantly and can not only be applied to high-risk pregnancies but can also be employed in low-risk pregnancies. Undoubtedly there lies a grey area between the benefit of IOL as opposed to the safe continuation of a pregnancy; however, the obstetrician has the means at hand to appropriately evaluate the likelihood of a successful outcome.

46.2 Historical Background

The history of induction of labour dates back to descriptions of mammary stimulation and mechanical cervical dilation as demonstrated by Hippocrates. Soranus, in the second century AD, implemented artificial rupture of the membranes. From the second to the seventeenth century the application of mechanical methods of labour induction were commonly employed [1, 2]. Thomas Denman, in 1756, recommended that labour induction may be a useful treatment for cephalopelvic disproportion, which at the time was a common cause of maternal and fetal mortality [3]. From the evolutionary point of view, cephalopelvic disproportion may have determined the appropriate gestational age in bipedal *Homo sapiens*, as obstruction of a large post-term neonate would exert significant natural selective pressure by elimination not only of the neonate but also of the mother [4]. Body size and dietary intake may have determined the appropriate gestational age in *Homo sapiens*. Obese women tend to have post-term pregnancies [5],

while low-weight women are at greater risk for preterm delivery [6].

The combination of both medical and surgical methods of labour induction was utilized by Bourgeois, who induced and augmented labour with strong enemas and herbal medicines. In 1906, Dale observed that extracts from the pituitary infundibular lobe caused myometrial contractions. Three years later, Bell reported the first experience of using pituitary extract for labour induction. Although pituitary extract initially gained acceptance for labour induction, the extract fell out of favour due to the fact that when large doses were employed, cases of uterine rupture ensued [1]. Page, in 1943, utilized an intravenous infusion of Pitocin for postpartum haemorrhage, and later on Theobald reported his initial results with controlled intravenous infusion of Pitocin for labour induction [1]. Karim et al reported the use of prostaglandins for labour induction [1]. More recently, the synthetic prostaglandin analogue misoprostol is gaining acceptance as an effective and safe method of labour induction [7].

46.3 Modern-day Labour Induction

Despite the widespread application of labour induction, caution is required as it is not without risk [8]. In the UK, induction of labour led to less than two thirds of women giving birth without further intervention, with 15% of induced mothers requiring instrumental deliveries and a further 22% requiring emergency caesarean section. Increased analgesia is required in induced labours. Uterine hyperstimulation can develop following prostaglandin and syntocinon induction of labour, resulting in fetal distress [9].

The rates of labour induction vary between countries and even within the national units themselves. The frequency of labour induction in French maternity units differs from 7.7% to 33% of deliveries [10]. In Germany, between 2005 and 2012, labour induction rates rose significantly from 16.5 to 21.9% [11]. Labour induction rates in the Republic of Ireland reached 25.0% (range 14.5–33.2%), whilst in the USA IOL rates increased from 9.5% in 1990 to 22.1% in 2004 [12]. Similarly, in 2004 and 2005, 1 in every 5 deliveries in the UK was induced [9].

The reasons for the increased rates of IOL vary from medical to social. The most common medical reason for induction of labour is post-dates pregnancy. Other medical reasons involve maternal conditions such as hypertension and diabetes, and fetal reasons including intrauterine growth restriction. The underpinning rationale for labour induction is the

Table 46.1 Pregnancy variables determining induction of labour

Favours labour induction	Await spontaneous onset of labour
Low-risk pregnancy >41+3 weeks' gestation	Low-risk pregnancy <41+3 weeks' gestation
Bishop score >8	Bishop score <8
Presence of medical conditions (e.g. hypertension, diabetes)	Absence of medical conditions
Maternal age > 40 years	Multiparous maternal age <40 years
Reduced fetal movements at term	Satisfactory fetal movements
Equivocal cardiocotograph (CTG) and amniotic fluid volume	Satisfactory CTG and amniotic fluid volume
Obstetric history of fetal loss	Satisfactory obstetric history

perception that the intrauterine environment appears less favourable for the mother and/or the child [8] (Table 46.1).

There also are management and patient safety issues with induction of labour. Labour induction exerts greater strain on delivery suites than spontaneous labour. Traditionally, induction is carried out during the daytime when labour wards are often already busy with other elective procedures such as planned caesarean sections [8].

46.4 Induction of Labour for Post-dates Pregnancy

Post-dates pregnancy is the commonest reason for IOL. Beyond term there is increased risk of intrauterine fetal death and perinatal death. The risks of prolonged gestation on pregnancy are better reflected by calculating fetal and infant losses per 1000 ongoing pregnancies. With the rare occurrence of post-dates stillbirth, large studies are required to discern the association between prolonged gestation and fetal loss [8].

Two large studies have assessed the stillbirth rates across the later weeks of pregnancy. Hilder et al [13] undertook an observational retrospective analysis of 171 527 births. Stillbirth rates per 1000 ongoing pregnancies indicate a progressive rise from 37 weeks' gestation OR (odds ratio) 0.35 (95% confidence intervals (CI) 0.26–0.44) until 40 weeks OR 0.86 (95% CI 0.68–1.05). Beyond 41 weeks' gestation, the odds ratio increases to 1.17 (95% CI 0.92–1.62) until it doubled at 43 weeks 2.12 (95% CI 0.55–5.43). Despite the large numbers of births, the confidence intervals in the later cohorts crossed unity. Moreover, in this study neonatal and post-neonatal mortality rates fell significantly with advancing gestation, reaching a nadir at 41 weeks of gestation (0.7 and 1.3 per 1000 live births, respectively).

Another study from Norway [14] also showed that in over 27 000 births, the stillbirth rate increase was noted at the 42 weeks' gestation. However, it was concluded that the number of inductions required before 41 weeks to avoid one fetal or neonatal death before 41 weeks was too high.

Randomized controlled trials suggest that elective induction of labour at 41 weeks of gestation and beyond may be associated with a decrease in both the risk of caesarean section rates and meconium-stained amniotic fluid. However, the evidence regarding elective induction of labour prior to 41 weeks of gestation is insufficient to draw any conclusion.

A meta-analysis of randomized controlled trials on elective IOL at 41 completed weeks of gestation showed that elective IOL was not associated with lower risk of perinatal mortality compared to expectant management (relative risks (RR) 0.33, 95% CI 0.10–1.09). Elective induction was, however, associated with a significantly lower rate of meconium aspiration syndrome (RR 0.43, 95% CI 0.23–0.79) [15].

A recent update of the Cochrane Database Review compared induction of labour and expectant management in term and post-term pregnancies. The majority of trials in this review adopted a policy of induction at ≥41 weeks' gestation for the intervention arm. This update confirmed the superiority of induction of labour in this particular cohort of patients [16].

The Cochrane Database update reconfirmed that a policy of labour induction at ≥41 weeks was associated with fewer perinatal deaths (RR 0.33, 95% CI 0.14–0.78). In the labour induction group, there were two perinatal deaths (no stillbirths) compared with 16 perinatal deaths (10 stillbirths) in the expectant management group. The risk ratio for caesarean section in the induction cohort was lower compared with expectant management (RR 0.92, 95% CI 0.85–0.99); and a corresponding marginal increase in operative vaginal births with labour induction (RR 1.07, 95% CI 0.99–1.16) [16]. A recent meta-analysis reported that IOL at 39 weeks in low-risk nulliparous women did not improve perinatal outcome, but it did result in significantly lower caesarean section rates. However, this meta-analysis was significantly weighted by one study that was open label and compared labour induction to expectant management up to 42+2 weeks' gestation [17].

Larger studies do not indicate any advantage of inducing women before 40 weeks' gestation to prevent stillbirth. Little et al carried out a large retrospective correlation of term delivery timing and stillbirth over a 6-year period. Over the period of 2005 till 2011, there was a decline in early-term deliveries across the USA. In 2005, the percentage of early term (37–39 weeks' gestation) deliveries was 31.8% compared to 28.5% in 2011 (1 123 467 of 3 533 233 term, singleton deliveries occurred in the early term in 2005 compared with 978 294 of 3 429 172 in 2011). There was no significant change in the term stillbirth rate; however, a significant increase in term stillbirths among women with diabetes was observed (from 238/100 000 to 300/100 000 births; P=.010) [18]. A similar finding was noted by MacDorman et al, indicating a static stillbirth rate in the USA of 6.05 stillbirths per 1000 deliveries despite the percent distribution of live births by gestational age changed considerably, with births at 34–38 weeks decreasing by 10–16%, and births beyond 39 weeks increasing by 17%. Fetal losses were noted to have risen under 38 weeks' gestation [19].

46.5 Predicting Antepartum Stillbirth

A key issue in allowing a pregnancy to continue up to 41weeks gestation is putting the obstetrician's mind at rest that antepartum surveillance is reliable enough to prevent stillbirth. Rates of stillbirth in the developed world, despite improvements in antenatal surveillance, have been static or actually rising in recent years.

Clinical prediction of stillbirth risk may require more rigorous antenatal surveillance. The most prevalent independent risk factors are nulliparity, advanced age and obesity. These risk factors have become increasingly prevalent in the developed world [20]. In 2011, a large retrospective study in the USA added more independent factors for stillbirth risk. This multivariate analyses analysis included 614 cases and 1816 control pregnancies [21].

This multivariate analysis [21] demonstrated the following factors were independently associated with stillbirth:

- previous stillbirth (adjusted odds ratio (aOR) 5.91, 95% CI 3.18–11.00);
- diabetes (aOR 2.50, 95% CI 1.39–4.48);
- maternal age 40 years or older (aOR 2.41, 95% CI, 1.24–4.70);
- maternal AB blood type (aOR 1.96, 95% CI, 1.16–3.30);
- history of drug abuse (aOR 2.08, 95% CI 1.12–3.88);
- smoking during the 3 months prior to pregnancy (aOR 1.55, 95% CI 1.02–2.35);
- not living with a partner (aOR 1.62, 95% CI 1.15–2.27);
- and multiple pregnancy (aOR 4.59, 95% CI 2.63–8.00) [21].

Obesity is particularly associated with stillbirth at term and after term. A fourfold increase in fetal death has been noted in relation to gestational diabetes. Obesity also correlates with an increased risk for fetal malformation [22]. Morbidly obese women (body mass index (BMI) >40 kg/m^2) are at particularly high risk. A prospective population-based cohort study indicated that both the ante-partum stillbirth rate (2.79, 95% CI 1.94–4.02) and neonatal death (3.41, 95% CI 2.07–5.63) were elevated for women with morbid obesity. For women with BMIs between 35.1 and 40, the associations were similar but to a lesser degree [23].

A recent study [24] confirmed previous preterm labour and small for gestational age as risk factors for stillbirth. A previous preterm birth or small-for-gestational-age neonate increased the risk of subsequent stillbirth as OR 1.70, 95% CI 1.34–2.16 and OR 1.98, 95% CI 1.70–2.31, respectively. The risk of stillbirth also varied with prematurity, increasing threefold following preterm labour (OR 2.98, 95% CI 2.05–4.34) and sixfold following growth restriction (OR 6.00, 95% CI 3.43–10.49) (24).

Stillbirth is strongly related to significant deviations of fetal growth from the norm. A population-based case-control study in the USA compared fetal growth of stillbirths and a representative sample of live births [25]. Among 527 singleton stillbirths and 1821 singleton live births studied, stillbirth was associated with small for gestational age noted on ultrasound, and individualized norms (OR 4.7, 95% CI 3.7–5.9; OR 4.6, 95% CI 3.6–5.9, respectively). Large for gestational age was also associated with increased risk of stillbirth utilizing ultrasound and individualized norms (OR 3.5, 95% CI 2.4–5.0; OR 2.3, 95% CI 1.73.1 respectively). This study emphasizes the importance of rigorous assessment and surveillance of fetal growth patterns during pregnancy [25].

46.6 Cerebral Palsy and Gestational Age at Birth Close to Term

Besides stillbirth and neonatal death, the issue of cerebral palsy has also been assessed in relation to gestational age. A population-based follow-up study utilized the Medical Birth Registry of Norway including 1 682 441 singleton children born in the years 1967–2001 between the gestational ages of 37 through to 44 weeks. Occurrence of cerebral palsy at the extremes of the gestational ages was at 37 weeks 1.91/1000 (95% CI 1.58–2.25) and 42+ weeks 1.44/1000 (95% CI 1.15–1.72) and least at 40 weeks 0.99/1000 (95% CI 0.90–1.08). Compared with delivery at 40+ weeks' gestation, delivery at 37 or 38 weeks or at 42 weeks or later was associated with an increased risk of cerebral palsy [26].

46.7 Maternal Age and Induction of Labour

Besides post-dates pregnancies, another increasing indication for labour induction is advanced maternal age. Over the past three decades, economic and social changes in the developed world have significantly increased the number of women who delay childbirth to their late 30s and beyond. More children are being born to women at the extremes of their reproductive life.

In just over a decade, between 1980 and 1993 in the European Union, the mean maternal age at first birth had risen by 1.5 years, from 27.1 to 28.6 years. In 2003, this increased to 29.7 years. For the older women cohort in the USA, between 1991 and 2001, the percentage of first births for women 35–39 years of age increased by 36% and for women 40–44 years of age, it increased by 70% [8].

A literature review of 913 studies [27] has shown that advanced maternal age was significantly associated with an increased risk of stillbirth. Across the studies assessed, the relative risks varied from 1.20 to 4.53 for older versus younger women. A study in Sweden also showed that stillbirth rates increased by maternal age: 25–29 years, 0.27%; 30–34 years, 0.31%; 35–39 years, 0.40%; and 40 years or older, 0.53%, with nullipara at greater risk. In multipara, stillbirth risk increased with maternal age in women in relation to the level of education [28]. The biological mechanism of this increase in stillbirth risk with advanced maternal age remains unknown. The direct effect of maternal aging may be related to inadequate uteroplacental perfusion caused by diminished uterine vasculature in older women. Older women are more likely to have higher BMIs, experiencing pregnancy-induced hypertension or gestational diabetes. Some of these medical conditions may at the time of pregnancy, be silent and remain undiagnosed [8].

46.8 Antenatal Surveillance in the Post-dates Period

In 1986, Boehm et al showed that cardiotocography was a commonly used modality for fetal well-being assessment in high-risk pregnancies. The rate of stillbirths with reactive cardiotocography performed once a week was 6.1 per 1000; however, when cardiotocography was performed on a twice weekly basis, the rate of stillbirths was reduced to 1.9 per 1000 [29]. While randomized controlled trials (RCTs) to evaluate an impact of cardiotocography in reducing stillbirth are lacking, apparent reductions in stillbirth rates have followed the incorporation of the cardiotocography into protocols for management of high-risk pregnancy in the USA [29]. Combined testing of a range of fetal biophysical variables was described as an excellent predictor of fetal acidaemia and risk of death or damage. Controversy persists regarding the optimal means of measuring amniotic fluid volume, some authors supporting the amniotic fluid index method while others favouring the maximal vertical pocket method.

It is becoming increasingly more evident that a spectrum of fetal testing modalities based on clinical interpretation of different aspects of fetal adaptive responses to adversity is preferable in fetal surveillance. Furthermore, it is evident that in some fetal conditions, such as intrauterine growth restriction, the fetal condition may change acutely, and accordingly the best outcome is achieved by much more frequent assessments.

Doppler ultrasonography has not been shown to provide any advantage for evaluating post-date or post-term pregnancies and should not be routinely used. A modified biophysical profile has been shown to be as sensitive as a full biophysical profile. Caughey et al conclude that the use of a nonstress test and an amniotic fluid index twice a week for pregnancies continuing past 41 weeks is reasonable. In addition, if any indication during antenatal surveillance leads the practitioner to question the intrauterine environment, delivery should be expedited [30].

Fetal movements as felt by the mother are routinely used as a corollary of fetal well-being. Ultrasonic investigation of fetal well-being has demonstrated an association between reduced fetal movements and poor perinatal outcome. Importantly, 55% of women experiencing fetal loss observed a reduction in fetal movements prior to diagnosis [31]. A Norwegian study assessing reduced fetal movements before and after standardized fetal movement detection in the third trimester demonstrated a reduction of stillbirths (OR 0.36, 95% CI 0.19–0.69) in the post-intervention period [32]. A Cochrane review, however, indicated that there are insufficient data from randomized trials to guide practice regarding the management of reduced fetal movements [33]. Crucially, the relevance of fetal movements as a mode of reducing stillbirths very much depends on standardized patient education and accentuating women's awareness in detecting reduction of fetal movements.

One observational study of routine ultrasound use suggested that ultrasound may help to identify some high-risk pregnancies especially in cases of growth restriction. Mahran and Omran reported that routine ultrasound (89.7% detection rate) was superior to symphysis fundal height (34.7% detection rate) in identifying fetal growth restriction [34]. Two Cochrane reviews [35, 36] adequately controlled trials of routine ultrasound imaging in early and late pregnancy. The study found that routine ultrasound examination was associated with reduced rates of induction of labour for post-term pregnancy. The Cochrane review also found no difference in antenatal, intrapartum and neonatal morbidity in those undergoing ultrasound screening late in pregnancy versus those not screened. Routine late pregnancy ultrasound was not associated with improvements in overall perinatal mortality. However, another randomized controlled trial [37] utilizing placental grading, resulted in a stillbirth rate of 0/1014 compared to 9/1011 in the control group (P<0.05) [37].

Currently, no single method of antenatal surveillance has been shown to be superior to any other. Options include a fetal kick count, nonstress test, contraction stress test, full biophysical profile, modified biophysical profile (nonstress test and amniotic fluid index) or a combination of these modalities. Evaluation of the amniotic fluid level has been shown to be especially important, as it has been associated with increased adverse pregnancy outcomes. Although there is no consensus on optimal protocol for fetal monitoring, Nageotte et al [38] suggested that it is reasonable to implement the modified biophysical profile (cardiotocography and amniotic fluid volume measurement only).

46.9 Induction for Vaginal Birth after Caesarean Section (VBAC)

Individualized assessment on the suitability of the patient for VBAC should be made based on the history of the previous reason for caesarean section, the risk of uterine rupture, the current obstetric history and the Bishop score. This discussion should be carried out with the patient, taking into consideration patients' wishes, including the pros and cons of a VBAC. It should be noted that the risk for rupture of an unscarred uterus is 2/10 000, whereas the risk of scar rupture with a previous caesarean section is 10 times greater. The risk of rupture with prostaglandin and oxytocin is 90/10 000 and 100/10 000, respectively. Intracervical Foley catheter application is an acceptable method of labour induction for a vaginal birth after caesarean section [39].

46.10 Modes of Induction of Labour

The Bishop score was developed as a tool for assessment of the cervix to predict the success of elective induction of labour. This helped to standardize the method of patient selection for successful induction of labour. The scoring system involved 5 cervical characteristics, each with a score from 0–3 for a maximum score of 13. If the total score was >9, the patient was deemed favourable for induction of labour.

Table 46.2 NICE Guideline for induction of labour

Pelvic score	0	1	2	3
Dilation (cm)	0	1–2	3–4	5–6
Length (cm)	>4	2–4	1–2	<1
Station	–3	–2	–1/0	+1/+2
Consistency	Firm	Medium	Soft	
Position	Posterior	Middle/anterior		

The National Institute for Health and Care Excellence (NICE) guideline for the induction of labour presents a different modified Bishop score, as seen in Table 46.2, where effacement has been replaced by length of cervix and the maximum score is 12. The favourable predictive score is stated to be >8 [9].

Poor Bishop scores at induction of labour have been repeatedly shown to result in increased caesarean section rates. A prospective study by Xenakis et al showed that low (4–6) and very low Bishop scores (0–3) resulted in the highest risk for caesarean section in both nulliparous and parous women [40]. Vrouenraets et al demonstrated that a Bishop score of 5 or less was a significant risk factor for caesarean section [41].

46.10.1 Non-medical Methods of Induction of Labour

Non-medical methods are not routinely used as they are not as effective as modern methods of labour induction. There is some evidence to suggest that sexual intercourse and mammary stimulation may be effective in ripening the cervix and inducing labour at term [1]. Purgatives such as castor oil and enemas were widely used by seventeenth century obstetricians such as Bourgeois, but have largely been abandoned; however, purgative-induced evacuation of a full rectum is desirable prior to labour. Acupuncture is an accepted method for labour induction in Asia and some parts of Europe [1].

The most common non-medical method of labour induction is membrane sweep. The procedure involves a vaginal examination, whereby the fetal membranes are separated from the cervix and lower uterine segment. If the cervix is closed, gentle stretching of the cervix or cervical massage may be attempted. These procedures release endogenous prostaglandins, soften the cervix and may encourage oxytocin-induced uterine contractions. After membrane sweep the plasma concentration of prostaglandin rises to 10% of the levels achieved in labour [8].

A Cochrane review assessed 22 trials involving sweeping of the membranes. Membrane sweep at term (38–41 weeks) reduced the frequency of pregnancies continuing after 41+0 weeks (RR 0.59, 95% CI 0.46–0.74) and after 42+0 weeks (RR 0.28, 95% CI 0.15–0.50 [42].

46.10.2 Induction of Labour with Prostaglandins

Prostaglandin E2 (PGE2) is the mainstay of treatment for pharmacological induction. A large meta-analysis analyzing 70 RCTs showed that PGE2 tablets, gel and pessary appear to be equally effective with minimal difference in their side-effect profile. When using the gel, it is given as a cycle, where one dose is given vaginally after assessment of the cervix followed by a second gel after 6 hours [9].

Prior to the administration of prostaglandin, the history of the pregnancy should be assessed. Obstetric contraindications to induction of labour include an abnormal lie, placenta praevia, presenting umbilical cord and prior classical uterine incision. The dating of the pregnancy should be confirmed by reviewing the first trimester ultrasound. The placental site as assessed from third trimester ultrasound should be confirmed, and any contraindication to the application of prostaglandin should be sought. Consent should be obtained from the patient and an abdominal examination performed to confirm the lie and the presentation of the fetus. The fetal heart should be auscultated for 1 minute.

As a good practice, nulliparous women with unfavourable Bishop scores should have an initial dose of 2 mg applied and after six hours the cervix be re-assessed. If uterine activity does occur and the cervix is still unfavourable, a second dose of 1 mg PGE2 should be administered vaginally. Following the second administration of PGE2, if there is minimal or no response, then 2 mg PGE2 should be administered vaginally. A maximum dose of 4 mg in 24 hours can be given in nulliparous women (Figure 46.1).

As the risk of hyperstimulation is greater in multipara, lower doses of prostaglandins should be utilized. Accordingly, if the Bishop score is unfavourable, an initial dose of 1 mg vaginally is administered and the cervix re-assessed after 6 hours. If following the initial administration uterine activity does ensue but the cervix is still unfavourable, 1 mg PGE2 should be administered vaginally. Alternatively, if there is no response to the initial dose, 2 mg PGE2 should be applied vaginally. In multipara a maximum dose of 3 mg PGE2 in 24hrs can be given. Cardiotocography should be performed 1 hour after every application of prostaglandin to check the fetal heart and uterine activity.

46.10.3 Misoprostol

A Cochrane review in 2003 indicated that doses not exceeding 25 mcg four-hourly appeared to have similar effectiveness and risk of uterine hyperstimulation to prostaglandin induction [7]. In 2009, a review article showed that low-dose oral misoprostol solution (20 micrograms) administered every 2 hours appeared as effective as both vaginal dinoprostone and vaginal misoprostol, with lower caesarean section rates and uterine hyperstimulation [8].

Another study on misoprostol use showed that 66% respondents (69% response rate) used misoprostol for induction of labour in viable term pregnancies while 34% never used misoprostol for labour induction. The reluctance to use misoprostol for labour induction was the lack of licence and medico-legal uncertainty of its usage for this indication [43]. As regards routine use of misoprostol for induction of viable pregnancies, there is need for the establishment of sanctioned guidelines, based on the best available evidence [44].

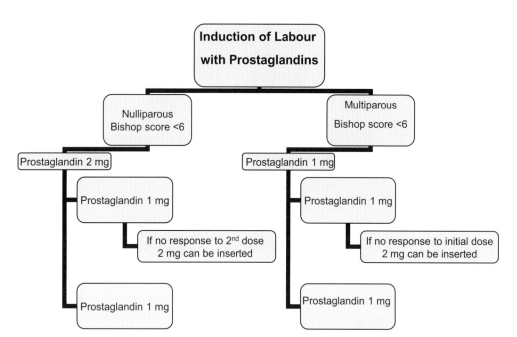

Figure 46.1 Induction of labour with prostaglandins

46.10.4 Balloon Induction of Labour

Mechanical methods of induction include balloon devices, such as a Foley catheter, which apply pressure on the internal os of the cervix, stretching the lower uterine segment and resulting in release of local prostaglandins. A size 18 Foley catheter is introduced under sterile technique past the internal os. The balloon is then inflated with 30–60 cc of water. It is then left in place for 24 hours. Traction can also be administered to the catheter. Balloon induction has been shown to be as effective as prostaglandins in achieving delivery within 24 hours of the start of the intervention, with fewer episodes of hyperstimulation, which is ideal in vaginal births after caesarean section. Caesarean section rates were similar to induction with prostaglandin [45].

46.10.5 Syntocinon

The mainstay of induction of labour is amniotomy followed by oxytocin infusion. Oxytocin's greatest disadvantage is that some patients will not respond well to it, especially those with a low Bishop score. On the other hand, in women with receptive uteri, oxytocin has the advantage of short half-life and the option for prompt cessation in case of hyperstimulation.

There are several regimes as to the application of syntocinon [46]. Higher-dose regimens of oxytocin (4 mU per minute or more) were associated with a reduction in the length of labour and in caesarean section, and an increase in spontaneous vaginal birth [47]; however, further studies are required to confirm this finding. The concentration of syntocinon is 10 IU in 1000 mL of 0.9% normal saline solution to start with. This solution is usually started at a low dose of 4 mL/hour (1.33 mU/minute) and increased by doubling the dose every 15 minutes up to 32 mL/hour. Thereafter the doubled dose is increased more gradually after 30 minutes to 1 hour until a maximum dose of 128 mL/hour is reached. Throughout the induction process, the maternal parameters and fetal heart are monitored (Figure 46.2).

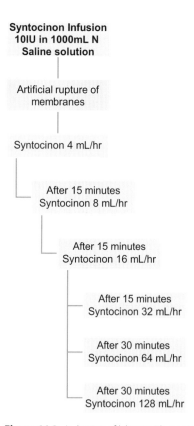

Figure 46.2 Induction of labour with oxytocin. Fetal heart monitored continuously, and contractions should not exceed 3 to 4 in 10 minutes. Proceed with caution in patients with previous caesarean section scar.

46.10.6 Uterine Hyperstimulation

One of the greatest risks of pharmacological labour induction is uterine hyperstimulation resulting in fetal distress and rarely, but most devastatingly, uterine rupture. In the event of tachysystole, the oxytoxic agent should be stopped or, in the case of dinoprostone, the prostaglandin should be removed

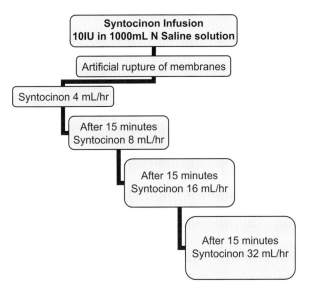

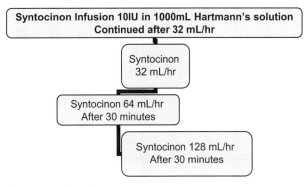

Figure 46.2 (cont.)

Figure 46.2 (cont.)

caesarean delivery rate; on the contrary, it may decrease the caesarean delivery rate.

from the vagina. Tocolytic agents may be considered by administering either terbutaline or nitroglycerine intravenously or via nasal spray [39].

46.11 Conclusion

The management of post-dates pregnancies frequently presents a dilemma between an expectant management with further antenatal surveillance or resorting to induction of labour. It appears from the most recent evidence that inducing labour at 41 weeks (maximum 41+3) in accurately dated low-risk pregnancy is currently the best strategy of managing the post-dates gestation. Prior to induction of labour between 40 and 41+3, antenatal testing with cardiotocography and amniotic fluid assessment may strengthen the safety net of antenatal surveillance. The combination of post-dates antenatal fetal surveillance and induction of labour between 41 and 41+3 does not increase the

46.12 Best Practice Points

- Induction of labour has a significant impact on pregnancy outcome and patient safety management in the delivery suite and should be employed judiciously.
- Induction of labour is associated with an increased intervention rate.
- Evidence-based recommendations for induction of labour for post-dates low-risk cases is 41+3 gestation.
- Pregnancy dating by first trimester ultrasound is highly recommended.
- Increased antenatal surveillance 40 to 41+3 with cardiotocography (CTG) and amniotic fluid (either deepest vertical pool (DVP) or amniotic fluid index (AFI)).
- Women may be offered the option of membrane sweeping commencing at 38 to 41 weeks.

References

1. Sanchez-Ramos L, Kaunitz, A. Induction of labour. In *The Global Library of Women's Medicine* (ISSN:1756–2228). 2009. doi: 10.3843/GLOWM.10130

2. Graham H. *Eternal Eve: The History of Gynecology and Obstetrics*. London: T. Brun; 1950.

3. Denman T. *An Introduction to the Practice of Midwifery*. London: J. Johnson; 1794.

4. Muscat Baron Y. Why did *Homo sapiens* develop a large brain? *Human Evolution*. 2016:31(4):229–36.

5. Usha Kiran TS, Hemmadi S, Bethel J, et al. Outcome of pregnancy in a woman with an increased body mass index. *BJOG*.2005;**112**:768–72.

6. Hickey CA, Cliver SP, McNeal SF, et al. Low pregravid body mass index as a risk factor for preterm birth: variation by ethnic group. *Obstet Gynecol*.1997;**89**:206–12.

7. Kundodyiwa TW, Alfirevic Z, Weeks AD. Low-dose oral misoprostol for induction of labour: a systematic review. *Obstet Gynecol*. 2009;**113**(2 Pt 1):374–83.

8. Muscat Baron, Y. (2012). *Clinical Practice Guideline on Induction of Labour and Antenatal Surveillance of the Post-Dates Pregnancy*. UMMS, Malta. 2011. [e-book publication]

9. NICE. *Inducing Labour*. Clinical Guideline 70. 2008.

10. Blanc-Petitjean P, Salomé M, Dupont C, et al. Labour induction practices in France: a population-based

declarative survey in 94 maternity units. *J Gynecol Obstet Hum Reprod*. 2018;**47**(2):57–62.

11. Schwarz C, Schäfers R, Loytved C et al. Temporal trends in foetal mortality at and beyond term and induction of labor in Germany 2005–2012: data from German routine perinatal monitoring. *Arch Gynecol Obstet*. 2016;**293**:335–43.

12. Sinnott SJ, Layte R, Brick A, Turner MJ. Variation in induction of labour rates across Irish hospitals; a cross-sectional study. *Eur J Public Health*. 2016;**26**:753–60.

13. Hilder L, Costeloe K, Thilaganathan B. Prolonged pregnancy: evaluating gestation-specific risks of foetal and infant mortality. *Br J Obstet Gynaecol*. 1998;**105**(2):169–73.

14. Heimstad R, Pål R, Romundstad O, Salvesen A. Induction of labour for post-term pregnancy and risk estimates for intrauterine and perinatal death. *Acta Obstet Gynecol Scand.*2008;**87**(2):247–9.

15. Wennerholm UB, Hagberg H, Brorsson B, Bergh C. Induction of labor versus expectant management for postdate pregnancy: is there sufficient evidence for a change in clinical practice? *Acta Obstet Gynecol Scand.* 2009;**88**(1):6–17.

16. Middleton P, Shepherd E, Crowther CA. Induction of labour for improving birth outcomes for women at or beyond term. *Cochrane Database Syst Rev.* 2018 May 9(5):CD004945.

17. Sotiriadis A, Petousis S, Thilaganathan B. Maternal and perinatal outcomes after elective induction of labor at 39 weeks in uncomplicated singleton pregnancy: a meta-analysis. *Ultrasound Obstet Gynecol.* 2019;**53**(1):26–35.

18. Little SE, Zera CA, Clapp MA, et al. A multi-state analysis of early-term delivery trends and the association with term stillbirth. *Obstet Gynaecol.* 2015;**126**(6):1138–45.

19. MacDorman M, Reddy U, Silver R. Trends in stillbirth by gestational age in the United States, 2006–2012. *Obstet Gynecol.* 2015;**126**(6):1146–150.

20. Smith GC. Predicting antepartum stillbirth. *Curr Opin Obstet Gynecol.* 2006 Dec;**18**(6):625–30.

21. Stillbirth Collaborative Research Network Writing Group. Association between stillbirth and risk factors known at pregnancy confirmation. *JAMA.* 2011 Dec 14;**306**(22):2469–79.

22. Savona-Ventura C. Secular trends in obstetric practice in Malta. *Int J Risk & Safety in Med.* 2004;**16**:211–15.

23. Cedergren, M. Maternal morbid obesity and the risk of adverse pregnancy outcome. *Obstet Gynecol.* 2004;**103**(2):219–24.

24. Malacova E, Regan A, Nassar N, et al. Risk of stillbirth, preterm delivery, and foetal growth restriction following exposure in a previous birth: systematic review and meta-analysis. *BJOG.* 2018;**125**(2):183–92.

25. Bukowski R, Hansen NI, Willinger M. Foetal growth and risk of stillbirth: a population-based case-control study. *PloS Med.* 2014;**11**(4):e1001633.

26. Moster D, Wilcox AJ, Vollset SE, et al. Cerebral palsy among term and postterm births. *JAMA.* 2010 Sep 1;**304**(9):976–82.

27. Huang L, Sauve R, Birkett N, et al. Maternal age and risk of stillbirth: a systematic review. *CMAJ.* 2008 Jan 15;**178**(2):165–72.

28. Waldenström U, Cnattingius S, Norman M, Schytt E. Advanced maternal age and stillbirth risk in nulliparous and parous women. *Obstet Gynecol.* 2015;**126**(2):355–62.

29. Boehm FH, Salyer S, Shah DM. Improved outcome of twice weekly nonstress testing. *Obstet Gynecol.* 1986 Apr;**67**(4):566–8.

30. Caughey AB, Nicholson JM, Cheng YW, et al. Induction of labour and caesarean delivery by gestational age. *Am J Obstet Gynecol.* Sep 2006;**195**(3):700–5.

31. Efkarpidis S, Alexopoulos E, Kean L, et al. Case-control study of factors associated with intrauterine foetal deaths. *Med Gen Med.* 2004;**6**:53.

32. Saastad E, Tveit JV, Flenady V, et al. Implementation of uniform information on foetal movement in a Norwegian population reduced delayed reporting of decreased foetal movement and stillbirths in primiparous women – a clinical quality improvement. *BMC Res Notes.* 2010;**3**(1):2.

33. Hofmeyr GJ, Novikova N. Management of reported decreased foetal movements for improving pregnancy outcomes. *Cochrane Database Syst Rev.* 2012 Apr 18;(4):CD009148.

34. Mahran M, Omran M. The impact of diagnostic ultrasound on the prediction of intrauterine growth retardation in developing countries. *Int J Gynaecol Obstet.*1988;**26**:375–8.

35. Neilson J. Ultrasound for foetal assessment in early pregnancy. *Cochrane Database Syst Rev.* 2000;(2):CD000182.

36. Bricker L, Neilson JP, Dowswell T. Routine ultrasound in late pregnancy (after 24 weeks' gestation). *Cochrane Database Syst Rev.* 2008 Oct 8;(4):CD001451.

37. Proud J, Grant AM. Third trimester placental grading by ultrasonography as a test of foetal wellbeing. *Br Med J (Clin Res Ed).*1987;**294**:1641–4.

38. Nageotte MP, Towers CV, Asrat T, Freeman RK. Perinatal outcome with the modified biophysical profile. *Am J Obstet Gynecol.* 1994;**170**(6):1672–6.

39. Leduc D, Biringer G, Lee L. Induction of labour review. *J Obstet Gynaecol Can.* 2013;**35**(9):840–857.

40. Xenakis EM, Piper JM, Conway DL, Langer O. Induction of labor in the nineties: conquering the unfavorable cervix. *Obstet Gynecol.* 1997;**90**(2):235–9.

41. Vrouenraets FP, Roumen FJ, Dehing CJ, et al. Bishop score and risk of caesarean delivery after induction of labor in nulliparous women. *Obstet Gyanecol.* 2005;**105**:690–7.

42. Boulvain M, Irion O. Stripping/sweeping the membranes for inducing or preventing post-term pregnancy. *Cochrane Database Syst Rev.* 2004;(3):CD001328.

43. Voigt, F., Goecke, T., Najjari L. et al. Off-label use of misoprostol for labor induction in Germany: a national survey. *Eur J Obstet Gynecol Reprod Biol.* 2015;**187**:85–9.

44. Hofmeyr GJ, Gülmezoglu AM. Vaginal misoprostol for cervical ripening and induction of labour. *Cochrane Database Syst Rev.* 2003;(1):CD000941.

45. Lim S, Tan T, Yang Huang Ng G, Patient satisfaction with the cervical ripening balloon as a method for induction of labour: a randomised controlled trial. *Singapore Med J.* 2018;**59**(8):419–24.

46. Clark SL, Simpson KR, Knox GE, Garite TJ. Oxytocin: new perspectives on an old drug. *Am J Obstet Gynecol.* 2009;**200**(1):35.

47. Kenyon S, Tokumasu H, Dowswell T, et al. High-dose versus low-dose oxytocin for augmentation of delayed labour. *Cochrane Database Syst Rev.* 2013 Jul 13;(7):CD007201.

Intrapartum Fetal Monitoring

Branka M. Yli, Jørg Kessler & Diogo Ayres-de-Campos

47.1 Introduction

The aim of intrapartum fetal monitoring is to identify fetal hypoxia and intervene appropriately before permanent damage occurs, while concomitantly avoiding unnecessary operative deliveries. Therefore, such monitoring needs to identify fetuses whose physiological defence mechanisms are becoming compromised, so that healthcare professionals can act before an uncontrolled phase leading to injury occurs.

Reports on the presence of fetal heart signals were first published in the eighteenth century, but continuous fetal heart monitoring did not become a reality until cardiotocography (CTG) was introduced into obstetric practice in the late 1960s. The technology rapidly gained wide acceptance in high-resource countries and was introduced into routine intrapartum care in many centres. However, from the beginning, there was wide disagreement on how CTG tracings should be interpreted. This, together with the high complexity of intrapartum CTG signals, led to a high interobserver variability and a limited specificity in detecting fetal hypoxia [1]. It was rapidly realized that adjunctive technologies were needed to increase the objectivity and specificity of CTG interpretation, thus limiting the use of unnecessary obstetric interventions. A range of strategies, including computer analysis of CTGs (cCTG), fetal blood sampling (FBS), ST interval analysis of the fetal electrocardiogram (STAN) and fetal scalp stimulation (FSS), were developed in this context.

47.2 The Physiology of Fetal Oxygenation in Labour

The fetus lives in a low oxygen (O_2) environment but is usually not hypoxic. The median value of the partial pressure of oxygen (pO_2) in the umbilical artery after normal labour is 2.1 kPa (range, 0.7–4.1 kPa) [2]. This is possible due to adaptive mechanisms that support fetal function and growth in a low-O_2 environment. Adult haemoglobin (HbA) is chemically different from fetal haemoglobin (HbF). HbF is a structure of the Hb tetramer molecule, which consists of γ-chains instead of the adult β-chains, in addition to the α-chains included in both molecules. The O_2-Hb dissociation curve for HbF is shifted to the left compared to that for HbA, since HbF has a greater affinity for O_2 at the same pO_2. This allows the saturation of fetal blood with O_2 at a lower pO_2. In addition, the haemoglobin level is higher in fetal blood than in adult blood, the fetal heart rate (FHR) is higher than the adult heart rate, and the cardiac output (i.e. volume of blood

per kilogram of body weight) is approximately four times higher than in adults. Thus, the fetal circulation overperfuses certain organs, including the brain and the myocardium. The higher pO_2 in the maternal circulation compared to that of the fetal circulation facilitates the maternal-to-fetal transfer of O_2 via diffusion across the placental membranes. In addition, respiratory changes during pregnancy decrease the partial pressure of carbon dioxide in maternal circulation, which facilitates the transfer of carbon dioxide from the fetus to the mother [3].

47.3 Fetal Defence Mechanisms against Oxygen Deficiency

Regulation of the FHR is controlled by the autonomic nervous system, with control centres located in the medulla oblongata, and which in turn are affected by the cerebral cortex and hypothalamus. Autonomic control of the FHR is coordinated via input from various sources, including chemoreceptors, baroreceptors, volume receptors, the medullary cardiorespiratory centre, and hormonal inputs.

The sympathetic system uses the hormone noradrenaline to accelerate FHR and improve fetal cardiac inotropy, via nerves distributed throughout the myocardium. The parasympathetic nervous system acts through the vagus nerve, which has terminations in the sinoatrial and atrioventicular nodes. These release the neurotransmitter acetylcholine that slows the FHR and increases baseline variability. The parasympathetic system exerts greater influences on the frequency as gestational age advances.

The heart is equipped with baroreceptors and volume receptors that sense changes in blood pressure and volume. The aortic arch and carotid bodies contain chemoreceptors that sense changes in the O_2 content of blood coming from the placenta. These send neuronal messages to the medulla oblongata, which result in slowing of the FHR via the parasympathetic nervous system. Arterial baroreceptors are sensitive to vessel distension caused by changes in blood pressure. These send neuronal messages to the medulla oblongata, which cause rapid slowing of the FHR via the parasympathetic nervous system. Thus, the autonomic nervous system is provided with continuous information on the circulatory and respiratory systems, adjusting the FHR to the needs of the fetus. In situations of hypoxaemia (decrease in blood O_2 level) of sufficient intensity and duration to cause hypoxia (decrease in tissue O_2 level), the fetus will reduce its O_2 consumption and, if necessary, switch to anaerobic cellular metabolism.

The mechanisms underlying the haemodynamic responses to chronic hypoxia are based on the activation of chemoreflexes, which results in an endocrine response via corticotropin-releasing hormone in the hypothalamus, and adrenocorticotropic hormone secretion from the anterior pituitary. The resulting catecholamine production in the adrenal glands increases FHR and regulates the vasoconstriction of peripheral vessels. Consequently, blood flow is redirected to maximize perfusion of the brain, heart and adrenal glands [4].

In summary, the fetal defence mechanisms operating to protect against a gradually developing O_2 deficiency are as follows:

1. Activation of the sympathetic adrenal system, increasing FHR and cardiac output.
2. Decrease in O_2 consumption.
3. Switch to anaerobic cellular metabolism.
4. Redistribution of cardiac output to preferentially perfuse vital organs such as the heart, brain and adrenal glands.

47.4 Methods for Fetal Heart Monitoring during Labour

47.4.1 Cardiotocography

Cardiotocography (CTG) refers to the method of continuous monitoring of FHR and uterine contractions. The use of CTG in labour increased dramatically in many high-resource countries, making it one of the most frequently used obstetric

procedures. FHR monitoring can be performed either by placing an external Doppler transducer on the mother's abdomen, or an internal fetal electrode on the presenting part to register the R-R interval in the fetal electrocardiogram (ECG). A pressure-sensitive external contraction transducer (called a tocodynamometer or tocotransducer) measures increased tension of the maternal abdominal wall, caused by underlying myometrial contractility. Alternatively, an intrauterine pressure catheter can be introduced into the uterine cavity.

Intrapartum CTG provides a complex signal and there has been wide variation in the way healthcare professionals interpret the resulting tracings. Recent guidelines, based on the largest worldwide consensus reached in the field, were promoted by the International Federation of Gynaecology and Obstetrics (FIGO) in 2015 [5]. However, many European countries still use the CTG classification promoted by ST-analysis experts in the 1990s, which was inspired in the FIGO guidelines of 1987 [6]. This classification was used in most studies where ST-analysis of the fetal ECG (STAN) was evaluated. Most of these studies also used fetal blood sampling (FBS). An updated version of this CTG classification was published in 2007 and will be referred to as STAN 2007 [7].

Cardiotocographic patterns are defined by evaluating the FHR baseline, variability, accelerations, decelerations and contractions, as described below. Based on these individual events, according to FIGO 2015, a CTG recording is then classified as normal, suspicious or pathological (Table 47.1). STAN 2007 classifies the recording as normal, suspicious, pathological or preterminal.

Table 47.1 FIGO 2015 cardiotocography classification criteria, interpretation and recommended management

	Normal	Suspicious	Pathological
Baseline	110–160 beats per minute (bpm)	Lacking at least one characteristic of normality, but with no pathological features	<100 bpm
Variability	5–25 bpm	Lacking at least one characteristic of normality, but with no pathological features	Reduced variability, increased variability, or sinusiodal pattern
Decelerations	No repetitive decelerations[1]	Lacking at least one characteristic of normality, but with no pathological features	Repetitive late[2] or prolonged decelerations during >30 min or 20 min if reduced variability, or one prolonged deceleration with >5min. Fetus with a high probability of hypoxia/acidosis
Interpretation	Fetus with no hypoxia/acidosis	Fetus with low probability of having hypoxia/acidosis	Fetus with high probability of having hypoxia/acidosis
Clinical management	No intervention necessary to improve fetal oxygenation state	Action to correct reversible causes if identified, close monitoring or additional methods to evaluate fetal oxygenation	Immediate action to correct reversible causes, additional methods to evaluate fetal oxygenation, or if this is not possible to expedite delivery. In acute situations (cord prolapse, uterine rupture, placental abruption) immediate delivery should be accomplished.

[1] The presence of accelerations denotes a fetus that does not have hypoxia/acidosis, but their absence during labour is of uncertain significance.
[2] Decelerations are repetitive in nature when they are associated with more than 50% uterine contractions.

47.4.1.1 FHR Baseline

The FHR baseline represents the mean level of a stable FHR and is expressed in beats per minute (bpm). It refers to the mean level of the most horizontal and less oscillatory FHR segments. It should preferably be measured between contractions. Normal baseline range, according to FIGO 2015, is between 110 and 160 bpm. STAN 2007 indicates a range between 110 and 150 bpm.

Fetal tachycardia refers to a baseline value above 160 according to FIGO 2015, and above 150 bpm according to STAN 2007. It should last at least 10 minutes (min). Tachycardia results from an increase in sympathetic and a decrease in parasympathetic activities. It may be a sign of early fetal hypoxia, especially when associated with decreased variability, late decelerations or a long deceleration area [8]. In this context, tachycardia is a compensatory mechanism to chronic hypoxaemia, caused by an increase in circulating catecholamines. Alternatively, tachycardia may just be the first sign of maternal fever, which may or may not be due to intrauterine infection [9]. Less frequently it is associated with fetal anaemia, maternal hyperthyroidism, increased maternal sympathetic tone, use of beta-sympathomimetic drugs or parasympathetic blockers, and fetal arrhythmias such as supraventricular tachycardia and atrial flutter.

Fetal bradycardia refers to a baseline below 110 bpm lasting more than 10 min according to FIGO 2015. According to STAN 2007, when the FHR is between 100 and 110 bpm or when it is below 100 bpm for less than 3 min, the CTG should be classified as suspicious. If the FHR is below 100 bpm for more than 3 min, this is called persistent bradycardia and the CTG should be classified as pathological (Table 47.2). Bradycardia may result from a vagal stimulus mediated by fetal chemoreflexes. It may also be caused by direct depression of myocardial activity due to reduced O_2 supply [10]. Less frequently, bradycardia occurs due to hypothermia, to the effect of beta-blockers, or to cardiac arrhythmias such as atrial-ventricular block.

47.4.1.2 Effect of Hypoxia on the Baseline

It is important to remember that there is a large variation between fetuses in baseline level, suggesting that each fetus should preferably be used as its own reference. With the development of chronic hypoxia, tachycardia occurs as a compensatory mechanism, while a lower baseline or bradycardia is a sign of possible cardiovascular decompensation. Recent studies have found that tachycardia is a better predictor of fetal acidaemia (cord artery pH <7.10) than late decelerations alone, with adjusted odds ratios of 3.68, 95% confidence interval (CI) 2.58–5.25 vs. 2.28, 95% CI 1.43–3.63 [11]. Acute hypoxia results in the sudden development of bradycardia. It is usually due to an excessive frequency of contractions, to aortocaval compression when the mother is in the supine position or to sudden hypotension after regional anaesthesia. More rarely, it occurs with an obstetric emergency, such as placental abruption, uterine rupture or umbilical cord prolapse.

47.4.1.3 Variability

Variability refers to the fine oscillations in the FHR signal, evaluated as the average bandwidth amplitude of the signal in one-minute segments. Normal variability occurs when the bandwidth amplitude is 5–25 bpm. Short-term or beat-to-beat variability is not reliably evaluated by the naked eye, so variability in clinical assessments usually refers to long-term variability, excluding accelerations and decelerations. Physiological conditions induce continuous small changes in the fetal beat-to-beat interval. Fetal heart rate variability is the result of a continuous balancing between the sympathetic and parasympathetic branches of the autonomic nervous system [12]. Normal FHR variability indicates that the fetus has an adequately functioning autonomous nervous system and thus is unlikely to be undergoing hypoxia.

Increased variability, or saltatory pattern, occurs when variability exceeds 25 bpm. According to FIGO 2015, it should not be valued unless it lasts longer than 30 min, while STAN 2007 does not define any time frame. There is limited research on the length of the saltatory pattern that increases the risk of acidosis [13]. The pathophysiology of this pattern is incompletely understood, yet it may be observed in conjunction with recurrent decelerations that develop rapidly during the initial phases of hypoxia. It is presumed to be caused by fetal autonomic instability or a hyperactive autonomic system.

Reduced variability refers to a bandwidth amplitude below 5 bpm. According to FIGO 2015, it needs to last more than 50 min in baseline segments, or more than 3 min during decelerations to be clinically relevant. According to STAN 2007, it is defined as reduced when lasting more than 40 min, and the CTG should be classified as suspicious. When lasting more than 60 min the CTG should be classified as pathological. When variability falls below 2 bpm, it should be classified as 'absent variability' and the tracing classified as preterminal, requiring immediate delivery (Table 47.2). Reduced variability is a consistent indicator of developing hypoxia, especially when combined with other FHR abnormalities, and indicates reduced central nervous system activity. However, it can also be due to infection, administration of central nervous system depressants or parasympathetic blockers. During the fetal behavioural state of 'deep sleep', which can last up to 50 minutes, variability is usually in the lower range of normality, but the bandwidth amplitude is seldom under 5 bpm.

The sinusoidal pattern is a smooth, sine-wave-like pattern of regular frequency and amplitude. The amplitude of oscillations is usually between 5 and 15 bpm (rarely higher) and the frequency of 2–5 cycles per min. According to FIGO 2015, it should last at least 30 min to be clinically relevant and have no areas of normal variability or accelerations. STAN 2007 does not define a minimum time frame for the sinusoidal pattern. The pathophysiological basis behind it is incompletely understood, but it occurs in association with severe fetal anaemia found in anti-D alloimmunization, fetal–maternal haemorrhage, twin-to-twin transfusion syndrome and ruptured vasa praevia. It has also been described in cases of acute fetal hypoxia, infection, cardiac malformations, hydrocephalus and gastroschisis [14].

It needs to be differentiated from the pseudo-sinusoidal pattern, which can appear similar but has a more jagged 'saw-tooth' appearance, its duration seldom exceeds 30 min, and it is characterized by normal CTG patterns before and after. This pattern is a normal part of CTG recordings and has been described after analgesic administration, and during periods of fetal sucking and other mouth movements. It is sometimes difficult to distinguish between the two, leaving the short duration of the pseudo-sinusoidal pattern as the most important discriminatory factor.

Effect of Hypoxia on Variability

The chronic development of hypoxaemia in both animal and human studies manifests with an increase in variability as the first sign of O_2 deficit [15, 16]. If hypoxia develops, variability will gradually decrease until it become almost imperceptible, but this is a late sign [17]. It may appear concomitantly with decelerations and an increase in FHR baseline. There is a high degree of subjectivity in visual evaluations of decreased or absent variability, and therefore careful re-evaluation is recommended.

47.4.1.4 Accelerations

These are abrupt increases in FHR above the baseline of more than 15 bpm in amplitude and lasting more than 15 seconds, but less than 10 min. An acceleration lasting more than 10 min is considered a baseline change. The amplitude and frequency of accelerations may be lower before 32 gestational weeks (10 seconds and 10 bpm). After 32–34 weeks, with the establishment of fetal behavioural states, accelerations rarely occur during periods of deep sleep. Most accelerations coincide with fetal movements and are a sign of a neurologically responsive and adequately oxygenated fetus. The absence of accelerations in an otherwise normal intrapartum CTG recording is of uncertain significance, but it is unlikely to indicate hypoxia or acidosis.

47.4.1.5 Decelerations

Decelerations are transient episodes of slowing of the FHR below the baseline of ≥15 bpm and lasting more than 15 seconds, but less than 10 min. A deceleration lasting more than 10 min and below 110 bpm is considered a bradycardia. They should be subdivided into different types, associated with different pathophysiological mechanisms, as delineated here:

Early decelerations are shallow, short-lasting decelerations, with normal variability within the deceleration, and occurring at the same time as the peak of the contraction. They are believed to be caused by fetal head compression and do not indicate fetal hypoxia. The early decelerations are a part of normal intrapartum CTG.

Variable decelerations (V-shaped) exhibit a rapid drop, rapid recovery to the baseline, normal variability within the deceleration, and are of varying size, shape and relationship to uterine contractions. According to STAN 2007, they can be further divided as being uncomplicated or complicated. Uncomplicated variable decelerations last less than 60 seconds and have an FHR drop of more than 60 bpm. Complicated variable decelerations last more than 60 seconds. Repeated

uncomplicated decelerations should lead to a CTG classification of suspicious and repeated complicated decelerations to a CTG classification of pathological (Table 47.2).

Variable decelerations constitute the majority of decelerations, and translate a baroreceptor-mediated response to increased arterial pressure, as occurs with umbilical cord compression.

Late decelerations (U-shaped) have a gradual onset, gradual return to the baseline or reduced variability within the deceleration. Late decelerations start more than 20 seconds after the onset of a contraction, nadir after the acme and return to the baseline after the end of the contraction. These are indicative of a chemoreceptor-mediated response to fetal hypoxaemia. In the presence of a tracing with no accelerations and reduced variability, the definition of late decelerations also includes those with an amplitude of 10–15 bpm.

FIGO 2015 defines 'prolonged decelerations' as those lasting more than 3 minutes. They are likely to include a chemoreceptor-mediated component and thus to indicate hypoxaemia. Decelerations exceeding 5 minutes, with FHR maintained <80 bpm and reduced variability within the deceleration are frequently associated with acute fetal hypoxia and require emergent intervention. According to STAN 2007 this pattern is defined as bradycardia.

Decelerations and Hypoxia

Although no pattern of repeated deep or late decelerations is necessarily benign, fetuses with normal reserve can withstand frequent decelerations for surprisingly long intervals, before the development of acidosis and hypotension. This reflects the remarkable ability of the fetus to adapt to repeated episodes of hypoxaemia [18]. Recent studies suggest that the deceleration area is the CTG pattern that better predicts acidaemia, and combined with tachycardia is associated with a significant risk of neonatal morbidity [8].

47.4.1.6 Contractions

Contractions can be evaluated based on their frequency, duration and amplitude, as well as the basal uterine tone between them. However, when using a tocodynamometer, only the frequency of contractions can be reliably assessed. The normal frequency of uterine contractions during labour is every 2–3 min, depending on the stage of labour. Contractions are necessary for the progression of labour, but they may compress the vessels running inside the myometrium and transiently decrease placental perfusion or cause umbilical cord compression. An excessive contraction frequency is defined as the occurrence of more than five contractions per 10 min, in two successive 10-min periods or averaged over 30 min. This is called tachysystole and is associated with an increased risk of the development of hypoxia; for example, more than five contractions per 10 min were found to result in fetal O_2 saturation decreasing by 29% after 30 min [19].

47.5 Tracing Classification

Tracing classification requires previous evaluation of the basic CTG features described above. Due to the changing nature of

CTG signals during labour, tracing re-evaluation should be carried out at least every 30 minutes.

Longitudinal evaluations of the CTG should be undertaken to understand the progression of fetal deterioration and to help decide the need for appropriate intervention. Cardiotocographic patterns during labour can quickly progress from normal to pathological in the presence of acute insults such as placental abruption, uterine rupture, ruptured vasa praevia or cord prolapse. However, it is more common for such progression to develop gradually over the course of a few hours. Starting from a normal CTG recording, compromised fetuses will often exhibit a progression in FHR patterns characterized by the sequential development of variable decelerations, loss of accelerations, short periods of increased variability, increased frequency and duration of decelerations, baseline rises with frequent episodes of tachycardia or continuous tachycardia, reduced variability in between and during decelerations and finally bradycardia.

47.6 Actions in Situations of Suspected Fetal Hypoxia

When fetal hypoxia is anticipated or suspected, actions are required to avoid adverse neonatal outcome, but this does not necessarily mean performing a caesarean section or instrumental vaginal delivery. The underlying cause can frequently be identified, and the situation reversed, with subsequent recovery of adequate fetal oxygenation and the return to a normal tracing.

Excessive uterine activity is the most frequent cause of fetal hypoxia, and this can be detected by documenting tachysystole in the CTG tracing or palpation of the uterine fundus. It can usually be reversed by reducing or stopping oxytocin infusion, removing administered prostaglandins, or starting acute tocolysis with beta-adrenergic agonists (salbutamol, terbutaline, ritodrine), atosiban, or nitroglycerine. During the second stage of labour, maternal pushing can also contribute to decreased placental perfusion and resulting fetal hypoxia. The mother should be asked to stop pushing, to push on alternate contractions or to start passive pushing with an open glottis, until the situation is reversed.

Aortocaval compression can occur when the mother is in the supine position and leads to reduced placental perfusion. In these cases, changing the maternal position is frequently followed by normalization of the CTG pattern. Transient cord compression is another common cause of CTG changes (variable decelerations), and these can sometimes be reverted by changing the maternal position or by performing amnioinfusion. Sudden maternal hypotension can also occur during labour, usually after epidural or spinal analgesia, and it is frequently reversible by rapid fluid administration or by an intravenous ephedrine bolus.

Administration of O_2 to the mother is widely used, with the objective of improving fetal oxygenation and normalizing CTG patterns, but there is no evidence that this intervention is useful when maternal oxygenation and circulation are adequate.

Other less frequent complications affecting the maternal respiration, maternal circulation, placenta, umbilical cord or fetal circulation can also result in fetal hypoxia. These include acute situations such as placental abruption, uterine rupture, ruptured vasa praevia and cord prolapse, all of which require emergent delivery.

Good clinical judgement is required to diagnose the underlying cause for a suspicious or pathological CTG, to judge the reversibility of the condition and to determine the timing of delivery, with the objective of avoiding prolonged fetal hypoxia, as well as unnecessary obstetric intervention. When a suspicious or worsening CTG pattern is identified, the underlying cause needs to be addressed before a pathological tracing develops. If the situation does not revert and the pattern continues to deteriorate, consideration needs to be given to rapid delivery. According to STAN 2007, a preterminal pattern requires immediate delivery.

47.7 Evidence from Randomized Controlled Trials

Continuous CTG monitoring has been compared to intermittent auscultation in several randomized controlled trials (RCTs). All were performed between 1976 and 1993, and they all used CTG monitors and interpretation criteria that are very different from current practice. Although RCTs are generally seen as the strongest evidence for the use of any technology, it is difficult to establish how the results of these RCTs relate to current clinical practice, given the evolution that occurred in technical characteristics of CTG monitors, increased knowledge on the pathophysiology of FHR events and response to CTG changes. With these limitations in mind, they indicate a limited benefit of continuous CTG for fetal monitoring in all women during labour. Several meta-analyses have determined that it reduces the incidence of neonatal seizures by about 50%, but has not been shown to affect overall perinatal mortality and cerebral palsy rates. However, it is widely recognized that the trials were underpowered to detect differences in these outcomes. Only a small proportion of perinatal deaths and cerebral palsies are caused by intrapartum hypoxia, so a very large number of cases is needed to show any benefit. In addition, continuous CTG was associated with a 63% increase in caesarean sections and a 15% increase in instrumental vaginal deliveries [20].

47.7.1 Computer Analysis of CTGs

The development of computer analysis of CTGs began in the 1980s, in an attempt to overcome the well-demonstrated poor reproducibility of visual analysis and subjectivity in the interpretation of parameters such as variability. The first systems could only perform analysis of antepartum CTGs, where reduced baseline instability, limited signal loss and artefacts and smaller tracing length pose lesser challenges for signal processing and algorithm development.

Over the last two decades, several systems were adapted for analysis of intrapartum signals, and some have been commercialized in association with fetal central monitoring stations. Continued improvements in computer memory and processing speed have allowed real-time display and analysis of several tracings on the same computer screen. Systems have also incorporated real-time visual and sound alerts, based on the results of computer analysis, to promote tracing re-evaluation and intervention, if necessary.

Four systems for computer analysis of CTG signals are currently commercially available [21]. Perhaps because of commercial issues, the available descriptions of system characteristics are usually limited. Despite different developers, there are some similarities between the systems. For instance, they all use relatively similar colour-coding and sound alarms, and they all refrain from providing clinical management recommendations. However, different mathematical algorithms are used, and analysis is based on different interpretation guidelines.

The SisPorto system (Speculum, Lisbon, Portugal) was developed at the University of Porto in Portugal. The system recently incorporated revised algorithms based on the FIGO 2015 guidelines. Combined alerts, integrating CTG and ST events, have also been introduced. A good agreement with experts on identification of basic CTG features, and a high accuracy in detection of neonatal acidaemia was reported [22]. The system was compared with visual analysis in a multicentre RCT evaluating 7730 women in the UK. Metabolic acidosis rates were lower in the computer analysis arm, but the difference did not reach statistical significance (0.40% vs. 0.58%, relative risk (RR) 0.69, 95% CI 0.36–1.31). In a subgroup of high-risk pregnancies, umbilical blood acidaemia (pH <7.10) was significantly reduced in the computer arm (4.05% vs. 5.85%, RR 0.69, 95% CI 0.50–0.96) [23]. In a large retrospective cohort of 38 466 deliveries, introduction of the system together with the STAN technology in a tertiary care hospital was associated with significant reductions in hypoxic-ischaemic encephalopathy (5.3% vs. 2.2%, RR 0.42, 95% CI 0.29–0.61) and overall caesarean section rates (29.9% vs. 28.3%, RR 0.96, 95% CI 0.92–0.99) [24].

The INFANT system (K2 Medical System, Plymouth, UK) was developed at the University of Plymouth and K2 Medical Systems in the UK, integrating mathematical algorithms and trained neural networks for CTG analysis. In a large observational study, the Infant system was found to be in good agreement with experts' opinions [21]. In a large RCT carried out in the UK, involving 46 042 participants, cOMPuter analysis with Infant System was compared with visual analysis of CTGs. Poor neonatal outcome (defined as intrapartum stillbirth, early neonatal death excluding malformations, neonatal encephalopathy, early neonatal intensive care unit admission for more than 48 hours with encephalopathy or respiratory illness) was similar in the two arms (adjusted risk ratio (aRR): 1.01, 95% CI 0.82–1.25), as were intervention rates (aRR for spontaneous cephalic vaginal delivery: 0.99, 99% CI 0.97–1.01) [25].

The PeriCALM system (LMS Medical systems, Montreal, Canada, and PeriGen, Princeton, USA) was developed at the University of Montreal in Canada. Computer analysis is based on the National Institute of Child Health and Human Development (NICHD) guidelines and incorporates mathematical algorithms and trained neural networks for CTG

interpretation. A good agreement in tracing classification between experts and the system was reported, and alerts showed a good capacity to predict metabolic acidosis and hypoxic-ischaemic encephalopathy [21]. Decelerations lasting more than 2 min with loss of internal variability and those with greater depth and duration were found to be good predictors of metabolic acidosis [26].

The Trium system (GE Healthcare, Little Chalfont, UK, and Trium Analysis Online GmbH, Munich, Germany) was developed by Trium, in association with the Technical University of Munich in Germany. Analysis of CTG tracings is based on the 1987 FIGO guidelines for fetal monitoring. A good agreement between the system and experts in classification of CTGs and a good accuracy in prediction of acidosis evaluated by FBS were reported [27].

In conclusion, computer analysis of intrapartum CTGs is a relatively new but promising technology, aimed at increasing the objectivity of interpretation and alerting healthcare professionals to CTG events associated with fetal hypoxia. Optimization of algorithms is likely to continue in the future and to result in improved results. Further research is required to evaluate the capacity of computerized CTG to detect impending fetal hypoxia and, in combination with adequate action, to reduce adverse outcomes and obstetric interventions.

47.7.2 Fetal Scalp Blood Sampling

Fetal blood sampling (FBS) of the scalp to evaluate capillary blood pH has been used since the 1960s as a diagnostic test for intrapartum fetal hypoxia in the presence of abnormal CTG patterns. The fetal presenting part is visualized through a cylindrical amnioscope inserted in the vagina, and capillary blood is obtained via a small stab wound. Obtained blood can be analyzed for pH or lactate. FBS use is mainly limited to Central and Northern Europe. The reason for the low global uptake of FBS may include the fact that it is not very patient-friendly and is time-consuming, with a median interval of 10 minutes between the decision to perform scalp pH and the result [28]. This interval is significantly shorter when using point-of-care devices, with a median sampling interval of 2 minutes for lactate. Given the dynamic nature of labour, the information provided quickly becomes outdated, requiring repetitions of the method. In a large RCT comparing pH with lactate measurements, the rate of operative deliveries was identical when cut-off values for intervention were set at pH less than 7.21 and lactate greater than 4.8 mmol/L, and the latter value is used to define the need for intervention [29]. These cut-off values ware established with a specific point-of-care monitor and have not been validated for others. However, both pH and lactate have low sensitivities and specificities for prediction of adverse neonatal outcome variables, such as low Apgar scores, low cord artery pH and neonatal encephalopathy [30].

A Cochrane systematic review looked at the use of FBS as an adjunctive method to continuous CTG that appeared to increase the rate of instrumental deliveries while decreasing the rate of neonatal acidosis [20]. More than 50 years after the introduction of FBS, a high-quality RCT is still needed to evaluate its effect on perinatal outcomes and intervention rates.

47.7.3 CTG with Automatic ST Analyses (STAN)

STAN technology is based on evaluating changes in the ST interval of the fetal ECG. For this purpose, a scalp electrode is attached to the fetal presenting part, and thus requires ruptured membranes. The ST interval of the ECG represents the phase of ventricular repolarization, an energy-consuming process that is sensitive to hypoxia. ST elevations occur as a specific sign of myocardial hypoxia, leading to a chemoreceptor-mediated adrenaline surge and β-adrenoceptor-mediated anaerobic metabolism with myocardial glycogenolysis. These are the main physiologic mechanisms behind a T-wave elevation.

The presence of a depression in the ST segment can be due to myocardial ischaemia but is also associated with a decrease in myocardial performance. Thus, basically all factors that affect the performance of the myocardial wall, such as prematurity, infections, fever, myocardial dystrophy and cardiac malformations, can result in this occurrence [31].

The STAN monitor (Neoventa, Gothenburg, Sweden) automatically evaluates and detects significant elevations of the T-wave (baseline or episodic T/QRS rises) and depressions in the ST-interval (grade 2 and 3 biphasic STs), which are displayed on the screen as 'ST events'. The STAN technology uses ST events in conjunction with CTG to predict situations of fetal hypoxia. Interventions due to ST events should only be performed in cases of a suspicious or pathological CTG recording. A normal CTG recording has a high negative predictive value for adequate fetal oxygenation, while a lack of variability and accelerations (i.e. a preterminal CTG pattern according to STAN 2007) should always prompt an intervention, irrespective of fetal ECG changes. The STAN technology has only been evaluated with the STAN 2007 CTG classification (Table 47.2).

The STAN technology is currently used in several labour wards throughout Europe, and its clinical introduction included education of the staff in fetal physiology and fetal monitoring as a prerequisite for certified use. Furthermore, the STAN 2007 guidelines defined specific time frames for intervention in cases of suspected fetal hypoxia. Delivery should be accomplished within 20 min during the first stage of labour, and immediate operative intervention should be performed during the active second stage. These are not arbitrary limits, since non-adherence to these guidelines has been shown to increase the risk of neonatal morbidity [32].

Six randomized studies evaluating the STAN technology, involving 26 446 women, have been published. Five of these trials compared CTG alone with STAN, having the option of FBS in both arms. The sixth trial did not use FBS in either arm. These six RCTs have been evaluated in several systematic reviews, all of which have demonstrated a reduction in the need for FBS, and a reduction in vaginal operative deliveries when STAN technology is used. There is seemingly conflicting evidence about whether the use of STAN technology reduces cord metabolic acidosis at delivery. Unfortunately, not all systematic reviews used revised cord acid-base data from the RCTs, or included methodologically correct cord blood data [33]. If statistics are based on correct data, the STAN technology reduces the frequency of cord metabolic acidosis by more than 30% [34].

Several large-scale observational studies with more than 50 000 deliveries performed over the past two decades have also consistently shown that the use of STAN methodology is associated with a decrease in neonatal cord metabolic acidosis [35].

47.7.4 Fetal Scalp Stimulation

Fetal scalp stimulation (FSS) is another intermittent test that can be used to assess fetal well-being. This technique involves the stimulation of the fetal scalp by rubbing it with the fingers. Digital scalp stimulation is the most widely used method, as it is the easiest to perform, less invasive than other methods and appears to have similar predictive value to the others. The main

Table 47.2 CTG classification according to STAN 2007

CTG classification	Baseline heart rate	Variability, reactivity	Decelerations
Normal	■ 110–150 bpm	■ 5–25 bpm ■ Accelerations present	■ Early decelerations ■ Uncomplicated variable decelerations with duration <60 seconds (s) and loss <60 bpm
Suspicious	■ 100–110 bpm ■ 150–170 bpm ■ Short episode of bradycardia <100 bpm <3 min	■ >25 bpm without accelerations ■ <5 bpm for >40 min	■ Uncomplicated variable decelerations with duration <60 s and loss >60 bpm
Pathological	■ >170 bpm ■ Persistent bradycardia <100 bpm >3 min	■ <5 bpm for >60 min ■ Sinusoidal pattern	■ Complicated variable decelerations with duration >60 s ■ Repeated late decelerations
	Combination of at least two characteristics of suspicious CTG		
Preterminal	■ Total lack of variability (<2 bpm) and reactivity with or without decelerations and/or bradycardia		

purpose of FSS is to evaluate fetuses showing reduced variability on the CTG in order to distinguish between deep sleep and hypoxia. It is of uncertain value in other patterns. Observational studies have shown that the appearance of an acceleration and subsequent normalization of the fetal heart pattern should be regarded as a reassuring feature, with a high negative predictive value for fetal hypoxia. A negative intrapartum FSS has limited positive predictive value. A meta-analysis comparing FBS with FSS, among other intrapartum fetal stimulation tests, found similar positive and negative likelihood ratios [36]. Holzmann and co-workers demonstrated that stimulation tests are only helpful when accelerations are present [37]. FSS is easy to perform, but the benefits of this technique have not been evaluated in RCTs, and therefore little is known about how FSS affects neonatal outcomes or intervention rates.

47.8 Conclusion

It is necessary to understand the pathophysiology of fetal responses to hypoxia during labour and their effect on the different intrapartum CTG patterns. Longitudinal evaluations of the CTG should be undertaken to understand the progression of fetal deterioration and to help decide the need for appropriate intervention. Regular staff training on CTG analysis is important to raise awareness and to maintain high levels of attention to the subtle details of FHR interpretation. There remains a need to further develop and investigate adjunctive technologies to remove the uncertainty that surrounds many of them, and to provide more robust evidence on how they affect intervention and adverse outcome rates.

References

1. Sabiani L, Le Dû R, Loundou A, et al. Intra- and interobserver agreement among obstetric experts in court regarding the review of abnormal foetal heart rate tracings and obstetrical management. *Am J Obstet Gynecol* .2015 Dec;**213**(6):856.e1–8.

2. Arikan GM, Scholz HS, Petru E, et al. Cord blood oxygen saturation in vigorous infants at birth: what is normal? *BJOG*. 2000 Aug;**107**(8):987–94.

3. Yli BM, Kjellmer I. Pathophysiology of foetal oxygenation and cell damage during labour. *Best Pract Res Clin Obstet Gynaecol*. 2016 Jan;**30**:9–21.

4. Jensen A, Roman C, Rudolph AM. Effects of reducing uterine blood flow on foetal blood flow distribution and oxygen delivery. *J Dev Physiol*. 1991 Jun;**15**(6):309–23.

5. Ayres-de-Campos D, Spong CY, Chandraharan E, FIGO Intrapartum Foetal Monitoring Expert Consensus Panel.FIGO consensus guidelines on intrapartum foetal monitoring: cardiotocography. *Int J Gynecol Obstet*. 2015 Oct;**131**(1):13–24.

6. Goesta Rooth O, Huch A, Huch R, et al. FIGO News. Guidelines for the Use of Foetal Monitoring* by the FIGO Subcommittee on Standards in Perinatal Medicine, November, 1986. *Int J Gynaecol Obstet*. 1987;**25**: 159–67.

7. Amer-Wahlin I, Arulkumaran S, Hagberg H, Marsál K, Visser GHA. Foetal electrocardiogram: ST waveform analysis in intrapartum surveillance. *BJOG*. 2007 Oct 12;**114** (10):1191–3.

8. Cahill AG, Tuuli MG, Stout MJ, López JD, Macones GA. A prospective cohort study of foetal heart rate monitoring: deceleration area is predictive of foetal acidemia. *Am J Obstet Gynecol*. 2018 May;**218**(5):523. e1–523.e12.

9. Ugwumadu A. Infection and foetal neurologic injury. *Curr Opin Obstet Gynecol*. 2006 Apr;**18**(2):106–11.

10. Williams KP, Galerneau F. Foetal heart rate parameters predictive of neonatal outcome in the presence of a prolonged deceleration. *Obstet Gynecol*. 2002 Nov; **100** (5 Pt 1): 951–4.

11. Cahill A, Tuuli MG, Stout MJ, et al. 345: Electronic foetal monitoring (EFM) patterns are associated with acidemia. *Am J Obstet Gynecol*. 2016 Jan 1;**214**(1): S194–5.

12. Dalton KJ, Dawes GS, Patrick JE. The autonomic nervous system and foetal heart rate variability. *Am J Obstet Gynecol*. 1983 Jun 15;**146** (4):456–62.

13. Nunes I, Ayres-de-Campos D, Kwee A, Rosén KG. Prolonged saltatory foetal heart rate pattern leading to newborn metabolic acidosis. *Clin Exp Obstet Gynecol*. 2014;**41**(5):507–11.

14. Modanlou HD, Murata Y. Sinusoidal heart rate pattern: reappraisal of its definition and clinical significance. *J Obstet Gynaecol Res*. 2004 Jun;**30** (3):169–80.

15. Ikenoue T, Martin CB, Murata Y, Ettinger BB, Lu PS. Effect of acute hypoxemia and respiratory acidosis on the foetal heart rate in monkeys. *Am J Obstet Gynecol*. 1981 Dec 1;**141** (7):797–806.

16. Lu K, Holzmann M, Abtahi F, et al. Foetal heart rate short term variation during labour in relation to scalp blood lactate concentration. *Acta Obstet Gynecol Scand*. 2018 Oct;**97** (10):1274–80.

17. Williams KP, Galerneau F. Intrapartum foetal heart rate patterns in the prediction of neonatal acidemia. *Am J Obstet Gynecol*. 2003 Mar;**188** (3):820–3.

18. Westgate JA, Wibbens B, Bennet L, et al. The intrapartum deceleration in center stage: a physiologic approach to the interpretation of foetal heart rate changes in labour. *Am J Obstet Gynecol*. 2007 Sep;**197**(3):236. e1–11.

19. Simpson KR, James DC. Effects of oxytocin-induced uterine hyperstimulation during labour on foetal oxygen status and fetal heart rate patterns. *Am J Obstet Gynecol*. 2008 Jul;**199**(1):34.e1-5.

20. Alfirevic Z, Devane D, Gyte GM, Cuthbert A. Continuous cardiotocography (CTG) as a form of electronic foetal monitoring (EFM) for foetal assessment during labour. *Cochrane Database Syst Rev*. 2017 Feb; (2):CD006066.

21. Nunes I, Ayres-de-Campos D. Computer analysis of foetal monitoring signals. *Best Pract Res Clin Obstet Gynaecol*. 2016 Jan;**30**:68–78.

22. Costa A, Ayres-de-Campos D, Costa F, Santos C, Bernardes J. Prediction of neonatal acidemia by computer analysis of foetal heart rate and ST event signals. *Am J Obstet Gynecol*. 2009 Nov;**201**(5):464.e1–6.

23. Nunes I, Ayres-de-Campos D, Ugwumadu A, et al. Central foetal monitoring with and without computer analysis. *Obstet Gynecol.* 2017 Jan;**129**(1):83–90.

24. Lopes-Pereira J, Costa A, Ayres-de-Campos D, et al. Computerized analysis of cardiotocograms and ST signals is associated with significant reductions in hypoxic-ischemic encephalopathy and cesarean delivery: an observational study in 38 466 deliveries. *Am J Obstet Gynecol.* 2019 Mar;**220**(3):269.31–269.e8.

25. Brocklehurst P, Field D, Greene K, et al. Computerised interpretation of foetal heart rate during labour (INFANT): a randomised controlled trial. *Lancet.* 2017 Apr 29;**389**(10080):1719–29.

26. Hamilton E, Warrick P, O'Keeffe D. Variable decelerations: do size and shape matter? *J Matern Neonatal Med.* 2012 Jun;**25**(6):648–53.

27. Schiermeier S, Pildner von Steinburg S, Thieme A, et al. Sensitivity and specificity of intrapartum computerised FIGO criteria for cardiotocography and foetal scalp pH during labour: multicentre, observational study. *BJOG.* 2008 Nov;**115**(12):1557–63.

28. Rimmer S, Roberts SA, Heazell AEP. Cervical dilatation and grade of doctor affects the interval between decision and result of foetal scalp blood sampling in labour. *J Matern Neonatal Med.* 2015 Oct 20;**29**(16):1–4.

29. Wiberg-Itzel E, Lipponer C, Norman M, et al. Determination of pH or lactate in foetal scalp blood in management of intrapartum foetal distress: randomised controlled multicentre trial. *BMJ.* 2008 Jun 7;**336**(7656):1284–7.

30. Ramanah R, Martin A, Riethmuller D, Maillet R, Schaal J-P. [Value of foetal scalp lactate sampling during labour: a comparative study with scalp pH]. *Gynecol Obstet Fertil.* 2005 Mar;**33**(3):107–12.

31. Yli BM, Källén K, Stray-Pedersen B, Amer-Wåhlin I. Intrapartum foetal ECG and diabetes. *J Matern Neonatal Med.* 2008; Apr;**21**(4):231–8.

32. Kessler J, Moster D, Albrechtsen S. Delay in intervention increases neonatal morbidity in births monitored with cardiotocography and ST-waveform analysis. *Acta Obstet Gynecol Scand.* 2014 Feb;**93**(2):175–81.

33. Neilson JP. Foetal electrocardiogram (ECG) for foetal monitoring during labour. *Cochrane Database Syst Rev.* 2015 Dec 21;(12):CD000116.

34. Vayssière C, Ehlinger V, Paret L, Arnaud C. Is STAN monitoring associated with a significant decrease in metabolic acidosis at birth compared with cardiotocography alone? Review of the three meta-analyses that included the recent US trial. *Acta Obstet Gynecol Scand.* 2016 Oct;**95**(10):1190–1.

35. Timonen S, Holmberg K. The importance of the learning process in ST analysis interpretation and its impact in improving clinical and neonatal outcomes. *Am J Obstet Gynecol.* 2018; Jun;**218**(6):620.e1–620.e7.

36. Skupski DW, Rosenberg CR, Eglinton GS. Intrapartum foetal stimulation tests: a meta-analysis. *Obstet Gynecol.* 2002 Jan;**99**(1):129–34.

37. Holzmann M, Wretler S, Nordström L. Absence of accelerations during labour is of little value in interpreting foetal heart rate patterns. *Acta Obstet Gynecol Scand.* 2016 Oct; **95**(10):1097–103.

Augmentation of Labour

Rumana Rahman & Neela Mukhopadhaya

48.1 Definition

Augmentation of labour is the process of stimulating the uterus to increase the frequency, duration and intensity of contractions after the onset of labour. Augmentation is used to treat delayed labour when uterine contractions are assessed to be insufficiently strong or inappropriately coordinated to effectively cause cervical dilation or effacement. Labour augmentation has traditionally been performed with the use of intravenous oxytocin infusion and/or artificial rupture of amniotic membranes. The procedure aims to shorten labour in order to prevent complications relating to undue prolongation and to avert caesarean section. It is central to the concept of active management of the first stage of labour, which was proposed about four decades ago as a strategy for expediting labour and reducing caesarean section rates [1].

There is wide disparity in labour augmentation protocols among different countries and also among different hospitals in the same country. The differences are usually related with the timing and indications for amniotomy, variations with the initiation and dosage of oxytocin and modifications based on the use of special procedures like epidural anaesthesia. This chapter will provide a consolidated review of evidence and guidance for effective labour augmentation.

48.2 WHO Guiding Principles and Recommendations for Labour Augmentation

The World Health Organization (WHO) has laid down a list of guiding principles and recommendations to help end-users and stakeholders adapt and implement guidelines for augmentation of labour guidelines. These principles were consensus-based and were not derived from a systematic process of evidence retrieval, synthesis and grading. They are intended to underscore the importance of respect for women's rights and dignity as recipients of care, and the need to maintain high ethical and safety standards in clinical practice.

The WHO guiding principles apply to

- singleton fetuses
- in cephalic presentations
- in an unscarred uterus

Augmentation should be carried out in a facility with the capacity to manage potential adverse outcomes including failure to achieve a vaginal delivery and fetal distress. There should be a valid medical indication for augmentation with

clear documentation of the expected benefits. Augmentation should entail continuous support and one-to-one care with regular monitoring of fetal heart rate and uterine contraction. Clinical assessment should aim to exclude cephalopelvic disproportion before starting augmentation.

Appendix 48.1, Table 48.1 presents the list of 20 recommendations from WHO laid down in 2014.

48.3 Women's Experiences in Labour

Maternity services support women and their families through a milestone moment in their lives. The quality of the care a woman receives during this life-changing period will influence not only the health of mother and child, but also their interactions with health services throughout the rest of their lives.

One of the main determining factors for a successful labour augmentation is involvement of the woman and family in decision making. Birth attendants who practise evidence-based maternity care need to review critically the potential risks, benefits, safety, effectiveness and cost of each tradition, practice, procedure or intervention selected by them and family. The effect on the encouragement and empowerment of the childbearing family unit, particularly the woman giving birth, must be assessed critically. Each intervention must be evaluated as part of the entire birth event, with the understanding that even small, seemingly insignificant interventions may have a cascade effect on the entire birth and family [2]. Women's experiences of childbirth are affected by their perceptions of support and care from relatives and obstetricians, sense of control, sense of security and involvement in decision making during labour [3]. A normal first childbirth with a positive experience is very important with regard to future pregnancies and childbirths. Women with a negative experience and a severe fear of childbirth often request an elective caesarean delivery [4] which is associated with increased risks for both mother and baby. A Swedish study reports on the development and testing of the Childbirth Experience Questionnaire (CEQ) to assess different aspects of women's experiences of first childbirth. The 22-item CEQ yielded four dimensions in the childbirth experience which were Own capacity, Perceived safety, Professional support and Participation [3]. The four dimensions were concordant with previous research into women's experience in childbirth. All four dimensions revealed significantly low scores for women on oxytocin augmentation of labour. Another relevant outcome that came out of this Swedish randomized controlled trial was that early oxytocin augmentation for slow labour progress does not appear to be more beneficial than expectant management regarding women's perceptions of childbirth 1 month postpartum [5]. Slow progress was defined as an arrest of cervical dilation for 2 hours or a dilation of less than 1 cm for 3 hours in the first stage of active labour. If labour progress was slow and membranes were intact, an amniotomy was performed. If there was still no progress after 1 hour of amniotomy, the woman was randomly allocated to one of the two approaches of labour augmentation: the early oxytocin group (oxytocin started in 20 minutes) and the expectant group (oxytocin postponed for another 3 hours). The authors recommend prudent expectant management to be a safe and viable alternative to earlier intervention and oxytocin augmentation to improve patient experience.

48.4 Methods of Augmentation of Labour

Although augmentation of labour can be achieved by natural means like nipple stimulation, the two principal methods have been artificial rupture of membranes and the use of oxytocin.

48.4.1 Artificial Rupture of Membranes

There are three main purposes of doing an amniotomy or deliberate rupture of membranes: reduction in time in labour, evaluation of the amniotic fluid for meconium or blood and application of internal monitoring devices such as fetal scalp electrodes. Potential adverse effects have been suggested, however, including cord prolapse, maternal or fetal infection, fetal laceration or scalp infection, fetal cephalohaematoma, increased caput and increased malalignment of fetal cranial bones [6]. The fetal head has been believed to be applying greater force for cervical dilation compared to bag of membranes. Most of the randomized controlled trials (RCTs) show that amniotomy performed between 3 and 6 cm dilation shortens labour by 1 to 2 hours and show a trend toward reduction in the use of oxytocin and 5-minute Apgar score of less than 7. There are some pre-requisites which should be fulfilled before embarking on an amniotomy. They include:

- Vertex presentation.
- Engagement in the pelvis. If there is polyhydramnios or an unengaged presenting part, it would be prudent to perform the amniotomy in a controlled fashion in theatre settings and/or using a small-gauge needle.
- Adequate cervical dilation.
- Checking fetal heart immediately before and after the procedure.

The amniotomy can be performed using a specialized tool like an amnihook or amnicot or with just the obstetrician's fingers. With the amnihook method, a sterile plastic hook is inserted into the vagina and used to puncture the membranes containing the amniotic fluid.

48.4.2 Oxytocin

Oxytocin is a nonapeptide synthesized in the supraoptic and paraventricular nuclei of the hypothalamus. It travels from the hypothalamus to the posterior pituitary via the nerve axons. It has a half-life of 3–4 minutes and a duration of action of approximately 20 minutes. It is rapidly metabolized and degraded by oxytocinase. The route of administration is intravenous or nasal. Oxytocin receptor activation triggers a number of signalling events to stimulate contraction, primarily by elevating intracellular calcium (Ca^{2+}). This includes inositol trisphosphate-mediated calcium release, store-operated Ca^{2+} entry and voltage-operated Ca^{2+} entry. Both the activation and the inhibition of the oxytocin receptor have long been targets in the management of dysfunctional and preterm labours, respectively [7].

In the 1950s, du Vigneaud and his colleagues were awarded the Nobel Prize for their ground-breaking work on the structure of oxytocin. They manufactured an exogenous version which had better administrative control and less potential risks [8].

In the 1960s, O'Driscoll and colleagues pioneered the active management of labour (AML). The optimal goal was a vaginal delivery within 12 hours of admission. Carefully outlining the protocol, the investigators included the diagnosis of active labour, early amniotomy, high-dose oxytocin and continuous labour support. Ever since then, there have been ongoing systematic reviews, randomized controlled trials and cohort studies to find the best protocol for the active management of labour.

While no single regimen of oxytocin administration has been demonstrated to be superior in terms of clinical outcomes, one of the most fundamental principles of quality improvement is that, in general, greater practice variation is associated with poorer outcomes than more uniform practice patterns.

48.4.3 Clinical Indications for Oxytocin

The following are clinical indications for the introduction of oxytocin:

- Induction of labour
- Augmentation of labour
- Active management of third stage of labour
- Management of major obstetric haemorrhage

48.4.4 Role of Oxytocin in Specific Scenarios

Oxytocin has a role in selected cases after a review of previous caesarean section operative notes, indication, stage in labour at which caesarean was performed and patient preferences. The Royal College of Obstetricians and Gynaecologists (RCOG) recommends counselling women about 2–3 times of increased risk of scar rupture and 1.5 times of increased risk of caesarean section.

There has been an increased need for oxytocin for labour augmentation in the cohort of women with a high body mass index (BMI) [9].

A complete assessment to rule out any cephalopelvic disproportion should be completed before commencing oxytocin. Usually a senior obstetrician is to be involved in the decision making. The aim should be a cautious titration of oxytocin dose to achieve 3–4 contractions in 10 minutes. There is a high risk of uterine rupture and postpartum haemorrhage.

48.4.5 Side Effects of Oxytocin

Side effects of oxytocin include the following:

- Nausea and vomiting
- Decreased blood pressure/hyponatraemia/water intoxication
- Increased heart rate
- Subarachnoid haemorrhage
- Cardiac arrhythmias and premature ventricular contraction
- Afibrinogenaemia leading to haemorrhage and death
- Anaphylaxis

Excessive or prolonged use of oxytocin can have deleterious effects. Clinical judgement is of paramount importance to prevent prolonged oxytocin use particularly in multiparous women and women with a BMI greater than 40 and trial of labour following caesarean section. The effects can be maternal or fetal.

Maternal effects are:

- Tetanic uterine contractions
- Uterine rupture
- Postpartum haemorrhage: prolonged use can be fatal as it can lead to water intoxication
- Hyponatraemia may occur in about 25% of labours.

Fetal effects can include:

- Increased uterine contractions can lead to poor fetal outcome with pathological cardiotocography (CTG), cardiac arrhythmia, brain damage, seizures and death
- Meconium aspiration syndrome <5% cases

48.5 Evidence behind Augmentation of Labour

In the 1990s, several important large clinical trials of AML were published. The two largest showed a significant reduction in labour lasting greater than 12 hours, from 19% to 5% [10] and from 26% to 9% [11]. The results from the studies as well as from subsequent meta-analyses have reassuringly not found an association between oxytocin use and neonatal outcomes regarding Apgar scores, neonatal intensive care unit (ICU) admission, neurological abnormalities or umbilical cord gases [12].

The studies differed in the dosing regimens of oxytocin and caesarean section rates. In 2013, a Cochrane review [13] demonstrated high-dose regimens reduced the rate of caesarean sections (relative risk (RR) 0.62, 95% confidence interval (CI) 0.44–0.86) and increased vaginal birth (RR 1.35, 95% CI 1.13–1.62). The Cochrane review was based on a small number of trials, some of which were quasi-randomized. However, the most recent study, a multi-centre parallel double-blinded randomized control trial in six labour wards in Sweden, concluded there was no advantage to high-dose oxytocin over a low-dose regimen in the management of delay in labour and the authors recommend a low-dose oxytocin regimen to avoid unnecessary events of tachysystole and fetal distress [14].

The same definition of high- and low-dose oxytocin regimens was used in both the Cochrane review in 2013 and the Swedish study in 2018. In the high-dose group, the infusion started with 6.6 mU oxytocin/minute (20 mL/hour), and could be increased every 20 minutes by 6.6 mU to a maximum dose of 59.4 mU/min. In the low-dose group, the infusion started with 3.3 mU of oxytocin/min, and could be increased every 20 min by 3.3 mU to a maximum dose of 29.7 mU oxytocin/min. In both groups, the infusion was increased until adequate uterine contractions were achieved or progress of labour was established. Adequate contractions were defined as a maximum of 5 contractions in 10 minutes. Progress of labour was established with progressive dilation of the cervix and descent of the fetal head. One of the reasons for the difference in the caesarean section rates between the Cochrane review and Swedish study may be that in Sweden a longer time in labour is permitted, compared with studies from other countries where women have a caesarean section for 'failure to progress' at a much earlier time.

48.6 Use of a Checklist for Labour Augmentation

In recent decades, the airline industry has established an enviable record of safety, due, in large part, to the extensive use of a uniform, checklist-based approach to the management of certain high-risk situations. Clark et al examined the effects of implementation of a conservative uniform checklist-based system of oxytocin administration in a large, tertiary level facility.

In 2007, Clark and colleagues [15] conducted a retrospective review and data extraction examining the effects of a checklist-based protocol for oxytocin administration. The checklist was based on maternal and fetal response to oxytocin administration. The study used a pre-oxytocin checklist and an in-use checklist. The checklists revealed a 17% reduction in maximum infusion rates (13.8 mU/min vs. 11.4 mU/min) without lengthening time to delivery (8.5 hours vs. 8.2 hours), and overall caesarean delivery rate declined (15% vs. 13%). The pre-oxytocin checklist consisted of 12 points, which ensured assessment and documentation of maternal and fetal status, physical examination findings and the ability to perform a caesarean section if indicated. During oxytocin administration, an in-use checklist consisted of fetal assessment based on fetal heart monitoring and uterine assessment based on tocometer readings and palpations between contractions. The authors strongly recommend using a checklist as the appropriate way of managing oxytocin administration.

48.7 Monitoring the Progress of Labour/ Partogram

To visualize the progression of labour, the status of the cervix dilation is recorded throughout labour on a graphic curve called a partogram. The partogram is widely used internationally and facilitates the ability of midwives and doctors to monitor labour progression and, together with criteria for labour dystocia, consequently carry out necessary interventions.

The WHO recommends an active-phase partogram with a 4-hour action line. It is the basis for the diagnosis of labour dystocia and identification of need for necessary interventions. It is based on the Friedman's curve, which was first established in the 1950s and has been adapted and adopted internationally. In 2002, Zhang et al presented a new labour curve based on data from 1329 low-risk women [16]. Zhang's findings were confirmed in a large cohort of 26 838 women in 2010 [17].

Friedman's curve is a linear progression curve in which cervical dilation is expected to be 1 cm/hour, whereas the Zhang curve is a dynamic progression curve. The Labour Progression Study (LaPS) was a multicentre, cluster randomized trial involving 14 birthing units in Norway to evaluate whether Zhang's curve for labour progression made any significant difference to the number of intrapartum caesarean sections without jeopardizing maternal and fetal outcomes when compared to the traditional Friedman's curve. The results of the trial showed there was an overall reduction in the number of intrapartum caesarean sections in both groups, possibly explained by the Hawthorn effect. A better focus on labour progression and assessment is suggested to have a stronger effect on reducing the number of intrapartum caesarean sections rather than adhering to the guidelines themselves [18].

48.8 Conclusion

Prolonged labour and difficult labour are known to be important causes of perinatal mortality and morbidity. Common underlying causes include inadequate uterine contractions, abnormal fetal presentation or position, bony pelvis or soft tissue abnormalities of the mother. A less invasive intervention is to start the augmentation of labour in order to achieve adequate uterine contractions. This can lead to a reduction in major interventions such as intrapartum caesarean section for 'failure to progress'.

Appendix 48.1

Table 48.1 WHO recommendations for required observations relating to augmentation of labour

Pre-oxytocin checklist

Name of midwife
Name of consultant
Indication for admission in labour ward
Gestational age
Induction
Indication for induction
Pelvic assessment prior to starting oxytocin- seems adequate or not
Growth charts
Cervix assessment
Number of uterine contractions
CTG

30-minute observation checklist

FETAL ASSESSMENT
CTG – note any new changes
MATERNAL ASSESSMENT
Number of uterine contractions
Uterus soft in between contractions
Measurement of intrauterine pressure in Montevideo units if using pressure catheters

Post-delivery observations

Normal delivery/instrumental delivery/caesarean section

Source: [19]

References

1. O'Driscoll K, Foley M, MacDonald D. Active management of labour as an alternative to caesarean section for dystocia. *Obstet Gynecol.* 1984;**63** (4):485–90.

2. Petrie K, Larimore WL. Management of labor. In Ratcliffe SD, Baxley EG, Cline MK, Sakornbut EL, eds. *Family Medicine Obstetrics*, 3rd ed. St Louis: Mosby, 2008. pp. 382–434.

3. Dencker A, Taft C, Bergqvist L, Lilja H, Berg M. Childbirth experience questionnaire (CEQ): Development and evaluation of a multidimensional instrument. *BMC Pregnancy Childbirth* [Internet]. 2010;**10**(1):81. Available from: www.biomedcentral.com/1471-2393/10/81

4. Pang MW, Leung TN, Lau TK, Hang Chung TK. Impact of first childbirth on changes in women's preference for mode of delivery: follow-up of a longitudinal observational study. *Birth.* 2008, **35** (2):121–8.

5. Bergqvist L, Dencker A, Ladfors L, Skaring Thorse'n L, Lilja H. Labor augmentation by means of oxytocin – women's experiences. *Amer J Obstet Gynecol.*2006;**195**. 10.1016/j .ajog.2006.10.346.

6. Petrie K, Larimore WL. Management of labor abnormalities. In Ratcliffe SD, Baxley EG, Cline MK, Sakornbut EL, eds. *Family Medicine Obstetrics*, 3rd ed. St Louis: Mosby, 2008. pp. 435–53.

7. Arrowsmith S, Wray S. Oxytocin: its mechanism of action and receptor signalling in the myometrium. *J Neuroendocrinol.*2014;**26**:356–69. doi:10.1111/jne.12154

8. du Vigneaud V, Ressler C, Swan J, et al. The synthesis of an octapeptide amide with the hormonal activity of oxytocin. *J Am Chem Soc.* 1953;**75**(19):4879–80.

9. Grotedut CA, Gunatilake RP, Feng L, et al. The influence of maternal body mass index on myometrial oxytocin receptor expression in pregnancy. *Reprod Sci.* 2013; **20**(12):1471–7.

10. Lopez-Zeno JA, Peaceman AM, Adashek JA, et al. A controlled trial of a program for the active management of labor. *N Engl J Med.* 1992;**326**(7):450–4.

11. Frigoletto FD Jr, Lieberman E, Lang JM, et al. A clinical trial of active management of labor. *N Engl J Med.* 1995;**333**(12):745–50.

12. Fraser W, Vendittelli F, Krauss I, et al. Effects of early augmentation of labour with amniotomy and oxytocin in nulliparous women: a meta-analysis. *Br J Obstet Gynaecol.* 1998;**105**(2):189–94.

13. Kenyon S, Tokumasu H, Dowswell T, et al. High-dose versus low-dose oxytocin for augmentation of delayed labour. *Cochrane Database Syst Rev* 2013;(7):CD007201.

14. Selin L, Wennerholm UB, Jonsson M, et al. High-dose versus low dose of oxytocin for labour augmentation: a randomised controlled trial. *Women Birth.* 2019;**32**(4):356–63.

15. Clark S, Belfort M, Saade G, et al. Implementation of a conservative checklist-based protocol for oxytocin administration: maternal and newborn outcomes. *Am J Obstet Gynecol.* 2007;**197**(5):480.e1-5.

16. Zhang J, Troendle JF, Yancey MK. Reassessing the labour curve in nulliparous women. *Am J Obstet Gynecol.* 2002;**187**(4):824–8.

17. Zhang J, Landy HJ, Branch DW, et al. Contemporary patterns of spontaneous labor with normal neonatal outcomes. *Obstet Gynecol.* 2010;**116**(6):1281–7.

18. Bernitz S, Dalbye R, Ahang J, et al. The frequency of intrapartum caesarean section use with the WHO partograph versus Zhang's guideline in the Labour Progression Study (LaPS): a multicentre, cluster-randomised controlled trial. *Lancet.* 2019;**393**:340–8.

19. WHO Recommendations for Augmentation of Labour. Geneva: WHO; 2014. https://apps.who.int/iris/ bitstream/handle/10665/112825/97892 41507363_eng.pdf;jsessionid=6E74F60 E7DA3BB10602DDC3561AA6F68? sequence=1

Chapter 49

Analgesia and Anaesthesia during Labour

Britt Ingjerd Nesheim

Childbirth is painful. During the first stage of labour, pain originates in the uterus and cervix. It is caused by ischaemia during contractions and traction on tissue fibres during distention of the cervix. Visceral sensory nerve fibres traverse into the pelvic plexus, and from there to the spinal cord at the level of T10 to L1. During the second stage, pain originates from distention of the vagina, perineum and the pelvic floor. The pudendal nerve transmits the pain signals to the spinal cord at the level of S2–S4.

Labour pain is described as abdominal contraction pain, but also includes low back pain. The low back pain may be intermittent with the contractions or continuous. Pain may also spread to the thighs and buttocks.

Pain is perceived differently. While some women are able to cope, others may feel a total loss of control. Unrelieved pain may contribute to postpartum depression, and even to post-traumatic stress syndrome symptoms.

Hyperventilation during painful contractions may lead to a low PCO_2, and to acute respiratory alkalosis. This causes a left-shift of the oxyhaemoglobin dissociation curve, and thus less release of oxygen to peripheral tissues – and the placenta. Hyperventilation during contractions may also lead to hypoxia due to a reduced respiratory drive between contractions [1]. Blood flow through the uterus to the placenta is normally inhibited during contractions [2]. A healthy fetus is able to tolerate this reduced oxygenation, but for a fetus already somewhat compromised from placental insufficiency, the reduced availability of oxygen between contractions might lead to fetal hypoxia and distress.

For the labouring woman, perceived control of the decision-making process correlates with greater satisfaction with labour, regardless of the degree of pain. Preparation for labour should include education of the stages and progress of labour, the pain that can be expected and the options for pain relief.

Local anaesthetics provide the most efficient pain relief. It is also the most resource-intensive method of analgesia in labour. Neuraxial analgesia, paracervical block and pudendal block will be described here.

In surroundings with fewer resources, or for the parturient who prefers less invasive pain relief, other methods – pharmacological and non-pharmacological – are available.

49.1 Neuraxial Analgesia

The use of continuous caudal analgesia for labour pain was first described in 1943 [3]. Since then, neuraxial analgesia has been used on an increasing scale, and is now the most commonly used method for pain relief during labour (Figure 49.1).

Neuraxial analgesia is the most efficient method of pain relief in labour. As a result of the relief of pain, there is less alteration in acid-base status during the first stage of labour compared to women managed conventionally [4].

Epidural, spinal and combined epidural-spinal are all techniques that are used. The local anaesthetic may be given as one shot, in pulses or continually through a catheter. During the last several years, a mixture of local anaesthetic and opioid has been used, which allows the dosage of local anaesthetic to be reduced and the patient to be able to move around. The opioids used are usually fentanyl or sufentanyl. Neuraxial analgesia is administrated by an anaesthesiologist. For an overview of neuraxial analgesia and a detailed description of techniques and references, see [5].

The indication for instituting analgesia is the woman's wish for pain relief and her consent to neuraxial analgesia. Neuraxial analgesia may be started at any stage during labour, regardless of cervical dilation, fetal descent or parity. The technique used should be individualized, taking the estimated time to delivery and the woman's needs into account.

There are few contraindications. Relative contraindications are coagulopathy, infection of the lower back and increased intracranial pressure due to an intracranial lesion.

49.1.1 Adverse Effects

For a full description of all possible adverse effects, see [6].

49.1.1.1 Hypotension

Epidural analgesia causes a sympathetic block in the lower extremities, leading to vasodilation. This may cause hypotension. The hypotension can be counteracted by fluid infusion. Therefore, it is obligatory that an intravenous line is established. The incidence of hypotension is reported as 12 – 27%. There is no difference in the incidence of hypotension between combined spinal epidural versus low dose or traditional epidural [7].

49.1.1.2 Headache

Post dural puncture headache is caused by leakage of cerebrospinal fluid through the punctured dura. This may be caused by accidental puncture during a traditional epidural or in conjunction with a combined spinal-epidural. The risk of accidental dural puncture is approximately 1.5%, and about half of these patients develop headache. The risk of developing headache after puncture with a spinal needle is 1.7%. The headache can occur from 1 to 7 days after the puncture and

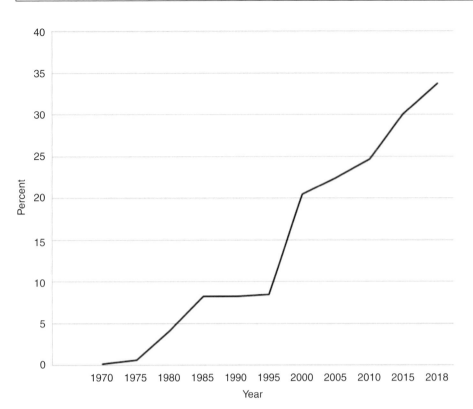

Figure 49.1 Epidural analgesia 1970–2018.
Percentage of vaginal births.
Data from The Medical Birth Registry of Norway,
comprising 3 008 781 births.

will last from 12 hours to 7 days [8]. Severe post dural puncture headache may be treated by administering a blood patch placed in the epidural space.

49.1.1.3 Pruritus

Pruritus is a rather common side effect of the administration of opioids in the epidural or spinal space. The pruritus is mostly located on the legs, the abdomen and thorax. The pruritus is not caused by the release of histamine, and antihistamines are not useful. Opioid antagonists may be useful. A systematic review concluded that naloxone, naltrexone, nalbuphine and droperidol were efficacious in the prevention of opioid-induced pruritus [9].

49.1.1.4 Fever

There is a frequent association between neuraxial analgesia and temperature rise. The aetiology is incompletely understood [10]. Neuraxial analgesia blocks both the adrenergic nerves regulating vasoconstriction and the cholinergic nerves regulating sweating. These changes might lead either to a loss of temperature or a temperature increase, dependent on the ambient temperature. At room temperature, the muscle work of labour might well lead to an increase in temperature.

Another possible explanation is a sterile inflammatory response in the epidural space, followed by secondary placental inflammation. This is reflected in an increased IL-6 level. There is no proven safe and effective method for preventing neuraxial analgesia/anaesthesia-related temperature elevation.

49.1.1.5 Urinary Retention

Urinary retention might be a side effect of neuraxial analgesia, although it is also not uncommon after labour in women who have not had this type of analgesia. Neuraxial analgesia might cause

a decreased ability to sense a full bladder. The possibility of an overfilled bladder should always be kept in mind and checked for.

49.1.2 Possible Effects on Labour

There has been much discussion about the possible effects of neuraxial analgesia on labour: on duration, a possible increase in caesarean sections and in assisted vaginal delivery. Observational studies are biased, because of the tendency to provide neuraxial analgesia for women who are considered to be at greater risk for a prolonged labour, have more pain early on in labour, and for women who are particularly anxious of childbirth. There are also problems in the interpretation of prospective randomized studies. Women who agree to be randomly assigned to either epidural or another form of anaesthesia, or perhaps no anaesthesia during labour, may represent a subgroup of women with less difficult labours or other characteristics that render them unrepresentative of the general population. There may also be a crossover in the groups, e.g. for women with very rapid labours, there is no time to administer an epidural.

49.1.2.1 Duration of Labour

A systematic review of controlled trials comparing epidural analgesia to systemic opioids or no analgesia concluded that both first and second stages of labour were shorter for the women who received opioids than for the women who received an epidural (mean difference 32.28 minutes, 95% confidence interval (CI) 18.34–46.22). Heterogeneity was particularly high for the second stage where three trials appeared to favour epidural [11]. A lower concentration of local anaesthetics, as is used at present, may lower this difference [6]. There seems to be no difference in the rate of oxytocin stimulation.

49.1.2.2 Assisted Vaginal Deliveries

Earlier studies have suggested an increased incidence in assisted vaginal deliveries in women who have neuraxial analgesia. However, when studies conducted after 2005 are analyzed separately, this observation is negated [11].

49.1.2.3 Caesarean Section

There is no difference in the rate of caesarean deliveries [6, 11].

49.2 Paracervical Nerve Block

Paracervical nerve block for labour pain was first described in 1945 [12]. Since then, the method has been refined by the use of a specially constructed guard-tube and needle. The needle does not protrude more than 7 mm from the guard-tube.

The afferent nerve fibres transmitting pain from the uterus to the spinal cord are located close to the cervix and the lateral ligament. They are easily accessed from the vaginal fornix.

Before administering a paracervical nerve block, the cervical dilation has to be at least 4 cm. A local anaesthetic is injected at two to six positions around the cervix. When two positions are used, it is usually at the three o'clock and nine o'clock positions, but this is not essential. A local anaesthetic with or without adrenaline may be used. As the uterine artery and vein are located very close to the nerve bundle, it is important to ascertain that there is no intravascular injection of the local anaesthetic.

The effect is almost immediate, and will last for 2 to 3 hours. A systematic review in 2012 concluded that local anaesthetic nerve blocks were more effective than placebo, opioid and non-opioid analgesia for pain management in labour based on randomized controlled trials of unclear quality and limited numbers [13].

There has been concern about fetal bradycardia associated with paracervical block, although the incidence was low (around 3%) and the bradycardia almost always transient [14]. At present, the method has gone very much out of use.

49.3 Pudendal Block

Pudendal block can be used to alleviate pain in the second stage of delivery. The lower vagina, vulva and perineum are innervated by the pudendal nerve, which conveys the afferent stimuli to S2, S3 and S4. The nerve is in proximity to the sacrospinous ligament where the ligament attaches to the ischial spine. Infiltration of these points with a local anaesthetic results in analgesia of the lower vagina, vulva and perineum. It does not influence contraction pain. A transvaginal approach is mostly used, but the pudendal nerve can also be reached from the perineum. For a more detailed description of the technique, see [15].

49.4 Pharmacological Methods of Pain Relief

49.4.1 Opioids

Opioids have been widely used as labour analgesia – a tradition going back to a time when evidence-based medicine was not established. In many settings they are administered by the midwife, without consulting a physician. A 2018 Cochrane review concluded that parenteral opioids provided only moderate or poor pain relief. The evidence was graded as low quality or very low quality regarding the analgesic effect of opioids [16]. The effect is more sedating rather than analgesic. Side effects include nausea, vomiting, and obstipation. Opioids may be administered by the intermittent bolus technique or by patient-controlled analgesia (PCA). In PCA, the drug is administered by the parturient herself in pre-set doses with minimum intervals.

Pethidine (meperidine) is a synthetic opioid, acting as an agonist on the μ-opioid receptor. It may be administered as subcutaneous, intramuscular or intravenous injections. It has been widely used during labour, but its popularity is decreasing. Pethidine is highly lipid soluble, and penetrates cell membranes quickly, including the placenta. It has a half-life of 2.5–5 hours. It is partly metabolized to norpethidine, which has convulsant and hallucinogenic effects, and a half-life of 8–12 hours. Plasma concentration in the infant is highest 1–4 hours after administration. Estimated time to delivery should therefore be taken into account when pethidine is administered. There may be a flattened cardiotocographic (CTG) pattern, due to less variations in the heart rate. Pethidine makes the infant drowsy, and sucking at the breast is inhibited. There may also be respiratory depression and a lower threshold for convulsions. The morphine antagonist naloxone should always be present when pethidine is used. Norpethidine is, however, not reversed by naloxone [17].

Remifentanil is a short-acting μ-opioid receptor agonist. It has a half-life of 4 minutes. In contrast to pethidine, it is metabolized by non-specific tissue and plasma esterases. Its metabolite has a very low potency. After intravenous injection, there is onset of the effect within 60 seconds, and maximum effect after 2.5 minutes. Placenta passage is rapid, but it is also rapidly metabolized in the fetus. When used as PCA, it will have effect on contraction pain if it is started at the beginning of the contraction. The main side effect is respiratory depression. Intense itching, especially in the face, is another – although less serious – side effect. A meta-analysis from 2012 concluded that remifentanil-PCA was superior to pethidine in providing analgesia and in patient satisfaction, with a comparable degree of adverse events [18]. There are case reports of respiratory and/or cardiac arrests connected to remifentanil in labour. The popularity of its use may be discussed, especially in light of its modest effects on pain relief [19].

Fentanyl is mainly a μ-opioid receptor agonist. It has a half-life of 3–4 hours, and no active metabolites. There are few studies comparing fentanyl to other opioids. It has been shown to provide either more effective analgesia or fewer side effects than morphine, pethidine or alfentanil when given as PCA [20]. Subcutaneous or intranasal fentanyl has been compared with intramuscular pethidine and been shown to be as efficacious in relieving labour pain, but with greater patient satisfaction [21].

49.4.2 Inhaled Analgesia

The inhalation of a subanaesthetic concentration of gases while the mother remains awake has been used to ease labour pain since the middle of the nineteenth century [22]. Only nitrous oxide is widely used in modern obstetric practice. Nitrous oxide (N_2O) is a colourless, non-flammable gas. It is usually delivered as a blend of 50% N_2O and 50% O_2 through a handheld mask, administered by the parturient herself. It has an onset time of approximately 30–60 seconds, and the inhalation should therefore be started at the beginning of a contraction, to achieve maximal effect at the top of the contraction. At this point, the patient is usually so sedated that she loses her hold on the mask, and the effect will wear off when the contraction is over. The gas is eliminated between contractions and does not accumulate. Nitrous oxide does not affect the contractions.

Although nitrous oxide is widely used, there are few studies of good quality addressing its effectiveness [23]. Nitrous oxide seems to have fairly good effect in most patients, but it does not provide complete analgesia [20, 22]. Side effects are nausea and drowsiness. It is not known whether nitrous oxide has any effect on the infant brain.

The use of nitrous oxide is controversial, due to concerns about the health of the personnel working in the delivery ward. Subfecundability and an increased incidence of spontaneous abortions among female staff have been shown. Therefore, many countries have standards as to the concentration of the gas in the air of the delivery ward, and the number of hours personnel should be working in surroundings where nitrous oxide is in use. The concentration of gas in the ambient air can be substantially reduced by using closed systems with gas scavengers, and by good ventilation [22]. Because of these problems, and because of the increasing accessibility of neuraxial analgesia, nitrous oxide has gone out of use in many hospitals.

49.5 Non-pharmacological Methods of Pain Relief

Non-pharmacological methods of pain relief have been classified according to the resources required [24].

- Low-resource interventions include movement, relaxation, breathing techniques, support from a companion or doula, stroking, application of heat or cold, showers, use of a birth ball, music.
- Moderate-resource interventions include aromatherapy, acupuncture/acupressure, sterile water injections, yoga, hypnosis, transcutaneous electrical nerve stimulation (TENS), biofeedback, water immersion.

There are few and small studies concerning the effects of several of the low-resource interventions, but support, care and a sense of safety will doubtlessly give the woman a better birth experience.

49.5.1 Movement

A review studying movement during the first stage of labour [25] concluded that walking and upright positions reduced the duration of the first stage, the risk of caesarean birth and the need for an epidural.

49.5.2 Relaxation and Breathing Techniques

There is low-quality evidence suggesting that relaxation may lead to greater satisfaction with pain relief, but without any difference in pain intensity [26]. Relaxation is usually combined with breathing techniques, where the woman concentrates on slow and controlled breathing during contractions. While this may help to give a feeling of control, there is little evidence as to its effect on pain perception.

49.5.3 Aromatherapy

Aromatherapy involves application of concentrated essential oils or essences. A systematic review concluded that there is insufficient evidence from randomized controlled trials about the benefits of aromatherapy on pain management in labour [27].

49.5.4 Acupuncture/Acupressure

Acupuncture involves inserting fine needles at specific points; acupressure involves exerting pressure on specified trigger points. Originating in traditional Chinese medicine, where it was thought that body energy was flowing through channels called meridians, acupuncture and acupressure points lie along these meridians. While the explanation of a possible effect of these methods is difficult to support with Western science, there is a possibility that the stimulation of the nervous system by acupuncture/acupressure through afferent nerves might modulate the perception of pain through the gating theory of pain [28]. There might also be an endorphin release. A systematic review from 2011 concluded that while it may be suggested that acupuncture and acupressure may give some pain relief, it cannot be safely concluded that the effect is different from that of placebo [29]. The points used in the different studies have varied. There are no known risks when acupuncture is practised by trained personnel.

49.5.5 Sterile Water Injections

Sterile water injections are used to relieve back pain. They can be placed intracutaneously or subcutaneously. Four injections of 0.05 to 0.1 mL of sterile water are placed in the lower back. The injections are painful, and the pain lasts for 1 or 2 minutes. The theory is that this would trigger an endorphin release. Alternatively, it is explained by the gating theory, where the somatic component of pain reduces the visceral component. A systematic review in 2012 concluded that there was little robust evidence that sterile water is effective for low back or any other labour pain [30].

49.5.6 Transcutaneous Nerve Stimulation (TENS)

Transcutaneous nerve stimulation (TENS) is applied using a device that emits a low-voltage current in pulses. The strength of the current can be manipulated by the parturient herself, or by a companion. It is usually applied to the low back, but may also be applied to acupuncture points and also directly to the head. The mechanism of action would be the same as for acupuncture and sterile water injections. A systematic review updated in 2009 [31] concluded that pain scores were similar in women using TENS and in control groups. There was some evidence that the women using TENS were less likely to describe their pain as severe, and many women stated that they were likely to use TENS again in their next labour. There were no effects on the length of labour, interventions or well-being of the mother and baby.

49.5.7 Immersion in Water

Immersion in water is popular, perhaps especially in settings of midwife-led births. The woman may be immersed in water during the first stage only, or again during the second stage. All published trials have taken place in hospital ward settings. The interpretation of the trials is difficult, because the

intervention cannot be blinded. A systematic review from 2018 [32] concluded that there might be a small reduction in the risk of using regional analgesia for women allocated to water immersion during the first stage of labour from 43% to 39%. There is probably no difference in the risk of instrumental vaginal delivery and caesarean section.

49.5.8 Biofeedback

Biofeedback is taught in some prenatal classes and aims to enable women to observe signals from their body in order to control the responses. A review to see whether biofeedback, as taught in prenatal classes, would have an effect in relieving pain during labour concluded that there is no evidence that this is an effective approach for the management of pain during labour [33].

References

1. Reed PN, Colquhoun AD, Hanning CD. Maternal oxygenation during normal labour. *Br J Anaesth.* 1989;**62**:316–18.
2. Janbu T, Koss KS, Nesheim BI, Wesche J. Blood velocities in the uterine artery in humans during labour. *Acta Physiol Scand.* 1985;**124**:153–61.
3. Hingson RA, Edwards WB. Continuous caudal analgesia in obstetrics. *JAMA.* 1943;**121**(4):225–9.
4. Pearson JF, Davies P. The effect of continuous lumbar epidural analgesia on the acid-base status of maternal arteial blood during the first stage of labour. *BJOG.* 1973;**80**:218–24.
5. Toledano R d'A. Neuraxial analgesia for labor and delivery (including instrumented delivery). In Hepner, DL, ed. *UpToDate.* Waltham, MA: UpToDate Inc.; [cited 2019 July 26]. www.uptodate.com/contents/neuraxial-analgesia-for-labor-and-delivery-including-instrumented-delivery?search=labor%20analgesia&source=search_result&selectedTitle=1~60&usage_type=default&display_rank=1.
6. Grant GJ. Adverse effects of neuraxial analgesia and anesthesia for obstetrics. In Hepner, DL, ed. *UpToDate.* Waltham, MA: UpToDate Inc.; [cited 2019 July 09]. www.uptodate.com/contents/adverse-effects-of-neuraxial-analgesia-and-anesthesia-for-obstetrics?search=labor+analgesia&topicRef=101803&source=related_link.
7. Simmons SW, Taghizadeh N, Dennis AT, Hughes D, Cyna AM. Combined spinal-epidural versus epidural analgesia in labour. *Cochrane Database Syst Rev.* 2012 Oct 17; (10): CD003401.

8. Choi PT, Galinski SE, Takeuchi L, et al. PDPH is a common complication of neuraxial blockade in parturients: a meta-analysis of obstetrical studies. *Can J Anaesth.* 2003;**50**(5):460–9.
9. Kjellberg F, Tramèr MR. Pharmacological control of opioid-induced pruritus: a quantitative systematic review of randomized trials. *Eur J Anaesthesiol* 2001;**18**(6):346–57.
10. Chen CT. Intrapartum fever. In Berghella, V, Hepner DL, eds. *UpToDate.* Waltham, MA: UpToDate Inc.; [cited 2019 July 10]. www.uptodate.com/contents/intrapartum-fever?search=labor+analgesia&topicRef=4469&source=see_link#H483714642.
11. Anim-Somuah M, Smyth RMD, Cyna AM, Cuthbert A. Epidural versus non-epidural or no analgesia for pain management in labour. *Cochrane Database Syst Rev.* 2018 May 21;(5): CD000331.
12. Rosenfeld SS. Paracervical anesthesia for the relief of labor pains. *Am J Obstet Gynecol.* 1945;**50**(5):527–32.
13. Novikova N, Cluver C. Local anaesthetic nerve block for pain management in labour. *Cochrane Database Syst Rev.* 2012 Apr 18;(4): CD009200.
14. Palomäki O, Huhtala H, Kirkinen P. A comparative study of the safety of 0.25% levobupivacaine and 0.25% racemic bupivacaine for paracervical block in the first stage of labor. *Acta Obstet Gynecol Scand.* 2005;**84**(10):956–61.
15. Vidaeff AC. Pudendal and paracervical block. In Berghella, V, Hepner DL, eds. *UpToDate.* Waltham, MA: UpToDate Inc.; [cited 2019 July 10]. www

.uptodate.com/contents/pudendal-and-paracervical-block?search=paracervical%20block&source=search_result&selectedTitle=1~39&usage_type=default&display_rank=1.
16. Smith LA, Burns E, Cuthbert A. Parenteral opioids for maternal pain management in labour. *Cochrane Database Syst Rev.* 2018 Jun;(6): CD007396.
17. Cowan A, Geller EB, Adler MW. Classification of opioids on the basis of change in seizure threshold in rats. *Science.* 1979;**206**(4417):465–7.
18. Schnabel A, Hahn N, Broscheit J, et al. Remifentanil for labour analgesia: a meta-analysis of randomised controlled trials. *Eur J Anaesthesiol.* 2012;**29**(4):177–85.
19. Muchatuta NA, Kinsella SM. Remifentanil for labour analgesia: time to draw breath? *Anaesthesia.* 2013;**68**(3):231–5.
20. Grant GJ. Pharmacologic management of pain during labor and delivery. In Hepner DL, Berghella V, eds. *UpToDate.* Waltham, MA: UpToDate Inc.; [cited 2019 June 26]. www.uptodate.com/contents/pharmacologic-management-of-pain-during-labor-and-delivery?search=labor%20analgesia&source=search_result&selec.
21. Fleet J, Belan I, Jones M, Ullah S, Cyna A. A comparison of fentanyl with pethidine for pain relief during childbirth: a randomised controlled trial. *BJOG.* 2015;**122**(7):983–92.
22. Klomp T, van Poppel M, Jones L, et al. Inhaled analgesia for pain management in labour. *Cochrane Database Syst Rev.* 2012 Sep 12;(9): CD009351.

23. Likis FE, Andrews JC, Collins MR, et al. Nitrous oxide for the management of labor pain: a systematic review. *Anesthesia Analgesia*. 2014;**118**(1):153–67.

24. Simkin P, Klein MC. Nonpharmacologic approaches to management of labor pain. In Lockwood CJ. ed. *UptoDate*. Waltham, MA: UpToDate Inc.; [cited 2019 June 27]. www.uptodate.com/contents/nonpharmacologic-approaches-to-management-of-labor-pain?search=labor%20analgesia&topicRef=4468&source=see_link.

25. Lawrence A, Lewis L, Hofmeyr GJ, Styles C. Maternal positions and mobility during first stage labour. *Cochrane Database Syst Rev*. 2013 Oct 9;(10): CD003934.

26. Smith CA, Levett KM, Collins CT, et al. Relaxation techniques for pain management in labour. *Cochrane Database Syst Rev*. 2018 Mar 28;(3): CD009514.

27. Smith CA, Collins CT, Crowther CA. Aromatherapy for pain management in labour. *Cochrane Database Syst Rev*. 2011 Jul 6;(7): CD009215.

28. Melzack R. Myofascial trigger points: relation to acupuncture and mechanisms of pain. *Arch Phys Med Rehab*. 1981;**62**(3): 114–17.

29. Smith CA, Collins CT, Crowther CA, Levett KM. Acupuncture or acupressure for pain management in labour. *Cochrane Database Syst Rev*. 2011 Jul 6;(7):CD009232.

30. Derry S, Straube S, Moore RA, Hancock H, Collins SL. Intracutaneous or subcutaneous sterile water injection compared with blinded controls for pain management in labour. *Cochrane Database Syst Rev*. 2012 Jan;(1).

31. Dowswell T, Bedwell C, Lavender T, Neilson JP. Transcutaneous electrical nerve stimulation (TENS) for pain management in labour. *Cochrane Database Syst Rev*. 2009 Apr 15;(2): CD007214.

32. Cluett ER, Burns E, Cuthbert A. Immersion in water during labour and birth. *Cochrane Database Syst Rev*. 2018 May;(5):CD000111.

33. Barragán Loayza IM, Solà I, Juandó Prats C. Biofeedback for pain management during labour. *Cochrane Database Syst Rev*. 2011 Jun 15;(6): CD006168.

Chapter 50

Preterm Labour

William C. Maina

50.1 Introduction

Preterm birth represents the single largest cause of morbidity and mortality for newborns and a major cause of morbidity for pregnant women. It affects about 9% of births in high-income countries and an estimated 13% of births in low- and middle-income countries. Babies born preterm have high rates of early, late and post-neonatal mortality, and the risk of mortality increases as gestational age at birth decreases. Babies who survive have increased rates of disability.

The major long-term consequence of prematurity is neurodevelopmental disability. Although the risk for the individual child is greatest for those born at the earliest gestational ages, the global burden of neurodevelopmental disabilities depends on the number of babies born at each of these gestations, and so is greatest for babies born between 32 and 36 weeks, less for those born between 28 and 31 weeks, and least for those born at less than 28 weeks' gestation [1].

50.2 Definition of Terms Used

- Preterm labour – onset of labour before 37+0 weeks of pregnancy
- Planned preterm labour – labour induced before 37+0 weeks of pregnancy
- Symptoms of preterm labour – a woman has presented before 37+0 weeks of pregnancy reporting symptoms that might be indicative of preterm labour (such as abdominal pain), but no clinical assessment (including speculum or digital vaginal examination) has taken place.
- Suspected preterm labour – a woman is in suspected preterm labour if she has reported symptoms of preterm labour and has had a clinical assessment (including a speculum or digital vaginal examination) that confirms the possibility of preterm labour but rules out established labour.
- Diagnosed preterm labour – a woman is in diagnosed preterm labour if she is in suspected preterm labour and has had a positive diagnostic test for preterm labour.
- Established preterm labour – a woman is in established preterm labour if she has progressive cervical dilation from 4 cm with regular contractions.
- 'Rescue' cervical cerclage – cervical cerclage performed as an emergency procedure in a woman with premature cervical dilation and often with exposed fetal membranes.
- ACTIM® Partus – a fast and reliable point-of-care test to identify women at real risk of preterm delivery.

50.3 Aetiology of Preterm Labour

The causes of preterm labour are poorly understood and identifying a cause may not be possible. Up to 40% of preterm deliveries before 32 weeks of gestation are associated with infection [2, 3]. Risk factors for preterm labour are listed in Table 50.1.

Labour, whether term or preterm, involves the synchronization of myometrial activity and structural changes in the cervix. The biochemical events involved in labour resemble an inflammatory reaction in which pro-inflammatory cytokines and prostaglandins play a crucial role. There are several mechanisms by which term or preterm labour may be initiated. Current treatment strategies aim to suppress these mechanisms. A detailed discussion of these mechanisms can be found in the review by Gibbs and Challis [4].

50.4 General Principles of Management

Women at increased risk of preterm labour, with suspected, diagnosed or established preterm labour, or having a planned preterm birth may be particularly anxious and should be provided both oral and written information describing signs and

Table 50.1 Risk factors for preterm labour

Maternal	Fetal
Infection (genital tract or extra-genital tract)	Fetal abnormalities
Preterm prelabour rupture of membranes	Multiple pregnancy
History of previous preterm birth	Intrauterine fetal death
Significant polyhydramnios	
Placental abruption	
Uterine anomalies	
Cervical incompetence	
Medical complications of pregnancy	
Smoking and other substance misuse	
Short inter-pregnancy interval	
Low body mass index	
Other risks	

symptoms of preterm labour and the care they may be offered. This should include:

- the likelihood of the baby surviving and other outcomes (including long-term outcomes) and risks for the baby;
- explaining the neonatal care of preterm babies, including location of care;
- explaining the immediate problems that can arise when a baby is born preterm; and
- explaining the possible long-term consequences of prematurity for the baby.

Women and families should be offered:

- ongoing opportunities to talk about and state their wishes about resuscitation of the baby;
- an opportunity to tour the neonatal unit; and
- an opportunity to speak to a member of the neonatal team.

50.5 Diagnosing Preterm Labour in Women with Intact Membranes

Explain to women reporting symptoms of preterm labour who have intact membranes about the clinical assessment and diagnostic tests that are available. Explain how the clinical assessment and diagnostic tests are carried out and what the benefits, risks and possible consequences of the clinical assessment and diagnostic tests are, including the consequences of false positive and false negative test results.

Offer a clinical assessment to women reporting symptoms of preterm labour who have intact membranes. This should include:

- clinical history taking;
- the observations for the initial assessment of a woman in labour; and
- a speculum examination (followed by a digital vaginal examination if the extent of cervical dilation cannot be assessed).

If the clinical assessment suggests that the woman is in suspected preterm labour and she is 29+6 weeks pregnant or less, advise treatment for preterm labour. If the clinical assessment suggests that the woman is in suspected preterm labour and she is 30+0 weeks pregnant or more, consider transvaginal ultrasound measurement (TVUS) of cervical length as a diagnostic test to determine likelihood of birth within 48 hours [5, 6].

Transvaginal ultrasound measurement of cervical length should be performed by healthcare professionals with training in, and experience of, TVUS of cervical length. Act on the results as follows:

- If cervical length is more than 15 mm, explain to the woman that it is unlikely that she is in preterm labour. Consider alternative diagnoses and discuss with her the benefits and risks of going home compared with continued monitoring and treatment in hospital. Advise her that if she does decide to go home, she should return if symptoms suggestive of preterm labour persist or recur.
- If cervical length is 15 mm or less, view the woman as being in diagnosed preterm labour and offer treatment.

If TVUS of cervical length is not possible, consider ACTIM® Partus testing as a screening test to determine likelihood of birth within 7 days for women who are 30+0 weeks pregnant. Be aware that ACTIM® Partus has a low positive predictive value and make women aware of this before undertaking the test. Use of ACTIM® Partus is likely to result in over-intervention.

Act on the results as follows:

- If ACTIM® Partus is negative, explain to the woman that it is unlikely that she is in preterm labour (98% negative predictive value) and think about alternative diagnoses.
- Discuss with her the benefits and risks of going home compared with continued monitoring and treatment in hospital. Advise her that if she does decide to go home, she should return if symptoms suggestive of preterm labour persist or recur.

If a woman in suspected preterm labour who is 30+0 weeks pregnant or more does not have TVUS of cervical length or ACTIM® Partus testing to exclude preterm labour, offer treatment for preterm labour. Women in established preterm labour should not have ACTIM® Partus testing.

Maternity units should have standard operating procedures for performing ACTIM® Partus testing.

50.6 Treatments Options for Diagnosed Preterm Labour

Treatment options for diagnosed preterm labour are shown in Figure 50.1.

50.6.1 Tocolysis

Tocolytic agents include a wide range of drugs that can inhibit labour to prolong pregnancy and potentially improve fetal outcome. Widely used agents include calcium channel blockers such as nifedipine and oxytocin antagonists such as atosiban. Limitations of tocolytic therapy include lack of clear benefit for neonatal health from the various systematic reviews published in the Cochrane Library and maternal side effects.

Consider tocolysis for women between 24+0 and 33+6 weeks of pregnancy with suspected or diagnosed preterm labour. Take the following factors into account when deciding about whether to start tocolysis:

- whether the woman is in suspected or diagnosed preterm labour;
- clinical features, such as bleeding or infection, which may suggest that stopping labour is contraindicated;
- gestational age at presentation;
- likely benefit of maternal corticosteroids, availability of neonatal care and possible need for transfer to another unit;
- local guidelines; and
- the preference of the woman.

50.6.2 Corticosteroids

Respiratory morbidity including respiratory distress syndrome (RDS) is a serious complication of preterm birth and the primary cause of early neonatal mortality and morbidity.

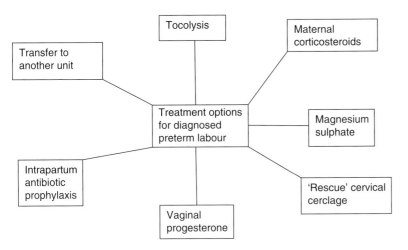

Figure 50.1 Treatment options for diagnosed preterm labour

While researching the effects of the steroid dexamethasone in premature parturition in fetal sheep in 1969, Liggins found that there was some inflation of the lungs of lambs born at gestations at which the lungs would be expected to be airless. Liggins and Howie published the first randomized controlled trial in humans in 1972 and many others followed.

50.6.2.1 Single Course of Prenatal Corticosteroids

In a recent systematic review [7] (339 studies, 7774 women and 8158 infants), treatment with antenatal corticosteroids, compared with placebo or no treatment, is associated with a reduction in the most serious adverse outcomes related to prematurity, as shown in Box 50.1.

When offering or considering maternal corticosteroids for women in diagnosed, suspected or established preterm labour or preterm prelabour rupture of membranes (PPROM) or those having planned preterm birth, discuss with the woman:

- how corticosteroids may help; and
- the potential risks associated with them.

Between 23+0 and 23+6 weeks, discuss the use of maternal corticosteroids in the context of her individual circumstances. Between 24+0 and 25+6 weeks, consider the use of maternal corticosteroids. Between 26+0 and 33+6 weeks, offer maternal corticosteroids. Between 34+0 and 35+6 weeks, consider the

use of maternal corticosteroids, particularly if delivery by caesarean section is planned or likely.

Administer 2 doses of either dexamethasone or betamethasone 12 milligrams intramuscularly 24 hours apart. Reassure the woman that a single course of corticosteroids is safe for her and her baby. Both steroids have very high glucocorticoid activity and insignificant mineralocorticoid activity, and readily cross the placenta. Recommend admission for women with diabetes in pregnancy for control of blood glucose with intravenous insulin. Advise close monitoring in women with fluid retention.

50.6.2.2 Repeat Courses of Prenatal Corticosteroids

In a systematic review in 2015 [8], the authors concluded that the short-term benefits for babies of less respiratory distress and fewer serious health problems in the first few weeks after birth support the use of repeat dose(s) of prenatal corticosteroids for women still at risk of preterm birth 7 days or more after an initial course. These benefits were associated with a small reduction in size at birth. The current available evidence reassuringly shows no significant harm in early childhood, although no benefit. In women, for the two primary outcomes, there was no increase in infectious morbidity of chorioamnionitis or puerperal sepsis, and the likelihood of a caesarean birth was unchanged.

Do not routinely offer repeat courses of maternal corticosteroids; consider the interval since the end of the last course, gestational age and the likelihood of birth within 48 hours.

50.6.3 Magnesium Sulphate

Antenatal magnesium sulphate therapy given to women at risk of preterm labour significantly reduces the risk of their infant developing cerebral palsy (risk ratio (RR) 0.68, 95% confidence interval (CI) 0.54–0.87; five trials, 6145 infants) and also significantly reduces the rate of gross motor dysfunction (RR 0.61, 95% CI 0.44–0.85) [9].

There is continuing debate on the gestational age at which magnesium sulphate has the greatest benefit. The number needed to treat to prevent cerebral palsy or severe motor dysfunction increases significantly with increasing gestational age. The number needed to treat at less than 30 weeks was 46 and rose to 56 at less than 32–34 weeks of gestation [10].

> **Box 50.1 Serious Adverse Outcomes Related to Prematurity That Are Improved by a Single Course of Maternal Corticosteroids**
>
> Perinatal death
>
> Neonatal death
>
> Respiratory distress syndrome
>
> Intraventricular haemorrhage
>
> Necrotizing colitis
>
> Need for mechanical ventilation
>
> Systemic infections in the first 48 hours of life

When early preterm birth is planned, commence magnesium sulphate as close to 4 hours before birth as possible. If delivery is anticipated to occur sooner than 4 hours, there continues to be some advantage from administration of magnesium sulphate; therefore, it should be given.

Between 24+0 and 29+6 weeks, offer magnesium sulphate to women in established preterm labour or having a planned preterm birth within 24 hours. Between 30+0 and 33+6 weeks, consider the use of magnesium sulphate for women in established preterm labour or having a planned preterm birth within 24 hours.

Administer magnesium sulphate in a place where there are appropriate staff and resources for adequate maternal and fetal monitoring. Explain to the woman the common side effects, which include feeling warm and flushing. Administer the drug slowly to minimize side effects. Administer the loading dose of 4 grams intravenously over 20 minutes via an infusion pump followed by a maintenance dose of 1 gram per hour as per local protocols. Continue this regimen until birth or 24 hours, whichever comes first. Advise monitoring of maternal pulse, respiratory rate, oxygen saturation and patellar reflexes hourly, and urine output 4 hourly. In the absence of complications, advise fetal monitoring every 6–8 hours. Serum levels of magnesium sulphate do not require monitoring in the absence of renal compromise. Serious complications of magnesium sulphate include muscle paralysis, respiratory arrest and cardiac arrest. Magnesium sulphate must be stopped if signs of toxicity occur, which include loss of tendon reflexes, fall in respiratory rate below 14, fall in oxygen saturation below 94% and fall in urine output below 50 millilitres in 2 consecutive hours.

50.6.4 Intrapartum Antibiotic Prophylaxis in Established Preterm Labour

Offer intrapartum antibiotic prophylaxis to women with known group B streptococcus (GBS) colonization in the current pregnancy as per local protocols. In women without known GBS colonization, there is currently no evidence to guide practice. The recommendation to offer intrapartum antibiotic prophylaxis to these women in the UK by the Royal College of Obstetricians and Gynaecologists [11] is based on expert opinion.

50.6.5 Cervical Stitch (Cerclage) for Preventing Preterm Birth in a Singleton Pregnancy

Box 50.2 shows the outcomes of the systematic review by Alfirevic et al [12] of 15 trials, comprising 3490 women.

Do not offer 'rescue' cervical cerclage to women with:

- signs of infection;
- active vaginal bleeding;
- uterine contractions; and
- ruptured fetal membranes.

Consider 'rescue' cervical cerclage for women between 16+0 and 27+6 weeks of pregnancy with a dilated cervix and exposed, unruptured fetal membranes, in consultation with a senior obstetrician. Explain to women for whom 'rescue' cervical cerclage is being considered about the risks of the procedure:

- premature contractions;
- rupture of membranes;

Box 50.2 Findings in the Systematic Review by Alfirevic et al [12]

Cerclage versus No Cerclage
- Risk of perinatal death not reduced (RR 0.82, 95% CI 0.65–1.04; 10 studies, 2927 women; moderate-quality evidence).
- Serious neonatal morbidity was similar with and without cerclage (RR 0.80, 95% CI 0.55–1.18; 6 studies, 883 women; low-quality evidence).
- Pregnant women with and without cerclage were equally likely to have a baby discharged home healthy (RR 1.02, 95% CI 0.97–1.06; 4 studies, 657 women; moderate-quality evidence).
- Pregnant women with cerclage were less likely to have preterm births compared to controls before 37, 34 and 28 completed weeks of gestation (average RR 0.77, 95% CI 0.66–0.89; 9 studies, 2415 women; high-quality evidence).
- In 5 subgroups (history-indicated; short cervix based on one-off ultrasound in high-risk women; short cervix found by serial scans in high-risk women; physical exam–indicated; and short cervix found on scan in low-risk or mixed populations), there were too few trials to make meaningful conclusions and no evidence of differential effects.

Cerclage versus Progesterone
- Two trials (129 women) compared cerclage to vaginal progesterone in high-risk women with short cervix on ultrasound; these trials were too small to detect reliable, clinically important differences for any review outcome.

History Indicated Cerclage versus Ultrasound Indicated Cerclage
- Evidence from 2 trials (344 women) was too limited to establish differences for clinically important outcomes.

Conclusion
- Cervical cerclage reduces the risk of preterm birth in women at high risk of preterm birth but does not reduce risk of perinatal death. There was no evidence of any differential effect of cerclage based on previous obstetric history or short cervix indications, but data were limited for all clinical groups. The question of whether cerclage is more or less effective than other preventive treatments, particularly vaginal progesterone, remains unanswered.

- cervical infection;
- cervical laceration if labour starts before the cerclage is removed; and
- risks associated with spinal or general anaesthesia.

50.7 Progesterone Therapy

A systematic review by Su et al in 2014 [13] concluded that there is insufficient evidence to advocate progesterone agents as a tocolytic therapy for women presenting with suspected preterm labour. A placebo-controlled randomized trial of vaginal progesterone by Norman et al [14] concluded that vaginal progesterone was not associated with reduced risk of preterm birth or composite adverse neonatal outcomes, and had no long-term benefit or harm on outcomes in children at 2 years of age.

50.8 Transfer to Another Unit

The neonatal or paediatric team must be informed of all women diagnosed with preterm labour, in a timely manner, to ensure optimal care for the baby. Depending on the gestation and capacity of the neonatal unit, the woman may need to be transferred to another unit.

50.9 Prediction and Prevention of Preterm Labour

Cervical length scans should be offered between 16+0 and 24+0 weeks of pregnancy to women with history of:

- spontaneous preterm birth or mid-trimester loss between 16+0 and 34+0 weeks of pregnancy. If they are found to have a cervical length of less than 25 mm, they should be offered prophylactic cervical cerclage.
- preterm prelabour rupture of membranes in a previous pregnancy. If they are found to have a cervical length of less than 25 mm, prophylactic cervical cerclage should be considered.
- physical injury to the cervix including surgery such as previous cone biopsy and large loop excision of the transformation zone. If they are found to have a cervical length of less than 25 mm, prophylactic cervical cerclage should be considered.

If they have none of the above risk factors and are found to have a cervical length of less than 25 mm, prophylactic cervical cerclage may be considered.

References

1. NICE. *Preterm Labour and Birth.* Guideline 25. November 2015. www .nice.org.uk/guidance/ng25.

2. Watts DH, Krohn MA, Hillier SL, Eschenbach DA. The association of occult fluid infection with gestational age and neonatal outcome among women in preterm labour. *Obstet Gynecol.* 1992;**79**:351–7.

3. Salafia CM, Vogel CA, Vintzileos AM, et al. Placental pathologic findings in preterm birth. *Am J Obstet Gynecol.* 1991;**165**:934–8.

4. Gibbs W, Challis JRG. Mechanism of term and preterm birth. *J Obstet Gynaecol Can.* 2002;**24** (11):874–83.

5. Schmitz T, Kayem G, Maillard F, et al. Selective use of sonographic cervical length measurement for predicting imminent preterm delivery in women with preterm labour and intact membranes. *Ultrasound Obstet Gynecol.* 2008 Apr;**31**(4): 421–6.

6. Tsoi E, Fuchs IB, Rane S, Geerts L, Nicolaides KH. Sonographic measurement of cervical length in threatened preterm labour in singleton pregnancies with intact membranes. *Ultrasound Obstet Gynecol.* 2005;**25**:353–6.

7. Roberts D, Brown J, Medley N, Dalziel SR. Antenatal corticosteroids for accelerating fetal lung maturation for women at risk of preterm birth. *Cochrane Database Syst Rev.* 2017 Mar 21;(3): CD004454.

8. Crowther CA, MacKinlay CJD, Middleton P, Harding JE. Repeat doses of prenatal corticosteroids for women at risk of preterm birth for improving neonatal health outcomes. *Cochrane Database Syst Rev.* 2015 Jul 5;(7): CD003935.

9. Doyle LW, Crowther CA, Middleton P, Marret S, Rouse D. Magnesium sulphate for women at risk of preterm birth for neuroprotection of the fetus. *Cochrane Database Syst Rev.* 2009. Jan 21;(1):CD004661.

10. Costantine MM, Weiner SJ, Eunice Kennedy Shriver; National Institute of Child Health and Human Development Maternal-Fetal Medicine Units Network. Effects of antenatal exposure to magnesium sulfate on neuroprotection and mortality in preterm infants: a meta-analysis.*Obstet Gynecol.* 2009;**114**:354–64.

11. *Prevention of Early-Onset Neonatal Group-B Streptococcal Disease*, Green-top Guideline No 36. London: Royal College of Obstetricians and Gynaecologists, 2017.

12. Alfirevic Z, Stampalija T, Medley N. Cervical stitch (cerclage) for preventing preterm birth in singleton pregnancy. *Cochrane Database Syst Rev.* 2017 Jun 6; (6):CD008991

13. Su L-L, Samuel M, Chong Y-S. Progestational agents for treating threatened or established preterm labour. *Cochrane Database Syst Rev.* 2014. Jan 20;(1):CD006770.

14. Norman JE, Marlow N, Messow CM, et al. Vaginal progesterone prophylaxis for preterm birth (the OPPTIMUM study): a multicentre, randomised, double-blind trial. *Lancet.* 2016 May 21;**387** (10033):2106–16.

Management of Multiple Pregnancy during Labour

Nikolaos Vrachnis, Dimitrios Zygouris & Asma Khalil

51.1 Introduction

Maternal morbidity and mortality are significantly higher in multiple pregnancies when compared to a singleton pregnancy. The main contributors to adverse outcome are haemorrhage, preterm labour, placental abruption, placenta praevia, hypertensive disorders, malpresentations and cord prolapse [1]. There is also increased risk of complications after delivery, such as postpartum haemorrhage, mainly due to uterine atony [1, 2].

Perinatal morbidity and mortality are also higher in comparison to singleton pregnancies. Moreover, preterm twins have lower survival rates compared to singletons of the same week of gestation [2].

For all these reasons, multiple pregnancies are characterized as high-risk pregnancies: thus, special attention and management are necessary during labour, which must take place in a well-equipped maternity unit. The presence of an experienced obstetrician and adequately trained staff as well as an experienced neonatologist in a highly equipped unit is essential [3].

Over the past few decades, there has been a steady increase in the rates of twins delivered by caesarean section (CS). In 1995, the rate was approximately 50%; this has risen to 70–75% in 2008. For triplets, it is currently estimated to be over 95%, significantly increasing the overall CS rates [4]. The main reasons for this trend are, first, the traditional belief that vaginal delivery increases adverse outcomes, especially for the second twin, and, second, the lack of adequate training of new doctors in vaginal delivery.

However, labour can be attempted in twin pregnancies after very careful case selection, taking into consideration that not all twin pregnancies will result in successful vaginal delivery [5, 6].

51.2 Epidemiology

Twin pregnancy rates have gone up steadily over the last few decades in developed countries, resulting in today's multiple birth rate constituting 1.5% of total births [4]. The main reason for this rise is the advent of assisted reproductive techniques along with the increased maternal age at first pregnancy. The increased rates chiefly concern dizygous twinning pregnancies, while monozygous rates are relatively constant and are estimated to comprise about 0.35% of births; of those, 80% of twin pregnancies are dizygous and 20% are monozygous [6].

51.3 Chorionicity

Even more important than determining monozygosity and dizygosity is establishing the chorionicity of a twin pregnancy, this ideally being determined by ultrasound scan before 14 weeks.

All dizygotic pregnancies develop two separate placentas and amniotic sacs (dichorionic-diamniotic (DCDA)). However, a monozygotic twin pregnancy has the following possibilities:

- Dichorionic-diamniotic twins (DCDA), 20–25% of monozygotic twin pregnancies
- Monochorionic-diamniotic twins (MCDA), 70–75% of monozygotic twin pregnancies
- Monochorionic-monoamniotic twins (MCMA), 1–5% of monozygotic twin pregnancies

51.3.1 Dichorionic-Diamniotic Twins (DCDA)

Perinatal care needs to be undertaken with utmost attention and the parents must be fully informed about labour and the possible consequences.

After the mother's admission, the following must be checked:

- gestational age
- maternal or fetal complications, which might indicate delivery by CS
- well-being of both fetuses
- presentation of first twin

The presentation of the second twin must also be checked, though it will not affect the decision for a vaginal birth. There is the possibility that the second twin will be cephalic before delivery of the first twin and subsequently change to breech presentation, or vice versa.

Continuous fetal heart monitoring using a twin monitor must be undertaken, and vaginal examination should be performed periodically to determine cervical dilation.

51.3.2 Monochorionic-Diamniotic Twins (MCDA)

In MCDA pregnancies, several antenatal complications may arise due to the unequally shared placenta and linked fetoplacental circulations, including selective fetal growth restriction (sFGR), twin-to-twin transfusion syndrome (TTTS) and twin anaemia polycythaemia sequence (TAPS). These events are normally identified and managed antenatally, CS usually being indicated in this setting. Conversely, when an MCDA pregnancy has proceeded to term without any such problems being identified, a common recommendation is to plan for a vaginal delivery, as for dichorionic twins, this is dependent on the presentation of the first twin. The reasoning behind a recommendation for CS in MCDA twins, even in the case of the first twin being cephalic, is based on the risk of acute intrapartum twin-to-twin transfusion, a condition hypothesized to result from acute transfusion due to uterine contractions or sudden changes in fetal position. The incidence of acute TTTS is reported to be 2.5% of MCDA pregnancies and 4.2% of twins delivered vaginally [4]. While the aetiology of acute TTTS is as yet unknown, it has not to date been determined whether CS could reduce the risk of perinatal morbidity as a result of this condition.

Pregnancies without any indication of TTTS or with successful laser treatment can be delivered vaginally [1].

51.3.3 Monochorionic-Monoamniotic (MCMA) Twins

Delivery is performed by CS because there is a very high possibility of umbilical cord problems, as well as abnormal presentation of the second twin. A CS is booked at 32–34 weeks of gestation (after corticosteroid administration) [2]. If there are signs of preterm labour, an emergency CS should be performed.

51.4 Presentation of Twins

The presentation of the first twin strongly influences the decision either for or against vaginal birth. The second twin could change its presentation after the birth of the first twin. This possibility increases significantly in multiparous women and when the gestational age is less than 34 weeks.

Types of presentations:
- Cephalic – cephalic, 40%
- Cephalic – non-cephalic, 40%
- Non-cephalic – cephalic, breech, vertex 20%

When both twins are cephalic, vaginal birth can be attempted in the absence of any indication for CS. When the first twin is non-cephalic, CS is indicated.

51.5 Indications for CS

There are absolute and relative indications for CS, which help determine whether or not a trial of labour in a twin pregnancy is possible (Table 51.1) [7].

51.6 Safety of Labour

Until 2013, a large number of retrospective studies had been carried out on twin vaginal delivery with, however, conflicting conclusions as well as significant selection bias. Some concluded that CS was beneficial in twin pregnancies, while others found no difference in outcomes [8–11].

However, in 2013, the Twin Birth Study was published, which was a randomized controlled trial comparing planned vaginal delivery and planned CS [12]. This study included 2804

Table 51.1 Indications for CS

Absolute indications for CS	Relative indications for CS
• Monoamniotic twins	• Monochorionic twins
• Conjoined twins	• Maternal request
• Twin 1 is non-cephalic	
• Triplets or higher-order pregnancies	
• Abnormal placental site, i.e. praevia	

women from 25 countries, with dichorionic and monochorionic twins, only monoamniotic twins being excluded. There was no significant difference between the two groups in the fetal and neonatal mortality and morbidity or maternal morbidity [12–14]. Moreover, these outcomes were not affected by presentation of the second twin, chorionicity, gestational age or maternal age.

It is therefore clear that in twin pregnancies, after 32 weeks, planned vaginal delivery is not associated with adverse maternal or neonatal outcome compared with CS, provided that the first twin is in vertex presentation. It is nevertheless essential that labour should be attempted in a well-equipped maternity unit with a very experienced obstetrician in case breech extraction or internal podalic version is needed.

51.7 Timing of Delivery

Twin pregnancies are planned for delivery earlier than singletons due to the increased risk of intrauterine fetal death. In dichorionic-diamniotic (DCDA) twin pregnancies, the risks are balanced at 37 weeks with an increase in the perinatal mortality in pregnancies continuing beyond 38 weeks, while in monochorionic pregnancies, the risk of intrauterine mortality seems to exceed the risk of neonatal mortality after 36 weeks. The aim is to strike a fine balance between the risk of prematurity and stillbirth; thus, the usual recommendations are [15–17] :

- Dichorionic-diamniotic: 37 weeks
- Monochorionic-diamniotic: 36 weeks

Labour can be induced either by artificial rupture of the membranes, with or without oxytocin, or via the use of prostaglandins. While a secondary analysis of the Twin Birth Study, including pregnancies from 32 weeks, observed no difference in outcome between the two methods, the risk of CS following labour induction amounted to 40% with both [8].

The choice of amniotomy for induction of labour is thought to be more common among multiparous women as well as in women with a higher Bishop score, since these groups are more likely to have vaginal delivery. The Twin Birth Study noted a strong association between advanced maternal age, nulliparity and a non-vertex second twin and higher rates of unplanned CS following induction of labour [8]. Thus, it is crucial for these factors to be taken into consideration when women are counselled concerning induction of labour.

51.8 Analgesia

During a trial of labour in twin pregnancy, regional anaesthesia is highly recommended. It will allow improved cooperation of the mother if breech extraction of the second twin is necessary, this being extremely difficult to perform with local anaesthesia or without any kind of anaesthesia. Furthermore, regional anaesthesia can facilitate better fetal monitoring during labour, while, in the case of an emergency CS, general anaesthesia can be avoided, thus decreasing the risk of aspiration.

51.9 Intrapartum Management

51.9.1 First Stage

A woman in the first stage of labour in twin pregnancy should be managed according to the protocols listed in Table 51.2. Ultrasound assessment is performed on admission (Table 51.3), and all relevant staff involved informed.

51.9.2 Second Stage

Delivery of the first twin takes place in the same manner as that of a fetus of a singleton pregnancy, with operative delivery and episiotomy performed when indicated.

After completing delivery of the first twin, a vaginal examination is carried out to determine the presentation of the second twin. Ultrasound assessment should be performed to determine presentation. Continuous evaluation of the CTG is also essential [18].

There are a few risks for the second twin at this stage, which, fortunately, are infrequent: transverse lie, compound presentation, umbilical cord accident, acute feto-fetal transfusion and placental abruption.

During all twin deliveries, ultrasound and a competent operator must be at hand for clarification of presentation and,

Table 51.2 First stage of labour management

- Admission to delivery unit

- Blood tests: full blood count, group & save
- Intravenous access (venflon)

• Continuous cardiotocography (CTG) for both twins	o Abnormal rate of 1st twin → fetal blood sampling
	o Abnormal rate 2nd twin → CS
	o Monitoring cannot be achieved →CS

Table 51.3 Ultrasound examination during 1st stage of labour

- Presentation of fetuses
- Amniotic fluid volume
- Placental site
- Viability of fetuses

when choice of a version is necessary, to aid the clinician in selecting which will be the more successful direction to take. While from the beginning of labour the second twin's presentation is known, in about 20% of cases, there is a change of presentation following delivery of the first twin. Thus, after the delivery of the first twin, palpation and ultrasound should be used whenever possible to assess presentation of the second twin.

51.9.2.1 Second Twin Cephalic

If the second twin is cephalic, then labour follows as the mother continues to push. Oxytocin may be increased or else administered if not already in use. Continuous fetal heart monitoring is necessary, while artificial rupture of membranes is made during a uterine contraction. Operative delivery should be performed depending on the findings.

51.9.2.2 Second Twin Breech or Transverse

If the second twin is breech or transverse, a breech extraction must be performed within a few minutes [18, 19]. More specifically, the fetal feet are grasped at the ankles and gentle traction is applied. If the membranes are not ruptured, artificial rupture is undertaken and the fetal breech at the introitus is awaited. When it is not possible to grasp both feet, one foot is pulled until it is delivered, after which delivery of the other foot follows. The umbilical cord is then slightly lengthened, and the baby is held by the hips carefully. The obstetrician places both hands around the buttocks and the fetus' hips, with the thumbs on the sacrum and index fingers on the anterior iliac spine.

There follows delivery of the fetal abdomen and chest with slight pulling, if needed, and concurrent rotation, either clockwise or counterclockwise, to dislodge the arms (Figure 51.1). The operator may help with the delivery of the arm by sweeping a thumb along the arm. The fetal head is delivered last using the Mauriceau–Smellie–Veit manoeuvre. The fingers of the dominant hand are placed on each side of the mouth and the palm on the chest. The other hand is placed on the upper back, with the middle finger on the occiput, pushing it down in order to flex the fetal head. The body is elevated gradually, and the head is delivered (Figure 51.2).

A nuchal arm (or arms) is a potentially serious situation that can arise during a breech extraction. The operator must stop pulling and start rotating the fetal body to release the arm. When the right arm is diagnosed as nuchal, rotation of the body must be counterclockwise, and vice versa.

Another potentially dangerous complication during extraction is head entrapment, i.e. inability to deliver the fetal head through the contracted cervix. This may be solved with good analgesia, forceps, rapid-acting uterine relaxant, suprapubic pressure and, last, Dührssen incisions of the cervix at two, six and ten o'clock. If all the previous manoeuvres are not successful, then emergency CS must be performed as soon as possible.

51.9.2.3 Second Twin Unengaged

In cases of an unengaged, vertex or oblique second twin, an internal podalic version should be tried until breech presentation is achieved, after which delivery can proceed as breech extraction.

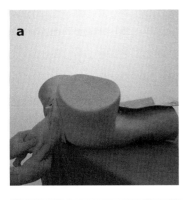
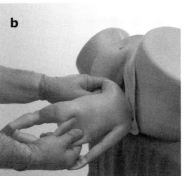
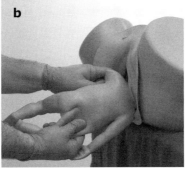
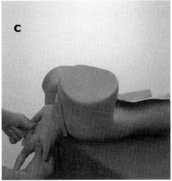
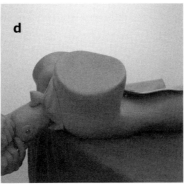

Figure 51.1 Demonstration of Lovset's manoeuvre for delivery of twin 2 (breech). (a) The obstetrician's thumbs are placed on the infant's sacrum and the other fingers hold the hips and the pelvis. (b) Turn the infant 90° so as to bring the anterior shoulder under the symphysis pubis; (c) engage the anterior arm and deliver it. (d) Then, continue with 180° counter rotation, and the posterior arm that is now moved under the symphysis pubis is delivered. A black and white version of this figure will appear in some formats. For the colour version, please refer to the plate section.

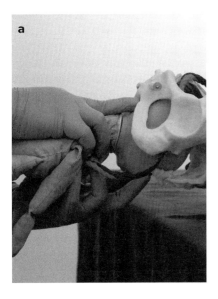
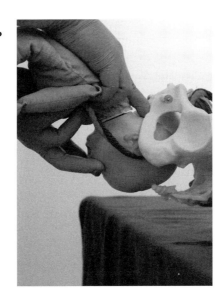

Figure 51.2 Mauriceau–Smellie–Veit manoeuvre for delivery of twin 2 (breech). (a) The obstetrician inserts the non-dominant hand into the vagina: he or she palpates the fetal maxilla with the index and middle fingers and places these fingers on the neonate's cheekbone. The index and ring fingers of other hand are used to hook the baby's shoulders, while the middle finger presses the occiput in order to flex the head. (b) The head is flexed gently towards the chest until the hairline is visible. Then the obstetrician continues to raise the baby, holding in place the non-dominant hand until the head is free. A black and white version of this figure will appear in some formats. For the colour version, please refer to the plate section.

The operator's hand in the opposite side of fetal back is placed in the vagina and elevates the vertex higher until he or she finds the fetal foot. The other hand is placed on the mother's abdomen and keeps the vertex elevated until the fetus is at breech presentation.

All these cases are at increased risk for cord or hand prolapse, and when these situations occur, it is not safe to attempt breech extraction. Consequently, an emergency CS may be required for delivery of the second twin if the attempt at podalic version is not successful.

51.9.2.4 Inter-twin Delivery Interval

It is important to record the inter-twin delivery time interval, since increased time is associated with adverse outcome. The existing data have shown that the risk for fetal acidosis and fetal distress are significantly higher when the twin-to-twin delivery time interval exceeds 30 minutes [20–23]. Acknowledging this, it is important to consider the clinical picture before intervening to hasten the delivery of the second twin since it is not proven that the interval is the cause of the fetal compromise, and hasty intervention may in fact precipitate more complications than it prevents [24].

51.9.3 Third Stage

Labour finishes with cord blood gas analysis, if this is available, delivery of the placenta, uterotonic injection and repair of any laceration, as in a singleton pregnancy.

Active management is recommended, using a bolus infusion of oxytocin (5 IU), followed by continuous infusion of 5–10 IU/hour for 4–6 hours.

As twin pregnancies have an increased risk for uterine atony (due to overdistended uterus), 2 units of red blood cells (RBCs) should be crossmatched on admission. Apart from the active management of the third stage, all other management measures can be followed as in the uterine atony algorithm of a singleton pregnancy [25].

51.10 Triplet Gestation

The rate of CS for triplet pregnancies is over 95% [26]. Although there are at present inadequate data to support this approach, it is a common practice. The existing studies are case series and retrospective studies due to the relatively rare incidence; thus, they cannot lead to any definitive conclusions [27, 28].

Though vaginal delivery could be an option in extreme prematurity, women who request this procedure should be well informed of the limited evidence. A very experienced obstetrician must be present.

51.11 Previous CS

The rates of trial of labour after prior CS (TOLAC) are extremely low in twin pregnancies. It is believed that TOLAC in twin pregnancy is associated with increased risk for uterine rupture, as the uterus is overdistended. However, the existing data from a large number of retrospective studies have not demonstrated this [29].

Trial of labour after prior CS has remarkably high success rates. For example, one study reports an 85% success rate, without increased rates of complications, compared with singleton pregnancies. Consequently, in carefully selected twin pregnancies with previous CS, TOLAC can be attempted, though there must be preparation for an emergency CS at any time [30].

51.12 Special Circumstances

51.12.1 Complicated Monochorionic Twin Pregnancies – Prenatal Treatment of Twin-to-Twin Transfusion Syndrome

A randomized control trial (RCT) studying fetoscopic laser treatment for TTTS reported that only 57% of cases treated were delivered by CS, while the mode of delivery was left to the discretion of the treating clinician [31]. A theoretical risk exists of uterine rupture at the trocar site; however, this risk is likely to be lower than that associated with prior CS, which is not a contraindication to vaginal delivery. Nevertheless, since thus far few data have been published, a precise risk quantification

is a challenge. Meanwhile, the option of vaginal delivery remains viable for twins treated by laser who show no evidence of fetal growth restriction, TAPs, or recurrent TTTS.

51.12.2 Growth Discordance

In both planned CS and planned vaginal delivery, an estimated difference in the twins' fetal weight of >20% has been associated with a higher risk of neonatal mortality and morbidity. It is proposed that in twin pregnancies, significant growth discordance is a predictor of failed operative vaginal delivery. An increase in the risk of combined delivery (CS for the second twin) is expected in cases where the second twin is larger; nonetheless, a successful vaginal delivery is still feasible [32].

51.12.3 Extreme Prematurity

In the Twin Birth Study, twins presenting prior to 32 weeks' gestation were excluded; meanwhile, there are as yet no randomized controlled data for CS or for vaginal birth. Therefore, in the latter cases, a decision must be made between an intrapartum CS and continuation with vaginal delivery. Furthermore, there is greater likelihood of success with a planned vaginal delivery in preterm twins than there exists in more mature pregnancies. Evidently, in this group such a choice reduces the maternal morbidity that is associated with emergency CSs [33]. In the case of vertex/vertex twins presenting in spontaneous preterm labour where no other indications for CS exist, we would, however, normally recommend attempted vaginal delivery. Regarding extremely preterm (23–28 weeks) singleton fetuses in breech presentation, CS has been associated with both significantly lower risk of intraventricular haemorrhage and of neonatal death [34]. Finally, the conclusions of a recent systematic review regarding vertex/non-vertex twin pairs were that there was little to no conclusive evidence of any significant difference between vaginal delivery and CS [35]. It is our belief that once the woman has been counselled concerning the increased surgical risks of CS and provided with an individualized gestation-based prognosis of her babies, CS may reasonably be offered to her during spontaneous labour in the case of an extremely preterm gestation where vaginal delivery is not immediately imminent.

51.12.4 Discordant Anomaly and 'Perinatal Switch'

It is estimated that 1–2% of twin pregnancies will be complicated by discordant anomalies that were detected using antenatal ultrasound screening. It is of note that the twin that presents first on ultrasound will not always be the first delivered. The latter, known as the 'perinatal switch phenomenon', is an event that occurs in approximately 6% of vaginal deliveries and 20% of CS deliveries and which is often not clinically apparent [36]. It is important for both parents and clinicians to be aware of this phenomenon, while it is of particular importance in cases where a fetal condition that is not externally obvious (e.g., congenital diaphragmatic hernia or hypoplastic left heart) requires immediate postnatal intervention. In such instances, there is the need for meticulous pre-delivery ultrasound identification as well as preparation for immediate postnatal differentiation, together with bedside echocardiography or imaging.

51.13 Key Messages

- The incidence of multiple pregnancies has increased in recent years.
- Planned vaginal delivery is not associated with adverse maternal or neonatal outcome in carefully selected cases.
- Labour should be attempted in a well-equipped maternity unit with an experienced obstetrician.

- There must be adequate space in the delivery room for all necessary birth attendants as well as easy access to the operating theatre facilities.
- The presenting twin should be cephalic in order to attempt vaginal delivery.
- For delivery of the second twin, either podalic version and breech extraction or only breech extraction may be needed. Alternatively, external cephalic version should be attempted. The choice will depend on the operator's experience.
- Adequate analgesia is vital.
- Prolonged intertwin delivery time increases the risk for adverse outcome.
- Active management is recommended for the third stage of labour.

References

1. American College of O, Gynecologists, Society for Maternal-Foetal M. ACOG Practice Bulletin No. 144: Multifoetal gestations: twin, triplet, and higher-order multifoetal pregnancies. *Obstet Gynecol.* 2014;**123**(5):1118–32.

2. Committee on Practice B-O, Society for Maternal-Foetal M.Practice Bulletin No. 169: Multifoetal gestations: twin, triplet, and higher-order multifoetal pregnancies. *Obstet Gynecol.* 2016;**128**(4):e131–46.

3. Melka S, Miller J, Fox NS. Labour and delivery of twin pregnancies. *Obstet Gynecol Clin North Am.* 2017;**44**(4):645–54.

4. Martin JA, Hamilton BE, Osterman MJ, Driscoll AK, Mathews TJ. Births: final data for 2015. *Nat Vital Stat Rep.* 2017;**66**(1):1.

5. Schmitz T, Carnavalet Cde C, Azria E, et al. Neonatal outcomes of twin pregnancy according to the planned mode of delivery. *Obstet Gynecol.* 2008;**111**(3):695–703.

6. Smith GC, Shah I, White IR, Pell JP, Dobbie R. Mode of delivery and the risk of delivery-related perinatal death among twins at term: a retrospective cohort study of 8073 births. *BJOG.* 2005;**112**(8):1139–44.

7. Vintzileos AM, Ananth CV, Kontopoulos E, Smulian JC. Mode of delivery and risk of stillbirth and infant mortality in triplet gestations: United States, 1995 through 1998. *Am J Obstet Gynecol.* 2005;**192**(2):464–9.

8. Barrett JF, Hannah ME, Hutton EK, et al. A randomized trial of planned cesarean or vaginal delivery for twin pregnancy. *N Engl J Med.* 2013;**369**(14):1295–305.

9. Asztalos EV, Hannah ME, Hutton EK, et al. Twin Birth Study: 2-year neurodevelopmental follow-up of the randomized trial of planned cesarean or planned vaginal delivery for twin pregnancy. *Am J Obstet Gynecol.* 2016;**214**(3):371 e1–e19.

10. Hutton EK, Hannah ME, Ross S, et al. Maternal outcomes at 3 months after planned caesarean section versus planned vaginal birth for twin pregnancies in the Twin Birth Study: a randomised controlled trial. *BJOG.* 2015;**122**(12):1653–62.

11. Tavares MV, Domingues AP, Nunes F, et al. Induction of labour vs. spontaneous vaginal delivery in twin pregnancy after 36 weeks of gestation. *J Obstet Gynaecol.* 2017;**37**(1):29–32.

12. Bauer C, Voutsos LJ. Preventing the first cesarean delivery: summary of a joint Eunice Kennedy Shriver National Institute of Child Health and Human Development, Society for Maternal-Foetal Medicine, and American College of Obstetricians and Gynecologists workshop. *Obstet Gynecol.* 2013;**121**(3):686–7.

13. Hofmeyr GJ, Barrett JF, Crowther CA. Planned caesarean section for women with a twin pregnancy. *Cochrane Database Syst Rev.* 2015(12):CD006553.

14. Dodd JM, Crowther CA, Grivell RM, Deussen AR. Elective repeat caesarean section versus induction of labour for women with a previous caesarean birth. *Cochrane Database Syst Rev.* 2017;(7): CD004906.

15. Monson M, Silver RM. Multifoetal gestation: mode of delivery. *Clin Obstet Gynecol.* 2015;**58**(3):690–702.

16. Arabin B, Kyvernitakis I, Liao A, Zugaib M. Trends in cesarean delivery for twin births in the United States: 1995–2008. *Obstet Gynecol.* 2012; **119**(3):657–8; author reply 8–9.

17. Leung TY, Tam WH, Leung TN, Lok IH, Lau TK. Effect of twin-to-twin delivery interval on umbilical cord blood gas in the second twins. *BJOG.* 2002;**109**(1):63–7.

18. Lindroos L, Elfvin A, Ladfors L, Wennerholm UB. The effect of twin-to-twin delivery time intervals on neonatal outcome for second twins. *BMC Pregnancy Childbirth.* 2018;**18**(1):36.

19. Breathnach FM, McAuliffe FM, Geary M, et al. Prediction of safe and successful vaginal twin birth. *Am J Obstet Gynecol.* 2011;**205**(3):237 e1–7.

20. Hoffmann E, Oldenburg A, Rode L, et al. Twin births: cesarean section or vaginal delivery? *Acta Obstet Gynecol Scand.* 2012;**91**(4):463–9.

21. Peaceman AM, Kuo L, Feinglass J. Infant morbidity and mortality associated with vaginal delivery in twin gestations. *Am J Obstet Gynecol.* 2009;**200**(4):462e1-6.

22. Chevreau J, Foulon A, Abou Arab O, et al. Management of breech and twin labour during registrarship: A two-year prospective, observational study. *J Gynecol Obstet Hum Reprod.* 2018; **47**(5):191–6.

23. Rabinovici J, Barkai G, Reichman B, Serr DM, Mashiach S. Randomized management of the second nonvertex twin: vaginal delivery or cesarean section. *Am J Obstet Gynecol.* 1987;**156**(1):52–6.

24. Vogel JP, Holloway E, Cuesta C, et al. Outcomes of non-vertex second twins, following vertex vaginal delivery of first

twin: a secondary analysis of the WHO Global Survey on maternal and perinatal health. *BMC Pregnancy Childbirth.* 2014;14:55.

25. Van Veelen AJ, Van Cappellen AW, Flu PK, Straub MJ, Wallenburg HC. Effect of external cephalic version in late pregnancy on presentation at delivery: a randomized controlled trial. *Br J Obstet Gynaecol.* 1989;96(8):916–21.

26. Fox NS, Silverstein M, Bender S, et al. Active second-stage management in twin pregnancies undergoing planned vaginal delivery in a U.S.population. *Obstet Gynecol.* 2010; 115 (2 Pt 1): 229–33.

27. Grobman WA, Peaceman AM, Haney EI, Silver RK, MacGregor SN. Neonatal outcomes in triplet gestations after a trial of labour. *Am J Obstet Gynecol.* 1998;179 (4):942–5.

28. Alran S, Sibony O, Luton D, et al. Maternal and neonatal outcome of 93 consecutive triplet pregnancies with 71% vaginal delivery. *Acta Obstet Gynecol Scand.* 2004; 83(6):554–9.

29. Varner MW, Thom E, Spong CY, et al. Trial of labour after one previous cesarean delivery for multifoetal gestation. *Obstet Gynecol.* 2007; 110(4):814–19.

30. Kabiri D, Masarwy R, Schachter-Safrai N, et al. Trial of labour after cesarean delivery in twin gestations: systematic review and meta-analysis. *Am J Obstet Gynecol.* 2019. Apr;220(4):336–47.

31. Senat M-V, Deprest J, Boulvain M, et al. Endoscopic laser surgery versus serial amnioreduction for severe twin-to-twin transfusion syndrome. *N Engl J Med.* 2004 Jul 8;351 (2):136–44.

32. Persad VL, Baskett TF, O'Connell CM, Scott HM. Combined vaginal-cesarean delivery of twin pregnancies. *Obstet Gynecol.* 2001 Dec;98(6):1032–7.

33. Sentilhes L, Oppenheimer A, Bouhours A-C, et al. Neonatal outcome of very preterm twins: policy of planned vaginal or cesarean delivery. *Am J Obstet Gynecol.* 2015;213:73.e1–73.e7.

34. Grabovac M, Karim J, Isayama T, Liyanage SK, McDonald S. What is the safest mode of birth for extremely preterm breech singleton infants who are actively resuscitated? A systematic review and meta-analyses. *BJOG.* 2018 May;125(6):652–63.

35. Dagenais C, Lewis-Mikhael A-M, Grabovac M, Mukerji A, McDonald SD. What is the safest mode of delivery for extremely preterm cephalic/ non-cephalic twin pairs? A systematic review and meta-analyses. *BMC Pregnancy Childbirth.* 2017 Dec 29; 17(1):397.

36. Dias T, Ladd S, Mahsud-Dornan S, et al. Systematic labeling of twin pregnancies on ultrasound. *Ultrasound Obstet Gynecol.* 2011 Aug;38(2):130–3.

Abnormal Obstetric Presentation

Chapter 52

Frank Louwen

52.1 Introduction

Abnormal obstetric presentation is a challenge for obstetricians when either birth of a viable fetus (>23 weeks of gestation) is imminent or when counselling expecting women. Vertex or cephalic presentation is the most common situation and is associated with the lowest complication rate during birth. It is important to screen for abnormal obstetric presentation in order to prevent adverse outcomes and to prepare for the appropriate perinatal management.

52.2 Breech Presentation

52.2.1 Definition

Breech presentation is a vertical position of the fetus with leading coccyx or feet of the baby. Differential leg posture presentations (Frank breech, complete breech, incomplete breech or footling presentation) of the fetus should only be diagnosed after onset of labour:

Frank breech: The coccyx is in leading position; the legs are stretched upwards.

Complete breech: The coccyx and both feet are in leading position.

Incomplete breech: The coccyx and one foot are in leading position.

Footling presentation: Both feet are in leading position, the legs are stretched downwards.

52.2.2 Epidemiology and Aetiology

Breech presentation at term is found in up to 4% of pregnancies, and the less advanced the gestational age, the higher the rate of breech presentation [1]. In most cases, a reason for the abnormal fetal presentation cannot be found, but breech presentation is associated with pelvic disproportion, uterine malformation and placenta praevia. Multiparous women have a higher incidence of a breech presentation at term. A frequently discussed reason for a breech position is umbilical cord entrapment, a nuchal cord or a short umbilical cord.

52.2.3 Counselling / Mode of Delivery

Women who have a breech presentation at term following an unsuccessful or declined offer of external cephalic version (ECV) should be counselled on the risks and benefits of planned vaginal breech delivery versus planned caesarean section. Counselling for expecting women with a baby in breech presentation should lead to an informed consent in the planned delivery approach. Pros and cons of the vaginal delivery approach as well as of the caesarean section have to be explained.

52.2.3.1 Preterm Delivery

In preterm delivery (<34 weeks of gestation, <2500 g) a caesarean section as mode of delivery is common practice. Studies comparing fetal outcome in accordance to the delivery mode are rare but available data show a trend towards a benefit of a caesarean section in terms of fetal morbidity [2, 3]. Clinicians are cautious in recommending a vaginal intended birth because of the risk of head dystocia when the cervix is not fully dilated. This complicates the conception of large prospective studies.

To date, caesarean section is not recommended by guidelines in spontaneous preterm deliveries. When a vaginal birth has progressed, the presence of a skilled obstetrician and continuing fetal well-being should be ensured. In cases of planned preterm deliveries, a caesarean section is recommended.

52.2.3.2 Term Delivery

In daily clinical practice, a caesarean section often is recommended in breech presentation. Vaginal breech delivery at term has been reported to be associated with a slightly greater early fetal morbidity in comparison to a planned caesarean section as well as compared to a vaginal intended delivery of a vertex presentation. Long-term morbidity is not affected by the mode of delivery [4]. The risks following a caesarean section, like wound infection, extensive bleeding, invasive placenta in the following pregnancy and uterine rupture in the following pregnancy, have to be considered.

National guidelines recommend intended vaginal delivery with some restrictions. There is no international consensus on conditions leading to a caesarean section indication [5].

The Royal College of Obstetricians and Gynaecologists (RCOG) guideline [6] proposes the following restrictions:

- Hyperextended neck on ultrasound.
- High estimated fetal weight (more than 3.8 kg).
- Low estimated weight (less than 10th centile).
- Footling presentation.
- Evidence of antenatal fetal compromise.

A large cohort study investigating the role of birthweight (>2500 g) could not show an association between birthweight and perinatal fetal morbidity [7].

52.2.3.3 Special Anamnestic Findings

There is a lack of evidence to recommend caesarean section in some additional situations. A prospective monocentre cohort study found that neonatal morbidity and mortality as well as maternal outcome were not significantly different in successful vaginal deliveries of women with prior caesarean compared to primiparous patients. A prior caesarean should not be taken as an exclusion criterion for a planned vaginal delivery out of a breech presentation at term [8].

A large prospective monocentre cohort study found neonatal morbidity and mortality not significantly different in deliveries of nulliparous versus multiparous women. Nulliparous women had a significantly higher rate of a caesarean section during labour than did multiparous women. Maternal birth-injury rates and the use of epidural anaesthesia were significantly higher when comparing vaginal births of nulliparous versus multiparous women. Nulliparity seems not be an exclusion criterion for intended vaginal breech birth at term [9].

A large prospective monocentre cohort study compared the short-term maternal and fetal outcome in intended vaginal breech deliveries before the estimated due date (until 40+0 weeks of gestation) to the outcome of deliveries carried out past the estimated due date (later than 40+1 weeks of gestation). No significant difference in maternal and neonatal short-term mortality and morbidity was found. The rate of caesarean sections was increased in the group of patients, who delivered later than 40+0 weeks of gestation. This study provided evidence that an elective caesarean section for breech presentations at term is not obligatory when the estimated due date has passed in singleton pregnancy [8].

52.2.3.4 Breech Presentation in Twin Pregnancy

In cases of a breech presentation of the leading twin, almost no evidence is available to base counselling on. Guidelines recommend caesarean sections in this case [6, 10]. A second twin in breech presentation is not an indication to perform a caesarean section.

52.2.4 Clinical Management

52.2.4.1 External Cephalic Version

External cephalic version (ECV) is the manipulation of the fetus to a cephalic presentation. Women with a breech presentation at term should be offered ECV unless there is an absolute contraindication. They should be advised on the risks and benefits of ECV and the implications for mode of delivery. (Grade of recommendation: A) [6]

Evidence discovering contraindications is limited. Pregnant women should be informed about a possible increased risk of an ECV when the following criteria apply:

- placental abnormality
- multiple pregnancy
- rupture of membranes
- vaginal bleeding

Success rates are reported to be below 50% [11].

Complications (e.g. disruption of the placenta) that lead to an emergency caesarean section can occur within 24 hours and happen in 0.5% of cases.

The RCOG published a guideline on ECV (Green-top Guideline No 20a [16]). The following is a summation of the recommendations and their grades:

- Women should be informed that the success rate of ECV is approximately 50%. – Grade of recommendation: A
- Women should be informed that after an unsuccessful ECV attempt at 36+0 weeks of gestation or later, only a few babies presenting by the breech will spontaneously turn to cephalic presentation. [New 2017] – Grade of recommendation: B
- Women should be informed that a few babies revert to breech after successful ECV. [New 2017] – Grade of recommendation: B
- Women should be informed that a successful ECV reduces the chance of caesarean section. – Grade of recommendation: A
- Women should be informed that labour after ECV is associated with a slightly increased rate of caesarean section and instrumental delivery when compared with spontaneous cephalic presentation. – Grade of recommendation: B
- ECV success can be predicted to some extent, but the use of models to predict success should not be used routinely to determine whether ECV can be attempted. [New 2017] – Grade of recommendation: B
- Use of tocolysis with betamimetics improves the success rates of ECV. – Grade of recommendation: A
- Routine use of regional analgesia or neuraxial blockade is not recommended, but may be considered for a repeat attempt or for women unable to tolerate ECV without analgesia. [New 2017] – Grade of recommendation: B
- ECV should be offered at term from 37+0 weeks of gestation. – Grade of recommendation: B
- In nulliparous women, ECV may be offered from 36+0 weeks of gestation. – Grade of recommendation: ✓
- There is no general consensus on the eligibility for, or contraindications to, ECV. – Grade of recommendation: C
- Women should be informed that ECV after one caesarean delivery appears to have no greater risk than with an unscarred uterus. [New 2017] – Grade of recommendation: C
- What are the risks of ECV? Women should be counselled that with appropriate precautions, ECV has a very low complication rate. – Grade of recommendation: B
- What measures are appropriate to ensure fetal safety? ECV should be performed where facilities for monitoring and surgical delivery are available. – Grade of recommendation: ✓
- The standard preoperative preparations for caesarean section are not recommended for women undergoing ECV. – Grade of recommendation: ✓
- Following ECV, EFM is recommended. – Grade of recommendation: ✓
- Women undergoing ECV who are D negative should undergo testing for fetomaternal haemorrhage and be offered anti-D. [New 2017] – Grade of recommendation: D

- ECV should only be performed by a trained practitioner or by a trainee working under direct supervision. [New 2017] – Grade of recommendation: ✓
- Although most women tolerate ECV, they should be informed that ECV can be a painful procedure. – Grade of recommendation: C
- The uptake of ECV is best increased by timely identification of the baby presenting by the breech and provision of evidence-based information. – Grade of recommendation: C
- There is no evidence to support any particular service model although larger institutions may consider a dedicated ECV clinic. [New 2017] – Grade of recommendation: ✓
- What is the role of non-ECV methods?
- Women may wish to consider the use of moxibustion for breech presentation at 33–35 weeks of gestation, under the guidance of a trained practitioner. [New 2017] – Grade of recommendation: C
- Women should be advised that there is no evidence that postural management alone promotes spontaneous version to cephalic presentation. – Grade of recommendation: B

52.2.4.2 Maternal Birth Position

Dorsal position: The natural birth line is directed onto the mother's belly. In order to support the natural birth direction within the birth canal, the obstetrician has to lead the baby's body upwards – opposing gravity. Here, most frequently, the **Bracht** manoeuvre is used. The lower abdomen and flexed upper legs of the baby are bent upwards. Delivery of the head can be assisted by flexing the baby's head with traction on the inner fetal chin (**Mauriceau–Smellie–Veit** manoeuvre).

Upright position / on all fours: When the mother delivers in the upright position during the second stage, they use the force of gravity to naturally support the fetal direction within the birth canal. Manipulations often are not necessary. Louwen et al have reported a beneficial effect on fetomaternal perinatal outcome of this birth position [12].

52.2.4.3 Delivery Progress Management

Breech-experienced obstetricians should attend birth. A vaginally intended breech delivery should take place in an obstetric institution where immediate caesarean section is possible.

The progression of birth with its basic features and time frames is not different when compared to a delivery from the vertex position. Progression of the cervical opening, fetal heart rate and progression of the leading fetal part should be monitored. It is of utmost importance that – independent from the leg posture – the position of the fetus' coccyx within the mother's pelvis poses the relevant diagnostic parameter. The baby's hip should be found in a digital vaginal examination in order to be able to assess birth progression and indicate a caesarean section when birth arrest is diagnosed. The use of a partogram to record the progress of labour is recommended (Figure 52.1). Women should be informed that while evidence is lacking, continuous electronic fetal monitoring may lead to improved neonatal outcomes [6].

52.2.4.4 Assisted Delivery

When arms are bent upwards besides the fetus' head, an arrest of birth occurs after delivery of the fetal coccyx. The faster the obstetrician recognizes the problem and initiates assistance / manual manoeuvres, the better the fetal outcomes will be. While assisting, the obstetrician never should enforce traction in any of the following manoeuvres:

Classical assisted arm delivery (dorsal position): Grab the baby by its feet and pull diagonally upwards and in the direction of the baby's front (ten or two o'clock). Glide with the free hand alongside the baby's back until you reach the posterior arm and release it through pressure at the lower upper arm. Lead the fetus' body back to the stating position and rotate 180°. Through pulling upwards again, the contralateral shoulder will be released.

Lovset's manoeuvre (dorsal position): Pull the feet upwards. When the shoulder presents itself underneath the symphysis, rotate 180°. Release the baby's torso slowly downwards. Then pull out the ventral arm with two fingers. Repeat this manoeuvre to assist delivery of the contralateral shoulder.

Mauriceau–Smellie–Veit manoeuvre (dorsal position): To assist delivery of the head, insert the index finger into the baby's mouth and pull at the chin in order to flex the baby's head. The other hand fixates the baby's shoulders. It is important to lead the baby's neck around the mother's symphysis.

Forceps: When the baby's head cannot be delivered, forceps can be used equivalently to forceps in vertex deliveries. The obstetrician should press the forceps away from the baby's head while inserting in order to avoid ocular injuries.

Louwen's manoeuvre: Delivery of arms (upright position): The obstetrician acts from behind the mother. Criterion for shoulder dystocia / birth arrest: The baby's delivery stops at the upper abdominal level; the baby is rotated 90°.

The shoulder dystocia sign [13] becomes visible in the upright maternal position and at the same time directly indicates the solution of the fetal arm fixed on the maternal symphysis. While in an uncomplicated vaginal breech birth, the child presents the obstetrician with his front side in spontaneous descending from the visibility of his navel; with the arm fixed on the symphysis, the body rotates 90° to the side. If the child shows his left side, the right arm is fixed on the maternal symphysis. As a solution, at the end of the manoeuvre, the fetal shoulders must be positioned across the pelvic entrance.

Grab both shoulders of the baby by reaching gently upwards with thumb and index finger (both hands). Rotate the baby's body 180° in the direction that the baby's front is turned towards you. Turn the baby's body 90°. Do not pull. Through the rotation process, both shoulders will be released from the pelvic entrance level [9].

Frank's nudge (dorsal position): To assist head delivery in a dorsal birth position, push both shoulders backwards and

Partogram in cephalic presentation

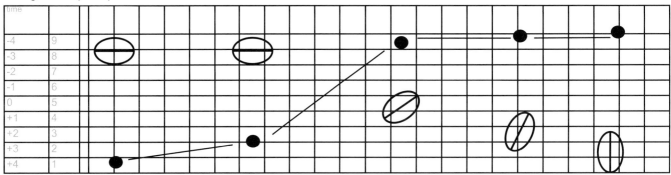

Partogram in breech presentation

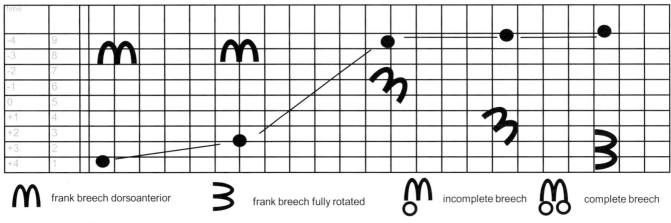

𝗠 frank breech dorsoanterior   Ƹ frank breech fully rotated   𝗠̥ incomplete breech   𝗠̥̥ complete breech

Figure 52.1 Use of the partogram

upwards. The impact will flex the baby's head (mother's pubis works as a fulcrum) (Figure 52.2).

Mother's position during second stage: It should be recognized that the mother's position during active second stage whether in dorsal position or in the upright position offers different approaches for conducting the birth of a baby.

While the mother is labouring in dorsal position, the obstetrician is in full control of various manoeuvres which may be required to deliver a breech baby. While in the dorsal maternal position, the child's body always requires assistance whether performing Bracht, or Lovset's or any other classical manoeuvre, all of which are more akin to assisting or pulling the baby.

Whereas when the mother is in the upright position, the whole process of birth seems more natural whether it is dealing with shoulder dystocia or applying Louwen's manoeuvre for breech birth, which recommends, 'only push by the mother' but not to pull the baby. There are data to show that this approach has significant advantages as regards neonatal morbidity [9].

52.2.4.5 Analgesia

The impact of epidural anaesthesia on perinatal outcome in breech deliveries is unknown. Women should be informed that the effect

of epidural analgesia on the success of vaginal breech birth is unclear, but that it is likely to increase the risk of intervention [6].

In cases of complete or incomplete breech, wedging of a leading leg within the birth canal could lead to increased pain during birth. Here, an early peridural anaesthesia may be indicated [13].

52.2.4.6 Augmentation and Birth Induction

There are not enough data on birth induction and breech presentation. Therefore, birth induction is not usually recommended. Pregnant women at term with an indication for birth induction otherwise applied in vertex cases (rupture of membranes, overdue pregnancy) should be counselled accordingly in order to support shared decision making. Contractions may be augmented when frequency declines.

52.2.4.7 Unplanned Breech Delivery

If a breech presentation is detected for the first time during labour, obstetricians and the patient should decide together on how to proceed. Resources (skills in vaginal breech birth of the present team, availability of immediate caesarean section) as well as birth progression (rupture of membranes, dilation of the cervix) should be considered. Fetal weight and exact fetal position should be determined by ultrasound if time permits.

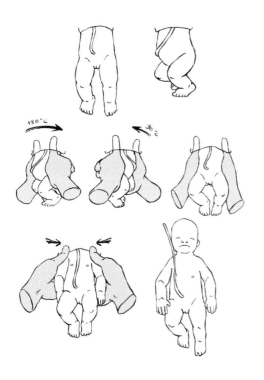

Figure 52.2 Dystocia sign and Frank's nudge manoeuvre

DYSTOCIA
SIGN

MANOEUVRE

FRANK'S
NUDGE

All obstetric departments, whether breech deliveries are routine or not, should employ a standardized way of managing breech presentations in order to limit perinatal morbidity.

A digital assessment of the pelvis, especially of the pubic angle (see also pelvic measurements) is recommended to initially exclude serious complications such as a lingering of the head after birth of the shoulders at breech birth.

52.3 Pelvic Measurements

In midwifery, pelvimetry already plays an important role prior to birth in order to estimate birth outcome. When expecting women are counselled on their baby in breech presentation, it would be helpful to be able to foresee the possibility of a vaginal birth through ruling out a pelvic disproportion. Pelvic measurement is not routinely recommended yet since data are insufficient. There are reports on an association of the mode of delivery and the obstetric conjugate (OC), distance between the sacral promontory and the pubic symphysis, the subpubic angle (PA), the distance between both ischial tuberosities (intertuberous distance, ITD) and the distance between both ischial spines (ISD).

Measurements reported to be in favour for a successful vaginal birth [10–13]

- OC >11.9 cm
- PA >70°
- ITD >10.9 cm
- ISD >10.5 cm

Pelvic measurement can be performed using magnetic resonance imaging (MRI) at the end of pregnancy and through a digital vaginal examination by an experienced obstetrician.

In the digital study, in particular, the conjugate vera obstetrica (OC) and the pubic angle are relevant [14, 15]. However, while OC only correlates with the likelihood of a successful vaginal delivery or caesarean section after onset of labour and rather plays a role in advising the patient, the determination of pubic angle by measuring the intertuberous distance is relevant. For this purpose, the examiner's fist is placed on the mother's perineum. The distance between both ischial tuberosities (intertuberous distance, ITD) can be deduced from the previously determined width of the fist. If the distance is less than 11 cm, the risk of maternal pelvic fixation is highly significant; in some cases, forceps on the head can save aftercoming the life and health of the baby. Therefore, a section is strongly recommended for ITD <11 cm.

52.4 Transverse Presentation

52.4.1 Definition

In transverse presentation, the infant's axis is orthogonal to the mother's axis. There is a dorsointerior and a dorsocranial transverse presentation.

52.4.2 Epidemiology and Aetiology

Transverse presentation at term is mostly found in multiparous women or when uterine malformation or myoma or a placenta praevia which favour abnormal obstetric presentation.

52.4.3 Clinical Management

Although there is not enough evidence, external cephalic version can be offered when there is a transverse presentation at term.

If transverse presentation is recognized after onset of labour, a caesarean section is indicated.

Clinicians should be cautious when rupture of membranes occurs, since there is a high risk for umbilical cord prolapse (especially in a dorsocranial transverse presentation).

52.5 Key Messages

- In breech presentation at term, counselling based on up-to-date data on breech delivery is essential.
- Breech teams should be made available in any greater obstetric department.

- An upright birth position can be preferred in order to enforce 'don't pull, only push'.

52.6 Key Guidelines to the Topic

- *Management of Breech Presentation* (Green-top Guideline No 20b) [6]
- *External Cephalic Version and Reducing the Incidence of Term Breech Presentation* (Green-top Guideline No 20a) [16]

References

1. Hickok DE, Gordon DC, Milberg JA, Williams MA, Daling JR. The frequency of breech presentation by gestational age at birth: a large population-based study. *Am J Obstet Gynecol.* 1992;**166**:851–2. doi: 10.1016/0002-9378(92)91347-d

2. Schmidt S, Norman M, Misselwitz B, et al. Mode of delivery and mortality and morbidity for very preterm singleton infants in a breech position: a European cohort study. *Eur J Obstet Gynecol Reprod Biol.* 2019;**234**:96–102. doi: 10.1016/j.ejogrb.2019.01.003

3. Bergenhenegouwen LA, Meertens LJE, Schaaf J, et al. Vaginal delivery versus caesarean section in preterm breech delivery: a systematic review. *Eur J Obstet Gynecol Reprod Biol.* 2014;**172**:1–6. doi: 10.1016/j.ejogrb.2013.10.017

4. Goffinet F, Carayol M, Foidart J-M, et al. Is planned vaginal delivery for breech presentation at term still an option? Results of an observational prospective survey in France and Belgium. *Am J Obstet Gynecol.* 2006;**194**:1002–1011. doi: 10.1016/j.ajog.2005.10.817

5. Tsakiridis I, Mamopoulos A, Athanasiadis A, Dagklis T. Management of breech presentation: a comparison of four national evidence-based guidelines. *Am J Perinatol.* 2020;**37**(11):1102–9. doi:10.1055/s-0039-1692391

6. Impey LWM, Murphy DJ GM. Management of breech presentation: Green-top Guideline No. 20b. *BJOG.* 2017;**124**:e151–e177. doi: 10.1111/1471-0528.14465

7. Jennewein L, Kielland-Kaisen U, Paul B, et al. Maternal and neonatal outcome after vaginal breech delivery at term of children weighing more or less than 3.8 kg: A FRABAT prospective cohort study. *PLoS One.* 2018;**13**:e0202760. doi: 10.1371/journal.pone.0202760

8. Paul B, Möllmann CJ, Kielland-Kaisen U, et al. Maternal and neonatal outcome after vaginal breech delivery at term after cesarean section – a prospective cohort study of the Frankfurt Breech at Term Cohort (FRABAT). *Eur J Obstet Gynecol Reprod Biol.* 2020;**252**:594–8.

9. Kielland-Kaisen U, Paul B, Jennewein L, et al. Maternal and neonatal outcome after vaginal breech delivery of nulliparous versus multiparous women of singletons at term – a prospective evaluation of the Frankfurt Breech at Term Cohort (FRABAT). *Eur J Obstet Gynecol Reprod Biol.* 2020;**252**:583–7.

10. American College of Obstetricians and Gynecologists; Society for Maternal-Fetal Medicine. ACOG Practice Bulletin No. 144: multifetal gestations: twin, triplet, and higher-order multifetal pregnancies. *Obstet Gynecol.* 2014;**123**:1118–32. doi: 10.1097/01.aog.0000446856.51061.3e

11. Melo P, Georgiou E, Hedditch A, Ellaway P, Impey L. External cephalic version at term: a cohort study of 18 years' experience. *BJOG.* 2019;**126**:493–9. doi:10.1111/1471-0528.15475

12. Louwen F, Daviss BA, Johnson KC, Reitter A. Does breech delivery in an upright position instead of on the back improve outcomes and avoid cesareans? *Int J Gynecol Obstet.* 2017;**136**:151–61. doi:10.1002/ijgo.12033

13. Jennewein L, Allert R, Möllmann CJ, et al. The influence of the fetal leg position on the outcome in vaginally intended deliveries out of breech presentation at term – a FRABAT prospective cohort study. *PLoS One.* 2019;**14**(12).

14. Klemt A-S, Schulze S, Brüggmann D, Louwen F. MRI-based pelvimetric measurements as predictors for a successful vaginal breech delivery in the Frankfurt Breech at term cohort (FRABAT). *Eur J Obstet Gynecol Reprod Biol.* 2019;**232**:10–17. doi: 10.1016/j.ejogrb.2018.09.033

15. Hoffmann J, Thomassen K, Stumpp P, et al. New MRI criteria for successful vaginal breech delivery in primiparae. *PLos One.* 2016;**11**. doi: 10.1371/journal.pone.0161028

16. [No authors listed]. External cephalic version and reducing the incidence of term breech presentation: Green-top Guideline No. 20a. *BJOG.* 2017;**124**: e178–e192. doi: 10.1111/1471-0528.14466

Chapter 53

Intrapartum Emergencies

Nikolaos Vrachnis, Vasilios Pergialiotis & Austin Ugwumadu

53.1 Massive Intrapartum Haemorrhage

Massive obstetric haemorrhage, defined as blood loss ≥1500 mL before or after the delivery of the fetus, occurs in approximately 2–5% of all deliveries [1]. It is the leading cause of maternal mortality worldwide [2]. The most common cause of intrapartum haemorrhage worldwide is obstetric trauma of the female reproductive tract; however, in the developed world, the most common causes are uterine atony, abnormal placentation (including placenta accreta and placenta praevia) and placental abruption. The reader is referred to the relevant chapters on this for more detailed discussions of the clinical problems.

Placental abruption complicates approximately 1% of deliveries and is usually associated with bleeding, abdominal pain, uterine tenderness, tetanic uterine contractions and fetal heart rate abnormalities. The severity of the presenting signs and symptoms correlates with the extent of the abruption; however, some cases of central abruption may be concealed, in which case vaginal bleeding may not be observed. The Royal College of Obstetricians and Gynaecologists (RCOG) proposes that vaginal bleeding be categorized into spotting, minor (blood loss is <50 mL), major (blood loss between 50 and 1000 mL) and massive (when it exceeds 1000 mL) [1]. Risk factors associated with placental abruption are presented in

Table 53.1. However, approximately 70% of cases of abruption occur in low-risk pregnancies.

When placental abruption is suspected, other causes of intrapartum haemorrhage including placenta praevia and trauma should be ruled out. The status of the woman should be evaluated using the ABCDE (Airway, Breathing, Circulation, Disability and Exposure) criteria and, following that, intrapartum evaluation of fetal well-being using cardiotocography (CTG) and, if possible, fetal ultrasound is recommended. Two large-bore intravenous catheters should be inserted and rigorous fluid resuscitation offered using crystalloids. Transfusion of red blood cells and blood products is guided by the results of full blood count (FBC) [3]. In most cases, placental abruption is diagnosed in the first stage of labour; hence, CTG will guide the decision concerning the optimal mode of delivery. However, when the mother is in hypovolaemic shock due to massive bleeding, caesarean section (CS) is the safest option. A Kleihauer–Betke test is necessary in rhesus-negative mothers to determine the optimal dose of anti-D immunoglobulin [1].

53.2 Rupture of the Uterus

Uterine rupture is a rare obstetric complication in developed countries, with an incidence of 1 in 3000–5000 [4] in contrast to low-income countries with an estimated incidence of 1 in 80 pregnancies. Common underlying factors that increase the risk for uterine rupture are presented in Table 53.2 [5]. Very rarely, uterine rupture may result from blunt or penetrating trauma to the abdominal cavity. The American College of Obstetricians and Gynecologists (ACOG) [6], the RCOG [7] and other international bodies have recently advocated vaginal birth after caesarean section (VBAC) and trial of labour after caesarean section (TOLAC) in an effort to reduce escalating caesarean section rates. These policies are expected to lead to a rise in the risk of uterine rupture in the coming years.

Depending on the severity of the defect, uterine rupture can result in variable degrees of maternal and/or fetal/neonatal

Table 53.1 Risk factors associated with placental abruption

Multiparity

Pre-eclampsia

Fetal growth restriction

Polyhydramnios

Non-vertex presentation

Assisted reproductive techniques

Intrauterine infection

Premature rupture of the membranes (PROM)

Abdominal trauma

Large intramural myomas

Smoking

Drug abuse

Low maternal body mass index (BMI)

Table 53.2 Risk factors for uterine rupture

Grand multiparity

Previous hysterotomy (caesarean section, myomectomy)

Obstructed labour

Operative obstetric manoeuvres (external cephalic version, inappropriate use of metallic forceps and rotational forceps manoeuvres)

Table 53.3 Signs and symptoms of uterine rupture

Abdominal pain

Presence of fetal parts intra-abdominally

Cessation of uterine contractions

Disengagement of the fetal part

Hypovolaemic shock (tachypnoea, tachycardia)

Fetal hypoxia

Fetal bradycardia

Maternal bradycardia

Asystole

morbidity and mortality. Mild defects that do not bleed may result in subtle signs and symptoms, including mild lower abdominal pain that is mainly perceived as tenderness at the site of a previous caesarean section. However, if the defect extends laterally, towards the ascending branches of the uterine vessels and the broad ligament, the symptomatology becomes severe (Table 53.3) [8]. Other suggestive signs of imminent pathology include bleeding through the vagina and gross haematuria, although these are rarer, as they are mainly associated with lower extension of the defect: the latter is generally not expected, unless this occurs in previous vertical scars (such as those of prior myomectomy).

Given the variable symptomatology, vigilance is essential in women with risk factors for uterine rupture to initiate emergency caesarean section and achieve good maternal and neonatal outcomes. Several reports have advocated the use of the double-layer closure technique to reduce the rate of rupture, although a recent meta-analysis does not seem to support this approach [9].

The principles of ABCDE resuscitation should be followed in the event of a uterine rupture. A large-bore vascular access should be inserted as soon as possible (16 G or wider). The need for a central venous line should be individualized and on a case-by-case basis. Blood group and crossmatching and a complete blood count should be undertaken and vigorous fluid resuscitation commenced using crystalloids. In most cases, a Pfannenstiel incision is sufficient to complete the caesarean section and repair the defect. However, in patients with haemodynamic collapse, a midline incision may be deemed more appropriate to achieve a better operating field. Exteriorization of the uterus is required to fully visualize the uterus and parametria and to repair the defect. In cases with extension of the scar to the broad ligament, care should be taken not to injure the ureter, which crosses the uterine artery and runs near the lateral border of the uterus. Operating safely in the retroperitoneal space is outside the remit of the average obstetrician, and if this is necessary assistance should be sought from general and/or vascular surgeons. If bleeding is profuse and prevents proper visualization of the surgical field, consideration should be given to compression of the lower aorta to minimize blood loss. In some cases, ligation of the internal iliac

vein may effectively control the bleeding. This should be performed below the level of the superior gluteal artery. Continuous oozing from the bleeding site may be seen. This may be managed by abdominal packing with a Bogota bag (a sterile plastic bag used for temporary closure of abdominal wounds), and second-look definitive surgery 24 hours later, provided that the patient is stable. Caesarean hysterectomy may be needed in uncontrollable haemorrhage. Bladder laceration may require the input of a urologist or repaired in two layers. Abdominal drains should be inserted and antibiotic prophylaxis and thromboprophylaxis given. Pregnancy should be avoided for at least 18 months after a uterine rupture and elective caesarean section offered after 34 completed weeks of gestation [10].

53.3 Perineal Trauma

Perineal trauma is a common complication of vaginal delivery, either from an episiotomy or the result of stretching and rupture of the soft tissues during delivery of the fetus. The incidence may be up to 85% of vaginal deliveries. Some factors such as primiparity, fetal macrosomia, gestational diabetes, previous vaginal surgery and operative vaginal delivery with forceps or vacuum appear to increase the risk of perineal trauma [11].

Perineal trauma is classified into four degrees (Table 53.4). Anal sphincter tear is termed obstetric anal sphincter injury (OASIS) in the literature and is associated with incontinence of faeces, fluid or flatus, and adverse effect on women's quality of life [12, 13]. Women with minor and intermediate degrees of tear have reduced risk of anal incontinence compared to women with tears of stage >3b. Anal sphincter tear should be sought and ascertained and, if this present, an evaluation of the integrity of the internal and external anal sphincters is paramount with a view to repairing them separately. To accomplish this, the index finger should be inserted into the anal canal to palpate the internal and external anal sphincter. Unfortunately, suboptimal clinical diagnosis of OASIS ranges between 20 and 40% of cases.

To repair the defect, appropriate analgesia should be provided (either local or regional) and an absorbable material used to reduce the risk of surgical site infection and persistent pain, which may arise as the result of excessive tissue fibrosis (polyglactin 910 sutures are preferred (Vicryl®)). End-to-end suturing of the anal sphincter using a continuous non-locking technique ensures tissue approximation and avoids excessive tension. When the trauma extends to the anal epithelium (fourth degree laceration), a 3/0 Vicryl® should be used, taking care to tie the knots within the anal canal to reduce the odds of the patient developing an anal fistula. Cases treated for OASIS should receive a 7-day course of antibiotics to lower the risk of developing surgical site infection, while stool softeners should be used to decrease the risk of wound disruption.

Women who have sustained OASIS have increased risk of developing anal incontinence. Previous studies have suggested that anal squeeze pressure and/or sonographic evidence of sphincter defects may be used as prognostic markers for recurrent complication in subsequent pregnancies; however, the implications for clinical practice are as yet undetermined.

Table 53.4 Categorization of perineal lacerations

First degree	Laceration of the superficial skin and/or vaginal epithelium that is limited to the vaginal introitus
Second degree	Tearing of underlying muscles (superficial transverse perineal muscle, the deep transverse perineal muscle and bulbocavernosus) with an intact anal sphincter
Third degree	• Tearing of the anal sphincter of variable severity • 3a: less than 50% of the external anal sphincter • 3b: more than 50% of the external anal sphincter • 3c: tearing of the internal anal sphincter
Fourth degree	Disruption of the anal epithelium

Several techniques have been described to reduce the risk of developing perineal trauma including episiotomy, antenatal perineal massage and perineal support; however, results of randomized trials of their efficacy are conflicting and their clinical utility doubtful.

53.4 Umbilical Cord Prolapse

Umbilical cord prolapse is associated with a high risk of fetal asphyxia and mortality may reach 10%. It is widely believed that exposure of the umbilical cord to the relatively cooler temperature of the vagina or external environment results in spasm of the umbilical cord vessels and compromise of the blood flow. Alternatively, the umbilical cord vessels may become occluded by mechanical compression against fetal or maternal structures. The risk of cord prolapse increases with abnormalities of fetal presentation such as transverse or oblique lie, footling and flexed breech presentation. Other risk factors include polyhydramnios, premature rupture of the membranes, preterm birth, multiple gestation and obstetric interventions such as amniotomy, external cephalic version and internal podalic version.

There are no reliable screening tests for cord prolapse; however, caution in the management of specific clinical situation, such as abnormal fetal lie, unengaged fetus, and low-lying placenta, may reduce the risk of cord prolapse. Immediate fetal compromise does not follow all cases of cord prolapse, and fetal heart abnormalities may be subtle in the early stages of the process. Obstetricians and midwives should aim to exclude cord prolapse or cord presentation whenever they undertake vaginal examination. Amniotomy should be performed after fetal head engagement to minimize the possibility of cord prolapse. If the umbilical cord is palpated below or by the side of the presenting part, amniotomy is contraindicated, and in the absence of fetal heart rate (FHR) abnormalities, there is no requirement to dislodge the fetal part as this may lead to the descent of further loops of cord.

Women with abnormal fetal lie are at increased risk of developing umbilical cord prolapse and a trial of external cephalic version should be offered at 37 weeks. If the lie is deemed to be unstable or when there is external cephalic version (ECV), it would be prudent to consider admission of these women at 38 weeks of gestation [14]. Otherwise, these women should be carefully instructed to return to the hospital immediately if they experience signs of labour or rupture of the membranes.

If umbilical cord prolapse is diagnosed, immediate call for help should be made and the anaesthetist and neonatologist summoned to attend the delivery of the fetus. Baseline blood count and serum save should be done if not already and a large-bore (14 or 16 G) venous cannula inserted. Caesarean section is required if the woman is in the first stage of labour, or not in labour at all, and the fetus is alive. On the other hand, it is reasonable to undertake assisted vaginal delivery if the woman is in the second stage of labour, particularly if she is parous, as this is likely to be a faster and safer alternative. If there is no CTG recording, the fetal heart rate should be evaluated with a handheld Doppler device or ultrasound scan to exclude fetal compromise. If none of these is available, the FHR may be determined with a fetal stethoscope or by gently palpating the cord, bearing in mind that this may induce cord spasm. If there are FHR abnormalities, the mother should be placed in a knee-chest position in an effort to use gravity to decompress the umbilical cord. Displacement (elevation) of the fetal part is also recommended when caesarean section is planned, and continuous transvaginal digital pressure is the best way to alleviate cord compression. The obstetrician should beware that replacing the umbilical cord back into the uterus may be accompanied by vasospasm. If this procedure is indicated, the clinician should be gentle and, ideally, cradle the cord with saline-soaked gauze. Alternatively, instilling normal saline into the urinary bladder via a catheter may be used to encourage dislodgement of the presenting part as the bladder distends.

Tocolytics may be administered if there is fetal bradycardia (preferably terbutaline 0.25 mg subcutaneously) to resuscitate the fetus whilst definitive management is in progress.

53.5 Shoulder Dystocia

Shoulder dystocia occurs when one or both fetal shoulders are impacted against the bony maternal pelvis following the delivery of the head. It complicates between 0.6 and 1.4% of vaginal deliveries [15] and is associated with fetal hypoxic and traumatic injury, and in rare cases mortality. Maternal morbidity may also occur. Shoulder dystocia occurs more frequently in macrosomic babies; however, it is also seen in a significant proportion of infants of average birthweight. Women with pre-existing or gestational diabetes or obesity, women who gained excessive weight during the index pregnancy (≥20 kg) and those with prior history of shoulder dystocia have increased risk of developing this complication [16]. Intrapartum factors associated with increased odds of shoulder dystocia include operative vaginal delivery and marked prolongation of the second stage of labour.

The diagnosis is suspected if the fetal head retracts back into the vagina between uterine contractions / maternal pushing ('turtle sign') or restitution of the fetal head fails to occur.

Shoulder dystocia should be resolved in a timely and efficient manner to avoid significant fetal hypoxia. However, the manoeuvres should be gentle to avoid injury to the fetus and/or the mother. Several manoeuvres have been described to overcome this complication and mnemonics have been developed to assist memory and a systematic approach to management. However, an individualized approach is generally considered, as each case is different and may not be resolved by any particular manoeuvre. First, help must be sought as soon as possible and a scribe should record the times of key events such as head-to-body delivery interval and the time and numbers of attempted manoeuvres. The woman should be instructed to discontinue pushing and any further traction should be ceased, as both increase the impaction of shoulders and render essential manoeuvres difficult to accomplish. Her buttocks should be placed at and just hanging beyond the edge of the bed so that the space beneath is available for manipulating the fetus. Although mnemonic rules have been described in the literature, most of the manoeuvres break down into disimpaction, simple, rotative and advanced [17].

- Disimpaction: This may be accomplished by hyperflexing the mother's hips by pulling her thighs over her abdomen (McRoberts manoeuvre) and applying gentle suprapubic pressure.
- Simple manoeuvres: Episiotomy is usually performed to make room for the hand for rotative manoeuvres.
- Rotative manoeuvres: Shoulder rotation is attempted to disengage the anterior shoulder and place it at the larger transverse pelvic diameter (Woods screw manoeuvre). the obstetrician uses the same hand to perform the Woods screw manoeuvre (right hand for right fetal shoulder and vice versa) and places it posteriorly by applying gentle pressure (Figure 53.1). If this fails, a reverse Woods screw manoeuvre is attempted by placing the opposite hand on the front side of the shoulder and applying counterpressure. Release of the posterior arm is undertaken following a successful screw manoeuvre by inserting a hand in the posterior vaginal wall and retrieving the fetal forearm by flexing it at the elbow and subsequently the shoulder. This is more safely done with the index finger and thumb only rather than with a grip and traction.
- Rotation of the mother on all four and trying to deliver.
- Advanced manoeuvres (to be used only when everything else fails): If the above manoeuvres fail to successfully deliver the baby, cleidotomy should be attempted by applying pressure with the index finger on the fetal clavicle in a cephalad direction (caudal direction may result in significant bleeding, as it may traumatize the subclavian vessels). Symphysiotomy has also been described as a solution; however, it may be accompanied by significant maternal morbidity as it can cause significant trauma to the female urogenital system (including the urethra) and, if appropriate care is not applied to support the pelvis during delivery of the fetus, severe fractures may occur. The Zavanelli procedure refers to repositioning the fetus back into the uterus and completion of the delivery with CS. This is not an atraumatic or risk-free procedure and it is associated with severe maternal and neonatal morbidity and mortality. It is therefore, reserved and/or attempted as a last resort.

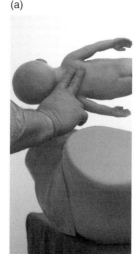
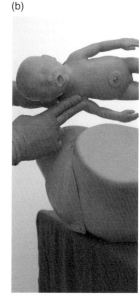

Figure 53.1 Woods screw manoeuvre for disengagement of the anterior shoulder. (a) Using the fingers of the right hand for the right fetal shoulder (and vice versa for the left) placed posteriorly and applying gentle pressure. (b) Assisting the back pressure using the fingers of the opposite hand on the front side of the shoulder to apply pressure. A black and white version of this figure will appear in some formats. For the colour version, please refer to the plate section.

53.6 Uterine Inversion

Uterine inversion is a rare obstetric complication of the third stage of labour and is associated with significant maternal morbidity and mortality. The incidence ranges from 1 in 2000 to 1 in 23 000 deliveries. Several risk factors have been implicated in the pathogenesis of this complication, including morbidly adherent placenta, cord traction prior to placental separation, manual removal of the placenta, uterine overdistention (multiple pregnancy and polyhydramnios), fetal macrosomia, precipitate delivery, use of tocolytics and a previous history of uterine inversion [18]. Uterine inversion results from the protrusion of the relaxed uterus through the dilated cervix. The condition may arise either within 24 hours postpartum (acute), or within 4 weeks from delivery (subacute), or even later (chronic). It is subdivided into:

- Grade 1: inversion of the uterine fundus with the uterine body in the peritoneal cavity
- Grade 2: protrusion of the uterine fundus from the ectocervix
- Grade 3: inversion of the uterus below the level of the vaginal introitus
- Grade 4: complete inversion of the uterus and the vagina

Of these, Grade 2 is most commonly seen, though the most severe form is by far that of complete inversion. The most common sign of uterine inversion is the presence of shock. During the early stages uterine inversion, neurogenic shock can result as the peritoneum, ligaments and ovaries progressively protrude below the level of the external cervical os, producing significant pain. As the process continues, the accumulation of blood in the uterine body, via the arterial supply, results in significant tissue oedema that renders the retraction of the uterine body through the cervical ring even more difficult (uterine entrapment). It is therefore easily understood that early management of uterine inversion is critical to avoid these effects, which may aggravate the morbidity. Help must be sought immediately, and aggressive fluid resuscitation initiated, as blood loss is usually significant and often underestimated. The neurogenic shock is reversed when the uterus is repositioned.

Several techniques to reposition the uterus and restore normal reproductive anatomy have been described. Manual replacement is the most commonly described and used. The obstetrician inserts his/her hand and forearm in the vagina and grasps the uterine fundus with the palm, taking care to palpate the isthmus with the fingertips (Figure 53.2). Gradual pressure of the uterine fundus towards the umbilicus helps dilate the cervical ring and reposition the uterus in its normal position. The success rate of this technique is variable and ranges between 40 and 90% of cases. Any attempt to remove a retained placenta should be performed after the uterus has been repositioned, to avoid exacerbating the morbidity further. The use of hydrostatic pressure to replace the inverted uterus has been described. This involves the instillation of 4–5 litres of fluid in the vagina to restore the uterus to its normal position. However, this technique is difficult to accomplish because fluid loss through the introitus makes the intravaginal pressure >150 mm Hg required to achieve replacement of the uterus difficult to achieve. The use of the Bakri balloon has also been described and may minimize blood loss after repositioning the uterus. Tocolysis is seldom used, as it may aggravate the blood loss and hypovolaemic shock; however, when necessary, terbutaline should be used (0.25 mg IV at a slow infusion rate). This allows rapid discontinuation and reversal of any adverse effect on the cardiovascular system given its short half-life. If these manoeuvres fail, laparotomy is performed, and the uterine fundus repositioned by Allis forceps or sutures. If the cervical ring is very constricted, hindering restoration of the uterus, its posterior aspect may be incised (Haultain manoeuvre). If all of

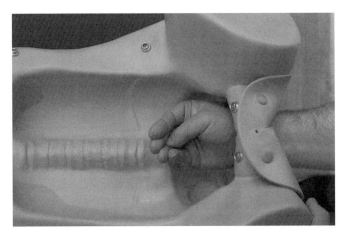

Figure 53.2 Proper placement of two thirds of the hand and the forearm in the vagina to perform elevation of the inverted uterine fundus towards the abdominal cavity. Keeping fingers as shown at the level of the uterine isthmus, proceed to lift the fundus of the uterus above the umbilicus. A black and white version of this figure will appear in some formats. For the colour version, please refer to the plate section.

the aforementioned procedures fail, then hysterectomy is the treatment of last resort.

Timing of the need for and administration of general anaesthesia is of great value in these patients. If manual replacement fails, the patient should be transferred to the operating room and general anaesthesia should be administered to eliminate pain and enable more manipulation and manoeuvres. This condition is rare and individual obstetricians are unlikely to have acquired extensive experience during the course of their careers.

53.7 Amniotic Fluid Embolism

The incidence of amniotic fluid embolism (AFE) is estimated to range between 1.25 in 100 000 and 12.5 in 100 000 maternities [19]. Survival rates have increased over time. In 1979, survival after AFE was reported to be only 14%, but had risen to 30% and 80% in 2005 and 2010, respectively [20]. Permanent neurological deficit following AFE still remains high, reported to occur in up to 85% of cases.

It was proposed and accepted for many decades that amniotic fluid debris escaped into the venous circulation, leading to pulmonary vascular obstruction and oedema. However, in 1995 Clark et al reported that a significant proportion of women who suffered AFE had a personal history of allergic reactions [20]. This is consistent with current thinking that the passage of minimal volumes of amniotic fluid (<1 mL) may induce an allergic-anaphylactoid response of variable severity. Several risk factors have been described, including operative delivery, cervical trauma, polyhydramnios, twin pregnancy, placental accreta or praevia, prostaglandin E_2 induction of labour excluding oxytocin administration for augmentation of labour. Given its rarity, AFE remains an unpredictable and unpreventable obstetric emergency.

In the full syndrome, AFE is characterized by haemodynamic shock, severe coagulopathy and tissue hypoxia (including myocardial and central nervous system ischaemia). The condition may develop within minutes or hours and is usually observed intrapartum or immediately postpartum. Sporadic cases of amniotic fluid embolism following dilation and evacuation have been reported. National registries were developed for centralized case reporting using diagnostic criteria of variable specificity resulting in heterogeneous interpretation of the disease and lack of consensus to guide research and practice. As a consequence, Clark et al in 2016 proposed a set of specific criteria for the case definition of AFE including:

- Acute hypotension (systolic blood pressure <90 mm Hg) and respiratory dysfunction (dyspnoea, cyanosis, SpO₂ <90% or cardiorespiratory arrest)
- Coagulopathy manifesting as disseminated intravascular coagulation or severe otherwise unexplained blood loss
- Establishment of these symptoms either intrapartum or within 30 minutes postpartum
- Absence of fever during labour (temperature <38°C) [21]

Amniotic fluid embolism has a progressive symptomatology beginning with pulmonary hypertension (attributed to debris or vascular constriction), ultimately leading to left ventricular dysfunction and failure [22]. Coagulopathy may be observed in survivors, with the haemorrhage exacerbating the cardiovascular instability. Cardiac arrest occurs as the result of either asystole, pulseless electrical activity or ventricular fibrillation [23].

53.8 Neonatal Resuscitation

Neonatal resuscitation may be required in a planned delivery because of an antenatal maternal and/or fetal pathology. In this scenario, detailed assessment of the perinatal risks is crucial and a multidisciplinary meeting may be required to decide the optimal time and mode of delivery. Outside of this context, the first question that needs to be addressed when considering neonatal resuscitation is the gestational age of the neonate. Following its delivery, a quick assessment may be attempted using the Apgar score, noting, however, that its use in premature fetuses is limited. An Apgar score >7 at 5 minutes is considered indicative of good neonatal outcome, and when the newborn has good tone and is breathing or crying it is generally accepted that it is safe for it to stay with the mother. However, when this is not the case, appropriate measures should be taken to keep it dry, clear the airway (usually using a bulb syringe or a suction catheter) and ensure that it is exposed to the appropriate temperature (generally between 36.5°C and 37.5°C). Special care should be taken of preterm newborns, as they are particularly prone to hypothermia, which in turn is associated with co-morbidity, including hypoglycaemia, increased risk of intraventricular haemorrhage and sepsis. The American Heart Association released an updated algorithm in 2015 that should be followed vigorously to optimize neonatal outcome of newborns at risk [24].

Special rules that need to be borne in mind during newborn resuscitation are the following:

- Chest compressions should be performed at the lower part of the sternum, seeking to reach a depth equal to one third of the anteroposterior chest diameter.
- Chest compressions should be performed along with ventilation at a ratio of 3:1. Proper neonatal ventilation requires adequate support of the mandible to ensure an open upper airway (Figure 53.3). Care should be taken to coordinate these manoeuvres in order to avoid their simultaneous delivery. The American Heart Association suggests that approximately 90 compressions and 30 ventilations should be delivered each minute to ensure appropriate resuscitation.
- The use of adrenaline is seldom required in neonatal resuscitation, as it is generally accepted that appropriate ventilation and chest compressions effectively reverse bradycardia. However, if the heart rate persists below 60 beats per minute (bpm), then intravenous administration of adrenaline should be considered at a dose of 0.01 to 0.03 mg/ kg of 1:10 000 epinephrine.
- Volume expansion should be restricted in cases of suspected blood loss (when the neonate is pale). Isotonic solutions are preferred and a recommended dose of 10 mL/kg is initially administered that may be repeated if needed.
- Resuscitated newborns are at risk of hypoglycaemia, intraventricular haemorrhage and sepsis and should be followed up during the first days of life to ensure their well-being.

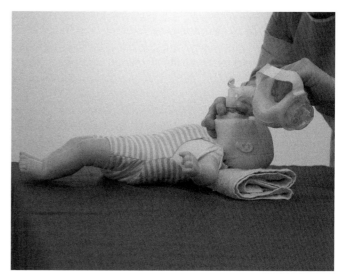

Figure 53.3 Proper neonatal ventilation requires adequate support of the mandible to ensure an open upper airway. A black and white version of this figure will appear in some formats. For the colour version, please refer to the plate section.

53.9 Key Messages

- Massive intrapartum haemorrhage is encountered in 2–5% of all deliveries. Early detection is critical in preventing haemodynamic instability and shock. Uterine atony, trauma, abnormal placentation and uterine rupture should be considered.
- Uterine rupture is relatively rare; however, this is expected to increase in the coming decades with increased uptake of VBAC and TOLAC.
- Given the variable symptomatology in uterine rupture, vigilance is mandatory in at-risk women.
- Perineal trauma occurs in up to 85% of vaginal deliveries. Severe trauma involving >50% of the anal sphincter may result in anal incontinence. Early identification and meticulous repair are essential to reduce the risks of anal incontinence.
- Umbilical cord prolapse is rare. However, clinicians should have raised awareness in women with risk factors such as non-cephalic presentation and prematurity.
- Manoeuvres to resolve shoulder dystocia may be classified into *disimpactive, simple,* and *rotative.* An understanding of how they work may help recall in an emergency.
- Uterine inversion is very rare, and most obstetricians are unlikely to encounter many such cases. Early identification is essential to reduce the risk of severe morbidity and mortality associated with inversion of the uterus below the introitus.
- Amniotic fluid embolism can be fatal. Further research is needed to reach a consensus concerning its management.
- Neonatal resuscitation should be primarily based on adequate oxygenation and chest compressions of the newborn. Fluid expansion and the use of vasotonic agents should be restricted for selected cases where aggressive cardiopulmonary resuscitation have failed.

53.10 Key Guidelines Relevant to the Topic

- Massive intrapartum haemorrhage remains the most common obstetric emergency and obstetric trauma represents the most common underlying cause.
- Aggressive resuscitation is of paramount importance in maternal and neonatal intrapartum emergencies.
- Risk factors for uterine rupture should always be taken into account when attempting a VBAC or TOLAC procedure.
- Specific criteria for the definition of amniotic fluid embolism are required to help future researchers reach firm conclusions regarding its management and, thus, reduce maternal morbidity and mortality rates.
- Uterine inversion remains an extremely rare obstetric emergency and its early identification is of high importance to minimize maternal complications and mortality.
- Whereas maternal resuscitation is mainly based on fluid replenishment, neonatal resuscitation primarily involves adequate tissue oxygenation that is mainly accomplished through chest compressions and ventilation support.

References

1. *Antepartum Haemorrhage*, Green-top Guideline No 63. London: Royal College of Obstetricians and Gynaecologists, 2011. Accessed from www.rcog.org.uk/en/guidelines-research-services/guidelines/gtg63/.

2. Say L, Chou D, Gemmill A, et al. Global causes of maternal death: a WHO systematic analysis. *Lancet Glob Health.* 2014 Jun;**2**(6):e323-33.

3. Alexander JM, Wortman AC. Intrapartum hemorrhage. *Obstet Gynecol Clin North Am.* 2013 Mar;**40**(1):15–26.

4. Kieser KE, Baskett TF. A 10-year population-based study of uterine rupture. *Obstet Gynecol.* 2002 Oct;**100**(4):749–53.

5. Zwart JJ, Richters JM, Ory F, et al. Uterine rupture in the Netherlands: a nationwide population-based cohort study. *BJOG.* 2009 Jul;**116**(8):1069–78; discussion 78–80.

6. American College of Obstetricians and Gynecologists. ACOG practice bulletin no. *115*: vaginal birth after previous cesarean delivery. *Obstet Gynecol.* 2010 Aug; **116**(2 Pt 1): 450–63.

7. *Birth after Previous Caesarean Birth*, Green-top Guideline No 45. London: Royal College of Obstetricians and Gynaecologists, 2015. www.rcog.org.uk/en/guidelines-research-services/guidelines/gtg45/.

8. Vlemminx MW, de Lau H, Oei SG. Tocogram characteristics of uterine rupture: a systematic review. *Arch Gynecol Obstet.* 2017 Jan;**295**(1):17–26.

9. Stegwee SI, Jordans I, van der Voet LF, et al. Uterine caesarean closure techniques affect ultrasound findings and maternal outcomes: a systematic review and meta-analysis. *BJOG.* 2018 Aug;**125**(9):1097–108.

10. Bujold E, Gauthier RJ. Risk of uterine rupture associated with an interdelivery interval between 18 and 24 months. *Obstet Gynecol.* 2010 May;**115**(5):1003–6.

11. *Management of Third and Fourth Degree Perineal Tears*, Green-top Guideline No 29. London: Royal College of Obstetricians and Gynaecologists, 2007.

12. Roos AM, Thakar R, Sultan AH. Outcome of primary repair of obstetric anal sphincter injuries (OASIS): does the grade of tear matter? *Ultrasound Obstet Gynecol.* 2010 Sep;**36**(3):368–74.

13. Norderval S, Rossaak K, Markskog A, Vonen B. Incontinence after primary repair of obstetric anal sphincter tears is related to relative length of reconstructed external sphincter: a case-control study. *Ultrasound Obstet Gynecol.* 2012 Aug;**40**(2):207–14.

14. Szaboova R, Sankaran S, Harding K, Shennan A. PLD.23 Management of transverse and unstable lie at term. *Arch Dis Child Fetal Neonatal Ed.* 2014;**99**(Suppl 1):A112–A13. doi: 10.1136/archdischild-2014-306576.324

15.. *Shoulder Dystocia*, Green-top Guideline No 42. London: Royal College of Obstetricians and Gynaecologists, 2012.

16. Committee on Practice Bulletins – Obstetrics. Practice Bulletin No 178: Shoulder Dystocia. *Obstet Gynecol.* 2017 May;**129**(5):e123–e33.

17. Hoffman MK, Bailit JL, Branch DW, et al. A comparison of obstetric maneuvers for the acute management of shoulder dystocia. *Obstet Gynecol.* 2011 Jun;**117**(6):1272–8.

18. Thakur M, Thakur A. Uterine inversion. In *StatPearls* [Internet]. Treasure Island, FL: StatPearls Publishing; 2018 Jan–. [Updated 2018 Oct 27]. www.ncbi.nlm.nih.gov/books/NBK525971/.

19. *Maternal Collapse in Pregnancy and the Puerperium*, Green-top Guideline No 56. London: Royal College of Obstetricians and Gynaecologists, 2011.

20. Clark SL, Hankins GD, Dudley DA, Dildy GA, Porter TF. Amniotic fluid embolism: analysis of the national registry. *Am J Obstet Gynecol.* 1995 Apr;**172**(4 Pt 1):1158–67; discussion 67–9.

21. Clark SL, Romero R, Dildy GA, et al. Proposed diagnostic criteria for the case definition of amniotic fluid embolism in research studies. *Am J Obstet Gynecol.* 2016;**215**(4):408–12.

22. Indraccolo U, Battistoni C, Mastrantonio I, et al. Risk factors for fatality in amniotic fluid embolism: a systematic review and analysis of a data pool. *J Matern Fetal Neonatal Med.* 2018 Mar;**31**(5):661–5.

23. Pacheco LD, Saade G, Hankins GDV, Clark SL. Amniotic fluid embolism: diagnosis and management. *Am J Obst Gynecol.* 2016;**215**(2):B16–B24.

24. *Part 13: Neonatal Resuscitation*. Web-based Integrated 2010 & 2015 American Heart Association Guidelines for Cardiopulmonary Resuscitation and Emergency Cardiovascular Care. https://eccguidelines.heart.org/index.php/circulation/cpr-ecc-guidelines-2/part-13-neonatal-resuscitation/

Caesarean Section

Charles Bircher & Edward Prosser-Snelling

54.1 Introduction

Caesarean section is the most commonly performed obstetric operation. A woman's first caesarean section is generally an easy operation. Obstetricians are the only surgeons who routinely operate on the same surgical scar, and a third or fourth caesarean section can be a very challenging operation indeed. There is no question that a caesarean section is a lifesaving operation, but in the modern world the expectation from the women we serve is that it will also be a safe one, with as few side effects as possible. It is hoped that some of the information in this chapter will help you to achieve that.

54.1.1 Epidemiology and Phenomenology

54.1.1.1 What Is the Safest Way to Deliver a Baby?

Historically, there has been an assumption that vaginal birth is safest for the mother and baby. While this may be true, good, reliable evidence as to the safest way to deliver a baby is sorely lacking. More than this, it is unfair to compare caesarean section with vaginal birth. No woman going into labour is guaranteed a vaginal delivery. When looking for the safest way to deliver a baby, you must compare planned caesarean section with planned vaginal delivery. When examining evidence, the National Institute for Health and Care Excellence (NICE) and the American College of Obstetricians and Gynecologists (ACOG) both point to this lack of evidence in this area [1, 2].

In terms of maternal outcomes, the only variables with moderate-quality evidence were that postpartum haemorrhage is less frequent with planned caesarean section, and the length of hospital stay is shorter with vaginal delivery (although in terms of length of stay, this is not a *planned* vaginal delivery, rather a vaginal delivery, so this is not a true comparison). Other maternal outcomes have poor-quality evidence, but in studies, when compared with planned vaginal delivery, planned caesarean section has a higher risk of cardiac arrest, wound haematoma, hysterectomy, major infections, anaesthetic complications and venous thromboembolism, and lower risks of obstetric sphincter damage, pelvic organ prolapse and stress urinary incontinence [1, 2].

When looking at neonatal outcomes, the only variable with moderate-quality evidence was transient neonatal respiratory morbidity, and this is gestation dependent and may not be true if the caesarean is done after 39 weeks. Other neonatal outcomes are from poor evidence, but studies show planned caesarean reduces the risk of low Apgar scores, neonatal intensive care admission and neonatal infection rates [1, 2].

In the long term, having a caesarean section certainly increases the risk of placenta praevia and accreta spectrum in subsequent pregnancies. When considering the safest mode of delivery for the mother, future plans need to be part of the discussion. This leads to a discussion about maternal-request caesarean section. Both NICE and the ACOG support the fact that vaginal birth is safe, but also support women when they make the choice to deliver by caesarean section. When offering a choice, you should not decline a woman's choice when you do not agree with it. The evidence does not support planned caesarean as the safest mode of delivery, but it also does not support planned vaginal delivery. A full discussion about why a woman makes the choice is vital. Some reasons may be addressed, such as a fear of pain. Others, such as a history of abuse or true fear of labour, may not. When discussing risks and benefits of any choice, it is important to individualize them to the woman and not just talk generally. Do not dismiss reasonable requests; rather, offer support and reassurance about the safety of vaginal delivery.

54.1.1.2 Global Perspective / Increasing Use

In 1985, the World Health Organization (WHO) proposed an ideal caesarean section rate between 10 and 15%. Since 1985, caesarean rates have significantly increased, in both developed and developing countries. In 2015, the WHO released a statement looking to revisit these increasing rates. Their statement recommends that at a population level, rates below 10% demonstrate inadequate access to healthcare, but rates greater than 10% do not improve maternal or neonatal mortality (they do not comment on morbidity). In the same year, it is estimated globally that 21% of births were by caesarean section, a number which has almost doubled since 2000 [3]. There is huge global variation in rates, with rates 10 times higher in Latin America and the Caribbean (44%) compared to West and Central Africa (4%). Within these rates, there is significant socio-economic variation, with rates higher in wealthier women in low- and middle-income countries. And worldwide caesarean sections are 1.6 times more common in private versus public healthcare facilities [3].

There remains great debate as to the 'correct' acceptable caesarean rate. In the WHO 2015 statement, they recommend avoiding specific target rates, rather focusing on offering caesareans to those who need it. In the *Lancet* paper looking at global epidemiology of the use of caesareans [3], the authors point out the stark difference in rates from country to country, suggesting there is an overuse in some, with 63% of the countries reporting rates greater than 15%, but poor access in others, with 28% reporting rates less than 10%. Rates were significantly higher in countries with higher levels of socio-economic development, higher levels of net female enrolment in secondary education, higher levels of urbanization, greater density of physicians and lower levels of fertility. These inequalities are complex and difficult to address. What remains clear is a caesarean section is a potentially lifesaving operation that all women should have access to, but it has significant risks associated with it, including long-term consequences. Therefore, it is a procedure to be instigated in correct situations.

54.2 Indications

The following list of indications is not exhaustive and decisions as to mode of delivery need to be made on an individual basis. There is no definitive algorithm for obstetricians to follow when deciding about caesarean section. There are relatively few absolute indications for caesarean section. However, there are a number of common indications where it is felt vaginal delivery poses higher risks, and generally these can be divided into maternal and fetal indications.

54.2.1 Relative Indications

54.2.1.1 Maternal

- More than two previous caesarean sections
- Previous classical uterine incision
- Other uterine surgery that involves full thickness of the myometrium and the upper segment, such as myomectomy or hysterotomy
- Obstructive lesions in lower genital tract, such as fibroids or a vaginal septum
- Maternal medical conditions that mean the pressure caused by pushing should be avoided, such as certain cardiac conditions or retinal detachment
- Previous vaginal or perineal corrective surgery that is likely to be damaged by vaginal delivery, such as vaginal prolapse repairs or some bowel surgeries; previous fourth degree perineal tear, and in some situations, previous third degree tear
- Maternal request

54.2.1.2 Fetal

- Abnormal lies or non-vertex presentation
- Monoamniotic twin pregnancy
- Triplets or greater
- Fetal congenital abnormality likely to cause true cephalon-pelvic disproportion, such as hydrocephalus
- Maternal infections with potential to transmit to the fetus, such as recent primary herpes outbreak or poorly controlled HIV
- Suspected fetal compromise in labour
- Previous shoulder dystocia, especially if internal manoeuvres were required, or the dystocia resulted in fetal injury

54.2.1.3 Both Maternal and Fetal

- Placenta praevia – minor
- Suspected placental abruption
- Failure to progress in labour or obstructed labour

54.2.1.4 Absolute Indications

- Placenta praevia – major – in labour
- Interlocking twins
- Failed instrumental delivery

54.3 How to Perform a Safe Lower Segment Caesarean Section

54.3.1 Preoperative Preparation

Ideally, the woman should have written consent prior to the day of her caesarean section, and this can be confirmed on the day of her surgery. The optimal timing of elective caesarean sections is after 39 weeks. A full blood count should be performed in the preoperative period. The woman should not eat for 6 hours and only drink clear fluids up to 2 hours prior to surgery. Prior to starting anaesthesia, a preoperative surgical safety checklist should be carried out, such as modification of the WHO version [4]. A single-shot spinal anaesthetic is ideal. The patient should receive antacid medication, such as ranitidine 150 mg, preoperatively. A urinary catheter is inserted. The table should be on a left lateral tilt of 15 degrees. Prior to skin incision, antibiotics that are effective against endometritis and urinary tract and wound infections should be administered intravenously, such as a cephalosporin and metronidazole, but not co-amoxiclav. Any hair that is likely to be in the way of the skin incision can be removed. This should be done with clippers and not a razor [5].

54.3.2 Operative Procedure

After confirmation the anaesthesia is effective, the Joel-Cohen incision should be used. This involves a straight transverse incision 3 cm above the symphysis pubis. This needs to be large enough to deliver the fetus, and therefore will be variable, but usually approximately 12 cm [6]. The subcutaneous tissue is incised in the medial 3 cm and extended bluntly. The rectus sheath incision is extended bluntly by the surgeon inserting his or her fingers into the deep space created by the incision. There is no evidence to promote the use of a second 'clean' scalpel from the initial scalpel used for the skin [1]. After the sheath is opened, it is then dissected from the underlying rectus muscles in both the cephalic and, if needed, caudal directions by a combination of blunt and sharp dissection. Once the sheath has been mobilized, the peritoneum should be exposed, staying in the midline. Blunt entry into the parietal peritoneum is then made, and the peritoneal incision is extended by the surgeon and the assistant stretching laterally. Confirmation of the location of the lower segment is made by finding where the visceral peritoneum is loosely attached. Adequate access to the lower uterine segment is required for delivery. Some dissection of the bladder off the lower segment is required, but this should be kept to a minimum, and only what is needed to access the lower segment. The peritoneum is grasped and lifted superiorly, opened with scissors and extended bluntly; the bladder is reflected with a retractor, usually a Doyen's, to expose the lower uterine segment. The surgeon then confirms the rotation of the uterus by palpating the round ligaments and corrects for this [6]. The lower segment of the uterus is then opened sharply transversely, either with scissors or a scalpel, 2 to 3 cm below the upper level of the uterovesical fold of peritoneum and the incision extended bluntly in an upwards curve, enough to deliver the fetus. Delivery should be performed by the surgeon placing his or her dominant hand below the fetal head and elevating it to the level of the uterine incision. The bladder retractor is removed, and delivery is facilitated with fundal pressure applied by an assistant. After delivery, early skin-to-skin contact between the mother and baby should be encouraged, and 5 international units of oxytocin should be given by slow intravenous injection [1]. The placenta is delivered by uterine massage and gentle cord traction. A manual removal is not recommended [6]. The uterine cavity should be examined to check there are no placental remnants. Identification of the angles of the uterine incision is vital, and these should be sutured securely. Any large bleeding vessels should be clamped with atraumatic forceps, such as Green-Armytage. A two-layer closure of the uterus should be performed using a short-term, absorbable, braided size 1 suture, such as Vicryl* 1. The first layer should include minimal decidua. The aim of the second layer is to bury the first layer. After uterine closure, a meticulous check of haemostasis should be made, especially checking the uterine angles and edges of the peritoneum. The paracolic gutters should be cleaned. Do not close either the parietal or visceral peritoneum [1]. The rectus sheath is then closed. Suture choice will depend on patient factors such as body mass index and pervious surgery, but often a similar absorbable, braided size 1 suture is used. The subcutaneous fat is only closed if it is greater than 2 cm in depth. There is a lack of evidence as to what suture should be used to close the skin [1]. Commonly, a non-braided 2/0 suture is used. This can be absorbable or non-absorbable, depending on the surgeon's preference.

54.3.3 Postoperative Care

As a minimum, maternal observations (respiratory rate, heart rate, blood pressure, pain and level of sedation) should be performed every half hour for 2 hours [1]. Regular pain relief with nonsteroidal anti-inflammatory drugs (e.g. ibuprofen 400 mg three times a day), paracetamol (1 g four times a day) and opioids (but not codeine if the woman is planning on breastfeeding). Early eating and drinking should be encouraged when the patient feels hungry or thirsty. The catheter can come out when the woman is mobile, and, if uncomplicated, she can be offered early discharge home after 24 hours [1]. Early mobilization should be encouraged, and consideration of low molecular weight heparin should be made.

54.4 Modification of Technique

54.4.1 Anaesthesia

Regional anaesthesia results in less maternal and neonatal morbidity than general anaesthetic. When using regional anaesthesia, women should be offered intravenous ephedrine or phenylephrine and volume pre-loading with crystalloid or colloid to reduce the risk of hypotension [1]. In planned caesarean sections, spinal anaesthetic is preferred, as an adequate block is achieved quicker and more reliably, and less anaesthetic is required [7]. If operative time is expected to exceed 90 minutes, a spinal anaesthetic alone may not be adequate. Combined spinal epidural anaesthetic may be required. If a woman has had a good working epidural for labour, it is often possible to utilize this without the addition of spinal anaesthetic.

General anaesthesia is reserved mainly for acute fetal or maternal compromise when it is felt it is the quickest way to achieve adequate anaesthesia. There is risk of aspiration of gastric contents, failed intubation and anaphylaxis [8]. Other indications would be maternal request or suspected invasive placenta. When using general anaesthetic, it should include preoxygenation, cricoid pressure and rapid sequence induction to reduce the risk of aspiration [1]. General anaesthetic is also used when it is felt the regional anaesthesia is not effective enough to continue with the surgery. General anaesthetic is not usually required for women undergoing caesarean for placenta praevia, although women should be advised that it may be necessary to convert regional anaesthesia to general [9].

54.4.2 Skin Incision

Generally, skin incisions can be divided into suprapubic, transverse incisions (e.g. Pfannenstiel and Joel-Cohen) and vertical incisions. Transverse incisions are associated with less pain, dehiscence, infection, and hernia formation, as well as being cosmetically more acceptable [6]. The Joel-Cohen is preferred due to less pain, shorter incision-to-delivery times, shorter total operating times, less blood loss and quicker mobilization [10]. However, when faced with significant adhesions and scar tissue, blunt dissection is not always possible. In this situation, sharp dissection is required, as used with a Pfannenstiel incision. Classically, a Pfannenstiel skin incision is made 2–3 cm above the pubic symphysis in a curvilinear direction. Dissection to the level of the rectus sheath is performed, which is opened with a scalpel. The sheath is then opened laterally with scissors or a scalpel. Care should be taken to avoid, or cauterize if damaged, the superficial epigastric veins.

There are circumstances when a vertical skin incision is recommended. Generally, this would be when access to the upper abdomen or uterine fundus is required, such as with significant lower segment fibroids or low-lying, invasive placenta, or when other significant surgery is likely, such as with invasive placenta when a caesarean hysterectomy is likely. The initial incision should be from below the umbilicus to just above the symphysis pubis. This can be easily extended if required. Sharp dissection down to the level of the sheath is performed, the sheath opened and the incision extended sharply with scissors. The rectus muscle is then dissected off the sheath sharply. In the case of midline incisions, a mass closure technique is recommended [11].

54.4.3 Abdominal Entry

Blunt entry into the peritoneum is preferred. With previous surgery, this is not always possible, so sharp entry is required. This can be performed by elevating the peritoneal membrane between two forceps and palpating the opposing pieces through the peritoneum to exclude entrapped bowel, then incising with a scalpel or scissors [6]. Closure of the visceral or parietal peritoneum may be appropriate where there is a need for haemostasis, or to isolate compartments (intra-abdominal, rectus sheath, subcutaneous) where needed (e.g. to place specific drains).

54.4.4 Uterine Incision

A low transverse uterine incision is used in up to 95% of caesareans [11]. However, there are occasions when a classical incision may be required. These would include situations where access to the lower segment is limited, such as lower segment fibroids, or dense adhesions over the lower segment, or when delivery is likely planned through a high uterine incision, such as invasive placenta or a very vascular lower segment seen with anterior placenta praevia. A classical incision is vertical on the uterus, and extends higher on the uterus into the thicker, contractive part of the uterus. A vertical incision is also required if the lower segment is poorly formed or not large enough to deliver the baby through, as with extreme preterm caesareans. In this case, the surgeon needs to decide if a low vertical incision is needed (De Lee incision) where the incision stops at the level of the round ligaments, or a true classical incision is required. Generally, the lower segment is formed well enough for a transverse incision by 28 weeks' gestation, but this will be influenced by factors such as fetal size and presentation. The risks of a classical incision include increased blood loss and increased risk of uterine rupture in subsequent pregnancies.

There are situations when a transverse uterine incision is made, but fetal delivery is not easily achieved. Commonly, this can be with transverse lie, especially with the back down and/or no fluid, or when the fetal head is deeply engaged. In these cases, the incision may need to be made. Commonly used methods are an inverted T incision, where a low vertical incision is made in the midline of the transverse uterine incision, or a J, where the vertical incision is at the lateral aspect of the uterine incision. The extension of the incision should remain low enough to stay within the lower segment and away from the thicker contractile part of the uterus. These extensions are associated with increased incidence of maternal blood loss, broad ligament haematoma and uterine artery laceration [6]. Although these extensions, as well as De Lee incisions, are associated with a decreased risk of rupture in subsequent pregnancies compared with true classical incisions, generally

an elective caesarean would be recommended in future pregnancies [11].

Careful consideration as to placement of uterine incision needs to be made when caesareans are done in advanced labour, especially the second stage. In the second stage of labour, the lower segment is stretched and the cervix is drawn up superiorly, meaning differentiation between the uterus and cervix is difficult, so a low incision risks lateral extension, bladder damage or opening of the vagina or cervix [6, 12]. As long as the visceral peritoneum is loosely attached to the uterus, the incision is in the lower segment. The incision can be made beneath the upper part of this loose attachment.

54.5 Special Circumstances

54.5.1 Obesity

Obesity alone is not an indication for caesarean section, even a body mass index (BMI) of greater than 50 [1]. It does increase the risk of emergency caesarean section due to failure to progress in labour or fetal heart rate concerns, and therefore poses challenges to obstetricians [13]. Historically, when presented with a significantly voluminous panniculus, surgeons retract the panniculus using different options, such as tape or surgical clips on the rectus sheath attached to a gauze roll. Despite this, access is challenging, and there are reported complications caused by the retraction of the panniculus [14]. A major modification to surgical technique can be made, described by Tixier et al [13]. Instead of retracting the panniculus, allow the patient to lie flat and leave the panniculus untouched in the 'apron' position. The symphysis pubis is then palpated, and a projection of where it would lie on the panniculus is determined. A transverse skin incision is then made two finger breadths above this projection, on the upper abdomen. This may be above or below the umbilicus. The rest of the caesarean section is performed as routine, as by using the symphysis as a body landmark, when the surgeon enters the peritoneal cavity, he or she enters at the level of the lower uterine segment. This helps with access and vision at the time of caesarean section, as the thickness of the adipose tissue is minimal at this level, and therefore reduces intraoperative complications, as well as keeping the skin incision away from the anaerobic fold under the panniculus [13]. A few considerations need to be made. The anaesthetist must be aware the surgeon is making a high incision so they can make sure their block is high enough to cover the correct dermatomes. And when dissecting down to the level of the rectus sheath, continuous palpation of the symphysis through the adipose tissue needs to be done in order to keep orientation and make sure the peritoneal cavity is entered at the usual level. The skin incision does not need to be any larger than a standard caesarean. There can be blood supply to panniculus laterally, so making a larger incision risks damaging this.

54.5.2 Placenta Praevia

The timing of delivery needs to be adapted with placenta praevia and needs to take into account individual circumstances. When praevia is combined with a history of vaginal bleeding or significant risk factors for preterm delivery, delivery should be considered between 34 and 36+6 weeks. With uncomplicated praevia, delivery should be considered between 36 and 37 weeks. Delivery should be planned in a unit with on-site blood transfusion, and a crossmatch of blood preoperatively should be performed. Cell salvage should be made available, and the woman should be counselled about the increased risk of bleeding and therefore caesarean hysterectomy. Spinal anaesthetic is considered safe initially. A vertical skin and/or uterine incision may be necessary to avoid transecting the placenta when the fetus is lying transversely. This is especially true before 28 weeks' gestation [9]. There is debate concerning uterine incision with term, longitudinal lie anterior placenta praevia caesareans. Avoiding the placenta with either a classical or even fundal incision reduces blood loss. But doing so increases risks in future pregnancies. A discussion should be had with the woman about her future fertility plans, including the option of sterilization. Immediately or even intraoperatively an ultrasound can be performed to precisely determine the location of the placenta, and therefore to plan for the incision site. If the placenta is transected, then immediately clamp and cut the umbilical cord after delivery of the fetus [9].

54.5.3 Placenta Accreta Spectrum

When placenta accreta spectrum is suspected, it is vital to avoid unplanned delivery. Therefore, in the absence of risk factors for preterm delivery, delivery should be planned between 35 and 36+6 weeks' gestation. When counselling women with suspected accreta, special mention needs to be made of the risk of major obstetric haemorrhage, blood transfusion, lower urinary tract damage and hysterectomy. The discussion should also involve interventional radiology and cell salvage. The most senior obstetrician and anaesthetist should be present, and if the obstetrician is not confident in caesarean hysterectomy, a gynaecologist should also be present. Spinal anaesthetic may be appropriate, but there is an increased risk of converting to general. Ureteric stents may be needed, especially if the invasion is thought to involve the bladder [9].

The major concern with accreta spectrum is what to do with the placenta after delivery of the fetus. Initially, it is vital to avoid transecting the placenta during fetal delivery. Uterine incision needs to be planned to avoid the placenta. The diagnosis of accreta spectrum antenatally is never 100% reliable. It is most important not to pull on the placenta. If after fetal delivery it separates on its own, then the caesarean can continue in a routine manner. If there are no signs of separation, caesarean hysterectomy with the placenta in situ is preferable to attempting to separate it manually. If the area of invasion is small in depth and surface area, and the whole of the placenta is visualized, consideration of uterine preserving techniques, such as myometrial resection or leaving part of the placenta in situ, can be made. In some cases, women may find it unacceptable to electively have a caesarean hysterectomy. In these cases, the placenta can be left in situ whole. Risks of haemorrhage and infection need to be discussed with the woman, including the risk of future hysterectomy, and easy access to regular planned

and emergency follow-up needs to be in place. When leaving all or part of the placenta in situ, methotrexate should not be used. It is of unproven benefit and has significant side effects [9].

In the presence of percreta, there is limited evidence to support uterine preserving surgery. When there is thought to be bladder involvement, uretic stents and cystoscopy are recommended [9].

54.5.4 Perimortem Caesarean Section

In maternal cardiac arrest, emptying the uterus will aid in the resuscitation of the mother. It may be lifesaving for the fetus, but this is not the aim. If there is no response to cardiopulmonary resuscitation after 4 minutes in a woman 20 weeks or more pregnant, a perimortem caesarean should be performed, and delivery achieved within 5 minutes of collapse. This should happen wherever the woman has collapsed. The only equipment needed is a scalpel and two clamps for the cord, as there will be minimal bleeding. If cardiac output is restored, then transfer to an appropriate operating theatre. The quickest way to deliver a baby may be through a midline abdominal incision and classical uterine incision. However, the surgeon should use whatever technique he or she is most familiar and practised with due to the stress of the situation [15].

54.5.5 Complications

The Royal College of Obstetricians and Gynaecologists publishes an example consent form for caesarean section [16]. Risks can be broken down by maternal/fetal/anaesthetic, or by timing (intraoperatively, short term, long term).

54.5.5.1 Short Term

- Need for further surgery at a later date, including curettage, 5 women in every 1000 (uncommon)
- Thromboembolic disease, 4–16 women in every 10 000 (rare)
- Persistent wound and abdominal discomfort in the first few months after surgery, 9 women in every 100 (common)
- Readmission to hospital, 5 women in every 100 (common)
- Haemorrhage, 5 women in every 1000 (uncommon)
- Infection, 6 women in every 100 (common) – this includes wound infection, endometritis, bacteraemia, pelvic abscess, necrotizing fasciitis, urinary tract infection [11].

54.5.5.2 Long Term

- Increased risk of repeat caesarean section when vaginal delivery attempted in subsequent pregnancies, 1 woman in every 4 (very common)
- Increased risk of uterine rupture during subsequent pregnancies/deliveries, 2–7 women in every 1000 (uncommon)
- Increased risk of antepartum stillbirth, 1–4 women in every 1000 (uncommon)
- Increased risk in subsequent pregnancies of placenta praevia and placenta accreta, 4–8 women in every 1000 (uncommon)

54.5.6 Return to Theatre

As surgeons, we all fear taking patients back to theatre feeling that we inherently have failed. If you are facing a situation where you think there is a need for a return to theatre, seek advice or a second opinion from a trusted colleague – you will be stressed, and this advice will be invaluable. Consider if you need additional assistance, as returns to theatre are invariable difficult. If available, consider asking the on-call gynaecologist or general surgeon, or at least informing them.

54.5.7 Indications for Returning to Theatre

- Haemorrhage, uterine or intra-abdominal
- Bowel or bladder injury suspected
- Pelvic collection (also consider percutaneous drainage under computed tomography (CT) or ultrasound guidance)

54.5.8 Procedure

Carefully explain to the patient and her family the reason for return to theatre. Consent should be taken for all foreseeable surgical eventualities including hysterectomy, blood transfusion and admission to intensive care unit for all cases. For some cases, bowel resection, stoma formation, long-term indwelling catheter or ureteric stenting may be appropriate. Ensure that the obstetric anaesthetist understands the nature of the case and make provision for rapid infusion of fluid via a Level 1 device or similar. A general anaesthetic, in the absence of contraindications, is appropriate. Understand the original operation as much as possible. Re-read the operation notes, speak to the original surgeon if it was not you. Use the original scar if possible, as further incisions can always be made later on if there are problems with surgical access. Remove old suture material as

you proceed; leaving this behind will increase the chance of infection. Identify and deal with problems as you discover them; if there is a complex problem you cannot deal with, ask an unscrubbed member of staff to note it down and make sure everything is dealt with before you close. You will need to have a good level of surgical experience to deal with this kind of case and a full explanation is outside the scope of this chapter. Understand and consider what haemostatic measures are available in your hospital. The authors have found absorbable haemostats in the form of activated fibrin matrices useful. If the situation is out of your control, call for additional help quickly. Do not finish the operation until all the problems have been resolved, and if even at this late stage, do not be tempted to close and 'hope for the best' if you are not certain that you have resolved the situation.

54.6 Conclusion

In an era in which obstetricians are increasingly scrutinized for our decisions, it is of paramount importance that we are clear with our patients when caesarean delivery is needed. There are many difficult decisions to be made around birth choices, and frequently these are being made in high-stress environments on the labour ward. Make sure that all of these complex decisions and your expert care are meticulously documented, so that the next obstetrician going through your old scar knows exactly what you did. It is of paramount importance to remember that the complex decisions belong to the woman and not the obstetrician, our role is to provide advice, guidance and support.

References

1. NICE. *Caesarean Section*, Guideline 32. 2011. www.nice.org.uk/guidance/cg132/evidence/full-guideline-pdf-184810861.

2. American College of Obstetricians and Gynecologists. Caesarean delivery on maternal request: ACOG Committee Opinion Number 761. *Obstet Gynecol.* 2019;**133**(1):e73-e77.

3. Boerma T, Ronsmans C, Melesse DY, et al. Global epidemiology of use of and disparities in caesarean sections. *Lancet.* 2018;**392**(10155):1341–8.

4. NPSA. WHO Surgical Safety Checklist: For Maternity Cases Only: National Patient Safety Agency; 2010. http://binarystore.wiley.com/store/10.1111/1471–0528.12041/asset/supinfo/bjo12041-sup-0001-AppendixS1.pdf?v=1&s=308472a88dac95ccf3475920c42b5115e0f927c3.

5. Tanner J, Norrie P, Melen K. Preoperative hair removal to reduce surgical site infection. *Cochrane Database Syst Rev.* 2011;**9**(11).

6. Naji O, Abdallah Y, Paterson-Brown S. *Cesarean Birth: Surgical Techniques.* Glob libr women's med. 2010.

7. IQWiG. *Pregnancy and Birth: Cesarean Sections: What Are the Pros and Cons of Regional and General Anesthetics?* Cologne, Germany: Institute for Quality and Efficiency in Health Care; 2008 [updated 22/03/18]. www.ncbi.nlm.nih.gov/books/NBK279566/.

8. Levy DM. Obstetric anaesthesia and analgesia. In Luesley DM, Baker PN, eds. *Obstetrics and Gynaecology: An Evidence-Based Text for MRCOG*, 2nd ed. London: Hodder Arnold; 2010. pp. 389–400.

9. Jauniaux E, Alfirevic Z, Bhide AG, et al. Placenta praevia and placenta accreta: diagnosis and management: Green-top Guideline No. 27a.*BJOG.* 2019;**126**(1):e1–e48.

10. Abuelghar WM, El-Bishry G, Emam LH. Caesarean deliveries by Pfannenstiel versus Joel-Cohen incision: A randomised controlled trial. *J Turk Ger Gynecol Assoc.* 2013;**14**(4):194–200.

11. Hayman R. Caesarean section. In Luesley DM, Baker PN, eds. *Obstetrics and Gynaecology: An Evidence-Based Text for MRCOG*, 2nd ed. London: Hodder Arnold; 2010. pp. 401–12.

12. Vousden N, Cargill Z, Briley A, Tydeman G, Shennan AH. Caesarean section at full dilatation: incidence, impact and current management. *Obstet Gynaecol.* 2104;**16**:199–205.

13. Tixier H, Thouvenot S, Coulange L, et al. Cesarean section in morbidly obese women: supra or subumbilical transverse incision? *Acta Obstet Gynecol Scand.* 2009;**88**:1049–52.

14. Norwitz ER, Zelop CM, Miller DA, Keefe DL. *Evidence-Based Obstetrics and Gynecology.* Oxford: Wiley-Blackwell; 2019.

15. *Maternal Collapse in Pregnancy and the Puerperium*, Green-top Guideline No 56. London: Royal College of Obstetricians and Gynaecologists, 2011.

16. *Caesarean Section*, Consent Advice No 7. London: Royal College of Obstetricians and Gynaecologists, 2009.

Chapter 55

Instrumental Operative Obstetrics

Jørg Kessler & Anke Reitter

55.1 Introduction and History

A number of factors have contributed to an increasing preference for caesarean delivery: maternal and neonatal morbidity related to instrumental vaginal delivery, fear of litigation, lack of practical skills and financial incentives in favour of caesarean delivery.

Conversely, the negative consequences of caesarean delivery for the mother and the child in subsequent pregnancies are extensively documented. Further, there is evidence that delivery by caesarean section may have detrimental effects on offspring health, including an increased risk of allergy, asthma and obesity.

The highest risk of complications relates to caesarean delivery during the second stage of labour [1]. It should therefore be a focus in obstetric training to acquire solid skills in instrumental vaginal delivery as a safe alternative for labouring women in need of delivery during the second stage.

Chamberlain described the first use of obstetric forceps around 1700. Numerous types of forceps were developed and came into use, designed for extraction and rotation of the fetal head (Figure 55.1).

It was not until 1954 that Malmstrøm introduced a basically different delivery instrument – the vacuum extractor – into clinical practice [2] (Figure 55.2). In parallel with forceps, the vacuum extractor has undergone plastic and silicone modifications.

The initial aim of operative vaginal delivery was to prevent maternal death, often at expense of the fetus and/or serious maternal morbidity. Nowadays, obstetric care, including operative delivery, is expected not only to prevent maternal and perinatal mortality but also to reduce morbidity in the mother and the neonate.

55.2 Epidemiology

In many European countries, the proportion of women delivered by caesarean section has continuously increased during the past five decades [3]. Data from the Peristat project indicate that the proportion of instrumental vaginal deliveries decreased from 10.1% in 2000 to 7.6% in 2015, with an increasing number of countries reporting data. The huge range in the prevalence of instrumental vaginal deliveries from 0.5 to 16% in European countries was not correlated with the respective frequency of caesarean deliveries [3].

The choice of instruments varies widely. For example, in Scandinavia, the Netherlands and Germany the vacuum extractor is almost exclusively used, while forceps accounts

for one third and half of the instrumental vaginal deliveries in France and England, respectively.

The exclusive use of a rigid plastic vacuum in many countries, seemingly demanding less skill and experience, has been found to result in failure rates up to 30% [4]. This highlights the necessity of skills training in both vacuum and forceps delivery so an informed choice can be made of the most appropriate instrument to be used for women in need of delivery.

55.3 Clinical Management

55.3.1 General Considerations

55.3.1.1 Types of Instruments

There are two types of instruments for vaginal operative delivery, forceps and vacuum, and both differ in material, design and, as a consequence, indications for their use (Figures 55.1 and 55.2).

Forceps designed for extraction (e.g. Nägele, Simpson) usually have blades with both a cephalic and a pelvic curvature, and a fixed lock (Figure 55.1A). In contrast, forceps for rotation (e.g. Kielland) have a cephalic but very little pelvic curvature and a sliding lock (Figure 55.1B). An extraction forceps can also be used in cases of malrotation of the head up to about 45 degrees. Biparietal application of the blades necessitates wandering of the more anterior blade, and rotation must not be done in the axis of the forceps, but rather as a semicircular movement of the handles. Rotational forceps of the Kielland type are also appropriate for extraction, but due to the lack of pelvic curvature, extensive elevation of the instrument is not recommended because of the risk of vaginal laceration.

Vacuum cups are either plastic (Kiwi OmniCup, Figure 55.2A) or metal type (Figure 55.2B–D). While the pulling handle and the suction tube are fused in the Malmstrøm model (Figure 55.2B), they are separated in the Bird modification (Figure 55.2C and D). To make the application of the vacuum cup easier in occiput transverse (OT) and occiput posterior (OP) presentation, the suction tube is moved to the lateral brim in the 'posterior cup' (Figure 55.2D).

55.3.1.2 Classification of Instrumental Deliveries

A synthesis of common classification systems is shown in Table 55.1. With the exception of the delivery of the second twin (only in rare circumstances), high instrumental deliveries are considered obsolete in modern obstetrics due to the high risk of fetal and maternal morbidity compared to caesarean delivery.

440

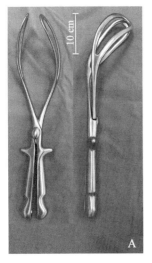
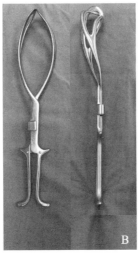
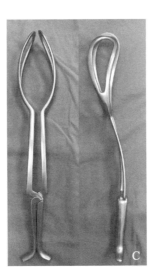

Figure 55.1 Different types of obstetric forceps. A: Simpson's traction forceps; B: Kielland's rotational forceps; C: Piper's forceps for delivery of after-coming head in breech presentation.

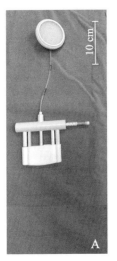
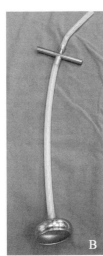
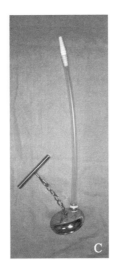
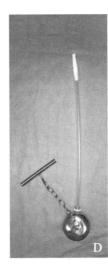

Figure 55.2 Vacuum cup varieties. A: Kiwi OmniCup; B: Malmstrøm model; C: Bird modification – use of vertex presentation; D: Bird modification for OP or OT presentation.

55.3.1.3 Indications for Instrumental Deliveries

Indications for vaginal operative deliveries are the following:

1. Prolonged labour, second stage
2. Fetal compromise, fetal distress
3. Maternal exhaustion
4. To shorten the second stage and reduce maternal expulsive effort due to:
   a. Cardiac disease New York Heart Association (NYHA) Grade 3/Grade 4
   b. Severe hypertension
   c. Retinopathy

55.3.1.4 Prerequisites

In all instrumental deliveries, independent of the instrument used, the items in the left column in Table 55.2 should be checked carefully. These universal examinations or procedures are not mentioned repeatedly for the different instrumental procedures unless specific comments are necessary.

55.3.1.5 Position of the Mother

The mother should be in a modified lithotomy position with the buttocks at the edge or end of the bed to allow space for the instruments, allow traction and follow the correct axis with lowering and elevating the instruments according to the station of the head. The legs of the mother should be supported, and the upper bed should be elevated so that the mother can still push.

55.3.1.6 Anaesthesia

Available methods of anaesthesia include local infiltration of the perineum, pudendal block, epidural and spinal block or general anaesthesia. In addition, inhalation of nitrous oxide should be possible.

An epidural can be helpful if already applied, but in prolonged labour at second stage and in fetal distress, it may be too late for it to be initiated if delivery is required.

General anaesthesia should be reserved for obstetric emergencies in need of urgent delivery by forceps – it will nullify the maternal expulsive effort and reduce uterine contractions.

For a vacuum extraction in experienced hands, there should be little discomfort and usually no extra analgesia is

441

Table 55.1 Modified classification for vaginal operative deliveries

Anatomical description	Classification for vaginal operative deliveries (ACOG)	Fetal head position	Part of the head palpable by abdominal palpation	Presenting part on view	Station (De Lee) distance to ischial spines (cm)	Which instrument	Modified classification for vaginal operative deliveries
Inlet Pubic brim	High	Floating or starting to engage	4/5 to 5/5	n.a.	−4	Vaginal operative delivery NOT recommended if head is more than 2/5 palpable	
					−3		
					−2		
			2/5		−1		
Mid-pelvis At or just below the level of the ischial spines	Mid	Engaged Sagittal suture often >45 degrees in right or left OA/OP	1/5	Deep in the vagina visible (be aware of caput)	0	Consider manual rotation if OP Vacuum – metal cup (In OP use posterior cup) Forceps for extraction or rotation	Vaginal operative delivery from Station: 1. Mid-pelvis 2. Low or 3. Outlet Type of procedure: 1. Rotational 2. Non-Rotational
					+1		Instrument: 1. Forceps 2. Vacuum
	Low	Deeply engaged Sagittal suture often in AP diameter (or <45 degrees in right or left OA/OP)	0/5	Separating labia, visible in the contraction	+2	Vacuum – metal cup or Kiwi* handheld vacuum Forceps for extraction or rotation	
					+3		
Outlet Below the ischial spines	Outlet			Stays visible outside of contractions Perineum stretching	+4	Vacuum Kiwi* handheld vacuum or metal cup Forceps for extraction	
Pelvic floor				Crowning Perineum stretched			

Adapted from [8], [19] and [20]

ACOG: American College of Obstetricians and Gynecologists; OA: occiput anterior; OP: occiput posterior; AP: anteroposterior

Table 55.2 Prerequisites for undertaking an operative vaginal delivery

Cervix	Fully dilated
Analgesia	Epidural/spinal, pudendal block or local infiltration of perineum
Position, mother	Modified lithotomy
Consent	Verbal consent
Abdominal palpation	<2/5 of the fetal skull palpable above the symphysis
Head station	At ischial spines or below
Head position and attitude	Must be known, use ultrasound if any doubt
Cephalopelvic disproportion	Not suspected
Maternal urinary bladder	Emptied
Staff/operator	Sufficient skills, experience and knowledge
Equipment	Check vacuum (building up of the pressure?) Forceps (blades locking?)
Failure	Plan for caesarean (or an alternative instrument)

required; however, in less experienced hands introducing and applying the cup may cause minimal discomfort. Local anaesthesia or pudendal block is usually sufficient in these cases.

The forceps blades are thin, but will add to the fetal circumference and so will require extra space. Application may therefore cause discomfort or pain.

Sometimes locking the blades causes brief pain or discomfort. If the lock does lock easily, this should be not be seen as unusual or worrying.

As a rule of thumb, a forceps delivery requires anaesthesia more so than local infiltration. While a pudendal block is sufficient for outlet forceps, rotational or midcavity procedures should be done under epidural or spinal anaesthesia.

Sufficient pain relief may prevent pelvic floor injuries by relaxation of the levator muscle.

55.3.1.7 Instrumentation

Prepare and check the instrument before use (vacuum: intact tubes and connections, vacuum device generating negative pressure; forceps: lock the blades, both fit as a pair).

Use a vacuum cup as large as possible (size 60 mm) to minimize the risk of detachment. Consider a smaller forceps for premature deliveries if the gestational age is below 32 weeks.

The vacuum should be inserted gently. It may be lubricated before insertion. It should be held with two or three fingers and manoeuvred/pushed into the space where the flexion point (3 cm anterior to the small fontanelle) is expected to be. Cup placement at the flexion point promotes flexion of the fetal

head and thus keeps the diameter of the head passing through the birth channel at a minimum.

In experienced hands, applying the forceps should be like 'cutting butter' with no force being applied. The blade should glide automatically in the right place – in inexperienced hands force may be used involuntarily. In case of any resistance when applying the forceps, or if the blades are not sitting correctly or the lock does not lock, remove the forceps, reassess, reapply, seek support and be prepared to abandon the procedure.

In rotational forceps, applying the blades will be more challenging but should follow the above-mentioned rules.

Always check and confirm the correct placement of the instrument after application.

Independent of the instrument being used, a key for success is a dynamic direction of traction, depending on the station of the head in the birth channel. This means pulling sharply downwards when starting a mid-pelvic delivery. At contrast, the instrument has to be elevated when the fetal head is finally crowning to allow for extension of the head. Pulling must *not* be augmented by a backwards move of the operator's upper body or stretching one or both feet.

Consider removal of the instrument when the head crowns. This may be useful in particular for forceps in order to minimize the maximum circumference passing the perineum.

Consider episiotomy in particular in primiparous women and forceps delivery to prevent obstetric anal sphincter injury (OASIS) [5, 6].

Deliver the shoulders, arms and body under continuous protection of the perineum.

55.3.1.8 Counselling

Informed consent should always be obtained. The mother and birth partner should be informed about the need to intervene and which instrument is used. This should be adapted according to the clinical situation and should include risks related to the instrument, risk of failure of the procedure and alternatives (e.g. caesarean section).

55.3.1.9 Post-procedure Management

After instrumental delivery, women and neonates are in need of extended care and special attention [7] (Table 55.3).

55.3.2 Non-rotational Delivery/Pelvic Outlet/De Lee Station +2 [8]

55.3.2.1 Vacuum

These deliveries are usually straightforward and without significant risk of morbidity or failure. Either Kiwi or metal cups may be used.

– Infiltration and/or pudendal anaesthesia.
– Insert the cup and place on the flexion point.
– Establish vacuum pressure (to 80 mm Hg).
– Check for interpolated vaginal tissue.
– Use one hand for traction. The other hand is placed with the thumb on the cup and two fingers on the fetal head to

Table 55.3 Checks required post-operative vaginal delivery intervention

Manage third stage carefully	Increased risk for postpartum haemorrhage
Assess mother	Tears: cervix, vagina, perineum (bleeding)
Assess neonate	Head (haematoma) Neurological abnormalities Marks, chignon, caput succedaneum – check for correct assessment of presentation and placement of the instrument for own learning or teaching involved staff
Debriefing	Mother, partner Immediate debriefing, further offer within days
Keep records	Use if available standardized forms
Urine	Be aware of urinary retention
Pain	Pain relief should be offered
Prevention of urinary incontinence/pelvic floor problems/prolapse	Early pelvic floor exercises

confirm descent of the head and to detect any possible cup detachment.

- The initial direction of traction depends on fetal station.
- Consider episiotomy in nulliparous women when the head starts crowning.
- Stop traction when the head crowns. Protect the perineum with one hand. Control the pace of the fetal head with the other hand.
- Release the vacuum pressure and remove the cup when the head is delivered.

55.3.2.2 Forceps

- Regional and/or pudendal anaesthesia.
- Perform a vaginal examination (confirm full dilation, station and sagittal suture anteroposterior or <45 degrees).
- Inform patient, explain the procedure and explain backup plan.
- Hold the pair of forceps in front of the introitus.
- Start with the left blade in the left hand, insert it on the left side of the woman, guide it with the right hand.
- The right hand/fingers will protect the maternal pelvic wall and the blade can be guided with the thumb.
- Repeat with change of hand; hold the right blade with the right hand and place it in the right side, guide with the left hand and with the thumb.
- Check that fenestration is just about visible.
- Do the blades the lock easily? Wait for the next contraction.
- Steadily pull using the pivot manoeuvre; using both hands, pull in the direction where the handles point.

- Expect steady progress; when the occiput is crowning, lift the handles and allow the head to deflex, using the hand to protect the perineum.

Extra technical skills are required for the occiput posterior position or minor malrotation (sagittal suture <45 degree deviating from straight anteroposterior position).

5.3.3 Rotational Delivery/Mid-pelvic/De Lee Station 0 to +1

55.3.3.1 Vacuum

These deliveries carry a higher risk of failure than non-rotational deliveries. There is some evidence that metal cups should be preferred in these cases due to a lower failure rate. A crucial point for success is the placement of the cup over the flexion point. In practical terms, the cup has to be positioned much more posteriorly (in case of occiput posterior) or laterally (for occiput transverse) than in the more frequent occiput anterior presentation. This is best achieved by using a posterior cup, where the vacuum tube is attached laterally at the rim of the cup (Figure 55.2C).

Unlike forceps, where the rotation of the instrument itself forces rotation of the fetal head, the vacuum cup should never be used for a direct rotational movement. In steady traction, force is thought to initiate autorotation of the head, which will occur in 50–75% of the cases with occiput posterior presentation.

- If the arrest of labour happens in the mid-pelvis, be aware of pulling sharply downwards.
- Be prepared to have the descent of the fetal head begin during the second or sometimes the third pull.
- Autorotation may occur at any time during delivery.

55.3.3.2 Forceps

In the mid-pelvis, the Kielland forceps is used to rotate and guide the head further down, to mimic head flexion and rotation as they occur in physiological labour [9].

In occiput transverse or occiput posterior position, using forceps may be necessary if the above-mentioned manoeuvres (manual rotation, vacuum) fail.

Kielland forceps have only a very small pelvic curve and are therefore suitable for larger (>45 degrees) rotational procedures in the mid-pelvis. Extraction type forceps cannot be used due to the very pronounced pelvic curve. Both forceps have a very similar cephalic curve (Figure 55.1).

Be aware in which direction to rotate; where the fetal back lies must be identified, because this will provide guidance on whether to turn clockwise or anticlockwise.

Usually the occiput has to be rotated to the fetal back (shortest turn).

In occiput posterior position, the blades will be applied directly in one of two ways:

a. Apply them the 'other way round', meaning holding the pair of forceps upside down (knobs pointing down). Apply the blade held in the left hand, which is originally the right blade into the left lateral fornix. Apply the remaining originally left blade into the right lateral fornix. Perform the rotation with very little force. With the successful turn the forceps are now in the 'right' way and the knobs form the sliding lock point upwards, the advantage being that the forceps are applied only once.

b. Scanzoni manoeuvre: Apply the blades directly and turn the head ('screwing out') in between the contractions using the forceps with a wide circle. If turning is successful (may need up to 135 degrees), take the blades out and reapply them again in the usual way to assist fetal descent.

In occiput transverse/occiput oblique presentation, the anterior blade is the one which will wander from the lateral fornix to the brow and the posterior blade is placed directly.

The sliding lock in Kielland forceps allows for application if there is an (anterior) asynclitism, typically in occiput transverse presentation. The asynclitism should be corrected for after application by sliding the blades until the two nobs meet each other.

Rotation should be attempted between the contractions using minimal force; it is usually achieved with lowering the hands and angling the forceps.

A more challenging technique for occiput transverse/occiput oblique presentation is to start with the anterior blade introduced behind the symphysis using the cephalic curve. It is then turned 180 degrees inside the uterus in the axial direction. It will then be side by side with the fetal head. Let the anterior blade wander towards the occiput and then apply the second blade directly. The forceps will be face down; rotation and reapplication follow according to the Scanzoni manoeuvre (described above).

55.3.4 Special Circumstances

55.3.4.1 Deflexed Presentations

In cases of a sinciput, the leading point (centrally placed at vaginal examination) is the large fontanelle. The deflexed fetal head increases the largest diameter to about 11 cm, compared to 9.5 cm in flexed occiput anterior. Virtually all cases of sinciput are in occiput posterior presentation. Due to the increased diameter, prolonged labour is common, the fetal skull is often configured with a substantial caput succedaneum and autorotation rarely occurs.

Instrumental delivery is challenging. The deflexed head increases risk of instrumental failure and perineal trauma. Even if the position is occiput posterior, rotation with forceps is not advantageous due to the severe configuration and caput succedaneum.

For obstetricians experienced with the instrument, forceps will be preferred.

Correct placement of the vacuum cup is challenging since the distance from the introitus to the flexion point is longer than in the commonly flexed occiput posterior position.

In face presentation, the fetal head is most deflexed and vaginal delivery is possible if the mentum is anterior. In fact, the largest diameter of the fetal head is comparable with the flexed occiput anterior position. Forceps remain the only option for instrumental delivery, and mannequins are used for training with them due to the rareness of cases. Forceps with a pelvic curvature (Nägele, Simpson) should be used with a different application technique to avoid brachial nerve plexus damage and to prevent flexion of the head.

- Insert first the left and then the right blade of the forceps as previously described for non-rotational forceps.
- Do **not** close the lock.
- Elevate both blades (unlocked) to an almost vertical position.
- Close the lock.
- Push on the shaft of the forceps with a shovel-like movement.

55.3.4.2 Forceps for the After-coming Head in Breech Presentation

Breech vaginal delivery can be offered to selected women as a safe option. However, due to the breech situations that are undiagnosed until the late second stage of labour, obstetricians have to be able to manage vaginal breech birth. The manual manoeuvres to deliver the breech fetus are dealt with elsewhere (Chapter 52, Abnormal Obstetric Presentation). During assisted vaginal delivery, the atraumatic delivery of the after-coming head is important in order to minimize neonatal morbidity. In the case of failure of manual manoeuvres to deliver the fetal head, application of forceps remains an effective alternative. Since the fetal lower extremities and body are delivered, forceps with little or no pelvic curvature should be used. The Piper forceps with long shanks (Figure 55.1 C) is specifically designed for that purpose. The Kielland forceps (Figure 55.1B) may also be used.

If the fetal neck is not visible in the introitus, the head has not descended to the pelvic floor. Check by digital examination:

- Station of the head.
- Position of the fetal chin.

A common reason for lack of descent is malrotation of the fetal head remaining in an oblique position. Place index and long fingers of your hand inserted on each side of the chin and rotate the fetal head to a sagittal (direct occiput anterior) position.

The angle of application for the Piper forceps is different from forceps with pelvic curvature:

- You need an assistant to elevate the fetal body and upper extremities (preferably wrapped in a towel) to get access to the perineum and the posterior part of the introitus, until the application of the forceps is completed.
- Starting with the *left* blade of the forceps in the *left* hand, hold it in a horizontal plane, at a 90-degree angle towards the maternal spine.
- Use your right hand to protect the left vaginal wall and guide the left blade around the fetal head.
- Continuing with the *right* blade in the *right* hand, hold it in a horizontal plane, at a 90-degree angle towards the maternal spine.

445

– Use your left hand to protect the right vaginal wall and guide the right blade around the fetal head.
– Close the lock.
– The direction of initial traction depends on the station of the fetal head, downwards if above the pelvic floor, horizontal if on the pelvic floor.
– Avoid extensive elevation due to the lack of the pelvic curvature (risk of vaginal tears by the toes of the forceps).

55.3.4.3 Use of Obstetric Instruments during Caesarean Delivery

If the head is deeply engaged and a vaginal operative delivery is not feasible, a caesarean section will be technically difficult and challenging. In those cases, there are different options to assist abdominal delivery. Instrumental options include

– Forceps (e.g. Sellheimlöffel, also known as 'elevating spoon' or a small Simpson forceps) – usually only one blade. It will be introduced lateral and below the head and then tilted in order to lift the head out. If the blade is introduced not far enough or too much force is applied there is a risk of skull fracture.
– Kiwi* handheld vacuum, which is easier to use and may be less harmful – apply the cup as close as possible to the occiput and deliver the head with gentle traction out of the pelvis.

Non-instrumental manoeuvres, which may be helpful:
– Digital vaginal push up of the fetal head
– Extraction as a breech: grasp a foot, extract and deliver the lower extremities and body of the fetus first, followed by the after-coming head.

55.4 Complications and Sequelae of Treatment –Prognosis

55.4.1 Failure and Sequential Use of Instruments

A common manifestation of vacuum failure is detachment of the cup due to a loss of negative pressure. Reasons for pop off are often wrong placement, non-appropriate direction of pull, a severe caput succedaneum and, rarely, a cephalopelvic disproportion. Except for the latter reason, reapplication of the vacuum (with appropriate placement and pull) is recommended and will often succeed. After a second or at the most third pop off, an instrumental failure should be recognized, and the course of labour and delivery including maternal and fetal risk factors assessed carefully.

Failure to apply the forceps is either due to lack of technical skills or incorrect assessment of fetal presentation. The blades of the forceps may not have been inserted sufficiently deep, or may not have been closed into the lock. A non-forceful correction of the blade position or a new clinical assessment and complete reapplication are then warranted.

Failure is more likely with BMI >30, fetal weight >4000 g and OP position. Failure is more likely with the vacuum compared to forceps [10]. The failure with the vacuum is more likely when using soft cups compared to metal rigids cups [11].

Lack of training or competence can result in a higher rate of complications and failure; therefore, senior staff should be available for rotational and mid-cavity procedures.

There is evidence that sequential use of instruments is associated with increased maternal and neonatal morbidity [12, 13]. Often the question will be whether to apply forceps after a failed vacuum extraction. This should only be considered by an experienced operator capable of balancing the risks of the repeated instrumental attempt or a rather difficult caesarean section (CS) with a deeply impacted head; both are associated with an increased risk to the mother and neonate.

Operative vaginal delivery should be abandoned when there is no evidence of progressive descent with moderate traction during each contraction or where delivery is not imminent following three contractions of a correctly applied instrument by an experienced operator.

55.4.2 Maternal Complications

Perineal and vaginal lacerations, and obstetric anal sphincter injuries (OASIS) occur more often in instrumental than spontaneous delivery or caesarean section [14, 15]. Forceps delivery is a stronger risk factor for levator muscle avulsions than vacuum delivery [16].

The Cochrane meta-analysis of randomized studies comparing vacuum and forceps deliveries indicates a doubled risk of OASIS using forceps. Of note, a study with exclusively junior doctors as operators, a highly selective practice of episiotomy, and an OASIS rate of 29 and 12% for forceps and vacuum use, respectively, contributes to 42% of the analytic weight. This is in contrast to recently published studies of OASIS rates below 5% even for rotational forceps deliveries [9]. Nevertheless, there are continuous controversies regarding the use of forceps because of pelvic floor injuries [17, 18].

A substantial and sustained decrease in OASIS rates on a national basis is achievable by continuous training and tight supervision of trainees and daily focus on the technique of instrumental delivery [19].

Recent research around birth injuries and the risk associated with vaginal delivery per se are focusing on the levator muscle avulsion and long-term sequelae and rising awareness of urinary incontinence and pelvic floor prolapse.

55.4.3 Neonatal Complications

Typical complications after vacuum delivery are:
– Chignon (caput succedaneum)
– Cup marks
– Bruising and cup discolouration
– Superficial scalp lacerations

Typical complications after forceps delivery are:
– Forceps marks
– Facial nerve palsy (almost always temporary/ transient)
– Skull fracture (rare)

Cephalohaematoma (usually limited to the area of one bone, most often the parietal (1–25%), may take a few weeks to dissolve), subcutaneous haematoma (may take a few days for resolution), retinal haemorrhage, subgaleal haematoma/haemorrhage (rare) and intracranial bleeding (rare) may occur after use of either instrument.

Haematoma and bruising may lead to a higher rate of jaundice. If the clinical observation of the neonate after vacuum or forceps delivery reveals abnormal neurological behaviour, early diagnosis and further investigation/treatment are mandatory.

55.5 Key Messages

Teaching in obstetrics should include extensive and supervised training in instrumental vaginal delivery. Profound skills, preferably in both vacuum and forceps delivery, are required to provide a safe alternative to second stage caesarean section.

55.6 Key Guidelines Relevant to the Topic

Operative Vaginal Delivery, Green-top Guideline No 26. London: Royal College of Obstetricians and Gynaecologists, 2011. www.rcog.org.uk/globalassets/documents/guidelines/gtg_26.pdf. [20]

Committee on Practice Bulletins – Obstetrics. ACOG Practice Bulletin No. 154: operative vaginal delivery. *Obstet Gynecol*. 2015 Nov;**126**(5):e56-65 [21]

References

1. Asicioglu O, Gungorduk K, Yildirim G, et al. Second-stage vs first-stage caesarean delivery: comparison of maternal and perinatal outcomes. *J Obstet Gynaecol*. 2014 Oct;**34**(7):598–604.

2. Malmstrom T. Vacuum extractor, an obstetrical instrument. *Acta Obstet Gynecol Scand Suppl*. 1954;**33**(4):1–31.

3. Macfarlane AJ, Blondel B, Mohangoo AD, et al. Wide differences in mode of delivery within Europe: risk-stratified analyses of aggregated routine data from the Euro-Peristat study. *BJOG*. 2016 Mar;**123**(4):559–68.

4. Groom KM, Jones BA, Miller N, Paterson-Brown S. A prospective randomised controlled trial of the Kiwi Omnicup versus conventional ventouse cups for vacuum-assisted vaginal delivery. *BJOG*. 2006 Feb;**113**(2):183–9.

5. Lund NS, Persson LK, Jango H, Gommesen D, Westergaard HB. Episiotomy in vacuum-assisted delivery affects the risk of obstetric anal sphincter injury: a systematic review and meta-analysis. *Eur J Obstet Gynecol Reprod Biol*. 2016 Dec;**207**:193–9.

6. van Bavel J, Hukkelhoven C, de Vries C, et al. The effectiveness of mediolateral episiotomy in preventing obstetric anal sphincter injuries during operative vaginal delivery: a ten-year analysis of a national registry. *Int Urogynecol J*. 2018 Mar;**29**(3):407–13.

7. Murphy DJ, Pope C, Frost J, Liebling RE. Women's views on the impact of operative delivery in the second stage of labour: qualitative interview study. *BMJ*. 2003 Nov 15;**327**(7424):1132.

8. De Lee J. *The Principles and Practice of Obstetrics*, 4th ed. Philadelphia, PA: WB Saunders; 1924.

9. Al Wattar BH, Al Wattar B, Gallos I, Pirie AM. Rotational vaginal delivery with Kielland's forceps: a systematic review and meta-analysis of effectiveness and safety outcomes. *Curr Opin Obstet Gynecol*. 2015 Dec;**27**(6):438–44.

10. Murphy DJ, Liebling RE, Verity L, Swingler R, Patel R. Early maternal and neonatal morbidity associated with operative delivery in second stage of labour: a cohort study. *Lancet*. 2001 Oct 13;**358**(9289):1203–7.

11. O'Mahony F, Hofmeyr GJ, Menon V. Choice of instruments for assisted vaginal delivery. *Cochrane Database Syst Rev*. 2010 Nov 10;(11):CD005455.

12. Demissie K, Rhoads GG, Smulian JC, et al. Operative vaginal delivery and neonatal and infant adverse outcomes: population based retrospective analysis. *BMJ*. 2004 Jul 3;**329**(7456):24–9.

13. Murphy DJ, Macleod M, Bahl R, Strachan B. A cohort study of maternal and neonatal morbidity in relation to use of sequential instruments at operative vaginal delivery. *Eur J Obstet Gynecol Reprod Biol*. 2011 May;**156**(1):41–5.

14. Gurol-Urganci I, Cromwell DA, Edozien LC, et al. Third- and fourth-degree perineal tears among primiparous women in England between 2000 and 2012: time trends and risk factors. *BJOG*. 2013 Nov;**120**(12):1516–25.

15. Muraca GM, Skoll A, Lisonkova S, et al. Perinatal and maternal morbidity and mortality among term singletons following midcavity operative vaginal delivery versus caesarean delivery. *BJOG*. 2018 May;**125**(6):693–702.

16. Friedman T, Eslick GD, Dietz HP. Delivery mode and the risk of levator muscle avulsion: a meta-analysis. *Int Urogynecol J*. 2019 Jun;**30**(6):901–7.

17. Fitzpatrick M, Behan M, O'Connell PR, O'Herlihy C. Randomised clinical trial to assess anal sphincter function following forceps or vacuum assisted vaginal delivery. *BJOG*. 2003 Apr;**110**(4):424–9.

18. Dietz HP. Forceps: towards obsolescence or revival? *Acta Obstet Gynecol Scand*. 2015 Apr;**94**(4):347–51.

19. Laine K, Rotvold W, Staff AC. Are obstetric anal sphincter ruptures preventable?– large and consistent rupture rate variations between the Nordic countries and between delivery units in Norway. *Acta Obstet Gynecol Scand*. 2013 Jan;**92**(1):94–100.

20. *Operative Vaginal Delivery*, Green-top Guideline No. 26. London: Royal College of Obstetricians and Gynaecologists, 2011, www.rcog.org.uk/globalassets/documents/guidelines/gtg_26.pdf

21. Committee on Practice Bulletins – Obstetrics. ACOG Practice Bulletin No. 154: operative vaginal delivery. *Obstet Gynecol*. 2015 Nov;**126**(5):e56-65.

Chapter 56

Maternal Collapse in Labour

William C. Maina

56.1 Introduction

Maternal collapse is defined as an acute event involving the cardiorespiratory systems and/or brain, resulting in a reduced or absent conscious level (and potentially death), at any stage in pregnancy and up to 6 weeks postpartum [1]. Causes and management of maternal collapse in labour are discussed, including adult basic life support. For detailed adult advanced life support, national resuscitation council and European Resuscitation Council guidelines should be consulted.

56.2 Epidemiology and Aetiology

The incidence of maternal collapse is unknown but the frequency in labour will depend on the number of deliveries and case mix in a maternity unit. It has a wide-ranging aetiology, as shown in Table 56.1, but vasovagal attacks and the postictal state following an epileptic seizure are the most common causes. Consider using the 5Hs to ascertain the cause [2].

56.3 Pathogenesis and Pathophysiology

This will depend on the underlying cause, but the common mechanisms are hypoxia, hypovolaemia, hypotension,

Table 56.1 Possible causes of maternal collapse in labour [2]

Head
- Eclampsia, epilepsy, cerebrovascular accident, vasovagal response

Heart
- Myocardial infarction, arrhythmias, peripartum cardiomyopathy, congenital heart disease, dissection of thoracic aorta, tamponade

Hypoxia
- Asthma, pulmonary embolism, pulmonary oedema, tension pneumothorax, anaphylaxis

Haemorrhage
- Abruption, placenta praevia, uterine rupture and rarely splenic or hepatic rupture

w**H**ole body and **H**azards
- Hypoglycaemia, amniotic fluid embolism, sepsis, complications of epidural analgesia, drug toxicity, hypothermia

hypoglycaemia and other metabolic disturbances, brain insults and drug toxicities. Prompt and effective resuscitation is key to reduction in maternal and fetal morbidity and mortality. The outcome of maternal collapse in labour will range from full recovery, single or multiple organ failure and, sadly, maternal and/or fetal demise.

Physiological and physical changes in pregnancy can exacerbate maternal and/or fetal response to maternal collapse and can make resuscitation more challenging [3]. These are listed in Tables 56.2, 56.3 and 56.4.

56.4 Approach to Management of Maternal Collapse in Labour

The first step is to assess whether it is safe for you to approach the woman, followed by assessment of whether she is responsive or unresponsive. If the woman is responsive, she should be placed in the recovery position and appropriate help should be summoned. If the woman is unresponsive, call for help and follow the standard ABCDE approach starting with Airway assessment followed by assessment of Breathing, Circulation, Disability (neurological status), Exposure and warming. The sequence shown in Box 56.1 should be followed with modification as appropriate to the circumstances.

Resuscitation should be conducted according to national resuscitation guidelines. This includes basic life support (Figure 56.1), adult advanced life support and automated external defibrillation (AED). European Resuscitation Council guidelines [4] and UK Resuscitation Council guidelines [5] are described in this chapter.

An individual who is unresponsive and not breathing normally is in cardiac arrest and requires CPR. In the maternity setting, cardiac arrest is a rare event. Most instances of maternal collapse in labour are associated with rapid deterioration in the clinical condition of the woman due to a potentially reversible course. Prompt and effective resuscitation is crucial to optimizing the outcome for the mother and her fetus or fetuses.

In the community setting, basic life support should be administered, and rapid transfer arranged, unless appropriate personnel and equipment are available.

From 20 weeks of gestation onwards, the pressure of the gravid uterus must be relieved from the inferior vena cava and aorta. Manual uterine displacement is preferred using an 'up, off and over' technique while maintaining the woman in a fully

Table 56.2 Cardiovascular changes in pregnancy and impact on resuscitation

Parameter	Change	Effect
Plasma volume	Increased by up to 50%	Dilutional anaemia
Heart rate	Increased by 15–20 bpm	Reduced oxygen-carrying capacity
Cardiac output	Increased by 40%	Increased CPR circulation demands
Uterine blood flow	Significantly reduced by pressure of gravid uterus on IVC	Increased CPR circulation demands
	10% of cardiac output at term	Potential for rapid massive haemorrhage
Systemic vascular resistance	Decreased	Sequesters blood during CPR
Arterial blood pressure	Decreased by 10–15 mm Hg	Decreased reserve
Venous return	Decreased by pressure of gravid uterus on IVC, in supine position, from 20 weeks' gestation onwards	Increased CPR circulation demands
		Decreased reserve

bpm = beats per minute; CPR: cardiopulmonary resuscitation; IVC inferior vena cava

Table 56.3. Respiratory changes in pregnancy and impact on resuscitation

Parameter	Change	Effect
Respiratory rate	Increased	Decreased buffering capacity, acidosis more likely
Oxygen consumption	Increased by 20%	Hypoxia develops more quickly
Functional residual capacity	Decreased by 25%	Decreased buffering capacity, acidosis more likely
Arterial PCO$_2$	Decreased	Decreased buffering capacity, acidosis more likely
Laryngeal oedema	Increased	Difficult intubation

PCO$_2$: partial pressure of carbon dioxide

Table 56.4 Changes in other systems and impact on resuscitation

Parameter	Change	Effect
Gastric motility	Decreased	Increased risk of aspiration
Lower oesophageal sphincter	Relaxed	Increased risk of aspiration
Uterus	Enlarged	Diaphragmatic splinting reduces residual capacity and makes ventilation more difficult
		Large breasts may interfere with intubation
Weight	Increases	Makes ventilation more difficult

Box 56.1 Steps in Resuscitation Guidelines: Primary and Secondary Surveys

Primary survey	Identify life-threatening problems
Resuscitation	Deal with these problems as you find them
Assess fetal well-being and viability	Consideration for delivery
Secondary survey	Top to toe, back to front examination
Definitive care	Specific management
Continuous re-evaluation	

supine position [6]. Alternatively, a left lateral tilt to an angle of at least 15% can be used, by sliding a solid wedge extending from the shoulder to pelvis under the woman to ensure effectiveness.

Early vascular access should also be obtained using 2 wide-bore cannulas (minimum 16 G) above the level of the diaphragm so that fluids administered are not affected by aortocaval compression [6]. Intraosseous access is a suitable alternative in situations where rapid access is required or where intravenous cannulation is difficult. Aggressive fluid resuscitation should be commenced as soon as practicable. Blood and blood products should be requested early and administered according to clinical need. Caution must be exercised in the presence of severe pre-eclampsia and eclampsia where fluid overload can contribute to poor outcome.

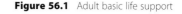

Figure 56.1 Adult basic life support

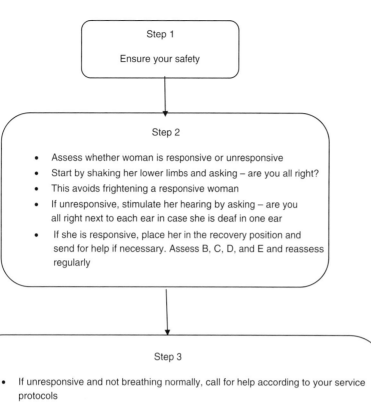

Step 1

Ensure your safety

Step 2

- Assess whether woman is responsive or unresponsive
- Start by shaking her lower limbs and asking – are you all right?
- This avoids frightening a responsive woman
- If unresponsive, stimulate her hearing by asking – are you all right next to each ear in case she is deaf in one ear
- If she is responsive, place her in the recovery position and send for help if necessary. Assess B, C, D, and E and reassess regularly

Step 3

- If unresponsive and not breathing normally, call for help according to your service protocols
- Follow ABCDE approach
- Open airway (head tilt, chin lift, remove any foreign bodies)
- Assess breathing (listen and feel for breaths, look for chest movements)
- If not breathing, commence CPR
- 30 chest compressions at a rate of 100–120 per minute to a depth of 5–6cm in the centre of the sternum followed by 2 rescue breaths. Continue until AED arrives. Do chest compressions alternately with colleagues to maintain efficiency and allow rest. Avoid interruptions
- As soon as AED arrives, switch it on and follow instructions

In most cases, delivery should be expedited to facilitate maternal resuscitation. An emergency caesarean section is preferred unless a vaginal delivery can be accomplished rapidly. If there is no return of spontaneous circulation after 4 minutes of effectively performed CPR, perimortem caesarean section should be commenced while continuing CPR. It should be performed in the delivery room or where resuscitation is taking place, as moving the woman to an operating theatre causes unnecessary delay and general anaesthesia is not required. However, with successful return of spontaneous circulation, general anaesthesia is required to allow the procedure to be completed.

Obstetricians, midwives, anaesthetists, theatre staff and all other personnel providing care in labour must be competent and confident in management of maternal collapse. The clinical governance team are responsible for ensuring that all staff attend annual training in management of obstetric emergencies.

56.4.1 Adult Advanced Life Support

In the hospital setting, adult advanced life support is guided by the cardiac arrest team. Precipitating cause is identified and treated. A detailed discussion of adult advanced life support is available in national resuscitation council and European Resuscitation Council guidelines.

56.4.2 Post-collapse Management Principles

- Ensure accurate documentation.
- Debrief patient (if alive) and relatives.
- Senior staff should offer staff support and debriefing.
- Review case through clinical governance process.
- Report the case to MBRRACE (UK and Ireland) or equivalent organization in your country. MBRRACE is an abbreviation for Mothers and Babies: Reducing Risk through Audits and Confidential Enquiries.

56.5 Some Key Points in CPR

- Chest compressions should be performed to a depth of 5 cm and not more than 6 cm.
- Perform chest compressions at a rate of 100–120/minute.
- Allow the chest to recoil completely after compression: do not lean on the chest.
- Chest compressions are tiring. They should be performed in turns and continued without interruptions.
- An experienced person should take the lead role.
- The duration of any individual resuscitation should be based on the individual circumstances of the case.
- Refer to key guidelines for more detailed description of CPR.

56.6 Key Messages

- The incidence of maternal collapse in labour is unknown
- The frequency of maternal collapse in labour will depend on the number of deliveries and the case mix in a maternity unit
- Maternal collapse is due to a wide range of aetiology, but cardiac arrest is a rare event
- Prompt and effective multidisciplinary care is crucial to the outcome for the woman and her fetus or fetuses.
- Survival of the collapsed pregnant woman in labour beyond 24 weeks gestation depends not only on effective CPR but also on relieving pressure of the gravid uterus on the inferior vena cava and aorta by appropriate techniques and timely perimortem caesarean section
- Resuscitation and post-collapse management must follow national guidelines
- All clinicians providing care to women in labour must be competent and confident in management of maternal collapse

References

1. *Maternal Collapse in Pregnancy and Puerperium*, Green-top Guideline No 56. London: Royal College of Obstetricians and Gynaecologists, 2011. www .rcog.org.uk.

2. Sowter M, Weaver E, Beaves M, eds. *Practical Obstetric Multi-Professional Training (PROMPT): Course Manual.*

Melbourne: RANZCOG, Highway Press; 2013.

3. Whittey JE. Maternal cardiac arrest in pregnancy. *Clin Obstet Gynaecol.* 2002;**45**:377–92.

4. European Resuscitation Council. Guidelines for Resuscitation. 2015. www .erc.edu

5. Resuscitation Council UK. 2015 Resusciatation Guidelines. 2015. www.erc.org.uk/resuscitation-guidelines

6. Paterson-Brown S, Howell C, eds. *The MOET Course Manual: Managing Obstetric Emergencies and Trauma*, 3rd ed. Cambridge: Cambridge University Press; 2014.

Management of Postpartum Haemorrhage

Emma Leighton & Edwin Chandraharan

57.1 Introduction

Postpartum haemorrhage (PPH) is one of the leading causes of maternal morbidity and mortality worldwide, with the World Health Organization (WHO) estimating 140 000 maternal deaths every year due to PPH [1]. Between 1990 and 2015 there has been a decrease in the number of women dying in the perinatal period (all-cause mortality) with 385 deaths per 100 000 live births in 1990 decreasing to 216 per 100 000 live births; however, a significant gap in the mortality in developed and developing countries persists [2]. In 2015, the maternal mortality rate in low-income countries was 479 per 100 000 live births versus 13 per 100 000 births in high-income countries [2]. In the UK, PPH is the third most common direct cause of maternal death and was attributable for 0.78 deaths per 100 000 maternities between 2014 and 2016 [3]. Maternal death, however, can only be seen as the tip of the iceberg, with 492 cases of morbidities reported in Scotland during 2012 and many other unreported cases of morbidities such as post-traumatic stress syndrome [4].

Despite the overall reduction in the global maternal deaths, the number of women dying from PPH in developed countries is actually increasing. This can be almost wholly attributable to an increase in the incidence of women dying from PPH secondary to morbidly adherent placenta (MAP): placenta accreta, increta or percreta. MAP itself is increasing in prevalence secondary to a rising caesarean section rate as well as advancing maternal age [5].

The 2012–2014 Confidential Enquiries into Maternal Deaths and Morbidity report (MBRRACE) identified a theme of 'too little done too late' among the women who died. It reported that improvements in care may have made a difference to the outcome for 38% of women who died and 74% of women with major obstetric haemorrhage who survived [3]. Failure to appreciate the severity of the PPH, inappropriate or delayed management, failure to seek senior support and lack of an multidisciplinary team (MDT) approach were all highlighted as contributing factors.

In this chapter, we will discuss the aetiopathogenesis, investigations and management of PPH.

57.2 Definition

Primary postpartum haemorrhage is the most common form of obstetric haemorrhage. The Royal College of Obstetricians and Gynaecologists (RCOG) Green-top guidelines define primary PPH as the loss of more than 500 mL of blood from the genital tract within 24 hours of giving birth [6]. For women

Table 57.1 Classification of severity of haemorrhage

Haemorrhage class	Blood loss	Percentage
Minor	500–1000 mL	8–16%
Major	>1000 mL	>16%
Moderate	1001–2000 mL	16–33%
Severe/Massive	>2000 mL	>33%

undergoing caesarean section, the cut-off is traditionally higher at 1000 mL of blood loss.

Secondary PPH takes place between 24 hours and 12 weeks postpartum and is most commonly caused by retained products of conception +/– endometritis. Primary postpartum haemorrhage is most commonly classified by the volume of blood lost into minor (500–1000 mL) and major (>1000 mL) blood loss.

Major PPH is further divided into moderate (1001–2000 mL) and severe (more than 2000 mL or more than 30–40% volume) (Table 57.1).

These definitions, however, are just a guide, and clinical judgement is needed to identify women who may become haemodynamically unstable with smaller volumes of blood loss (e.g. women with low body mass index (BMI) or baseline anaemia). Therefore, the definition of massive obstetric haemorrhage should also include any woman who has lost more than 30% of her blood volume, is bleeding more than 125 mL/minute or has developed haemodynamic instability. As volume of blood loss can be difficult to estimate, tools such as the shock index and the rule of 30 can be used to aid clinical judgement [7].

57.3 Epidemiology and Aetiology

57.3.1 Epidemiology

Worldwide, 6% of deliveries are affected by PPH [6]. Between 2014 to 2016, 18 women in the UK died due to PPH. This accounts for 0.78 deaths per 100 000 maternities and makes PPH the second most common direct cause of death following thrombosis and thromboembolism [3]. In developed countries, the rate of PPH is increasing and there was a near doubling of the maternal death rate from 2010–12 to 2013–15. This can be almost entirely attributed to haemorrhage secondary to morbidly adherent placenta [3].

57.3.2 Risk Factors

Risk factors for PPH can develop both antenatally and intrapartum. A frank discussion regarding place of delivery should be had with all women who have risk factors for PPH. The Confidential Enquiry into Maternal and Child Health have advised that women with risk factors for PPH should be delivered in a hospital with a blood bank on site.

Despite the risk factors in Table 57.2, the majority of PPH occurs in those with no risk factors and therefore clinicians need to be prepared for PPH in all individuals [8].

57.3.3 Managing Risks

57.3.3.1 Antenatally

Identification of anaemia in the antenatal period allows for treatment with iron and subsequent reduction in risk of postpartum morbidity.

57.3.3.2 Intrapartum

Active Management of the Third Stage

Active management of the third stage of labour with a combination of the use of uterotonics and controlled cord

traction has been shown to reduce the risk of PPH. However, early cord clamping is associated with reduced birthweight and therefore the National Institute for Health and Care Excellence (NICE) recommends waiting at least 1 minute after birth before clamping the cord if there are no concerns regarding the baby [9].

The RCOG recommendations for uterotonics in the third stage are as follows:

- Low-risk women delivering vaginally – oxytocin 10 IU by intramuscular injection
- Women delivering by caesarean section – oxytocin 5 IU by slow intravenous injection
- Women at increased risk of PPH – consider using ergometrine-oxytocin in the absence of hypertension (reduces the risk of minor PPH)
- Women at increased risk of PPH delivering by caesarean section – consider the use of tranexamic acid (0.5–1 g)

57.3.3.3 Placenta Praevia

Women who have placenta praevia as well as a history of previous caesarean section delivery have a high incidence of abnormal placentation [6]. The location and anatomy of the

Table 57.2 Risk factors for PPH [6]

Antenatal	Risk (OR/95% CI)	Intrapartum	Risk (OR/95% CI)
Age >40 years		Instrumental delivery	
Anaemia		Episiotomy	4.70 (2.60–8.40) 2.18 (1.68–2.76) 1.7 (1.20–2.50)
High BMI		Retained placenta	7.83 (3.78–16.22) 3.50 (2.10–5.80) 6 (3.50–10.4)
Asian and African ethnicity		Suspected or proven placental abruption	
Placenta praevia		Prolonged third stage of labour	7.6 (4.2–13.5) 2.61 (1.83–3.72)
Anaemia and grand multiparity		General anaesthetic	2.9 (1.9–4.5)
Pre-eclampsia	5 (3–8.5) 2.20 (1.3–3.7)	Prolonged second stage	3.4 (2.4–4.70) 1.9 (1.2–2.9)
Hypertension		Perineal laceration	1.40 (1.04–1.87) 2.4 (2–2.80) 1.7 (1.1–2.5)
Previous caesarean section			
Previous PPH	3.6 (1.2–10.20)		
Macrosomia	2.1 (1.62–2.76) 2.4 (1.9–2.9)		
Multiple pregnancy	3.3 (1–10.6) 4.7 (2.4–9.1)		
Placenta accreta	3.30 (1.70–6.40)		

OR: odds ratio; CI: confidence interval

Table 57.3 Causes of PPH with incidence [10]

4Ts	Cause	Approximate incidence
Tone	Uterine atony	80%
Tissue	Retained tissue, invasive placenta	5%
Trauma	Genital tract laceration or tear, uterine rupture, uterine inversion	13%
Thrombin	Coagulopathy, disseminated intravascular coagulation (DIC)	2%

Table 57.4 Rule of 30 for massive obstetric haemorrhage

Systolic blood pressure (BP)	Falls by 30 mm Hg
Pulse	Increase by 30 beats/minute
Hb	Falls by 30% (approx. 3 g/dL)
Haematocrit	Falls by 30%
Estimated blood loss	30% of normal (70 mL/kg in adults) (100 mL/kg during pregnancy)

placenta need to be clearly defined with a high suspicion for placentae accreta, increta and percreta. Those with suspected abnormal placental invasion should be managed in a tertiary centre with the appropriate level of expertise.

57.3.4 Aetiology

The causes of PPH can be summarized as the 4Ts: tone, tissue, trauma and thrombin (Table 57.3). Every woman needs to have a systematic examination of the external genitalia, vaginal walls, cervix and uterus to ensure timely identification of PPH and its cause. Any personal or family history of clotting abnormalities should be sought as well as a clotting screen (thrombin).

57.4 Clinical Features

At term, the blood supply to the uterus is approximately 1 L per minute; therefore, women can lose a lot of blood very quickly if not identified and managed appropriately. Signs and symptoms secondary to PPH are those attributed to anaemia and haemodynamic instability as well as the cause of the PPH.

Symptoms
- dizziness
- shortness of breath
- palpitations
- anxiety
- confusion/lethargy

Signs
- visible blood loss – volumes often poorly estimated
- sweating
- decreased Glasgow Coma Scale (GCS) score
- falling oxygen concentrations
- tachycardia
- tachypnoea
- hypotension
- signs of peripheral shut down – cold extremities and oliguria
- biochemical evidence of metabolic acidosis
- clinical features specific to cause of PPH

The symptoms and signs of PPH that develop at worsening severities can be seen in Table 57.4. However, the blood loss at which signs and symptoms develop can vary greatly between individuals. Young fit pregnant women can compensate for a very long time before becoming hypotensive and showing signs of shock. Furthermore, those with co-morbidities or low BMI have less compensatory reserve and the use of medications e.g. labetalol in pre-eclampsia can blunt tachycardia. Tools such as the rule of 30 and the shock index have been identified to help clinicians quantify the volume of blood loss and degree of haemodynamic compromise in different individuals [10].

57.5 Shock Index

The shock index is calculated by dividing heart rate by systolic blood pressure. The normal shock index is between 0.5 and 0.7. An obstetric shock index in the pregnant population has been described in which a shock index >1 is associated with a significant increase in incidence of blood transfusion [11].

57.6 Investigations

- Bloods tests: full blood count (FBC), urea and electrolytes, clotting profile, lactate group and save (crossmatch at least 4 units in massive PPH) in all patients. A rapid haemoglobin (Hb) result can be obtained by venous blood gas (VBG) or haemocue; however, it can be falsely reassuring if the patient has not undergone adequate fluid resuscitation.

Further investigations are dependent upon response to initial resuscitation and likely cause of bleeding.

- Abdominal ultrasound (US) to identify uterine rupture or intraperitoneal bleeding
- Exteriorization and inspection of uterus during caesarean section
- Examination under anaesthesia if retained products of conception are suspected

57.7 Clinical Management

A systematic approach to the management of PPH is needed, starting with assessment and resuscitation and then progressing through medical to surgical management dependent on the cause. Approaches such as the haemostasis algorithm have been developed in order to ensure timely and stepwise management. Local systematic MDT protocols such as 'code blue' should be developed in all hospitals with regular simulation training to ensure a systematic approach to PPH is employed [12] (Box 57.1).

57.7.1 Ask for Help and Hands on the Abdomen (uterine massage)

In all cases of PPH, the first step should be to alert members of the MDT team to ensure optimal monitoring and management of the patient. In massive obstetric haemorrhage, the switchboard can be used to put out a 'code blue' call to ensure all members of the MDT including the haematologist and porter are contacted. As 80% of PPH is secondary to uterine atony, uterine massage should be commenced immediately.

57.7.2 Assess and Resuscitate

The main objectives of resuscitation are to replace the circulating volume, oxygen-carrying capacity and coagulability of blood. The patient should be managed with a systematic ABCDE approach; however, with an MDT team the steps of assessment and resuscitation should happen in tandem.

Airway – Ensure patency of the airway and apply 15 L of oxygen via non-rebreathe mask regardless of oxygen saturations.

Breathing – Respiratory rate, oxygen saturation, work of breathing and air entry should be monitored at least every 15 minutes.

Circulation – Heart rate, capillary refill time, blood pressure monitoring at least every 15 minutes. Position the patient flat on the back, insert two large-bore cannulas, take blood samples and crossmatch at least 4 units of blood in massive PPH. Start resuscitation with crystalloid fluids and progress to blood products if needed. The volume and rate of fluid resuscitation are dependent on blood loss and haemodynamic instability.

Box 57.1 Haemostasis Algorithm for Management of PPH [12]

H - Ask for **h**elp and **h**ands on the uterus (uterine massage)
A - **A**ssess (ABCDE) and resuscitate (intravenous (IV) fluids)
E - **E**stablish aetiology, **e**nsure availability of blood and ecbolics
M - **M**assage the uterus
O - **O**xytocin infusion (10 units/hour) or intramuscular prostaglandins (250 ug)
S - **S**hift to theatre, with aortic compression, bimanual compression or anti-shock garment (for low-resource settings before transfer to a tertiary centre) as appropriate
T - **T**amponade by balloon or uterine packing after exclusion of retained tissue and trauma. Administer IV tranexamic acid (1 g)
A - **A**pply compression sutures on the uterus (B-Lynch or modified technique)
S - **S**ystematic pelvic devascularization (uterine, ovarian, quadruple or internal)
I - **I**nterventional radiology and, if appropriate, uterine artery embolization
S - **S**ubtotal or total abdominal hysterectomy

Disability – Disability can be assessed using the AVPU criteria (alert, voice, pain, unresponsive).

Exposure – Systematic examination of abdomen and genital tract to identify the cause of PPH; keep the patient warm to prevent coagulopathy.

57.7.3 Establish Aetiology, Ensure Availability of Blood, Ecbolics (bolus of oxytocin, syntometrine, ergometrine)

The cause of the PPH needs to be identified by investigating for each of the 4Ts (tone, tissue, trauma and thrombin).

1. Tone: palpate the uterus for contraction and retraction
2. Tissue: examination of the placenta. If any evidence of retained tissue, then take the patient back to theatre and perform an examination and manual removal of placenta under anaesthesia.
3. Trauma: thorough examination of the vulva and vagina.
4. Thrombin – identify any history of personal or family history of coagulopathy, blood tests should be taken for coagulation studies.

57.7.3.1 Ecbolics

If an atonic uterus is identified as the primary cause of PPH then rapid administration of uterotonic medication should be commenced:

1. Oxytocin: 5 units of syntocinon injected intramuscularly (this can be repeated)
2. If bleeding persists, syntometrine (combination of oxytocin 5 units and ergometrine 0.5 mg) or ergometrine 0.5 mg by slow intravenous or intramuscular injection should be administered (use with caution in women with hypertension/ pre-eclampsia)

57.7.3.2 Ensure Availability of Blood and Blood Products

Blood and blood products are important to restore the oxygen-carrying capacity of blood and correct coagulopathy. Blood transfusion is required in patients with massive obstetric haemorrhage or those who have lost smaller volumes but are displaying signs of haemodynamic compromise. Initiating blood transfusion is a clinical decision that should be based on multiple factors including the patient's demographics, estimated volume of blood loss and haemodynamic signs and symptoms (Table 57.5). An obstetric shock index of more than 1 can help aid in the decision to start transfusion. Rapid point of access tests such as haemocue can be taken to help monitor response to resuscitation; however, they should not dissuade staff from initiating transfusion. A blood transfusion should not be held up if formal blood test results are not available. Each unit of red blood cells transfused is estimated to raise a patient's haemoglobin by 10 g/L and the haematocrit by 3%. As well as red cells, other blood products may also be required (e.g. clotting factors, fibrinogen and platelets). Early involvement of a haematologist is essential in all women with massive PPH to guide the administration of red blood cells and other blood products [13, 14].

Table 57.5 Therapeutic aims of management of massive blood loss, guidance from British Committee for Standards in Haematology [14]

Haemoglobin	>8 g/dL
Platelets	>75 x 10^9/L
Fibrinogen	1 g/L
Prothrombin time	<1.5 x mean control
Activated prothrombin time	<1.5 x mean control

Coagulopathy in PPH is secondary to two main phenomena: 1) dilution of clotting factors by fluid and red cell infusions and 2) activation of disseminated intravascular coagulation (DIC),which is characterized by widespread activation of the clotting cascade and subsequent consumption of clotting factors. In the obstetric setting, it is associated with sepsis (e.g. secondary to chorioamnionitis, placental abruption, amniotic fluid embolization). It can also be triggered by massive blood loss independent of other factors. The dilution of clotting factors is likely once 80% of the blood volume has been lost (e.g. 4.5 L in a 60 kg woman). However, this may begin much earlier in the presence of other predisposing factors (e.g. pre-eclampsia or low BMI). It is normally recommended that 1 litre of fresh-frozen plasma (FFP) is transfused for every 6 units of red cells.

57.7.4 Massage the Uterus

Stimulation of uterine contraction and retraction by uterine massage should be commenced as early as possible. Additionally, temporary compression of the aorta can help control rapid bleeding. The heel of the hand should be placed firmly in the midline just above the uterus and umbilicus.

57.7.5 Oxytocin Infusion/Prostaglandins

1. Oxytocin: Syntocinon can be administered as an infusion (40 units in 500 mL at a rate of 125 mL/hour) unless the patient is at high risk of fluid overload (e.g. severe pre-eclampsia). If oxytocin is infused in large amounts, then fluid balance needs to be carefully monitored due to the risk of significant dilutional hyponatraemia and subsequent pulmonary oedema, cerebral oedema and convulsions.

2) Prostaglandins: Hemabate (15-methyl prostaglandin 2 alpha) 250 μg can be administered intramuscularly. The dose can be repeated every 15 minutes for a maximum of 8 doses (2 mg). If bleeding persists after administering 3 doses of Hemabate, consider transferring the patient to theatre to continue further doses and consider surgical management. Caution should be exercised if administering Hemabate to a patient with asthma.

3. Misoprostol: 800 μg sublingually or 600–1000 μg rectally can be tried, particularly if an oxytocin infusion was not commenced earlier. Misoprostol is particularly useful in developing countries as it is low cost and easy to store.

4. Fibrinolytics: Tranexamic acid is a competitive inhibitor of plasminogen activation and can reduce bleeding by

inhibiting the breakdown of fibrinogen and fibrin clots. The WOMAN trial showed that the use of tranexamic acid decreased mortality secondary to PPH, regardless of cause, leading to the recent amendment of the WHO guidelines [15]. One gram of tranexamic acid in 10 mL (100 mg/mL) should be administered over 10 minutes (i.e. 100 mg/minute). A second dose of tranexamic acid can be administered if bleeding continues after 30 minutes. Tranexamic acid should be administered as soon as possible after bleeding starts and within 3 hours of birth.

57.7.6 Shift to Theatre

If bleeding continues despite medical management, the patient should be transferred to theatre. In theatre the patient can be continuously monitored, and examination can be performed under local or general anaesthesia to rule out any retained placental tissue or membranes. Bimanual compression can be employed at this stage. One hand is placed on the abdomen and the other inside the vagina and the uterus compressed between the two.

On transferring the patient to theatre, consent should be obtained for anaesthesia, tamponade balloon, laparotomy and hysterectomy to ensure that each procedure can be swiftly initiated if needed. When performing laparotomy, it is vital to involve the anaesthetist and seek their advice on the ability of the patient to withstand further blood loss if conservative methods were to fail. This helps avoid 'too little being done too late'. If the patient is stable, then conservative procedures can be attempted.

There are no randomized clinical trials investigating the best way to manage PPH after medical management fails. A systematic review of the different surgical procedures available to manage PPH showed good efficacy of balloon tamponade (84%), arterial embolization (90.7%), compression sutures (91.7%) and pelvic devascularization (84.6%) in managing PPH [16]. There was no significant difference seen between the different methods; therefore, it would be logical to begin with the least invasive procedure first.

57.7.7 Tamponade Balloon

A uterine balloon can be used as the next line in management when medical management fails to halt bleeding. Different types of balloons used include Sengstaken–Blakemore oesophageal catheter (SBOC) (most common), Rusch urological hydrostatic balloon and the 'Bakri SOS' balloon. Uterine balloons inhibit bleeding by exerting counterpressure on blood vessels in the uterine sinuses. A volume of approximately 300–400 mL is commonly used to provide a pressure equal to or above systolic pressure. It is a quick and relatively easy method and therefore can be initiated by even very junior staff. It inhibits bleeding, provides time for the correction of coagulopathy and prevents the need for more invasive surgical procedures in the vast majority of cases. The use of a uterine balloon has been referred to as the tamponade test. If the tamponade effect of the balloon stops bleeding, there is an 87% chance that no further surgical management will be required [17]. In developing countries where balloons are not widely available, an alternative option is to pack the uterus with sterile gauze to produce a tamponade. This technique is no longer advised in developed countries, as it is more difficult and traumatic compared with balloons.

57.7.8 Apply Compression Sutures

Failure of a tamponade balloon to stop bleeding requires immediate laparotomy. Direct bimanual compression of the uterus can be tried initially to determine whether compression sutures will be effective. The first compression sutures were described by Christopher B. Lynch, with further adaptations including the horizontal, vertical sutures and Cho's multiple square technique developed later. Compression sutures work by opposing the anterior and posterior walls of the uterus together, aiming to halt bleeding from the placental site.

The B-Lynch suture involves hysterotomy and the placement of vertical brace sutures. It enables the exploration of the uterus at the same time as suture placement; however, it requires a skilled surgeon to perform it, as areas close to the ureters and uterine vessels are involved. Alternatives to B-Lynch sutures includes the placement of separate vertical compression sutures. This type of suture allows for increased tension to be applied to the walls of the uterus and also negates the need for the uterus to be opened. Horizontal full-thickness sutures can be used at the time of caesarean section to control bleeding from the placental site in placenta praevia and can also be placed in the lower uterine segment. Cho et al developed a technique in which multiple squares are sutured to approximate the anterior and posterior uterine walls and virtually eliminate the uterine cavity; however, this technique may interfere with the drainage of inflammatory exudate from the uterus leading to pyometra. Vertical compression sutures (Figure 57.1) can be performed by less experienced surgeons and often take less time than the traditional B-Lynch sutures.

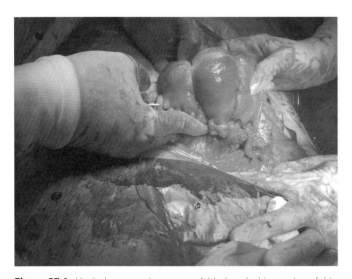

Figure 57.1 Vertical compression sutures. A black and white version of this figure will appear in some formats. For the colour version, please refer to the plate section.

57.7.9 Systematic Pelvic Devascularization

Ligation of blood vessels supplying the uterus can be attempted in a stepwise fashion. Initially, uterine arteries are ligated and if bleeding persists, the surgeon can proceed to a 'quadruple ligation' involving ligation of both ovarian arteries. Arterial ligation can be technically challenging as well as very time consuming. It is therefore essential that the patient is haemodynamically stable and able to tolerate a possibly lengthy procedure. Additionally, failure of arterial ligation and subsequent hysterectomy are associated with higher levels of morbidity compared to hysterectomy as the primary procedure. To achieve uterine artery ligation, the uterovesical fold of the peritoneum needs to be identified and incised and the bladder reflected down. A window is then made in the broad ligament just lateral to the uterine vessels and the needle is passed through this window. The needle should then be passed through the myometrium approximately 2 cm from the lateral border and a double knot then tied [18]. The same procedure should be repeated on the opposite side. If bleeding persists, both tubal branches of the ovarian artery in the mesosalpinx can be ligated as part of the quadruple ligation. If bleeding continues, ligation of the internal iliac artery can be attempted. This procedure will also arrest the bleeding arising from the lower segment, the broad ligament or the vagina. This procedure, however, requires an experienced surgeon with good anatomical knowledge of the pelvic sidewall. Success rates of this procedure range from 40–75% and it is an invaluable option for avoiding a hysterectomy. Two different techniques may be used dependent on the surgeon's skills and preference. Complications include injury to the ureters, haematoma of the pelvic sidewall or accidental ligation of the external iliac artery and subsequent lower limb ischaemia. Ligation of the main trunk of the internal iliac artery instead of the anterior branch can lead to intermittent claudication of the gluteal region.

57.7.10 Interventional Radiology

Arterial embolization can be considered in women who are not haemodynamically compromised in an attempt to preserve fertility. A catheter is passed into the femoral artery to reach the target vessel (internal iliac, uterine or ovarian) which is occluded using material such as gelatine sponge, polyurethane foam or polyvinyl alcohol particles. Alternatively, balloons can be inflated in the artery to provide temporary occlusion and then deflated hours later. Arterial embolization is particularly useful in the presence of coagulopathy. It can also be used prophylactically in women undergoing a planned caesarean section anticipated to have a PPH (e.g. cases of placenta accreta or increta). Success rates as high as 85–95% have been reported as well as successful subsequent pregnancies [19]. Complications include vessel perforation, infection, haematoma and tissue necrosis. Unfortunately, due to the need for expert interventional radiology input, this procedure is only available in specialized centres.

57.7.11 Subtotal or Total Hysterectomy

Hysterectomy is the last resort in order to save a woman's life. It should be a decision made by the most senior clinician and ideally two senior clinicians if available. It should be performed if all other procedures have failed or significantly earlier if the woman is haemodynamically unstable and not able to tolerate more conservative management. Although devastating, the life of the woman should not be risked in order to preserve her fertility.

If the bleeding is mainly from the upper segment due to an atonic uterus, then a subtotal hysterectomy can be performed. It is quicker and easier to perform as well as having lower morbidity and mortality rates compared to total hysterectomy. If the bleeding is predominantly from the lower segment, as seen in a morbidly adherent placenta, or when cervical or upper vaginal tears contribute to PPH, a total abdominal hysterectomy should be performed. Although similar to a standard transabdominal hysterectomy, the anatomical changes of pregnancy present additional difficulties for the surgeon including high rates of urinary tract damage. A 25-year review reported a maternal mortality rate of 11.6% [18]. This reflects the difficulties involved, the importance of involving experienced clinicians early and the need to consider a hysterectomy before it becomes too late to save the woman's life.

In cases where a morbidly adherent placenta have been identified early in pregnancy, then an MDT-discussed management plan, additional procedures (e.g. uterine artery embolization) and additional members of staff can be arranged for the delivery. Traditionally, the majority of women underwent elective caesarean section with peripartum total abdominal hysterectomy; however, newer procedures (e.g. the Triple P Procedure) developed to avoid hysterectomy and reduce blood loss have shown very promising results.

Hysterectomy can have long-term medical as well as psychological sequelae for a patient due to loss of perceived 'femininity' as well as fertility. It is therefore of paramount importance to provide a thorough debrief to all patients and their partners. This should involve discussions soon after the procedure as well as an opportunity to return to clinic following discharge to discuss events further.

57.8 The Other 3Ts

Postpartum haemorrhage caused by tissue, thrombin and trauma is significantly less common; however, it can lead to large blood loss by itself or worsen atonic PPH. It is therefore important to identify and effectively manage these underlying conditions.

57.8.1 Tissue

If active management of the third stage of labour with administration of oxytocin and controlled cord traction fails to deliver the placenta or if there is any evidence of an incomplete placenta, then the woman should be transferred to theatre. Manual removal of the placenta should be attempted under anaesthesia (regional or general) with the aid of ultrasound guidance to ensure an empty cavity.

57.8.2 Thrombin

Congenital or acquired clotting disorders (e.g. factor VIII or factor IX deficiency, von Willebrand disease) can cause or contribute to PPH. Coagulopathy can be identified with FBC and clotting studies as well as rapid bedside testing. Whether there is history of heavy nose bleeds, periods or with tooth extraction or a family history of clotting disorders should be confirmed. Coagulopathy can be acquired secondary to dilution, sepsis, pre-eclampsia or DIC. Local transfusion policies should be followed to help prevent secondary coagulopathy and advice from a haematologist should be sought early and is essential in all cases of blood loss of >2000 mL or any case of ongoing bleeding suspected to be caused by coagulopathy.

57.8.3 Trauma

Trauma includes bleeding from tears to the genital tract or episiotomy, uterine rupture, extension of uterine angles or tears during caesarean section extragenital, and very rare causes include subcapsular liver rupture or rupture of ovarian or splenic vessels.

Over 85% of women who give birth vaginally will endure some degree of perineal trauma, either in the form of a tear or episiotomy. From 60–70% of these women will require suturing. Systematic inspection of the vagina, cervix and perineum, under good light with adequate exposure, is paramount in order to grade and repair tears and episiotomies. It is advised that first and second degree tears are repaired with continuous absorbable sutures. Third and fourth degree tears should be repaired under direct supervision of a senior clinician. Anterior vaginal tears may be particularly prevalent in women with previous female genital cutting. These tears can bleed profusely, and, if close to the urethral orifice, a catheter should be inserted during repair to avoid inadvertent injury to the urethra. Multiple shallow vaginal lacerations may be difficult to suture and therefore can be managed with insertion of a vaginal pack. It is very important to exclude any arterial bleeding before insertion of the pack. Lubrication with flavin or povidone iodine or insertion of the pack inside sterile plastic bags can be used to reduce trauma on removal of the vaginal pack.

Any tears of the upper vagina should be repaired by a senior clinician due to the presence of multiple anatomical structures (e.g. bladder, urethra, ureters, bowel and rectum) in the vicinity. A stay suture can be used to help pull the tear downwards and enable easier suturing. Cervical tears are uncommon postdelivery. The cervix should be fully explored and only tears that are profusely bleeding or bigger than 2 cm need to be repaired.

57.8.4 Perineal and Pelvic Haematomas

Up to 50% of women giving birth develop small, self-limiting vulvar or infra-levator haematomas. As long as the haematoma is less than 5 cm and is not rapidly expanding, it can be managed conservatively [18]. Larger haematomas or those expanding quickly should be managed surgically. Large vulvar or infra-levator haematomas (>5 cm) should be incised through the vagina and drained and bleeding points identified and ligated using figure of eight sutures. If no discernible bleeding points can be seen, a vaginal pack or Foley catheter balloon can be inserted to treat persistent oozing. Antibiotic cover should be provided as well as an indwelling Foley catheter to prevent urinary retention. Supra-levator haematomas should be suspected in any woman with haemodynamic instability out of proportion to perceived blood loss or with an upper vaginal tear. Presentation can be either immediately after delivery or after the first 24 hours. Ultrasound should be used to visualize supra-levator or broad ligament haematomas. If the patient is stable and the haematoma is not increasing in size, then conservative management can be employed with IV fluids, blood transfusion, antibiotics, vaginal pack for tamponade as well as close monitoring of the patient. In the author's experience, the use of a Bakri balloon coated with the haemostat 'Floseal' was found to be effective in arresting haemorrhage in four cases of para-vaginal, supra-levator haematomas. If the haematoma is increasing in size or the patient is unstable, then surgical management is required. Exploratory laparotomy with ligation of the bleeding vessel or ligation of the anterior internal iliac artery should be performed. Alternatively, if expertise is available, selective arterial emobilization may be attempted in order to avoid a laparotomy.

57.9 Management of PPH in Special Circumstances

Morbidly adherent placenta (MAP) (placenta accreta, increta or percreta) is abnormal invasion of the placenta into the uterine myometrium. It carries a mortality rate of 7–10% worldwide due to PPH and damage to surrounding pelvic organs. The incidence of morbidly adherent placenta is increasing worldwide due to an increasing rate of caesarean section. Other risk factors include uterine surgery (e.g. myomectomy), increasing maternal age and in vitro fertilization (IVF). Early diagnosis, multidisciplinary planning and patient-specific management are crucial to ensure good maternal and perinatal outcomes. Traditionally, MAP is managed by caesarean section and either conservative retention of the placenta or hysterectomy +/– resection of placenta adherent to adjacent structures. Intentional retention of the placenta is used in an attempt to avoid massive PPH and its sequelae; however, this carries the risk of secondary PPH, DIC, sepsis, emergency caesarean section and the development of fistulae. Women undergoing conservative management also require frequent follow-up with βhCG levels and ultrasound scanning.

The most drastic management of MAP is a caesarean hysterectomy and resection of affected organs in cases of placenta percreta (Figure 57.2). This can be performed either electively or as an emergency surgery if other, more conservative methods fail to control bleeding. The advantage of an elective peripartum hysterectomy is that it prevents the possibility of having to perform an emergency caesarean section and therefore reduces the risk of massive blood loss. The disadvantages include continuing blood loss after caesarean due to bleeding from placental blood supply provided by adjacent organs (placenta percreta), damage to adjacent organs as well as the long-term loss of fertility, risk of vaginal prolapse and psychological sequelae.

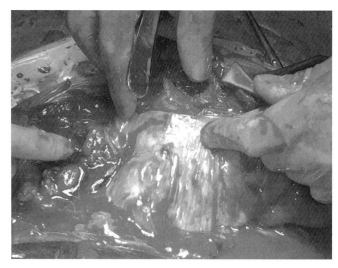

Figure 57.2 Placenta percreta. A black and white version of this figure will appear in some formats. For the colour version, please refer to the plate section.

The Triple P Procedure has been developed as a conservative surgical alternative to a peripartum hysterectomy to reduce maternal morbidity and mortality [20]. It has been shown to have reduced levels of peripartum blood loss, maternal morbidity [21]. The Triple P Procedure involves 1) perioperative placental localization 2) pelvic devascularization and 3) placental nonseparation. It has been reported that the Triple P Procedure reduced the incidence of postpartum haemorrhage with no cases of peripartum hysterectomy [21].

57.9.1 Placental Localization

All patient with suspected MAP should undergo transabdominal ultrasound and Doppler scanning to identify the placental location as well as the classical features of MAP such as placental lacunae, thinning of the myometrial border and disruption of the posterior wall of the bladder. Magnetic resonance imaging (MRI) scanning is not routinely indicted in MAP; however, it may be used if the placenta is posterior or to help determine the extent of lateral extension into the broad ligament. Transabdominal ultrasound is also used perioperatively to delineate the placental location. A transverse incision can then be made above the upper border of the placenta to avoid incising the placenta.

57.9.2 Pelvic Devascularization

Interventional radiology is used to place occlusive balloons in the internal iliac arteries prior to surgery. After delivery of the baby, the balloons are inflated to reduce blood loss. The balloons are deflated after 6 hours to prevent ischaemia or thrombosis of the pelvic structures. Uterine artery embolization can also be used if bleeding is persistent after the inflation of occlusive balloons.

57.9.3 Placental Nonseparation

The myometrium and attached placenta are removed without placental separation, and the myometrium is reconstructed. A 2 cm margin of myometrium (with invading placenta) must be left in the lower uterine lip to allow repair of the myometrial defect. In cases of percreta with placenta invasion of the bladder, haemostatic agents (e.g. PerClot) and sutures should be used to control bleeding from the retained placenta. After achieving haemostasis, the myometrial defect is repaired in two layers, the first with interrupted sutures and the second in a continuous layer. By leaving the bladder essentially 'untouched' maternal morbidity is minimalized. The average blood loss is 2 L with no reported cases of peripartum hysterectomy, bladder or ureter injuries reported so far.

57.10 Secondary Haemorrhage

Secondary postpartum haemorrhage occurs between 24 hours and 12 weeks postpartum. The most common time for women to present is in the second week postpartum. Secondary PPH is most likely due to retained products and infection (endometritis). All women with secondary PPH should undergo transvaginal ultrasound to identify retained products. Products measuring >2 cm should be removed. A high vaginal swab should be taken, and broad-spectrum antibiotics should be started in all women with endometritis.

57.11 Secondary PPH

Bleeding occurs after the first 24 hours of birth, usually due to infection (endometritis) or retained products of conception. Rare causes such as coagulopathy and pseudo-aneurysm of the uterine artery may also cause a secondary postpartum haemorrhage. Investigation and management should be aimed at identifying and treating the specific cause of secondary PPH.

Infographics may aid the management of primary and secondary PPH [22].

57.12 Key Messages

- Forty per cent of women who suffer PPH have no previously identifiable risk factors; therefore, clinicians need to be vigilant concerning the possibility of PPH in all women.
- The uterus receives 1 L of blood/minute at term; therefore, women can lose very large amounts of blood quickly if not managed in a timely fashion.
- Pregnant women can compensate for large volumes of blood loss before becoming hypotensive; clinicians can use tools such as rule of 30 and shock index to help quantify blood loss and degree of haemodynamic instability.
- A stepwise approach to the management of PPH should be initiated with algorithms such as HAEMOSTASIS available.
- Remember the maxim: 'too little too late'.

57.13 Key Guidelines Relevant to the Topic

Prevention and Management of Postpartum Haemorrhage, Green-top Guideline No 52. London: Royal College of Obstetricians and Gynaecologists, 2016. [6]

FIGO Consensus Guidelines on Placenta Accreta Spectrum Disorders, www.figo.org/news/now-available-figo-consensus-guidelines-placenta-accreta-spectrum-disorders-0015836

References

1. Abouzahr C. Global burden of maternal death and disability. *Br. Med Bull.* 2003;**67**(1):1–11. doi: org/10.1093/bmb/ldg015

2. https://data.worldbank.org/indicator/SH.STA.MMRT

3. Knight M, Bunch K, Tuffnell D, et al. eds., on behalf of MBRRACE-UK. *Saving Lives, Improving Mothers' Care: Lessons Learned to Inform Maternity Care from the UK and Ireland Confidential Enquiries into Maternal Deaths and Morbidity 2014–16.* Oxford: National Perinatal Epidemiology Unit, University of Oxford; 2018

4. Health Improvement Scotland. Scottish Confidential Audit of Severe Maternal Morbidity. 7th Report, 2011.

5. Wu S, Kocherginsky M, Hibbard JU. Abnormal placentation: twenty-year analysis. *Am J Obstet Gynecol.* 2005 May;**192**(5):1458–61.

6. *Prevention and Management of Postpartum Haemorrhage*, Green-top Guideline No 52. London: Royal

College of Obstetricians and Gynaecologists, 2009.

7. Mavrides E, Allard S, Chandraharan E, et al. Prevention and management of postpartum haemorrhage: Green-top Guideline No 52. *BJOG.* 2016;**358**:e106-49.pmid:27981719.

8. Carroli G, Cuesta C, Abalos E, Gulmezoglu A. Epidemiology of postpartum haemorrhage: a systematic review. *Best Pract Res Clin Obstet Gynaecol.* 2008; **22**(6):999–1012.

9. NICE. *Intrapartum Care: Care of Healthy Women and Their Babies during Childbirth.* Clinical Guideline 190. 2014

10. Chandraharan E, Arulkumaran S. Massive postpartum haemorrhage and management of coagulopathy. *Obstet, Gynaecol Reprod Med.* 2007 Apr; **17**:119e22.

11. Le Bas A, Chandraharan E, Addei A, Arulkumaran S. Use of the 'obstetric shock index' as an adjunct in identifying significant blood loss in patients with massive postpartum hemorrhage. *Int J Gynaecol Obstet.* 2014 Mar;**124**(3):253–5.

12. Chandraharan E, Arulkumaran S. Management algorithm for atonic postpartum haemorrhage. *J Paediatr Obstet Gynaecol.* 2005;**31**(3):106–12.

13. Pinas Carillo A, Chandraharan E. Postpartum haemorrhage and haematological management. *Obstet Gynaecol Reprod Med.* 2014;**24**(10):291–5. ttps://doi.org/10.1016/j.ogrm.2014.07.004

14. Hunt BJ, Allard S, Keeling D, et al.; British Committee for Standards in Haematology. A practical guideline for the haematological management of major haemorrhage. *Br J Haematol.* 2015;**170**: 788–803.

15. WOMAN Trial Collaborators. Effect of early tranexamic acid administration on mortality, hysterectomy, and other morbidities in women with post-partum haemorrhage (WOMAN): an international, randomised, double-blind, placebo-controlled trial. *Lancet.* 2017; May 27;**389** (10084):2105–16.

16. Doumouchtsis S K, Papageorghiou A T, Arulkumaran S. Systematic review of conservative management of postpartum hemorrhage: what to do when medical treatment fails. *Obstet Gynecol Surv.* 2007;**62**(8): 540–7.

17. Condous GS, Arulkumaran S, Symonds I, et al. The 'tamponade test' in the management of massive postpartum hemorrhage. *Obstet Gynecol.* 2003;**101**: 767–72.

18. Chandraharan E, Arulkumaran S. Surgical aspects of postpartum haemorrhage. *Best Pract Res*

Clin Obstet Gynaecol. 2008 Dec;**22** (6):1089–102. doi: 10.1016/j. bpobgyn.2008.08.001

19. Ratnam LA, Gibson M, Sandhu C, et al. Transcatheter pelvic arterial embolisation for control of obstetric and gynaecological haemorrhage. *J Obstet Gynaecol.* 2008 Aug;**28** (6):573–9. doi: 10.1080/ 01443610802273374

20. Chandraharan E, Rao S, Belli AM, Arulkumaran S. The triple-P procedure as a conservative surgical alternative to peripartum hysterectomy for placenta percreta. *Int J Gynaecol Obstet.* 2012 May;

117(2):191–4. doi: 10.1016/j. ijgo.2011.12.005

21. Teixidor Viñas M, Belli AM, Arulkumaran S, Chandraharan E. Prevention of postpartum hemorrhage and hysterectomy in patients with morbidly adherent placenta: a cohort study comparing outcomes before and after introduction of the triple-P procedure. *Ultrasound Obstet Gynecol.* 2015 Sep;**46**(3):350–5.

22. Chandraharan E, Krishna A. Diagnosis and management of postpartum haemorrhage. *BMJ.* 2017 Sep 27;**358**: j3875. doi: 10.1136/bmj.j3875

Chapter 58

Birth Injuries and Perineal Trauma

Katariina Laine & Sari Räisänen

58.1 Introduction

Perineal injury during vaginal birth is common, and most of the nulliparous women need suturing after childbirth. Among parous women perineal injuries are less frequent.

Obstetric perineal trauma is classified to degrees from 1 to 4 regarding the severity of trauma and to what extent the pelvic floor muscles and tissues are injured. First degree injuries are superficial tears without involvement of the pelvic floor muscles. In second degree injury, pelvic floor muscles are injured but the anal sphincter muscles are intact. In a third degree injury, the external anal sphincter is injured (degrees 3A and 3B). In a fourth degree injury, the entire perineum is ruptured, including the anal sphincter muscles and the rectal mucosa.

Obstetric anal sphincter injury is the most important risk factor for female anal incontinence. Pain, discomfort, sexual dysfunction and psychological complaints are also associated with obstetric anal sphincter injuries (OASIS) [1]. Due to the many complaints associated with OASIS, it is obviously worth trying to avoid OASIS with best possible clinical practice.

58.2 Definition and Classification of Perineal Injuries

58.2.1 Anatomy

58.2.1.1 Perineum

The perineum is the surface region between the pubic symphysis and the coccyx, the inferior part of the pelvic outlet. This diamond-shaped structure is anteriorly bordered by the pubic arch, posteriorly by the coccyx and laterally by the ischiopubic rami, ischial tuberosities and the sacrotuberous ligaments. The deep border of the perineum is the inferior surface of the pelvic floor and the superficial border is the skin. The pelvic floor contains superficial and deep muscles. The superficial compartment of the perineum contains three muscles: transverse perineal muscle, the bulbospongiosus (bulbocavernosus) muscle and the ischiocavernosus muscle (Figure 58.1). The perineal body is the central area between the urogenital and anal triangles, interlocking fibres from the superficial transverse, bulbospongiosus and external anal sphincter muscles.

Figure 58.1 Pelvic floor (Figure by S. Sahlstein)

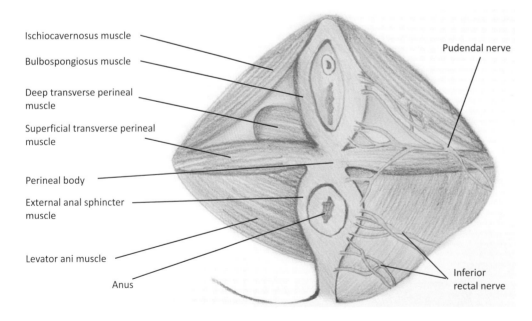

Ischiocavernosus muscle

Bulbospongiosus muscle

Deep transverse perineal muscle

Superficial transverse perineal muscle

Perineal body

External anal sphincter muscle

Levator ani muscle

Anus

Pudendal nerve

Inferior rectal nerve

58.2.1.2 Anal Sphincter Muscles

The anal sphincter contains two muscles: the external and internal anal sphincter muscles. The external anal sphincter (EAS) is a striated muscle and is further divided into three parts: subcutaneous, superficial and deep (Figure 58.2). The internal anal sphincter muscle (IAS) is a smooth muscle partly covered by the EAS. The longitudinal smooth muscle of the rectum lies between these two structures (Figure 58.2). The EAS is innervated by the pudendal nerve (somatic nerve) and contributes most of the squeezing pressure, as IAS is innervated by autonomic nerves and provides most of the resting pressure of the anal canal.

58.2.2 Classification of Perineal Injuries

Different classification methods for perineal injuries have been used, the most well-known of which are the Martius, Williams Obstetrics Textbook and Sultan. Martius defined perineal injury in three degrees, Williams and Sultan contain degrees from 1 to 4 and Sultan presented a classification wherein the third degree is further subdivided to three sub-degrees (Table 58.1). First degree tears are similarly defined in these three systems. Martius' second degree tear also involves a partial tear of the anal sphincter muscle, and the third degree tear includes complete anal sphincter tearing. In Williams' and Sultan's classification, the second degree involves the superficial perineal muscles but not the anal sphincter muscle. Williams' third degree tears are also called partial tears and include any injury of the anal sphincter muscle, while a fourth degree tear includes a tearing of rectal mucosa, also called a complete tear. Sultan divides the third degree tears into three subgroups (3A, 3B and 3C), as fourth degree tears consist of tearing of the sphincter muscles together with the rectal mucosa tear (Figure 58.3). The definition created by Sultan is adopted by the Royal College of Obstetricians and Gynaecologists (RCOG) and also recommended by the World Health Organization (WHO). Isolated internal anal sphincter tears occur rarely, and such injuries are not included in these classification systems. The so-called buttonhole injury in the rectal mucosa may occur without

injury in the perineal body or sphincter muscles, and may not be detected if rectal exploration is not performed after vaginal birth. Several other terms have been used across decades, such as different combinations of words denoting perineal or anal sphincter damage, including *laceration, injury, tear, rupture, trauma, disruption* as well as *damage*. Numerous abbreviations have been used as shorthand to describe anal sphincter injury: AST, OAST, ASR, OASR, OASI and OASIS. In the International Statistical Classification of Diseases and Related Health Problems (ICD-10), perineal injuries are classified in four degrees, as presented in Table 58.1.

58.2.3 Diagnosis and Repair

All women should be carefully examined after vaginal birth to identify possible perineal injuries, and the findings should be registered in patient records and in local patient quality registries to be able to follow up the quality of the obstetric healthcare provided. Primary diagnosis of OASIS is crucial to performing a correct primary repair. An unrepaired anal sphincter muscle injury increases the risk of anal incontinence.

Rectal exploration is needed to evaluate and determine the degree and depth of the perineal injury, as recommended in the RCOG Green-top Guideline [2]. With the index finger in the anal canal, and using a 'pill-rolling' movement with the sphincter muscle between thumb and index finger, a possible defect in the sphincter can be palpated. With careful examination, all anal sphincter injuries should be detected. Occult injuries are rare [3]. OASIS repair should be conducted in the operating theatre where proper pain relief for the patient is available, as well as a lithotomy position to achieve good visualization and conditions for surgery. Also, adequate lighting, instruments and assistance are important and often better in the operation theatre than in the labour room. The physician performing the repair should be well trained and educated for this kind of surgery. An unexperienced doctor should be carefully guided by a more experienced colleague. External and internal anal sphincter muscle defects should be repaired separately, as well as buttonhole injuries in the rectal mucosa. A defect in any of the muscles increases the risk of anal incontinence. Two main

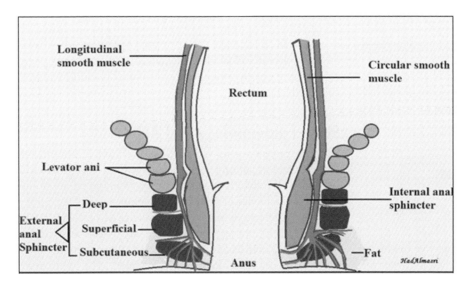

Figure 58.2 Coronal section of the anorectal structures
(Fig by Hadeel A. Masri)

Table 58.1 Classification of perineal injuries

	Martius	Williams Obstetrics	Sultan	ICD-10
Injured structure		Degree of injury		
Perineal skin and/or vaginal mucosa	1	1	1	O 70.0
Perineal muscles and fascia, excluding anal sphincter	2	2	2	O 70.1
External anal sphincter muscle <50%	2	3	3A	O 70.2
External anal sphincter >50%	3	3	3B	O 70.2
External and internal anal sphincter	3	3	3 C	O 70.2
Anal sphincter muscles and rectal mucosa	3	4	4	O 70.3

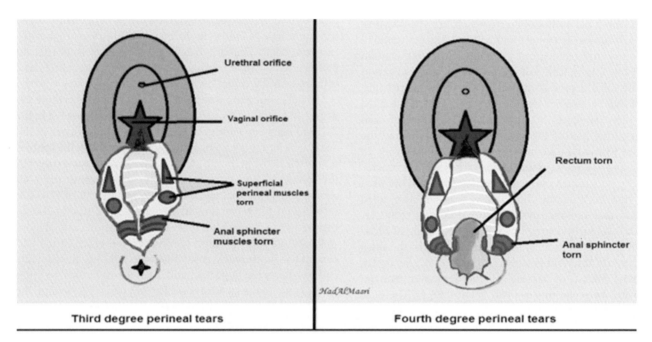

Figure 58.3 Third and fourth degree perineal injuries.

methods of anal sphincter repair are described; studies have shown that end-to-end and overlapping techniques have similar results according to anal incontinence. Therefore, the technique that the surgeon/gynaecologist is most familiar with should be chosen.

First and second degree injuries are mostly easier to repair, and the repair may be conducted in the labour room. However, large second degree injuries may be challenging to repair and may 'hide' an OASIS and therefore repair in the operation theatre should be considered.

58.3 Complications and Sequelae of Disease – Prognosis

58.3.1 Anal Incontinence

Anal incontinence cannot be measured by objective methods. The woman's subjective reporting of frequency and type of

incontinence can be classified in St. Mark's score (from 0–24) (Table 58.2). A high score indicates anal incontinence, and a low score (0) indicates no experience of anal incontinence, or complete continence. Obstetric anal sphincter injury is the most important risk factor for female anal incontinence. Many studies have assessed the prevalence of anal incontinence after childbirth.

58.4 Epidemiology and Aetiology

Perineal trauma during vaginal birth is common, and notably more common among nulliparous women compared with women with previous vaginal delivery. Many previous studies report the incidence of obstetric anal sphincter injuries, but few previous publications report the incidence of first and second degree perineal injuries. Samuelsson et al reported an incidence of 73.3% first and second degree perineal injuries among nulliparous and 59.4% among parous women. The same study

Table 58.2 Obstetric history and prevalence (%) of reported anal incontinence in St. Mark's score, based on study of Laine et al [4]

Obstetric history Score	Nulliparous n=1792 %	Previous caesarean only n=140 %	Parous, no previous OASIS n=873 %	Previous OASIS n=41 %
St. Mark's 0	81.1	85.7	78.8	58.5
St. Mark's 1–2	11.1	7.9	12.0	17.1
St. Mark's 3–16	7.8	6.4	9.2	24.4
St. Mark's 5–16	2.7	1.4	4.4	12.2

reported intact perineum among 6.6% of the nulliparous and 34.2% among parous women. Consequently, more than half of the women needed suturing after vaginal delivery [5].

The incidence of OASIS varies between countries and even between birth units, and an increasing trend has been described [6–10]. A large European study reports high variation in OASIS incidence, from 0.1 to 4.9% in different European countries [11]. Reasons for the variations and increasing trends are unknown but may be explained by different routines during vaginal birth, different obstetric interventions or differences in reporting and diagnostic qualities in delivery units. Studies from Finland reveal large differences between delivery units – the largest and the smallest delivery units had the highest incidences of OASIS. Large units presumably have more high-risk pregnancies and more complicated deliveries, which could explain the higher risks of OASIS. However, the finding of higher incidences of OASIS in the smaller delivery units with less complicated deliveries may indicate different policies in the management of the second stage of labour [12, 13].

58.5 Risk Factors and Prevention

Many studies have described risk factors for OASIS. Most studies report nulliparity, large baby and instrumental delivery as the most important risk factors. Additionally, a prolonged second stage of labour and persistent occiput posterior presentation are often described as risk factors for OASIS [10, 13, 14]. OASIS is also reported to be more common in women with a previous caesarean section [15].

Some of the previously listed risk factors are identifiable pre-delivery, but the importance of such factors in the prevention of OASIS has been shown to be poor. Predicting OASIS by identified risk factors has not been shown to be helpful to reduce the risk or occurrence of OASIS.

The risk factors can be classified as maternal, fetal, obstetric and administrative and personnel factors. Risk factors can also be classified as modifiable and non-modifiable. Maternal and fetal risk factors (or characteristics) are mostly non-modifiable: parity, maternal age and infant birthweight. Some obstetric factors are modifiable, such as choice of the instrument in vaginal assisted delivery or whether or not using manual perineal protection

methods. Administrative factors associated with OASIS risk may be lacking a focus in providing education in clinical routines that reduce the risk of OASIS.

58.5.1 Risk Factors

58.5.1.1 Parity

Nulliparous women are at higher risk of both OASIS and perineal injury in general compared with parous women with previous vaginal delivery. OASIS incidence among nulliparous women is 4-fold compared with parous women with previous vaginal delivery, and the risk of OASIS reduces with increasing vaginal birth number. Women with previous caesarean delivery only and no vaginal deliveries have a notably increased risk of OASIS, even higher than nulliparous women [5, 10, 12, 13]. Women with previous OASIS during vaginal delivery have a 4-fold risk of recurrent OASIS. This risk increases notably with increasing birthweight in subsequent delivery. An infant birthweight >4000 g in a second delivery after previous OASIS increases the risk of recurrent OASIS 10-fold, and if the birthweight is >4500 g, the increased risk of OASIS is 17 times higher compared with a birthweight less than 3000 g [16, 17].

58.5.1.2 Infant Birthweight

Increasing infant birthweight is associated with increased risk of OASIS. A linear increase in the OASIS incidence is described for every 500 g increase in birthweight. Several studies describe a 3- to 4-fold increased risk of OASIS when the birthweight is >4000 g compared to infants of 3000 g birthweight. Large head circumference and occiput posterior presentation also increase the risk of OASIS [10, 14, 18, 19].

58.5.1.3 Delivery Method

Mode of the operative vaginal delivery is a modifiable risk factor. The risk of OASIS in vacuum-assisted deliveries is 2- to 4-fold compared with spontaneous vaginal delivery. OASIS risk in forceps delivery is 6-fold compared with spontaneous vaginal deliveries [10, 14, 20, 21]. When instrumental delivery is indicated, a careful consideration of the choice of instrument is important to avoid unnecessary risk for OASIS.

58.5.1.4 Second Stage Duration

The risk of OASIS is positively correlated with the length of the second stage of labour. Almost linearly, increased risk is described with increasing duration of second stage of labour. Prolonged duration of the second stage is also associated with macrosomia, but large population studies reveal that second stage duration is an independent risk factor for OASIS [13, 14, 18]. Prolonged second stage of delivery also indicates a 'difficult' delivery.

58.5.2 Prevention of OASIS

Obstetric anal sphincter injury is chosen to be one of the patient safety quality indicators in OECD countries. A quality indicator is an outcome that presumably can be avoided with good clinical practice. Several interventions aimed to prevent severe perineal tears have been introduced.

58.5.2.1 Manual Perineal Protection

Tradition of routine use of manual perineal protection seems to result in lower OASIS incidence [6, 22–25]. Large observational studies from Denmark and Norway show reduced OASIS incidence after re-introduction of manual perineal protection during the last phase of the second stage (when the head is crowning), simultaneous slowing of the speed of head expulsion and communication with the mother. When the head is delivered, manual perineal protection should continue while the shoulders are delivered. All these studies describe a careful educational programme of the manual perineal protection method for the delivering staff [23–27].

A study from the UK shows a significant reduction in OASIS rates in two hospitals after implementation of RCOG guidelines to reduce OASIS risk; manual perineal protection was one of the components in this project [28]. Another study from the UK showed a reduction of OASIS risk with simply slowing the delivery of the baby's head [29].

The effect of manual perineal protection on OASIS has not been tested in well-designed randomized controlled trials (RCTs). Most of the published RCTs regarding perineal injuries have not had OASIS as a primary outcome, but instead had perineal pain, intact perineum or need for suturing (including all perineal tears) and are therefore underpowered to assess OASIS [30].

58.5.2.2 Episiotomy

Episiotomy is the most common surgical intervention performed on women. It was introduced in the eighteenth century to aid in difficult births such as prolonged second stage of delivery or to expedite delivery in cases of maternal or fetal distress. In the nineteenth century, it was used more routinely to prevent severe perineal tears, urine and faecal incontinence and to allow better sexual function. The evidence on the effect of episiotomy in prevention of perineal tear has been conflicting. The recent literature review covering literature from 1989 to 2014 concluded that episiotomy with correct technique should be considered as an effective method in prevention of perineal tears.

Several episiotomy types are described in textbooks, and the most well-known types are median, mediolateral and lateral, as reviewed by Kalis et al in 2012 [31]. The median type of episiotomy begins in the posterior fourchette and runs along the midline through the central tendon of the perineal body; this type is preferred in the USA. The technique beginning in the midline and directed laterally and downwards away from the rectum is the mediolateral type. Mediolateral episiotomy is probably the most common technique used especially in Europe. Lateral episiotomy begins laterally 1 or 2 cm from the midline and is directed downwards towards the ischial tuberosity. Based on the evidence from large observational studies, mediolateral and lateral techniques reduce the risk of OASIS, especially among nulliparous women and in instrumental deliveries [10, 14, 20, 21, 32, 33].

Correct technique is important; the episiotomy cutting angle should be large enough to achieve a protective effect of episiotomy. A small episiotomy angle may increase the risk of OASIS [34, 35]. It is of note that the suture angle is smaller than the cutting angle, and it is recommended that at least an angle of 60 degrees should be used when cutting episiotomy [36]. A 60-degree angle is easier to conduct with Episcissors, an instrument guiding the user to the correct cut for the episiotomy [28, 37].

The WHO recommendation from 2018 is the following: 'Routine use of episiotomy is not recommended for women undergoing spontaneous vaginal delivery, and if episiotomy is performed mediolateral incision should be used' [38]. This guideline does not comment on episiotomy use during instrumental vaginal delivery.

Women with episiotomy and women with second degree perineal injury reported similar experiences of pain, and women with OASIS reported more pain than women without OASIS 1 year after delivery. Women with OASIS postponed sexual activity after birth more often than women with episiotomy or second degree perineal injury [39].

58.5.2.3 Warm Compresses and Perineal Massage

A Cochrane review from 2017 describes many interventions during the second stage of delivery that were tested in randomized controlled trials, such as warm perineal compresses, perineal massage and using oils during delivery. Most of these studies were conducted to study other outcomes than OASIS, such as intact perineum, need for suturing in general (including first and second degree injuries) or postpartum perineal pain, and are therefore underpowered to assess the risk of OASIS. Many studies have weaknesses that hamper the quality, and therefore the evidence is classified weak or moderate [30]. The main conclusion was that warm compresses and perineal massage may reduce the risk of OASIS, but the evidence is unclear. The techniques described in the review have not been verified in a large population with any effect in reducing OASIS.

58.6 Key Messages

Careful clinical examination, including rectal exploration, immediately after vaginal delivery is important to define the degree of perineal injury, and to be able to perform a correct primary repair.

Obstetric anal sphincter injury is the most important risk factor for female anal incontinence and efforts should be made to avoid this injury during vaginal delivery. Pain and discomfort are associated with OASIS.

To reduce the occurrence of OASIS, the delivering staff should be educated and trained to use perineal protection techniques to slow and control the delivery of the baby's head and shoulders. Without education, training and guidance, the effect of manual perineal protection cannot be achieved.

The leaders in a delivery unit should take the responsibility for training all healthcare personnel to optimal delivering techniques.

References

1. Lindqvist M, Persson M, Nilsson M, Uustal E, Lindberg I. 'A worse nightmare than expected' – a Swedish qualitative study of women's experiences two months after obstetric anal sphincter muscle injury. *Midwifery.* 2018;**61**:22–8.

2. *The Management of Third- and Fourth-Degree Perineal Tears,* Green-top Guideline No 29. London: Royal College of Obstetricians and Gynaecologists, 2015. www.rcog.org.uk/globalassets/documents/guidelines/gtg-29.pdf

3. Andrews V, Sultan AH, Thakar R, Jones PW. Occult anal sphincter injuries–myth or reality? *BJOG.* 2006;**113**(2):195–200.

4. Laine K, Skjeldestad FE, Sandvik L, Staff AC. Prevalence and risk indicators for anal incontinence among pregnant women. *ISRN Obstet Gynecol.* 2013;**2013**:947572.

5. Samuelsson E, Ladfors L, Lindblom BG, Hagberg H. A prospective observational study on tears during vaginal delivery: occurrences and risk factors. *Acta Obstet Gynecol Scand.* 2002;**81**(1):44–9.

6. Laine K, Gissler M, Pirhonen J. Changing incidence of anal sphincter tears in four Nordic countries through the last decades. *Eur J Obstet Gynecol Reprod Biol.* 2009;**146**(1):71–5.

7. Ampt AJ, Ford JB, Roberts CL, Morris JM. Trends in obstetric anal sphincter injuries and associated risk factors for vaginal singleton term births in New South Wales 2001–2009. *Aust N Z J Obstet Gynaecol.* 2013;**53**(1):9–16.

8. Ekeus C, Nilsson E, Gottvall K. Increasing incidence of anal sphincter tears among primiparas in Sweden: a population-based register study. *Acta Obstet Gynecol Scand.* 2008;**87**(5):564–73.

9. Gurol-Urganci I, Cromwell DA, Edozien LC, et al. Third- and fourth-degree perineal tears among primiparous women in England between 2000 and 2012: time trends and risk factors. *BJOG.* 2013;**120**(12):1516–25.

10. Baghestan E, Irgens LM, Bordahl PE, Rasmussen S. Trends in risk factors for obstetric anal sphincter injuries in Norway. *Obstet Gynecol.* 2010;**116**(1):25–34.

11. Blondel B, Alexander S, Bjarnadottir RI, et al. Variations in rates of severe perineal tears and episiotomies in 20 European countries: a study based on routine national data in Euro-Peristat Project. *Acta Obstet Gynecol Scand.* 2016;**95**(7):746–54.

12. Räisänen S, Vehviläinen-Julkunen K, Gissler M, Heinonen S. Hospital-based lateral episiotomy and obstetric anal sphincter injury rates: a retrospective population-based register study. *Am J Obstet Gynecol.* 2012;**206**(4):347.e1–347.e6.

13. Räisänen S, Vehviläinen-Julkunen K, Gissler M, Heinonen S. High episiotomy rate protects from obstetric anal sphincter ruptures: a birth register-study on delivery intervention policies in Finland. *Scand J Public Health.* 2011;**39**(5):457–63.

14. Laine K, Skjeldestad FE, Sandvik L, Staff AC. Incidence of obstetric anal sphincter injuries after training to protect the perineum: cohort study. *BMJ Open.* 2012;**2**(5):10.1136/bmjopen-2012-001649.

15. Räisänen S, Vehviläinen-Julkunen K, Gissler M, Heinonen S. Smoking during pregnancy is associated with a decreased incidence of obstetric anal sphincter injuries in nulliparous women. *PLoS One.* 2012;**7**(7):e41014.

16. Baghestan E, Irgens LM, Bordahl PE, Rasmussen S. Risk of recurrence and subsequent delivery after obstetric anal sphincter injuries. *BJOG.* 2012;**119**(1):62–9.

17. Spydslaug A, Trogstad LI, Skrondal A, Eskild A. Recurrent risk of anal sphincter laceration among women with vaginal deliveries. *Obstet Gynecol.* 2005;**105**(2):307–13.

18. de Leeuw JW, Struijk PC, Vierhout ME, Wallenburg HC. Risk factors for third degree perineal ruptures during delivery. *BJOG.* 2001;**108**(4):383–7.

19. Räisänen S, Vehviläinen-Julkunen K, Gissler M, Heinonen S. Up to seven-fold inter-hospital differences in obstetric anal sphincter injury rates – a birth register-based study in Finland. *BMC Res Notes.* 2010;**3**(1):345.

20. de Leeuw JW, de Wit C, Kuijken JP, Bruinse HW. Mediolateral episiotomy reduces the risk for anal sphincter injury during operative vaginal delivery. *BJOG.* 2008;**115**(1):104–8.

21. Jangö H, Langhoff-Roos J, Rosthöj S, Sakse A. Modifiable risk factors of obstetric anal sphincter injury in primiparous women: a population-based cohort study. *Am J Obstet Gynecol.* 2014;**210**(1):59.e1–59.e6.

22. Pirhonen JP, Grenman SE, Haadem K, et al. Frequency of anal sphincter rupture at delivery in Sweden and Finland–result of difference in manual help to the baby's head. *Acta Obstet Gynecol Scand.* 1998;**77**(10):974–7.

23. Laine K, Rotvold W, Staff AC. Are obstetric anal sphincter ruptures preventable?- Large and consistent rupture rate variations between the Nordic countries and between delivery units in Norway. *Acta Obstet Gynecol Scand.* 2012;**92**(1):94–100.

24. Laine K, Pirhonen T, Rolland R, Pirhonen J. Decreasing the incidence of anal sphincter tears during delivery. *Obstet Gynecol.* 2008;**111**(5):1053–7.

25. Leenskjold S, Hoj L, Pirhonen J. Manual protection of the perineum reduces the risk of obstetric anal sphincter ruptures. *Dan Med J.* 2015;**62**(5):A5075.

26. Hals E, Øian P, Pirhonen T, et al. A multicenter interventional program to reduce the incidence of anal sphincter tears. *Obstet Gynecol.* 2010;**116**(4):901–8.

27. Stedenfeldt M, Oian P, Gissler M, Blix E, Pirhonen J. Risk factors for obstetric anal sphincter injury after a successful multicentre interventional programme. *BJOG.* 2014;**121**(1):83–91.

28. Mohiudin H, Ali S, Pisal PN, Villar R. Implementation of the RCOG guidelines for prevention of obstetric anal sphincter injuries (OASIS) at two

London Hospitals: A time series analysis. *Eur J Obstet Gynecol Reprod Biol*. 2018;**224**:89–92.

29. Basu M, Smith D. Long-term outcomes of the Stop Traumatic OASI Morbidity Project (STOMP). *Int J Gynaecol Obstet*. 2018;**142**(3):295–9.

30. Aasheim V, Nilsen ABV, Reinar LM, Lukasse M. Perineal techniques during the second stage of labour for reducing perineal trauma. *Cochrane Database Syst Rev*. 2017;(6):CD006672.

31. Kalis V, Laine K, de Leeuw JW, Ismail K, Tincello DG. Classification of episiotomy: towards a standardisation of terminology. *BJOG*. 2012;**119**(5):522–6.

32. Räisänen S, Vehviläinen-Julkunen K, Gissler M, Heinonen S. Hospital-based lateral episiotomy and anal sphincter injury rates: a retrospective population-based register study. *Am J Obstet Gynecol*. 2012;**206**(4):P347.

33. Verghese TS, Champaneria R, Kapoor DS, Latthe PM. Obstetric anal sphincter injuries after episiotomy: systematic review and meta-analysis. *Int Urogynecol J*. 2016;**27**(10):1459–67.

34. Eogan M, Daly L, O'Connell PR, O'Herlihy C. Does the angle of episiotomy affect the incidence of anal sphincter injury? *BJOG*. 2006;**113** (2):190–4.

35. Stedenfeldt M, Pirhonen J, Blix E, et al. Episiotomy characteristics and risks for obstetric anal sphincter injuries: a case-control study. *BJOG*. 2012;**119** (6):724–30.

36. Kalis V, Karbanova J, Horak M, et al. The incision angle of mediolateral episiotomy before delivery and after repair. *Int J Gynaecol Obstet*. 2008;**103**(1):5–8.

37. Sawant G, Kumar D. Randomized trial comparing episiotomies with Braun-Stadler episiotomy scissors and EPISCISSORS-60 . *Med Devices (Auckl)*. 2015;**8**:251–4.

38. WHO. WHO recommendation on episiotomy policy. 2018. https://extranet.who.int/rhl/topics/preconception-pregnancy-childbirth-and-postpartum-care/care-during-childbirth/care-during-labour-2nd-stage/who-recommendation-episiotomy-policy-0.

39. Fodstad K, Staff AC, Laine K. Episiotomy preferences, indication, and classification – a survey among Nordic doctors. *Acta Obstet Gynecol Scand*. 2016;**95**(5):587–95.

Chapter 59

Management of Stillbirth

Martin Cameron

59.1 Introduction

Stillbirth for many couples will be a catastrophic event. This chapter aims to equip the clinician with a sound grasp of this problem. It generally deals with stillbirth occurring in developed countries such as Europe and the USA, rather than exploring the global and the challenges of stillbirth in the developing world, accepting that progress in reducing stillbirth rates in poorer economic countries would have the greatest reduction in worldwide stillbirth rates.

59.2 Definition

In the UK, MBRRACE defines a stillbirth as a baby delivered at or after 24+0 weeks' gestational age showing no signs of life, irrespective of when the death occurred [1]. MBRRACE divides stillbirth into antepartum stillbirth (a baby delivered at or after 24+0 weeks' gestational age showing no signs of life and known to have died before the onset of care in labour) and intrapartum stillbirth (a baby delivered at or after 24+0 weeks' gestational age showing no signs of life and known to have been alive at the onset of care in labour).

The definition recommended by the World Health Organization (WHO) for international comparison is a baby born with no signs of life at or after 28 weeks' gestation [2].

There is much debate in the literature regarding classification systems for stillbirth. A systematic review identified 81 systems for classification of causes of stillbirth (SB) and neonatal death (NND) between 2009 and 2014 [3].

59.3 Incidence

In the UK there were 3200 stillbirths in 2017, equating to a stillbirth rate of 4.2 per 1000 total births. This was the lowest UK rate ever recorded [4]. The recent European Perinatal Health Report states, 'Almost all countries have stillbirth rates between 2.0 and 3.5 per 1000 total births at and after 28 weeks of gestation and between 2.5 and 4.5 per 1000 total births at and after 24 weeks of gestation. Accordingly, there were around 60–80% more stillbirths in the countries with the higher rates than in those with the lower rates' [5]. They state that stillbirth rates fell between 2010 and 2015, but trends were very heterogeneous. Some countries experienced significant reductions in their stillbirth rates, including the Netherlands, Poland, Scotland, and England and Wales, whereas rates were stable or increased elsewhere.

59.4 Risk Factors

Exact causes of stillbirth are explored under the investigation section. However, there are certain well-recognized risk factors for stillbirth in the European population. Important to consider are body mass index (BMI), smoking, age, previous stillbirth and socio-economic background.

In women with high BMI (>25) there is around a 20% increase in stillbirth risk for every 5 additional BMI points [6]. Smoking increases the risk of stillbirth and appears to be related to the number of cigarettes consumed with an increase of around 50% in women who smoked 10 or more cigarettes [7]. Poorer socio-economic background is related to increased risk for stillbirth in European countries [8].Older maternal age is also recognized as a risk factor for stillbirth [9]. Compared with women who had a live birth in their first pregnancy, those who experienced a stillbirth are almost five times more likely to experience a stillbirth in their second pregnancy [10].

59.5 Presentation and Diagnosis

Stillbirth may be antenatal or intrapartum. Antenatal presentation is often with a history of reduced or no fetal movements with half of women with stillbirth reporting slowing down of movements beforehand [11]. A further common antenatal presentation is for the woman to attend a routine midwifery appointment and for the midwife to fail to auscultate a fetal heartbeat, consequently sending the patient to hospital for confirmation of whether or not the pregnancy is ongoing. Other antenatal presentations are acutely with abruption or chorioamnionitis and sepsis (sometimes following known pre-labour preterm rupture of membranes).

Intrapartum stillbirth may occur with inadequate monitoring of the fetal heart rate in labour or with cord prolapse or acute abruption in labour.

The UK has produced guidance for the optimal method of diagnosis of late intrauterine fetal death (IUFD) with its guidance reproduced here [12]:

1. Auscultation and cardiotocography (CTG) should not be used to investigate suspected IUFD.
2. Real-time ultrasonography is essential for the accurate diagnosis of IUFD.
3. Ideally, real-time ultrasonography should be available at all times.
4. A second opinion should be obtained whenever practically possible.

5. Mothers should be prepared for the possibility of passive fetal movement. If the mother reports passive fetal movement after the scan to diagnose IUFD, a repeat scan should be offered.

Diagnosis presents a challenge to clinicians because women and family members may often either be shocked with the news or experience severe grief reactions. Discussions should aim to support parental choice. Clinicians need to be good communicators and empathetic and have experience in how to break bad news.

59.6 Management (including the puerperium)

For women presenting with an acute problem such as placental abruption or sepsis, treatment may involve the initial haemodynamic stabilization of the patient. The reader should refer to other chapters of this textbook for the basic principles of treating these conditions. In addition, if a patient is unwell with an IUFD following one of these conditions the clinician should remember disseminated intravascular coagulopathy (DIC) may be present.

Fortunately, most women with IUFD in the antenatal period will not present in extremis, and their management is covered here.

Around 85% of women with IUFD will labour within 3 weeks, although there is around a 10% risk of developing DIC within 4 weeks of IUFD. If the woman has evidence of sepsis, rupture of membranes or pre-eclampsia, then expediting delivery is advised. For well women with intact membranes, a more individualized approach may be taken, although in the author's experience most women will wish for an active approach to be taken in managing birth.

In an unscarred uterus, a combination of mifepristone 200 mg followed by a prostaglandin is commonly used [12]. The addition of mifepristone to the prostaglandin shortens the labour duration. In controlled trials, oxytocin infusions have been shown to be not as effective as the use of a prostaglandin. Misoprostol within the UK is generally considered the preferred prostaglandin because it is highly efficacious, can be stored at room temperature and is inexpensive. Misoprostol can be given orally or vaginally, although there is some evidence that the vaginal route is superior in terms of reducing length of labour and reducing the use of oxytocin augmentation. There is some evidence for the dose of misoprostol to be gestation dependent:

1. <27+0: Consider 100 micrograms 6 hourly
2. 27+0 and later: Consider 25–50 micrograms 4 hourly up to 24 hours

For women with a scarred uterus, care needs to be individualized. There are few data on the safety of induction of labour (IOL) for intrauterine death (IUD) for women with two or more lower segment caesarean sections (LSCS). For women with one previous LSCS, the UK Royal College of Obstetricians and Gynaecologists (RCOG) guidance suggests misoprostol can be used but in lower doses of 25–50 micrograms [12].

Pain relief is important to consider during labour. Opiates such as diamorphine (which is superior to pethidine in analgesic effects) can be used. Regional anaesthesia will be useful for some women and should be available. Before siting regional anaesthesia, the clinicians should exclude DIC.

Antibiotics are not routinely administered for prophylaxis purposes but should be given to women with symptoms and signs of sepsis or chorioamnionitis.

During a woman's care through labour, there should be some discussion with her about whether she wishes to see and hold the baby after birth. Initially, many couples may not wish to do this, but in the author's experience initial views often change and at the time of birth many couples do wish to see the baby. Conversations should also include a discussion of whether the couple wish to have mementos made or a memory box. Photographs, prints of hands and feet, pieces of hair are things that some couples will wish for while others may not. The couple may wish to name the baby.

The healthcare professionals should also gently explore with the couple whether they wish for any spiritual or faith support. This needs to be individualized to the couple's needs. Couples often have questions about what happens to the baby after birth, both in the short term (immediately after birth) and the longer term. Some hospitals will have developed hospital chaplaincy services who will have links with all faiths in their local community and they may be helpful in exploring options with the couple. As an example, at the Norfolk and Norwich University Hospital (NNUH) the couple can be given contacts for arrangements for either a funeral or cremation and the hospital chaplains have contact with all local faiths and with funeral service directors and the local crematory. If the couple do not wish to organize their own service, they can delegate responsibility to the hospital, and in that situation the NNUH has an agreement with a local cemetery where babies can be buried at no cost to the parents [13].

After delivery, suppression of lactation should be considered. Around a third of women will experience severe breast pain if they use non-pharmacological options such as support bras and simple analgesia. Options for pharmacological treatment include single-dose carbergoline 1 mg or bromocriptine 2.5 mg twice daily for up to 14 days. Both are equally efficacious, but the author prefers carbergoline because of the need for only one dose. These drugs are contraindicated in women with hypertension, as they can increase blood pressure and have been associated with intracerebral bleeding, so care needs to be taken with women with pre-eclampsia.

Some thought needs to be placed on where these women are cared for during the delivery and postnatal stay. In the UK, women are generally cared for on the delivery suite, with an experienced midwife providing one-to-one care. Many units have appointed a bereavement midwife and she may have a role in delivering this care and in the ongoing follow-up with the couple. Some units have built a bereavement suite associated with the delivery suite. This area may have a separate entrance to the main delivery suite, a large room with emergency equipment often hidden in cupboards to make the area look more homely, en suite facilities, space for other family members to stay (including a double bed to accommodate the patient and her partner) and a kitchen area so that the family members can make beverages or even meals if they wish. Whilst in this bereavement room the couple should not be able to hear other activity going on in the delivery suite.

Before discharge, a sensitive discussion about contraception should be made as fertility can return rapidly and before the next menstrual period. Women should also be assessed for the need of thromboprophylaxis against national or local guidelines, although IUFD is not in itself an increased risk factor for venous thromboembolic problems.

59.7 Communication with Associated Healthcare Providers

It is important that the maternity staff communicate with other healthcare professionals who have responsibility for the patient. The community midwife needs to be informed (as well as the health visitor if she has made contact with or was planning to contact the patient). The family practitioner/general practitioner should also be informed. Ideally, all appointments (e.g. scan and antenatal clinic) should be cancelled by the time of discharge from hospital.

59.8 Registration of the Stillbirth

This will be dependent on the legal framework of each country. Within the UK, a stillbirth certificate is issued to the couple by a medical practitioner or midwife attending them at the birth or who has seen the baby post-delivery. The parents are responsible in law for registering the birth but can delegate the task to a healthcare professional. Currently, if there was a stillbirth it does not need to be referred to a coroner, but this is an area where there is discussion about a change in the law in England and Wales with Parliament seeking consultation in 2019 [14]. However, since 2018 all intrapartum stillbirths in England are being investigated by the Healthcare Safety Investigation Branch (HSIB) of the NHS [15].

59.9 Emotional Support and Psychological Sequelae

A systematic review and meta-analysis states that 'stillbirth is a distressing experience that can result in high levels of psychological symptoms including anxiety, depression, distress, and negative well-being. Symptoms appear to be highest in the first few months' post loss although there is evidence to suggest that for some, symptoms may persist up to 3 years' [16]. Men and women experience grief differently and this may contribute to the increased risk of relationship breakup after perinatal loss [17]. Recommendations from the RCOG are reproduced in Box 59.1.

It should be noted that from the literature debriefing services for birth trauma may increase harm and generally do not demonstrate a beneficial effect.

Support groups may be beneficial for the woman and her partner. In the UK charitable organizations such as Sands provide this much needed support [18].

Box 59.1 Recommendations from RCOG for Psychological Issues in Stillbirth [12]

- Carers must be alert to the fact that mothers, partners and children are all at risk of prolonged severe psychological reactions including post-traumatic stress disorder but that their reactions might be very different.
- Carers should be aware of and responsive to possible variations in individual and cultural approaches to death.
- Counselling should be offered to all women and their partners.
- Other family members, especially siblings and grandparents, should also be considered for counselling.
- Debriefing services must not care for women with symptoms of psychiatric disease in isolation.
- Parents should be advised about support groups.
- Bereavement officers should be appointed to coordinate services.

59.10 Investigations for Stillbirth

The WHO [2] describes the major causes of stillbirth as

- childbirth complications;
- post-term pregnancy;
- maternal infections in pregnancy (malaria, syphilis and HIV);
- maternal disorders (especially hypertension, obesity and diabetes)
- fetal growth restriction;
- congenital abnormalities.

It should be remembered that round 60% of stillbirths are unexplained [19]. However, Man and Hutchinson ranked the following as explanations for stillbirths:

- Ascending infection in 17%
- Placenta factors, including placental abruption and pre-eclampsia in 12%
- Congenital abnormality in 5%
- Fetal growth restriction in 2%
- Complications with twins in 2%

Investigation for the cause of stillbirth is important for several reasons. First, it can be helpful for the woman and her partner in their recovery process after the stillbirth. Second, it can inform the clinician and the parents about recurrence risk, and if any issues need to be addressed in preparation for a further pregnancy. Third, it can provide details about whether the care given to the woman prior to the diagnosis of stillbirth was appropriate. Finally, it can be useful in terms of collecting local, national and international data in classifying stillbirth. It should be noted that there are multiple suggested classification schemes for stillbirth [3].

The RCOG Green-top guidance has a very clear table for investigations for stillbirth. Table 59.1 is a modified version. the tests in the upper part of the table are key tests to be considered. The tests listed under Selective Tests should be considered in certain clinical situations or groups of patients.

Table 59.1 Investigations for late IUFD (adapted from RCOG Green-top guidance [12])

Test	Underlying reason for test	Additional comments
Routine biochemical and haematological bloods	Pre-eclampsia Organ failure from sepsis or haemorrhage	
Bile acids	Obstetric cholestasis	
C-reactive protein (CRP)	Sepsis	
Kleihauer–Betke	Fetomaternal haemorrhage	Offer to all women
Random blood sugar and HbA1c	Diabetes mellitus	
Thyroid function tests	Thyroid disease	
Maternal viral serology	Maternal fetal infection	Toxoplasmosis, parvovirus B19, cytomegalovirus (CMV), herpes simplex (rubella if not immune, syphilis if serology not already know in the pregnancy)
Fetal & placental microbiology (placental & fetal swabs, fetal blood)	Fetal infections	Written consent advised for fetal blood (cord or cardiac)
Fetal & placental tissue for karyotype	Aneuploidy Single gene defects	Written consent
Postmortem examination	See main text	Written consent

Selective tests	Underlying reason	Additional comments
Clotting/fibrinogen	DIC	Pre-eclampsia, abruption and sepsis risk factors for DIC
Maternal bacteriology (blood cultures, midstream specimen urine, cervical and vaginal swabs)	Maternal bacterial infection	Indicated if there is: Fever Flu-like symptoms Abnormal amniotic fluid Prolonged rupture of membranes before IUFD
Maternal thrombophilia screen	Maternal thrombophilia	Indicated if fetal growth restriction/placentation disease. Repeat at 6 weeks if positive
Anti-red cell antibody	Haemolytic disease	If hydrops
Anti-Ro and anti-La antibodies	Autoimmune disease	If hydrops or endomyocardial fibro-elastosis
Alloimmune antiplatelet screen	Alloimmune thrombocytopenia	If intracranial haemorrhage on PM
Maternal urine for cocaine	Occult drug use	If suspected by history, with consent
Parental bloods for karyotype	Parental balanced translocation Parental mosaicism	Indicated if: fetal unbalanced translocation other fetal aneuploidy fetal genetic testing fails and history suggestive of aneuploidy (fetal abnormality on postmortem, previous unexplained IUFD, recurrent miscarriage)

The wishes of the couple as to postmortem should always be respected, but postmortem is a very important investigation and provides the most information to inform recurrence risk. Discussions about postmortem should be led by a clinician who has been trained in explaining options to the couple. Written consent is required. There are four main options for postmortem:

1. A full post-mortem in which there is an external examination, measurements of length and weight, x-rays. The chest, abdomen and skull are opened to examine the internal organs. Small specimens from each organ are taken for microscopy.

2. A limited or selective examination. In this situation, the parents would limit what could and could not be done. In the author's experience some parents do not wish the skull opened and so may wish for a limited postmortem rather than a full postmortem.

3. An external examination only, usually with x-rays.

4. Examination of the placenta and cord only.

Clearly, as one moves from option 1 to 4, there is less information gathered to determine cause and to estimate recurrence risk.

Imaging modalities such as magnetic resonance imaging (MRI) appear in studies to have similar diagnostic accuracy as full postmortem, although in the UK such imaging is not widely adopted as a replacement for traditional postmortem [20]. In the future it may become a more routine option and may offer options for couples who do not want a conventional postmortem.

59.11 Follow-up and Review after IUFD

There is no clear consensus on when to offer follow-up to these patients. It usually takes 6 to 8 weeks for postmortem results to become available, and so many clinicians will offer to review around that time. The purpose of follow-up is to find out how the patient is recovering both physically and emotionally, to review the past pregnancy care and the results of any investigations performed and to offer pre-pregnancy advice for any future pregnancy the couple may be considering. Before this appointment, the obstetrician should ensure all results to investigations are known and should have read the hospital records and be able to summarize the key findings and implications of the stillbirth and its investigation. Specific general issues to be considered include offering assistance in smoking cessation when needed, considering weight reduction if BMI is increased and ensuring the couple are aware of the need for pre-pregnancy folic acid in those countries that do not fortify common foodstuffs such as bread. Couples will often ask how long they should wait before trying to conceive. At this point, the most important issue is that they need to have given time to recover from the severe emotional distress of the stillbirth, as any future pregnancy is likely to provoke significant anxiety. Given there are some data showing that in the general population, pregnancy intervals of less than 6 months are associated with a slightly increased risk of adverse events, it would seem sensible to suggest that a pregnancy interval of 6 months or more is ideal. If the patient is being seen at around 2 months after stillbirth, this also allows them to obtain and commence folic acid for the 3 months required pre-pregnancy. At the end of the consultation, a letter should be written to the patient and copied to the family practitioner outlining the results of the investigations and detailing a suggested plan for a future pregnancy.

59.12 The Next Pregnancy Following an IUFD

Clearly, if a cause is known then an appropriate management plan based on need for exclusion of recurrence can be instigated. However, how should the woman with a previously unexplained stillbirth be managed?

These women should be booked under obstetric care. The RCOG Green-top guidance advises that they be screened for gestational diabetes in subsequent pregnancies. If the woman has combined screening, the clinician should look at the pregnancy-associated plasma protein-A (PAPP-A) result, as a low

multiple of the median is associated with fetal growth restriction. Many clinicians (including the author) offer third trimester growth scans looking for evidence of fetal growth restriction, although the evidence for benefit is not strong. Additional scanning may give the couple assurance and support that the pregnancy is progressing well.

Timing of birth is controversial. Women often ask for early delivery, and the clinician should be cognitive of the gestation of the previous stillbirth. Some studies in women with previous IUFD have suggested iatrogenic harm of increased caesarean section and instrumental delivery rates through early induction of labour. In the clinical scenario of a previous late, unexplained IUFD with a pregnancy progressing well with normal growth scans, it would be the author's practice to consider induction of labour from 39 weeks, given recent studies in low-risk nulliparous women showing no adverse effects, if the couple wished to consider delivery before 40 weeks [21]. Some couples will request delivery by elective lower-segment caesarean section and the obstetrician should consider this request.

Following the birth of a successful pregnancy, caregivers should be aware that some mothers may have unresolved grief issues and are more prone to postnatal depression and difficulties bonding with their child.

59.13 Prevention

In 2015, NHS England embarked on an ambitious programme to reduce stillbirth and infant deaths by 50% by 2030, subsequently moved to 2025 [22]. This initiative has concentrated on a stillbirth safety bundle, concentrating on five issues (originally four) associated with stillbirth [23], namely:

1. Reducing smoking in pregnancy
2. Risk assessment, prevention and surveillance of pregnancies at risk of fetal growth restriction (FGR)
3. Raising awareness of reduced fetal movement (RFM)
4. Effective fetal monitoring during labour
5. Reducing preterm birth

Although this programme has merit in terms of what it is trying to achieve, it remains controversial [24]. It was introduced in the UK with minimal prior evaluation on the effects of the programme as a whole.

1. The one modifiable risk factor for stillbirth is smoking and so it could be argued that helping those 12% of women in the UK who smoke in pregnancy to reduce their intake would likely result in a stillbirth reduction.
2. The issue of fetal growth is more complex. There remains controversy about whether to use customized or non-customized growth charts (GROW, WHO, INTERGROWTH), which women should screen for growth restriction (high risk vs. all women), how to screen (schedule of ultrasound scan appointments) and how to reduce the number of women who are diagnosed with a small baby but who have a constitutionally small fetus rather than a growth-restricted fetus [25]. This area contains much contention.

3. The issue of promotion of awareness of reduced fetal movements could be considered even more controversial because the RCOG Green-top guidance is full of good clinical practice points rather than randomized control trial evidence, and one recent paper does not show any benefit to this [26].

4. The fourth element of the programme – promotion of education and assessment of fetal heart rate interpretation by healthcare professionals – also seems weak, given the lack of evidence about the effectiveness of CTG in improving perinatal outcome and given the INFANT study demonstrating that even with computerized decision support there are no improvements in clinical outcomes [27].

5. Given that for the prevention of antenatally detected at-risk fetuses the obstetrician's main intervention is iatrogenic delivery (either induction of labour or caesarean section) and, given that there is some evidence that delivery at 37

compared to 38 compared to 39 weeks increases the risk of special educational needs in children, there are concerns that these interventions increase early-term births and could be harmful [28].

It therefore remains to be proven whether this package of care will on balance promote more benefit than harm or even whether it can reduce stillbirth rates in 2025 by 50% from baseline.

59.14 Conclusions

Stillbirth continues to be a tragic health problem for women and their families throughout the world. More research is needed to work out the optimal strategies to reduce stillbirth incidence in countries such as the UK. Care for these women requires the clinician to be empathetic to their needs and to individualize care.

References

1. Manktelow BN, Smith LK, Prunet C, et al. *MBRRACE-UK Perinatal Mortality Surveillance Report: UK Perinatal Deaths for Births from January to December 2015.* Leicester: Department of Health Science University of Leicester; 2017. www.npeu.ox.ac.uk/downloads/files/mbrrace-uk/reports/MBRRACE-UK-PMS-Report-2015%20FINAL%20FULL%20REPORT.pdf

2. World Health Organization. Stillbirths. www.who.int/maternal_child_adolescent/epidemiology/stillbirth/en/

3. Leisher SH, Teoh Z, Reinebrant H, et al. Classification systems for causes of stillbirth and neonatal death, 2009–2014: an assessment of alignment with characteristics for an effective global system. *BMC Pregnancy Childbirth.* 2016;**16**:269.

4. Office of National Statistics. *Vital Statistics in the UK: Births, Deaths and Marriages – 2018 Update* [Data set].2018. www.ons.gov.uk/peoplepopulationand community/populationandmigrati.

5. Euro-Peristat Project. *European Perinatal Health Report. Core Indicators of the Health and Care of Pregnant Women and Babies in Europe in 2015.* November 2018. www.europeristat.com/images/EPHR2015_Euro-Peristat.pdf

6. Aune D, Saugstad OD, Henriksen T, Tonstad S. maternal body mass index and the risk of fetal death, stillbirth, and infant death: a systematic review and meta-analysis. *JAMA.* 2014;**311**(15):1536–46. doi: 10.1001/jama.2014.2269

7. Marufu TC, Ahankari A, Coleman T, Lewis S. Maternal smoking and the risk of still birth: systematic review and meta-analysis. *BMC Public Health.* 2015;**15**:239 https://doi.org/10.1186/s12889-015-1552-5

8. Zeitlin J, Mortensen L, Prunet C, et al. Socioeconomic inequalities in stillbirth rates in Europe: measuring the gap using routine data from the Euro-Peristat Project. *BMC Pregnancy Childbirth.* 2016;**16**:15.

9. Page JM, Silver RM. Interventions to prevent stillbirth. *Semin Fetal Neonatal Med.* 2017;**22**(3):135–45.

10. Lamont K, Scott NW, Jones GT, Bhattacharya S. Risk of recurrent stillbirth: systematic review and meta-analysis. *BMJ.* 2015 Jun 24;**350**: h3080. doi: 10.1136/bmj.h3080

11. *Reduced Fetal Movements*, Green-top Guideline No. 57, London: Royal College of Obstetricians and Gynaecologists, 2011. www.rcog.org.uk/globalassets/documents/guidelines/gtg_57.pdf

12. *Late Intrauterine Fetal Death and Stillbirth*, Green-top Guideline No 55. London: Royal College of Obstetricians and Gynaecologists, 2010. www.rcog.org.uk/globalassets/documents/guidelines/gtg_55.pdf

13. Colney Woods. Babies and children. www.greenacresgroup.co.uk/park/colney/options-prices/saying-goodbye-to-children/

14. Fairbairn C, Bate A, Hawkins O. The investigation of stillbirth. (2017 HC 08167). https://researchbriefings

.files.parliament.uk/documents/CBP-8167/CBP-8167.pdf

15. Maternity Investigations. www.hsib.org.uk/maternity/

16. Campbell-Jackson L, Horsche A. The psychological impact of stillbirth on women: a systematic review. *Illn Crisis Loss.* 2014;**22**(3):237–56.

17. Kersting A, Wagner B. Complicated grief after perinatal loss. *Dialogues Clin Neurosci.* 2012 Jun; **14**(2):187–94. www.ncbi.nlm.nih.gov/pmc/articles/PMC3384447/

18. Sands: Stillbirth and Neonatal Death Charity. www.sands.org.uk/

19. Man J, Hutchinson JC. Stillbirth and intrauterine fetal death: factors affecting determination of cause of death at autopsy. *Ultrasound Obstet Gynecol.* 2016;**48**:566–73. doi: 10.1002/uog.16016

20. Thayyil S, Sebire NJ, Chitty LS, et al. Post-mortem MRI versus conventional autopsy in fetuses and children: a prospective validation study. *Lancet.*2013 Jul 20;**382** (9888):223–33. doi: 10.1016/s0140-6736(13)60134-8

21. Grobman WA, Rice MM, Reddy, UM, et al. Labor induction versus expectant management in low-risk nulliparous women. *N Engl J Med.* 2018;**379**:513–23 doi: 10.1056/NEJMoa1800566 www.nejm.org/doi/full/10.1056/NEJMoa1800566

22. New ambition to halve rate of stillbirths and infant deaths. 13 November 2015. www.gov.uk/government/news/new-

ambition-to-halve-rate-of-stillbirths-and-infant-deaths

23. NHS England. Saving Babies' Lives Version Two: A care bundle for reducing perinatal mortality. March 2019. www.england.nhs.uk/wp-content/uploads/2019/07/saving-babies-lives-care-bundle-version-two-v5.pdf

24. Widdows K, Roberts SA, Camacho EM, Heazell AEP. *Evaluation of the Implementation of the Saving Babies' Lives Care Bundle in Early Adopter NHS Trusts in England.* Manchester, UK: Maternal and Fetal Health Research Centre, University of Manchester; 2018. www.manchester.ac.uk/discover/news/

action-plan-can-prevent-over-600-stillbirths-a-year/

25. McCowan LM, Figueras F, Anderson NH. Evidence-based national guidelines for the management of suspected fetal growth restriction: comparison, consensus, and controversy. *Am J Obstet Gynecol.* 2018 Feb;**218**(2S):S855–68. doi: 10.1016/j.ajog.2017.12.004 www.ncbi.nlm.nih.gov/pubmed/29422214

26. Norman JE, Heazell AEP, Rodriguez A, et al. Awareness of fetal movements and care package to reduce fetal mortality (AFFIRM): a stepped wedge, cluster-randomised trial. *Lancet.* 2018; **392**(10158):1629–38.www

.thelancet.com/journals/lancet/article/PIIS0140-6736(18)31543–5/fulltext

27. INFANT Collaborative Group. Computerised interpretation of fetal heart rate during labour (INFANT): a randomised controlled trial. *Lancet.* 2017 Apr 29;**389**(10080):1719–-29.DOI: 10.1016/s0140-6736(17)30568-8 https://www.thelancet.com/journals/lancet/article/PIIS0140-6736(17)30568–8/fulltext

28. MacKay DF, Smith GCS, Dobbie R, Pell JP. Gestational age at delivery and special educational need: retrospective cohort study of 407,503 schoolchildren. *PLoS Med.* 2010;7(6):e1000289. https://doi.org/10.1371/journal.pmed.1000289

Intrapartum Asphyxia and Its Sequelae

Simon Attard Montalto

60.1 Introduction

Asphyxia describes any condition that results in oxygen deprivation and, in the unborn or soon-to-be-born infant, may occur prenatally in utero, during delivery or postnatally [1]. In cases of intrapartum asphyxia, the duration of oxygen deprivation may vary and is critical to the ensuing insult to the infant's vital organs and, especially, to the brain. Oxygen deficiency at tissue level (hypoxia, see Box 60.1) is often accompanied by glucose and nutrient deprivation, and is further compounded by pre-existing or complicating factors in the mother, especially pyrexia, and in the infant such as sepsis or congenital anomalies, the concomitant degree of metabolic derangement (e.g. extent of hypoglycaemia or metabolic acidosis), and the time to delivery and effective resuscitation. All of these factors will potentially compound any hypoxic injury and the extent of any ensuing brain damage, described as hypoxic ischaemic encephalopathy (HIE, Box 60.1). Attempts to assign an HIE 'grade' may help to correlate early symptoms and signs with the degree and likelihood of long-term sequelae [2], although accurate prognostication of asphyxial brain damage remains difficult.

Unfortunately, the introduction of obstetric measures such as fetal monitoring during labour, have had little effect on the incidence of HIE [3] and, worldwide, asphyxia accounts for almost 25% of all neonatal deaths. Although 'modern' neonatal intensive care, including therapeutic hypothermia, has improved the outcome of some asphyxiated newborns, intrapartum asphyxia remains one of the most common causes of long-term sequelae, neurodisability and cerebral palsy [4]. Worldwide, the incidence of neonatal encephalopathy (NE, see Box 60.1) from all causes has been estimated at around 3 in 1000 live births, and half of these are due to HIE [5]. Indeed, 1.2–2.5 in 1000 infants in developed countries and up to 6 in 1000 infants born in developing countries will develop HIE [6]. Of those, approximately 40–60% will die before their second birthday, usually from complications of cerebral palsy, or survive with severe disability [7]. The World Health Organization (WHO) estimates that a million children survive birth asphyxia every year and go on to develop cognitive difficulties and/or cerebral palsy [8]. Greater vigilance to anticipate and prevent cases of intrapartum asphyxia is required.

60.2 Epidemiology and Aetiology

The fetal heart is well developed by 3 weeks in utero, whereas nephrogenesis starts at 4 weeks, and although complete at birth, nephrons continue to mature thereafter. The neural plate appears at 2–3 weeks, and although the embryonic structures that go on to form the brain and spinal cord appear as early as 4–6 weeks, these organs are still immature at birth. Indeed, brain myelination and growth continue so that the number of neurones double by 3 years of age. All these developing organs are constantly dependent on a good supply of oxygen, glucose as well as nutrients including amino acids, and are very vulnerable to hypoxia. The central nervous system (CNS), in particular, is still highly immature at delivery, has little propensity for neuronal repair and recovery and is extremely sensitive to hypoxic damage.

Any insult that significantly alters perfusion and oxygenation to delicate embryonic tissues may result in ischaemic damage. Such insults may occur acutely as 'sentinel' events or over a period during gestation, and may involve problems in the mother, uterus, placenta or fetus (Table 60.1). Sudden 'catastrophic' events include maternal collapse, uterine rupture or massive abruption, cord prolapse and shoulder dystocia, as well as circulatory collapse from any cause in the fetus. Maternal illness such as severe anaemia, hypertension, poorly controlled diabetes or systemic lupus erythematosus (SLE), obstructed labour, placental insufficiency and congenital anomalies may result in chronic underperfusion of the developing embryo.

Box 60.1 Definitions

Asphyxia: any condition where the body is deprived of oxygen
Hypoxia: deficiency of oxygen reaching body tissues
Hypoxaemia: deficiency of oxygen in the circulation
Neonatal encephalopathy (NE): a condition with disordered brain function in the neonate resulting from several causes, including hypoxia
Hypoxic ischaemic encephalopathy (HIE): neonatal encephalopathy due to impaired oxygen delivery (±decreased perfusion) to the brain that results in an insult due to primary or secondary energy failure

Table 60.1 Causes of intrapartum asphyxia

	Acute, sentinel	Chronic
Maternal	Collapse from any cause maternal haemorrhage, shock	Pre-eclampsia, hypertension Severe anaemia SLE, diabetes, epilepsy Thrombotic disorder
Uterus-placenta	Uterine rupture abruption Cord prolapse, obstruction Amniotic fluid embolism	Obstructed labour Placental insufficiency
Fetus	Shock, arrest Acute blood loss Arrhythmia Antenatal stroke	Complex congenital heart disease Vascular anomaly Arrhythmia

60.3 Pathophysiology and Pathogenesis

60.3.1 Pathophysiology

The initial response to severe hypoxia is a redistribution of the circulation without developing acidosis in order to perfuse the heart and CNS. This is followed by increasing de-oxygenation and a build-up of acidosis in underperfused organs such as the skeletal muscle and bowel and, finally, hypoxia and significant acidosis in vital organs. This pathophysiological sequence was demonstrated in the early 1960s, via eloquent studies that mimicked an acute asphyxial insult and are unlikely to be reproduced today [9, 10]. The vital parameters of a sheep fetus were monitored after it was removed from the ewe's womb, but it had its head immersed in a bag of water whilst the umbilical cord was clamped. The sudden cessation in oxygen delivery initially resulted in tachycardia and hyperventilation, followed by bradycardia and deep, gasping 'agonal' respiration as hypoxia, hypercarbia and metabolic acidosis ensued. The sheep's vital parameters including blood pressure were sustained at this point, when simple intervention such as opening the airway and giving a few assisted breaths could resuscitate the fetus. Without any attempt at 'rescue', and after a few minutes of sustained hypoxia, primary apnoea set in. This cessation of respiratory efforts was soon followed by more infrequent, irregular gasps associated with ever-worsening metabolic milieu. After a few more minutes, respiration stopped altogether – secondary or terminal apnoea – and this was rapidly associated with profound bradycardia and hypotension, leading to cardiac arrest (Figure 60.1). Fetuses allowed to reach this stage of hypoxic deterioration could only be resuscitated by means of sustained artificial ventilatory support and, in the more severe cases, additional external cardiac compressions. Current training on resuscitation of the compromised newborn is largely based on the knowledge obtained from these experiments, whereby the all-important clinical signs, especially heart rate and respiratory effort, together with body colour and tone, determine the need, timing and degree of resuscitative support required after birth (see below).

Hypoxia at the cellular level results from decreased levels of oxygen in the air supplied, or due to a problem with the lungs or circulation. Apart from those newborns with severe congenital anomalies affecting the heart and lungs, hypoxia is almost always secondary to decreased oxygen delivery 'at source' and, in the newborn, this equates to the mother, placenta or umbilical cord.

60.3.2 Histopathology

Hypoxia causes energy failure in cells and triggers a number of mechanisms that, in turn, result in cell degeneration and cell death. These include oxidative stress, inflammatory cascades and activation of cell-death pathways resulting in apoptosis. Histologically, cell damage leading to cell death, especially in neurones after a significant ischaemic insult, is the complex combined result of overt cell necrosis, apoptosis and autophagy [11].

60.3.3 Macro-pathology

The 'watershed' areas of the brain where circulation is provided by fewer end-vessels are particularly vulnerable to hypoxia. Hence, the periventricular regions, basal ganglia, thalamus and internal capsule are prime candidates for hypoxic damage, reflecting the prevalence and type of cerebral palsy in survivors. The micro-histological changes, especially if extensive, may be associated with visible changes on imaging of the brain, even if a relatively crude modality such as ultrasound is employed [12]. The latter is non-invasive, relatively inexpensive, easily available on most neonatal units and shows changes at an early stage of asphyxia. Periventricular increased brightness, 'flares', may denote areas of altered perfusion (Figure 60.2a) and, with regular sequential scans, may proceed to show overt cystic changes, leukomalacia, with eventual brain atrophy and secondary ventricular hydrocephaly (Figure 60.2b & c). Good-quality and sequential ultrasound scans have been shown to correlate with the clinical status and future degree of neurodisability [12].

The changes on ultrasound are mirrored by corresponding changes on computerized tomography (CT) and, preferably, magnetic resonance imaging (MRI) that is considered the

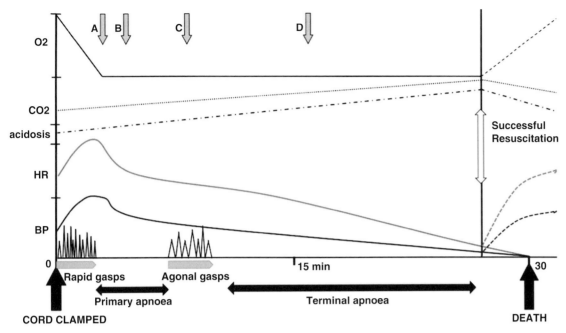

Figure 60.1 Pathophysiology of asphyxia in the fetus

An infant born at point A [the arrow at the top of the figure] is not unduly compromised such that simple assistance at birth, including stimulation, drying and opening the airway, may suffice. Those born at point B are more likely to require inflation breaths, whilst those born at point C will almost certainly need inflation and a period of ventilatory breaths. Infants born during terminal apnoea at point D are likely to be severely hypoxic and acidotic, often requiring cardiac compressions ±drugs in addition to ventilation. Reproduced with kind permission of the Resuscitation Council (UK).

O2=oxygen level; CO2=carbon dioxide level; HR=Heart rate and BP=blood pressure

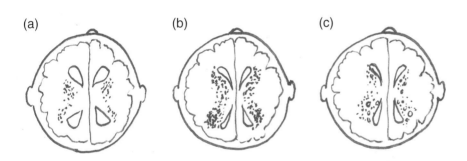

Figure 60.2 Ultrasound in (a) mild, (b) moderately, (c) severely asphyxiated newborns. Perihilar and ventricular 'flares' are seen in the mildly asphyxiated brain (a), with marked enhancement, compressed ventricles and periventricular cystic changes with increasingly severe asphyxia (b and c).

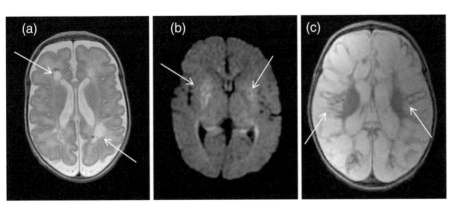

Figure 60.3 MRI showing (a) PVL, (b) BGTL, (c) MCE in asphyxiated newborns.

MRIs showing (a) extensive bilateral cystic periventricular leukomalacia with haemosiderin deposition within the cystic spaces (arrows); (b) damage to the basal ganglia and thalamus with restricted diffusion around the occipital horns of the lateral ventricles and basal ganglia (arrows), plus oedema in the corpus callosum; and (c) multi-cystic encephalomalacia with multiple cystic cavities of variable size separated from one another by glial septations (arrows), and preservation of the immediate periventricular white matter. Images kindly provided courtesy of Dr Andre S. Gatt, Medical Imaging Department, Mater Dei Hospital, Malta.

gold standard, and where derangement of the brain cytoarchitecture can be better defined [12]. Nuclear imaging describes three patterns of hypoxic-ischaemic injury (Figure 60.3a–c) including periventricular leukomalacia (PVL), basal ganglia thalamic lesions (BGTL) and multi-cystic encephalopathy (MCE) [13].

60.4 Clinical Features

Asphyxiated newborns will manifest a host of symptoms and signs, some of which may indicate the degree of asphyxia. Simple scoring methods, such as the sentinel score devised by Virginia Apgar in 1953, provide a snapshot of the condition of the baby at the time the score was calculated (Table 60.2) [14]. Although around 10% of infants with a low Apgar score of ≤3 at 5 minutes may have signs of cerebral palsy at 1 year of age, compared with just 0.1% of those with a score of 9 [15], the correlation is too non-specific to help prognosticate in individual cases. Indeed, these scores are useful as indicators of the need and urgency for intervention, and the Apgar score, like others, do not correlate closely with the degree of asphyxia and are of limited long-term prognostic value [16].

Asphyxiated infants manifest a host of symptoms that may vary from mild irritability and reluctance to feed to poor handling, abnormal movements, seizures and somnolence to outright coma. These symptoms correlate with varying clinical signs that may include, with increasing severity, irritability on handling, poor suck reflex, increased jitteriness and reflexes, excessive head lag and hypotonia, overt seizures, decerebrate posturing, profound stupor to outright coma. With increasing severity of hypoxia, these symptoms and signs are indicative of brain injury, from mild cerebral irritability to a severe brain insult, and often associated with multi-organ failure [17]. Indeed, it is not unusual for severely asphyxiated infants to also develop an acute renal insult, usually acute tubular necrosis (ATN) with oliguria or anuria, acute lung injury requiring oxygen and respiratory support, myocardial insult with heart failure and, at times, bone marrow and liver dysfunction resulting in haematological and metabolic derangements (e.g. thrombocytopenia, clotting abnormalities, hypoglycaemia, lactic acidosis, and abnormal liver enzymes) [17]. Except in the most severe cases, the associated organ damage is, with appropriate support, recoverable, leaving irreversible brain damage as the single most important cause for long-term disability in those who survive.

Several attempts to develop an 'Encephalopathy Score' that identifies and grades symptoms and signs according to the severity of the asphyxia and, ultimately, the extent of tissue insult including HIE with a view towards prognostication have been reported [15, 16]. These are helpful as they assess developing encephalopathy over a period of 24–48 hours, as opposed to a brief snapshot taken a few minutes after birth. One of the most commonly applied is that proposed by Sarnat and Sarnat 1976 (modified, Levene 1986) [18, 19], but all grading classifications simplify a complex condition that changes with time, and there is marked overlap of the artificially set grades. Nevertheless, they do help to guide therapy and provide an overview of outcome. Probably, these scoring systems are best used to describe the 'degree' of encephalopathy in terms of severity rather than using a computed and highly artificial number (Box 60.2). Hence, in so doing, it is more helpful to equate Grade I HIE as defined by Sarnat with an approximate 10% chance of long-term neurodisability, Grade II with a 25% risk, whereas Grade III is likely to be linked with a high risk of mortality and severe problems in >80% of survivors.

60.5 Differential Diagnosis

Generally, the predisposing clinical scenario is one known to be at high risk for asphyxia and, therefore, the suspicion for asphyxia is not in doubt in, for example, those infants who are clearly in trouble after loss of the heart rate in utero, cord prolapse, shoulder dystocia, severely prolonged second stage of labour and so forth. Others may not have undergone such an overt clinical insult, yet may still manifest clinical symptoms and signs of asphyxia and, for those, the possibility of unrecognized asphyxia should still be entertained.

Conversely, all infants with an encephalopathic picture, and possibly a presumptive diagnosis of asphyxia, should be assessed for and covered against sepsis, especially group B streptococcus. Other congenital infections like toxoplasmosis, rubella, cytomegalovirus and herpes viruses (TORCH) will also result in neonatal encephalopathy that may mimic asphyxia. Intracerebral anomalies, trauma including intracerebral and intraventricular haemorrhage and congenital lung anomalies including diaphragmatic hernia may also result in

Table 60.2 The Apgar score

Score	0	1	2
Heart rate	Nil	<100	>100
Respiratory effort	Nil	Irregular, gasps	Regular, strong
Colour	White/blue	Blue peripheries	Pink
Tone	Flaccid, none	Hypotonic	Good, flexed
Activity	None	Little	Vigorous

Box 60.2 Grading of HIE by Severity

Mild (Grade I)	normal activity, alert, minor irritability, poor feeding, reduced suck, exaggerated reflexes and Moro, normal tone
	pupils dilated, tachycardia, normal respiration
Moderate (Grade II)	decreased activity, lethargic, marked irritability, poor feeding, weak suck, exaggerated reflexes, weak Moro, hypotonia, some seizures
	pupils constricted, bradycardia, irregular respiration
Severe (Grade III)	no activity, coma, no suck, absent Moro, flaccid, variable/intractable seizures, decerebrate posturing
	pupils dilated/non-reactive, variable heart rate, apnoea

a significantly depressed infant. Rare genetic neurometabolic conditions, neuronal migration defects and thrombotic disorders may also present with symptoms and signs similar to asphyxia. Hence, infants with a diagnosis of asphyxia should have blood cultures taken as well as a TORCH screen. In addition, they should undergo a chest x-ray and brain imaging with a brain ultrasound scan as a minimum. More detailed CT or MRI scanning of the brain (and lung in cases of lung-airway abnormalities), and neurometabolic and genetic screening would be indicated especially in those with a positive family history, parental consanguinity and associated dysmorphic or syndromic features (Box 60.3).

Box 60.3 Investigations in Asphyxiated Newborns

Haematology	haemoglobin, white cell count, differential
	platelet count, clotting profile
Biochemistry	urea, electrolytes (Na^+, K^+, Cl^-, Ca^{2+}, Mg^{2+}, PO_4^{3-})
	creatinine
	glucose
	blood gas, base deficit, lactate
	liver function (aspartate aminotransferase (AST), alanine aminotransferase (ALT))
Inflammatory markers	C-reactive protein (CRP), erythrocyte sedimentation rate (ESR)
Microbiology	blood culture (±lumbar puncture)
Radiology	chest x-ray
	ultrasound brain, kidneys
	MRI brain
Other tests	electrocardiograph (ECG), echocardiogram (ECHO)
	continuous electroencephalography (CEEG)/cerebral function monitor (CFM)

Investigations to consider with other causes of neonatal encephalopathy

	congenital infection screening (Toxoplasma gondii, rubella, cytomegalovirus, herpes (TORCH))
	genetic testing (e.g. Prader-Willi syndrome, thrombophilia)
	neurometabolic screening (metabolic acidaemias, congenital myotonia, mitochondrial disorders, myopathies)
	imaging for neuronal migration defects
	CT lungs (congenital airway anomalies)

60.6 Clinical Management

Birth asphyxia is a serious complication in newborns with major implications for future prognosis, neurodisability and survival. All infants with this suspected or confirmed diagnosis need to be managed appropriately with timely investigations, and a management plan that aims to support the infant to maintain homeostasis, encourage healing and limit brain damage.

60.6.1 Investigations

Fetal scalp blood samples collected pre-delivery may herald intrapartum ischaemia and acidosis. Shortly after delivery, paired venous and arterial umbilical cord blood pH and lactate levels may give a good indication of the degree of hypoxia and acidosis. The arterial sample reflects fetal blood, and has a lower pH than the venous sample that is 'improved' by placental action. A pH reading below 7.2 is assumed to be abnormal, but a pH below 7.0 is increasingly associated with HIE [20]. Hence, up to 12% of infants with a cord pH of ≤7.0 may develop HIE, compared with 33% with a pH <6.9, and 80% with a pH <6.7. When both arterial and venous pH samples are poor, this suggests that the ischaemic result was prolonged and could not be corrected by placental filtration.

Although further tests may vary according to individual cases, in general, asphyxiated infants require investigation to assess the degree of asphyxia and the extent of organ involvement and damage, and to help guide management (Box 60.3).

60.6.2 Treatment

60.6.2.1 Resuscitation

Severely compromised infants will require immediate resuscitation at birth, even before any investigations have been undertaken. The heart rate and breathing effort are the two most important parameters, with the heart rate being the best indicator of the infant's condition and the most sensitive in responding to effective resuscitation. Tone, activity and even body colour may vary widely and may appear 'poor' even in babies who are perfectly fine. Indeed, in 25% of entirely normal babies, oxygen saturation and, therefore, body colour make take up to 10 minutes to rise above 90% (Table 60.3) [21]. Those with an inadequate respiratory effort – irregular and gasping breaths – and those with an inadequate heart rate (less than 60 beats per minute) require immediate support. Even the now-accepted practice of delayed cord clamping for at least 1 minute needs to be forgone in these critical infants who must be transferred without delay onto the resuscitaire where effective resuscitation can commence.

Table 60.3 25th percentile for oxygen saturation in normal newborns

Time (minutes)	1	2	3	4	5	10
O_2 saturation (%)	40	60	70	80	85	90

Pre-ductal oxygen saturation in entirely normal newborns.

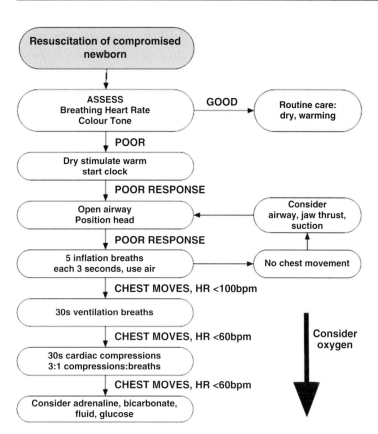

Figure 60.4 Algorithm for newborn resuscitation

Several guidelines for newborn resuscitation exist but essentially follow the same format (Figure 60.3). The European Resuscitation Council (ERC) and UK Resuscitation Council both emphasize the assessment of the infant's respiratory effort and heart rate, less so muscle tone and body colour. This assessment can be improved by obtaining oxygen saturation and the heart rate via a pulse oximeter attached to the right upper limb (i.e. pre-ductally, before any shunting of blood may occur through a still-open ductus arteriosus). Senior assistance should be called for earlier rather than later, and anticipated during all high-risk deliveries. Intervention follows the sequence airway-breathing-circulation (ABC) and, in practice for most newborns, once the airway and breathing are addressed, the circulation corrects itself. Opening airway manoeuvres alone may suffice in mildly compromised infants, whereas those with a greater asphyxial insult are likely to require help in expanding their lungs and initiate normal respiration (see Section 60.3.1, Figure 60.1). For those, five initial inflation breaths that are sustained for 3 seconds each are delivered, with the observation of chest expansion being the best guide to confirm lung inflation (and more sensitive than listening for 'air entry'). Resuscitation using air rather than oxygen is generally adequate and, in those where the chest has inflated but the heart rate/baby's condition remain poor, 30 seconds of ventilation breaths is required. Severely asphyxiated infants, particularly those born in secondary/terminal apnoea and those whose heart rate remains less than 60 beats per minute (bpm) despite adequate ventilation, will require cardiac compressions at a rate of 3:1 compressions to ventilations. The situation is reviewed at 30-second intervals and, if there is still no response, resuscitative

drugs such as adrenaline and bicarbonate, possibly glucose and a saline bolus, should be considered. An umbilical venous line would need to be inserted with urgency at this stage.

In reality, almost 10% of newborn infants require a degree of assistance at birth mostly to support the 'transition' period, but few will need prolonged ventilation beyond the initial five inflation breaths and very few require cardiac compressions, with or without drugs. No return of spontaneous circulation after 10 minutes of appropriate resuscitation is indicative of an extreme hypoxic insult, and is associated with an extremely high mortality and severe morbidity in any survivors. At this stage, and after due consultation with parents and the whole team, difficult decisions relating to the discontinuation of resuscitative efforts will need to be taken by senior and experienced staff.

60.6.2.2 General Medical Support

As with any seriously ill newborn, asphyxiated infants may require intensive and extensive support, preferably undertaken in a dedicated neonatal unit [22]. Often some form of respiratory support, including nasal continuous positive airway pressure (CPAP) and intubation with ventilation in the worst cases, is required. Settings need to be adjusted to maintain, as far as possible, normal oxygenation with saturations in the mid- to high 90s, normocapnia and a normal arterial blood pH. Hyperoxaemia and hypocapnia that reduces cerebral blood flow are associated with increased brain damage and should be avoided.

Fluids including dextrose and electrolytes should ensure adequate perfusion, blood pressure and perfusing pressure for the kidneys. Correction of any electrolyte or glucose disturbance and acidosis should be carried out promptly, again to maintain normal homeostasis and not exacerbate brain injury. Due attention to warmth (except for those eligible for therapeutic hypothermia, see below) usually necessitates incubator care in a suitably heated unit.

Heart failure and liver and renal dysfunction due to acute tubular necrosis will commonly accompany infants who have experienced a significant asphyxial event, but usually resolve. These complications may necessitate inotropic support, diuretics and, rarely, peritoneal dialysis. Seizures are a common complication of HIE and often necessitate anticonvulsant therapy, including phenobarbitone and midazolam. Neuroprotection is augmented by means of adequate and continuous sedation, often with opiate and benzodiazepine infusions, whereas any concomitant anaemia, thrombocytopenia and clotting abnormalities need to be treated to improve oxygen delivery to damaged tissues and prevent secondary haemorrhages.

Since it is almost always impossible to categorically exclude sepsis as a confounding complication in this cohort, almost all asphyxiated infants will receive broad-spectrum antibiotics (according to individual protocols customized to cover the most likely pathogenic organisms encountered on any given unit). Finally, since many of these sick infants are unable to feed as a result of their poor condition, with or without an ileus and the possible associated risk of necrotizing enterocolitis, they require total parenteral feeds via central line access (initially, usually an umbilical arterial line, followed by some form of tunnelled, long-term indwelling line).

60.6.2.3 Therapeutic Hypothermia

In the 1990s, animal studies showed that levels of neurotoxic and neuroprotective mediators altered after an initial hypoxic event, with delayed apoptosis within the first 12 hours confirming an optimal period spanning a few hours after birth [23]. Similarly, in animal models, induced hypothermia during this ideal period was shown to have a neuroprotective effect and subsequently reduced neurological damage. Encouragingly, these findings were also reproduced in human subjects. After extensive inter-country multicentre trials and a convincing meta-analysis that confirmed reduced neurological sequelae in survivors at 18 months [24] and reduced changes on MRI [25], therapeutic hypothermia was established as the standard therapy for significantly asphyxiated infants. In practice, asphyxiated infants should be resuscitated and then immediately assessed for eligibility for this treatment, according to clinical criteria, an HIE score and blood gas parameters, in line with the individual unit's protocol. Ideally, cooling should start within 6 hours of birth and may be induced passively by removing heat sources. The infant is then cooled rapidly over 2 hours to around 33.5°C for 72 hours using a customized head or whole-body cooling device, and gradually rewarmed to 37.5°C over the next 6–8 hours. This therapy has few and reversible side effects such as thrombocytopenia, hypercalcaemia and fat necrosis [26]. Optimal results have been obtained in term infants who have suffered a moderate hypoxic insult, and hypothermia will avoid significant long-term neurodisability in one out of every nine patients treated. It

has been estimated to reduce health expenditure by about €1,000,000 for every successfully treated child [31].

60.6.2.4 Surgical Interventions

Asphyxiated infants may require surgical intervention to insert central lines, deal with the complications of associated necrotizing enterocolitis and insert ventriculoperitoneal shunts to relieve complicating hydrocephalus in those with associated haemorrhages.

60.6.3 Preventive Measures

Clearly, HIE and its sequelae may have disastrous effects on neurodevelopment, and interventions including therapeutic hypothermia certainly do not result in a significant improvement in the majority of cases. Therefore, prevention must be the priority and, at all times, awareness and, whenever possible, avoidance of all those causes of intrapartum asphyxia (see Table 60.1) must be maintained. Good practice must, therefore, include vigilant anticipation and prompt intervention in all perinatal obstetric emergencies.

60.6.4 Research and Developments

Approximately 50% of infants who have been cooled still have abnormal long-term neurology. The combination of cooling with xenon-gas ventilation has been shown to be feasible, but is expensive and early results showed little enhancement of the neuroprotection achieved with cooling [27]. Several other modalities and medications, sometimes in combination, are currently under assessment within research settings, with variable results [28]. These include erythropoietin, magnesium sulphate, melatonin, monogangliosides, N-acetyl cysteine, immunobiotin, endocannabinoids, azithromycin and topiramate, amongst others [28]. Stem cells may offer the possibility of nerve cell repair and regeneration and, in theory, may reverse brain damage, but this option is still a long way from becoming reality [29]. Unfortunately, research on many of these 'new' agents is still at the pre-clinical stage, often limited to small, underpowered studies and, as a result, collated data via meta-analyses or review bodies (e.g. Cochrane) are often inconclusive.

60.7 Complications, Prognosis and Sequelae

Accurate prognostication is difficult but infants with more severe encephalopathy fare worse, and if they survive, they do so with severe cerebral palsy [30]. Hence, those with mild HIE with fewer symptoms and signs (see Box 60.2) have a 10% chance of long-term neurodisability, moderate HIE carries a 25% risk, whereas severe HIE is associated with up to 60% mortality and severe neurological sequelae in >80% of survivors. Strong indicators for a severe asphyxial insult include cardiac arrest pre-delivery, and late and prolonged decelerations on cardiotocography, with or without meconium staining, and an arterial cord pH of ≤7.0 [30]. Infants who manifest severe stupor, intractable seizures, multi-organ failure and a slow response to resuscitation such that they do not establish effective, self-ventilation by 15–20 minutes have a poor prognosis. Survivors are left with problems including severe spastic

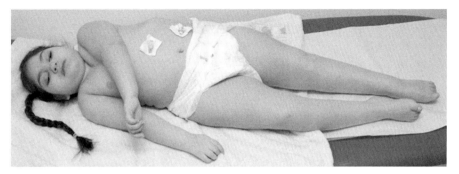

Figure 60.4 School-age child with post-HIE severe spastic tetraplegia.
A 10-year old with post-HIE spastic cerebral palsy, who is failing to grow appropriately, had recurrent chest infections, feeding difficulties (has a gastrostomy tube to clear secretions in view of severe oesophageal reflux and an ileostomy for feeds) and seizures. She also has limited awareness, communication and cognition, and global developmental delay (e.g. still requires nappies), generalized spasticity, muscle atrophy, contractures and immobility (hence, she is lying on a soft fleece rug to prevent pressure sores). A black and white version of this figure will appear in some formats. For the colour version, please refer to the plate section.

tetraplegia; global developmental delay; loss of special senses such as speech, sight and hearing, often associated with complications such as frequent seizures. Bulbar or pseudobulbar palsy will result in feeding difficulties and an increased risk of aspiration and the latter, in conjunction with immobility and hypostasis, may lead to secondary pneumonia (Figure 60.4).

60.8 Key Messages

- Birth asphyxia causes 25% of all neonatal deaths.
- Hypoxic encephalopathy amounts to 50% of all neonatal encephalopathies.
- Survivors of HIE may have devastating long-term effects, including cerebral palsy.
- Obstetric complications contribute significantly to birth asphyxia and HIE.
- Vigilance during pregnancy and, especially after labour, may reduce the incidence.
- Affected infants require general supportive measures.
- Therapeutic hypothermia is now the 'standard of care' for asphyxiated infants.
- Therapeutic hypothermia may avoid 1 in 9 cases developing a neurodisability.
- New treatments, although promising, are still experimental.

References

1. Long M, Brandon DH. Induced hypothermia for neonates with hypoxic-ischaemic encephalopathy. *J Obstet Gynaecol Neonatol Nurs.* 2007;**36**:293–8.

2. Robertson NR, Groenendaal F. Neurological syndrome and encephalopathy scores. In *Rennie and Roberton's Textbook of Neonatology*, 5th ed. London: Churchill Livingstone; 2012. pp. 1135–6.

3. Alfiveric Z, Devane D, Gyte GM. Continuous cardiotocography (CTG) as a form of electronic fetal monitoring (EFM) for fetal assessment during labour. *Cochrane Database Syst Rev* 2006Jul 19;(3):CD006066.

4. Rocha-Ferreira E, Hristova M. Plasticity in the neonatal brain following hypoxic-ischaemic injury. *Neural Plast.* 2016;**2016**:4901014. http://dx.doi.org/10.1155/2016/4901014

5. Kurinczuk J, White-Koning M, Badwani N. Epidemiology of neonatal encephalopathy and hypoxic-ischaemic encephalopathy. *Early Hum Develop.* 2010;**86**:329–38.

6. Badwani N, Kurinczuk JJ, Keogh JM, et al. Intrapartum risk factors for newborn encephalopathy: the Western Australian case-control study. *BMJ.* 1998;**317**:1554.

7. Allen KA, Brandon DH. Hypoxic ischaemic encephalopathy: Pathophysiology and experimental treatments. *Newborn Infant Nurs Rev.* 2011;**11**(3):125–33.

8. World Health Organization. World Health Report: make every mother and child count. 2005.

9. Cross KW. Resuscitation of the asphyxiated infant. *Brit Med Bull.* 1966;**22**:73–78.

10. Dawes G. Birth asphyxia, resuscitation and brain damage In *Foetal and Neonatal Physiology.* Chicago:Year Book Publisher; 1968; pp. 141–59.

11. Northington FJ, Chavez-Valdez R, Martin LJ. Neuronal cell death in neonatal hypoxia-ischaemia. *Ann Neurol.* 2011;**69**(5):743–58.

12. Salas J, Tekes A, Hwang M, Northington FJ, Huisman TAGM. Head ultrasound in neonatal hypoxic-ischaemic injury and its mimickers for clinicians. A review of patterns of injury and the evolution of findings over time. *Neonatology.* 2018;**114**:185–97.

13. Cabaj A, Bekiesinska-Figatowska M, Madzik J. MRI patterns of hypoxic-ischaemic brain injury in preterm and full term infants – classical and less common MR findings. *Pol J Radiol.* 2012;**77**(3):71–6.

14. Apgar V. A proposal for a new method of evaluation of the newborn infant. *Anesth Analg (Clev).* 1953;**32**:260–7.

15. Lie KK, Groholt EK, Eskild A. Association between cerebral palsy and Apgar score in low and normal birthweight infants – a population-based cohort study. *Br Med J.* 2010;**341**: c4990.

16. Thompson CM, Puterman AS, Linley LL, et al. The value of a scoring system for hypoxic-ischaemic encephalopathy in predicting neurodevelopmental outcome. *Acta Paediatr.* 1997 **86**;757–61.

17. LaRosa D, Ellery S, Walker DW, Dickinson H. Understanding the full spectrum of organ injury following intrapartum asphyxia. *Front Pediatr.* 2017;00016. https://doi.org/10.3389/fped.2017.00016

18. Sarnat H, Sarnat M. Neonatal encephalopathy following fetal distress. A clinical and

electroencephalographic study. *Arch Neurol.* 1976;**33**:696–705.

19. Levene M, Sands C, Grindulis H, Moore JR. Comparison of two methods of predicting outcome in perinatal asphyxia. *Lancet.* 1986;**1**:67–9.

20. Goodwin TM, Belai L, Hernandez P, Durand M, Paul RH. Asphyxial complications in the term newborn with severe umbilical acidaemia. *Am J Obstet Gynecol.* 1992;**167**:1506–12.

21. Dawson JA, Kamlin CO, Vento M, et al. Defining the reference range for oxygen saturation for infants after birth. *Pediatrics.* 2010;**125**:e1340–47.

22. Azzopardi D. Clinical management of the baby with hypoxic ischaemic encephalopathy. *Semin Fetal Neonatol Med.* 2010;**86**:345–50.

23. Thoresen M, Penrice J, Lorek A, et al. Mild hypothermia after severe transient hypoxic-ischaemia ameliorates delayed cerebral energy failure in the newborn piglet. *Pediatr Res.* 1995;**37**:667–70.

24. Edwards A, Brocklehurst P, Gunn A, et al. Neurological outcomes at 18 months of age after moderate hypothermia for perinatal hypoxic ischaemic encephalopathy: synthesis and meta-analysis of trial data. *BMJ.* 2010;**340**:c363. https://doi.org/10.1136/bmj.c363

25. Rutherford M, Ramenghi L, Edwards A, et al. Assessment of brain tissue injury after moderate hypothermia for perinatal hypoxic ischaemic encephalopathy: a nested sub-study of a randomised controlled trial. *Lancet Neurol.* 2010;**9**:39–45.

26. Shankaran S, Pappas A, Laptook AR, et al. Outcomes of safety and effectiveness in a multicentre trial of whole-body hypothermia for neonates with hypoxic-ischaemic encephalopathy. *Pediatr.* 2008;**122**(4):e791.

27. Azzopardi D, Robertson NJ, Bainbridge A, et al. Moderate hypothermia within 6 h of birth plus inhaled xenon versus moderate hypothermia alone after birth asphyxia (TOBY-Xe): a proof-of-concept, open-label, randomised controlled trial. *Lancet Neurol.* 2016;**15**(2):145–53.

28. Nair J, Kumar VHS. Current and emerging therapies in the management of hypoxic ischaemic encephalopathy in neonates. *Children.* 2018;**5**(7):99.

29. Van Velthoven CT, Kavelaars A, van Bel F, Heijnen CJ. Repeated mesenchymal stem cell treatment after neonatal hypoxia-ischemia has distinct effects on formation and maturation of new neurons and oligodendrocytes leading to restoration of damage, corticospinal motor tract activity, and sensorimotor function. *J Neurosci.* 2010;**30**:9603–11.

30. Cowan F. Outcome after intrapartum asphyxia in term infants. *Semin Neonatol.* 2000;**5**:127–40.

31. Azzopardi D, Strohm B, Linsell L, et al., on behalf of TOBY Register. Implementation and conduct of therapeutic hypothermia for perinatal asphyxia encephalopathy in the UK – analysis of National Data. *PLoS* One. 2012;7(6):e38504. doi: 10.1371/journal.pone.0038504

Chapter

61

Short- and Long-Term Challenges of Neonatal Care

Omobolanle Kazeem & Rahul Roy

61.1 Introduction

Neonatal service specializes in the care of preterm or seriously ill newborns and plays a critical role in ensuring the best possible start in life for these infants. In spite of the irrefutable progress in neonatal care, however, challenges remain vast. This chapter outlines the short- and long-term challenges of neonatal care.

The first part of this chapter is two pronged, examining the short-term challenges in both preterm and term neonates, while the second part addresses the long-term challenges of neonatal care.

61.2 Short-term Challenges

61.2.1 Preterm Neonates

61.2.1.1 Background

Infants born prior to 37 weeks' completed gestation are classified as *premature* [1]. Prematurity is further subdivided by gestational age and birthweight (Table 61.1).

Short-term complications or challenges of neonatal care in preterms (Table 61.2) are due to immaturity and poor postnatal adaptation [2].

61.2.1.2 Respiratory System

Respiratory Distress Syndrome (RDS)

Epidemiology and Risk Factors – – Respiratory distress syndrome (RDS), also called hyaline membrane disease, is an acute respiratory disorder caused by pulmonary surfactant insufficiency. It is the most frequent complication in premature infants and a major cause of morbidity and mortality, correlating with morphological and functional lung immaturity [3, 4].

Table 61.1 Classification of prematurity [1]

Gestational age	
Late preterm (LPT)	34 weeks to 36+6 weeks
Very preterm (VPT)	⩽ 32 wks.
Extremely preterm (EPT)	⩽ 28 weeks
Birthweight	
Low birthweight (LBW)	<2500 g
Very low birthweight (VLBW)	<1500 g
Extremely low birthweight (ELBW)	<1000 g

The incidence of RDS inversely relates to gestational age [5]. While it is a rare occurrence in term infants, RDS affects approximately 50% of infants born <30 weeks, and it is almost inevitable in infants born at <28 weeks' gestation [3–5].

Although prematurity is the greatest risk factor for RDS, there are several other factors that increase the risk of RDS (Table 61.3) [3, 4].

On the other hand, there is reduced risk of RDS with certain factors (Table 61.4), all of which have been described to stimulate surfactant production [5, 6].

Pathophysiology of RDS [5, 7] – – Surfactant, a mixture of phospholipids and proteins, is produced in type 2 pneumocytes from 24 weeks' gestation and acts to reduce alveolar surface tension, thus preventing alveolar collapse.

Respiratory distress syndrome is due to defective or delayed surfactant production by structurally immature lungs with the immature type 2 pneumocytes. Immediate consequences are increase in alveolar surface tension, decrease in lung compliance, atelectasis and impaired ventilation. Resultant hypoxaemia with acidosis orchestrates pulmonary vascular constriction, hypoperfusion and, ultimately, lung tissue ischaemia. Finally, cell debris of sloughed epithelium and proteinaceous exudates form hyaline membranes which line the alveolar sacs (Figure 61.1).

Table 61.2 Short-term challenges of prematurity [2]

Systems	Challenges
Respiratory	Respiratory distress syndrome (RDS) Bronchopulmonary dysplasia (BPD)
Cardiovascular	Patent ductus arteriosus
Gastrointestinal	Necrotizing enterocolitis
CNS	Intraventricular haemorrhage Periventricular leukomalacia Apnoea of prematurity
Eyes	Retinopathy of prematurity
Metabolic problems of prematurity	Hypothermia Hypoglycaemia Hyperbilirubinaemia Electrolyte derangements
Immune system	Sepsis

Clinical Presentation of RDS [5, 7] – – Respiratory distress syndrome usually manifests immediately after birth, but may be up to 4 hours after birth, with:

- Tachypnoea (respiratory rate >60 breaths/min)
- Grunting respirations (exhaling against a closed glottis to maintain a high residual air volume in the lungs in order to prevent alveolar collapse)
- Retractions (subcostal, intercostal and sternal retractions) – due to compliant chest wall and non-compliant lungs
- Nasal flaring
- Apnoea and cyanosis (in severe cases).

Diagnosis of RDS [8] – – Chest x-ray (CXR) is diagnostic with ground glass appearance, atelectasis and air bronchograms (Figure 61.2). Of note, ultrasound scan of the chest has been shown to have high diagnostic sensitivity, even though it is not frequently used [9].

Treatment of RDS – – The treatment of RDS is broadly divided into delivery room stabilization, general and specific treatments.

Delivery room stabilization: These treatments include delayed cord clamping, use of plastic bags or occlusive wrapping (if <28 weeks' gestation) and use of continuous positive airway pressure (CPAP) in spontaneously breathing patients. Where inflation breaths are needed, air or blended air with oxygen (30–40%) should be used rather than 100% oxygen. Intubation and surfactant administration are reserved for those preterms that fail CPAP [10, 11].

General: Treatments focus on thermoregulation, fluid management, antibiotic treatment, nutritional support and oxygen supplementation [10, 11].

Specific: Treatments largely involve the underlying cause of RDS (surfactant treatment), and provision of respiratory support [10, 11].

Exogenous Surfactant Therapy

By improving lung compliance, functional residual capacity and oxygenation, exogenous surfactant has substantially reduced RDS-related morbidity and mortality [12]. Surfactant is even more effective when combined with antenatal steroids.

There are both natural (containing apoproteins SP-B & SP-C) and synthetic (containing no proteins) surfactants. However, modified natural surfactants are commonly used in clinical practice, as they have been shown to have greater efficacy [13].

Table 61.3 Factors that Increase the risk of RDS [3, 4]

Risk factors	Description
Perinatal asphyxia	Resulting hypoxia/acidosis inhibits synthesis of surfactant
Gender and race	RDS is common in male Caucasian infants. Androgenic effects on type 2 pneumocytes delay surfactant synthesis
Twin pregnancy	The risk of RDS is increased in the second twin due to increased risk of hypoxia/acidosis
Infant of diabetic mother	Insulin delays maturation of type 2 pneumocytes resulting in delayed surfactant synthesis
Caesarean section (CS)	There is lack of cortisol response associated with normal delivery process which stimulates surfactant secretion
Genetic disposition	Partial or complete deficiency of SP-B (a component of surfactant). <1% of reported cases of familial RDS in term babies is due to genetic reasons

Table 61.4 Factors associated with reduced risk of RDS

Chronic fetal stress due to premature rupture of membrane (PROM), maternal hypertension, and maternal drug abuse
Intrauterine growth restriction (IUGR) / small for gestational age (SGA)
Antenatal glucocorticoids

Figure 61.1 Pathophysiology of RDS

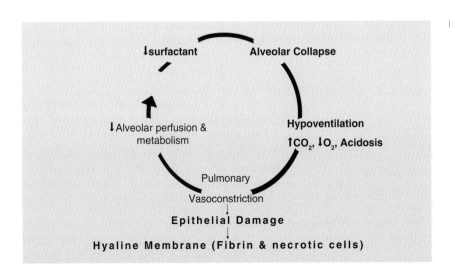

487

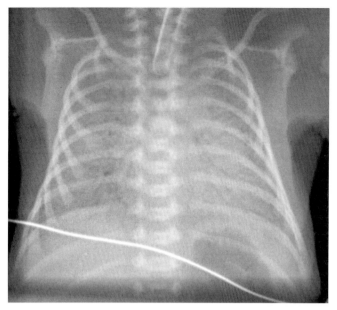

Figure 61.2 CXR of RDS in a very preterm neonate showing 'ground glass' appearance, air bronchograms and reduced lung volume. Source: (https://commons.wikimedia.org/w/index.php?curid=71691505) by Mikael Häggström, August 16, 2018. No Creative Commons License

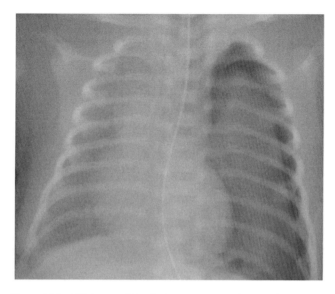

Figure 61.3 CXR showing left-sided tension pneumothorax with mediastinal shift, air in the pleura and collapsed left lung. (Image courtesy of Daniels Rob)

In the UK, for example, Curosurf* and Survanta* are the only surfactants currently licensed for use.

The two approaches to surfactant administration are prophylactic and rescue . The prophylactic approach involves giving surfactant soon after birth to preterm at risk of RDS, and the rescue approach involves giving surfactant to infants with established RDS. However, prophylactic surfactant is no longer recommended, as nasal CPAP (nCPAP) is used routinely from birth [10]. Transient adverse effects of exogenous surfactant shown in clinical studies include bradycardia, obstruction of endotracheal tube and pulmonary haemorrhage [14].

The INSURE technique, which consists of an Intubation SURfactant Extubation sequence, is regarded as the gold standard for surfactant administration in intubated infants [14]. However, there are newly emerging, minimally invasive techniques such as LISA (Less Invasive Surfactant Administration) and MIST (Minimally Invasive Surfactant Therapy), as alternatives to INSURE in non-ventilated infants [10, 15, 16]. Repeated surfactant dosing may be required if a significant oxygen requirement persists.

Respiratory Support [10, 17–20]

Non-invasive methods: Respiratory support can be provided by non-invasive methods such as nCPAP, high-flow nasal cannulae (HFNC) and non-invasive positive-pressure ventilation (NIPPV). CPAP provides a continuous level of positive pressure (PEEP) to distend the lungs, thereby improving functional residual capacity (FRC) as well as lung function. Complications of CPAP include nasal trauma, CPAP belly syndrome (gaseous distention of stomach), air leak syndromes and CPAP failure.

Mechanical ventilation is indicated when there is CPAP failure and respiratory acidosis (PaCO$_2$ >60 mm Hg, PaO$_2$ <50 mm Hg or SaO$_2$ <90%) with an FiO$_2$ >0.4, or severe frequent apnoea.

Prevention of RDS [10, 21, 22] –– The use of antenatal steroid in women at risk of preterm delivery at <34 weeks is recommended. The premise for doing so is that antenatal steroid induces surfactant production and accelerates lung maturation in addition to reducing the risk of necrotizing enterocolitis (NEC) and intraventricular haemorrhage (IVH).

Complications of RDS [23] – – Acute complications of RDS include air leaks, pulmonary haemorrhage, IVH, NEC and persistent ductus arteriosus (PDA). Chronic adverse outcomes of RDS include chronic lung disease (CLD) and retinopathy of prematurity (ROP).

Air Leaks [24-26]

Air leaks are characterized by alveolar rupture from poor lung compliance requiring high ventilator pressures. Air can leak into the pleura, mediastinum, pericardium or extra thoracic areas. Pneumothorax and pulmonary interstitial emphysema (PIE) are the commonest air leaks.

Pneumothorax: In pneumothorax, air leaks into the pleural cavity. It may present with sudden collapse, hypoxaemia, reduced ipsilateral breath sounds and chest movement. Transillumination or CXR is diagnostic and treatment is by needle thoracentesis and chest drain insertion (Figure 61.3)

Pulmonary interstitial emphysema (PIE): PIE is a well-recognized complication of RDS characterized by tracking of air into the interstitium (between the alveoli) and perivascular sheaths, resulting in poor gas exchange. CXR is diagnostic (Figure 61.4).

Pulmonary Haemorrhage

Pulmonary haemorrhage may occur after surfactant therapy or with heart failure secondary to a large PDA. It may present

Table 61.5 Stages of lung development

Stages	Lung development	Effect of abnormal development
Embryonic (3–6 weeks)	Formation of lung bud Differentiation into trachea and bronchi	Errors lead to tracheoesophageal fistula
Pseudo-glandular (5–16 weeks)	Branching of the terminal bronchioles	Respiration is impossible, incompatible with life
Canalicular (16–26 weeks)	The terminal bronchioles subdivide into two or more respiratory bronchioles that divide into three to six alveolar ducts	Fetus born at this stage may or may not survive
Saccular sac (26 weeks to birth)	Primitive alveoli form and alveolar capillaries establish close contact with the alveoli Pneumocytes develop	Fetus born at this stage survive
Alveolar (birth to childhood)	Alveoli mature and divide further to reach adult numbers	At birth: 20–70 million alveoli By 8 years: 300–400million alveoli

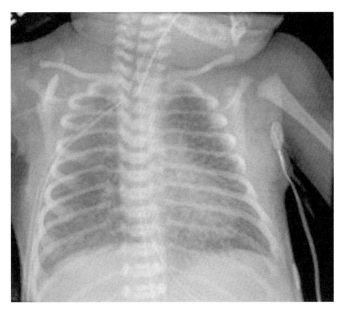

Figure 61.4 CXR showing pulmonary interstitial emphysema (PIE): 'Salt and pepper' appearance is due to the linear lucencies that are present. {Image by Rivard. M – own work / September 3, 2012 / CC BY-SA 3.0/https://creativecommons.org/licenses/by-sa/3.0}

with sudden collapse, blood-stained tracheal aspirate, gross pulmonary haemorrhage with respiratory failure and CXR evidence of dense consolidation. The mainstay of treatment includes vigorous resuscitation, increased ventilator pressures, ibuprofen to close PDA and management of heart failure. Paradoxically, re-treatment with surfactant may help to improve oxygenation.

Intraventricular Haemorrhage

An increased incidence of intraventricular haemorrhage is seen in ventilated premature infants with RDS due to intravascular pressure swings.

Patent Ductus Arteriosus (PDA)

Patent ductus arteriosus closes with oxygen. However, in RDS, there is hypoxaemia (low PaO_2) which causes persistent PDA

Necrotizing Enterocolitis

Hypoxaemia (low PaO_2) resulting from RDS causes intestinal ischaemia and entry of gut bacteria into intestinal wall.

Retinopathy of Prematurity (ROP) and Bronchopulmonary Dysplasia (BPD)

Oxygen toxicity from oxygen treatment orchestrates free radical (superoxide) damage of the retina (ROP) and small airways (BPD).

Prognosis of RDS [27] –– Respiratory distress syndrome classically peaks in severity within 2–3 days, with the recovery phase beginning at 72 hours. The recovery phase, which is usually heralded by spontaneous diuresis, occurs as a result of increased production of endogenous surfactant. RDS in very low birthweight (VLBW) or extremely low birthweight (ELBW) infants may have a protracted course. Severe cases of RDS evolve into bronchopulmonary dysplasia.

Chronic Lung Disease (CLD) or Bronchopulmonary Dysplasia (BPD) [28–31]

Epidemiology and Risk Factors –– Chronic lung disease, also called BPD, is defined as oxygen dependency for at least 28 days from birth, and at 36 weeks corrected gestational age. It is a multifactorial condition, albeit prematurity constitutes the greatest risk factor. Other demographic risk factors associated with BPD include male sex, low birthweight, white race and family history of asthma.

Pathophysiology –– Briefly summarized, lung development is a dynamic process that begins at 4 weeks' gestational age and continues postnatally into childhood. It progresses in five developmental stages: embryonic, pseudo-glandular, canalicular, saccular and alveolar (Table 61.5).

Each step during fetal lung development is critical to establishing a mature respiratory system [32].

Bronchopulmonary dysplasia occurs as a result of disrupted lung development in the late canalicular or early saccular stage of lung development, in the setting of preterm birth. Lung injury (from barotraumas, hyperoxia, inflammation,

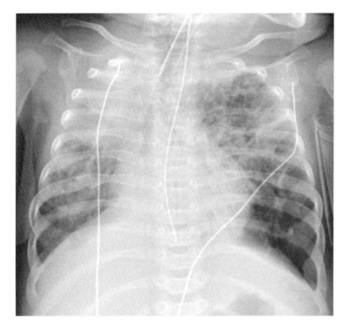

Figure 61.5 CXR showing areas of over-inflation, widespread coarse interstitial markings and atelectasis typical of BPD {Image by Pulmonological – Own work, January 23, 2006, CC BY-SA 3.0, https://commons.wikimedia.org/w/index.php?curid=18189316CC}

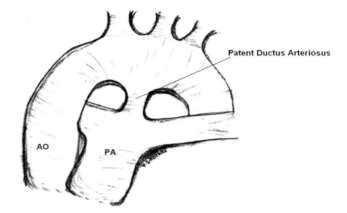

Figure 61.6 Heart cross section with patent ductus arteriosus.

infection and volume overload) acts on the susceptible lung, leading to arrested alveolar development and impaired pulmonary vasculature growth. These culminate in alveolar structural simplification and reduced lung function. This pathology of alveolar simplification with fewer and larger alveoli, coined the new BPD, has been attributed to advances in medical therapy (use of surfactant and steroids). In contrast, the old BPD described by Northway before surfactant and antenatal steroids, characteristically demonstrates inflammation and fibrosis.

Clinical Presentation – – Bronchopulmonary dysplasia may present with respiratory distress, desaturations, feeding problems, cor pulmonale and right heart failure. Further, BPD may have lifelong consequences such as abnormal respiratory function, asthma-like symptoms, exercise intolerance, recurrent respiratory infections and/or require more frequent hospitalization later in childhood.

Diagnosis of CLD/BPD [33] – – The diagnosis of BPD is made clinically based on the gestational age, and oxygen requirement at 36 weeks postmenstrual age (PMA). The chest radiograph may show areas of cystic changes, hyperinflation and atelectasis (Bubble lungs) (Figure 61.5). Occurrence of BPD in the absence of mechanical ventilation is called Wilson–Mikity syndrome [34].

Treatment of CLD/BPD – – In established CLD, fluid restriction, diuretics, nutrition optimization, permissive hypercapnia, oxygen therapy, steroids and vaccination against respiratory pathogens may relieve symptoms and prevent exacerbations. Indications for steroids (low-dose dexamethasone) in infants with CLD include failure to wean from ventilator or persisting oxygen and ventilation requirements after more than 7 days of age. Possible benefits and harms of

steroids must be discussed with the parents before treatment is given.

Prevention of CLD/BPD – – Preventive strategies such as prevention of prematurity, PDA closure, use of antenatal steroids in women at risk of preterm delivery and exogenous surfactant therapy in neonatal RDS may reduce the severity of BPD.

Prognosis of CLD/BPD – – The majority of infants with BPD survive, and chest radiographic findings appear to improve with time. Improvement occurs slowly over time, with less and less respiratory support.

In severe cases, however, infants can have 'BPD exacerbation', require tracheostomy and develop cor pulmonale with poor neurodevelopmental outcomes.

61.2.1.3 Cardiovascular System

Patent Ductus Arteriosus (PDA) [35, 36, 37]

The ductus arteriosus (DA) is a fetal communicating vessel between the pulmonary artery and the descending aorta, which allows blood to bypass the fetal non-functioning lungs. Normally, this vessel closes after birth. However, failure of the spontaneous closure of the DA postnatally results in PDA (Figure 61.6).

PDA is more common in female preterm neonates. It affects more than 70% of infants born at less than 28 weeks' gestation, and the incidence varies inversely with the gestational age.

The most common risk factor for PDA is prematurity. Other risk factors include:

- Low birthweight (<1500 g)
- Respiratory distress syndrome
- Fluid overload
- Sepsis/perinatal stress
- Genetics
- High altitude
- Maternal rubella

Pathophysiology – – Oxygen and endothelin are very strong vasoconstrictors, while nitric oxide and prostaglandins (E2 and I2) are strong vasodilators of the DA.

In utero, ductal patency is maintained by low oxygen tension ($\downarrow$PaO$_2$) and elevated levels of prostaglandins ($\uparrow$PGE2 and $\uparrow$PGI2). Prostaglandin levels are elevated in the fetal circulation because of placental production and decreased metabolism in the fetal lungs.

At birth, however, the rapid increase in PaO$_2$ mediated by lung inflation and the drop in the prostaglandins, from the cutoff of the placenta, result in the biphasic closure of the duct:

- Functional closure occurs within 72 hours of birth due to constriction of the smooth muscle structure.
- Anatomical closure, due to fibrosis of the smooth muscle structure, occurs by 2–3 weeks.

This normal physiological adaptation is delayed or interrupted in preterm infants, placing them at increased risk for PDA. Contributing factors include the following:

- There are a greater number of circulating prostaglandins because of poor clearance by the immature lungs.
- The immature tissue of the DA is less sensitive to the increased PaO$_2$ and more sensitive to the vasodilatory effects of prostaglandins.

Substantial left-to-right shunt through PDA ('ductal steal') results in:

- Hyperperfusion of the lung circulation: This predisposes the development of pulmonary congestion, right heart volume overload.
- Hypoperfusion of the systemic circulation (brain, kidneys, guts): This haemodynamic effect is presumed to cause morbidities including renal dysfunction, necrotizing enterocolitis (NEC), intraventricular haemorrhage or periventricular leukomalacia (IVH/PVL), chronic lung disease (CLD).

Clinical Presentation – – Small PDAs are asymptomatic but large PDAs can cause hypotension, feeding intolerance, respiratory compromise and congestive heart failure.

Bounding peripheral pulses with widened pulse pressure, hyperdynamic precordium and continuous 'machinery murmur' at the left upper sternal border (the diastolic component of the murmur is not heard in preterm infants) are some of the physical examination findings of PDA.

Diagnosis of PDA – –

Electrocardiogram (ECG): *left ventricular hypertrophy*

CXR: *cardiomegaly and pulmonary congestion*

Echocardiography: *identifies ductal size, degree of shunt and left heart volume loading (gold standard).*

Treatment – – Treatment of PDA is a function of its haemodynamic significance. There are three treatment options for PDA:

Conservative approach (watchful waiting): The goal here is to allow time for the PDA to close spontaneously.

Pharmacotherapeutic: Indomethacin and ibuprofen remain the mainstay of medical treatment for PDA. They are both cyclo-oxygenase inhibitors and act by downregulating PGE2, a potent relaxant of the PDA. Further, both are of proven efficacy in the management of PDA. However, due to concerns about the high complication risk of indomethacin (NEC, platelet dysfunction and renal toxicity), ibuprofen is favoured as it has similar efficacy but fewer side effects and a better toxicity profile. Enteral and intravenous (IV) ibuprofen are equally effective. Ibuprofen is given as an initial dose of 10 mg/kg followed at 24 hour intervals by two doses of 5 mg/kg.

Recently, oral acetaminophen has gained increasing attention as an alternative pharmaceutical agent for PDA closure in premature infants. Acetaminophen is postulated to exert its action through inhibition of the peroxidase enzyme thereby leading to downregulation of PGE2 production.

Surgical ligation is reserved for PDA refractory to medical treatment. Complications of PDA ligation include laryngeal nerve paralysis, chylothorax, scoliosis and pulmonary contusion.

In neonates with adequate weight and beyond infancy, percutaneous transcatheter closure can now be done with a success rate close to 100%.

Prognosis of PDA – – Generally, the prognosis of PDA is excellent, but it is poor in preterm infants with other prematurity-related co-morbidities.

61.2.1.4 Gastrointestinal System

Necrotizing Enterocolitis (NEC) [38–40]

Epidemiology and Risk Factors – – Necrotizing enterocolitis is an acquired disease of the gastrointestinal system characterized by inflammation and necrosis of the mucosal layers. It is a disease that occurs almost exclusively in preterm (<32 weeks), low birthweight infants (<1500 g), with the incidence inversely related to gestational age and birthweight.

Although prematurity remains the greatest NEC risk factor, other well-established risk factors for NEC include:

- *Enteral feeding:* 90% of infants with NEC have been fed milk enterally. Formula feedings, rapid advancement of feeding and hyperosmolar stress from hypertonic formula have been implicated. Poor gastrointestinal (GI) motility results in stasis and bacterial overgrowth. Of note, breast milk is protective compared to formula milk.
- *Bowel hypoperfusion and ischaemia:* This can result from PDA, hypotension, cardiac failure, exchange transfusion, indomethacin treatment and sepsis.
- *Infection:* Impaired host defence of the immature GI tract predisposes it to bacterial overgrowth and pathogenic organisms. Though a variety of viral and bacterial pathogens have been associated with NEC, infection of ischaemic mucosa is mainly by gas-forming or gram-negative organisms. Additionally, NEC can occur in clusters (epidemics).

Pathophysiology – – Although the pathogenesis of NEC remains elusive, the combined effect of the above-named risk factors (i.e. infection, enteral feeding and bowel compromise) in at-risk preterm neonates breaches the bowel mucosal barrier. The breach of the mucosal barrier is believed to be the sentinel pathogenic event allowing for bacterial translocation from the bowel lumen into the bowel wall. This, in turn, activates an

Table 61.6 Modified Bell's staging for NEC

Bell's staging	Clinical findings	Radiographic findings	Gastrointestinal findings
Stage 1	Apnea + bradycardia, temperature instabillity	Normal gas pattern or mild ileus	Gastric residuals, occult blood in stool, mild abdominal distension
Stage II A	Apnea + bradycardia, temperature instability	Ileus gas pattern +> 1 dilated loops + focal pneumatosis	Grossly bloody stools, prominent abdominal distension, absent bowel sounds
Stage II B	↓Platelets & mild metabolic acidosis	Widespread pneumatosis, ascites & portal venous gas	Abdominal wall oedema with palpable loops and tenderness
Stage IIIA	Mixed acidosis, oliguria, ↓ blood pressure (BP), coagulopathy	Prominent bowel loops, worsening ascites, no free air	Worsening wall oedema erythema & induration
Stage IIIB	Shock, deterioration in laboratory values & vital signs	Pneumoperitoneum	Perforated bowel

Adapted from Kliegman and Walsh [43].

inflammatory cascade (release of proinflammatory mediators: platelet-activating factor, nitric oxide and interleukin-8) with resultant ulcerative inflammation and necrosis of the intestinal wall. Any part of the bowel can be affected, but more often than not, the terminal ileum and proximal colon are involved.

Clinical Presentation –– The clinical presentation of NEC ranges from subtle non-specific systemic signs (apnoea, bradycardia, temperature instability) to localized gastrointestinal signs (abdominal distension, bilious vomiting, gastric residuals, haematochezia) and, worse still, haemodynamic collapse.

Diagnosis of NEC – – Necrotizing enterocolitis is diagnosed clinically and radiographically. The abdominal x-ray (AXR) is the modality of choice for diagnosis and follow-up of NEC. Characteristic findings on abdominal radiographs include abnormal persistent dilated loops, thickened bowel wall, pneumatosis intestinalis [41] (air in the intestinal wall) (Figure 61.7), portal venous gas and pneumoperitoneum (abdominal free air). Recent studies have shown the potential of abdominal ultrasound scan (USS) as an adjunct to the AXR in the diagnosis of NEC [42].

Additional laboratory studies include a blood culture, coagulation studies (evidence of disseminated intravascular coagulation: ↓fibrinogen, ↑partial thrombin time (PTT), complete blood count (thrombocytopenia, leukocytosis, anaemia) and serial blood gases (acidosis).

Treatment of NEC – – Treatment depends on NEC severity, measured by Bell's staging of NEC (Table 61.6) [43]. Treatment measures include keeping the neonate nil by mouth for bowel rest, nasogastric decompression, fluid resuscitation, total parenteral nutrition, parenteral antibiotics and cardiorespiratory support as required. Surgical intervention is indicated in advanced cases of NEC.

Prevention of NEC –– Protective strategies include use of antenatal steroids, enteral probiotics in at-risk neonates and use of human milk as well as GI priming with cautious advancement of milk.

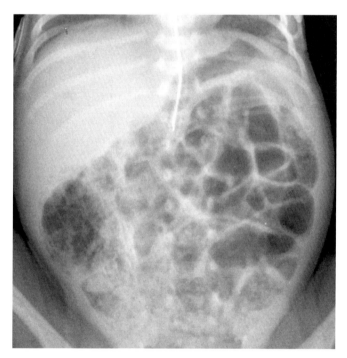

Figure 61.7 AXR showing pneumatosis intestinalis in an infant with NEC. Pneumatosis intestinalis – air within the bowel wall (bubbly appearance). {image by Radswiki, January 21, 2008, CC BY-SA 3.0, https://commons .wikimedia.org/w/index.php?curid=3429446}

Differential Diagnosis of NEC – – The differential diagnosis includes sepsis, intestinal obstruction, omphalitis, isolated intestinal perforation (IIP).

Prognosis of NEC – – Necrotizing enterocolitis can be a life-threatening disease, but most babies make a complete recovery once treated. Nonetheless, the mortality rate of NEC is approximately 40% in premature infants.

NEC survivors may develop complications such as intestinal stricture with bowel obstruction, short bowel syndrome, cholestasis (if prolonged dependence on total parenteral nutrition

(TPN)), poor growth and long-term neurodevelopmental impairments.

61.2.1.5 Central Nervous System

Germinal Matrix/Intraventricular Haemorrhage (GM/IVH) [44–46]

Epidemiology and Risk Factors – – Intraventricular haemorrhage is the most common neurological complication of preterm births. It occurs in approximately 10–25% of preterm infants born before 32 weeks, with an incidence that increases with decreasing gestational age.

Prematurity is the most important risk factor for GM/IVH. In addition to prematurity, any perinatal or neonatal event that increases the chances of hypoxia or cerebral blood flow disturbance amplifies the risk of GM/IVH.

Pathophysiology –– The principal initiating pathogenetic factor relates to bleeding from thin-walled vessels in the germinal matrix. The latter is a richly vascularized fetal structure located in the caudothalamic groove.

The germinal matrix is the site of origin of neuronal-glial precursor cells, and it generally involutes by term age. However, in the very preterm infant, the inherent fragility of the immature germinal matrix vasculature, along with fluctuation in cerebral blood flow, sets the ground for GMH (Table 61.7).

Clinical Presentation – – Intraventricular haemorrhage has diverse clinical presentations, including non-specific symptoms (refusal of feeds, vomiting, abnormal tone and bulging anterior fontanelle), and acute clinical deterioration (increased ventilatory requirements, seizures and unconsciousness). More often than not, however, GM/IVH is clinically silent and is only picked up on transcranial ultrasound.

The severity of IVH is often graded according to Papile's classification (Table 61.8) (Figure 61.8).

Table 61.7 Fate of germinal matrix haemorrhage

Fate of germinal matrix haemorrhage	Description
Germinal matrix haemorrhage	Blood is restricted to the germinal matrix and gradually resolves forming a sub-ependymal pseudocyst.
Intraventricular haemorrhage	GMH extends to the lateral ventricle.
Post-haemorrhagic hydrocephalus	This results from blockage of cerebrospinal fluid (CSF) flow or reabsorption at the level of the third ventricle (non-communicating) or at the arachnoid villi (communicating), respectively.
Haemorrhagic parenchymal infarction (HPI)	A large IVH can obstruct the venous drainage from the cerebral cortex, resulting in parenchymal venous infarction. Breakdown of the clot results in a porencephalic cyst.

Table 61.8 Papile's classification of GM/IVH

Grade	Description	Outcomes
I	Isolated germinal matrix haemorrhage	Resolves without major long-term disability, can form sub-ependymal pseudocyst
II	IVH without ventricular dilation	Resolves without major long-term disability
III	IVH with ventricular dilation	Risk of developing posthaemorrhagic hydrocephalus
IV	IVH with parenchymal haemorrhage	Risk of developing posthaemorrhagic hydrocephalus, can evolve into a porencephalic cyst.

Figure 61.8 Diagrammatic representation of Papile's staging of IVH (cross section of the brain) PPHN: persistent pulmonary hyperstension of the newborn

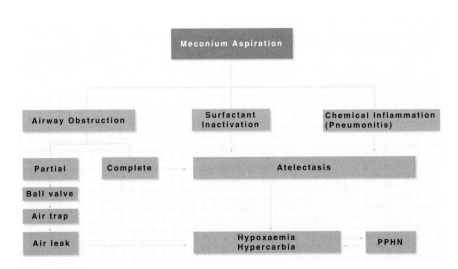

493

Diagnosis of GM/IVH --
Transcranial ultrasound is the modality of choice [47]. Preterm babies born at <32 weeks' gestation are serially scanned at birth, at 3 and 7 days of age, and at 36–40 weeks postmenstrual age. This is based on the premise that majority of haemorrhages occur in the first week of life. In addition, weekly transcranial ultrasonography is indicated to monitor for progression of GM/IVH and the development of hydrocephalus.

Treatment of GM/IVH -- There is no cure for IVH. Treatment is generally supportive, and prevention of preterm birth is the key. Ventriculo-peritoneal shunt may be necessary in post-haemorrhagic hydrocephalus.

Prognosis of GM/IVH -- The severity of IVH is an important factor in the clinical outcome; infants with grades III and IV IVH have a significant risk of developing post-haemorrhagic hydrocephalus (PHH) and often suffer from significant neurodevelopmental deficits in the long term. In contrast, grades I and II IVH tend to resolve without major long-term disability.

Periventricular Leukomalacia (PVL) [48–51]

Epidemiology and Risk Factors -- Periventricular leukomalacia, characterized by coagulation necrosis, is a predominant form of white matter injury typical for preterm (<32 weeks' gestation), low birthweight (<1500 g) infants and is associated with a high risk of cerebral palsy.

The aetiology of PVL is multifactorial and involves prenatal and perinatal factors that amplify the chances of hypoxia-ischaemia and inflammation (Table 61.9).

Pathophysiology of PVL -- Characteristically, preterm infants, by virtue of their unique immature cerebrovascular anatomy and physiology (e.g. watershed zones, impaired autoregulation), are susceptible to ischaemia and inflammation. These two upstream mechanisms cause activation of two principal downstream mechanisms: excitotoxicity and free radical attack, leading to death of the vulnerable premyelinating oligodendrocytes (pre-OL). The vulnerability of pre-OL associated with immature antioxidant defences is central to the pathogenesis of PVL. Consequent death and/or maturational arrest of pre-OLs lead to periventricular focal necrosis and diffuse white matter reactive gliosis which are underlying substrates of cerebral palsy and cognitive deficits, respectively.

Clinical Presentation of PVL -- Remarkably, PVL presents silently and typically evolves over weeks or months with variable severity of spastic paraparesis, as well as visual and cognitive impairment.

Diagnosis of PVL -- Periventricular leukomalacia can be detected by transcranial ultrasonography (CrUSS) as initial periventricular echodensities or flare, followed later by cystic formation (by age 6 weeks). The ultrasound can underestimate the incidence of PVL, in which case magnetic resonance imaging (MRI) is more sensitive, especially in detecting non-cystic PVL.

Table 61.9 Risk factors for PVL

Period	Risk factors
Prenatal	Preterm premature rupture of membranes (PPROM)
	Chorioamnionitis
Perinatal	Birth asphyxia
	Maternal haemorrhage
Neonatal	Recurrent apnoea
	Hypocarbia
	PDA
	Hypotension
	NEC
	Sepsis

Treatment of PVL -- Currently there are no specific treatments for PVL. Management is limited to prevention, early recognition, supportive treatment and close neurodevelopmental follow-up.

Prognosis of PVL -- Depending on severity, infants with PVL are at risk for neurodevelopmental deficits.
Mild PVL: Spastic diplegia cerebral palsy
Severe PVL: May lead to quadriplegic cerebral palsy, visual defects or intelligence deficiencies.

Apnoea of Prematurity (AOP) [52–55]

Epidemiology and Risk Factors -- Apnoea of prematurity is defined as a pause in breathing for >20 seconds or a shorter pause in breathing with concomitant bradycardia (<100 beats per minute (bpm)), cyanosis or pallor in preterm infants.

The frequency or severity of AOP inversely correlates to gestational age: while it is almost universal in infants born at <28 weeks, it is rare after 36 weeks of gestation.

Types of AOP -- Apnoea of prematurity can be classified as one of three types: central, obstructive or mixed.
Central apnoea:(40%): In central apnoea, there is cessation of both the airflow and respiratory effort and airflow (absence of chest wall movement and airflow).
Obstructive apnoea (10%): This type is characterized by absence of airflow in the presence of inspiratory efforts (presence of chest wall movement but no airflow).
Mixed apnoea (50%): Central apnoea is either preceded or followed by airway obstruction. It is the most common type in preterm infants.

Pathophysiology of AOP -- The pathophysiology of AOP is not fully understood but it has been attributed to immaturity of the central respiratory drive and/or mechanical function of the respiratory system.

Clinical Presentation of AOP -- Apnoea of prematurity usually presents after 1–2 days of life and within the first week of life. Irrespective of type, however, prolonged AOP can present with hypoxaemia, cyanosis and bradycardia.

Table 61.10 Features and description of ROP

Features of ROP	Description
ICROP classification	Based on 4 parameters: Zones, Extent, ± Plus disease, Severity/Stages (Table 61.11)
Screening for ROP	Birthweight <1500 g and/or GA <32 weeks. ROP examination 4–7 weeks after birth
Treatment of ROP	Cryotherapy (outdated) Laser treatment (gold standard) Anti-VEGF, omega-3, vitamin E (adjuvant before laser & surgery) Surgery for advanced retinal detachment

ICROP: International Classification of ROP

Table 61.11 Stages of ROP

Stages	Characteristics of ROP
1	Demarcation line
2	Ridge
3	Ridge + extra retinal fibrovascular proliferation
4	Subtotal retinal detachment 4A: Extra foveal 4B: Detachment including fovea
5	Total retinal detachment

Diagnosis of AOP –– Apnoea of prematurity is a diagnosis of exclusion and should be considered only after secondary causes of apnoea such as infection, anaemia, RDS, intraventricular haemorrhage (IVH), gastroesophageal reflux and hypoglycaemia have been excluded.

Treatment of AOP –– Treatment measures for AOP include:

- Tactile stimulation
- Proper positioning to maintain a patent airway
- Use of methylxanthine: caffeine citrate. Routinely, extremely preterm infants are treated prophylactically with caffeine citrate until 34 weeks.
- Respiratory support: supplemental oxygen, CPAP, and mechanical ventilation.

Differential Diagnosis of AOP ––

Seizures and Periodic Breathing

Periodic breathing is characterized by recurring cycles of normal breathing lasting 5 to 20 seconds, alternating with brief (<20 seconds) periods of apnoea, without change of heart rate or colour. This is common in preterm infants and has little or no clinical relevance

Prognosis –– Resolution of AOP occurs by 37 weeks postmenstrual age in most preterm infants. Nonetheless, AOP may be protracted in extremely premature infants (e.g., 23 to 27 weeks' gestation). The effect on neurological outcome is not yet clarified. Death is rare.

61.2.1.6   Eyes

Retinopathy of Prematurity (ROP) [56–59]

Epidemiology and Risk Factors –– Retinopathy of prematurity is disorganized growth of retinal blood vessels in preterm infants. It is a significant cause of preventable childhood visual loss with an incidence that varies inversely with birthweight and gestational age. Its classification is based on the International Classification of ROP (Table 61.10).

Pathophysiology –– Retinopathy of prematurity occurs in two phases:

Phase 1 (vaso-obliterative) (birth to 32 weeks postmenstrual age) occurs due to:

- Arrest of normal retinal vascularization in preterm infants
- Reduced maternally derived angiogenic factors for normal vascular development in preterm infant
- Exposure of the developing retina to hyperoxic environment (ambient and supplemental)

Phase 2 (vasoproliferative phase) (after 32 weeks PMA): Resultant hypoxia from vaso-obliteration induces overproduction of angiogenic factors, especially VEGF. This causes aberrant retinal neovascularization with fragile friable retinal vessels which can become tortuous, leak and form a ridge of scar tissue with the attendant risk of retinal detachment and visual loss (Table 61.11).

61.2.1.7   Metabolic Problems of Prematurity

Hypothermia [60–62]

Epidemiology and Risk Factors –– Preterm infants are uniquely at risk of hypothermia (<36.5°C) because of rapid heat loss through the mechanisms of conduction, evaporation, radiation and convection (Table 61.12), and too little heat production. The preterm infant has a poor thermoregulatory balance due to:

- Immaturity of the hypothalamic regulatory centre
- High ratio of skin surface area to weight and highly permeable thin epidermis: preterm infants have 4 times the surface area to body mass of an adult, which increases surface area exposure to cold
- Poor vasomotor control and a naturally extended position: increases surface area exposure to cold
- Decreased subcutaneous fat for insulation
- Less brown fat: brown fat is an important organ of non-shivering thermogenesis in newborns. Anatomically, it accumulates around the fetal groin, kidneys, adrenal gland, para-aortic areas and the interscapular and axillary areas in the last trimester of pregnancy. The implication is that the more preterm a baby is, the less brown fat the baby will have, making non-shivering thermogenesis difficult, if not impossible

Table 61.12 Heat loss

Mechanism	Description
Convection	Heat loss by being near a source of cool air, e.g. open doors, fan, window, air conditioning
Conduction	Heat loss by coming in contact with a cold surface, e.g. scale, cold hands, cold stethoscope
Evaporation	Heat loss through moisture on the skin, e.g. during birth, insensible water loss, wet linens
Radiation	Heat loss by being near a cold surface, not directly in contact with it, e.g. baby in a cot near the cold walls of the nursery

Pathophysiology of Hypothermia –– In an attempt to conserve or increase heat, the cold-stressed or hypothermic preterm infant signals the hypothalamus to activate the sympathetic centres' release of norepinephrine, resulting in several responses, including:

- Peripheral vasoconstriction, which results in metabolic acidosis. Pulmonary vasoconstriction and impairment of surfactant resulting from metabolic acidosis further lead to hypoxaemia and metabolic acidosis.
- Brown fat oxidation or lipolysis in an attempt at non-shivering thermogenesis causes release of free fatty acids, which compete with bilirubin for albumin-binding sites causing hyperbilirubinaemia.
- Increased metabolic rate leads to increased consumption of oxygen and glucose, causing hypoxia and hypoglycaemia.

Summarily, the poor thermoregulatory adjustments to cold in preterm infants result in hypoglycaemia, metabolic acidosis, hypoxaemia and hyperbilirubinaemia.

Clinical Presentation of Hypothermia –– Mottled skin, lethargy, poor feeding and bradycardia are all indications of hypothermia.

Prevention of Hypothermia –– Prevention of hypothermia by maintaining preterm infants in a neutral thermal environment (conditions at which metabolic demands are minimal) is imperative in the management of preterm infants. Plastic bags, radiant warmers, hats, appropriate clothing and warm delivery rooms are some hypothermia preventive strategies in preterm infants. Moreover, professional alertness of healthcare providers is essential.

Hypoglycaemia [63–66]

Epidemiology and Risk Factors –– Hypoglycaemia is the commonest metabolic disorder encountered in preterm infants in the neonatal intensive care unit (NICU). It is defined as glucose concentration <2.6 mmol/L or 47 mg/dL in the first 72 hours of life. Preterm neonates are uniquely vulnerable to hypoglycaemia due to:

- Limited glycogen and fat stores
- Impaired gluconeogenesis and immature hepatic responses
- Higher metabolic demands due to a relatively increased ratio of brain to body mass. Glucose turnover is greatest in premature neonates (5–6 mg/kg/min) compared with term neonates (3–5 mg/kg/min) and adults (2–3 mg/kg/min)
- Inability to mount a counter-regulatory response to hypoglycaemia

Treatment of Hypoglycaemia –– Treatment of hypoglycaemia is with enteral feeds in asymptomatic mild cases. However, in severe symptomatic cases or where the neonate is unable to tolerate enteral feeds, intravenous 10% dextrose (2.5 mL/kg) is usually used, followed by a continuous infusion of 5–8 mg/kg/minute and thereafter graded feeds as tolerated by the infant.

Prognosis of Hypoglycaemia –– Severe and profound hypoglycaemia can cause devastating neurological sequelae.

Hypocalcaemia [67–69]

Early hypocalcaemia occurs due to immaturity of the hormonal control system.

Fluid and Electrolyte Imbalance [70, 71]

This imbalance is due to immaturity of the kidneys. In addition, the immature skin and the large body surface area cause insensible water loss by mechanisms such as evaporation, which often results in hypernatremia.

Hyperbilirubinaemia [72, 73]

The occurrence of physiological jaundice in preterm neonates is well recognized. This is attributed to shorter red blood cell half-life, immaturity of the liver enzymes and poor gut motility promoting increased enterohepatic circulation. Further, there is increased risk of kernicterus at relatively lower bilirubin levels in preterm infants.

61.2.1.8 Infection

Sepsis [74–76]

Preterm infants are highly susceptible to infections due to suboptimal or absence of the protective maternal IgG, as the placental transfer occurs during the last trimester. Further, poor skin barrier and delicate mucous membranes predispose the infants to infections. Moreover, indwelling catheters also increase the risk of infections.

Sepsis is further classified as:

- Early-onset sepsis: sepsis onset within 72 hours of life
- Late-onset sepsis: sepsis onset after 72 hours of life

Group B streptococcal (GBS) infection and coliforms cause early-onset sepsis in preterm infants. Coagulase-negative staphylococci (CONS) are a common cause of nosocomial infection in these infants. Fungi can also occur, especially after the first week of life.

61.2.2 Term Neonates [27, 77–79]

61.2.2.1 Respiratory System

Neonatal respiratory disorders account for the majority of term newborn admissions to NICU and result in significant morbidity and mortality.

The causes of respiratory distress in term neonates can be usefully subclassified on the basis of aetiology into common, less common and rare (Table 61.13).

Transient Tachypnoea of the Newborn (TTN) [80]

Epidemiology and Risk Factors –– Transient tachypnoea of the newborn, also known as 'wet lung', is a benign respiratory disorder of the term or late-term newborn related to retained fetal lung fluid. It is the most common neonatal respiratory disorder, accounting for 5.7 to 5.9 per 1000 term singleton births.

Well-known risk factors for TTN include caesarean section without labour, maternal diabetes, maternal asthma, male sex, macrosomia and late prematurity.

Pathophysiology –– The fetal lung is filled with fluid. This fluid is actively secreted by the alveolar epithelial cells through a chloride channel dependent process. Fetal lung fluid plays a crucial role in normal lung development and it also contributes to the amniotic fluid. Clearance of the lung fluid, however, occurs during late gestation, during labour and after delivery – as part of pulmonary adaptation to extrauterine life.

During late gestation, fetal lung fluid production gradually decreases.

With the onset of labour, a perinatal increase in maternal cortisol and a surge in catecholamine change the fetal alveolar epithelium from a chloride-secreting membrane to a primarily sodium-absorbing membrane. Thoracic compression during vaginal delivery also plays a minimal role in fetal lung liquid clearance.

Postnatal lung distension with air further enhances the resorption of lung fluid by pulmonary vasculature and lymphatics.

Transient tachypnoea of the newborn occurs due to respiratory maladaptation at birth, with delayed clearance of the lung fluid causing ineffective gas exchange and consequent respiratory distress.

Clinical Presentation of TTN –– An infant with TTN typically presents within a few minutes to hours after birth with mild respiratory distress. Tachypnoea is the predominant feature.

Diagnosis of TTN –– Transient tachypnoea of the newborn is a clinical diagnosis, but a chest radiograph classically demonstrates perihilar markings and fluid in the horizontal fissure (Figure 61.9).

Treatment of TTN –– Transient tachypnoea of the newborn is managed conservatively with oxygen supplementation or non-invasive respiratory support as required.

Prognosis of TTN –– Transient tachypnoea of the newborn has an excellent prognosis. The condition is self-limiting and resolves generally within 2–3 days. It is therefore imperative to consider alternative diagnoses in cases requiring prolonged treatment.

Respiratory Distress Syndrome (RDS)

Although RDS is primarily a clinical entity of premature infants, it may also affect term newborns. Contrary to the situation in premature infants, however, term infants develop RDS due to inadequate surfactant, resulting from exposure to factors promoting delayed surfactant synthesis (such as maternal diabetes, MAS) or from dysfunctional surfactant stemming from a genetic mutation.

Management –– Management is the same as in preterm infants.

Meconium Aspiration Syndrome (MAS) [80–83]

Epidemiology and Risk Factors – – Meconium aspiration syndrome is defined as respiratory compromise in neonates born through meconium-stained amniotic fluid (MSAF). It

Table 61.13 Causes of respiratory distress in term neonates

Common	Less common	Rare
Transient tachypnoea of the newborn (TTN)	RDS	Airway obstructions
	Pneumonia	Congenital malformations
	Meconium aspiration syndrome (MAS)	Metabolic and haematological derangements
Persistent pulmonary hypertension of the newborn (PPHN)		
Pneumothorax		
Cardiac failure		

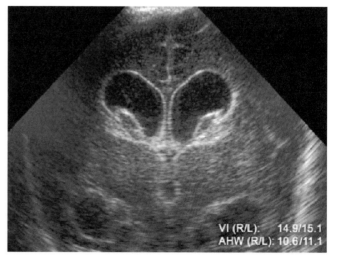

Figure 61.9 TTN on CXR (anterior – posterior): increased pulmonary interstitial markings ('wet lung') and fluid in the interlobar fissure.

accounts for 10% of all deliveries and is usually a clinical entity of the term, post-term or growth-restricted infants.

Meconium aspiration syndrome occurs secondary to meconium aspiration in utero or during delivery, in the setting of fetal distress. The latter may be due to uteroplacental insufficiency from post-maturity, cord compression and maternal risk factors including maternal pre-eclampsia, diabetes, chronic cardiovascular disease, drug abuse and smoking.

Pathophysiology – – Meconium is sterile, viscous, greenish-tinged fetal bowel content, which is composed of lanugo, intestinal epithelial cells, bile, water, mucus and amniotic fluid. It is not produced by the fetus until later in pregnancy, suggesting that meconium production is developmentally regulated. This may explain why MAS is frequently found in term or near-term babies. Furthermore, meconium is usually passed within 48 hours post-delivery, but in utero passage of meconium can occur in fetal distress.

Fetal stress causes neural stimulation, resulting in peristalsis of a mature GI tract with consequent passage of meconium into the amniotic fluid. Thereafter, fetal gasping respirations in response to the distress cause meconium aspiration into the fetal lung. The inhaled meconium can affect the lungs by obstructing the airways, irritating the lungs and inactivating surfactant production.

Airway obstruction: Total or partial airway obstruction may occur. With total obstruction, atelectasis develops while a ball-valve effect with air trapping occurs in areas of partial obstruction.

Chemical pneumonitis: As the inhaled meconium progresses distally, chemical pneumonitis may develop.

Inactivation of surfactant: When the inhaled meconium reaches the alveolar level, it may inactivate surfactant.

The final common pathway, consisting of atelectasis, hypoxia, acidosis and intra-pulmonary shunting, results in secondary persistent pulmonary hypertension (Figure 61.10).

Clinical Presentation of MAS – – Presentation may range from mild to severe respiratory distress, often complicated by air leaks or persistent pulmonary hypertension of the neonate (PPHN).

Diagnosis of MAS – – Diagnosis is based on an infant's history of meconium-stained amniotic fluid, signs of respiratory distress and classic chest radiographic findings of hyperinflation and heterogeneous opacities (Figure 61.11) [83].

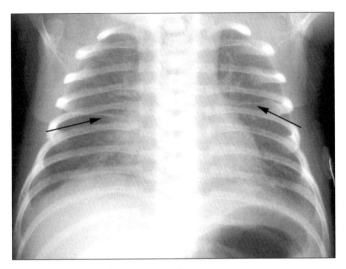

Figure 61.10 Pathophysiology of MAS

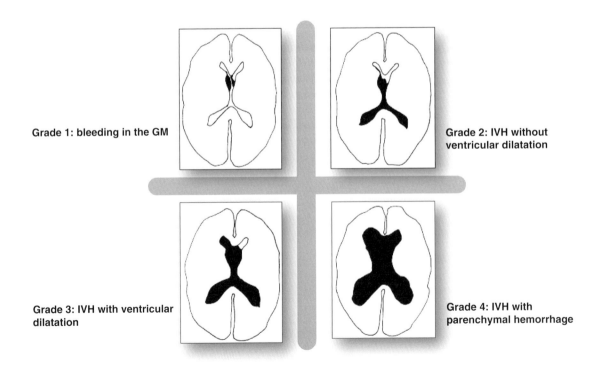

Grade 1: bleeding in the GM

Grade 2: IVH without ventricular dilatation

Grade 3: IVH with ventricular dilatation

Grade 4: IVH with parenchymal hemorrhage

Figure 61.11 MAS on CXR (anterior-posterior): hyperinflation and heterogeneous opacities. {Image by Kinderradiologie Olgahospital Klinikum Stuttgart, July 25, 2013, CC BY-SA 4.0, https://commons.wikimedia.org/w/index.php?curid=44865908}

Treatment of MAS –– The treatment of MAS consists of treatment in the delivery room and the NICU, respectively.

Delivery room treatment depends on how vigorous the newborn is at birth (Figure 61.12).

Treatment in the NICU includes supportive therapies, assisted ventilation, nitric oxide and extracorporeal membrane oxygenation (ECMO) in severe cases.

Prognosis of MAS –– Meconium aspiration syndrome generally has a good prognosis except in severe cases complicated by PPHN. Also, there are studies to suggest that newborns with MAS may be at greater risk of asthma later in life.

Pneumothorax

Pneumothorax in term neonates can occur spontaneously or as a result of vigorous resuscitation, infection, meconium aspiration, congenital lung malformation or barotrauma (from ventilation).

Management –– Management is the same as in preterm infants (see above).

62.2.2 Cardiovascular System

Persistent Pulmonary Hypertension of the Newborn (PPHN) [84–87]

Epidemiology and Risk Factors –– Persistent pulmonary hypertension of the newborn is a clinical syndrome which complicates transition to extrauterine life. It results from elevated pulmonary vascular resistance that causes right to left intracardiac shunting of blood and hypoxaemia.

PPHN can be idiopathic but more often than not, it occurs in association with meconium aspiration syndrome, pneumonia, RDS, and congenital lung malformations. Maternal use of selective serotonin reuptake inhibitors, especially in the third trimester, has also been implicated.

Pathophysiology of PPHN –– Varied aetiology notwithstanding, striking pulmonary vasoconstriction is the predominant pathophysiological feature of PPHN.

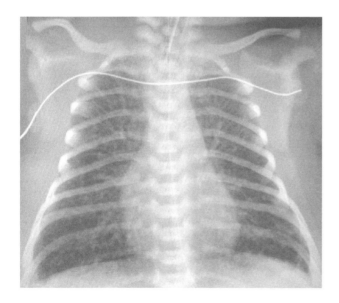

Figure 61.12 Management of MAS in the delivery room

Clinical Presentation of PPHN – – Clinical presentation of PPHN includes respiratory distress, labile hypoxaemia and differential cyanosis.

Differential Diagnosis of PPHN –– Most importantly, cyanotic heart disease is a differential diagnosis. A series of non-invasive bedside tests can be performed using arterial blood gas determinations to differentiate between cyanotic heart disease and pulmonary parenchymal disease. These include the hyperoxia test, preductal and postductal saturations and echocardiography.

In the hyperoxia test, oxygenation will markedly improve with supplemental oxygen in PPHN but minimally or not at all in cyanotic congenital heart disease. Further, a difference of >10% in the pre- and post-ductal saturation suggests left-to-right shunt and a diagnosis of PPHN.

Diagnosis of PPHN –– Echocardiography is the gold standard.

Treatment of PPHN –– Modalities of PPHN treatment include optimal oxygenation, mechanical ventilation, pressure stabilization, pulmonary vasodilator (NO) therapy and ECMO in severe cases.

61.3 Long-Term Challenges [88–90]

61.3.1 Cerebral Palsy (CP)

61.3.1.1 Epidemiology and Risk Factors

Cerebral palsy describes a group of permanent motor dysfunction (tone, posture and movement) due to non-progressive injury in the developing fetal or infant brain. With a prevalence of at least 2–3 in 1000 births, CP is the most common cause of permanent childhood neurodisability

The cerebral insult that gives rise to the motor impairment in CP can occur prenatally, perinatally or postnatally (Table 61.14).

61.3.1.2 Pathophysiology

The pathophysiological mechanisms include hypoxia, hypoperfusion and cortical or subcortical atrophy. Injuries can occur within the white and grey matter of the brain. In preterm infants, however, white matter injury in the form of periventricular leukomalacia is the leading cause of CP. Other pathologies include intraventricular haemorrhage and ventriculomegaly.

Table 61.14 Risk factors for cerebral palsy

Prenatal (70–80%)	Prematurity/low birthweight (LBW)
	Intrauterine infections: *Toxoplasma gondii*, other viruses, rubella, cytomegalovirus, herpes simplex (TORCH)
	Brain malformations
	Placental insufficiency
	Idiopathic, maternal conditions
Perinatal (10%)	Perinatal asphyxia
	Birth asphyxia
Postnatal (10%)	Central nervous system infections
	Head injuries, non-accidental
	Stroke

499

Table 61.15 Types of cerebral palsy

Type	Lesion	Description
Spastic (70%)	Cerebral cortex (pyramidal), e.g. prematurity, infarction of middle cerebral artery	Stiff and jerky movements, hypertonia
Dyskinetic • Choreoathetoid • Dystonia	Basal ganglia (extrapyramidal), e.g. kernicterus	Involuntary movements that disappear during sleep and increase with stress *Choreoathetoid:* Wormlike, writhing movements (face, extremities and torso) *Dystonia:* sustained muscle contractions
Ataxic	Cerebellum (extrapyramidal), e.g.cerebellar hypoplasia	Poor balance, lack of coordination, wide-based gait, hypotonia, intention tremor
Mixed (20%)	Diffuse	Most common combination is spastic and athetoid

61.3.1.3 Clinical Presentation of CP

Cerebral palsy presents as abnormality of posture and movement, which may be spastic, ataxic, choreoathetoid, or dystonic (Table 61.15). Subclassifications for spasticity are hemi, di, quadri, mono and triplegia.

More often than not, the motor dysfunction of CP is accompanied by disturbances of sensation, cognition, communication, perception and behaviour or by a seizure disorder.

61.3.1.4 Diagnosis of CP

Cerebral palsy is a clinical diagnosis based on the thorough history, developmental assessment and physical and neurological examinations. The diagnosis is usually established by the age of 18 months. If there are no possible aetiology or risk factors for CP, this warrants further diagnostic tests such as:

• Neuroimaging – CT/MRI
• Metabolic screening
• Chromosomal study

61.3.1.5 Differential Diagnosis

This includes congenital structural lesions, muscle disorders (myopathies, dystrophies).

61.3.1.6 Treatment

Management of CP is via the multidisciplinary team (MDT) with goals of maximizing function and minimizing impairment. The team includes the general paediatrician, physiotherapist, occupational therapist, language therapist, neurologist and social and educational support services.

61.3.1.7 Prognosis

This is related to the severity of the disorder.

61.4 Other Long-Term Challenges of Neonatal Care

Early detection through follow-up, anticipatory guidance and treatment of these problems offers the best opportunity to the health and developmental outcomes of high-risk infants, especially those born prematurely (Table 61.16).

Table 61.16 Other long-term challenges of neonatal care

Long-term challenges	Description
Impaired cognitive skills	Upon school age through to adulthood, preterm babies are at increased risk of poor academic performance and learning disabilities than full-term babies.
Sensory impairment	Blindness remains the most damaging impact of ROP. Other potential complications include strabismus, amblyopia, glaucoma and impaired visual acuity. Babies born preterm may also have some degree of sensorineural hearing loss and conducive hearing impairment loss. The impact of hypoxic-ischaemic encephalopathy in term babies may include cortical visual impairment and sensorineural deafness.
Behavioural and psychological problems	Increased risk of behavioural & psychological problems including impaired social skills, & attention-deficit /hyperactivity disorder (ADHD) in preterm than in full-term infants. The risk increases with decreasing gestational age and birthweight.
Chronic health issues	Premature babies are more likely to require recurrent hospital admittance due to chronic health issues than their full-term counterparts. These chronic health issues include but are not limited to recurrent chest infections, asthma, feeding problems and poor weight gain.

References

1. Howson CP, Kinney MV, Lawn JE, eds.; March of Dimes, PMNCH, Save the Children, WHO. *Born Too Soon: The Global Action Report on Preterm Birth.* Geneva: World Health Organization; 2012.

2. Eichenwald EC. Care of the extremely low-birthweight infant. In *Avery's Diseases of the Newborn.* Philadelphia: WB Saunders;2012. pp. 390–404.

3. Pramanik AK, Rangaswamy N, Gates T. Neonatal respiratory distress: a practical approach to its diagnosis and management. *Pediatric Clinics.* 2015 Apr 1;**62**(2):453–69.

4. Warren JB, Anderson JM. Newborn respiratory disorders. *Pediatr Rev Am Acad Pediatr.* 2010;**31**(12):487–95.

5. Carlo WA, Ambalavanan N. Respiratory distress syndrome. In Kliegman RM, Stanton BMD, St. Geme J, Schor NF, eds. *Nelson Textbook of Pediatrics*, 20th ed. Philadelphia: Elsevier; 2016.

6. Ley D, Wide-Swensson D, Lindroth M, Svenningsen N, Marsal K. Respiratory distress syndrome in infants with impaired intrauterine growth. *Acta Pædiatrica.* 1997 Oct;**86**(10):1090–6.

7. Pickerd N, Kotecha S. Pathophysiology of respiratory distress syndrome. *Paediatr Child Health (Oxford)* 2009; **19**:153–7.

8. Do P. Respiratory distress syndrome imaging. Medscape. March. 2018.

9. Hiles M, Culpan AM, Watts C, Munyombwe T, Wolstenhulme S. Neonatal respiratory distress syndrome: chest x-ray or lung ultrasound? A systematic review. *Ultrasound.* 2017 May; **25**(2):80–91.

10. Sweet DG, Carnielli V, Greisen G, et al. European consensus guidelines on the management of respiratory distress syndrome – 2019 update. *Neonatology.* 2019;**115**(4):432–50.

11. Sakonidou S, Dhaliwal J. The management of neonatal respiratory distress syndrome in preterm infants (European Consensus Guidelines – 2013 update). *Arch Dis Child Educ Pract Ed.* 2015 Oct 1;**100**(5):257–9.

12. Liechty EA, Donovan E, Purohit D, et al. Reduction of neonatal mortality after multiple doses of bovine surfactant in low birth weight neonates with respiratory distress syndrome. *Pediatrics.* 1991 Jul 1;**88**(1):19–28.

13. Ardell S, Pfister RH, Soll R. Animal derived surfactant extract versus protein free synthetic surfactant for the prevention and treatment of respiratory distress syndrome. *Cochrane Database Syst Rev.* 2015 Aug 24;8:CD000144.

14. Lopez E, Gascoin G, Flamant C, et al. Exogenous surfactant therapy in 2013: what is next? who, when and how should we treat newborn infants in the future? *BMC Pediatr.* 2013 Dec;**13**(1):165.

15. Aldana-Aguirre JC, Pinto M, Featherstone RM, Kumar M. Less invasive surfactant administration versus intubation for surfactant delivery in preterm infants with respiratory distress syndrome: a systematic review and meta-analysis. *Arch Dis Child Fetal Neonatal Ed.* 2017 Jan 1; **102**(1):F17–23.

16. Lau CS, Chamberlain RS, Sun S. Less invasive surfactant administration reduces the need for mechanical ventilation in preterm infants: a meta-analysis. *Glob Pediatr Health.* 2017 Mar 22;4:2333794X17696683.

17. Perlman JM, Wyllie J, Kattwinkel J, et al. Part 7: neonatal resuscitation: 2015 international consensus on cardiopulmonary resuscitation and emergency cardiovascular care science with treatment recommendations. *Circulation.* 2015 Oct 20;**132**(16 Suppl 1):S204–41.

18. Gregory GA, Kitterman JA, Phibbs RH, Tooley WH, Hamilton WK. Treatment of the idiopathic respiratory-distress syndrome with continuous positive airway pressure. *N Engl Med.* 1971 Jun 17;**284**(24):1333–40.

19. Niknafs P, Faghani A, Afjeh SA, Moradinazer M, Bahman-Bijari B. Management of neonatal respiratory distress syndrome employing ACoRN respiratory sequence protocol versus early nasal continuous positive airway pressure protocol. *Iranian J Pediatr.* 2014 Feb;**24**(1):57.

20. Göpel W, Kribs A, Härtel C, et al. Less invasive surfactant administration is associated with improved pulmonary outcomes in spontaneously breathing preterm infants. *Acta Paediatr.* 2015 Mar;**104**(3):241–6.

21. Martin R. Prevention and treatment of respiratory distress syndrome in preterm infants. In Kim MS, ed. *UpToDate* 2017.

22. McPherson C, Wambach JA. Prevention and treatment of respiratory distress syndrome in preterm neonates. *Neonatal Netw.* 2018 May 1;**37**(3):169–77.

23. Pramanik AK, Rosenkrantz T, Clark DA. Respiratory distress syndrome. *Medscape*, updated Jan 2015;**16**.

24. Yoon HK. Interpretation of neonatal chest radiography. *J Korean Soc Radiol.* 2016 May 1;**74**(5):279–90.

25. Morisot C, Kacet N, Bouchez MC, et al. Risk factors for fatal pulmonary interstitial emphysema in neonates. *Eur J Pediatr.* 1990 Apr 1;**149**(7):493–5.

26. Thibeault DW, Lachman RS, Laul VR, Kwong MS. Pulmonary interstitial emphysema, pneumomediastinum, and pneumothorax: occurrence in the newborn infant. *Am J Dis Child.* 1973 Nov 1;**126**(5):611–14.

27. Gallacher DJ, Hart K, Kotecha S. Common respiratory conditions of the newborn. *Breathe.* 2016 Mar 1;**12**(1):30–42.

28. Baraldi E, Filippone M. Chronic lung disease after premature birth. *N Engl J Med.* 2007 Nov 8;**357**(19):1946–55.

29. Principi N, Di Pietro GM, Esposito S. Bronchopulmonary dysplasia: clinical aspects and preventive and therapeutic strategies. *J Transl Med.* 2018 Dec;**16**(1):36.

30. Sahni M, Mowes AK. Bronchopulmonary dysplasia. In StatPearls Internet. Treasure Island, FL: StatPearls Publishing;2019 May 4

31. Pasha AB, Chen XQ, Zhou GP. Bronchopulmonary dysplasia: Pathogenesis and treatment. *Exp Ther Med.* 2018 Dec 1;**16**(6):4315–21.

32. Joshi S, Kotecha S. Lung growth and development. *Early Hum Dev.* 2007 Dec 1; **83**(12):789–94.

33. Semple T, Akhtar MR, Owens CM. Imaging bronchopulmonary dysplasia – a multimodality update. *Front Med.* 2017 Jun 29;4:88.

34. Hoepker A, Seear M, Petrocheilou A, et al. Wilson–Mikity syndrome: updated diagnostic criteria based on nine cases and a review of the literature. *Pediatr Pulmonol.* 2008 Oct;**43**(10):1004–12.

35. Dice JE, Bhatia J. Patent ductus arteriosus: an overview. *J Pediatr Pharmacol Ther.* 2007;**12**(3):138–46.

36. Gillam-Krakauer M, Reese J. Diagnosis and management of patent ductus arteriosus. *NeoReviews.* 2018 Jul 1; **19** (7):e394-402.

37. Subramaniam KG, Solomon N. The basis of management of congenital heart disease. In *Principles and Practice of Cardiothoracic Surgery.* London: IntechOpen; 2013 Jun 12.

38. Neu J, Walker WA. Necrotizing enterocolitis. *N Engl J Med.* 2011 Jan 20;**364**(3):255–64.

39. Niño DF, Sodhi CP, Hackam DJ. Necrotizing enterocolitis: new insights into pathogenesis and mechanisms. *Nat Rev Gastroenterol Hepatol.* 2016 Oct;**13** (10):590.

40. Alganabi M, Lee C, Bindi E, Li B, Pierro A. Recent advances in understanding necrotizing enterocolitis. *F1000Res.* 2019 Jan 25;**8**: F1000 Faculty Rev-107.

41. Epelman M, Daneman A, Navarro OM, et al. Necrotizing enterocolitis: review of state-of-the-art imaging findings with pathologic correlation. *Radiographics.* 2007 Mar;**27** (2):285–305.

42. Bohnhorst B. Usefulness of abdominal ultrasound in diagnosing necrotising enterocolitis. *Arch Dis Child Fetal Neonatal Ed.* 2013 Sep 1;**98**(5):F445–50.

43. Kliegman RM, Walsh MC. Neonatal necrotizing enterocolitis: pathogenesis, classification, and spectrum of illness. *Curr Prob Pediatr.* 1987 Apr 1;**17** (4):219–88.

44. Volpe JJ. Neurologic outcome of prematurity. *Arch Neurol* 1998 Mar 1;**55**(3):297–300.

45. Inder TE, Perlman JM, Volpe JJ. Preterm intraventricular haemorrhage/ posthemorrhagic hydrocephalus. In *Volpe's Neurology of the New-Born.* Philadelphia: Elsevier;2018 Jan 1. pp. 637–98.

46. de Vries LS, Leijser LM, Nordli DR Jr. Germinal matrix hemorrhage and intraventricular hemorrhage (GMH-IVH) in the newborn: prevention, management, and complications. In Kim MS, ed. *UpToDate*; 2018.

47. Brouwer MJ, De Vries LS, Pistorius L, et al. Ultrasound measurements of the lateral ventricles in neonates: why, how and when? A systematic review. *Acta Paediatr.* 2010 Sep;**99**(9):1298–306.

48. Huang J, Zhang L, Kang B, et al. Association between perinatal hypoxic-ischemia and periventricular leukomalacia in preterm infants: A systematic review and meta-analysis. *PLoS One.* 2017 Sep 20;**12**(9):e0184993.

49. Hatzidaki E, Giahnakis E, Maraka S, et al. Risk factors for periventricular leukomalacia. *Acta Obstet GynecolScand.* 2009 Jan;**88**(1):110–15.

50. Zaghloul N, Ahmed M. Pathophysiology of periventricular leukomalacia: what we learned from animal models. *Neural Regen Res.* 2017 Nov;**12**(11):1795.

51. Folkerth RD. Periventricular leukomalacia: overview and recent findings. *Pediatr Devl Pathol.* 2006 Jan;**9**(1):3–13.

52. Lemyre B, Davis PG, De Paoli AG. Nasal intermittent positive pressure ventilation (NIPPV) versus nasal continuous positive airway pressure (NCPAP) for apnea of prematurity. *Cochrane Database Syst Rev.* 2002(1): CD002272.

53. Gileles-Hillel A, Erlichman I, Reiter J. Apnea of prematurity: an update. *J Child Sci.* 2019 Jan;**9**(01):e50-8.

54. Kesavan K, Parga J. Apnea of prematurity: current practices and future directions. *NeoReviews.* 2017 Mar 1;**18**(3):e149-60.

55. Eichenwald EC; Committee on Fetus and Newborn. Apnea of prematurity. *Pediatrics.* 2016;**137**(1):1–7.

56. Sapieha P, Joyal JS, Rivera JC, et al. Retinopathy of prematurity: understanding ischemic retinal vasculopathies at an extreme of life. *J Clin Invest.* 2010 Sep 1;**120** (9):3022–32.

57. Hellström A, Smith LE, Dammann O. Retinopathy of prematurity. *Lancet.* 2013 Oct 26;**382**(9902):1445–57.

58. International Committee for the Classification of Retinopathy of Prematurity. The international classification of retinopathy of prematurity revisited. *Arch Ophthalmol.* 2005 Jul;**123**(7):991.

59. Early Treatment for Retinopathy of Prematurity Cooperative Group. Revised indications for the treatment of retinopathy of prematurity: results of the early treatment for retinopathy of prematurity randomized trial. *Arch Ophthalmol.* 2003 Dec;**121**(12):1684.

60. Nimbalkar SM, Khanna AK, Patel DV, Nimbalkar AS, Phatak AG. Efficacy of polyethylene skin wrapping in preventing hypothermia in preterm neonates (<34 weeks): a parallel group non-blinded randomized control trial. *J Tropical Pediatr.* 2018 May 23;**65** (2):122–9.

61. Kumar V, Shearer JC, Kumar A, Darmstadt GL. Neonatal hypothermia in low resource settings: a review. *J Perinatol.* 2009 Jun;**29**(6):401.

62. Alderdice F, Halliday HL, Vohra S, Johnston L, McCall EM. Interventions to prevent hypothermia at birth in preterm and/or low birth weight infants. *Cochrane Database Syst Revs.* 2018 Feb;**2018**(2):CD004210.

63. Sharma A, Davis A, Shekhawat PS. Hypoglycemia in the preterm neonate: etiopathogenesis, diagnosis, management and long-term outcomes. *Transl Pediatr.* 2017 Oct;**6**(4):335.

64. Alsaleem M, Saadeh L, Kamat D. Neonatal hypoglycemia: a review. *Clin Pediatr.* 2019 Nov;**58**(13):1381–6.

65. Wackernagel D, Gustafsson A, Edstedt Bonamy AK, et al. Swedish national guideline for prevention and treatment of neonatal hypoglycaemia in newborn infants with gestational age≥ 35 weeks. *Acta Paediatr.* 2020 Jan;**109**(1):31–44.

66. McKinlay CJ, Alsweiler JM, Ansell JM, et al. Neonatal glycemia and neurodevelopmental outcomes at 2 years. *N Engl J Med.* 2015 Oct 15;**373** (16):1507–18.

67. Vuralli D. Clinical approach to hypocalcemia in newborn period and infancy: who should be treated? *Int J Pediatr.* 2019;**2019**.

68. Jain A, Agarwal R, Sankar MJ, Deorari A, Paul VK. Hypocalcemia in the newborn. *Indian J Pediatr.* 2010 Oct 1;**77**(10):1123–8.

69. Venkataraman PS, Tsang RC, Steichen JJ, et al. Early neonatal hypocalcemia in extremely preterm infants: high incidence, early onset, and refractoriness to supraphysiologic doses of calcitriol. *Am J Dis Child.* 1986 Oct 1;**140**(10):1004–8.

70. Black MJ, Sutherland MR, Gubhaju L. Effects of preterm birth on the kidney. In *Nephrology and Acute Kidney Injury.* London: InTech; 2012; pp. 61–88.

71. Bhatia J. Fluid and electrolyte management in the very low birth weight neonate. *J Perinatol.* 2006 Apr 25;**26**(S1):S19.

72. Watchko JF, Maisels MJ. Jaundice in low birthweight infants: pathobiology and outcome. *Arch Dis Child Fetal Neonatal Ed.* 2003 Nov 1;**88**(6):F455-8.

73. Maisels MJ, Watchko JF. Treatment of jaundice in low birthweight infants. *Arch Dis Child Fetal Neonatal Ed.* 2003 Nov 1;**88**(6):F459-63.

74. el Hassani SE, Berkhout DJ, Niemarkt HJ, et al. Risk factors for late-onset sepsis in preterm infants: a multicenter case-control study. *Neonatology.* 2019;**116**(1):42–51.

75. Craft A, Finer N. Nosocomial coagulase negative staphylococcal (CoNS) catheter-related sepsis in preterm infants: definition, diagnosis, prophylaxis, and prevention. *J Perinatol.* 2001 Apr;**21**(3):186.

76. Simonsen KA, Anderson-Berry AL, Delair SF, Davies HD. Early-onset neonatal sepsis. *Clin Microbiol Rev.* 2014 Jan 1;**27**(1):21–47.

77. Reuter S, Moser C, Baack M. Respiratory distress in the newborn. *Pediatr Rev.* 2014 Oct;**35**(10):417.

78. Gouyon JB, Ribakovsky C, Ferdynus C, et al. Burgundy Perinatal Network. Severe respiratory disorders in term neonates. *Paediatr Perinat Epidemiol.* 2008 Jan;**22**(1):22–30.

79. Jing LI, Yun SH, Dong JY, et al. Clinical characteristics, diagnosis and management of respiratory distress syndrome in full-term neonates. *Chin Medi J.* 2010 Oct 1;**123**(19):2640–4.

80. Aly H. Respiratory disorders in the newborn. *Pediatr Rev.* 2004 Jun;**25**(6):201.

81. Yeh TF. Core concepts: meconium aspiration syndrome: pathogenesis and current management. *Neoreviews.* 2010 Sep 1;**11**(9):e503–12.

82. Chettri S, Bhat BV, Adhisivam B. Current concepts in the management of meconium aspiration syndrome. *Indian J Pediatr.* 2016 Oct 1;**83**(10):1125–30.

83. Dargaville PA. Respiratory support in meconium aspiration syndrome: a practical guide. *Int J Pediatr.* 2012 Feb 23;**2012**.

84. Roberts JD Jr, Polaner DM, Zapol WM, Lang P. Inhaled nitric oxide in persistent pulmonary hypertension of the newborn. *Lancet.* 1992 Oct 3;**340**(8823):818–19.

85. Kinsella JP, Neish SR, Shaffer E, Abman SH. Low-dose inhalational nitric oxide in persistent pulmonary hypertension of the newborn. *Lancet.* 1992 Oct 3;**340**(8823):819–20.

86. Andrade SE, McPhillips H, Loren D, et al. Antidepressant medication use and risk of persistent pulmonary hypertension of the newborn. *Pharmacoepidemiol Drug Saf.* 2009 Mar;**18**(3):246–52.

87. Mathew B, Lakshminrusimha S. Persistent pulmonary hypertension in the newborn. *Children.* 2017 Aug;**4**(8):63.

88. Patel RM. Short- and long-term outcomes for extremely preterm infants. *Am J Perinatol.* 2016 Feb;**33**(03):318–28.

89. Glass HC, Costarino AT, Stayer SA, et al. Outcomes for extremely premature infants. *Anesth Analg.* 2015 Jun;**120**(6):1337.

90. Moster D, Lie RT, Markestad T. Long-term medical and social consequences of preterm birth. *N Engl J Med.* 2008 Jul 17;**359**(3):262–73.

The Placenta and Its Association with Fetal Growth

Gwendolin Manegold-Brauer, Olav Lapaire & Irene Hösli

62.1 Introduction

The placenta is a unique organ of pregnancy that plays a key role in the normal development and normal growth of the fetus. It creates the intrauterine environment, which, as we know today, has a long-term impact on the health of the developing human being. Its ability to take over functions of the liver, lung, gastrointestinal tract, kidneys and endocrine organs illustrates its multi-organ function. The placenta has two main components – one is of maternal origin, one belongs to the fetus – and interaction between these two parts needs to be optimal for a successful pregnancy, controlling optimal exchange of nutrients, oxygen and removal of carbon dioxide. This chapter will give further insight into the structure, blood supply and metabolic transfer of the normal placenta and will present today's concepts of its role in long-term health.

62.2 Placental Morphology and Function

62.2.1 Development and Structure

At term, the placenta is a discoid organ that connects the circulation of the fetus with the circulation of the mother. An average placenta is approximately 22 cm in diameter and 500 g in weight. The placenta is perfused with 500 mL/min of blood, and the maternal blood in the placenta changes 2–3 times/ minute at the end of pregnancy.

The development of the placenta begins at the time of fertilization and it continuously expands in parallel to the growing fetus. The fetal tissue stems from the chorionic sac, whereas the maternal tissue is derived from the endometrium or decidua. Five days after fertilization the blastocyst develops the trophoblast, which is responsible for the formation of the placenta and the fetal membranes. At day 6 the blastocyst implants in the uterus, continues to grow and invades the maternal decidua. The cytotrophoblast differentiates along two pathways into the villous cytotrophoblast and the extra-villous cytotrophoblast. The villous cytotrophoblast later forms the specialized epithelium of the placenta, the syncytio-trophoblast, whereas the extravillous cytotrophoblast is key to the transformation of the maternal spiral arteries into the low resistance uteroplacental arteries (Figure 62.1).

Although it has been believed that the circulation starts between 10 and 12 gestational weeks and endometrial glands provide histotrophic nutrition until the end of the first trimester, recent evidence suggests that there is blood flow in the intervillous space as early as 6 gestational weeks [1]. The villous cytotrophoblast forms the primary villi, which are protrusions

covered by the syncytiotrophoblast and a cytotrophoblast core. In the third week, mesenchymal cells proliferate in the cyto-trophoblast (secondary villi) from which fetal capillaries evolve that form the tertiary villi. At the beginning, the villi are formed surrounding the entire embryo, but later the villi and the attached decidua regress at the luminal side of the fetus and the discoid shape is formed. In the mature placenta, the fetal umbilical cord vessels branch out on the chorionic plate into 30 to 40 chorionic villi, referred to as the fetal side of the placenta. The space between the maternal decidua and the chorionic plate, the intervillous space, is filled with maternal blood from the spiral arteries, which surround the chorionic villi. The surface of the chorionic villi is covered by the syncytio-trophoblast, which creates part of the placental barrier. The umbilical arteries carry deoxygenated blood into the chorionic villi where they come into contact with the maternal nutrients over a 12–14 m^2 large surface in the terminal villi, which consist of a complex arterio-capillary-venous system. The oxy-genated blood is then distributed to the fetus over the umbilical cord vein. On the maternal side, the endometrium transforms into the decidua with the uterine spiral arteries that carry the oxygenated maternal blood into the intervillous space where it comes into contact with the chorionic villi under low-pressure conditions. After exchange of nutrients and oxygen, it later flows back into the endometrial veins [2, 3]. Figure 62.2 shows a schematic drawing of the mature placenta.

62.2.2 Placental Structure of Twin Pregnancies

Twin pregnancies are high-risk pregnancies and require special prenatal and intrapartum care, which is discussed in earlier chapters of this book (Chapter 18 and Chapter 50). While the placentas of dichorionic twins have a similar structure com-pared to singleton placentas where one placenta supplies one fetus, the placentas of monochorionic twins often present with vascular anastomosis (Figure 62.3) on the placental surface that influence volume and blood supply of the twins. These anasto-moses can be the underlying cause of certain diseases unique to monochorionic twin pregnancies such as twin-to-twin transfusion syndrome (TTTS), twin anaemia polycythaemia sequence (TAPS) and selective growth restriction. Three differ-ent types of anastomoses have been described: arterioarterial (AA), arteriovenous (AV) and venovenous (VV). While the AA and VV anastomoses are bidirectional, the AV anastomosis are unidirectional, connecting the artery of one fetus with a vein of the other fetus. Arterioarterial anastomosis are present in about 87% of monochorionic placentas, while VV anastomosis are

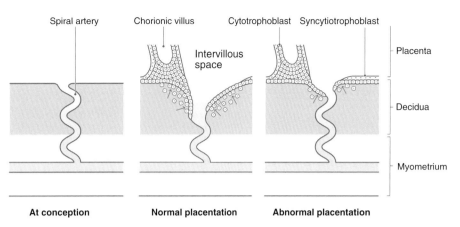

Figure 62.1 Development of blood supply to the human placenta

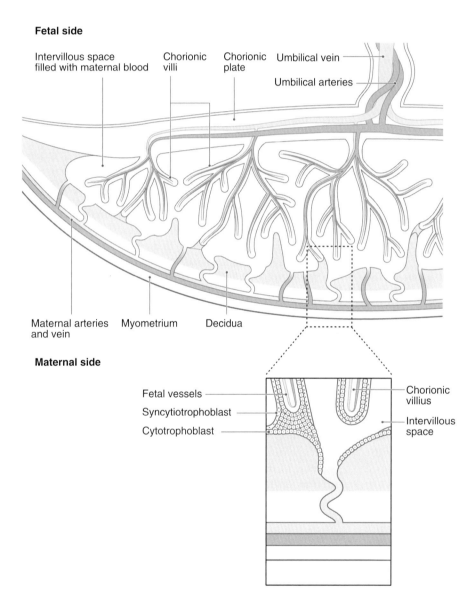

Figure 62.2 Placental morphology

much less frequent, presenting in 25% of the cases, and their role is not well understood. Arteriovenous anastomosis are the most common type, seen in 94% of monochorionic twin pregnancies. The AV anastomoses seem to be the underlying cause of TTTS, leading to a discrepancy in volume between the two fetuses. They are the targets of today's TTTS therapy with fetoscopic laser. Since AA anastomoses are frequently seen together with AV anastomoses in pregnancies not affected

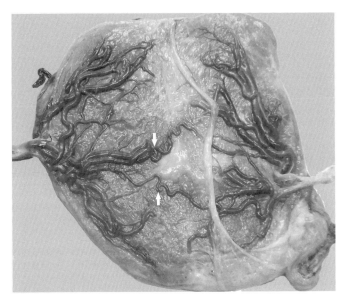

Figure 62.3 Monochorionic twin placenta with vascular anastomosis (arrows). Courtesy of Prof. Dr. Elisabeth Bruder. A black and white version of this figure will appear in some formats. For the colour version, please refer to the plate section.

with TTTS, it is believed that they have an protective effect with the flexibility of compensating volume imbalances between the fetuses. The anastomoses in pregnancies complicated by TAPS seem to be smaller than in TTTS, leading mainly to a transfusion of red blood cells rather than volume. Another finding occurring in monochorionic twin pregnancies is selective growth restriction. Growth is determined by the functional division of the single placenta between the twins as well as by the vascular anastomoses. These two factors determine the venous return upon which the fetus depends for its oxygen and nutritional supply. Unequally shared placentas have larger AA anastomoses, a larger net flow over AV anastomoses and a larger diameter of all anastomoses taken together than equally shared placentas. This may reduce the impact of their placental territory discordance and result in reduced birthweight discordance. So, if compensated, the intertwin blood exchange can fulfil a beneficial role by increasing the availability of oxygen and nutrients to the twin with the smaller placental share [4].

62.2.3 Endocrine Function

Since the placenta does not contain a nervous innervation, the maternofetal communication functions over humoral agents. There is a local regulation by paracrine or autocrine secretion of signalling molecules or via endocrine secretion into the maternal or fetal bloodstream. In the following the most important molecules and their roles are described [5].

62.2.3.1 Peptide Hormones

There are numerous different peptide hormones influencing fetal development, the most important of which are mentioned in the following sections.

Human Chorionic Gonadotropin (hCG)

Human chorionic gonadotropin (hCG) is secreted mainly by the syncytiotrophoblast and is found in the maternal

circulation from day 8 after conception. It is used for pregnancy testing in the blood and urine since it is almost exclusively produced in pregnancy (apart from some tumour cell types). Human chorionic gonadotropin is a glycoprotein consisting of an α- and β-chain. The β-chain is characteristic to hCG whereas the α-chain is identical with luteinizing hormone (LH), follicle-stimulating hormone (FSH) and thyroid-stimulating hormone (TSH). Human chorionic gonadotropin supports progesterone synthesis in the corpus luteum and plays a key role for cell fusion in the syncytiotrophoblast. Human chorionic gonadotropin binds to the LH-hCG receptor, which is expressed in the trophoblast, syncytiotrophoblast and in the extravillous trophoblast and influences a variety of signalling pathways in the cells. Furthermore, it supports a relaxing effect on the myometrium [6] and controls trophoblast invasion. Human chorionic gonadotropin levels rise at the beginning of pregnancy, reach their maximum at week 10 and drop to a low level after the 13th week when the placenta takes over the production of progesterone. Human chorionic gonadotropin can also bind to the maternal TSH receptor, which stimulates thyroid function at the beginning of pregnancy [5].

Pregnancy-Associated Plasma Protein-A (PAPP-A)

Pregnancy-associated plasma protein-A (PAPP-A) is a large glycoprotein produced by the placenta and is clinically used as one important component of combined first trimester screening for the assessment of the risk of aneuploidy. Low levels (i.e. below 0.4 multiples of the median (MoM) for a given gestational age) in maternal blood at 11–14 gestational weeks are also associated with an increased risk of fetal growth restriction, pre-eclampsia, preterm birth and stillbirth in fetuses with normal chromosomes. It is thought to be involved in several processes of placental function including local proliferative processes, angiogenesis, matrix mineralization and prevention of recognition of the fetus by the maternal immune system [7].

Human Placental Lactogen (HPL)

Human placental lactogen (HPL) is mainly synthesized in the syncytiotrophoblast. Its main function seems to be the regulation of maternal lipid and carbohydrate metabolism, and it is found in the maternal and fetal circulation. It has similarities to human growth hormone and to prolactin and binds to both of their receptors. The levels of HPL continue to rise over the course of pregnancy and correlate with the mass of the syncytiotrophoblast. Human placental lactogen increases the supply of glucose to the fetus by reduction of fatty acid storage in the mother but also stimulates the production of insulin-like growth factor, insulin and adrenocortical hormones and may also play a role in angiogenesis [8].

Insulin-Like Growth Factors (IGFs)

Insulin-like growth factors (IGFs) are important for fetal growth throughout gestation. IGF-I regulates placental cell differentiation while IGF-II is responsible for trophoblast invasion. Both regulate metabolism, differentiation and growth through interaction with the IGF receptors (IGFRs). IGF-binding proteins in the blood regulate the bioactivity of IGFs. Both IGFs support fibroblast proliferation in the placenta and increase placental uptake and transfer of glucose and amino acids [9].

Corticotropin-Releasing Hormone (CRH)

Corticotropin-releasing hormone is an amino acid peptide synthesized by the syncytiotrophoblast. Although the mechanisms are complex and still not fully understood, CRH plays an important role in the induction of physiological labour by coordinating the mechanisms that activate contractions. Women with preterm contractions show higher levels of CRH compared to women without contractions at the same gestational age. Placental CRH rises continuously during pregnancy but is inactivated by being bound to CRH-binding protein (CRHBP). CRHBP levels decrease prior to term. Another mechanism is that of cortisol stimulating placental CRH expression, explaining the transient pro-contractile effect after fetal lung maturation [10].

Vascular-Endothelial Growth Factor (VEGF) and Placental Growth Factor (PlGF)

Vascular-endothelial growth factor (VEGF) is produced in the trophoblast and in the macrophages where it is secreted into the maternal blood and functions over two tyrosine kinase receptors: VEGFR1 (FLT) and VEGFR2 (KDR), which are found in the villous vascular endothelium. VEGF promotes angiogenesis and trophoblast differentiation. Circulating VEGF bioactivity is blocked by binding to the soluble binding protein soluble fms-like tyrosine kinase 1 (sFlt1). Therefore sFlt1 promotes antiangiogenic function. Another hormone that shares homology with VEGF is placental growth factor (PlGF), which is expressed in the villous syncytiotrophoblast and in the media of larger placental vessels [11]. Both sFlt1 and PlGF alterations are known to be associated with pre-eclampsia and placental dysfunction and can be used clinically for pre-eclampsia prediction [12].

62.2.3.2 Steroid Hormones

Steroid hormones belong to a group of molecules that are all derived from the common precursor cholesterol. Steroid hormones are lipophilic molecules that are bound to proteins in the circulation but can easily cross the bilipid membranes of cells and can then alter the genetic activities of the cells and influence biochemical events.

Oestrogens

At the beginning of pregnancy, the corpus luteum is responsible for the production of oestrogens. As soon as the placenta takes over, four different types of oestrogens are produced in the placenta: oestrone (E1), 17β-oestradiol (E2), oestriol (E3) and oestetrol (E4). Levels rise continuously throughout pregnancy and are highest at term. However, for oestrogen production the placenta is dependent on the mother and on the fetus since the placenta cannot hydroxylate C21 steroids at the 17 position. So, the maternal and fetal bloodstream provide dehydroepiandrosterone sulphate (DHEAS) and 16-hydroxy DHEAS so that the production of oestrogens in the placenta is possible. Most of the DHEAS is produced in the fetal adrenal glands. Oestrogens can modulate gene expression via nuclear oestrogen receptors ER-α and ER-β. Other effects are modulated by receptors in the cell membranes that activate the adenylyl cyclase, mobilize Ca2+ and induce activity of the mitogen-activated protein kinase (MAPK). Oestradiol is the most frequent oestrogen in the placenta, fulfilling multiple functions. Oestradiol promotes endometrial growth and differentiation, is important for implantation and plays a role in uterine and placental angiogenesis and vasodilation. It ensures the adaptation of the maternal circulation to pregnancy by influencing volume retention, blood volume, coagulation, lipolysis and growth of the uterus and the breast glands. At term, oestrogens (oestradiol and oestriol) lead to the formation of gap junctions and activate the expression of oxytocin receptors [5].

Progesterone

Progesterone is essential for the continuation and maintenance of pregnancy. It keeps the uterus noncontractile. Like oestrogens, progesterone mediates effects through genomic and nongenomic signalling. It protects rejection of the fetus by the mother by anti-inflammatory and immunosuppressive functions. At the beginning of pregnancy, progesterone is produced by the corpus luteum that is stimulated by β-hCG of the developing embryo. The nuclear progesterone receptors PRα and PRβ are expressed in the maternal reproductive tract and in the placenta. Other actions are signalled by the membrane-associated progesterone receptors (MPRs). Binding leads to MAPK activation, reduction of cAMP production and intracellular Ca2+ mobilization [13]. Progesterone production is controlled and influenced by several other hormones such as oestradiol, IGF-1 and calcitriol that stimulate production, while leptin and CRH inhibit its production in the placenta [5].

Glucocorticoids

Glucocorticoids are needed for the regulation of organ development and for organ maturation but they can also lead to fetal growth restriction and hypertension later in life. Glucocorticoids are not produced in the human placenta, but the syncytiotrophoblast controls fetal exposure to maternal cortisol by oxidation via the enzyme 11-β-hydroxy-steroid-dehydrogenase (11-β-HSD) or by reduction via 11β-HSD2. It can, for example, convert cortisol to the inactive cortisone. This expression of 11β-HSD2 is reduced in pregnancies with pre-eclampsia or intrauterine growth restriction.

62.2.4 Transfer of Nutrients

The main site of exchange is the intervillous space where maternal blood is flowing around the chorionic villi. For exchange of nutrients, these must cross the microvilli on the maternal side of the syncytiotrophoblast, pass through the chorionic stromata and finally enter the fetal blood vessels. The placenta has a number of different mechanisms by which this transfer is regulated, including passive transfer, active transport and facilitated transport. The transfer further is influenced by the concentration of the individual substances in maternal and fetal blood, the surface area of the placenta for transfer, maternal blood flow to the placenta and the presence of specific binding proteins. The transfer of fatty acids, glucose and amino acids, which are the main classes of nutrients, are discussed in the following sections.

62.2.4.1 Fatty Acid Transport

Essential fatty acids cannot be synthesized by the human body. The fetus is dependent on maternal supply and placental transfer. Fatty acids serve as a source of energy, are important in cell signalling but most importantly play a key role in fetal brain development. For neurodevelopment, long-chain polyunsaturated fatty acids (LC-PUFAs) such as arachidonic acid and especially docosahexaenoic acid (DHA) seem to play a key role in the composition of cell membranes. In vivo studies have shown a preferential uptake of LC-PUFAs compared to other fatty acids, which is known as the biomagnification process. However, not all mechanisms of fatty acid transfer across the placenta are fully understood.

In the maternal bloodstream, over 97% of fatty acids are esterified forms and are bound in lipoproteins (e.g. triglycerides, phospholipids, cholesterol-esters). Non-esterified fatty acids (NEFAs) form only 3% of the maternal fatty acid content. These esterified fatty acids need to be transformed into NEFAs for uptake into the syncytiotrophoblast and finally transfer across the placenta to the fetus [14]. Two lipases in the placenta have been identified for the release of fatty acids and form the circulating lipoproteins: lipoprotein lipase and endothelial lipase [15]. The NEFAs can enter the syncytiotrophoblast by diffusion or fatty acid transport proteins (fatty acid translocase, fatty acid transport protein, plasma membrane fatty acid binding protein). From there, fatty acids can enter the various metabolic routes, including β-oxidation, conversion into eicosanoids and re-esterification to form phospholipids and triglycerides. The latter may then be stored in lipid droplets in the syncytiotrophoblast [16].

62.2.4.2 Amino Acid Transport

In contrast to glucose transport, the transfer of amino acids needs to be accomplished by active transport against a gradient. The concentration of amino acids is much higher in the fetus compared to the mother. Amino acids are required for protein synthesis and play an important role for growth. As they are large molecules, size is the limiting factor for uptake into the placenta and transfer to the fetus. The transfer needs to be accomplished with transports on both sides of the trophoblast. The families of amino acid carriers are numerous, but there are two basic types of amino acid transporters in the placenta: accumulative transporters and exchange transporters. While accumulative transporters ensure uptake of specific molecules into the syncytiotrophoblast, exchange transporters trade between amino acids and thus alter the content but not the number of amino acids in maternal plasma and the trophoblast. A third transporter system, amino acid efflux carriers, has recently been reported that transports from the placental cytoplasm to the fetal circulation. The regulation of the amino acid supply is mediated by needs of the fetus. For example, insulin, oxygen and amino acids influence the activity of the signalling polypeptide mammalian target of rapamycin (mTOR) and thus influence cell proliferation and growth and metabolism [17]. This is just one of many examples of how maternal nutritional and endocrine signals including insulin, insulin-like growth factors, adipokines and steroid hormones regulate placental amino acid transport against the background of growth signals originating from the fetus [18].

62.2.4.3 Glucose Transport

The fetus uses glucose as its main source of energy, and the fetal production of glucose is minimal. Glucose follows a concentration gradient from the mother to the fetus since the concentration of glucose is lower in the fetus compared to the mother. Members of the glucose transport family (GLUT) transport glucose via facilitated transport without the need for energy. At least seven GLUT transporters are known to be expressed in the placenta. The placental transport of glucose is buffered by the placenta itself that stores glucose in the form of glycogen or lactate.

Due to the high capacity and high threshold for downregulation of the glucose transporters, glucose transfer is almost unlimited. So glucose transport seems to be largely unchanged in cases of fetal growth restriction and in gestational diabetes [17].

62.2.4.4 Transport of Oxygen and Carbon Dioxide

Since the fetal lung does not take over its complete function until the first breathing after delivery and after clamping of the umbilical cord, the supply of oxygen and the return of fetal carbon dioxide via the placenta is essential for the development of life. The barrier between maternal and fetal blood, however, is much thicker than the lung and the surface area is smaller. The placental membranes are permeable for the small respiratory gas molecules that passively diffuse from the mother to the fetus and vice versa. The transfer of oxygen to the fetus depends on the content of oxygen in maternal blood, the flow rate in the uterine and umbilical vessels as well as the diffusing capacity of the placenta. Oxygen consumption by the placenta is a significant factor and a potential limitation on availability to the fetus. The oxygen transport across the placenta to the fetal circulation is aided by fetal haemoglobin (subunit α2γ2), which has a lower affinity for 2,3-diphosphoglycerate than adult haemoglobin (α2β2), promoting a higher oxygen affinity and thereby supporting a greater arterial oxygen saturation in fetal blood, compared with maternal blood, for any given arterial oxygen pressure. At the same time the carbon dioxide affinity is lower in fetal haemoglobin compared to maternal haemoglobin supporting the transfer of carbon dioxide from the fetus to the mother [19].

62.3 The Linkage between Placenta and Long-Term Health

62.3.1 Concept of Fetal Programming

The concept that the placenta plays a key role in the origin of chronic disease in adulthood was developed by Barker et al [20], who showed an inverse relationship between cardiovascular disease and birthweight in a large population-based epidemiological study in men born in the early twentieth century. They showed that newborns with a birthweight below 5 pounds had the highest rates of death from ischaemic heart disease later in life. Subsequently, a wide range of other cohort studies has demonstrated that lower birthweight correlates with adult morbidity and mortality, and specifically with increased risks of cardiovascular disease, hypertension, type 2 diabetes mellitus, stroke, chronic lung disease and chronic renal disease. The underlying mechanisms of these associations are referred to as 'fetal programming' where influences during in utero development form the structure and function of the organs for life.

It is believed that some alterations occur in a critical time period of development that established a permanent physiological response [21]. For example, adverse conditions such as poor maternal nutrition, chronic hypoxia, high levels of thyroid hormones or glucocorticoids are associated with alterations in fetal organ structures including reduced coronary arterial dimensions, low arterial elastin, reduced endowment of beta cells in the pancreas, decreased numbers of nephrons in the kidney and changes in brain structure and function. The sum of these alterations leads to a higher vulnerability for chronic diseases such as heart disease, diabetes, obesity and strokes [22]. Many of these mechanisms are not fully understood but are linked to the placenta as the key source of nutrients for the fetus.

One hypothesis is that normal variations in the process of development lead to variations in the supply of nutrients during critical periods via the many different systems of transport mentioned earlier. Although placental size and birthweight correlate with placental weight, another clue to the concept of individual nutrient supply is supported by the fact that there is a wide variety in placental weight among newborns of the same birthweight [23]. There are data from animals that placental growth can be stimulated by fasting in early pregnancy, resulting in heavier offspring. This, however, cannot be reproduced in later stages of pregnancy, indicating that there is a period of time when the placenta is able to respond to the demands of the fetus and loses this potential later during pregnancy.

Women with increased levels of glucocorticoids due to, for example, social stress can cause reduced fetal growth. Active cortisol is normally inactivated in the placenta by 11 β -HSD and 11 β -HSD2 but will cross the placenta in the active form when certain threshold levels are exceeded. The expression of 11 β -HSD and 11 β -HSD2 are downregulated by sex steroids and hypoxia and upregulated by glucocorticoids and cAMP. So, either increased levels of cortisol in maternal circulation or decreased levels of 11 β -HSD will lead to programming in the fetus. Higher glucocorticoid levels will then influence the fetus and are associated with hypertension, hyperinsulinaemia, hyperglycaemia and hyperactivity of the hypothalamic-pituitary-adrenal axis [24].

62.3.2 Placental Origin of Cardiovascular Disease

The Helsinki birth cohort comprises over 20 000 men and women born between 1924 and 1944 from which unique data

from over 6000 placentas were preserved. It was shown that the risk of sudden cardiac death was associated with a thin placenta. One possible explanation is that inadequate trophoblast invasion comprises nutrient exchange and the development of the autonomic nervous system, which could be associated with ventricular fibrillation often seen with sudden cardiac death [25]. Further, the cohort showed that chronic heart failure was associated with a small placental surface area, and coronary artery disease was associated with three different types of maternal placental phenotypes of placental deviation from roundness, placental surface area and placental efficiency [22].

Comparing growth restricted (IUGR) fetuses and appropriately grown (AGA) fetuses in utero with follow-up until 18 months of age showed that maximum aortic intima media thickening, as a surrogate marker for a predisposition to arteriosclerosis, was significantly higher in the IUGR fetuses and infants compared with the AGA infants. The systolic blood pressure at 18 months of age was significantly increased in the IUGR children. These findings may predispose the infants to hypertension early in life and cardiovascular risk later in life [26, 27]. Other studies have investigated the potential renal mechanisms that lead to adaptations in glomerular and tubular function that initiate hypertension of developmental origin [28].

62.3.3 Placental Origin of Metabolic Diseases

Placental function is regulated by maternal metabolic factors. About 5–10% of women today are affected by gestational diabetes (GDM) and another 1–2% have pre-existing diabetes. From what we know today, the diabetic state is associated with long-term consequences for both the mother and the fetus. Maternal diabetes affects fetal growth and leads to a higher rate of fetuses with macrosomia. While maternal hyperglycaemia stimulates fetal overgrowth, maternal vasculopathy, which can be associated especially with diabetes type 1, can lead to a deficiency in nutrient transfer and subsequently to fetal growth restriction. The placentas of women with pre-existing diabetes and GDM show changes in nutrient transfer and oxidative/inflammatory pathways. The offspring is at increased risk of metabolic syndrome and type 2 diabetes.

There are a number of structural changes found in the placentas of women with pre-existing diabetes and gestational diabetes. Among these are an increase in placental weight, pathological changes of maturation of the chorionic villi as well as enhancement in angiogenesis and fibrinoid necrosis [29]. The offspring shows a different phenotype with a higher proportion of adipose tissue even when the newborns have a weight appropriate for gestational age and this puts these children at risk for childhood obesity.

The underlying concept is that maternal hyperglycaemia (as well as excess of amino acids and fatty acids) leads to fetal hyperglycaemia, which stimulates the fetal pancreas to produce more insulin, resulting in fetal hyperinsulinaemia. Interestingly, it seems that glucose influx cannot be influenced in the second and third trimesters of pregnancy once hyperinsulinaemia is established. Consequences of hyperinsulinaemia include glycogen deposition in the placenta, growth of the fetal heart, aerobic fetal metabolism that increases the need for oxygen leading to erythropoietin stimulation and increased erythropoiesis. Additionally, glucose uptake into the fetal tissue (fat deposition, triglyceride synthesis) steepens the concentration gradient between the mother and the fetus, leading to an even higher influx of glucose to the fetus (glucose steal phenomenon). The increased transfer of glucose in GDM leads to an increase in glucose, lipid and amino acid levels in the fetus, stimulating insulin secretion and insulin-like growth factors 1 and 2 in the placenta and thereby increasing fetal growth. These effects explain why good glucose level controls in the mother cannot prevent the altered fetal phenotype once hyperinsulinaemia has occurred. It seems that earlier treatment before stimulation of the pancreatic fetal islet cells has occurred would be a window of opportunity for intervention [30].

62.4 Conclusion

Although the placenta has the vital functions that have been described in this chapter, many of these mechanisms are not fully understood at present since research has focused on the evaluation of the placenta after delivery. In 2014, however, the National Institute of Child Health and Human Development (NICHD) funded an ambitious project, the Human Placenta Project, which aims to develop innovative approaches and technologies to investigate the human placenta in a safe real-time monitoring of the organ during pregnancy. While this chapter is being written, the 10-year Human Placenta Project is ongoing. It received funding of over $46 million in 2015 in over 30 research centres in the USA. If successful, it may change how we understand and manage pregnancy and influence all that grows from pregnancy [31].

References

1. Roberts VHJ, Morgan TK, Bednarek P, et al. Early first trimester uteroplacental flow and the progressive disintegration of spiral artery plugs: new insights from contrast-enhanced ultrasound and tissue histopathology. *Hum Reprod.* 2017;**32**:2382–93.

2. Gude NM, Roberts CT, Kalionis B, King RG. Growth and function of the normal human placenta. *Thromb Res.* 2004;**114**:397–407.

3. Charnock-Jones DS, Burton GJ. Placental vascular morphogenesis. *Best Pract Res Clin Obstet Gynaecol.* 2000;**14**:953–68.

4 Lewi L, Deprest J, Hecher K. The vascular anastomoses in monochorionic twin pregnancies and their clinical consequences. *Am J Obstet Gynecol.* 2013;**208**:19–30.

5 Costa MA. The endocrine function of human placenta: an overview. *Reprod Biomed Online.* 2016;**32**:14–43.

6 Slattery MM, Brennan C, O'Leary MJ, Morrison JJ. Human chorionic gonadotrophin inhibition of pregnant human myometrial contractility. *BJOG.* 2001 [cited 2019 Jan 21];**108**:704–8.

7 Grill S, Rusterholz C, Zanetti-Dällenbach R, et al. Potential markers of preeclampsia – a review. *Reprod Biol Endocrinol.* 2009;**7**:70.

8 Handwerger S, Freemark M. The roles of placental growth hormone and placental lactogen in the regulation of human fetal growth and development. *J Pediatr Endocrinol Metab.* 2000 [cited 2019 Jan 21];**13**:343–56.

9 Forbes K, Westwood M. The IGF axis and placental function. *Horm Res Paediatr.* 2008;**69**:129–137.

10 Vannuccini S, Bocchi C, Severi FM, Challis JR, Petraglia F. Endocrinology of human parturition. *Ann Endocrinol (Paris).* 2016;**77**:105–113.

11 Hod T, Cerdeira AS, Karumanchi SA. Molecular mechanisms of preeclampsia. *Cold Spring Harb Perspect Med.* 2015;**5**: a023473.

12 Zeisler H, Llurba E, Chantraine F, et al. Predictive value of the sFlt-1: PlGF ratio in women with suspected preeclampsia. *N Engl J Med.* 2016;**374**:13–22.

13 Goldman S, Shalev E. Progesterone receptor profile in the decidua and fetal membrane. *Front Biosci.* 2007 [cited 2019 Jan 21];**12**:634–48.

14 Lewis RM, Childs CE, Calder PC. New perspectives on placental fatty acid transfer. *Prostaglandins Leukot Essent Fatty Acids.* 2018;**138**:24–9.

15 Gil-Sánchez A, Koletzko B, Larqué E. Current understanding of placental fatty acid transport. *Curr Opin Clin Nutr Metab Care.* 2012;**15**:265–72.

16 Herrera E, Desoye G. Maternal and fetal lipid metabolism under normal and gestational diabetic conditions. *Horm Mol Biol Clin Investig.* 2016;**26**:109–27.

17 Larqué E, Ruiz-Palacios M, Koletzko B. Placental regulation of fetal nutrient supply. *Curr Opin Clin Nutr Metab Care.* 2013;**16**:292–7.

18 Vaughan OR, Rosario FJ, Powell TL, Jansson T. Regulation of placental amino acid transport and fetal growth.

Prog Mol Biol Transl Sci. 2017;**145**: 217–51.

19 Murray AJ. Oxygen delivery and fetal-placental growth: Beyond a question of supply and demand? *Placenta.* 2012;**33**: e16–e22.

20 Barker DJ, Osmond C, Golding J, Kuh D, Wadsworth ME. Growth in utero, blood pressure in childhood and adult life, and mortality from cardiovascular disease. *BMJ.* 1989 [cited 2019 Feb 25];**298**:564–7.

21 Nelson DM. How the placenta affects your life, from womb to tomb. *Am J Obstet Gynecol.* 2015;**213**: S12-3.

22 Thornburg KL, Marshall N. The placenta is the center of the chronic disease universe. *Am J Obstet Gynecol.* 2015;**213**:S14–S20.

23 Alwasel SH, Abotalib Z, Aljarallah JS, et al. Secular increase in placental weight in Saudi Arabia. *Placenta.* 2011;**32**:391–4.

24 Cottrell EC, Seckl JR, Holmes MC, Wyrwoll CS. Fetal and placental 11 β -HSD2: a hub for developmental programming. *Acta Physiol.* 2014;**210**:288–95.

25 Barker DJP, Larsen G, Osmond C, et al. The placental origins of sudden cardiac death. *Int J Epidemiol.* 2012;**41**:1394–9.

26 Zanardo V, Visentin S, Trevisanuto D, et al. Fetal aortic wall thickness: a marker of hypertension in IUGR children? *Hypertens Res.* 2013;**36**:440–3.

27 Veit J, Lapaire O. Preeclampsia and its impact on long-term cardiovascular risk. *Ann Clin Exp Hypertens.* 2018; **6**(1):1053.

28 Singh RR, Denton KM. Role of the kidney in the fetal programming of adult cardiovascular disease: an update. *Curr Opin Pharmacol.* 2015;**21**:53–9.

29 Huynh J, Dawson D, Roberts D, Bentley-Lewis R. Current topic: a systematic review of placental pathology in maternal diabetes mellitus. *Placenta.* 2015;**36**:101–14.

30 Desoye G, van Poppel M. The feto-placental dialogue and diabesity. *Best Pract Res Clin Obstet Gynaecol.* 2015;**29**:15–23.

31 Guttmacher AE, Spong CY. The human placenta project: it's time for real time. *Am J Obstet Gynecol.* 2015;**213**:S3–S5.

Placental Pathology

Olav Lapare, Irene Hösli & Gwendolin Manegold-Brauer

Chapter

63

63.1 Introduction

The aim of this chapter is to summarize the most important placental pathologies that may affect pregnancy outcome and that have an important impact on the clinical management. The evaluation of the placenta requires a profound understanding of the problems and circumstances concerning both the fetus and the pregnant woman.

63.2 Abnormal Placentation

The abnormally invasive placenta (AIP) is one of the most important life-threatening conditions, which can lead to a high perinatal morbidity and mortality. The incidence varies (1:533 up to 1:2510 deliveries). The rising incidence goes along with the increasing rate of caesarean sections [1].The highest risk is observed in cases of placenta praevia and previous caesarean deliveries.

The high morbidity and mortality can be lowered with prenatal detection by ultrasound assessment in the second/third trimester and an interdisciplinary planning and delivery in an experienced perinatal centre. In some cases, the use of magnetic resonance imaging (MRI) is of added value. Due to missing data, the European Working Group on Abnormally Invasive Placenta – EW-AIP – was established in 2012, followed five years later by the International Group (www.is-aip.org).

Since the 1990s, a 10-fold increase of AIP has been observed. A projection estimates a total number of more than 4500 cases in the USA in 2020 [2, 3].

63.2.1 Placenta Praevia and Abnormally Invasive Placenta

The increasing number of caesarean sections being performed has been identified as a risk factor for placenta praevia and abnormally invasive placenta. Beside this major risk factor, other uterine surgeries, such as curettage, myomectomy and resection of scar tissue, as well as previous infections, seem to be relevant [4]. Other factors, such as advanced maternal age or reproductive therapy, may play an additional role [5, 6].

The most frequent condition for an AIP is a placenta praevia after a previous caesarean delivery.

Histologically, AIP can be split into placenta accrete, increta and percreta. Placenta accrete is defined as an invasion of trophoblast cells into the myometrium and a missing decidua layer. Placenta increta shows an invasion of tropho-blast cells deeply into the myometrium, whereas placenta

percreta is demonstrated by a trophoblast invasion up to the serosa or beyond that layer.

The exact pathogenesis remains unclear. However, a missing decidua basalis may play an important role. Furthermore, an exaggerating, non-regulated trophoblast invasion or a disturbed remodelling of maternal vessels may also play an important role.

The antenatal diagnosis of AIP has been a challenge in obstetric care. Up to 70% percent of cases with AIP are not detected during antenatal visits. However, an antenatal diagnosis significantly increases an interdisciplinary approach and improves maternal and fetal outcome.

The ultrasound criteria in Table 63.1 help to detect an AIP.

An additional method used to examine AIP is MRI, particularly in unclear cases after prenatal ultrasound, or in cases of a suspicion of infiltration of adjoining structures, to depict posterior placenta with the aim to improve interdisciplinary management [9]. Similar to an ultrasound examination, an experienced radiologist is essential.

In some case control studies, the authors were able to demonstrate an association between elevated alpha-fetoprotein and AIP. However, the sensitivity and specificity of this biomarker are too low to diagnose the presence of an AIP only with the biomarker.

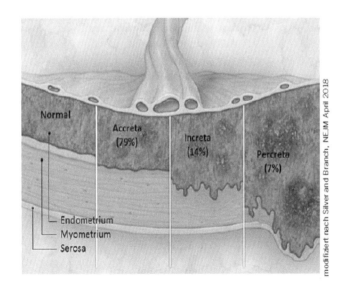

Figure 63.1 Schematic presentation of abnormally invasive placenta with its incidence. A black and white version of this figure will appear in some formats. For the colour version, please refer to the plate section.
Source: according to Hürter et al 2017 [7].

Table 63.1 Abnormally invasive placenta: ultrasound criteria

2D greyscale	2D colour Doppler
Loss of 'clear zone'	Uterovesical hypervascularity
Myometrial thinning	Sub-placental hypervascularity
Abnormal placental lacunae	Bridging vessels
Bladder wall interruption	Placental lacunae feeder vessels
Placental bulge	
Focal exophytic mass	

Source: Collins et al 2016 [8].

Table 63.2 Risk factors that may lead to placental abruption

Previous caesarean delivery	+
Previous placental abruption	++++
Previous intrauterine fetal death	++
Placental insufficiency (intrauterine growth restriction (IUGR))	++
Twin pregnancy	++
Hypertensive disorders	++
Rupture of membranes	++
Thrombophilia	++
Bleeding in early pregnancy	+
Smoking	++
Cocaine	+++
Invasive procedures (e.g. amniocentesis)	+
Polyhydramnios	++
Uterine anomaly	+
Trauma	+++
Bronchial asthma	+
Maternal age >35 years	+

Source: according to Ghaheh et al 2013 [12]

An essential step is the interdisciplinary round table after prenatal diagnosis of AIP, with the interprofessional attendance of obstetricians, anaesthetists, neonatologists, interventional radiologists, urologists and additional specialists, to plan the peripartal management and to plan the individual blood patient management [10].

63.2.2 Placental Abruption

The incidence of a placental abruption varies between 0.5 and 1% of all pregnancies [11]. Cross-sectional studies have shown a rising incidence, most likely due to the rising incidence of pregnancies with risk factors, or due to an increased awareness. The clinical presentation includes vaginal bleeding – especially in cases of placenta praevia or bleeding from the placental edge.

Placental abruption is defined as abruption of the placenta after 21 weeks of gestation. Pathophysiologically, a retroplacental haematoma proliferates and separates the placenta from the trapping centre. Immunological, ischaemic or inflammatory stimuli may lead to a rupture of decidua vessels. This event leads to a haematoma that detaches the placenta from the uterine wall. Other risk factors include trauma, uterine scars or myoma, which contribute to an insufficient decidua. Another risk factor is cocaine, leading to a vasoconstriction and consecutive acute ischaemic perfusion of the decidua. The same pathophysiological process is imaginable in cases of chronic maternal hypertension or maternal smoking (Table 63.2).

An abruption involving more than half of the placental surface is commonly associated with intrauterine fetal death. The continuous bleeding may also lead to a loss of coagulation factors and may be complicated by a disseminated intravascular coagulopathy. Furthermore, a uterine atony may complicate the clinical situation.

Approximately 80% of all placental abruptions are associated with vaginal bleeding. In two thirds of all cases, the clinical examination reveals an adamant uterus. Furthermore, a pathological cardiotocographic (CTG) reading is observed in 60% of all cases and shows tachycardia; bradycardia, decelerations or reduced variability may also occur [13]. Typical clinical signs include abdominal and back pain or an acute maternal hypotension. Similar to the clinical examination,

the ultrasound picture may also vary. The haematoma may present as a hypo-, hyper-, or isogenic mass. The specificity of ultrasound examination in case of a placenta abruption is high at 93%, whereas the sensitivity is much lower at 28% [14].

Pregnancy-associated plasma protein-A (PAPP-A) (decreased), alpha-fetoprotein (elevated) and inhibin A (decreased) might serve as biomarkers in the first and second trimesters. However, the sensitivity and specificity of those markers are too low to serve as biomarkers alone in clinical practice, and so far, no algorithms have been established. In the case of a placental abruption, the clinical management is dependent on gestational age, fetal condition (fetal hazard vs. intrauterine fetal death) and maternal status (stable vs. insecure).

63.2.3 Umbilical Cord and Placental Tumours

Umbilical cord and placental tumours are both rare conditions. On both localizations, the majority of tumours are benign.

63.2.3.1 Tumours of the Umbilical Cord

Most of the detected haemangiomas are incidental findings and are located in the proximity of the fetus [15]. Rarely, they can be associated with polyhydramnios or elevated alpha-fetoprotein values. Similarly, to haemangiomas, angiomyxomas (Figure 63.2A) are seen by chance. Cysts of the umbilical cord are another entity and are rare, too, and should be differentiated from omphalocele (Figure 63.2B) [16].

63.2.3.2 Tumours of the Placenta

A chorangioma is defined as a benign tumour, arising from vessels of the chorionic villi (Figure 63.2C). Its growth is most likely triggered by angiogenic factors. Most of these are incidental findings, feature a microscopic size and do not have a clinical significance. In contrast, large chorangiomas are detectable by ultrasound and may have a clinical significance, especially those larger than 4–5 cm [17]. According to the morphology, different types (cavernous, capillary and endotheliomatous) can be discriminated. Large chorangiomas may lead to polyhydramnios, placental insufficiency, fetal anaemia and hydrops fetalis.

Rarely, metastasis of a maternal neoplasia is histologically detected.

63.2.4 Umbilical Cord Abnormalities and Vasa Praevia

Physiologically, the umbilical cord insertion is located centrally or laterally. Even a marginal insertion is an anomaly, because the umbilical cord is in close contact with the amniotic membrane and therefore the placental vessels are less protected (Figure 63.3A). A direct insertion into the membrane is called velamentous cord insertion (Figure 63.3B). Dependent on the degree of the anomaly, a disturbance of the circulation may be relevant in the second or third trimester. Therefore, frequent ultrasound examinations are recommended to rule out an impending intrauterine growth retardation. Furthermore, the exposed vessels are not well protected by Wharton's jelly and hence are vulnerable to rupture, especially during labour. The incidence in singleton pregnancies is about 1:100, whereas in twin pregnancies and triplets, the incidence is dramatically higher at 1:4 [18]. To rule out a velamentous cord insertion, an ultrasound examination is recommended in the first or second trimester to localize and document the cord insertion. Furthermore, an elective caesarean section is not indicated in case of a velamentous cord insertion.

Vasa praevia are velamentous vessels, localized above the ostium internum or nearby (Figure 63.3C). They are clinically relevant, because rupture of the membrane and consecutive bursting of these vessels may lead to a significant fetoplacental bleeding. The incidence of vasa praevia is about 1:2500 deliveries and sometimes higher (up to 1:365 [19]).

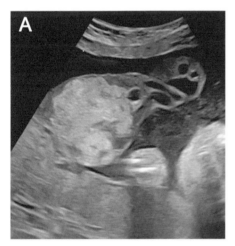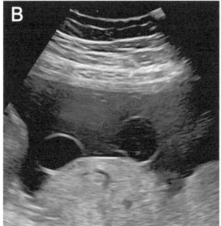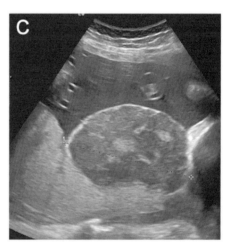

Figure 63.2 Tumours of the placenta and umbilical cord – A: angiomyxoma; B: placental cysts; C: chorangioma.

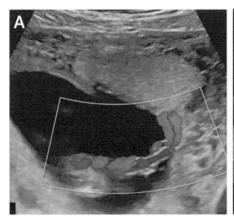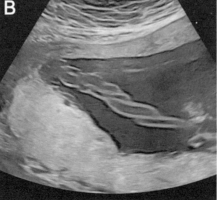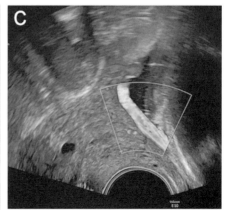

Figure 63.3 Umbilical cord abnormalities and vasa praevia – A: marginal cord insertion; B: velamentous cord insertion; C: vasa praevia. A black and white version of this figure will appear in some formats. For the colour version, please refer to the plate section.

Risk factors are the following:

- Multiple pregnancy
- In vitro fertilization
- Low-lying placenta
- Retracted placenta praevia
- Placenta bipartite
- Velamentous insertion of the umbilical cord in the lower part of the uterus

Prenatal ultrasound together with colour Doppler imaging in the second trimester (20–22nd week of gestation) is recommended to rule out vasa praevia [20]. Hospitalization or management as outpatients and caesarean delivery in a tertiary centre with experienced clinicians are the main recommendations [21].

63.3 Placental Biomarkers and Adverse Pregnancy Outcome

The early identification of patients with an increased risk for pre-eclampsia or IUGR is one of the most important goals in obstetrics. The availability of highly sensitive and specific physiological and biochemical markers would not only allow the detection of patients at risk but also permit a close surveillance, an exact diagnosis and timely intervention (e.g. lung maturation), as well as simplified recruitment for future studies looking at therapeutic medications and additional prospective markers. Today, several markers may offer the potential to be used, most likely in a combinatory analysis, as predictors or diagnostic tools [22].

Furthermore, when evaluating new screening strategies, not only sensitivity, specificity and predictive values should be taken into account but also costs, patient's acceptability and quality control. Thus, the implementation of clinical tests will require close collaboration between medical institutions, optimally in a worldwide network, together with the pharmaceutical industry in order to develop functional and, as best as possible, affordable tests which could be a bonus to pregnant women worldwide.

Placental angiogenesis requires the complex interplay between the pro-angiogenic factors vascular endothelial growth factor (VEGF) and placental growth factor (PlGF) with their cognate receptors VEGF receptor-1 (VEGFR-1, which is alternatively called fms-like tyrosine kinase (Flt)-1) and VEGFR-2. Interestingly, the placenta is a rich source of these factors. In addition to regulating blood vessel homeostasis, VEGF, PlGF and the Flt-1 receptor have been shown to be key components in regulating trophoblast cell survival and function.

Placental cells also secrete a soluble isoform of Flt1, which is generated through alternative splicing of the messenger RNA and acts as an anti-angiogenic factor by interacting with, and thereby neutralizing, PlGF and VEGF. There is strong evidence for the occurrence of higher placental expression of sFlt1 and repeated findings of elevated circulating levels of sFlt1 and reduced free bioactive PlGF and VEGF in pre-eclamptic patients. It was thus suggested that a part of this excess of circulatory sFlt1 may stem from the placenta.

Studies have shown that the ratio of soluble fms-like tyrosine kinase-1 (sFlt1) to placental growth factor (PlGF) is elevated in pre-eclampsia, and is raised even before clinical onset of the disease. The ratio has been used successfully in clinical trials to improve prediction of pre-eclampsia for women at risk of this condition. The sFlt1/PlGF ratio showed better predictive ability compared with using a single parameter (e.g. PlGF alone) [23].

The PRediction of short-term Outcome in preGNant wOmen with Suspected preeclampsIa Study (PROGNOSIS) is a previously reported, international, multicentre, prospective, double-blind, non-interventional study, evaluating the sFlt1/PlGF ratio as a tool for short-term prediction of pre-eclampsia in pregnant women with suspected pre-eclampsia [24]. Cut-offs for the sFlt1/PlGF ratio were derived and validated to rule out (for up to 4 weeks; sFlt1/PlGF ratio ≤38) or rule in (within 4 weeks; sFlt1/PlGF ratio >38) the occurrence of pre-eclampsia [25].

The results suggest that use of the sFlt1/PlGF ratio may enable better patient management for women with suspected pre-eclampsia, as clinicians can identify low- and high-risk patients and ensure that they are managed appropriately.

Furthermore, alterations in sFlt1 and PlGF are also more pronounced in early-onset in comparison to late-onset pre-eclampsia. However, it was also shown that increased levels of sFlt1 were also associated with IUGR (see also Chapter 25, Hypertensive Disorders in Pregnancy and Eclampsia).

63.3.1 Pathophysiology (abnormal placentation in pre-eclampsia)

The precise origin of pre-eclampsia remains elusive, but it is believed to be likely multifactorial. A certainty is the central role played by the placenta in its pathology. A long-standing hypothesis has been that pre-eclampsia develops as a consequence of some kind of immune maladaptation between the mother and the fetus during the very first weeks of pregnancy, leading to a two-step disorder progression that can be summarized as following: in a first – asymptomatic – step, local aberrant fetomaternal immune interactions within the uterine wall lead to impaired tissue and arterial invasion by trophoblast cells. This results in failed transformation of the uterine spiral arteries and subsequently worsened placental perfusion. Chronic hypoxia or alternate periods of hypoxia/reoxygenation within the intervillous space is expected to trigger tissue oxidative stress and increase placental apoptosis and necrosis. The clinical disorder arises, in a second step, when the maternal vascular and immune systems can no longer handle the increased shedding of placentally produced debris and the aberrant expression of pro-inflammatory, anti-angiogenic and angiogenic factors, leading to a systemic endothelial cell dysfunction and an exaggerated inflammatory response. Recently, this hypothesis has been challenged. It was proposed instead that intrinsic failure in trophoblast differentiation at different time points of ontogeny may lead to either a mild disorder with late-onset appearance, or IUGR complicated or not with the maternal symptoms [26]. However, the origin of pre-eclampsia might not be restricted to an alteration of trophoblast differentiation, but may also in some cases depend on underlying maternal constitutional factors such as genetic, obesity, dysfunctional maternal clearance or inflammatory systems (see also Chapter 25, Hypertensive Disorders in Pregnancy and Eclampsia).

References

1. Silver RM. Abnormal placentation: placenta previa, vasa previa, and placenta accreta. *Obstet Gynecol.* 2015 Sep;126(3):654–68.

2. Solheim KN, Esakoff TF, Little SE, et al. The effect of cesarean delivery rates on the future incidence of placenta previa, placenta accreta, and maternal mortality. *J Matern Fetal Neonatal Med.* 2011 Nov;24(11):1341–6. doi: 10.3109/ 14767058.2011.553695. Epub 2011 Mar 7.

3. Jauniaux E, Ayres-de-Campos D, Langhoff-Roos J, Fox KA, Collins S; FIGO Placenta Accreta Diagnosis and Management Expert Consensus Panel. FIGO classification for the clinical diagnosis of placenta accreta spectrum disorders. *Int J Gynaecol Obstet.* 2019 Jul;146(1):20–4.

4. Henrich W, Surbek D, Kainer F, et al. Diagnosis and treatment of peripartum bleeding. *Perinat Med.* 2008;36 (6):467–78.

5. Kaser DJ, Melamed A, Bormann CL, et al. Cryopreserved embryo transfer is an independent risk factor for placenta accreta. *Fertil Steril.* 2015 May;103 (5):1176–84.

6. Nageotte MP. Always be vigilant for placenta accreta. *Am J Obstet Gynecol.* 2014 Aug;211(2):87–8.

7. Hürter H, Manegold-Brauer G. Sonographische Kriterien zur Diagnostik von Plazentationsstörungen. 06_ 2017_ info@gynäkologie

8. Collins SL, Ashcroft A, Braun T, et al.; European Working Group on Abnormally Invasive Placenta (EW-AIP). Proposal for standardized ultrasound descriptors of abnormally invasive placenta (AIP). *Ultrasound Obstet Gynecol.* 2016 Mar;47(3): 271–5.

9. Palacios Jaraquemada JM, Bruno CH. Magnetic resonance imaging in 300 cases of placenta accreta: surgical correlation of new findings. *Acta Obstet Gynecol Scand.* 2005 Aug;84(8):716–24.

10. Palacios Jaraquemada JM, Pesaresi M, Nassif JC, Hermosid S. Anterior placenta percreta: surgical approach, hemostasis and uterine repair. *Acta Obstet Gynecol Scand.* 2004 Aug;83(8):738–44.

11. Downes KL, Shenassa ED, Grantz KL. Neonatal outcomes associated with placental abruption. *Am J Epidemiol.* 2017 Dec 15;186(12):1319–28.

12. Ghaheh HS, Feizi A, Mousavi M, et al. Risk factors of placental abruption. *J Res Med Sci.* 2013 May;18(5):422–6.

13. Hurd WW, Miodovnik M, Hertzberg V, Lavin JP. Selective management of abruptio placentae: a prospective study. *Obstet Gynecol.* 1983 Apr;61(4):467–73.

14. Glantz C1, Purnell L. Clinical utility of sonography in the diagnosis and treatment of placental abruption. *J Ultrasound Med.* 2002 Aug;21 (8):837–40.

15. Papadopoulos VG, Kourea HP, Adonakis GL, Decavalas GO. A case of umbilical cord hemangioma: Doppler studies and review of the literature. *Eur J Obstet Gynecol Reprod Biol.* 2009 May;144(1):8–14.

16. Zangen R, Boldes R, Yaffe H, Schwed P, Weiner Z. Umbilical cord cysts in the second and third trimesters: significance and prenatal approach. *Ultrasound Obstet Gynecol.* 2010 Sep;36 (3):296–301.

17. Fan M, Skupski DW. Placental chorioangioma: literature review. *J Perinat Med.* 2014 May;42(3):273–9.

18. Sepulveda W, Rojas I, Robert JA, Schnapp C, Alcalde JL. Prenatal detection of velamentous insertion of the umbilical cord: a prospective color Doppler ultrasound study. *Ultrasound Obstet Gynecol.* 2003 Jun;21(6):564–9.

19. Hasegawa J, Nakamura M, Ichizuka K, et al. Vasa previa is not infrequent. *J Matern Fetal Neonatal Med.* 2012 Dec;25(12):2795–6.

20. Cipriano LE, Barth WH Jr, Zaric GS. The cost-effectiveness of targeted or universal screening for vasa praevia at 18–20 weeks of gestation in Ontario. *BJOG.* 2010 Aug;117(9):1108–18.

21. Tsakiridis I, Mamopoulos A, Athanasiadis A, Dagklis T. Diagnosis and management of vasa previa: A comparison of 4 national guidelines. *Obstet Gynecol Surv.* 2019 Jul;74 (7):436–42.

22. Grill S, Rusterholz C, Zanetti-Dällenbach R, et al. Potential markers of preeclampsia – a review. *Reprod Biol Endocrinol.* 2009 Jul 14;7;70.

23. Verlohren S, Herraiz I, Lapaire O, et al. New gestational phase-specific cutoff values for the use of the soluble fms-like tyrosine kinase-1/placental growth factor ratio as a diagnostic test for preeclampsia. *Hypertension.* 2014 Feb;63(2):346–52.

24. Zeisler H, Llurba E, Chantraine F, et al. Predictive value of the sFlt-1: PlGF ratio in women with suspected preeclampsia. *N Engl J Med.* 2016 Jan 7;374(1):13–22.

25. Stepan H, Herraiz I, Schlembach D, et al. Implementation of the sFlt-1/ PlGF ratio for prediction and diagnosis of pre-eclampsia in singleton pregnancy: implications for clinical practice. *Ultrasound Obstet Gynecol.* 2015 Mar;45(3):241–6.

26. Huppertz B. Placental origins of preeclampsia: challenging the current hypothesis. *Hypertension.* 2008 Apr;51 (4):970–5.

Chapter 64

Placenta Accreta Spectrum Disorders

Edwin Chandraharan, Sabaratnam Arulkumaran & Amarnath Bhide

64.1 Introduction

Placenta accreta spectrum disorders (PASDs) are on the increase. Histologically, the placenta may be adherent to the myometrium without intervening decidua (accreta), invade the myometrium (increta) and/or extend beyond the myometrium and seen via the serosa of the uterus or invade into adjacent tissues like the bladder or parametrium (percreta). Since there are difficulties in defining each entity by ultrasound or by histology and also due to the possibility of histology showing different degrees of invasion in the same case, PASD is the term now commonly used and the previous terminology of morbidly adherent placenta is no longer used. The main contributor towards PASD is previous caesarean section (CS). With the global increase in CS, the incidence of PASD and related morbidity and mortality is on the increase.

Where facilities exist, the placental position should be visualized on ultrasound and the degree of invasion noted, especially if the placenta is in the lower segment. Placenta implanted over a previous scar increases the incidence of PASD. A large number of studies from different countries have shown a progressive increase in incidence of PASD over the years and the increased likelihood of PASD in a patient with an increasing number of uterine surgeries.

Due to limited length of this chapter, the reader is directed to five International Federation of Gynaecology and Obstetrics (FIGO) publications that provide an extensive introduction to the problem [1]; epidemiology [2]; prenatal diagnosis and screening [3]; conservative management [4]; and non-conservative surgical management [5]. In this chapter we give a summary of the above issues.

64.2 Risk Factors for Placenta Accreta Spectrum Disorders

The risk factors for placenta accreta spectrum (PAS) are well described and outlined here [6, 7]:

- Previous uterine surgery (e.g. myomectomy, hysteroscopic surgery, dilation and curettage)
- Caesarean delivery
- Placenta praevia
- First trimester diagnosis of pregnancy in the uterine scar of previous caesarean delivery
- Advanced maternal age
- Multiparity

- In vitro fertilization (IVF) pregnancies
- Previous intrauterine infection

The more caesarean sections a woman has had, the greater the chance of her having a placenta praevia and adherence to the scar. The possibility of various factors influencing the placental adherence to the scar has been studied – for example, single- versus double-layer closure, locked sutures for closure, use of monofilament suture, excision of fibrous uterine scar tissue and reconstructing. More studies are needed to draw definite conclusions. Similarly, there is a need to evaluate the influence of expectant management versus dilation curettage or suction curettage in cases of incomplete miscarriage and the use of prophylactic antibiotics with these procedures.

64.3 Diagnosis

Ultrasound is the mainstay of prenatal diagnosis of PAS. The prenatal ultrasound features of PAS are best described in the setting of placenta praevia and one or more previous caesarean sections. A combination of placenta praevia and previous caesarean delivery increases the risk of PAS several fold. In a systematic review of PAS [3, 8], the prevalence of PAS in cases with placenta praevia and previous caesarean delivery/uterine surgery was 19.3%.

Several ultrasound signs of PAS spectrum have been described [9] and are listed here:

- Abnormalities of the placental echo-structure, presence of lacunae [10] (Figure 64.1)

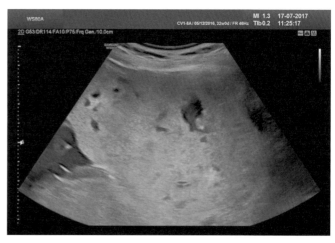

Figure 64.1 Presence of multiple lacunae in the placenta

- Abnormalities of the placental-uterine interface – loss of the retroplacental hypoechoic zone between the placenta and myometrium
- Interruption of the echogenic bladder border (Figure 64.2)
- Increased vascularity of the lower segment/abnormal vessels
- Vessel(s) that extends from the placenta across the myometrium and beyond the uterine serosa
- Increased vascularity in the parametrium
- Direct visualization of placental tissue beyond the uterine cavity. This is an uncommon sign but is associated with a high degree of positive predictive value.
- Increased placental thickness in the lower uterine segment [11] (Figure 64.3)

A lacuna is defined as an irregular hypoechoic space [5] within the placenta containing flow (which can be seen on greyscale and/or colour Doppler). This is one of the first ultrasound signs identified in PAS cases. Lacunae are graded as follows [10]:

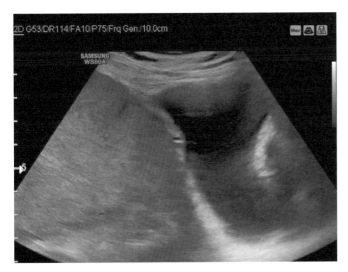

Figure 64.2 Interruption of the echogenic bladder border

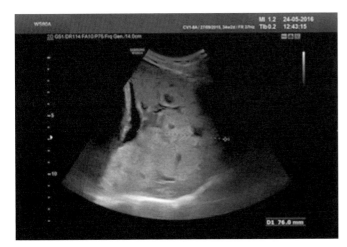

Figure 64.3 Increased placental thickness

Grade 0 – No lacunae seen

Grade 1 – One to three lacunae, generally small

Grade 2 – Four to six lacunae, generally larger and more irregular

Grade 3 – Many throughout the placenta, some appearing large and bizarre

The risk for PAS increases with increasing number, size and irregularity.

It is recommended that the evaluation be carried out using a high-frequency transducer, and a transvaginal approach is preferred. Imaging should be performed with a partially filled maternal bladder.

Referral to a centre of excellence is recommended for the following indications [1]:

64.3.1 Clinical

- Prior caesarean delivery, particularly multiple
- Placenta praevia
- Prior endometrial surgery (e.g. ablation/myomectomy)
- First/second trimester bleeding
- Current or previous CS scar pregnancy

64.3.2 Sonographic Risk Factors

- Multiple vascular lacunae within the placenta
- Loss of normal hypoechoic retroplacental zone
- Abnormalities of uterine serosa–bladder interface (interruption of line, thickening of line, irregularity of line and increased vascularity)
- Extension of villi into myometrium, serosa or bladder
- Retro-placental myometrial thickness of <1 mm
- Turbulent blood flow through lacunae on Doppler ultrasonography
- Increased subplacental vascularity
- Vessels bridging from placenta to uterine margin
- Gaps in myometrial blood flow

64.3.3 Other Investigations

The MRI signs of abnormally invasive placenta (AIP) are as follows [7]:

- Uterine bulging
- Heterogeneous signal intensity
- Dark intra-placental bands on T2-weighted magnetic resonance imaging (MRI)
- Focal interruption of myometrium
- Tenting of the bladder

An MRI is not absolutely necessary for the prenatal diagnosis of invasive placentation. It may be used to complement ultrasound imaging to assess the depth of invasion and lateral extension of myometrial invasion, especially with posterior placentation and/or in women with ultrasound signs suggesting parametrial invasion [12].

64.4 Clinical Management

Management of placenta accreta spectrum disorders depends on the degree of placental invasion (i.e. placenta accreta, increta or percreta), the site of placental invasion (i.e. lower uterine segment, cervix, anterior myometrium, posterior myometrium or the cornua) and the adjacent organs which have been invaded (i.e. urinary bladder, ureter, bowel, the broad ligament or the lateral pelvic sidewall), as well as the wishes of the patient for future fertility. Irrespective of the management option, it is vital to ensure appropriate surgical expertise as well as multidisciplinary and multiprofessional involvement in formulating a management plan to optimize maternal outcome. If PSAD is diagnosed in the antenatal period, then the patient should be transferred to a centre with all the facilities to deal with massive obstetric haemorrhage (i.e. availability of cell savers, blood bank, anaesthetists, intensivists and facilities for interventional radiology) as well as surgical expertise to control haemorrhage. Both conservative and radical surgical measures (Figure 64.4) should be considered, depending on the individual clinical circumstances and the availability of expertise.

Forcible extirpation of the placenta during delivery should be avoided at all costs because it can result in torrential haemorrhage leading to serious maternal morbidity and mortality. The preoperative Care Plan should include the type of proposed surgery as well as measures that may be required in an emergency (i.e. peripartum hysterectomy, uterine artery embolization or pelvic packing) in cases of massive obstetric haemorrhage to save the patient's life.

64.4.1 Expectant Management (intentional retention of the placenta (IRP))

Intentional retention of the placenta (IRP) involves leaving the entire placenta in situ after the delivery of the fetus, and ligating the umbilical cord very close to the placental mass to ensure a spontaneous reabsorption of the placenta by secondary necrosis of the villous tissue as a result of the progressive reduction in the blood flow to the uterine myometrium, parametrium and the placental bed [13]. The obvious aim of IRP is to avoid the morbidity and mortality associated with a peripartum hysterectomy, as well as excessive blood loss associated with forcible separation of the adherent placenta.

A transabdominal ultrasound scan immediately prior to the operation is recommended to delineate the upper border of the placenta so as to incise the myometrium above the upper border of the placenta to avoid inadvertently incising the placenta. The access to the upper myometrium may be achieved through a 'St George's boat incision' (please see the Triple P Procedure below) or via a midline abdominal incision. In a case of placenta praevia with abnormal invasion of the myometrium, a transverse incision should be made above the upper border of the placenta. However, if the placental site is in the upper segment, a midline 'fundal incision' on the myometrium may be required to avoid cutting through the placenta. If there is no evidence of percreta, and if attempts are made to determine whether placental separation is possible, all preparations should be made for an immediate peripartum hysterectomy as well as immediate blood transfusion, if massive

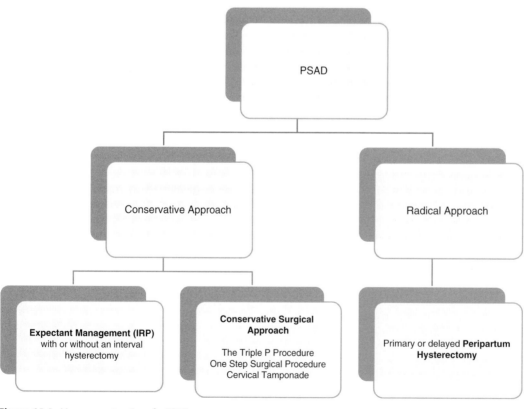

Figure 64.4 Management options for PSAD.

obstetric haemorrhage occurs during the attempted separation of the placenta.

It is important to avoid administration of uterotonic drugs, as this may lead to partial separation of the non-adherent part of the placenta, precipitating significant bleeding from the placental site. Antibiotics should be administered for approximately 7 days to avoid infection. Methotrexate is not recommended because placenta at term has very few rapidly dividing cells. Moreover, methotrexate may suppress the bone marrow, leading to sepsis. It is also important to avoid embolization of the internal iliac or the uterine arteries because a sudden reduction of the blood supply may result in rapid ischaemic necrosis, leading to secondary postpartum haemorrhage or sepsis. It is essential to allow a gradual necrosis of the placental tissue secondary to a progressive reduction in the blood supply. Embolization may be considered if the woman presents with massive secondary postpartum haemorrhage during the expectant management. A literature review on intentional retention of the placenta (IRP) found that of the 26 women managed without the use of additional therapies, 22 (85%) had a favourable outcome. Expectant management failed in 15% of cases, and secondary hysterectomy had to be performed owing to massive obstetric haemorrhage or infection [14]. In addition to secondary postpartum haemorrhage, severe sepsis with increased morbidity and mortality, disseminated intravascular coagulation (DIC) and the need for a delayed peripartum hysterectomy, even the development of a utero-cutaneous fistula, have been reported with IRP [15].

Intentional retention of placenta remains a viable option in centres where facilities and expertise to manage a massive postpartum haemorrhage are not available, and in cases where there is abnormal invasion of the placenta into the broad ligament invading vital structures such as the ureters and the lateral pelvic sidewall [16, 17]. In addition, if future fertility is desired after appropriate counselling, IRP may be attempted to avoid a peripartum hysterectomy. However, in such cases, patient compliance and facilities for regular monitoring and follow-up of patients to detect and timely manage

the potential complications of a retained and progressively necrotic placenta are essential.

64.4.2 Conservative Surgical Management: The Triple P Procedure

The Triple P Procedure was developed to avoid severe maternal morbidity and mortality associated with a peripartum hysterectomy [18]. It consists of three steps: perioperative placental localization by a transabdominal ultrasound scan immediately prior to surgery to delineate the upper border of the placenta; pelvic devascularization by inflation of pre-positioned pelvic arterial occlusive balloon catheters to reduce the blood supply to the placental bed, and placental nonseparation and myometrium excision (i.e. excising the placenta along with the underlying adherent myometrium without separating), followed by reconstruction of the myometrial defect [18]. Access to the myometrium above the upper border of the placenta is achieved through the 'St George's boat incision', whereby, the subcutaneous tissue overlying the rectus sheath is reflected upwards, and the rectus sheath is incised like a 'boat' so that the base of the incision is at a higher level (Figure 64.5) to enable access above the upper border of the placenta (Figure 64.6).

In cases of placenta percreta, the part of the placenta invading the bladder wall is left in situ, and a copious amount of local haemostat (PerClot) is applied to the bleeding placental venous sinuses at the area of invasion of the urinary bladder (Figure 64.7) to achieve haemostasis [19, 20]. The use of prophylactic occlusive pelvic arterial balloon catheters has been reported to be beneficial in avoiding massive obstetric haemorrhage as well as peripartum hysterectomy [21]. A comparative study has concluded that the Triple P Procedure is associated with a statistically significant reduction in postpartum haemorrhage as well as inpatient hospital stay, with no cases of peripartum hysterectomy [22]. The presence of an anterior placenta with invasion of the urinary bladder and/or the cervix (i.e. cervical invasion) has been reported to be associated with a longer hospital stay [23].

Recently, modifications of the Triple P Procedure, which included the use of temporary clamping of the internal iliac artery prior to the myometrial excision[24] or the application

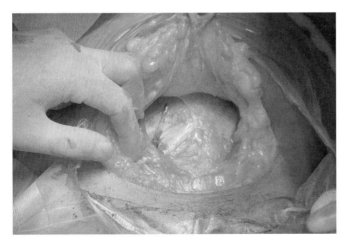

Figure 64.5 The rectus sheath is incised like a 'boat' so that the base of the incision is at a higher level. A black and white version of this figure will appear in some formats. For the colour version, please refer to the plate section.

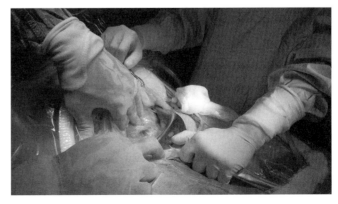

Figure 64.6 Access above the upper border of the placenta. A black and white version of this figure will appear in some formats. For the colour version, please refer to the plate section.

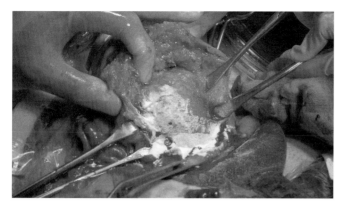

Figure 64.7 Copious amount of local haemostat (PerClot) is applied to the bleeding placental venous sinuses at the area of invasion of the urinary bladder. A black and white version of this figure will appear in some formats. For the colour version, please refer to the plate section.

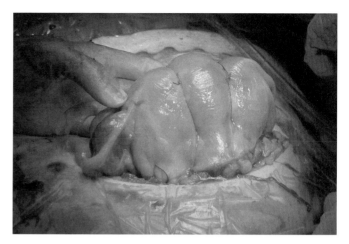

Figure 64.8 Two vertical compression sutures inserted immediately above the balloon, prior to its inflation to avoid the migration of the uterine tamponade balloon into the upper segment. A black and white version of this figure will appear in some formats. For the colour version, please refer to the plate section.

of tourniquet just about the cervix [25] prior to the myometrial excision, have been described with good outcomes. In cases of abnormal placental invasion in the upper uterine segment, the Triple P Procedure can be safely performed by ligating both the uterine arteries prior to the planned myometrial excision. If there is evidence of cervical invasion (i.e. a J-shaped placenta praevia with abnormal invasion of anterior and/or posterior myometrial invasion as well as the invasion of the cervix), a uterine tamponade balloon should be inserted after myometrial excision to avoid bleeding from cervical venous sinuses. Two vertical compression sutures should be inserted immediately above the balloon, prior to its inflation to avoid the migration of the uterine tamponade balloon into the upper segment (Figure 64.8). This will enable continuous pressure on the bleeding cervical venous sinuses to ensure an effective haemostasis.

Recent Green-top guidelines produced by the Royal College of Obstetricians and Gynaecologists (RCOG) on placenta praevia and accrete [7] as well as the International Consensus Guidelines on Placenta Accreta Spectrum Disorders produced by the International Federation of Gynaecology and Obstetrics (FIGO) [5] have included the Triple P Procedure as a conservative surgical alternative to a peripartum hysterectomy. Although the original intention of the Triple P Procedure was to avoid serious maternal morbidity and mortality associated with a peripartum hysterectomy, and not fertility preservation, the first case report of a successful pregnancy after the Triple P Procedure, with no recurrence of abnormal invasion of the placenta, was reported in 2018 [26].

64.5 Other Conservative Surgical Approaches

64.5.1 One Step Surgical Resection

The one step surgical resection technique is mainly useful when there is no evidence of placenta percreta, and it involves the resection of the areas of placental invasion (partial myometrial resection) followed by immediate uterine reconstruction and bladder reinforcement [27].

64.5.2 Cervical Tamponade

The cervical tamponade involves inverting the cervical lips into the uterine cavity and suturing the anterior and/or the posterior cervical lips into the areas of placental invasion in the anterior and/or posterior walls of the lower uterine segment [28]. This technique may be useful in localized areas of abnormal invasion of the placenta in the lower uterine segment, especially in a low-resource setting. The long-term implications including the effect on preterm labour or late miscarriage due to the suturing of the cervical length remain unknown.

64.6 Radical Surgery: Peripartum Hysterectomy

Peripartum hysterectomy should be performed as a lifesaving measure in all cases of placental adhesive disorders in the presence of haemodynamic instability and continuing bleeding. It may also be performed as an interval procedure (i.e. after intentionally leaving the placenta for spontaneous resorption to reduce vascularity or after transferring a woman to a tertiary referral centre). Peripartum hysterectomy has been associated with significant maternal morbidity and mortality, which include massive blood loss, which may exceed 10 000 mL in up to 13% of patients [29], injury to the urinary bladder in 6 to 29% [30, 31], injury to the ureters in up to 7% of cases [32, 33] as well as the maternal mortality rate of 1 to 6% [33–35]. It is important to note that injury remains a risk even in intentional hysterectomy, and it has been reported that intentional cystotomy and a partial cystectomy may be required in up to 33% of cases of delayed hysterectomy [36].

Therefore, in the light of the reported complications, serious maternal morbidity and increased risk of mortality, peripartum hysterectomy should be undertaken by a competent surgeon who is familiar with the procedure. Neovascularization that occurs as a result of abnormal invasion of the placenta results in formation of blood vessels with poor development of tunica media (i.e. the muscle layer), which may render standard measures of haemostasis (i.e. application of sutures and cautery) ineffective. Invasion of the placenta into the lateral uterine wall and into the broad ligament may not only lead to ureteric injury, but may also lead to profuse haemorrhage as a result of feeding vessels within the broad ligament.

64.7 Summary of Clinical Management

Although there is an ongoing debate with regard to the ideal management option in abnormal invasion of the placenta [37] in view of the heterogeneity of the condition, as well as varying degrees of placental invasion, the cornerstone of management should be to reduce serious maternal morbidity and mortality. Except in cases of emergencies, a conservative approach should be undertaken, with a ready recourse to an emergency peripartum hysterectomy if there is excessive bleeding. This is because unlike performing a peripartum hysterectomy for an atonic postpartum haemorrhage (i.e. where the placental site is usually in the upper segment with no neovascularization), abnormal invasion of the placenta poses additional surgical challenges due to involvement of adjacent vital organs as well as formation of blood vessels without tunica media. A multidisciplinary, multiprofessional approach, with involvement of the patient in the decision-making process prior to surgery, is essential in choosing the optimal management option.

64.8 Key Messages

PSAD should be suspected as a possibility when risk factors are present.

Women with previous CS should have placental localization early in pregnancy.

Pregnancies with placenta praevia, especially those with previous scarring, should be scanned by an expert to exclude PSAD.

Anaemia in the mother should be detected and treated early.

Those diagnosed or have high suspicion of PSAD should be referred for delivery in a regional centre with expertise.

A multidisciplinary team should plan the management and it should be documented in the notes.

The gestation at which delivery is planned should be determined to maximize the expertise and the needed facilities.

A consultant obstetrician with expertise and a consultant anaesthetist should be present and provide direct care with assistance from the team – they should meet with the woman and the family and explain what is planned and the possible complications and what is being prepared to minimize or avoid adverse outcome.

The blood bank and the haematologist should be alerted and blood should be readily available in case of massive haemorrhage; cell saver facilities should be utilized if such services are available.

The help of the urologist and/or oncologist should be available in theatre if invasion into bladder or adjacent tissue is suspected.

Interventional radiologists with facilities for arterial balloon occlusion or embolization should be utilized if available.

Corticosteroids should be administered to promote lung maturity if the CS is planned at 35 to 36 weeks; the neonatal unit should be informed to reserve a cot and a senior neonatal paediatrician should be available to care for the baby.

Intensive care facilities should be available to look after the mother should the need arise.

Debriefing with the mother, birth partner and staff should take place and future pregnancies discussed if the uterus was preserved.

64.9 Key Guidelines Relevant to the Topic

Jauniaux E, Alfirevic Z, Bhide AG, et al.; Royal College of Obstetricans and Gynaecologists. *Placenta Praevia and Placenta Accreta: Diagnosis and Management*: Green-top Guideline No. 27a. *BJOG*. 2019; **126**: e1-e48. doi: 10.1111/ 1471-0528.15306

References

1. Jauniaux E, Ayres deCampos D. FIGO consensus guidelines on placenta accreta spectrum disorders: introduction. *Int J Gynaecol Obstet*. 2018 Mar;**140** (3):261–4.

2. Jauniaux E, Chantraine F, Silver RM, et al. FIGO consensus guidelines on placenta accreta spectrum disorders; epidemiology. *Int J Gynaecol Obstet*. 2018 Mar;140(3):265–72.

3. Jauniaux E, Bhide A, Kennedy A, et al. FIGO consensus guidelines on placenta accreta spectrum disorders; prenatal

diagnosis and screening. *Int J Gynaecol Obstet*. 2018 Mar;**140**(3):274–80.

4. Allen L, Jauniaux E, Hubinent R, et al. FIGO consensus guidelines on placenta accreta spectrum disorders; non conservative surgical management. *Int J Gynaecol Obstet*. 2018 Mar;**140**(3): 281–90.

5. Sentilhes L, Kayem G, Chandraharan E, Palacios-Jaraquemada J, Jauniaux E. FIGO consensus guidelines on placenta accreta spectrum disorders; conservative management. *Int J Gynaecol Obstet*. 2018 Mar;**140**(3):291–8.

6. Silver RM, Fox KA, Barton JR, et al. Center of excellence for placenta accreta. *Am J Obstet Gynecol*. 2015;**212**:561–8. doi: 10.1016/j.ajog.2014.11.018

7. Jauniaux E, Alfirevic Z, Bhide AG, et al.; Royal College of Ostetricians and Gynaecologists. Placenta praevia and placenta accreta: diagnosis and management: Green-top Guideline No. 27a. *BJOG*. 2019;**126**: e1-e48. doi: 10.1111/1471-0528.15306

8. D'Antonio F, Iacovella C, Bhide A. Prenatal identification of invasive placentation using ultrasound:

systematic review and meta-analysis. *Ultrasound Obstet Gynecol.* 2013;**42**:509–17. doi: 10.1002/uog.13194

9. Comstock CH, Love JJ Jr, Bronsteen RA, et al. Sonographic detection of placenta accreta in the second and third trimesters of pregnancy. *Am J Obstet Gynecol* 2004;**190**:1135–40. doi: 10.1016/j.ajog.2003.11.024

10. Finberg HJ, Williams JW. Placenta accreta: prospective sonographic diagnosis in patients with placenta previa and prior cesarean section. *J Ultrasound Med.* 1992;**11**:333–43.

11. Bhide A, Laoreti A, Kaelin Agten A, et al. Lower uterine segment placental thickness in women with abnormally invasive placenta. *Acta Obstet Gynecol Scand.* 2019;**98**:95–100. doi: 10.1111/aogs.13422

12. D'Antonio F, Iacovella C, Palacios-Jaraquemada J, et al. Prenatal identification of invasive placentation using magnetic resonance imaging: systematic review and meta-analysis. *Ultrasound Obstet Gynecol.* 2014;**44**:8–16. doi: 10.1002/uog.13327

13. Sentilhes L, Goffinet F, Kayem G. Management of placenta accreta. *Acta Obstet Gynecol Scand.* 2013;**92**:1125–34.

14. Timmermans S, van Hof AC, Duvekot JJ. Conservative management of abnormally invasive placentation. *Obstet Gynecol Surv.* 2007;**62**:529–39.

15. Athanasias P, Krishna A, Karoshi M, Moore J, Chandraharan E. Uterocutaneous fistula following classical caesarean delivery for placenta percreta with intentional retention of the placenta. *J Obstet Gynaecol.* 2013;**33**(8):906–7.

16. Fox KA, Shamshirsaz AA, Carusi D, et al. Conservative management of morbidly adherent placenta: Expert review. *Am J Obstet Gynecol.* 2015;**213**:755–60.

17. Meyer NP, Ward GH, Chandraharan E. Conservative approach to the management of morbidly adherent placentae. *Ceylon Med J.* 2012 Mar;**57**(1):36–9.

18. Chandraharan E, Rao S, Belli A-M, Arulkumaran S. The Triple-P procedure as a conservative surgical alternative to peripartum hysterectomy

for placenta percreta. *Int Journal of Obstet & Gynecol.* **117**;2012:191–4.

19. Pinas Carrillo A, Chandraharan E. Management of morbidly adherent placenta. *Obstet Gynaecol Reproduc Med.* 2016;**26**(10):283–90.

20. Doncheva P, Chandraharan E. Effectiveness of PerClot: a topical haemostatic agent to reduce intra-operative bleeding during 'triple P procedure' for morbidly adherent placentae: a case series. *BJOG.* 2013;**120**:s1:17–18.

21. Teixidor Viñas M, Chandraharan E, Moneta MV, Belli AM. The role of interventional radiology in reducing haemorrhage and hysterectomy following caesarean section for morbidly adherent placenta. *Clin Radiol.* 2014 Aug;**69**(8):e345–51.

22. Teixidor Vinas M, Belli AM, Arulkumaran S, Chandraharan E. Prevention of postpartum hemorrhage and hysterectomy in patients with morbidly adherent placenta: a cohort study comparing outcomes before and after the introduction of the Triple P procedure. *Ultrasound Obstet Gynecol.* 2015;**46**:350–5.

23. El Tahan M, Carrillo AP, Moore J, Chandraharan E. Predictors of postoperative hospitalisation in women who underwent the Triple-P procedure for abnormal invasion of the placenta. *J Obstet Gynaecol.* 2018 Jan;**38**(1):71–3.

24. Tskhay VB, Yametov PK, Yametova NM. The use of modified triple-p method with adherent placenta long-term results. *MOJ Womens Health.*2017;**4**(2):00079.

25. Wei Y, Cao Y, Yu Y, Wang Z. Evaluation of a modified 'Triple-P' procedure in women with morbidly adherent placenta after previous caesarean section. *Arch Gynecol Obstet.* 2017 Oct;**296**(4):737–43.

26. Cauldwell M, Chandraharan E, Pinas Carillo A, Pereira S. The first reported case of successful pregnancy outcome following conservative management of placenta percreta using the Triple P Procedure. *Ultrasound Obstet Gynecol.* 2017. doi: 10.1002/uog.17566

27. Palacios-Jaraquemada JM, Pesaresi M, Nassif JC, Hermosid S. Anterior placenta percreta: Surgical approach, hemostasis and uterine repair. *Acta Obstet Gynecol Scand.* 2004;**83**:738–44.

28. El Gelany SA, Abdelraheim AR, Mohammed MM, et al. The cervix as a natural tamponade in postpartum hemorrhage caused by placenta previa and placenta previa accreta: a prospective study. *BMC Pregnancy Childbirth.* 2015;**15**:295.

29. Wright JD, Pri-Paz S, Herzog TJ, et al. Predictors of massive blood loss in women with placenta accreta. *Am J Obstet Gynecol.* 2011;**205**:38e1

30. Hoffman MS, Karlnoski RA, Mangar D, et al. Morbidity associated with nonemergent hysterectomy for placenta accreta. *Am J Obstet Gynecol.* 2010;**202**: e1–5.

31. Eller AG, Bennett MA, Sharshiner M, et al. Maternal morbidity in cases of placenta accrete managed by a multidisciplinary care team compared with standard obstetric care. *Obstet Gynecol.* 2011;**117**:331.

32. Awan N, Bennett MJ, Walters WA. Emergency peripartum hysterectomy: a 10-year review at the Royal Hospital for Women, Sydney. *Aust N Z J Obstet Gynaecol.* 2011;**51**:210.

33. Wright JD, Devine P, Shah M, et al. Morbidity and mortality of peripartum hysterectomy. *Obstet Gynecol.* 2010;**115**:1187.

34. Knight M. Peripartum hysterectomy in the UK: management and outcomes of the associated haemorrhage. *BJOG.* 2007;**114**:1380.

35. Yucel O, Ozdemir I, Yucel N, Somunkiran A. Emergency peripartum hysterectomy: a 9-year review. *Arch Gynecol Obstet.* 2006;**274**:84.

36. Tam Tam KB, Dozier J, Martin JN Jr. Approaches to reduce urinary tract injury during management of placenta accreta, increta, and percreta: A systematic review. *J Matern Fetal Neonatal Med.* 2012;**25**:329–34.

37. Perez-Delboy A, Wright JD. Surgical management of placenta accreta: to leave or remove the placenta? *BJOG.* 2014;**121**:163–70.

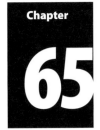

Chapter 65

Social and Cultural Aspects Affecting Pregnancy Outcomes in Migrant Populations

Pauline L. M. de Vries & Thomas van den Akker

65.1 Introduction

Over the last decades, the number of international migrants worldwide has not stopped growing. In 2017, there were 258 million international migrants worldwide, half of them women. Asia and Europe currently host 60% of all international migrants with 80 million and 78 million migrants each, followed by North America with 58 million [1]. With a growing number of migrants, healthcare workers in high-income countries will encounter them more frequently in their practice. Migrants, on the other hand, will encounter health professionals with sometimes very different cultural values and beliefs. These differences may cause misunderstandings and delays in accessing appropriate medical care during pregnancy and childbirth.

Conflicting findings regarding pregnancy outcomes in migrants are present in the literature. Both increased adverse pregnancy outcomes as well as a 'healthy migrant effect' have been described. The healthy migrant effect suggests that migrants sometimes have better pregnancy outcomes compared to native women. The idea behind this theory is that, in general, healthier people and those of higher economic status migrate more frequently and are accepted more readily into the country of arrival. These migrants consequently may have better pregnancy outcomes compared to native-born women since their health status was superior prior to conception.

For many migrants, however, this healthy migrant effect is an illusion. Although maternal morbidity in high-income countries has been reduced remarkably over the past decades leading to improved pregnancy outcomes in native women, outcomes in women with a migration background often lag behind. The Dutch LEMMoN study found that migrant women are at increased risk of severe acute maternal morbidity (SAMM), with non-Western background being an independent risk factor, and asylum seekers having the highest risk [2, 3]. Gibson-Helm et al found that migrants with a refugee background had a higher risk profile, worse pregnancy care attendance and more frequently a late first antenatal visit compared to non-refugee migrants [4]. Refugees and undocumented migrants have often survived extreme stress, violence and poor living circumstances, and their health status prior to pregnancy may be less favourable. In other words, the migrant population is highly heterogeneous, and this heterogeneity is likely to be reflected in pregnancy outcomes that differ between groups (Table 65.1).

Table 65.1 Definitions of populations

Migrant	Someone who is moving or has moved across an international border or within a state away from his/her habitual place of residence, regardless of (1) the person's legal status; (2) whether the movement was voluntary or involuntary; (3) what the causes for the movement were; or (4) what the length of the stay will be.
Refugee	A person who is outside the country of his/her nationality and is unable or, owing to fear of conflict, generalized violence or other circumstances that have seriously disturbed the public, is unwilling to avail him- or herself of the protection of that country.
Asylum Seeker	A person who seeks safety from persecution or serious harm in a country other than his/her own and awaits a decision on the application for refugee status under relevant international and national instruments.
Undocumented Migrant	People who enter, stay or work in a country without authorization or documentation under immigration regulations.

Adapted from the International Organization for Migration (IOM) [1].

In this chapter, we will focus on pregnancy outcomes in different subtypes of migrants settling from low- and middle-income countries into high-income countries. We will begin by discussing pregnancy outcomes in migrant women, and then describe risk factors contributing to adverse pregnancy outcomes. Last, recommendations are given with regard to improving clinical management of migrant women.

65.2 Pregnancy Outcomes in Migrants

65.2.1 Maternal Outcomes

65.2.1.1 Hypertensive Disorders

Women from sub-Saharan Africa are at the highest risk of developing hypertensive disorders during pregnancy [5]. Analyses from the United Kingdom (UK) obstetric surveillance system (UKOSS) indicated that black African or black

Caribbean women in the UK had a twofold risk of SAMM compared with white women [6]. Very few studies, however, have explored the pathophysiology that could explain this elevated risk. Different hypotheses suggest there might be a genetic predisposition as well as suboptimal care during pregnancy and labour. This last hypothesis was investigated in France, where prenatal care for migrants appeared to be of lower quality. Screening tests such as detection of proteinuria by dipstick or measurements of blood pressure were more often repeated before moving on to diagnostic tests such as 24-hour collection of urine or laboratory tests. Doctors also failed to take action on abnormal values. Both women and medical doctors did not recognize symptoms as being pre-eclampsia related. This was partly due to a different presentation of symptoms in these women compared to native women. For example, 'pain from my bra' was used to describe epigastric pain and 'vertigo' was specified rather than 'headache'. Low awareness about alarm symptoms in both women and health workers may have led to delay in diagnosis and the development of severe pre-eclampsia or eclampsia [7].

65.2.1.2 Postpartum Haemorrhage (PPH)

In the Netherlands and Germany, higher risks of postpartum haemorrhage (PPH) in non-Western migrants were found, in the Netherlands this was a threefold risk [2, 8]. Pregnant women from several migrant groups in several countries had higher rates of anaemia, rendering these women more vulnerable to adverse outcomes from PPH [9]. Anaemia may result from vitamin deficiencies because of poor nutritional status, haemoglobinopathies as well as short pregnancy-intervals due to lack of access to family planning.

65.2.1.3 Uterine Rupture

Uterine rupture may be primary (in case of unscarred uterus) or secondary (most often the result from caesarean section in a previous pregnancy). Risk factors include previous caesarean section(s), type of uterine incision used during these procedures, with transverse incisions in the lower uterine segment carrying the lowest risk, uterine overdistention (polyhydramnios, large for gestational age, multiple pregnancy), intrapartum oxytocin use or persistent and intense uterine contractions. Outcomes can be severe, and uterine rupture is one of the leading causes of maternal and fetal morbidity and mortality. The incidence of uterine rupture in high-income countries varies between 0.2 and 1.5% in the non-migrant population. Maternal mortality after uterine rupture in high-income countries, however, is low. A UK study found a maternal mortality ratio of 1.3%, 95% confidence interval (CI) 0.2%–4.5%, after uterine rupture [10]. Zwart et al found no maternal deaths in a population-based cohort study in the Netherlands. They found an 8.7% risk of perinatal death [11]. Maternal morbidity after uterine rupture is important. Of the 158 women with a uterine rupture, 15 (9%) women had a hysterectomy following uterine rupture and 69 (43%) women had other or additional morbidity following their uterine rupture such as blood transfusion due to PPH or ventilation [10].

According to the LEMMoN study, asylum seekers are at higher risk of SAMM (31.0 per 1000, compared with 6.8 per 1000 for the total LEMMoN population (risk ration (RR) 4.5, 95% CI 3.3–6.1). In 15% of asylum seekers with SAMM, uterine rupture occurred compared to 8.4% in the whole LEMMoN population with SAMM. This high percentage might be (partly) explained by the high number of prior caesarean section (CS) in asylum seekers (40%) compared to the entire LEMMoN population (18.6%) [3]. Similar findings in Canada among sub-Saharan African migrants showed that these women had higher rates of uterine rupture compared to the native population [12].

65.2.1.4 Sepsis

In pregnant women, infections commonly leading to sepsis are pyelonephritis, chorioamnionitis, septic abortion and puerperal infection. Case fatality is high if diagnosis and treatment are delayed ('golden hour of sepsis'). Sepsis accounts for 2.1% of all maternal deaths in high-income countries. A retrospective cohort study in the USA showed that women had significantly increased adjusted odds ratios (aOR) of progressing to severe sepsis if they were black, aOR = 2.09 (95% CI 1.34–2.26); Asian, aOR = 1.59 (95% CI 1.07–2.37); Hispanic, aOR = 1.42 (95% CI 1.09–1.83); or had public/no-insurance, aOR = 1.52 (95% CI 1.19–1.94) [13]. In contrast, a study in Sweden did not find sepsis to be more common among migrants [14]. The Global Obstetric Sepsis Study (GLOSS) from the World Health Organization (WHO) will elucidate risks of sepsis in migrant women.

65.2.1.5 Caesarean Section

The *Lancet* series on optimizing the use of caesarean section highlighted the fact that access to caesarean section is unequally distributed. Rates above 10–15% at the population level have not been associated with better pregnancy outcomes [15, 16]. This is an important conclusion since caesarean sections are associated with an increased risk of infection, haemorrhage, thromboembolism (especially in African women since protein S and antithrombin deficiencies are more common in this group [17]), laparotomy [18], peripartum hysterectomy and even maternal death. In subsequent pregnancies, risks of uterine rupture, placenta praevia or abnormally invasive placenta and placental abruption are increased. A large systematic review found that caesarean section rates in migrants are often above the population threshold. They also vary for different subpopulations of migrants, with women from sub-Saharan Africa generally having higher rates of particularly emergency caesarean section and women from Eastern Europe often having lower rates compared to native women [19]. Factors contributing to the higher rate of caesarean section in African women are poor maternal health, gestational diabetes mellitus (GDM), high body mass index (BMI), female genital mutilation (FGM), language barriers and women's cultural attitudes and expectations regarding labour [19, 20].

65.2.1.6 Maternal Mortality

Maternal death is defined by the WHO as the death of a woman during pregnancy or within 42 days of childbirth. Maternal death in Europe has been decreasing over the past decades due to improved antenatal care. Unfortunately, inequality exists and maternal mortality rates are higher in migrant women.

In France, the risk of postpartum maternal death was twice as high for foreign women, with an odds ratio of 5.5 (95% CI 3.3–9.0) for women from sub-Saharan Africa and 3.3 (95% CI 1.7–6.5) for those from Asia and North and South America. They found more substandard care among foreign women who died [21].

A large meta-analysis including 13 studies found that migrant women had a higher risk of maternal mortality compared to non-migrants, with a pooled relative risk of 2.00 (CI 1.72–2.33) [22].

Again, heterogeneity amongst migrants seems to reflect the different rates of mortality. For example, maternal mortality among asylum seekers in the Netherlands was found to be extremely high (RR 10.08, 95% CI 8.02–12.83) [23].

The recent MBRRACE-UK report of 2018 showed that black African women in the UK had a fivefold higher risk of maternal death.

65.2.2 Fetal Outcome

65.2.2.1 Low Birthweight

Low birthweight is an important pregnancy outcome and one of the leading causes of infant morbidity and mortality. Findings related to low birthweight in migrant populations are diverse and inconsistent [24]. Low birthweight is probably increased in specific subtypes of migrants. A 2019 review indicated that a larger proportion of low birthweight in undocumented compared to documented migrants was found, potentially because of social deprivation, poor living conditions, chronic fear and stress as well as impaired access to healthcare [25]. Obtaining permanent resident status was found to reduce risk of perinatal morbidity in non-documented immigrants [26].

65.2.2.2 Preterm and Post-term Birth

Preterm birth is a leading cause of neonatal mortality and morbidity. Chronic stress, depression and anxiety are associated with preterm birth and it is unsurprising that preterm birth is increased in undocumented migrants [24]. Data from the Swedish medical birth registry show that migrants from South Asia, sub-Saharan Africa and East Asia had an increased risk of preterm birth. North African and Middle Eastern, Somali and Ethiopian/Eritrean groups, on the other hand, had increased risk of post-term birth. Migrant women staying in Sweden for less than 3 years had higher risk for early preterm birth as well as post-term birth compared to those staying more than 10 years, suggesting that duration of residence has an impact on pregnancy outcomes [27].

65.2.2.3 Congenital Malformations

Findings related to congenital malformations in migration populations are heterogeneous. Risk appears to be increased in women from the Middle East, North Africa and Pakistan. Plausible explanations are consanguinity and socio-economic factors, both of which are independent risk factors for congenital anomalies. Children of Pakistani origin had an almost twofold risk of congenital anomalies compared to children born to native women. Infant death due to congenital anomalies in this group was also more frequent [28]. Consanguinity is frequent (>30% of marriages) in Pakistan, Afghanistan, the Middle East and many North African countries. The risk of congenital anomalies grows if consanguinity is present in multiple generations since recessive disorders are selected more easily [29].

65.2.2.4 Stillbirth

A study in Belgium found that migrants from North Africa, Egypt, sub-Saharan Africa and Turkey had a doubled risk of stillbirth compared to native-born women [30]. In Spain, a similarly increased risk of stillbirth was reported in women from sub-Saharan Africa and Eastern Europe [31]. In Denmark, an increased risk of stillbirth was found in women from Pakistan, Somalia and, to a lesser extent, Turkey, an increase not associated with income or education level [32]. Although findings reflect heterogeneity and may be confounded by lower socio-economic status, many report increased stillbirth rates in migrants, especially from sub-Saharan Africa, Pakistan and Turkey. A study in Rotterdam, the Netherlands, found a higher rate of stillbirth in women of non-Western origin, even after correcting for socio-economic status. Suboptimal pregnancy care appeared to play an important role [33].

65.3 Risk Factors in the Migrant Population

65.3.1 Poor Maternal Health

The health profile of migrant women differs from native-born women and varies greatly among subpopulations of migrants. According to the healthy migrant effect hypothesis, the health status of migrants may sometimes be superior to that of native-born women upon arrival. However, this hypothesis seems plausible only for certain groups of migrants.

In asylum seekers and non-documented migrants, general health is often poor. They are at increased risk of having had diseases such as tuberculosis, rheumatic heart disease, poliomyelitis and measles, which may impact negatively on pregnancy outcome. Other risk factors more common in asylum seekers include scarred uterus, anaemia, HIV-positive serostatus, single-parent household, language barriers and short stay since arrival [2, 3, 4].

Higher prevalence of obesity was found in subgroups of migrant women, including women from sub-Saharan Africa and North Africa, as well as migrant women arriving from 'humanitarian' source countries, probably a result of adopting a more Western lifestyle. Gestational diabetes is more frequent in certain groups of migrants, most likely due to genetic predisposition, childhood malnutrition and lower socio-economic status resulting in an unhealthier diet. Obesity is an independent risk factor for caesarean section [19, 20].

65.3.2 Substandard Care

Substandard care was found to be an important contributor to the higher risk of maternal mortality in migrant women in the Netherlands. There were important delays in recognition of symptoms and onset of treatment, due to late referrals and insufficient risk awareness among health professionals. Substandard care also includes patient-related factors, with migrant women more often refusing medical advice [34]. Migrants more frequently have late first antenatal visits and fewer visits than the eight recommended by the WHO. Although migrant women's wishes with regard to medical care are similar to those of native women (safe, attentive and individualized) they often rate their care as being of insufficient quality [35, 36].

65.3.3 Language Barriers

Language is an important component of maternity care since reports from women on symptoms of a complicated pregnancy and fetal movements are crucial in the assessment of the woman's health and that of the fetus. Pregnancy is an important life event, and it can be traumatizing for a woman to feel her concerns are not responded to. Since obstetrics is a field of medicine often dealing with acute complications that require quick access to care, language barriers as well as unfamiliarity with the healthcare system contribute to delays and adverse pregnancy outcomes.

Many women experience not being taken seriously or feeling unwelcome due to language barriers [35]. Language barriers may also increase anxiety during labour.

Use of interpretation services has been associated with improved pregnancy outcomes, and use of family members as interpreters should be avoided [7, 34, 35].

65.3.4 Low Socio-economic Status

Low socio-economic status is an important and independent risk factor for adverse neonatal outcomes such as low birthweight and preterm birth. Other risk factors such as young maternal age, smoking and being overweight are more common in people of low socio-economic status.

Low socio-economic status is unlikely to explain all disparities in adverse outcome. For example, in the UK, Bangladeshi parents were found to have a similar socio-economic profile to Pakistanis, whereas infant mortality rates differed significantly between these groups, with infant mortality higher in Pakistani groups. By contrast, a study conducted in Brussels did not find any influence of ethnicity on pregnancy outcomes after adjusting for socio-economic status [26, 30].

65.3.5 Social Deprivation

Social deprivation is the reduction of culturally normal interaction with society at large. Factors leading to social deprivation include unconducive living environment, single-parent household, lack of social participation and having experienced violence and stress, and such factors may reinforce each other. Social deprivation is an important risk factor of adverse pregnancy outcome, and was found to be more common among non-Western compared to Western women [33].

65.3.6 Cultural Attitudes

Women's ideas on prenatal care are often shaped by perspectives obtained in their countries of origin and traditional practices, which sometimes may lead to maternal morbidity [33, 34]. Women may be anxious about having to give birth in a birthing position they do not prefer, and may even shun intrapartum care for this reason [33]. Many Somali women associate caesarean sections with maternal mortality and some may avoid or refuse surgery [37].

65.3.7 Female Genital Mutilation (FGM)

Female genital mutilation (FGM) compromises all procedures that involve partial or total removal of the external female genitalia, or other injuries to the female genitalia for non-medical reasons. It is a form of gender inequality that may lead to severe complications.

Female genital mutilation is practised in a large part of the world and has become a global problem through migration. Although risks of complications during childbirth are higher in countries with limited health service, risks in high-income countries can be due to healthcare workers being unfamiliar with this practice [38]. If no adequate de-infibulation is performed, obstruction during labour can occur, leading to fetal death and fistulae. The slightly higher risk of caesarean section in high-income countries in this group is often initiated by healthcare workers not knowing how to perform a de-infibulation and not because of incapacity of the woman to deliver vaginally.

Tokopobia (fear of childbirth) is frequent and should be discussed during prenatal visits. A de-infibulation during the second trimester can be discussed and performed if this is the patient's preference. Healthcare workers should be aware of the risk of FGM for the neonate [38].

65.4 Ethics and Healthcare for Migrants

Article 12 of the International Covenant on Economic, Social and Cultural Rights (ICESCR) affirms the right of everyone to enjoy the highest attainable standard of physical and mental health. The Council of Europe Resolution 1509 on Human Rights of Irregular Migrants, Article 13.2, declares that as a minimum right, emergency care should be available for undocumented migrants. Cuadra states that these rights are not met uniformly throughout Europe. She compared the policies of 27 European countries to find that 10 member states do not grant access to emergency care for undocumented migrants. Twelve countries offer such access, and only five countries offer a broader range of medical care. Importantly, she finds that these differences do not seem to result from differences in health financing or the volume of migrants a country receives. Countries with more restrictive policies on healthcare for, especially, non-documented migrants seem not to rely on regularization practices [39].

An ethical question pertains to whether or not a health system of a particular country has the duty to accommodate cultural differences and, if so, to what extent. Since substandard care, language barriers and low socio-economic status contribute to adverse pregnancy outcomes, it is ethical to provide migrant-sensitive healthcare. Samanta et al state that 'the expression of faith-based values and their recognition by healthcare providers within a public healthcare system is a moral right' and recognition of religion and faith-based values should be recognized and incorporated at all levels [quoted in 40].

Xenophobia in Europe is a growing problem. Doctors of the World reported 'alarming increases in xenophobic violence' throughout Europe. Migrants, Roma and sex-workers are victims of such explicit xenophobic violence, and of more implicit forms of discrimination. This leads to dangerous delays in seeking medical care, and particularly in obstetrics.

In light of recent terroristic attacks and the migrant influx in Europe, xenophobic feelings appear to be on the rise and are exploited by populist politicians throughout the Continent. Migrants are held responsible for unemployment and financial insecurity of natives. Some claim that providing healthcare to migrants will increase costs and impact negatively on care received by natives. Feelings of self-interest may reinforce social deprivation and suboptimal healthcare in migrants [41].

65.5 Clinical Management of the Migrant Population

In 2004, the European initiative 'Migrant Friendly Hospitals' published a declaration [42] with several recommendations on how to develop migrant-friendly health services. Based on these recommendations and technical guidance provided by the WHO, we formulate several clinical tools, outlined below, to improve pregnancy outcomes among migrant women [43].

65.5.1 Provide Individualized Care

– *Be aware of a woman's background*

Try not to stereotype but do try to be aware of how cultural background, religion, migrant status and ethnicity may impact complications and clinical care during pregnancy.

– *Low socio-economic status*

Identify risk factors related to low socio-economic status and collaborate with social services at facility and/or community level.

– *Specific diseases*

Provide screening tests for infectious diseases such as syphilis and tuberculosis in risk groups. Screen for HIV, if this is not included in the standard screening programme. Provide screening for gestational diabetes to high-risk groups if this is not done routinely. Be aware of the increased risks of congenital anomalies. Always look for anaemia; identify the underlying cause and treat it.

65.5.2 Guarantee Access to Care

– *Free access*

Everyone should have free access to maternity care, regardless of legal status and insurance.

– *Organizational structures*

Try to provide maternal and neonatal healthcare in the areas where underserved populations live. Take into account the role of general practitioners, community centres and midwives. Try to share responsibilities between hospitals and primary care providers, who are often more accessible.

– *Health promotion*

Workshops can be organized or brochures can be created and distributed to raise awareness of health risks of consanguineous parenting, FGM, nutrition, breastfeeding, and so forth.

A tool addressing language barriers can be found on the website www.zanzu.be. This initiative, created by the Flemish Expertise Centre for Sexual Health and the German Federal Centre for Health Education, offers information for migrants about different topics such as family planning and pregnancy in many languages, illustrated by pictograms.

An interesting example of a health promotion programme is the MaMAACT trial in Denmark. In this trial, researchers developed, using input from migrant women, an application and folder on warning signs in pregnancy, illustrated by pictograms. They trained midwives on intercultural collaboration and they adjusted 5 minutes in the first prenatal consultation to see whether all of these measures help midwives to adequately manage warning signs and whether migrants respond better to warning signs of pregnancy. Results of this trial are currently being analyzed [44].

– *Communication*

Use interpreter services rather than family members to improve communication. Programmes exists in which healthcare workers can use telephone assistance provided by an interpreter. This can be cost-effective and very helpful, especially where there are no face-to-face interpreting services available.

65.5.3 Quality of Care

– *People-centred and migrant-sensitive healthcare*

Migrant women should receive the same level of care that native women receive. Healthcare providers should be responsive to social and cultural differences. The questionnaire in Table 65.2 is an example of a tool that may help healthcare workers and enhance responsiveness [45].

– *Referral*

Several studies showed that severe maternal morbidity and mortality were caused by late recognition and late referral. Migrant woman should therefore be referred more promptly [35].

– *Mutual trust*

Mutual trust between women and healthcare providers is very important. Explore the wishes of the migrant woman early during the pregnancy and try to inform her repeatedly concerning alarm symptoms during pregnancy.

– *Communication*

See above. Invest in your first consultation by taking more time in order to establish a good medical workup and confidence in the local health system.

Table 65.2 Questionnaire to gain responsiveness [45]

What do you call your problem?

What causes your problem?

Why do you think it started when it did?

How does it work – What is going on in your body?

What kind of treatment do you think would be best for this problem?

How has this problem affected your life?

What frightens or concerns you most about this problem and its treatment?

65.5.4 Healthcare Policy and Financing Systems

– *Financing systems*

Healthcare should be provided to all pregnant women and their newborns regardless of their migration and financial status. Barriers for seeking healthcare should be minimized.

– *Advocacy*

Women should be given the space to empower themselves through health education, through ethnically diverse health staff or promoting advocacy.

– *Family planning*

Since teenage pregnancy, short intervals between pregnancies and grand multiparity are more common in migrants (and risk factor for adverse pregnancy outcomes (APO)), it is of utmost importance to ensure access to reliable contraception. Midwives, obstetricians, general practitioners and other healthcare workers working with migrants should inform proactively and take a leading role in providing information. It can be helpful to use pictures or workshops with ethnically diverse staff.

– *Evaluation of healthcare in migrant population*

Following the Minority Humanitarian Foundation (MHF) project, the ROAM (Reproductive Outcomes And Migration)

collaboration developed a Migrant Friendly Maternity Care Questionnaire (MFMCQ). This validated questionnaire aims to assess migrant-friendly care in hospitals and aims to help the healthcare worker in providing questions that address the challenges migrant women might face.

Another interesting project is the Operational Refugee And Migrant Maternal Approach (ORAMMA) project, funded through the European Union's health programme, in which new recommendations for improvement of healthcare for pregnant migrant women based on scientific evidence will be evaluated in several pilot countries.

65.6 Key Messages

- Migrant factors influence maternal and fetal outcomes in pregnancy. Refugees, undocumented migrants and asylum seekers are especially vulnerable to adverse pregnancy outcomes.
- Literature on pregnancy outcomes in migrants is conflicting, most likely due to heterogeneity of the migrant population with some groups having higher risks than others.
- Important migrant factors influencing pregnancy outcomes are substandard care, communication barriers, socio-economic status and poor maternal health.
- Improving healthcare for migrants includes attention paid to a woman's background and the specific health problems related to this background.
- Good accessibility of care, including interpreter services and health promotion efforts, improves pregnancy outcomes in migrants.
- Migrant status should not affect the quality of healthcare women receive. We should strive for mutual trust and be responsive to social and cultural differences.
- Be aware of the clinical presentation in migrant women that might be different from native women.

References

1. United Nations. International migration reports. 2017.
2. Zwart J, Richters J, Öry F, et al. Severe maternal morbidity during pregnancy, delivery and puerperium in the Netherlands: a nationwide population based study of 371 000 pregnancies. *BJOG.* 2008;**115**:842–50.
3. Van Hanegem N, Miltenburg AS, Zwart JJ, Bloemenkamp KW, Van Roosmalen J. Severe acute maternal morbidity in asylum seekers: a two-year nationwide cohort study in the Netherlands. *Acta Obstet Gynecol Scand.* 2011 **90**(9):1010–16.
4. Gibson-Helm ME, Teede HJ, Chen I-H, et al. Maternal health and pregnancy

outcomes comparing migrant women born in humanitarian and nonhumanitarian source countries: a retrospective, observational study. *Birth.* 2015;**42**(2):116–24.
5. Knuist M, Bonsel GJ, Zondervan HA, Treffers PE. Risk factors for preeclampsia in nulliparous women in distinct ethnic groups: a prospective cohort study. *Obstet Gynecol.* 1998;**92**:174–8.
6. Knight M, Kurinczuk JJ, Spark P, et al. Inequalities in maternal health: national cohort study of ethnic variation in severe maternal morbidities. *BMJ.* 2009;**338**: b542.
7. Sauvegrain P, Azria E, Chiesa-Dubruille C, Deneux-Tharaux C. Exploring the hypothesis of differential care for African immigrant and native women in

France with hypertensive disorders during pregnancy: a qualitative study. *BJOG.* 2017;**124**(12):1858–65.
8. Reime B, Janssen PA, Farris L, et al. Maternal near-miss among women with a migrant background in Germany. *Acta Obstet Gynecol Scand.* 2012;**91**: 824–9.
9. Van den Akker T, van Roosmalen J. Maternal mortality and severe morbidity in a migration perspective. *Best Pract Res Clin Obstet Gynaecol.* 2016;**32**:26–38.
10. Fitzpatrick KE, Kurinczuk JJ, Alfirevic Z, et al. Uterine rupture by intended mode of delivery in the UK: a national case-control study. *PLoS Med.* 2012;**9**(3):e1001184.

11. Zwart J, Richters J, Ory F, et al. Uterine rupture in the Netherlands: a nationwide population-based cohort study. *BJOG.* 2009;**116**:1069–80.

12. Urquia ML, Glazier R, Mortensen L, et al. Severe maternal morbidity associated with maternal birthplace in three high immigration settings. *Eur J Public Health.* 2015;**25**(4):620–5.

13. Acosta CD, Knight M, Lee HC, et al. The continuum of maternal sepsis severity: incidence and risk factors in a population-based cohort study. *PLoS One.* 2013;**8**(7):e67175.

14. Wahlberg A, Rööst M, Moussa K, et al. Increased risk of severe maternal morbidity (near miss) among immigrant women in Sweden: a population register-based study. *BJOG.* 2013;**120**(13):1605–11.

15. Boerma T, Ronsmans C, Y Melesse D. Global epidemiology of use of and disparities in caesarean sections. *Lancet.* 2018 Oct 13; **392**(10155):1341–8.

16. Betran AP, Torloni MR, Zhang JJ, Gulmezoglu AM, for the WHO Working Group on Caesarean Section. WHO statement on caesarean section rates. *BJOG.* 2016;**123**:667–70.

17. Philipp C, Faiz A Beckman M, et al. Differences in thrombotic risk factors in black and white women with adverse pregnancy outcome. *Thromb Res.* 2014; **133**:108–11.

18. Witteveen T, Kallianidis A, Zwart JJ, et al. Laparotomy in women with severe acute maternal morbidity: secondary analysis of a nationwide cohort study. *BMC Pregnancy Childbirth.* 2018;**18** (1):61.

19. Merry L, Vangen S, Small R. Caesarean births among migrant women in high-income countries. *Best Pract Res Clinl Obstet Gynaecol.* 2016;**32**:88e9.

20. Merry L, Semenic S, Gyorkos TW. International migration as a determinant of emergency caesarean. *Women Birth.* 2016 Oct;**29**(5):e89-e98.

21. Philibert M, Deneux-Tharaux C, Bouvier-Colle M.-H. Can excess maternal mortality among women of foreign nationality be explained by suboptimal obstetric care?*BJOG.* 2008;**115** (11):1411–18.

22. Pedersen GS, Grøntved A, Mortensen LH, et al. Maternal mortality among migrants in Western Europe: a meta-analysis.*Maternal Child Health J.* 2014;**18**(7):1628–38.

23. van Oostrum IEA, Goosen S, Uitenbroek DG, et al. Mortality and causes of death among asylum seekers in the Netherlands, 2002–2005. *J Epidemiol Community Health.* 2011;**65**:376–83.

24. Gagnon AJ, Zimbeck M, Zeitlin J, et al. Migration to western industrialised countries and perinatal health: a systematic review. *Soc Sci Med,* 2009; **69**:934e46.

25. Gieles N, Tankink J, van Midde M. Maternal and perinatal outcomes of asylum seekers and undocumented migrants in Europe: a systematic review. *Eur J Public Health.* 2019 Aug; **29** (4):714–23.

26. Minsart A, Englert Y, Buekens P. Naturalization of immigrants and perinatal mortality. *Eur J Public Health.* 2013 Apr; **23**(2):269–74.

27. Khanolkar AR. Preterm and postterm birth in immigrant- and Swedish-born parents: a population register-based study. *BJOG.* 2002 Feb; **109**(2):212–13.

28. Sheridan E, Wright J, Small N, et al. Risk factors for congenital anomaly in a multiethnic birth cohort: an analysis of the Born in Bradford study. *Lancet.* 2013;**382**:1350e9.

29. Nybo Andersen A., Gundlund A, Fredsted Villadsen S. Stillbirth and congenital anomalies in migrants in Europe. *Best Pract Res Clin Obstet Gynaecol.*2016;**32**:50e59.

30. Racape J, De SM, Alexander S, et al. High perinatal mortality rate among immigrants in Brussels. *Eur J Public Health.* 2010;**20**:536e42.

31. Luque-Fernandez MA, Franco M, Gelaye B, et al. Unemployment and stillbirth risk among foreign-born and Spanish pregnant women in Spain, 2007–2010: a multilevel analysis study. *Eur J Epidemiol.* 2013;**28**:991–9.

32. Villadsen SF, Mortensen LH, Andersen AM. Ethnic disparity in stillbirth and infant mortality in Denmark 1981–2003. *J Epidemiol Community Health.* 2009;**63**:106–12.

33. Poeran J, Maas AF, Birnie E, et al. Social deprivation and adverse perinatal outcomes among Western and non-Western pregnant women in a Dutch urban population. *Soc Sci Med.* 2013;**83**:42e9.

34. Van Roosmalen J, Schuitemaker NW, Brand R. Substandard care in immigrant versus indigenous maternal deaths in the Netherlands. *BJOG.* 2002 Feb;**109**(2): 212–13.

35. Small R, Roth C, Raval M, et al. Immigrant and non-immigrant women's experiences of maternity care: a systematic and comparative review of studies in five countries. *BMC Pregnancy Childbirth.* 2014;**14**:1 52.

36. Benza S, Liamputtong T. Pregnancy, childbirth and motherhood: A meta-synthesis of the lived experiences of immigrant women, *Midwifery.*2014;**30**:575–84.

37. Essén B, Binder P, Johnsdotter S. An anthropological analysis of the perspectives of Somali women in the West and their obstetric care providers on caesarean birth. *J Psychosom Obstet Gynecol.* 2011 Mar;**32**(1):10–18.

38. Toubia N. Female circumcision as a public health issue. *N Engl J Med.* 1994 Sep 15;**331**(11):712–16.

39. Cuadra C. Right of access to health care for undocumented migrants in EU: a comparative study of national policies. *Eur J Public Health.* 2012; **22**(2):267–2.

40. Klingler C, Odukoya D, Kuehlmeyer K. Migration, health, and ethics.*Bioethics.* 2018;**3**(2):330–3.

41. Doctors of the World International Network. Report: Access to healthcare in Europe in times of crisis and xenophobia: an overview of the situation of people excluded from the health care system. n.d.

42. The MFH Project Group. The Amsterdam Declaration towards Migrant-Friendly Hospitals in an Ethno-Culturally Diverse Europe. n.d.

43. World Health Organization. *Improving the Health Care of Pregnant Refugee and Migrant Women and Newborn Children.* Technical guidance. Geneva: WHO; 2018.

44. Villadsen SF, Hvas Mortensen L, Nybo Andersen A-M. Care during pregnancy and childbirth for migrant women: how do we advance? The case of the MAMAACT intervention in Denmark. *Best Pract Res Clin Obstet Gynaecol.*2016;**32**:100e112.

45. Johnson TM, Hardt EJ, Kleinman A. Cultural factors in the medical interview. In Lazare A, ed. *The Medical Interview: Clinical Care, Education and Research.* New York: Springer;1995.

531

Chapter

66

Immunization in Pregnancy

Babill Stray-Pedersen, Kirsten Maertens, Elke Leuridan & Gilbert G. G. Donders

66.1 Introduction

Immunization is one of the most effective preventive health measures; it reduces the incidence and severity of vaccine-preventable infectious diseases, saving millions of people from illness, disability and death every year. According to the World Health Organization (WHO), safe and effective vaccines protecting against 26 different diseases are currently available, while another 24 vaccines are under development (Figure 66.1) [1, 2].

Pregnant women, fetuses and neonates are especially vulnerable to infectious diseases due to altered immune responses. Vaccine-preventable infectious diseases are responsible for significant maternal, neonatal and infant morbidity and even mortality. Vaccination during pregnancy (maternal vaccines) provides protection of the mother through active immunization, and leads to transplacental transfer of maternal antibodies providing protection

of the developing fetus, the neonate and the young infant during early life [3].

Ideally, vaccination should be given prior to conception, but administration during pregnancy is indicated in some situations. The decision whether to vaccinate a woman during pregnancy requires assessment of benefits and risks. In order to facilitate the decision, the healthcare practitioner and the woman should determine the potential risk of exposure to the specific disease and the effect this disease could have on the mother–infant pair. These risks must be weighed against the efficacy and the safety profile of the vaccine itself. No vaccine has ever proven any teratogenic effect until now. Side effects of vaccination during pregnancy are in general considered negligible and do not differ much from those outside pregnancy. Undesired vaccine-related fever reactions can rarely occur, as well as very rare complications such as anaphylactic reactions, which can cause hazard for both mother and child. Adequate use

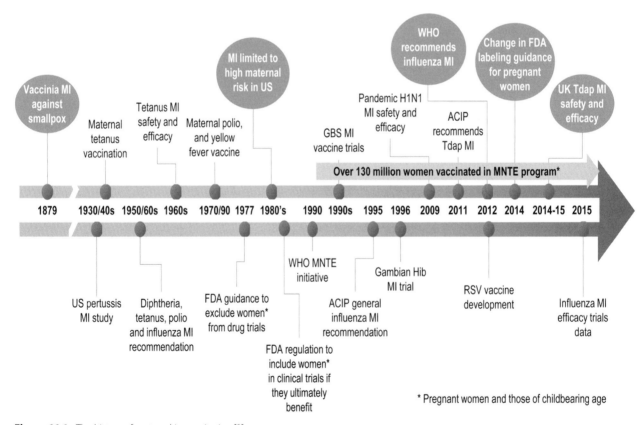

Figure 66.1 The history of maternal immunization [3]

of antipyretic medication should therefore be advised at vaccination. No higher incidence of anaphylactic reactions has been recorded after maternal immunization [4].

Importantly, some vaccines are recommended to be administered in pregnancy because of epidemiological reasons: tetanus, pertussis and influenza. Many countries have implemented this vaccination strategy in addition to vaccination of other age groups, or in view of specific vulnerability of the woman (influenza), neonate (tetanus) or infant (pertussis). Also, many other vaccines that have the potential to be used during pregnancy, such as vaccines against respiratory syncytial virus, cytomegalovirus, group B streptococcus, are currently under development and could theoretically be implemented in the maternal immunization programme in the near future.

In addition, today, pregnant women are more likely to travel for business or recreation, often to areas that have an infectious panorama that is unfamiliar to them. Therefore, before deciding upon remote travel, pregnant women should be recommended to visit a clinic specialized in travelling advice, as they offer vaccination packages which are adapted to pregnant women and to travel to different parts of the world.

66.2 Types of Vaccines

The main challenge in vaccine development is to create a vaccine strong enough to ward off the specific infection, without causing serious illness in the individual. There are four different types of vaccines in use today [5]:

1. *Live-attenuated vaccines* consist of live microorganisms that have lost the ability to cause serious disease but are able to stimulate immunity. They may produce a mild or subclinical form of the disease. Examples of live-attenuated vaccines are those for measles, mumps, rubella, varicella, rotavirus, (oral) polio, tuberculosis and yellow fever.
2. *Inactivated vaccines* contain organisms that have been killed or inactivated with chemicals or by heating. Inactivated vaccines produce a less pronounced immune response than the live-attenuated vaccines. Therefore, more doses of inactivated vaccines have to be administered to obtain a protective immune response. Vaccines against pertussis (whole cell pertussis), (injectable) polio, some forms of influenza and cholera are made from inactivated organisms.
3. *Subunit, recombinant, polysaccharide and conjugate vaccines* are made from the antigenic parts of the pathogen, necessary to elicit a protective immune response. These vaccines can be protein-based (e.g. acellular pertussis and hepatitis B vaccines), polysaccharide-based (meningococcal and pneumococcal vaccines) or conjugate vaccines (pneumococcal vaccines and *Haemophilus influenzae* type B).
4. *Toxoid vaccines* contain inactivated toxoids as the metabolic by-products of infectious organisms (toxins).

These toxoids are used to stimulate immunity against, for example, tetanus and diphtheria.

66.3 Safety of Vaccines in Pregnancy

The Global Advisory Committee on Vaccine Safety (GACVS) has evaluated data on the safety of immunization in pregnant women for several vaccines [6]. There is **no evidence** of adverse pregnancy outcomes from any vaccination with inactivated, subunit or toxoid vaccines. Therefore, pregnancy should not exclude women from receiving these vaccines, if medically indicated or recommended for epidemiological reasons. Growing evidence on the safety and efficacy of influenza and tetanus, diphtheria, and pertussis (Tdap) vaccinations in pregnancy has highlighted maternal immunization as an important strategy to reduce morbidity and mortality in pregnant women, fetuses and infants [7].

Theoretically, live vaccines may pose a teratogenic risk to the fetus by the viremia they cause and should be avoided in pregnancy. However, there is a substantial body of literature confirming the safety of live-attenuated vaccines, including monovalent rubella vaccines, combined measles-mumps-rubella (MMR) vaccines, oral poliovirus vaccines and yellow fever vaccines during pregnancy. Never has there been a significant adverse effect reported on a fetus following administration of any of these live-attenuated vaccines. The Pan American Health Organization (PAHO) data indicate, however, that the attenuated rubella vaccine strain could cause an immune response in the unborn child, confirming transplacental transport of the vaccine virus strain, without, however, causing congenital rubella disease [8]. In general, the ban on administering MMR vaccines in pregnancy can be seen as a precautionary measure. As a consequence, inadvertent vaccination of pregnant women with MMR-containing vaccines is not considered an indication for termination of the pregnancy. When vaccinating non-pregnant women of childbearing age with an MMR vaccine, 1 month of contraception is required after vaccination.

66.4 Mechanism of Vaccination in Pregnancy

Upon vaccination of the pregnant woman, the maternal immune system is challenged to produce IgG antibodies (humoral immune response) that will be transferred across the placenta and through the breast milk and thus protect the newborn before birth and during the first months of life. Evidence is consistent that the humoral immune response in pregnancy is equal to the humoral response in a non-pregnant woman [9].

Circulating maternal antibodies are transported across the placenta with the help of the FcRn receptor, present in the syncytiotrophoblast of the placenta. This transplacental transport starts from week 13 and gradually increases as the pregnancy proceeds. The placental transport system is highly selective for immunoglobulin G (IgG) antibodies and essentially excludes the transport of other major immunoglobulin classes

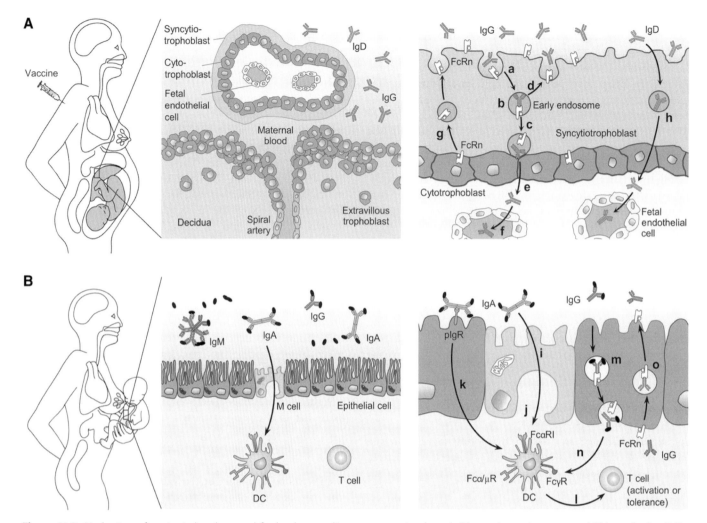

Figure 66.2 Mechanisms of vaccine-induced maternal, fetal and neonatal immune protection through (A) transplacental transport and (B) breastfeeding [10]

including immunoglobulin M (IgM), immunoglobulin E (IgE) and immunoglobulin A (IgA). Within the IgG antibodies, preferential transport of the IgG$_1$ and IgG$_3$ antibodies is seen over the IgG$_2$ and IgG$_3$ antibodies. Vaccines containing protein antigens eliciting predominantly IgG$_1$ and IgG$_3$ subclasses are more efficient during pregnancy than vaccines containing polysaccharide antigens eliciting IgG$_2$ antibodies (Figure 66.2).

Mucosal antibodies, on the other hand, including IgA, IgM and IgG, are secreted into colostrum and breast milk and are thus ingested by the neonate during breastfeeding, providing mucosal protection in the gastrointestinal tract [10].

66.5 Vaccines Recommended in Pregnancy

Some vaccines are routinely recommended in pregnancy [11, 12]. These vaccines are very well tested and can be given without any risk to pregnant women on usual indications (Table 66.1).

Vaccine against tetanus. The bacterium *Clostridium tetani* flourishes worldwide in the environment and the disease therefore cannot be eradicated. In some countries, deliveries still

take place in unhygienic circumstances, putting mothers and newborns at risk for maternal and neonatal tetanus (MNT). Tetanus is particularly serious in newborns (neonatal tetanus) and their mothers when the mothers are inadequately protected [13]. Immunizing pregnant women with tetanus toxoid-containing vaccines is a very inexpensive and efficacious way to prevent MNT.

As in some developing countries where neonatal tetanus is still the leading cause of neonatal death, the tetanus toxoid vaccine (monovalent or in combination with diphtheria) should be administered to all pregnant women, as included in many national Expanded Programs on Immunization (EPI).

In Europe, special attention should be paid to immigrants with unknown tetanus vaccination status [14]. The tetanus immunization programme comprises 3 doses: starting dose, dose after 4 weeks and dose after 6–12 months. Ideally, the full Tdap vaccine should replace the Td vaccine given as a single dose in the third trimester of pregnancy.

In special circumstances, like wound management, protection against tetanus is important, and thus immediate vaccination should be provided if necessary. If Td booster is indicated at

Table 66.1 Summary of vaccines that may be considered pre-pregnancy, during pregnancy and post-pregancy

Disease	Vaccine Type	Vaccination pre-pregnancy	Vaccination in pregnancy	Vaccination postpartum
MMR (mumps, measles, rubella)	Live	Yes Avoid conception 1 month	No	Yes
Varicella	Live	Yes Avoid conception 1 month	No	If necessary
Yellow fever	Live	Yes	To be avoided if travelling to endemic areas	Not during lactation
BCG tuberculosis	Live	Yes	If high risk Treatment treats fetus	If necessary
Polio (OPV)	Live	If high risk	If high risk	If high risk
Influenza	Live	Yes	No	If necessary
Tdap (tetanus, diphtheria, pertussis)	Inactivated	If necessary	Yes in every pregnancy according to country recommendations	If necessary
Influenza	Inactivated	If high risk	Yes	If necessary
Polio (IPV)	Inactivated	If high risk	If high risk	If high risk
Hepatitis A	Inactivated	Yes	Yes if needed	Yes
Hepatitis B	Inactivated	Yes	Yes if needed	Yes
HPV	Inactivated	Yes	No	Yes if not been in the young adult vaccination programme
Rabies	Inactivated	Yes	Yes if needed	Yes
Tick-borne encephalitis	Inactivated	Yes	Yes if needed	Yes
Japanese encephalitis	Inactivated	Yes	Yes if needed	Yes
Meningococcal vaccines	Inactivated	Yes	Yes	Yes
Cholera	Inactivated	Yes	Yes	Yes

any time in pregnancy, pregnant women should preferably be given Tdap.

Vaccine against influenza. Pregnant women are at increased risk for influenza-associated complications and are recognized as a priority group for seasonal and pandemic influenza vaccination. During both seasonal and pandemic influenza episodes, especially those of 1919, 1958 and 2010, pregnant women had up to four times higher risk of hospitalization and admission to intensive care units for acute cardiorespiratory illness and had even higher mortality than non-pregnant women and the general population. The disease severity increases with each trimester and is the highest for pregnant women with medical co-morbidity conditions such as asthma, diabetes mellitus and obesity [15].

Before an upcoming flu season, vaccination of pregnant women with co-morbidities are without discussion recommended worldwide. To better protect pregnant women, the WHO, the Centers for Disease Control and Prevention (CDC) and other national bodies recommend that every healthy pregnant women should be vaccinated with one dose of an inactivated influenza vaccine before the flu season [2, 11, 12]. None of the multiple studies evaluating safety has demonstrated an increased risk of either maternal complications or adverse fetal outcomes due to influenza vaccination [7]. So far, the uptake of the vaccine in pregnancy has been poor and strategies to improve the vaccination coverage have been stressed.

Although recently the full effect of the vaccination has been questioned [16], there is a clear benefit on morbidity in pregnant women including preterm deliveries, and on the birthweight of the neonates as well as the percentage of small-for-gestational-age infants [17].

Vaccine against tetanus, diphtheria, pertussis (Tdap vaccine). Due to universal immunization programmes for different age groups in the general population, tetanus and diphtheria have almost been eradicated in Europe. Still, the respiratory infection pertussis (whooping cough) is today an emerging public health problem in industrialized countries, with cyclic epidemiology affecting persons of all ages. Severe disease is especially observed in very young infants under 2 months of age, as they are too young to be protected by vaccination and experience the more severe symptoms of respiratory distress. Maternal immunization seems to be the key strategy to protect these neonates, with the currently available vaccines [18]. One has to be aware that pertussis-specific antibodies in adults are short-lived after maternal vaccination, which led to the recommendation that Tdap vaccine should be given every pregnancy in order to maximize the transport of antibodies towards the fetus and to maximize passive neonatal immunity.

The Tdap vaccines (combined inactivated tetanus toxoid, diphtheria toxoid and acellular pertussis vaccine) are safe and well tolerated in pregnant women and their infants. Multiple studies show Tdap vaccination, given in the second and third trimesters, prevents pertussis in at least 9 out of 10 infants younger than 2 months of age [19].

66.6 Vaccination of Pregnant Women in Case of Infection Risk

Cholera vaccine. Pregnant women are vulnerable to complications induced by cholera, and maternal infection with cholera may adversely affect pregnancy outcomes. In general, pregnant women should avoid travelling to cholera-affected areas. The oral cholera vaccines (OCVs) contain inactivated cholera bacteria. In mass vaccination campaigns during cholera outbreaks, the vaccine has been administered to pregnant women and have turned out to be safe [20].

Hepatitis A vaccine. Hepatitis A may be a serious infection in pregnancy with several reported cases of liver failure in pregnant women. Hepatitis A vaccine is a killed virus vaccine that has now been used extensively, and the safety risks of vaccination during pregnancy must be considered negligible[12]. As vaccination against hepatitis A in pregnancy is primarily meant to reduce the concomitant risk of infection with hepatitis B, a combined vaccine against hepatitis A and B is indicated.

Hepatitis B vaccine. Acute maternal hepatitis B infection in the third trimester can endanger the offspring. Vertical transmission rate is up to 60% and the risk to develop chronic hepatitis B infection is up to 90% in newborns born to infected mothers. Hepatitis B vaccine is safe for the fetus/newborn when it is given during pregnancy. Although hepatitis B childhood immunization is now routine in many European countries, many women have not been immunized [21].

Hepatitis B vaccination during pregnancy is indicated in the following cases:

Unvaccinated, uninfected women (hepatitis B surface antigen (HBsAg) negative) who are at high risk for acquiring hepatitis B virus in pregnancy (e.g. healthcare workers, women exposed to sexually transmitted infections and injection drug users).

Pregnant women who are in the middle of an immunization programme begun prior to conception.

The hepatitis B vaccination programme consists of 3 doses given at month 0, month 1 and month 4–6. In some countries, screening for hepatitis B surface antigen is a routine pregnancy screening test because of the potential reduction of vertical transmission of HBV by active immunization of the neonate immediately after birth. A woman found to be HBsAg positive in pregnancy should be monitored carefully to ensure that the infant receives HBIG (hepatitis B immune globulin) and begins the hepatitis B vaccine programme no later than 12 hours after birth. Some countries have implemented this birth dose in the general population, but in many countries, only infants of carrier mothers receive this first dose as an extra dose. It should be ensured that the infant also completes the regular hepatitis B vaccine series on schedule. The effect of giving pre-birth HBIG to mothers with active HBV infection to prevent mother-to-child transmission of HBV has been questioned and is not recommended [22].

HPV vaccine. In Europe, bi-, quadri- and nonavalent HPV vaccines are now available for the prevention of infection by HPV strains that are mainly responsible for cervical cancers and genital warts. The available HPV vaccines are manufactured using recombinant technology, ending up in a non-infectious virus-like vaccine. Although the vaccine is not yet recommended for use during pregnancy, there is no evidence that it is teratogenic. The *Cochrane Database of Systematic Reviews* recently published that the occurrence of severe adverse events or adverse pregnancy outcomes was not higher in pregnant recipients of HPV vaccines than in the controls [23]. In addition, a huge population-based Danish study reported no increased risk of spontaneous abortion, stillbirth or infant mortality following unintended HPV vaccination during pregnancy. In fact secondary analysis showed no association between number of doses and timing of administration (i.e. vaccination before or during pregnancy) and an increased risk of spontaneous abortion. However, as there is still insufficient experience in pregnancy, and the disease it can cause rarely, if ever, affects a pregnant woman (with the exception of very rare cases of neonatal laryngeal condyloma), the current recommendation is that if a woman becomes pregnant during the vaccine series, the rest of the series should be postponed. It is important to stress to women who conceive around the time of an HPV vaccination that therapeutic pregnancy termination is not indicated.

Pneumococcal vaccine. Pneumococcal diseases are a common cause of infant morbidity and mortality worldwide, mainly in countries where the pneumococcal vaccine is not yet part of the routine immunization programme. The disease is most common in young children and the elderly, especially persons with chronic medical conditions. Pregnancy is not a risk factor, but unvaccinated pregnant women with medical co-morbidities like cardiovascular diseases and diabetes should be counselled to start the pneumococcal vaccination programme. The currently available pneumococcal polysaccharide vaccines are safe and efficacious for pregnant women and are able to prevent infection and perhaps carriage in the newborn in the first months of life [24].

Polio vaccine. Poliomyelitis has been eradicated from most high- and middle-income countries worldwide, but cases are still reported in Pakistan, Afghanistan, Nigeria, Somalia, Papua New Guinea, Democratic Republic of the Congo and Niger. Endemic transmission is also continuing in Afghanistan, Nigeria and Pakistan. If possible, pregnant women should avoid travelling to polio outbreak regions [12, 25]. If travel is unavoidable, a polio vaccine should be given before departure. Both live-attenuated oral polio vaccine (OPV) and injectable inactivated polio vaccine (IPV) are available. The latter is preferred during pregnancy, even though in mass immunization programmes OPV was observed to be safe and not associated with perinatal death, preterm birth, growth restriction or any congenital anomalies [26].

Rabies vaccine. Rabies poses a 100% risk for death to pregnant women and is an indeterminate risk to the fetus. However, death by human rabies is entirely preventable through prompt administration of post-exposure prophylaxis (PEP) with rabies immunoglobulin and rabies vaccination. The rabies vaccine contains killed virus and is considered safe in pregnancy [27]. In Vietnam, 6 deaths due to rabies after animal bites were reported in pregnant women who were afraid to take the vaccine [28]. So, there is clearly a need for public health information about the safety and effectivness of PEP and rabies vaccination in preventing rabies among all persons with exposures, including pregnant and breastfeeding women.

Typhoid fever vaccine. Typhoid fever acquired from contaminated food or water creates outbreaks in Asia, Africa and Latin America. A single case report with pregnancy loss has been described, but few data exist [6]. Typhoid vaccination is partially protective and is recommended for persons travelling to typhoid-affected areas for longer stays. Preferably, pregnant women should not travel to such areas. If exposure is unavoidable, the inactive, capsular polysaccharide vaccine (Typhim Vi) should be given. The oral live-attenuated typhoid vaccine (Ty21a) should be avoided [29].

66.7 Vaccinations Contraindicated in Pregnancy

Measles, mumps, rubella vaccine. Maternal rubella is very teratogenic and can cause the devastating congenital rubella syndrome (CRS), resulting in severe affection of ears, eyes, heart and brain. Moreover, after several years the infected children may present with diabetes or a progressive encephalopathy. Congenital rubella syndrome can be eradicated almost completely by vaccinating all women before getting pregnant. Initially, vaccination was only recommended to schoolgirls aged 10–12, but today rubella vaccine is offered as part of the routine MMR childhood vaccination programme. Several European countries have completely eliminated rubella and CRS, but globally there are still challenges due to the lack of vaccination programmes [30]. The current recommendation is that all young susceptible women and women without rubella antibodies should be vaccinated before pregnancy. Pre-pregnancy healthcare should therefore include testing of rubella vaccination status by measuring rubella-specific antibodies.

The rubella vaccines are based on the live-attenuated RA 27/3 strain that produced an immune response of 95–100%. Rubella vaccines are available either as monovalent formulations or as combination vaccines against measles (MR), measles and mumps (MMR), or measles, mumps and varicella (MMRV). The vaccine is contraindicated in pregnancy [6]. Therefore, women are advised to delay pregnancy for 1 month following rubella vaccination. Conversely, despite the vaccine being on the market for more than 50 years, no cases of CRS have been reported in more than 1000 susceptible women who were inadvertently vaccinated against rubella during the early stages of pregnancy. Still, due to the theoretical teratogenic risk, rubella vaccination of pregnant women should be avoided. Although women should be asked about the possibility being pregnant prior to rubella vaccination, pregnancy tests to exclude pregnant women are usually not required. Also, rubella vaccination of unknowingly pregnant women is not an indication for abortion.

If a pregnant woman is identified as not immune to rubella, she should receive the MMR vaccine postpartum, ideally prior to discharge from the birth centre. The vaccine can be given safely to postpartum women who are breastfeeding. In fact, rubella virus may be excreted by breast milk, but no serious infection has been reported in breastfeeding infants [30]. Rarely, vaccinated women can show absence of rubella antibodies, even upon repeated vaccination, but there is evidence that they can be considered to be properly protected if it can be ascertained that they have received the vaccine.

Varicella vaccine. Varicella or chickenpox is a common, mild childhood disease with more than 90% seropositivity (VZV IgG) among pregnant women in Europe. Women from tropical and subtropical areas are more likely to be seronegative and thus more susceptible. Although rare, varicella can cause severe infection in pregnant women, complicated by pneumonia, hepatitis and encephalitis and even death. Maternal varicella in early pregnancy is associated with a 1% risk of the devastating congenital varicella syndrome, whereas infection during last 4 weeks before delivery may cause neonatal varicella with a case fatality rate as high as 31%. Acyclovir orally should be given immediately to pregnant woman with varicella infection, and via intravenous application to those with severe disease. Application of hyperimmune globulins was proposed for several years, but the difficulty of getting it in time and in sufficient quantities caused so many practical constraints that this approach has been abandoned.

The ideal approach to avoid the morbidity and mortality associated with varicella in pregnancy would be to screen and vaccinate all susceptible women prior to pregnancy. In Western Europe, the seropositivity and hence protection of pregnant women against varicella is in general high [31]. High-risk groups for infection include seronegative women working with young children, healthcare workers and women who emigrated from tropical regions. If these seronegative high-risk women get pregnant, they should immediately be removed from their working environment.

As the varicella vaccine contains live-attenuated virus, it should not be given in pregnancy. Preferably, it is provided pre-conceptionally or in the postpartum period. If a woman is identified as susceptible (seronegative) in pregnancy, she should receive varicella vaccine after birth. Breastfeeding is not a contraindication. Immunity from the vaccine persists for up to 20 years. Any woman vaccinated should be advised to avoid pregnancy for 1 month after completing the two-dose vaccination programme. The current recommendation is that termination of pregnancy due to unintended varicella vaccination in early gestation is not needed. Registration of more than 900 pregnant women vaccinated in the first trimester or just before showed no cases of congenital varicella and no increased prevalence of other birth defects [32].

BCG vaccine. Tuberculosis (TB) is still one of the world's deadliest communicable diseases. Live-attenuated bacteria are used in the BCG vaccine. WHO recommends BCG vaccination of all neonates in countries or settings with a high incidence of TB with the exception of children who got infected with HIV through vertical transmission from their mother, as these children are at risk of developing severe vaccine-related disease [33]. No harmful effects of BCG vaccination on the fetus have yet to be observed. However, insufficient evidence about the safety of BCG vaccination during pregnancy is available. Therefore, BCG vaccination is contraindicated for pregnant women [34].

Yellow fever vaccine. The yellow fever vaccine is also to be avoided in pregnancy, since it is a live-attenuated vaccine. The vaccination is obligatory in order to enter countries with yellow fever endemicity. Primary vaccination of pregnant women travelling to yellow fever endemic regions is sometimes performed, but reports on the safety of this vaccine during pregnancy are not conclusive. Therefore, travel to endemic areas should be discouraged during pregnancy [29].

66.8 Vaccination Prior to Planned Pregnancy

Antenatal care ideally begins before conception. Nowadays, almost half of all women plan pregnancy, and the pre-conceptional care aims to identify and modify lifestyle, behavioural, medical and social risks to a woman's health or pregnancy outcome through prevention and management. The ultimate aim of pre-conceptional care is to reduce maternal and perinatal morbidity and mortality. Thus, all women of childbearing age including those treated for infertility should have their immunization history assessed to ensure they have been immunized accordingly (see Table 66.1). In many cases, women who present for antenatal care have not had their immunization status reviewed since they had completed the school-age vaccination programme. Immunizations for rubella, varicella or hepatitis B should be offered to women who are susceptible, and women should avoid pregnancy for 1 month after receiving a live-attenuated vaccine (e.g., rubella or varicella), even though the evidence does not suggest that they are harmful [35].

66.9 Breastfeeding and Vaccines

Breastfeeding is almost never a barrier to vaccination. All vaccines, both inactivated, toxoid vaccines and live-attenuated, can be administered safely to lactating women without interruption in infant feeding patterns.

The live-attenuated yellow fever vaccine is an exception. Two reports state that yellow fever vaccine–associated neurological disease has appeared in breastfed infants after maternal vaccination [6, 36]. Therefore, breastfeeding women should not be vaccinated against yellow fever unless the risk for yellow fever acquisition is very high.

66.10 Conclusion

No vaccine has ever been proven to be embryotoxic or teratogenic when used in pregnancy.

Advantages and theoretical risks are to be weighed when vaccination is considered in pregnancy.

Some vaccines are recommended during pregnancy, such as tetanus, pertussis and influenza. In view of the protection of pregnant women against influenza disease, healthcare professionals should be vaccinated in order not to be a source of infection to more susceptible people.

Some vaccines can be considered to reduce personal risk for a woman or her offspring, in case of travelling or close contact to a source of infection.

References

1. World Health Organization. Immunization, vaccines and biologicals. Vaccines and diseases. 2018. www.who.int/immunization/diseases/en/ (Accessed on 13/ 02/2019.)

2. World Health Organization Europe. European Vaccine Action Plan 2015–2020. 2014. www.euro.who.int/_data/assets/pdf_file/0007/255679/WHO_EVAP_UK_v30_WEBx.pdf?ua=1 (Accessed on 13/ 02/2019.)

3. Sobanjo-Ter Meulen A, Duclos P, McIntyre P, et al. Assessing the evidence for maternal pertussis immunization: a report from the Bill & Melinda Gates Foundation Symposium on Pertussis Infant Disease Burden in Low- and Lower-Middle-Income Countries. *Clinical Infect Dis.* 2016;63: S123–S33.

4. Vaccine Adverse Event Reporting System. 2019. https://vaers.hhs.gov/ (Accessed on 13/02/2019.)

5. US Department of Health & Human Services. Vaccine Types 2017. www.vaccines.gov/basics/types/index.html

6. Global Advisory Committee on Vaccine Safety. Safety of immunization during pregnancy. A review of the evidence. 2014. www.who.int/vaccine_safety/publications/safety_pregnancy_nov2014.pdf (Accessed on 13/ 02/ 2019.)

7. McHugh L, Marshall HS, Perrett KP, et al. The safety of influenza and pertussis vaccination in pregnancy in a cohort of Australian mother-infant pairs, 2012–2015: the FluMum Study. *Clin Infect Dis.* 2019;68:402–8.

8. Castillo-Solorzano C, Reef SE, Morice A, et al. Guidelines for the documentation and verification of measles, rubella, and congenital rubella syndrome elimination in the region of the Americas. *J Infect Dis.* 2011;204 (Suppl 2):S683–9.

9. Huygen K, Cabore RN, Maertens K, Van Damme P, Leuridan E. Humoral and cell mediated immune responses to a pertussis containing vaccine in pregnant and nonpregnant women. *Vaccine.* 2015;33:4117–23.

10. Faucette AN, Unger BL, Gonik B, Chen K. Maternal vaccination: moving the science forward. *Hum Reprod Update.* 2015;21:119–35.

11. Committe on Obstetric Practice. Committee Opinion No. 718: Update on Immunization and Pregnancy: Tetanus, Diphtheria, and Pertussis Vaccination. *Obstet Gynecol.* 2017;130: e153–e7.

12. Castillo E, Poliquin V. No. 357 – immunization in pregnancy. *J Obstet Gynaecol Can.* 2018;40:478–89.

13. World Health Organization. Maternal and Neonatal Tetanus Elimination (MNTE). 2019. www.who.int/immunization/diseases/MNTE_initiative/en/ (Accessed on 13/ 02/2019.)

14. World Health Organization. Tetanus vaccines: WHO position paper – February 2017. *Wkly Epidemiol Rec.* 2017;92:53–76.

15. Grohskopf LA, Sokolow LZ, Broder KR, et al. Prevention and control of seasonal influenza with vaccines. *MMWR Recomm Rep.* 2016;65:1–54.

16. Demicheli V, Jefferson T, Ferroni E, Rivetti A, Di Pietrantonj C. Vaccines for preventing influenza in healthy adults. *Cochrane Database Syst Rev.* 2018;(2): CD001269.

17. Giles ML, Krishnaswamy S, Macartney K, Cheng A. The safety of inactivated influenza vaccines in pregnancy for birth outcomes: a systematic review. *Hum Vaccin Immunother.* 2019:15 (3):687–99.

18. World Health Organization. Pertussis vaccines: WHO position paper – September 2015. *Wkly Epidemiol Rec.* 2015;90:433–58.

19. McMillan M, Clarke M, Parrella A, et al. Safety of tetanus, diphtheria, and pertussis vaccination during pregnancy: a systematic review. *Obstet Gynecol.* 2017;129:560–73.

20. Khan AI, Islam MT, Qadri F. Safety of oral cholera vaccines during pregnancy in developing countries. *Hum Vaccin Immunother.* 2017;13:2245–6.

21. World Health Organization. Hepatitis B vaccines: WHO position paper – July 2017. *Wkly Epidemiol Rec.* 2017;92:369–92.

22. Eke AC, Eleje GU, Eke UA, Xia Y, Liu J. Hepatitis B immunoglobulin during pregnancy for prevention of mother-to-child transmission of hepatitis B virus. *Cochrane Database Syst Revi.* 2017;(2): CD008545.

23. Arbyn M, Xu L. Efficacy and safety of prophylactic HPV vaccines. A Cochrane review of randomized trials. *Expert Rev Vaccines.* 2018;17:1085–91.

24. Clarke E, Kampmann B, Goldblatt D. Maternal and neonatal pneumococcal vaccination – where are we now? *Expert Rev Vaccines.* 2016;15:1305–17.

25. World Health Organization. Polio vaccines: WHO position paper – March, 2016. *Wkly Epidemiol Rec.* 2016;91:145–68.

26. Harjulehto-Mervaala T, Aro T, Hiilesmaa VK, et al. Oral polio vaccination during pregnancy: no increase in the occurrence of congenital malformations. *A J Epidemiol.* 1993;138:407–14.

27. Fayaz A, Simani S, Fallahian V, et al. Rabies antibody levels in pregnant women and their newborns after rabies post-exposure prophylaxis. *Iran J Reprod Med.* 2012;10:161–3.

28. Nguyen HTT, Tran CH, Dang AD, et al. Rabies vaccine hesitancy and deaths among pregnant and breastfeeding women – Vietnam, 2015–2016. *MMWR Recomm Rep.* 2018;67:250–2.

29. Centers for Disease Control and Prevention. Guidelines for vaccinating pregnant women. 2017. www.cdc.gov/vaccines/pregnancy/hcp/guidelines.html#typhoid (Accessed on 15/ 02/ 2019.)

30. World Health Organization. Rubella vaccines: WHO position paper. *Wkly Epidemiol Rec.* 2011;86:301–16.

31. Vilibic-Cavlek T, Ljubin-Sternak S, Kolaric B, et al. Immunity to varicella-zoster virus in Croatian women of reproductive age targeted for serology testing. *Arch Gynecol Obstet.* 2012;286: 901–4.

32. Marin M, Willis ED, Marko A, et al. Closure of varicella-zoster virus-containing vaccines pregnancy registry – United States, 2013. *MMWR Recomm Rep.* 2014;**63**:732–3.

33. World Health Organization. BCG vaccines: WHO position paper – February 2018. *Wkly Epidemiol Rec.* 2018;**93**:73–96.

34. Loto OM, Awowole I. Tuberculosis in pregnancy: a review. *J Pregnancy.* 2012;**2012**:379271.

35. Shawe J, Delbaere I, Ekstrand M, et al. Preconception care policy, guidelines, recommendations and services across six European countries: Belgium (Flanders), Denmark, Italy, the Netherlands, Sweden and the United Kingdom. *Eur J Contracept Reprod Health Care.* 2015;**20**:77–87.

36. World Health Organization. Global vaccine safety: yellow fever vaccine and breastfeeding. 2010. www.who.int/vaccine_safety/committee/topics/yellow_fever/Jun_2010/en/ (Accessed on 15/02/2019.)

67

Saving Lives, Improving Mothers' Care

UK and Ireland Confidential Enquiries into Maternal Deaths and Morbidity

Rohan Chodankar, Ruth Howie, Chu Chin Lim & Tahir A. Mahmood

67.1 Introduction

The UK Confidential Enquiries into Maternal Deaths (CEMD) has set a gold standard to improve quality and safety in maternity services for over 60 years. It recognizes the importance of learning from every woman's death, occurring during or after pregnancy, not only for the clinical staff and services involved in the care, but also for the family and friends she leaves behind.

The latest MBRRACE-UK report (November 2018) is the fifth MBRRACE-UK annual report of the Confidential Enquiry into Maternal Deaths and Morbidity. It includes surveillance data on women who died during or up to one year after pregnancy between 2014 and 2016 in the UK. In addition, it also includes Confidential Enquiries into the care of women who died between 2014 and 2016 in the UK and Ireland [1].

Readers are urged to visit the MBRRACE-UK website to access the most recent annual report published by the organization: *Mother and Babies: Reducing Risk through Audits and Confidential Enquiries across the UK* (www.npeu.ox.ac.uk/mbrrace-uk/reprts).

A maternal death is defined as the death of a woman while pregnant or within 42 days of the end of the pregnancy from any cause related to or aggravated by the pregnancy or its management and not from accidental causes [2]. The World Health Organization (WHO) categorizes maternal deaths as direct, indirect, coincidental or late.

A *direct maternal death* is caused by an obstetric complication during pregnancy, labour or the puerperium. *An indirect death* is due to a condition or disease, that may or may not have been pre-existing, that is exacerbated by pregnancy. A *coincidental death* occurs during pregnancy or the puerperium but is unrelated to pregnancy. A *late death* is one which occurs between 42 days and 1 year after the pregnancy ended and is due to either direct or indirect causes. Table 67.1 summarizes the causes of maternal deaths since 2012.

The MBRRACE-UK report calculates Maternal Mortality Rate (MMR) by using the number of maternities as the denominator (birth at or beyond 24 weeks) per 100 000 maternities. Internationally the MMR uses live births as the denominator.

67.2 Salient Findings of 'The Women Who Died' (2014–16) Report [1]

Overall, 259 women died in 2014–16 during or within 42 days of the end of pregnancy (direct, indirect and coincidental causes) in the UK. The deaths of 34 of these women were classified as coincidental. The maternal death rate was 9.78 per 100 000 maternities (95% confidence interval (CI) 8.54–11.14).

Of the 225 women who died from direct and indirect causes in 2014–16, 28% (64 women) were still pregnant at the time of their death and of these women, 63% were ≤20 weeks' gestation.

The risk of maternal death in 2014–16 was almost fivefold higher among women from black ethnic minority backgrounds compared with white women (risk ratio (RR) 4.93, 95% CI 3.27–7.26). Women from Asian backgrounds were also at higher risk than white women (RR 1.81, 95% CI 1.16–2.73). A quarter of women who died in 2014–16 (24%) were born outside the UK. Sixteen per cent of women who died were known to social services, highlighting further the vulnerability of many of these women who died.

More than two thirds (68%) of the women who died in 2014–16 were known to have pre-existing medical problems, 24% were known to have pre-existing mental health problems, 8% had pre-existing cardiac problems and 37% of the women were obese.

In terms of the level of care, 26% of women, received the recommended level of care [3]. Of the 233 women whose case notes had sufficient information for an in-depth review, 28% were assessed to have received good care, but it also showed that for another 38% women, improvement in care may have made a difference to their outcome.

67.3 Salient Findings of 'The Previous Reports' [4–6]

There were 240 maternal deaths between 2013–15 in the UK and Ireland. In this triennium, 202 (84%) women died from direct and indirect causes and 38 (16%) deaths were classified as coincidental. The maternal death rate was 8.76 per 100 000 maternities (95% CI 7.59–10.05).

Between 2011 and 2013, there were 240 maternal deaths; 214 (89%) of these were due to either direct or indirect causes. The remaining 26 (11%) deaths were classified as coincidental. This is equivalent to a maternal death rate of 9.02 per 100 000 maternities (95% CI 7.85–10.31). This report showed a statistically significant reduction compared to a maternal death rate of 10.12 per 100 000 maternities reported between 2010 and 2012.

Between 2012 and 2014, 241 women died during or within 42 days of the end of the pregnancy in the UK. 200 women died

Table 67.1 A comparison of causes of maternal mortality, 2012–2016

Cause of death	2012–2014	2013–2015	2014–2016
	n	n	n
Direct deaths	**81**	**88**	**98**
Pregnancy-related infections – sepsis	7	10	11
Pre-eclampsia and eclampsia	2	3	6
Thrombosis and thromboembolism	20	26	32
Amniotic fluid embolism	16	8	9
Early pregnancy deaths	7	4	3
Haemorrhage	13	21	18
Anaesthesia	2	2	1
Psychiatric causes – suicides	14	12	16
Malignancy – direct	-	-	1
Unascertained – direct	-	2	1
Indirect	**119**	**114**	**127**
Cardiac disease	51	54	55
Indirect sepsis – influenza	1	1	2
Indirect sepsis–pneumonia/ others	14	3	6
Other indirect causes	23	26	26
Indirect neurological conditions	22	19	24
Psychiatric causes – drugs/alcohol/others	4	4	6
Indirect malignancies	4	7	8
Coincidental	**41**	**38**	**34**
Homicide	9	9	10
Other coincidental	32	29	24
Late deaths	323	326	286

from direct and indirect causes and 41 were classed as coincidental. In this triennium (2012–14), a maternal death rate of 8.54 per 100 000 maternities (95% CI 7.40–9.81) was reported.

There has been a statistically significant reduction (35%) in maternal mortality rates between 2003–05 and 2011–13. Maternal deaths due to direct causes continue to reduce but there has been no significant reduction in rates of indirect deaths since 2003 except deaths due to influenza.

The above data show that the overall maternal death rate has decreased despite incremental increase in the number of pregnancies since 2003. In addition, during this time there has been an increase in the number of women giving birth with risk factors such as raised maternal age, obesity and those born outside the UK.

All maternal deaths are reported, and local case reviews are held to ensure lessons are learnt for improving care. The Royal

College of Obstetricians and Gynaecologists (RCOG) regularly produces guidance, and local policies should be reviewed to ensure they are up to date and reflect new findings and recommendations.

67.4 Causes of Death

67.4.1 Direct Deaths

Maternal deaths from direct causes are unchanged with no significant change in the rates between 2009 to 2016. Thrombosis and thromboembolism continue to be the leading cause of direct deaths occurring within 42 days of the end of pregnancy, followed by deaths due to obstetric haemorrhage and deaths by suicide.

Thrombosis and thromboembolism were the leading cause of direct maternal death in the 1985–1987 triennial report. Since then, there has been a steady decline in MMR secondary to thromboembolic disease, essentially following the first publication of the RCOG Green-top guideline in 2004 and subsequent updates [7, 8]. The immediate positive impact of the implementation of this clinical guideline in routine clinical practice has not been sustained. It is likely that maternal obesity plays a significant role in making thrombosis and thromboembolism the leading cause of maternal death.

The maternal death rate from **pre-eclampsia and eclampsia** continues to be low. There was no statistically significant change in the rate of direct maternal deaths from any cause between 2009 and 2015. This is related to changes in management following updated guidance as the result of large randomized controlled trials.

Maternal suicide is the third largest cause of direct maternal deaths occurring during or within 42 days of the end of pregnancy. However, it remains the leading cause of direct deaths occurring within a year after the end of pregnancy.

67.4.1.1 Haemorrhage

Obstetric haemorrhage is the leading cause of maternal death globally. In both the UK and worldwide, rates of postpartum haemorrhage (PPH) are increasing. A PPH is defined as blood loss equal or greater than 500 mL following delivery. Major obstetric haemorrhage (MOH) is blood loss equal or greater than 2500 mL.

In the UK and Ireland, 22 women died from obstetric haemorrhage between 2013–15. The overall MMR was 0.88 (95% CI 0.55 to 1.33). Of note, 9 women died from haemorrhage in association with abnormal placentation, 8 of whom had placenta accreta, increta or percreta. In 2014–16, 18 women died of obstetric haemorrhage. The mortality rate was 0.78 (96% CI 0.46–1.24). There was a near doubling in the maternal death rate from haemorrhage between 2010–12 and 2013–15 (RR 1.99, 95% CI 0.96–4.92).

Anaemia is a risk factor for haemorrhage and therefore should be identified and investigated antenatally to allow haemoglobin to be optimized. A haemoglobin of 11.0 g/dL or less at booking or 10.5 g/dL or less at 28 weeks should be investigated and treated. Three of the women who died were anaemic antenatally; however, only one received iron therapy. In addition, risk groups such as Jehovah's Witnesses should be identified antenatally to allow appropriate planning for their care.

Intrapartum risk factors for haemorrhage such as uterine hyperstimulation should be avoided by appropriate use of oxytocics early. Almost half of the deaths from haemorrhage are due to uterine atony. Risk factors for PPH are listed in Table 67.2.

Messages for Improvement of Care

It is vital that the blood loss be accurately measured, as failure to recognize the seriousness of the blood loss occurred in more than half the women who died. Blood loss should be considered in context to the patient's size and the representative circulating volume they have lost. Regular observations should be recorded on the modified early obstetric warning system (MEOWS) chart. Abnormal observations should be escalated appropriately. Pregnant and postnatal woman may compensate for large blood loss very well prior to acute deterioration; therefore, normal observations in the presence of ongoing bleeding should not provide false reassurance.

An isolated haemoglobin result could be falsely reassuring and can cause delay in administrating fluid or blood products. Acid-base and lactate are much more accurate as an indicator of hypovolaemia and tissue hypoxia. Disordered coagulation is a late sign, and therefore a coagulopathy should be pre-empted with the administration of appropriate blood products.

Hysterectomy should be performed without delay if other medical and surgical management options are ineffective and considered early if blood products are refused or there has been a delay in diagnosis.

Retained placenta, once diagnosed, warrants close observations and prompt transfer to theatre when appropriate, as it can be associated with concealed bleeding and significant maternal deterioration.

When there has been a massive haemorrhage and the bleeding is ongoing, or there are clinical concerns, then a major obstetric haemorrhage call (MOH) should be activated.

Clear documentation in the notes should be undertaken after an informed discussion with women who are Jehovah's Witnesses about which fractions of blood products are acceptable.

The RCOG has issued excellent guidance on PPH management [9].

67.4.1.2 Sepsis

In 2013–15, 10 women died from pregnancy-related infections (direct cause) and 4 women died from indirect sepsis (influenza,

Table 67.2 Risk factors for postpartum haemorrhage

Antenatal risk factors	Approximate odds ratio	Intrapartum risk factors	Approximate odds ratio
Placental praevia	12	Emergency caesarean section	4
Multiple pregnancy	5	Retained placenta	5
Pre-eclampsia/gestation hypertension	4	Mediolateral episiotomy	5
Previous PPH	3	Induction of labour	2
Anaemia	2	Elective caesarean section	2
Obesity	2	Operative vaginal delivery	2

pneumonia and others). In 2014–15, 11 women died from pregnancy-related infections (direct cause) and 8 women died from indirect sepsis (influenza, pneumonia and others).

Between 2009 and 2012, 83 women died of sepsis, and less than a quarter of these were due to genital tract sepsis, which was a marked reduction from the previous report. Genital tract sepsis deaths were classed as direct deaths, whilst other infective causes were classified as indirect. Group A streptococcus (GAS) was the most significant organism in genital tract sepsis. Deaths occurred most commonly in the postnatal period (82%). There was a further reduction in deaths due to genital tract sepsis in the 2011–13 report. In the 2012–14 report, seven maternal deaths were attributed to sepsis.

The *influenza A/H1N1 pandemic* occurred during the time of the 2009–12 report. One in 11 of all maternal deaths were due to influenza. Twenty-nine deaths occurred secondary to influenza. Some of these occurred prior to immunization; however, over half were women who had not received a vaccine despite the introduction of the immunization campaign. All deaths after the introduction of the vaccine were in non-vaccinated women. There was a statistically significantly decrease in maternal deaths in 2011–13 due to influenza when compared with 2009–10. This may be due to a low level of influenza activity.

It has been recommended that the vaccine should be offered routinely to all pregnant women and health professionals.

Sepsis is defined as features of systemic inflammatory responses (SIRs) associated with infection or suspected infection. The addition of a single organ dysfunction, hypotension or lactic acidosis signifies the development of severe sepsis. Persistent hypotension despite adequate fluid resuscitation signifies the onset of septic shock. The SIRs criteria have been modified to consider the impact of pregnancy on physiology.

In general, pregnant women are young and fit and therefore can compensate for widespread sepsis. Thus, they often present in an advanced state of sepsis. Sepsis may present with many different symptoms. In particular, upper respiratory tract symptoms should raise concern regarding a possible GAS or influenza infection. All women attending community or hospital settings should have a detailed history and examination performed. Performing a set of basic observations in any unwell women is essential. Any abnormal results should trigger a thorough review. In the women who died, a lack of basic observations was noted in several cases, particularly during the postnatal period.

Sepsis in pregnant or postnatal women can progress quickly with disastrous consequences. Early detection and rapid treatment of sepsis has been shown to reduce morbidity and mortality associated with sepsis. The introduction of the Surviving Sepsis Campaign raised awareness of the importance of sepsis. Several guidelines on the management of sepsis and in particular GAS in maternity settings as well as RCOG guidance on bacterial sepsis related to pregnancy have been produced [10, 11].

Table 67.3 Care Bundle – Sepsis 6

Give high-flow oxygen	Take blood cultures	Administer IV antibiotics
Administer IV fluid bolus	Take bloods including lactate	Monitor urine output

A care bundle (Sepsis 6; see Table 67.3) has been introduced to ensure vital treatment is administered within 1 hour. Sepsis 6 involves administration of high-flow oxygen, rapid intravenous (IV) fluid resuscitation and appropriate IV antibiotic, monitoring of urine output, measurement of serum lactate, FBP and obtaining blood cultures. All of these should be achieved within 1 hour of identifying a woman as septic. For every hour that antibiotic treatment is delayed, mortality increases by 8%. Antibiotic choice should be focused on suspected source of infection and local policy. If a woman does not respond to initial antibiotics, advice should be obtained from a microbiologist or infectious disease physician.

Following immediate management, women require a consultant review and a detailed ongoing plan. Response to treatment should be assessed to ensure deterioration is not missed. Women should be cared for in a high-dependency area as a minimum. Access to critical care should be readily available to allow appropriate escalation and optimal care. Pregnant women have a much higher chance of requiring hospital admission and admission to intensive treatment unit (ITU) compared with the general population. Appropriate imaging to identify the source of sepsis should be performed and surgical intervention considered.

In a pregnant woman with signs of influenza, anti-viral treatment should be commenced as soon as possible. The majority of women who died did not receive timely treatment with anti-viral medication.

67.4.1.3 Thrombosis and Thromboembolism

All the recent reports (2010–12, 2011–13, 2012–14 and 2014–16) cite venous thromboembolism (VTE) as the leading cause of direct maternal death. The relative risk of VTE is increased in both pregnancy (4–6 times) and is even higher during the postpartum period. However, the overall absolute risk of a VTE in pregnancy or the postpartum period is 1 in 1000.

The RCOG have produced guidance for the prevention and the acute management of VTE [7, 8].

Between 2009 and 2013, there were 64 maternal deaths due to VTE. Forty-eight of these deaths were due to VTE during pregnancy or in the first 6 weeks postpartum. This included 43 women who died of a pulmonary embolism (PE) and 5 women who died of a cerebral vein thrombosis. In addition, 13 women died of a PE between 6 weeks and 6 months postnatally. There were a further 3 late deaths due to cerebral vein thrombosis.

Of the 48 deaths due to VTE during pregnancy or in the first 6 weeks postpartum during 2012–14, 24 deaths (50%) occurred antenatally and 24 (50%) occurred postnatally. In the antenatal group, 50% of these were in the first trimester and 25% in both the second and third trimesters. Twelve of these women died before their booking appointment. In the postnatal group, 12 women (50%) had been delivered by caesarean section, 10 had vaginal deliveries and 2 had surgical procedures early in pregnancy. Of these 48 women, 83% had one or more identifiable risk factors for VTE.

In 2013–15 and 2014–16, 26 (95% CI 0.74–1.65) and 32 (95% CI 0.95–1.96) women died due to known thrombosis and thromboembolic causes, respectively.

Risk factors for VTE are summarized in Table 67.4.

During antenatal risk assessment, women who stopped smoking immediately prior to pregnancy or in early pregnancy should be considered as smokers.

At the booking visit women should be assessed for VTE risks. Risk assessment should be repeated throughout pregnancy, especially if a woman is admitted to hospital. Subsequently, a further assessment should be done either during intrapartum or immediately postpartum and prior to discharge. The dose of thromboprophylaxis is weight dependent and obese women in particular should be weighed again prior to discharge. Patients should be offered information leaflets describing the prevention, signs and symptoms as well as diagnosis and treatment of venous thromboembolism.

Plans for postnatal thromboprophylaxis should be clearly documented in the antenatal notes and women should be informed of these recommendations. Postnatal women should receive their first dose of low molecular weight heparin (LMWH) within 6–8 hours of delivery if there are no contraindications. This allows for a minimum of 4 hours after regional anaesthesia. Following operative deliveries, the timing of thromboprophylaxis administration should be discussed in the WHO surgical safety checklist. If there are contraindications to LMWH administration, mechanical methods and intermittent pneumatic compression devices should be used to reduce VTE risk until it is safe to give LMWH. Anti-embolism stockings need to be appropriately fitted. In addition, women should be kept hydrated and

encouraged to mobilise as soon as possible. In the current Green-top Guideline 37a, all women with a body mass index (BMI) ≥40 should receive postnatal thromboprophylaxis, irrespective of mode of delivery.

At the time of discharge from secondary care women should be provided with the entire course of LMWH required. This reduces any barriers to accessing an ongoing prescription from their GP. The community midwife should further check the prescription in the community to ensure there is compliance and the duration of treatment is adequate.

Women attending the emergency department who are pregnant or postpartum should be discussed with the obstetric team to ensure they receive appropriate LMWH prophylaxis or undergo investigation and treatments for possible venous thromboembolism.

There should be a high clinical suspicion of VTE in pregnancy or the puerperium with a low threshold for investigations. Venous thromboembolism should be considered even if women are receiving the appropriate dose of LMWH thromboprophylaxis or even treatment dose. Pregnancy, the immediate postpartum period and following a caesarean section are not absolute contraindications to thrombolysis.

Risk scoring such as the Wells Score should not be used in pregnancy. However, if a D-dimer is performed, a very high result should not be presumed to just be related to pregnancy. In addition, a negative D-dimer should not be relied on in pregnancy to exclude a DVT.

Women on long-term anticoagulation or with medical comorbidities should receive pre-pregnancy counselling regarding the need for thromboprophylaxis or treatment dose LMWH in pregnancy.

Postnatal prescription for the combined oral contraceptive should consider all risk factors. The current Medical Eligibility Criteria for Contraceptive Use (UKMEC) considers only one risk factor at a time and therefore should be used with caution and the whole clinical picture assessed.

Cerebral venous thrombosis (CVT) should be considered when a maternity patient presents with a headache. In addition, CVT should be included in the differential diagnosis of a patient with seizures, despite eclampsia being the most likely cause. To diagnose a CVT women require magnetic resonance imaging (MRI) or computed tomography (CT) venogram rather than a plain CT brain.

67.4.1.4 Hypertensive Disorders of Pregnancy

The Confidential Enquiries into Maternal Death has grouped the following into one group as hypertensive disorders of pregnancy:

> Eclampsia; pre-eclampsia; haemolysis, elevated liver enzymes, low platelet syndrome (HELLP); elevated liver enzymes, low platelet syndrome (ELLP); and liver disorders associated with pregnancy (acute fatty liver of pregnancy, AFLP).

There has been a significant decrease in the mortality rate from hypertensive disorders of pregnancy in the period between 2009–11 and 2012–14. In the UK and Ireland, 11 women died between 2009 and 2011 (95% CI 0.21–0.76) whereas

Table 67.4 Risk factors for VTE

Antenatal risk factors		Intrapartum/ postnatal risk factors
Previous VTE	Co-morbidities	Immobility or dehydration
Thrombophilia	Family history	Instrumental delivery
Obesity	Pre-eclampsia	Prolonged labour >24 hours
Parity 3 or more	Age over 35 years	PPH
Smoking	Hyperemesis	Caesarean section
Multiple pregnancy	Surgical procedure in pregnancy	Current systemic infection

only 3 women died between 2012 and 2014 (95% CI 0.02–0.34). Six women died in 2014–16 due to hypertensive causes as per the latest report (95% CI 0.10–0.57), and intracranial haemorrhage was the most common cause of death followed by hepatic complications. Reassuringly, no women died in relation to inappropriate fluid management (pulmonary oedema and renal failure).

Although deaths from the hypertensive disorders of pregnancy have significantly reduced, the assessors felt that improvements in care may have made a difference to outcome for a majority of the women who died. Most recommendations made in the report to improve outcomes are in keeping with the NICE guideline [12].

67.4.1.5 Anaesthesia

In the 2009–11 and 2012–14 reports, three and two deaths, respectively, were attributed to anaesthetic causes. In the UK and Ireland, there were 2 women who died directly from complications of anaesthesia between 2013 and 2015. In 2014–16, one death was attributed to anaesthetic causes. Deaths due to anaesthesia have reduced significantly over the last few decades. Pregnant women are high-risk anaesthetic candidates and therefore anaesthetic staff should be capable of managing airway complications such as failed intubation. Prolonged hypoventilation during or following general anaesthesia resulted in the death of two women. Inadequate ventilation may occur due to accidental intubation of the oesophagus or bronchospasm. Anaesthetists should be confident to manage these complications, gaining experience through regular airway drills.

Themes for Improvement of Care

Local anaesthetic toxicity should also be considered in the differential diagnosis in an unwell or collapsed woman. Intralipids should be available for treatment of intravenous local anaesthetic toxicity.

Anaesthetic complications such as subdural haematoma and cerebral venous sinus thrombosis following dural puncture should be considered in women with a persistent headache.

Accidental dural tap during epidural insertion resulted in two deaths. These women died a few weeks postnatally and did not have follow-up in place. They failed to receive appropriate imaging and specialist referral in a timely manner. Subdural haematoma is a recognized complication of dural puncture. Cerebral venous sinus thrombosis is also a recognized postpartum cause of headache. These should be considered in the differential diagnosis of headache in a postnatal woman.

All patients should receive routine post-anaesthetic monitoring. Use of early warning scoring sheets is useful, and abnormal observations should be acted upon. Effective teamwork with clear and concise communication is essential in emergency situations.

Confirmation of a cardiac arrest by assessment of breathing and pulse by trained healthcare professionals is not always accurate, and hence a delay in commencing cardiopulmonary resuscitation (CPR) is likely to adversely affect survival, and

should be avoided. Even if a patient is not in cardiac arrest, chest compressions are unlikely to be harmful.

After induction of anaesthesia, despite the pregnant woman being on a lateral tilt, if severe hypotension ensues, aortocaval compression should be suspected. The woman should be put into left lateral position if the hypotension is refractory to conservative measures.

Women should be seen by an obstetrician and anaesthetist at a joint antenatal clinic if they are predicted to have significant airway problems. If rapid sequence induction is considered inappropriate, a clear management plan should be agreed antenatally.

Pregnant women with a booking BMI $\geq$40 kg/m^2 are at a high risk of difficulties with venous access and regional or general anaesthesia. An anaesthetic management plan for labour and delivery should be documented in the medical records after an antenatal anaesthetic review.

67.4.1.6 Amniotic Fluid Embolism (AFE)

Amniotic fluid embolism (AFE) occurs when amniotic fluid or other pregnancy-related debris enters the maternal circulation and causes a severe allergic reaction. It usually presents with maternal collapse. It is a clinical diagnosis following exclusion of other causes. The incidence of AFE is 1 in 50 000 women giving birth. It is associated with a significant mortality rate. The risk factors are summarized in Table 67.5.

There were 7 deaths during the period of the 2009–11 report and 16 deaths attributed to AFE during the 2012–14 report, with a mortality rate of 0.36 (95% CI 0.16–0.68) between 2014 and 2016.

Themes for Improvement of Care

Following maternal collapse, advanced life support should be commenced immediately, and all possible causes considered. In the event of a maternal cardiac arrest in women over 20 weeks' gestation, a perimortem caesarean section should be achieved within 5 minutes to improve maternal outcome.

Major obstetric haemorrhage protocol should be activated when the decision is made for a perimortem caesarean or in a postnatal woman after 4 minutes of CPR. Definitive surgical management should not be delayed, and blood products should be given early and in appropriate quantities.

All maternity staff should be up to date and competent with resuscitation and advanced life support, as well as managing an MOH.

Uterine hyperstimulation following induced labour was frequently identified among the women who died from haemorrhage or amniotic fluid embolism. Stimulating or augmenting uterine contractions should be done in accordance with current guidance and paying particular attention to avoiding

Table 67.5 Risk factors for AFE

Induction of labour	Advanced maternal age
Uterine hyperstimulation	Pre-eclampsia
Polyhydramnios	Operative delivery

uterine tachysystole or hyperstimulation. Lower dosages of oxytocics should be used in women with a previous uterine scar.

67.4.2 Indirect Deaths

Indirect causes still remain the major cause of (56%) maternal deaths in the UK. *Cardiac disease* remains the leading cause of indirect maternal death during or up to 6 weeks after the end of pregnancy with a rate of 2.34 per 100 000 maternities (95% CI 1.76–3.06) in 2013–15, and 2.39 per 100 000 maternities (95% CI 1.80–3.11) in 2014–16.

Deaths from *neurological causes* were the second most frequent cause of indirect maternal death.

There has been a decrease in indirect maternal mortality due to influenza deaths and deaths from indirect causes of maternal sepsis since 2012.

The constant nature of indirect maternal deaths highlights the need for specialist training in maternal medicine across several specialities, both in primary and secondary care.

67.4.2.1 Cardiac Disease

Cardiac disease has been the leading cause of overall maternal mortality in the UK since the 2000–02 triennium. Deaths from cardiac disease have increased and this has been attributed to increasing maternal age, increasing levels of obesity, and more precise recognition of cardiac pathology by pathologists at autopsy.

Between 2009 and 2014, 189 women died from heart disease associated with or aggravated by pregnancy. Of these, 108 occurred during pregnancy or within 42 days of delivery. The deaths of 153 women from cardiac disease were reviewed in detail. The following causes of deaths were identified in this group:

- Sudden arrhythmic cardiac death with a normal heart (SADS) was the most common cause of death (35%).
- Ischaemia was the next most common cause (22%).
- Seventy-seven per cent were not known to have pre-existing cardiac problems.

There is a need for all clinicians to be alert to the possibility of undiagnosed cardiac disease.

Key Messages Regarding Cardiac Deaths

Pre-Pregnancy Counselling – – Pre-pregnancy counselling should be available both within the paediatric cardiology transition service and to women of childbearing age with known cardiac disease, including the provision of appropriate contraceptive advice.

Cardiac Risk Factors –– A robust mechanism should be in place to identify women with cardiac risk factors or at higher risk of developing cardiac disease in pregnancy:

> The obese, those who smoke or who have existing hypertension and/or diabetes, a family history of heart disease and those over the age of 35 should have a cardiac assessment prior to receiving assisted reproductive technology or other infertility treatment.

Multidisciplinary Working –– Lack of joint obstetric and cardiac services jeopardizes multidisciplinary working and communication. Measures such as joint obstetric cardiac clinics, multidisciplinary care plans, copying letters to the woman and all clinicians involved in her care, as well as staff from all specialties writing in the woman's handheld notes may mitigate inadequate communication between specialists. Where time-dependent intervention is needed, clinicians should make direct contact with each other. Early involvement of senior clinicians from the obstetric and cardiology multidisciplinary team is important, particularly if she presents to the Emergency Department.

Delay in Diagnosis –– A raised respiratory rate, chest pain, persistent tachycardia and orthopnoea are important signs and symptoms that should always be fully investigated. All consultant-led maternity units should have ready access to an electrocardiogram (ECG) machine and someone who can interpret ECGs. Similarly, echocardiography should be available 7 days a week.

Medication and Investigation –– Pink frothy sputum is very suggestive of pulmonary oedema and should be investigated and treated accordingly.

Women should not be denied relevant investigations or treatments for life-threatening conditions, simply because they are pregnant or breastfeeding.

Angiotensin-converting enzyme (ACE) inhibitors are a mainstay of the management of patients with heart failure and should be restarted in the early postpartum period. They are safe to use when breastfeeding.

Important investigations such as CT scans should not be withheld because a woman is pregnant or breastfeeding or because of fears of the long-term increase in risk of breast cancer.

Perimortem Caesarean Section –– Perimortem caesarean section is an important part of the resuscitation of a pregnant woman. Ambulance crews should not delay this by prolonged attempts at resuscitation in the community before transferring the woman to hospital. The Joint Royal Colleges Ambulance Liaison Committee Guidelines (Joint Royal Colleges Ambulance Liaison Committee and Association of Ambulance Chief Executives 2016) state that there should be a time-critical transfer as soon as ventilation is achieved, and CPR commenced.

Specific Cardiac Diseases – Key Messages

Cardiac Ischaemic Disease ––
- consider myocardial ischaemia in any woman presenting with chest pain, particularly if it is associated with breathlessness, feeling faint, sweating and/or nausea.
- If an acute coronary syndrome is excluded, other causes for chest pain should be considered including aortic dissection or pulmonary embolism.
- It should be noted that ECG changes and elevated troponin levels can be associated with both these conditions.

- A normal ECG and/or a negative troponin does not exclude the diagnosis of an acute coronary syndrome.

Sudden Arrhythmic Cardiac Death with a Morphologically Normal Heart (SADS/MNH) --
- SADS/MNH is an emerging entity in which people (usually under 50 years of age) collapse from cardiac arrest; some may survive with prompt resuscitation.
- No gross or histopathological abnormality of the heart (or any other organ) is identified to account for their death.
- Drug screens for cardioactive drugs are negative.
- These deaths are presumed to be arrhythmic and the majority result from a malignant ventricular arrhythmia and are the end result of a complex interaction between an abnormal cardiac substrate and emotional, environmental or physiological triggers.
- Women should be asked at booking whether a close relative has died from their heart stopping unexpectedly due to an abnormal rhythm. There is an immediate need to determine the cardiac rhythm at cardiac arrest and attempt defibrillation as soon as possible for women in cardiac arrest with a shockable rhythm.
- All women who die from sudden cardiac arrest and who have a morphologically normal heart should have molecular studies at post-mortem with the potential for family screening.

Valvular Heart Disease -- All women of childbearing age referred for a valve operation before pregnancy should receive pre-pregnancy counselling by a team (cardiologist, obstetrician and relevant others) with expertise in managing patients with valvular heart disease during pregnancy about the risks and benefits of all options for operative interventions, including mechanical prosthesis, bioprosthesis and valve repair.
- Women with prosthetic valves in pregnancy are at extremely high risk and should be referred to specialist centres at the earliest opportunity. They need expert obstetric, haematology, cardiology and anaesthetic input.
- Onset of new cardiorespiratory symptoms and/or absence of valve clicks in women with prosthetic heart valves should prompt careful echocardiography and early review by a senior cardiologist to exclude the possibility of valve thrombosis.

Aortic Dissection -- Any woman presenting with chest pain which is severe enough to require opiate analgesia, justifies further investigations for a definite diagnosis. When aortic dissection occurs in a young person, the underlying diagnosis should be assumed to be an inherited aortopathy, with a need for family screening until proven otherwise. Future sudden deaths amongst relatives may then be prevented.

67.4.2.2 Neurological Conditions

One per cent of the UK population have **epilepsy**, with a significant number being women in their reproductive years. The major cause of death in pregnant or postnatal women with epilepsy is sudden unexpected death in epilepsy (SUDEP). The postpartum period is thought to be at high risk

of SUDEP. Women should be advised appropriately, in particular regarding not bathing or sleeping alone.

All women with epilepsy should have pre-conception counselling so that medications are reviewed and the safest regime is in place. Close liaison with epilepsy specialists, in particular nurse specialists should be routine and referral should be prompt.

Fourteen deaths were caused by seizures or epilepsy-related events in 2012–14. Twelve of these deaths were due to SUDEP. There were a further 12 late maternal deaths attributed to epilepsy. Of the women who died, few had pre-conception counselling and no input antenatally from epilepsy specialists. In addition, there was a general lack of understanding that women with epilepsy are high-risk patients. For example, women should not be accommodated in single rooms due to the increased risk of SUDEP.

Following the publication of the MBRRACE-UK 2014 report, the RCOG have published Green-top Guideline *Epilepsy in Pregnancy* [13] to standardize care and ensure effective multidisciplinary input.

Intracranial haemorrhage caused the death of 26 women during the 2012–14 report period. These women presented with severe headaches progressing to a rapid deterioration or with sudden collapse.

Full neurological examination should be performed in pregnant or postnatal women with neurological symptoms and should include examination for neck stiffness. Pregnancy should not alter the management of a suspected or confirmed stroke, this should be in a specialist hyperacute stroke unit. In addition, pregnancy or the postpartum period are not absolute contraindications for lifesaving thrombolytic procedures such as thrombolysis.

67.4.2.3 Medical Conditions/Complications

An increasing number of women with co-morbidities are becoming pregnant. It is vital that these women receive pre-conception counselling by experienced staff. Antenatal care should be coordinated in a multidisciplinary clinic to improve continuity and communication including senior physicians to agree on an individualized care plan. Coordination of care in women with pre-existing medical conditions should be the responsibility of one professional to ensure continuity and optimal communication between disciplines.

Other than deaths attributable to H1N1 influenza, there were 10 deaths during the 2013–15 period due to **respiratory causes**. The most common cause is *asthma*, accounting for 3 of these deaths. It is essential that women are counselled regarding the safety of asthma medications throughout pregnancy and the importance of being compliant with treatment. There should be a low threshold for admission and senior review in pregnant women with an exacerbation of asthma. Two women died of *cystic fibrosis*. The remaining deaths were related to rare conditions, and there was a lack of communication between specialties and failure to recognize the severity of the condition. Women with *severe lung disease* should be screened for pulmonary hypertension prior to pregnancy and counselled regarding the significant risks of becoming pregnant with this condition. Acute respiratory compromise is a medical emergency and patients should be reviewed urgently by a physician and anaesthetist.

Six of the women who died had type 1 **diabetes mellitus** (DM). Four of these women had long-standing DM with poor control pre-pregnancy. They engaged with the joint antenatal clinic but had difficulty gaining good glycaemic control. Women with DM should be made aware of the increased risk of hypoglycaemia and their families should be educated about the management of hypoglycaemia.

Liver disease resulted in the death of 5 women. Two of these women had fulminant liver failure, including one case associated with accidental paracetamol overdose. Two women died of a phaeochromocytoma. The diagnosis was not considered until late in their care. It should be considered in women with atypical severe hypertension.

Severe hyperemesis with thyrotoxicosis caused 2 deaths. One of the patients was poorly managed with failure to correct significant hypokalaemia or administer antiemetics.

67.4.2.4 Maternal Mental Health

Puerperium is the time when women are at the highest risk of new-onset severe mental illness. Pre-existing mental health problems may recur or deteriorate postnatally. Women with a history of bipolar affective disorder or schizophrenia are at the highest risk of a recurrent illness postpartum. There is evidence of a clear link between bipolar affective disorder and postpartum psychosis.

At booking, routine enquiry should be done about any history of any previous or current mental health problems. General practitioners should be aware of a woman's pregnancy to allow full information to be shared regarding a previous history of mental health problems. Women should be managed in specialist perinatal mental health services; however, these are not widely accessible throughout the UK and Ireland.

Pregnant or postnatal women with red flag symptoms (see Table 67.6) should have early senior input in their assessment and management. Acute assessment should be by teams with experience and training in perinatal mental health conditions with an understanding of their potential for rapid deterioration. Perinatal mental healthcare is best delivered within a network that provides specialist multidisciplinary input with clear referral and management protocols. Each perinatal mental health network should have designated inpatient services to allow admission of both mother and baby. Staff should be experienced in perinatal mental healthcare as well as be able to provide care for the babies. There should be access to a full range of therapeutic services and good integration with community mental health services.

Table 67.6 Perinatal mental health red flag symptoms

Recent significant change in mental state or emergence of new symptoms

New thoughts or acts of violent self-harm

New and persistent expressions of incompetency as a mother or estrangement from the infant

Risk Identification in Mental Illness

Seventy-one women died by suicide during pregnancy or up to one year after pregnancy in 2014–16 in the UK and Ireland, a mortality rate of 2.9 per 100 000 maternities (95% CI 2.2–3.6).

The first year after delivery has the highest risk of suicide compared to the antenatal period (88% vs. 12%). Onset of severe mental illness can be sudden with rapid deterioration. The onset of illness for the majority of women occurred in the weeks or months before their deaths. It is essential that any red flag symptoms are taken seriously and acted upon. In addition, previous presentations should be considered to assess if there is a pattern of evolving concern. Almost 1 in 5 of the women who committed suicide had new thoughts or acts of violent self-harm.

In some of the deaths there was no consideration of inpatient admission despite clear evidence of significant risk. This was even in the context of some women requesting admission. Admission to a mother and baby unit (MBU) should be considered for women with any of the following:

- A rapidly changing mental state
- Suicidal ideation
- Feelings of guilt or hopelessness
- Significant estrangement from their baby
- New or persistent beliefs of inadequacy as a mother
- Evidence of psychosis

Following discharge from a MBU, women remain at high risk and a comprehensive plan should be made for their ongoing care.

When there are child safeguarding concerns and a child is removed from the mother's care, it is vital that the increased risk to the mother's mental health is recognized. In addition, women who experience loss through stillbirth, neonatal death or miscarriage are increasingly vulnerable and require extra support.

Any concerns expressed by family members regarding the mental health of a woman should be taken seriously and acted upon. Family members may require education regarding mental illness to allow a better understanding of the seriousness of the illness and thus better support for the woman.

The women whose deaths were due to *substance misuse* were more likely to be from socially deprived backgrounds compared to those who died from suicide. In addition, 50% of the women booked late in pregnancy and were less likely to receive the minimum recommended levels of antenatal care. They tended to abuse multiple substances rather than alcohol alone. All but one of the women who died due to substance misuse was identified during pregnancy. All women should be asked at booking about the use of drugs or alcohol. Women identified to have substance misuse problems should be referred for specialist advice and treatment as well as offered brief interventions. Commitment to a methadone programme improves outcomes for the baby. In contrast, detoxification programmes are of little benefit and may increase risks to the baby.

Women with multiple medical and social factors may be engaged with many services. It is essential that each of these services communicate and there is a coordinated care plan for all to follow. The National Institute for Health and Care Excellence (NICE) guideline on pregnancy and complex social factors discusses management of women in pregnancy with substance misuse but does not give guidance for the postnatal period [14].

Clear communication between primary and secondary services is essential for women with a history of mental health illness. A booking notification of pregnancy should be sent to the GP and, in response, the GP should send a summary of the woman's medical history. If a woman is already known to mental health services, they should be informed of her pregnancy.

All deaths due to psychiatric causes during pregnancy or in the first postnatal year should be fully reviewed by all agencies that cared for the woman. The findings should be publicized so that lessons can be learnt from their deaths to improve future care given to pregnant and postnatal women with mental health problems.

67.4.2.5 Cancer in Pregnancy or the Puerperium

Diagnosis of cancer in pregnancy is rare with incidence varying between 1 in 1000 and 2 in 10 000 maternities worldwide. Most cancers do not directly affect fetal growth and therefore fetal outcomes should be good if inappropriate preterm iatrogenic delivery is avoided. Evidence is limited for long-term outcomes of fetal exposure to chemotherapy; however, short-term data are reassuring. This topic has been covered in other chapters (72–75).

There are only a few guidelines in the UK to guide management of cancer in pregnancy. Therefore, care is usually guided by expert opinion within a multidisciplinary team, resulting in variation in the treatment of cancer in pregnancy. The RCOG has produced a Green-top guideline on pregnancy and breast cancer [15].

Pregnant women with suspected cancer should be investigated and treated in the same way as non-pregnant women with caution of any specific risks to the fetus. Radiological investigations and treatment should not be inappropriately delayed. Care should be multidisciplinary, with a clear lead clinician, for pregnant women with a new diagnosis of cancer or a previous cancer.

Symptoms in pregnancy thought to be due to 'common' pregnancy causes should be further investigated if women present repeatedly or require increasing levels of opiate analgesia. A full neurological examination including fundoscopy should be performed in women presenting with headaches.

A diagnosis of malignancy within 6 months of becoming pregnant is a significant risk factor for venous thromboembolism. Guidance should be followed for thromboprophylaxis antenatally and postnatally.

It is possible for metastases to affect the placenta with rare transplacental spread to the fetus. This is most commonly seen with a malignant melanoma. In women with known or suspected metastatic disease, the placenta should be sent for urgent histopathology.

67.4.2.6 Homicide and Domestic Abuse

Women who are pregnant or in the puerperium are at an increased risk of domestic abuse and homicide. Domestic violence first begins in pregnancy for a third of all women who experience domestic violence. The women's partner is the most common offender.

Women who are being domestically abused may be at a higher risk of this during pregnancy and suffer from adverse pregnancy outcomes. These include low birthweight babies, preterm labour, antepartum haemorrhage and stillbirth.

Women should be asked routinely if they have experienced domestic abuse. Information about support services available should be displayed in appropriate places. This information should also be provided in the maternity handheld notes and at booking.

Risk factors for domestic abuse include alcohol abuse by one or both partners, previous sexual or physical abuse, young age and having had children from a previous relationship.

A woman should be considered high risk if she has a history of domestic violence. Staff caring for maternity patients should have basic training to allow them to confidently identify signs of domestic abuse and be aware of the pathway of referral and escalation. Women who experience domestic abuse should have a named midwife and receive the majority of their antenatal care from this person. There must be good communication between different agencies involved in the care of these women to allow coordinated care. There is a lack of evidence about interventions that could prevent or reduce domestic abuse against pregnant women.

Pregnant and postnatal women with repeated attendances to the Emergency Department or unusual injuries should be discussed with maternity staff and their GP. Women should also be asked again about domestic abuse, even if this has previously been done.

Female genital mutilation (FGM) is also considered as a form of domestic abuse and is associated with obstetric complications. Female genital mutilation was not considered a contributory factor in the death of any women reviewed in this report, including those who were murdered.

Between 2009 and 2013, 36 women were murdered during pregnancy or up to 1 year postnatal. This is a homicide rate of 0.97 per 100 000 maternities. In 2014–16, 10 homicides were recorded with an MMR of 0.43 (95% CI 0.21–0.80).

A third of the women had been victims of domestic abuse but did not have a history documented of this during their antenatal care. It was unclear whether they had been given adequate opportunity to disclose this information in confidence. A professional interpreter rather than a family member or friend should be used if required.

A multiagency *domestic homicide review* should be performed to assess the care of any woman murdered by her partner or a family member during pregnancy or up to 1 year afterwards to allow a full assessment.

67.4.3 Late Maternal Deaths

Late maternal deaths are those due to direct or indirect causes occurring between 42 days and 1 year after the end of the pregnancy. In 2014–16, there were 286 late maternal deaths, representing an MMR of 12.4 per 100 000 maternities (95% CI 11.0–14.0). This represents a 12% reduction compared to the triennium of 2011–13. Malignancy and maternal suicides represent an important cause of death in this group of women.

Maternal mortality rate was significantly increased in women aged over 35 years, reflecting age-related trends in the general female population. The majority of women who had late maternal deaths had at least one medical or mental health condition or a social factor, in addition to the cause of death, which complicated their care. Recognizing these conditions pre-pregnancy allows discussion of the increased risk of complications in pregnancy and the potential for deterioration of any pre-existing medical conditions. This is especially relevant among women seeking infertility treatment.

A full history at booking will allow identification of any risk factors and time for referral to necessary specialists. There should be dynamic, ongoing risk assessment during pregnancy to allow detection of any evolving problems. There should be individualized care if women are unable to attend routine antenatal care due to complex social issues. Often women have multiple medical morbidities and social factors requiring input from several agencies. Care by the various agencies should be coordinated to make services as accessible to the woman as possible. A named individual must take overall responsibility for coordinating the woman's care.

The risk factors for maternal death are summarized in Table 67.7.

During any hospital admission if a woman requires input from various specialties, it may be more appropriate for her to remain in one clinical area with input from the required specialties rather than repeatedly transferring the patient for better continuity of care. This should involve input from senior staff and good communication between the hospital teams, ideally using a structured communication tool.

A full summary of the maternity care should be completed in a timely manner by a senior obstetrician and sent to the GP after discharge from maternity services. There should be a clearly documented plan of the ongoing care required of these women, highlighting their specific medical or social needs.

67.4.4 Early Pregnancy Care

Early pregnancy complications (all types of miscarriages, ectopic pregnancies, trophoblastic disease) account for the largest

Table 67.7 Risk factors for maternal deaths

Age over 35 years	Substance misuse	Medical co-morbidities
Social deprivation	Alcohol dependency	Previous pregnancy complications
Obesity	Mental health problems	Domestic abuse

proportion of emergency work performed in gynaecology departments throughout the UK.

In 2009–14, 191 women died at less than 24 weeks' gestation in the UK and Ireland whilst still pregnant or after their pregnancy ended at less than 24 weeks. Twelve of these women died from early pregnancy-associated causes (nine died as a direct result of an ectopic pregnancy and three died from complications associated with termination or attempted termination of pregnancy). The assessors concluded that 7 of the 12 women received suboptimal care.

In 2014–16, the deaths of three women were classified as being early pregnancy deaths.

67.4.4.1 Lessons for Early Pregnancy Care

- Women of reproductive age who present with collapse or shock, in whom a pulmonary embolism is suspected, should have a Focused Assessment with Sonography in Trauma (FAST) units, and a scan should be performed to exclude intra-abdominal bleeding from a ruptured ectopic pregnancy.
- In any woman of reproductive age who presents with collapse, acute abdominal/pelvic pain or gastrointestinal symptoms, particularly diarrhoea, vomiting and dizziness, a diagnosis of ectopic pregnancy should be considered by performing a urine pregnancy test at the bedside.
- Providers and commissioners of care must ensure that there are safe pathways of transfer of care for women undergoing termination of pregnancy if complications develop in non-NHS facilities to local NHS services.

67.4.5 Critical Care

In December 2013, ICNARC (Intensive Care National Audit and Research Centre) and the OAA (Obstetric Anaesthetists' Association) published data on 6793 obstetric admissions to critical care over a 4-year period ending in December 2012. The data revealed that a majority of critical care admissions that occur in the postpartum period are attributed to obstetric haemorrhage and only a smaller proportion of women had pneumonia as the leading cause of critical care admissions.

67.4.5.1 Key Messages for Critical Care

It is important to have a high degree of suspicion for sepsis in women who are pregnant or within 6 weeks of a recent termination of pregnancy, miscarriage or birth.

67.4.5.2 Sepsis

Women at higher risk of sepsis include

- those who have impaired immunity secondary to illegal drug use or illness,
- have diabetes or other co-morbidities,
- needed obstetric intervention (i.e. caesarean section, forceps delivery),
- needed removal of retained products of conception,
- had prolonged rupture of membranes,
- currently suffer from or have had a significant exposure to group A streptococcal infection, and

- have continued vaginal bleeding or an offensive vaginal discharge.

Multidisciplinary team working is crucial to the success of critical care. Health professionals must work collaboratively with colleagues, respecting their skills and contributions.

Reduced or altered conscious level is a red flag indicating established illness. When a decision is made to admit to intensive care, this should occur within 4 hours of the decision.

Diagnoses of critical illnesses that are easy to make in a non-pregnant woman can be much more difficult when the woman is pregnant. There must be a balance between appropriate clinical suspicion and a conclusive diagnosis; not all cases of hypertension are pre-eclampsia, and shortness of breath is not always diagnostic of a pulmonary embolism.

An urgent medical review and portable echocardiogram or CT pulmonary angiography within 1 hour of presentation of a life-threatening pulmonary embolism should be arranged.

Early advice should be sought from an extracorporeal membrane oxygenation (ECMO) centre if a woman is failing to respond to standard respiratory support.

The clinical management of women with obstetric-specific conditions should involve a multidisciplinary team of obstetricians, midwives and obstetric anaesthetists. These conditions are rarely seen on the general critical care unit but are common problems on maternity units.

67.5 Caring for Women with Epilepsy (MBRRACE 2013–15 Report)

This section should be read in conjunction with the RCOG Green-top guideline *Epilepsy in Pregnancy* [13].

In 2013–15, eight women with epilepsy died during pregnancy or in the immediate postpartum period, and five women died between 6 weeks and 1 year after delivery. The commonest cause of death was sudden unexplained death in epilepsy (SUDEP). One woman drowned in the bath.

67.5.1 Themes for Improvement of Care

67.5.2 Drug Management in Women with Epilepsy

Discontinuation of anti-epileptic drugs (AEDs) without specialist advice in pregnancy is a very serious event and can be life threatening. Obstetric teams should act when such an event occurs, and urgent attempts should be made by all clinicians involved in care to offer the woman immediate access to an appropriately trained professional to review her medication and prescribe AEDs if appropriate.

67.5.3 Inadequate Medical Knowledge

In 2013–15, two women died because they were given the wrong advice from their doctor regarding AEDs in pregnancy. GPs, secondary care providers and commissioners should work together to ensure that women with epilepsy have access to appropriately specialized care, before, during and after pregnancy.

67.5.4 Care of Highly Vulnerable Women

In 2013–15, four women who died had socially complex lives or were vulnerable. Sociobiological factors associated with death in these women included poor English language skills, forensic issues (including some obstetric care in prison), domestic violence, contact with social services, older children in care and learning disability. Women with challenging circumstances should have access to additional care and this should consider interpersonal dynamics to provide multidisciplinary/multiagency integrated support.

67.5.5 Patient Education and Engagement

A woman with idiopathic generalized epilepsy had been highly resistant to multiple AEDs, and following extensive counselling with her epilepsy team had decided to stop all of her AEDs other than clobazam prior to pregnancy and died of SUDEP in pregnancy. Obstetric and epilepsy services should take women's choices into account, but frank and difficult discussions with women should be undertaken when appropriate.

67.5.6 Syndromic Diagnosis

The diagnosis of epilepsy and epileptiform seizures should be made by a neurologist. Women who have remained seizure-free for at least 10 years (with the last 5 years off AEDs) and those with a childhood epilepsy syndrome who have had no seizures or epilepsy treatment as adults can be considered no longer to have epilepsy and can be managed as low risk provided there are no other risk factors. In women with a clear diagnosis of non-epileptic attack disorder (NEAD), AED administration and iatrogenic early delivery should be avoided.

67.5.7 Birth Planning

A birth plan should consider epilepsy and its management in the intrapartum and immediate postpartum period, as failure of such consideration may result in seizure activity due to pain and sleep deprivation in the intrapartum and postpartum period.

67.5.8 Epilepsy Risk Advice

Women with epilepsy should be provided with verbal and written information on prenatal screening and its implications, the risks of self-discontinuation of AEDs and the effects of seizures and AEDs on the fetus, pregnancy, breastfeeding and contraception. Women should also be advised regarding intake of a higher dose of folic acid.

67.5.9 Contraception

Women with epilepsy should be offered effective contraception to avoid unplanned pregnancies. Women taking enzyme-inducing AEDs (carbamazepine, phenytoin, phenobarbital, primidone, oxcarbazepine, topiramate) should be counselled about the risk of failure with some hormonal contraceptives.

All methods of contraception may be offered to women taking non-enzyme-inducing AEDs (e.g. sodium valproate, leve-tiracetam, gabapentin, vigabatrin, tiagabine and pregabalin).

67.5.10 Baby Care

The care of neonates and infants by women with epilepsy requires specific guidance. Postpartum safety advice and stra-tegies should be part of the antenatal and postnatal discussions with the mother alongside breastfeeding, seizure deterioration and AED intake.

67.5.11 Epilepsy and Pregnancy Registers

The UK Epilepsy and Pregnancy Register has vastly improved our knowledge and understanding of the effects of AEDs in pregnancy and has allowed us to give advice to women about the effects of AEDs in pregnancy. The most recent MBRRACE 2017 review recommends that all pregnant women with epi-lepsy should be provided with information about the UK Epilepsy and Pregnancy Register and invited to register.

67.5.12 Mode of Delivery

Epilepsy is not an indication for a caesarean section or induc-tion of labour, and vaginal delivery as a mode of birth should be supported when appropriate.

67.6 Caring for Women with Stroke

There were 12 women who died from intracranial haemor-rhage during or up to 6 weeks after pregnancy, 7 from sub-arachnoid haemorrhage and 5 from intracerebral haemorrhage during 2013–15. A further 16 women died from stroke between 6 weeks and 1 year after the end of pregnancy.

67.6.1 Messages for Improvement of Care

67.6.1.1 Neurological Examination

Neurological examination and fundoscopy including assess-ment for neck stiffness is mandatory in all new-onset headaches or headache with atypical features, particularly focal symptoms. One woman died due to lack of a neurological examination as she was presumed to have hyperemesis gravidarum, which should only be diagnosed if its onset is in the first trimester and other causes of nausea and vomiting have been excluded.

67.6.1.2 Delayed Diagnosis

A change in mental state and new seizures should lead to prompt neurological assessment in conjunction with referral to psychiatric services when appropriate. Red flag symptoms that should prompt immediate intervention include headache of sudden onset, described as the 'worst ever'; headaches with additional symptoms not usually experienced – neck stiffness, fever, weakness, double vision, drowsiness, seizures; and a headache that takes longer to resolve than usual or persists longer than 48 hours.

67.6.1.3 Delayed Transfer

Pregnancy should not alter the standard of care for stroke as recommended by the Society of British Neurological Surgeons. All women, pregnant or not, should be admitted to a hyperacute stroke unit when appropriate.

67.6.1.4 Communication

A comprehensive summary by the senior obstetrician of the maternity care episode should be sent to the GP, who should be responsible for coordinating care after discharge from mater-nity services. The report cites a case of lack of communication between hospital and GP that resulted in the death of a postpartum woman from intracerebral haemorrhage due to lack of prescription of labetalol and regular blood pressure monitoring.

67.7 Caring for Women with Psychosis

Postpartum psychosis affects 1–2 per 1000 women after child-birth, with the majority of those affected having an onset within the first 12 weeks postpartum. However, there is a significantly increased risk for a woman to develop psychosis of 25–50%, when she has a past history of postpartum psycho-sis or bipolar disorder. If there is, in addition, a first degree relative with either disorder, the risk for the woman is even higher. This section should be read in conjunction with the NICE guideline on antenatal and postnatal mental health [16].

67.7.1 Messages for Improvement of Care

67.7.1.1 Early Identification of Risk

At a woman's first contact with services in pregnancy and the postnatal period, inquiries should be made about any past or present severe mental illness, past or present treatment by a specialist mental health service, including inpatient care and any severe perinatal mental illness in a first degree relative (mother, sister or daughter).

It is preferable for such women (who have or are suspected to have severe mental illness and have any history of severe mental illness during pregnancy or the postnatal period or at any other time) to be seen at a specialized perinatal mental health service.

67.7.1.2 Risk in the Early Postpartum Period

A significant change in mental state during late pregnancy or early postpartum, or emergence of new symptoms, is a red flag that should prompt further assessment by a consultant perina-tal psychiatrist.

67.7.1.3 Timeliness of Mental Health Service Responses

Mental health services should respond in a timely fashion when a pregnant or postpartum woman is becoming acutely unwell by following clear pathways of referral and response. If a woman has sudden onset of symptoms sug-gesting postpartum psychosis, referral to a secondary men-tal health service (preferably a specialist perinatal mental health service) for immediate assessment (within 4 hours of referral) is recommended.

67.7.1.4　Use of Interpreters and Mental Capacity

Family or friends should not be used as interpreters and, when possible, women should be seen in a private setting to discuss mental health issues. All healthcare staff have a duty to ensure that women have the capacity to make decisions regarding their physical and mental healthcare.

67.7.1.5　Narrow Interpretation of Risk

If there is a family history of postpartum psychosis or bipolar disorder, healthcare services should be alert for change in mental state in late pregnancy and the early postpartum period with a view to refer for urgent psychiatric assessment if needed. Referral for specialist psychiatric assessment in pregnancy should be considered for women with current mood disorder of mild or moderate severity who have a first degree relative with a history of bipolar disorder or postpartum psychosis. Any past history of psychosis should prompt psychiatric referral and assessment in pregnancy. Failure to assess and interpret risk can result in women becoming acutely unwell with delays in accessing psychiatric help.

67.7.1.6　Counselling on Future Risk

All women experiencing postpartum psychosis should receive a clear explanation of future risk, including the availability of risk minimization strategies, and the need for re-referral during subsequent pregnancies. This should be undertaken by the mental health team involved in the care of the woman and should be communicated to the relevant health professionals.

67.7.1.7　Late Pregnancy and Postpartum Care Plan

Care providers should ensure that a late pregnancy and early postnatal care plan is completed, jointly with the woman, usually at 28–32 weeks of pregnancy, and an input from a psychiatrist is sought when medication is involved.

67.7.1.8　Continued Neonatal and Maternity Care

When both baby and the mother require inpatient psychiatric care, neonatal and maternal services should ensure that visits to the baby are appropriately facilitated.

67.7.1.9　Joint Management of Diagnostic Overshadowing

Where there is diagnostic uncertainty by obstetric and/or medical specialists, there should be close liaison between, and regular review by, senior medical staff from obstetrics, medicine and psychiatry. Treatment with antipsychotic medication should not be delayed while investigations are undertaken.

67.7.1.10　Consideration of Mother and Baby Unit (MBU) Care

Joint admission of mother and baby is overwhelmingly recognized as best practice. It is important to consider routine monitoring of the proportion of women and babies who are unnecessarily separated when the mother is admitted for psychiatric care. With the woman's consent, families should be made aware at an early stage of the benefits of joint mother–infant admission.

67.7.1.11　Early Discharge and Readmission

Treating teams should be aware of fluctuating symptom patterns in postpartum psychosis and tailor management accordingly.

67.7.1.12　Prescribing in Pregnancy and Breastfeeding

Professional and patient resources on medicines in pregnancy, and professional resources on medicines in breastfeeding exist and should be routinely used.

- Pregnancy – for professionals: Toxbase (www.toxbase.org)
- Pregnancy – for women and families: Better Use of Medicines in Pregnancy (BUMPS) (www.medicinesinpregnancy.org)
- Breastfeeding – for professionals: LactMed (https://toxnet.nlm.nih.gov/newtoxnet/lactmed.htm)

67.8　Caring for Women with Medical and Surgical Disorders

The care of 43 women who died from other indirect causes was analyzed in the 2013–15 review.

67.8.1　Messages for Improvement of Care

Pre-pregnancy counselling by an appropriate specialist is an important pillar of ongoing healthcare provision for women with pre-existing medical disorders. Contraceptive advice should be offered to these women, both in a pre- and post-pregnancy setting. In pregnant or postpartum women with complex medical problems involving multiple specialties, the consultant obstetrician must show clear leadership for coordinating care and liaising with the multidisciplinary team (MDT).

67.8.1.1　Arterial Aneurysms

Ten women died from spontaneous intra-abdominal bleeding, and nine had a ruptured splenic artery aneurysm. In most instances, this was an unexpected event in the absence of clear risk factors except being pregnant, although two women were known to have portal hypertension. The report cites a case of a woman of reproductive age who presented at the emergency department collapsed, in whom a pulmonary embolism was suspected. There is also an association between splenic artery rupture and pregnancy, although rare. Healthcare professionals should have a high index of suspicion of intra-abdominal bleeding in pregnant women presenting acutely, and such woman should have a Focused Assessment with Sonography in Trauma (FAST) scan to exclude intra-abdominal bleeding.

67.8.1.2　Respiratory Causes

Nine women died from respiratory causes, including two from cystic fibrosis, two from asthma, two from other known lung diseases, two from non-specific respiratory failure and one from acute airway obstruction. The report recommends that screening for pulmonary hypertension should be undertaken prior to pregnancy in women with pre-existing severe lung disease.

67.8.1.3 Haematology

Two women died from thrombotic thrombocytopenic purpura (TTP) and one from an acute sickle cell crisis. Four women died from haemophagocytic lymphohistiocytosis (HLH). This condition is fatal without treatment with immunosuppression, etoposide-based chemotherapy, alemtuzumab and bone marrow transplantation. The clinicians should be aware of this potentially fatal disease to ensure timely diagnosis and treatment.

67.8.1.4 Connective Tissue Disorders

Six women died from connective tissue disorders in this report. Connective tissue disorders are frequently associated with reduced fertility, but it is important that fertility treatments should not be offered without expert counselling about the risks of pregnancy.

67.8.1.5 Deaths Related to Endocrine Issues

One woman died in the postnatal period from liver disease due to failure of communication of abnormal liver function tests to her GP. One woman died from Addison's disease and one from diabetic ketoacidosis. In all these cases, there was a serious lapse in organizing postnatal care. Two women died from pancreatitis, and in both instances admission to critical care was delayed.

67.8.1.6 Obesity

The MBRRACE 2017 report identified several instances of suboptimal care for obese women related to a lack of equipment, a reluctance to operate, or technical difficulties: anaesthetic, operative or radiological, solely due to a woman's body habitus. The report advocates strategies for reducing BMI to improve reproductive and pregnancy outcomes, and hence research into the most effective way to encourage obese women to normalize their weight before conception should be supported.

67.9 Caring for Women with Malignancy

During 2014–16 in the UK and Ireland, 104 women died during or up to 1 year after pregnancy from malignant disease. Twenty-six women died during or up to 6 weeks after the end of pregnancy, a mortality rate of 1.04 per 100 000 maternities (95% CI 0.68–1.53). Of these 26 women, 8 died from breast cancer, 6 from brain or cental nervous system (CNS) tumours, 5 from gastrointestinal tumours, 1 from choriocarcinoma and 4 from tumours in other sites. Two women had an unknown primary.

67.9.1 Messages for Improvement of Care

- Repeated presentation with pain and/or pain requiring opiates should be considered a red flag.
- Cervical cancer may present with recurrent vaginal bleeding (e.g. postcoital bleeding) or vaginal discharge. In such cases, a gentle speculum examination should be undertaken to exclude cervical abnormalities even in women with diagnosed placenta praevia. Women with a clinically suspicious cervix should be referred for colposcopy evaluation.

- Women with suspected pulmonary embolism should be advised that, compared with CTPA, ventilation-perfusion (V/Q) scanning may carry a slightly increased risk of childhood cancer but is associated with a lower risk of maternal breast cancer; in both situations, the absolute risk is very small. Occasionally a malignancy of the respiratory system may present as a PE.
- If a cancer diagnosis is suspected, investigations should proceed in the same manner and on the same timescale as for a non-pregnant woman, but with caution when there is evidence of specific risks to the fetus.
- Thrombosis, particularly migratory or in an unusual location, should be fully investigated as it may be a presenting sign of cancer in pregnancy or postpartum.
- Neurological examination including fundoscopy is mandatory in all women with new-onset headaches or headache with atypical symptoms, as it may indicate the presence of an underlying neurological malignancy.
- There should be an early multidisciplinary discussion about the care of any woman with complex medical conditions in pregnancy including cancer.
- All pregnant or postpartum women who are diagnosed with cancer should have the possibility of an underlying familial syndrome considered with appropriate investigations, including tumour testing performed and family testing offered as appropriate.

67.10 Caring for Vulnerable Women

The MBRRACE-UK 2018 report describes 'vulnerable women are those who died by homicide as a result of domestic violence, and those who died as a result of drug and alcohol misuse'. Fourteen women were murdered, all by a partner or a former partner, 10 of whom died during pregnancy or up to 6 weeks after pregnancy. Overall, 43 women died in relation to drug and alcohol misuse.

67.10.1 Messages for Improvement of Care

- Healthcare professionals need to be alert to the symptoms or signs of domestic abuse.
- Services should develop or adapt clear protocols and methods for sharing information, both within and between agencies, about people at risk of, experiencing or perpetrating domestic violence and abuse.
- All health professionals caring for women should be aware of the pathway of care once domestic abuse is disclosed and escalate to senior staff if necessary.
- With regard to substance misuse, offer the woman a named midwife or doctor who has specialized knowledge and provide a direct-line telephone number.
- Women with complex problems require additional care following discharge from hospital after birth for the postnatal period. This should include the timing of follow-up appointments, which should be arranged with the appropriate services before the women are discharged.

References

1. Knight M, Tuffnell D, Jayakody H, et al. eds. *Saving Lives, Improving Mothers' Care: Lessons Learned to Inform Maternity Care from the UK and Ireland Confidential Enquiries into Maternal Deaths and Morbidity 2014–16.* Oxford: National Perinatal Epidemiology Unit, University of Oxford; 2018.

2. World Health Organization. *Trends in Maternal Mortality: 1990 to 2008.* Geneva: WHO; 2010.

3. NICE. *Antenatal Care for Uncomplicated Pregnancies*, Clinical Guideline CG62, 2008. www.nice.org.uk/guidance/cg62/chapter/1-Guidance.

4. Knight M, Nair M, Tuffnell D, et al. eds., on behalf of MBRRACE-UK. *Saving Lives, Improving Mothers' Care: Lessons Learned to Inform Maternity Care from the UK and Ireland Confidential Enquiries into Maternal Deaths and Morbidity 2013–15.* Oxford: National Perinatal Epidemiology Unit, University of Oxford; 2017. pp. 24–36.

5. Knight M, Kenyon S, Brocklehurst P, et al. eds. *Saving Lives, Improving Mothers' Care: Lessons Learned to Inform Future Maternity Care from the UK and Ireland Confidential Enquiries into Maternal Deaths and Morbidity 2009–2012.* Oxford: National Perinatal Epidemiology Unit, University of Oxford; 2014.

6. Knight M, Tuffnell D, Kenyon S, et al. eds. *Saving Lives, Improving Mothers' Care: Surveillance of Maternal Deaths in the UK 2011–13 and Lessons Learned to Inform Maternity Care from the UK and Ireland Confidential Enquiries into Maternal Deaths and Morbidity 2009–13.* Oxford: National Perinatal Epidemiology Unit, University of Oxford; 2015.

7. *Reducing the Risk of Venous Thromboembolism during Pregnancy and the Puerperium*, Green-top Guideline No 37a. London: Royal College of Obstetricians & Gynaecologists, 2015. www.rcog.org.uk/globalassets/documents/guidelines/gtg-37a.pdf

8. *Thromboembolic Disease in Pregnancy and the Puerperium: Acute Management*, Green-top Guideline No 37b. London: Royal College of Obstetricians & Gynaecologists, 2015. www.rcog.org.uk/globalassets/documents/guidelines/gtg-37b.pdf

9. *Prevention and Management of Postpartum Haemorrhage*, Green-top Guideline No 52. London: Royal College of Obstetricians & Gynaecologists, 2009. https://obgyn.onlinelibrary.wiley.com/doi/epdf/10.1111/1471-0528.14178

10. *Bacterial Sepsis in Pregnancy*, Green-top Guideline No 64a. London: Royal College of Obstetricians & Gynaecologists, 2012. www.rcog.org.uk/globalassets/documents/guidelines/gtg_64a.pdf

11. *Bacterial Sepsis Following Pregnancy*, Green-top Guideline No 64b. London: Royal College of Obstetricians & Gynaecologists, 2012. www.rcog.org.uk/globalassets/documents/guidelines/gtg_64b.pdf

12. NICE. *Hypertension in Pregnancy: Diagnosis and Management*, Guideline No 133, 2019. www.nice.org.uk/guidance/ng133

13. *Epilepsy in Pregnancy*, Green-top Guideline No 68. London: Royal College of Obstetricians & Gynaecologists, 2016. www.rcog.org.uk/globalassets/documents/guidelines/green-top-guidelines/gtg68_epilepsy.pdf

14. NICE. *Pregnancy and Complex Social Factors*, Clinical Guideline 110, 2010. www.nice.org.uk/guidance/cg110

15. *Pregnancy and Breast Cancer*, Green-top Guideline No 12. London: Royal College of Obstetricians & Gynaecologists, 2011. www.rcog.org.uk/globalassets/documents/guidelines/gtg_12.pdf

16. NICE. *Antenatal and Postnatal Mental Health*, Clinical Guideline 192, 2014. www.nice.org.uk/guidance/cg192/evidence/full-guideline-pdf-4840896925

Clinical Governance in Obstetric Practice

William C. Maina

68.1 Introduction

Clinical governance is about all the processes and systems that ensure quality and safety of patient care are maintained and continuously improved. These processes can be divided into domains of practice that promote clinical effectiveness, patient safety and patient experience.

Most pregnant women in developed countries will have a normal outcome of their pregnancy, but a significant proportion will experience an adverse outcome. Obstetric clinical governance aims to minimize adverse pregnancy outcome and promote a positive experience for patients and staff.

68.2 Key Domains of Clinical Governance

The key principles of clinical governance are shown in Figure 68.1.

68.2.1 Clinical Effectiveness

Clinical effectiveness comprises the processes and systems that promote high standards of clinical care and include:

competent workforce;

evidence-based practice;

audit and quality improvement;

research; and

local performance monitoring.

68.2.1.1 Competent Workforce

Robust recruitment processes, training, retention and supervision are key to establishing an effective multidisciplinary team. Skill mix and numbers of staff should match local needs and complexity of patients.

Staff should maintain competencies by attending local and regional educational meetings and external courses where such need is identified. Competencies in management of obstetric emergencies should be maintained by attending mandatory drills and skills training. Accreditation with relevant professional bodies must be maintained as appropriate.

Clinicians and clinical teams are directly responsible and accountable for quality and safety of the care they provide. The senior management team is responsible and accountable for ensuring appropriate processes and systems are in place to support clinical teams. The Hospital Trust Board is ultimately responsible for quality and safety.

68.2.1.2 Evidence-based Practice

Practice should be based on assessment of patients' needs, and care and treatment provided in line with current legislation, standards and evidence-based guidance to achieve optimal outcomes.

68.2.1.3 Audit and Quality Improvement

Audit and quality improvement are used to provide assurance regarding the quality of services as well as identify where improvements are needed. An audit can also assist to benchmark services against other providers.

In an audit, the care provided is measured against existing defined quality standards. If a shortfall is identified, appropriate actions are taken to bring practice in line with the standard. As an example, elective caesarean sections should be performed between 39 and 40 weeks' gestation. An audit is performed which reveals that 95% were performed as per the

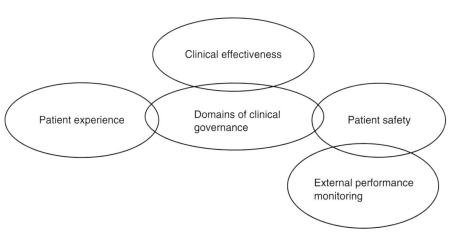

Figure 68.1 Key principles of clinical governance

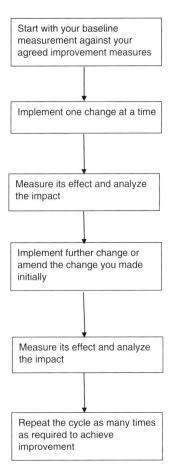

Start with your baseline measurement against your agreed improvement measures

Implement one change at a time

Measure its effect and analyze the impact

Implement further change or amend the change you made initially

Measure its effect and analyze the impact

Repeat the cycle as many times as required to achieve improvement

Figure 68.2 Principles of audit and quality improvement

standard and further analysis reveals that 5% were performed before 39 weeks for valid clinical reasons. This provides assurance that the quality standard has been met.

The 'Model for Improvement' which uses the Plan-Do-Study-Act (PDSA) technique [1] is an effective and quicker method for improving quality of care. The key principles of this method are shown in Figure 68.2.

As an example, a quality improvement project was performed in a maternity unit in the UK to improve detection of *Clostridium difficile* infection (CDI). Baseline assessment over a 3-month period identified 3 cases of CDI with delay in sending stool samples >24 hours. Seventeen stool samples were sent during this period. The project team aimed to improve the number of stool samples sent in symptomatic women and reduce delay in sending the samples. Multidisciplinary teaching on CDI was undertaken. Practice was assessed again over a 3-month period. Twenty-four stool samples were sent, resulting in detection of 1 case of CDI and no delays in sending samples were observed.

Projects may be selected locally or nationally. Engagement with stakeholders (team members and/or service users) is encouraged and the local audit and quality improvement team should be contacted for support and guidance.

68.2.1.4 Research

Maternity services should promote participation in multicentre research trials and other projects to address gaps in evidence. Support may be available from local, national or international research bodies and organizations that fund research.

68.2.1.5 Local Performance Monitoring

Validated and reliable indicators, and tools for collecting such indicators, are essential for monitoring performance of maternity services. A critical review of the literature by Escuriet et al in 2015 [2] identified 388 indicators and 7 tools specifically designed for capturing aspects of maternity care. Intrapartum care was the most frequently measured feature, through the application of process and outcome indicators. Postnatal and neonatal care of mother and baby were the least appraised areas.

The tools and indicators identified largely enable measurement of technical interventions and undesirable health outcomes. A need was identified for indicators that capture non-intervention, reflecting the reality that most births are low risk, requiring few, if any, obstetric interventions. It should be noted that this study was limited to countries within Europe. The 10 most frequently measured outcomes and processes are shown in Box 68.1.

The Maternity Dashboard [3] is a tool that can be used to monitor the performance of a maternity service against the standards agreed locally. This is achieved by setting local goals for each parameter as well as upper and lower thresholds. A suggested approach is to use the traffic light system:

- Green is used when the goals are met (parameter within lower threshold);
- Amber is used when the parameter is above the lower threshold but still within the upper threshold. Action is needed to avoid entering the red zone.
- Red is used when the upper threshold is breached. Immediate action is needed to restore safety and maintain quality.

Dashboards have been adopted in many maternity units in the UK to monitor clinical activity, workforce issues and clinical outcome indicators on a monthly basis. This enables local boards, clinical commissioning groups and the Care Quality Commission to assess compliance with standards of care.

Box 68.1 The 10 Most Frequently Measured Outcomes and Processes in Maternity Care [2]

Mode of onset of labour

Induction and augmentation of labour

Caesarean section

Vaginal delivery with instruments

Vaginal delivery without instruments

Maternal postnatal complications

Perineal tears

Method of infant feeding

Apgar scores

Other neonatal complications

68.2.2 Patient Safety in Maternity Services

The Care Quality Commission (CQC), the independent regulator of health and social care in England [4], standard on safety requires providers to ensure that no one is given unsafe care or treatment or put at risk of harm that could be avoided. All maternity services, irrespective of location, should aim to meet this standard.

The Care Quality Commission recommends the following approach to safety:

safeguarding and protection from abuse;

managing risks;

safe care and treatment; and

learning when things go wrong.

68.2.2.1 Safeguarding and Protection from Abuse

Maternity services provide care to adults and children. They are responsible for putting processes and systems in place to safeguard children and vulnerable adults. This is achieved through collaborative working with partner organizations within the community they serve. To ensure effective and high standards of professional practice, staff should be competent in recognition of vulnerability and abuse, and what to do about it.

Safeguarding is about protecting adults or children who may be in vulnerable circumstances which expose them to risk of abuse or neglect. Abuse can fall into any of the categories shown in Box 68.2.

Maternity services have responsibilities to ensure that all staff:

- are familiar with policies relating to safeguarding children and adults;
- know how to recognize abuse and how to report and respond to it; and
- have access to training that is appropriate for their level of responsibility.

Box 68.2 Types of Abuse

Physical

Domestic

Sexual

Psychological

Modern slavery

Discriminatory

Organizational

Neglect and acts of omission

Self-neglect

68.2.2.2 Managing Risks

This involves assessment and management of risks to minimize risks to patients and service users. Priority should be given to assessment and management of risks relating to the following areas:

- staffing levels and skill mix;
- arrangements for using bank, agency and locum staff;
- arrangements for handovers and shift changes;
- service users;
- how staff identify and respond to changing risks to people, including deteriorating health and well-being, medical or obstetric emergencies or behaviour that challenges;
- support from senior staff; and
- changes to service and staff.

Please note that this list is not exhaustive.

There are five steps that should be undertaken when carrying out a risk assessment [5]:

1. identify the risk or hazard;
2. decide who might be harmed and how;
3. evaluate the risks and decide on precautions;
4. record your significant findings; and
5. review your assessment and update if necessary.

68.2.2.3 Safe Care and Treatment

To ensure safe care and treatment, maternity services should ensure that:

- patients' care records, including clinical data, are recorded and managed in a way that keeps patients safe;
- all the information needed to deliver safe care and treatment is available to relevant staff in a timely and accessible manner;
- when patients move between teams, services and organizations, all the information needed for their ongoing care is shared appropriately, in a timely manner and in line with relevant protocols;
- there is good coordination between different electronic and paper-based systems, and appropriate access for staff to records;
- medicines are managed safely;
- robust infection control measures are available; and
- equipment and environment are managed appropriately to minimize harm to patients and staff.

Please note that this list is not exhaustive.

68.2.2.4 Learning When Things Go Wrong

Maternity services have a responsibility to ensure that lessons are learned and improvements made when things go wrong. They should put in place appropriate processes and systems that include:

- a no blame culture that encourages reporting of incidents and near misses;
- robust and effective processes for recording, reviewing and investigation of incidents and near misses in a timely manner;
- effective mechanisms for organizational learning and improvement of care;
- a culture that encourages openness and honesty to patients and the public when things go wrong and when complaints are made; and

- effective arrangement for responding to relevant external safety alerts, recalls, inquiries, investigations or reviews.

Management of incidents [6] includes the following:

- Thank staff for reporting incidents and near misses.
- The risk management team are responsible for monitoring, prioritization of investigation, escalation to senior management, dissemination of lessons learned and implementation of changes to local practice with support from senior management.
- Incidents are prioritized for root cause analysis by the level of severity of harm to the woman and the likelihood of recurrence. Root cause analysis (Box 68.3) is a technique for undertaking a systematic investigation that looks beyond the individuals concerned and seeks to understand the underlying causes and environmental context in which the incident occurs. Figure 68.3 shows the steps involved in a root cause analysis.

68.3 Patients' Experience

Maternity services have an obligation to ensure that patients' human rights are respected by putting in place processes and systems that encourage:

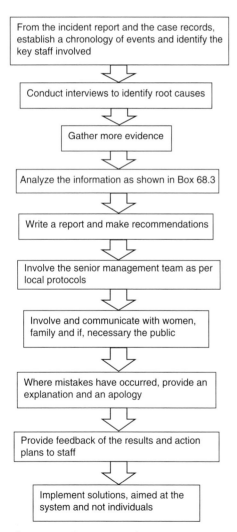

Figure 68.3 Root cause analysis process

Box 68.3 A Root Cause Analysis of an Incident

Patient factors

- Consider language or cultural barriers, unrealistic birth plans or case complexity.

Individual factors

- Consider stress and fatigue factors and work relationships.

Task factors

- Are policies up to date, useable, relevant and correct?

Communication factors

- Consider written, verbal and non-verbal communication issues.
- Were they adequate, effective, confusing or timely?
- Is there a robust handing-over culture?

Education and training factors

- Do staff have regular training in obstetric emergencies, cardiotocography and neonatal and adult basic life support?
- Are training targets met (percentage of staff trained annually)?

Equipment and resource factors

- Is equipment adequate, fit for purpose, maintained, stored appropriately and do staff know how to use it?
- Is budget allocation enough?
- Is staff allocation and skill mix appropriate?

Working conditions and environmental factors

- Are there effective policies and procedures for management of health and safety?
- Do staff demonstrate appropriate personal responsibility for their own health and safety, and that of others?

- kindness, respect and compassion;
- involving patients in decisions about their care; and
- privacy, dignity and choice.

Monitoring of patients' experience, through feedback, complaints and compliments is an essential strategy for maintaining and improving quality of services.

68.4 External Performance Monitoring

External performance monitoring is important to provide reassurance about the quality of local services. Participation in regional and national quality assurance programmes is encouraged such as:

- national confidential enquiries into maternal deaths and stillbirths;
- regulatory bodies; and
- national audits.

References

1. Institute for Healthcare Improvement. Plan-Do-Study-Act (PDSA) worksheet. www.ihi.org/resources/Pages/Tools/PlanDoStudyActWorksheet.aspx. (Accessed January 2019.)

2. Escuriet R, White J, Beeckman K, et al. Assessing the performance of maternity care in Europe: a critical exploration of tools and indicators. *BMC Health Serv Res.* 2015; **9**:491.

3. *Maternity Dashboard Clinical Performance and Governance Score Card*, Good Practice No 7. London: Royal College of Obstetricians and Gynaecologists, January, 2008.

   www.rcog.org.uk/globalassets/ documents/guidelines/goodpractice7 maternitydashboard2008.pdf. (Accessed January 2019.)

4. Care Quality Commission. The independent regulator of health and social care in England. www.cqc.org.uk. (Accessed January 2019.)

5. Health and Safety Executive. www.hse.gov.uk. (Accessed January 2019.)

6. Strachan KB. Reducing risk on the labour ward. *Obstet Gynaecol*, 2011;7:103–7.

Ethical Issues and Conflict in Maternal-Fetal Medicine and Obstetrics

Pierre Mallia

69.1 Introduction – Fidelity and What Is Ethics?

George E. Moore, one of the founders of the analytic tradition in philosophy, defines ethics as what we ought and ought not to do. It is a deliberation and although feelings such as empathy come into most decisions, ethics is not only a feeling but has to be supported by reason. In fact, saying that ethics is only a feeling or an intuition, not needing any reason, has to be supported by argument itself, annulling the very assertion.

Moore also put forward the 'naturalistic fallacy' – namely, that an *is* does not make an *ought* – which is to say that just because something 'is' like so in nature does not dictate that we 'ought' to always respect this. This argument is valid, for example, for in vitro fertilization (IVF) where it is generally reasoned (although not accepted by moral theology) that just because in nature babies are born through the conjugal act between a couple, it does not follow that we cannot treat infertile couples by IVF. Of course, there are slippery slopes to this argument, such as the use of IVF for same-sex couples.

There are conflicting arguments to this, but certainly we do treat disease even though in nature men can die of them and indeed make the human race more fit. Medicine therefore goes against natural law. This begs the argument on whether 'natural law' actually exists. It is important not to confuse natural law with *divine* law, although many do associate them together. But what interests us is its scientific value. Natural laws *have* been described, from physical laws to chemical laws. Biological laws have been more fragile, as it were, as they challenged certain cultural values. Certainly, science accepts laws such as Darwin's survival of the fittest and the struggle for survival. In fact, it can also be asserted that humanity organized itself around moral rules in order to survive. Primitive societies that need to protect themselves and hunt together may make utilitarian rules of not killing each other for simple reasons. Other punishments may be imposed. This automatically creates two rules (do not kill and do not steal) and a system of justice which prescribes punishments. This is area of evolutionary anthropology. In time, what was first a utilitarian rule can become so embedded in a society that it becomes what Immanuel Kant describes as a categorical imperative – if one can apply a rule universally, then it must be a principle.

Normative values in a community are formed by culture and reactions to the environment. Although values ought not to be considered a statistic, they do change in time and geographically (a space–time continuum in change, so to speak).

Today we speak more about rights and obligations, and their applicability is becoming more valued. The important distinction is that rights, be they defined as natural rights or not, are given to us by the state and there needs to be a general consensus for agreeing to what rights a country ought to allow and what not. This has found much discussion within the area of maternal-fetal medicine, which is the scope of this chapter.

The four principles of respect for autonomy, beneficence, non-maleficence and justice (made popular by Beauchamp and Childress [1]) have become a mantra. Although they are useful for ethical discussion and deliberation, and are certainly referred to here, they are lacking in applicability in a clinical situation, even though the authors say that they can be applied by specification to the situation and balancing of the principles, for example, whether autonomy ought to trump the best interests of a patient. Certainly, the principle of respecting autonomy is very important and meritorious in most societies, especially when dealing with maternal-fetal conflict. But one can argue either way of a moral dilemma using principles depending on which principle is given more weight. Therefore, they become difficult to be applied in a clinical situation unless guidelines have been clearly laid down.

69.1.1 The Principle of Double Effect and Its Reliability – the Case of Savita Halappanavar

Another important principle in moral discussion is the principle of double effect – when can one, in order to obtain a good, be able to commit a non-intentional harm.

The case of Savita Halappanavar, a 31-year-old Indian dentist who was refused termination after premature rupture of membranes and who died on 28 October 2012 at the University Hospital Galway in Ireland due to complications of a septic miscarriage at 17 weeks' gestation, is important. The case illustrates the importance of a revised approach to maternal-fetal conflict (if we should be speaking about a conflict at all) and also to illustrate the lack of clinical applicability of the principle of double effect in situations where hindsight suggests that the principle could have been applied. These arguments, especially when there is disagreement, also show the legal unsuitability of some established philosophical tools unless there are more clear legal guidelines.

The principle of double effect has four conditions relating to when a harm, which is foreseen, indirect and unintentional, is allowed according to moral theory. The principle was devised by Thomas Aquinas and therefore finds strong application within religious (especially Catholic) morality. The conditions to be fulfilled are the following:

> In obstetrics and gynaecology, the principle of 'double effect' finds application mostly with ectopic pregnancy and cancer of the uterus. With the former, the pathology is considered to be the damaged fallopian tube containing the still viable fetus and therefore the removal of the fetus is foreseen and an indirect consequence of removing the deceased organ – the fallopian tube. Due to the potentially dangerous nature of the condition, removal of the fetus is also considered proportional. With cancers, the woman is allowed to receive treatment, such as chemotherapy or radiotherapy, even if this causes harm to the fetus. If hysterectomy is necessary as part of the management of the malignancy, then this is also permitted even though it would result in removal of the fetus as well. Of course, the woman's wishes are always given priority.

The problems with the principle of double effect are mostly twofold. In the first instance, advancing technology can make one of the conditions obsolete. For example, it is today possible in cases of ectopic pregnancy to remove the fetus laparoscopically, conserving the fallopian tube. This makes the removal a *direct* killing of the fetus rather than an indirect one and therefore loses the double effect condition. For example, in the UK where abortion is allowed only through the application of the Abortion Act, this procedure is not considered under the terms of the legislation. The Royal College of Obstetricians and Gynaecologists (RCOG) have issued guidelines for the use of this procedure, which recommend, amongst others, that it can be used if the woman has already had another ectopic pregnancy and has had the other tube removed.

Of course, performing a salpingectomy with a fetal presence instead of simply removing the fetus does not make clinical or moral sense. To choose to do so simply to satisfy the principle of double effect is claiming the Shakespearian 'pound of flesh'.

But the more concerning doubt about the principle of double effect is its difficulty to be applied in non-prescribed situations. Even the presence of a clinical ethicist may not guarantee any legal implications. This certainly was the case with Savita. Although many theorists claimed in retrospect that the four conditions of double effect could have been satisfied, how can a clinician make that conclusion in such a situation especially when in most cases the death of the mother from such a situation does not generally result? Even experts may disagree on the applicability of the principle. This happened in the literature following the separation of the Maltese Siamese twins in Manchester in 2000. Certainly, one needs a more useable standard which does not put at risk the mothers concerned. In the case of Savita, even if the development of sepsis could have been detected, as the investigation maintained, one can question the rationale of putting such mothers through a distressing situation and potential clinical risks when it is known that the death of the baby in such cases at this gestation is inevitable and foreseen. The future will certainly see more discussion on the actually clinical applicability of this principle. Even in accepted situations such as giving pain relief at the end of

life, which may or may not hasten the demise of a dying patient, creates problems amongst doctors due to fear of litigation or moral correctness. It is better to have clear clinical guidelines and standards of care.

In Savita's case, the medical team may have been criticized for not diagnosing sepsis early enough and for not using established screening tools. However, why should a patient be put through such a risk when the outcome is known to be inevitable? Induction of delivery would have simply hastened the inevitable outcome with the intention of decreasing the risks to the mother. There certainly is proportionality and the (earlier) death of the baby is foreseen and can be argued to be indirect and unintended because of the high risk involved to the mother. This can be considered as the moral equivalent of using pain relief in terminally ill patients even if this hastens death. The intention in both is not to kill but to relieve a grave circumstance. What is disconcerting is that the doctors, working in a Catholic hospital, could not apply the principle, even if they wished to, because there may not have been sufficient time for debate – such as whether it is truly indirect. This case contributed to Ireland's revisions of its abortion laws.

69.2 General Issues

There are in actual fact two types of conflict that one may describe. There is the genuine conflict between the gestational mother and the fetus when, unfortunately, the pregnant woman acts in a way that is not conducive to a healthy pregnancy, thus harming the child [2]. There also exists the conflict between the rights of the gestational mother and the healthcare system which is looking after her during her pregnancy. While this has also been dubbed a maternal-fetal conflict, it is in reality a misnomer, as it bypasses the fact that the problem is really a conflict between society and the mother. Society can refer to the political system, the religious/cultural norms and, indeed, the doctor–patient relationship itself. Pregnant women are expected to bear babies and have no further responsibility other than the well-being of their child. Their own health maintenance is often viewed as conducive to bearing a healthy baby. Whilst this is indeed the accepted case by most women, there are genuine health cases in which the woman ought to be given the rights of her well-being as well. The scope of this section is to discuss the ethical implications of this course of action.

The medical and legal communities have now established *the patient's absolute right to refuse treatment*; a principle particularly relevant to end-of-life situations. In pregnancy, this right has become somewhat obscured by the fact that there seems to be a competition between the mother-as-patient and the fetus-as-patient. When two patients are involved, such as in the donation of organs for transplant, it is usually considered ethical that the physician responsible for the donor (who can be a dying patient) and the physician of the recipient be separate so as to avoid competing interests. This is not the case in pregnancy where the same clinician is the 'advocate' for both the mother and fetus. Under normal circumstances, this arrangement works well. But it is often assumed that when conflicts occur, one can override decisions made by the mother – decisions that may not be in the best interests of the developing child.

When a woman abuses some potentially harmful substance (drugs, alcohol etc.) and disregards the doctor's advice, she is endangering the life of the fetus. The past decades have seen the increasing trend to refer such situations to the courts of law [3]. How far can a government go to direct a pregnant woman's behaviour based on the interests of the state? Physicians are obliged to respect the pregnant woman's wishes, but what of the duty to the fetus who has been placed in a vulnerable state by the mother's decision? The question arises whether women can have management forced upon them for the benefit of the fetus. In situations of substance abuse, can mothers be forcefully admitted into hospital for the well-being of the fetus? Many would instinctively think that once the mother is abusing alcohol or drugs, then she may be less competent to make decisions on behalf of her baby. Indeed, pregnancy does confer a duty on the part of the mother towards the fetus being carried, and, assuming that the mother has agreed to continue with the pregnancy, a decision to embark on a pregnancy carries responsibilities, which, if defaulted upon, put into question her rights to an unhealthy lifestyle over the rights of safety to the fetus.

Situations may arise where the woman refuses proposed management to the potential detriment of the fetus. Is a woman entitled to refuse delivery by a caesarean section, which risks her own life in the process, potentially putting the fetus at risk? Or should she undergo a forced caesarean section for the benefit of the fetus, as some courts of law have pronounced in Western countries?

Finally, one has considerations of maternal-fetal conflict in occupational health. Can employers institute fetal protection policies that limit the work of a woman in certain risk areas? Should this be a public health policy?

Certainly, the acceptance to carry a pregnancy does put a moral onus on the woman to protect her fetus. Not all women will agree on the details and sometimes general policies may need to be instituted. One cannot, for example, receive treatment or vaccines that can be harmful to the fetus, even if beneficial to the mother. This has generally been accepted, and most women would want to receive information on whether a treatment can harm their baby.

69.3 Refusal of Treatment and Forced Caesarean

There are many cases from the legal literature which describe women who were forced to receive treatment. One compelling case is that of Angela Carder (District of Columbia. Court of Appeals. IN re A.C. (Docket No. 87–609), 26 April, 1990). Mrs. Carder was dying and 26 weeks into her pregnancy. She had agreed to life-prolonging treatment to give her baby a better chance. When her death was imminent, however, she appeared to refuse a caesarean section. The hospital referred the case to a Superior Court judge who, after hearing all the arguments brought forward, ruled in favour of the operation. The family appealed, but the Appeals Court concurred with the

decision. The baby died two hours after the operation and the mother two days later. In 1990 (cited above), the Appeals Court ruled that the lower court should not have given orders for surgery as there was not enough evidence that this is what the mother wanted [2].

There has been great discussion on the issue of forced treatment. Law scholars have argued that the law should uphold the woman's right to refuse surgery even if this is in the fetus' best interests [4]. Others have argued that one needs to balance the rights of the fetus with those of the mother. Some consider that once the baby reaches viability, it must be considered a person and fetal rights should prevail [5]. Of course, arguments as to when a fetus becomes a person are not very strong ones, but the case for viability does make more sense. Once a child is viable and there is no danger to the woman's health, society may have a duty to invoke people's responsibilities to each other. The fear and the risk of surgery on the part of the mother are often brushed aside by those who think it reasonable that society may expect the mother to make a decision in the best interests of her baby at this stage. Some have even said that at the stage of viability, the court should take over in a conflict [6].

However, it should be noted that many religious positions refute the notion on a decision based on viability. The Catholic Church and other religions state that the moral status of the fetus is the same from conception to birth [7]. Of course, many women, based on their normative values, go into this self-sacrificing mode without the need of the physician's advice.

Conversely, it is argued that women owe a reasonable duty to their fetuses to try to prevent disease or handicap but, given the uncertainties of modern medicine and the lack of adequate prenatal care in many communities, women cannot be held responsible for situations that are largely due to society's shortcomings [8]. In these cases, it is not justified that judges and physicians override women's decisions.

69.3.1 Rights of the Fetus

It is interesting to note that Iseminger and Lewis [7] point out that in the USA the *Roe* v. *Wade* case did not recognize that the fetus has any rights. Rather, these rights were recognized by court orders that overrode the rights of the woman such as in cases of caesarean sections and blood transfusions. In the UK, the fetus does not have any rights at law and the gestational mother has a right to an abortion for any health reason. Court-ordered caesarean sections have been ordered for severely mentally ill mothers, however.

Some authors argue that the fetus acquires progressively increasing moral status with advancing gestation, and is also marked by the increasing bonding that takes place between the mother and child [3]. British law supports the view that the fetus is not a person and that one has to obtain the consent of the mother for any intervention. However, arguments on moral status are more philosophical than legal, although the latter often bases reasoning on pragmatic philosophical arguments. Whilst it is difficult to argue that a non-born viable child has no moral status, which it then acquires a day later when it is born, it is also difficult to argue that the moral status of a fertilized egg or a morula is the same as that of an eight-month fetus. This does not mean that morality increases with gestational age, however. Rather, one seems to point out that this increase takes place only in the first few weeks in which some form of organ activity can be measured and we have an early stage that people can identify with. Religious and conservative positions do not take this view. Whilst it is true that the maternal-fetal attachment increases with gestational age [9], this cannot be connected to the moral status of the embryo, as at most it is based on subjective perception.

69.3.2 Rights of the Mother

What is at issue is whether women can have their basic right to refuse treatment so society can protect their fetus is justified. Some argue that withdrawal of these rights is a means of using pregnancy to control women [10], and that the state should not attempt to transform pregnant women into *ideal* baby-making machines – women ought to be helped to have healthy babies rather than be forced to have them [11]. Intrusion into women's rights should only occur in very narrow circumstances. It is argued that it is better to allow a few unfortunate consequences to fetuses or mothers than to introduce force into therapeutic relationships between physicians and their patients. The problems should be anticipated and discussed before conflict arises, recording the mental status of the mother, and explaining the possible scenarios of outcomes [12].

69.3.3 The Caregiver–Patient Relationship

Court-ordered decisions have created conflict between physicians and their patient (the mother) [13]. This raises the question of who the patient is. It is obviously normally assumed that the patient is primarily the mother or at most mother-and-baby. For the mother, the fetus is also a patient, but some have argued that this holds only when the mother confers such a status on it [14]. It is argued that directive counselling for fetal benefit can only be resorted to when this stage has been reached. When the fetus is as yet not seen as a patient, then non-directive counselling ought to be resorted to. As naïve as this may sound to a conservative world, it actually does make sense if one is to respect women's health rights. Of course, personhood is not conferred by the mother. But it is the mother who approaches the health system as a patient. When this system suddenly turns against her, there is reason for concern. Healthcare relationships are fiduciary relationships; they are based on trust. Losing this public trust is key to understanding these conflicts.

To explain this more clearly, consider why we treat young people for substance abuse and sexually transmitted infections. If we do not confer them their rights to confidentiality and treatment, they will not come forward with issues, potentially compounding their problems. Moreover, they will tell their friends of their experiences and encourage them not to come forward for care because professional trust will be questioned. This is unlikely to happen with pregnant women, as at first they have no confidentiality issues and come forward for help. But

the fact that they still come forward only shows their vulnerability. They assume society respects a pregnant woman *because* she is pregnant and that the pregnancy will not be used against her. The fact that physicians and courts act against their wishes when their health or life is in danger is cause for concern. Ethical dilemmas that arise in these situations create potential adversaries out of the pregnant woman and her fetus, when in reality it is the societal health system which has become her adversary [15].

Indeed, it is argued that there is a point at which the obstetrician's concerns appear to be more with the unborn fetus than with the mother – in other words, where the value of the fetus outweighs that of the mother [16]. This is not so much against the right to the life of the mother but to her right to free self-determination. It is a denial of autonomy and the use of law to coerce people. Certainly, it is not an easy question, but obstetricians and other healthcare providers must continue to uphold their fidelity to the mother unconditionally. The Hasting Center in New Jersey sees legislators and court orders increasingly being called upon to restrict the autonomy of pregnant women. This runs counter to helping women make less constrained and more informed choices for their babies. Punishing women is coercing them, which removes the voluntary choice in the informed consent process [17]. Society is thus stating that a woman's autonomy at a certain point does not count. There are even those who continue to advocate against the principle of so-called Western autonomy in order to continue to exert and influence healthcare.

Until a mother *gives* birth, that child is still dependent on her, even if it has the full moral status we can adorn it with. If one is to criticize autonomy, it is in its overpowering the phenomenon of beneficence in healthcare; beneficence is not without its faults, when, as explained in the introduction, it is difficult to balance principles. Rather than trumping autonomy of the woman over the rights of the child, or the rights of the child over autonomy of the mother, we should trump beneficence towards both mother and child together over individual autonomy and beneficence to the baby. This would mean that acting on the refusal of treatment on the part of the mother would mean acting on unreliable clinical judgement as a physician would have resisted the patients' exerting a positive right [18].

69.4 Recommendations of Professional Bodies

If the ethical debate is still unclear as to whether the law should interfere or not [19], there are sufficient guidelines to show that the profession bows towards a more understanding and respectful approach to the pregnant woman's choice, she being the primary patient with whom the doctor contends with.

The Committee on Ethics of the American College of Obstetricians and Gynecologists recommends that pregnancy is not an exception to the principle that a patient has a right to refuse treatment – even that needed to maintain life. Coercion is never acceptable, and differences ought to be resolved by a team approach which recognizes the life of the mother and her beliefs, and to consider seeking advice from ethics consultants. The College opposes the use of coerced medical intervention for pregnant women, including the use of courts to mandate medical interventions for unwilling patients [20].

The International Federation of Gynaecology and Obstetrics (FIGO) regulations state that 'no woman who has the capacity to choose among health care options should be forced to undergo an unwished-for medical or surgical procedure in order to preserve the life or health of her foetus, as this would be a violation of her autonomy and fundamental human rights. Resort to the courts or to judicial intervention when a woman has made an informed refusal of medical or surgical treatment is inappropriate and usually counter-productive.' Also, 'If maternal capacity to choose for medical decision-making is impaired, health care providers should act in the best interests of the woman first and her foetus second. Information from the family and others may help to ascertain what she would have wished. The wishes of pregnant minors who are competent to give informed consent regarding medical and surgical procedures should be respected' [21].

Cases of refusal of treatment are distressing for the healthcare team but the statutory rights to an informed choice cannot bypass pregnant women. Professionals should respect this right. At most they can provide further information, and make sure the patient has understood her position well. Persistence and other forms of persuasion remove the validity of a voluntary choice, as it is presumed that someone who needs persuasion is not yet ready to make a voluntary choice.

In view of the Carder case, there is now general agreement in the West about forced interventions – namely, that fully competent adults do not lose their constitutional rights to privacy and health. This does not mean that pregnant women do not have responsibilities, but these should remain separate arguments [22].

69.5 Other Considerations

69.5.1 Brain Death

A pregnant woman who is diagnosed as brain dead may be kept on life support to deliver the baby when viable by a caesarean section. Ethically, just because the technology is possible and the medical expertise exists, it need not be employed in every case [23]. Economic considerations must also be considered. In such cases, the wishes of the mother cannot always be obtained. It seems more reasonable to keep dead mothers on life support when the fetus is viable, and moralists have pointed out that keeping someone on a life support for more than two months may not be reasonable [24]. It is important that the interests of all concerned be taken into account – that of the dead mother, the fetus and the father or partner. Allowing a person to die a natural death is never morally wrong, and it would seem reasonable that the ethical concerns of the father/birth partner are taken into consideration, especially in cases where the fetus is not viable yet. Hospitals ought to have policies on these eventualities, even though rare. For example, whether one ought to transfer decision rights to the father/birth partner is

more difficult and emotionally laden than following a pre-established, morally permitted outcome following the principle of double effect. Indeed, if the father/birth partner feels it is in the best interests of the mother to be allowed to die, the death of the fetus becomes indirect. The situation may change if the fetus is, of course viable, and it would be reasonable, conditions permitting, that the mother be kept alive until delivery is possible.

There are great financial burdens in such situations and the end-of-life norm of not needing to give extraordinary treatment would not be inappropriate. However, each case has to be determined individually, not least due to the availability of the resources.

FIGO recommends that the goal to rescue the fetus should not exonerate physicians from the duty to care for the mother and to respect her right to die in dignity. Decisions must be taken with the family and partner and, in the absence of expressed wishes previously from the mother, a substitute must be found to act in her interests. When brain death occurs, an assessment must be made with regard to viability of the fetus should the mother be kept on support systems; no lower limit is recommended on gestational age but the best interests of the fetus must be taken into account once the decision on the mother has taken place, as explained above. Allowing a fetus to die a natural death when the mother is brain dead and the efforts needed are 'conspicuous', and inappropriate or disproportionate [21]. Conversely, it is pointed out that maternal mortality remains high worldwide and, where abortion is not against the law, services such as surgical abortion or access to medication should be available.

69.5.2 Substance Abuse and Lifestyle Issues

Substance abuse is another area of concern to obstetricians that raises a conflict between the lifestyle of the mother and the well-being of the baby. Indeed, it has been argued that the state may interfere to provide legal protection of the fetus [25]. To what extent this interference should be implemented is a different matter. In general, it would seem prudent that the state ought to provide programmes and rehabilitation services, but obligatory measures may have pushed these pregnant women further away from the healthcare system [26].

The question arises whether one can raise fetal abuse issues against a pregnant woman and whether the state ought to protect an unborn child to the point of prosecution. It would be unreasonable to hold the woman responsible; given the stigma against drug and alcohol abuse, it is easy for healthcare professionals to forget that such disorders are indeed psychiatric diagnoses. The mother is already ill and at most one can offer support, including prevention of pregnancy when possible. This does not, however, preclude her capacity to make decisions. Otherwise, it is easy to fall into the trap having been argued by some philosophers and legislators that a woman's right to abuse her own body does not give her the right to deliver these substances to the baby within her. The arguments will make sense only to those who see substance abuse as a vice and a responsibility of the abuser. Where possible, the mother should be offered the support necessary – especially providing the availability and quality of prenatal care. Criminalizing maternal behaviour to protect the fetus is an extreme measure and will not improve long-term solutions, as deterrents do not work much in these groups.

69.5.3 Occupational Health (and public policy)

Occupational medicine is usually of a non-discriminatory nature and boasts neutral health and public policies. Genetics has changed the debate somewhat and the example of employers requesting female workers to take a *BRCA* gene test in order to either disown responsibility for exposure to substances that can be associated with breast cancer or indeed refuse employment has become problematic. Obstetricians also face this issue when the occupational health and safety issues can militate against the pregnancy at hand. Public policy discourse will, of course, bring in the issue of discrimination.

These health issues are by no means resolved. Some authors believe that any fetal protection policies should be made on a bona fide argument and be fashioned narrowly so as to avoid impermissible discrimination [27]. Some law advisors suggest that policies should balance the interests of the other, the employer and the health of future generations [28]. Ethical opinions range from giving priority to women's rights over the health of future generations and vice versa. Obstetricians, however, ought to be frank about these issues, giving objective advice and not seeing them from the discriminatory point of view during consultations. Given background and socio-economic situations, potential mothers usually make the right decisions in the interest of their family.

69.6 Abortion: Right to Life vs. Right to Choice

From a purely biological point of view, life begins with the fertilization of the first cell. From a moral point of view, it would be reasonable to assume the same; however, many contest this and see the moral value starting at some other point, such as when there is a form or a primitive brain. This remains a point of contention and will therefore always be relative or subjective. Religions, which traditionally have been the normative force for many believers, have a right to guide their followers on their respective moral positions. In this regard, the Muslim community agrees that up to 21 days post-conception the fetus can be aborted in special circumstances. In the Catholic religion, this remains illicit and any person who agrees with abortion automatically excommunicates himself or herself according to the Catechism. It is acceptable only within the concept of the principle of double effect where the harm to the fetus (be it physical harm or death) is foreseen but indirect and unintended. This is usually applied to ectopic pregnancies, removal of a pathological uterus (usually as part of the management of malignancy) or chemotherapy. No moral provision is at present available within the Catholic tradition concerning a point at which the fetus is deemed to be causing harm to the mother.

Other issues with abortion are whether one should allow abortions for disabled or defective fetuses. Again, this is a point of contention and one must follow local laws. The main paradigm shift has occurred not so much as for the status of the embryo, but the balancing of the rights of the woman with the rights of the fetus. Assuming that the rights are equal, it is difficult to make an argument that one should force a woman to remain pregnant. Would this be ill-treating a person to protect an embryo which depends on that person? When, for instance, the argument of rape is considered from a status-of-embryo point of view, the argument remains the same. But when considered from the rights-of-the-woman point of view, one has to question whether anyone has the right to tell her to remain pregnant, especially in view of the psychological trauma she has gone through (and will then have to pay for) and the difficulties faced with motherhood in the future.

Requests for abortion in clinical practice ought to be seen by obstetricians or competent family doctors who, according to the Royal College of General Practitioners Clinical Skills Assessment, ought to be evaluated through a proper history, which includes whether the woman has considered other options, such as adoption. The social background of the woman should be considered, and she should be asked whether she thinks that she may suffer psychologically in the future.

FIGO notes that abortion for non-medical reasons remains controversial to obstetricians and the medical team and not least the mother. In countries where this has been measured, half of unintended pregnancies result in termination. In countries where abortion is restricted or prohibited, unsafe abortions are widely practised, and this has given rise for concern resulting in a recommendation by this body to governments to consider measures to prevent unintended pregnancies and to improve women's rights and services. However, abortion should never be promoted as a method of family planning.

69.7 Disabled Fetuses and Screening

Human development may be affected by many factors that cause malformations. There is no medical threshold of what constitutes a severe congenital malformation. However, a severely malformed and disabled child may have a very high impact on the physical, mental and social life of the woman and her family. Termination of a pregnancy, even in the presence of a malformation, still falls under the categories of abortion and brings up issues related to sanctity of life in many cultures, religions and the personal beliefs of many women. FIGO expresses the opinion that women ought to be counselled and that termination for severe malformation ought to be an acceptable option given the negative impact it can have [21]. Some countries have lists of diseases that fall under the category of choice for termination. Although abortion is technically legal in the UK, for example, the Abortion Act allows termination for biopsychosocial reasons and for genetic anomalies and prenatal tests provide an early diagnosis of the presence of severe congenital anomalies, no woman should undergo these tests without being counselled on why the test is being done and what the possibilities offered are. Some women may decide that this is not necessary if they believe they will raise even a severely disabled child.

It ought to be mentioned that disability groups have strong reservations about termination for reasons of disability, even though they may agree to abortion for general reasons. Of course, the reasoning behind this is the general outlook on disabled people. It is true that the lists for disabilities may include conditions such as Down syndrome, which many do not consider as a severe congenital malformation. FIGO recommends that couples should never be compelled to accept a medical termination, whatever the severity of the abnormality. Couples should be counselled accordingly and the impact this termination would have on their future mental well-being should be also considered [21].

Finally, the need for organs for children has raised the question of whether mothers who have anencephalic babies can be given the option to maintain the pregnancy with the view that the born baby is kept on life support for potential organ donation when it dies a natural death. Legal guidelines for death ought to be followed and competing interests to hasten decisions will amount to euthanasia, which is unacceptable. FIGO accepts organ donation from anencephalic babies who are defined as legally dead [21], but local ethical guidelines ought to be clearly available due to the cultural and social sensitivities that this raises. Certainly, where termination is available, mothers ought to be encouraged to maintain the pregnancy but it may be an altruistic option for those who believe in the sanctity of life.

References

1. Beauchamp TL, Childress JF. *Principles of Biomedical Ethics*, 4th ed. Oxford: Oxford University Press; 1994.

2. Carrington Coutts M. *Maternal-Fetal Conflict: Legal and Ethical Issues*, 14th ed. Washington, DC: The Joseph and Rose Kennedy Institute of Ethics; 1990.

3. Paintin D. Ethical issues in maternal – fetal medicine. *J R Soc Med.* 2002;**95**(7):371–2.

4. Annas GJ. Forced cesareans: the most unkindest cut of all. *Hastings Cent Rep.* 1982;**12**(3):16–17.

5. Kluge EW. When cesarean section operations imposed by a court are justified. *J Med Ethics.* 1988;**14**(4):206–11.

6. Peterfly A. Fetal viability as a threshold to personhood. a legal analysis. *J Leg Med.* 1995;**16**(4):607–36.

7. Iseminger KA, Lewis MA. Ethical challenges in treating mother and fetus when cancer complicates pregnancy. *Obstet Gynaecol Clin North Am.* 1998;**25**(2):273–85.

8. Purdy LM. Are pregnant women fetal containers? *Bioethics.* 1990;**4**(4):273–91.

9. Teixeira MI, Raimundo FM, Antunes MC. Relation between maternal fetal attachment and gestation age and parental memories. *J Nurs Referencia.* 2016;**8**(Jan/Feb):85–92.

10. Field MA. Controlling the woman to protect the fetus. *Law Med Health Care.* 1989;**17**(2):114–29.

11. Dawn J. A new threat to pregnant woman's autonomy. *Hastings Cent Rep.* 1987;**17**(4):3–40.

12. Nelson LJ. Compulsory treatment of pregnant women. *Clin Ethics Rep.* 1987;**1**(5):5–8.

13. Lindgren K. Maternal-fetal conflict: court-ordered cesarean section. *J Obstet Gynecol Neonatal Nurs.* 1996;**25**(8):653–6.

14. Chervanak FA, McCullough LB. The fetus as a patient: an essential ethical concept for maternal-fetal medicine. *J Matern Fetal Med.* 1996;**5**(3):115–19.

15. Flagler E, Baylis F, Rodgers S. Bioethics for clinicians: 12. Ethical dilemmas that arise in the care of pregnant women: rethinking 'maternal-fetal conflicts'. *CMAJ.* 1997;**156**(12):1729–32.

16. Cahill H. An Orwelian scenario: court ordered caesarian section and women's autonomy. *Nurs Ethics.* 1999;**6**(6):494–505.

17. Johnsen D. A new threat to pregnant women's autonomy. *Hastings Cent Rep.* 1987;**17**(4):33–40.

18. Mahowald MB. Maternal-fetal conflict: positions and principles. *Clin Obstet Gynaecol.* 1992;**35**(4):729–37.

19. Hollander M, Van Dillon J, Lagro-Janssen T, et al. Women refusing standard obstetric care: materno-fetal conflict or doctor-patient conflict? *J Pregnancy Child Health.* 2016;**3**:251.

20. American College of Obstetricians and Gynecologists. *Refusing of Medically Recommended Treatment during Pregnancy.* Committee Opinion No 664. 2016.

21. International Federation of Gynaecology and Obstetrics (FIGO). *Ethical Issues in Obstetrics and Gynecology* by the FIGO Committee for the Study of Ethical Aspects of Human Reproduction and Women's Health, October, London 2012.

22. Kukla R, Wayne K. Pregnancy, birth, and medicine. In *Stanford Encyclopaedia of Philosophy*. Stanford University; 2016.

23. Field DR, Gates EA, Greasy RK, Jonsen AR, Laros RK. Maternal brain death during pregnancy. *JAMA.* 1988;**260**(6):816–22.

24. Field DR'L, R.K., Reilly P, Shannon T. Keeping 'dead' mothers alive during pregnancy. In Evan MI, Dixler AO, Fletcher JC, Schulman JD, eds. *Fetal Diagnosis and Pregnancy.* Philadelphia: J.B. Lippincott; 1989. pp. 296–316.

25. Balisy S. Maternal substance abuse: the need to provide legal protection for the fetus. *South Calif Law Rev.* 1987;**60**(4):1209–38.

26. Jessup M, Roth R. Clinical and legal perspectives on prenatal drug and alcohol use: guidelines for individual and community response. *Med Law.* 1988;**7**(4):377–89.

27. Duncan AK. Fetal protection and the exclusion of women from the toxic workplace. *N C Centl Law J.* 1989;**18**(1):67–86.

28. Sor Y. Fertility or unemployment – should you have to choose? *J Law Health.* 1986–87;**1**(2):141–228.

70 Legal Considerations in Obstetric Practice

George Gregory Buttigieg

70.1 Introduction

The popular connotation that obstetrics is one of the hardest hit specialties by the suing epidemic is often true. The UK's £1.7 billion payout for obstetric negligence in 2016/17 also reflects that much of the 'epidemic' does in fact involve *avoidable* mishaps [1]. Furthermore, it is not infrequent for the *perception* of malpractice to underlie legal litigation and this often implies poor communication between obstetrician and patient. Legal confrontation is not automatically synonymous with medical injury or medical error. In a series of 1452 closed malpractice claims, 3% of patients had no verifiable medical injuries [2]. *Why* patients sue obstetricians is a question very worth asking. One fact is certain: most obstetricians need to raise *constructive* awareness (as distinct from defensive practice) of the legal aspects of their practice.

70.2 The European Scenario

In contrast to the well-published UK and US obstetric medico-legal scenario, an impressive lack of publications exists on the European front, coupled with a worrying lack of realization of effects on daily clinical practice [3]. Liability cases in general and in obstetrics are increasing everywhere, including Europe. France has seen a significant increase since the 1990s [4]. In Germany, the rise is clear, with appeal cases rising by 127% from 2004 to 2011 in Cologne alone [5]. In Italy, where OBGYN is the second most highly sued specialty, over €10 billion are now spent annually in litigation compensation [6]. In Malta, in spite of an excellent record of European level of healthcare, no relevant records are available, although the sharp increase in court cases is merely the tip of an unexplored iceberg [7]. There is also an evident lack of medical malpractice law, and medical indemnity only became a legal requirement by the Medical Council of Malta, as enforced by subsidiary legislation on the 14 March 2014. In Greece, where OBGYN also places second in medico-legal activity, a 2017 World Health Organization (WHO) report revealed a lack of central authority reporting and subsequently no significant litigation data are available [8]. In Portugal, not only do we have information of an increase in obstetric litigation, but the University of Coimbra also reports the breakdown of causes, with, as expected, birth management constituting the great proportion: perinatal asphyxia (50%), traumatic injuries of the newborn (24%), maternal sequelae (19%) and issues related to prenatal diagnosis and/or obstetric ultrasound (5.4%) [9]. Ireland has a mounting litigation rate, with brain damage or stillbirth constituting 38% of the claims and heralded by the record total payouts of £Ir 4.5 million for four major claims in 1999.

70.3 What Constitutes Obstetric Medical Negligence?

'Obstetric medical negligence' refers to substandard obstetric practice leading to an adverse outcome. Proving medical negligence in court requires proof that:

I.   The obstetrician owed the patient a duty of care.
II. This duty of care was breached/violated.
III. This breach was the cause of the patient's injuries as claimed.
IV. These injuries led to a damage, which will then be quantified.

Proving substandard practice alone is insufficient. In the cerebral palsy case of *Palmer* v. *Portsmouth Hospitals NHS Trust* (EWHC 2460, U.K., 2017), breach of care through substandard practice was confirmed, but the link of this to the causation of cerebral palsy was not.

70.3.1 Classifying Obstetric Litigation

Obstetric litigation is usually grouped into breach of the obstetric standard of care as relating to disclosure, diagnosis and the treatment administered. This does not exclude the possibility that a case presents multiple fronts of liability. Some examples are quoted.

70.3.1.1 Disclosure of Information to Obtain Consent

In the landmark case of *Montgomery* v. *Lanarkshire Health Board* (UKSC 11, Scotland, 2015), the defendant was, among other issues, found guilty of failing to disclose the 9–10% risk of shoulder dystocia in a case of elective vaginal breech delivery, complicated by maternal short stature and diabetes and fetal macrosomia. The complication did ensue and resulted in severe cerebral palsy. The ruling in this case helped to strengthen patient autonomy, further decrying the maxim that doctor knows best [10].

73.3.1.2 Diagnosis

In the appeal case *Lillywhite and another* v. *University College London Hospitals' NHS Trust* (EWCA Civ 1466, U.K., 2005), substandard practice was ruled for when the obstetrician failed to diagnose fetal holoprosencephaly on ultrasound screening.

70.3.1.3 Treatment

Breach of duty through failure to administer proper antenatal care was ruled in *MJ (a Minor)* v. *Dr Jonathan McLean*

Hayward (1) and The Royal Berkshire NHS Foundation Trust (2). The claimant suffered permanent brain damage in the form of periventricular leukomalacia (PVL) and an intraventricular haemorrhage (IVH) as a result of intrauterine hypoxia resulting from mismanaged pre-eclamptic toxaemia [11].

70.3.2 Two Landmark Cases

Before 2015, the UK and many other jurisdictions judged alleged medical negligence along the *Bolam* principle or its variants. This considers whether the judged practice, irrespective of the existence of other practices, is one accepted by a body of responsible peers. In such instances, no negligence can be deemed to have occurred. This 1957 ruling from *Bolam* v. *Friern Hospital Management Committee* (1 WLR 582, U.K., 1957) was further qualified in 1997 by the *Bolitho* ruling in *Bolitho* v. *City & Hackney Health Authority* (3WLR 1151, U.K., 1997) which added that the management must make *logical case* to the court and thus be defensible.

Bolam's near six decades of influence was seriously dented in 2015, by the landmark ruling in *Montgomery*. The UK High Court rejected the *Bolam* principle and ruled for the plaintiff awarding her £5.25 million. Since then, cases alleging obstetric negligence and related to disclosure are not dependent on peer standard of care but as per any trade or profession (and in this case, the highest standards in obstetrics). Although *Bolam* still rules in diagnosis and treatment, the *Montgomery* case has hammered a major nail in its coffin [12].

70.3.3 Causes of Litigation

In most countries, claims for obstetric litigation generally involve management during labour. In the UK, according to the report *Ten Years of Maternity Claims – An Analysis of NHS Litigation Authority 2000–2010*, the main subdivisions of intrapartum litigation target intrapartum management with cardiotocography (CTG) misinterpretation accounting for 14.05%, caesarean section issues at 13.24% and cerebral palsy at 10.65%. These litigation issues are looked at in greater depth below.

70.3.3.1 Fetal Morbidity and Mortality

Stillbirth, and early neonatal deaths, cerebral palsy, brachial plexus injuries, facial scars, skull and limb fractures are all massive disappointments to parents expecting a perfect newborn. Serious and prolonged intrapartum hypoxia (IPH) may lead to stillbirth at worst or at best organ damage such as cerebral palsy. From a liability point of view, a stillbirth involves much less quantum than brain damage where life expenses and money-not-earned will go into the calculation. However shocking and inhumane this sounds, this outlook is the norm with most court decisions.

A plethora of fetal morbidity effects have driven court claims. These range from clavicle fractures in cases of shoulder dystocia, to limb fractures in cases of assisted breech delivery, to skull fractures with or without underlying brain damage in cases of instrumental deliveries and manual rotations. In *D's parent and guardian* v. *Greater Glasgow Health Board,* (S.C.L.R. 124, 2012), a Kielland's rotational forceps delivery led to a rare spinal cord compression-torsion damage at C1/2, resulting in total paralysis from the head down including inability to breathe spontaneously.

Brachial plexus damage is not unknown even in caesarean section (CS) deliveries with too small an incision for adequate delivery. It may also occur spontaneously in labour, when the posterior shoulder forcefully abuts against the sacral promontory, propelled by uterine contractions. In shoulder dystocia, one aspect of litigation should scrutinize any antenatal or intrapartum warning and another seeks the details of the manoeuvres performed to free the shoulders.

Many other situations, such as metabolic disorders, chemical exposure and failure of rhesus immunization, may lead to fetal damage. Wrongful abortion and termination of a viable pregnancy (e.g. at hysterectomy) have led to litigations. An increasing element of litigation, however, concerns what is known as wrongful birth where the diagnosis of a malformation or the effects of disease such as rubella are missed, thus depriving the parents of a chance to terminate what they consider to be an abnormal pregnancy.

70.3.3.2 Antenatal Ultrasonography

The credentials of the ultrasonographer involved in the case are likely to be questioned in court. Sound training and an effective machine with good resolution, suitably sensitive callipers and an adequate transducer are basic musts in ultrasound investigations. To avoid litigation, one should ensure that patient consent is specifically asked for and full disclosure effected, including, if relevant, one's training particularly if incomplete. The limitations of ultrasound as a diagnostic tool should also be briefly discussed during the session. Questions must be carefully and honestly answered, and the written report must be immediately given to the patient while a copy is held in the notes. Any photographs given should show what is actually described, whether this shows normal or abnormal anatomy and possibly describing the type of the machine and the printer used.

Many basic missed obstetric diagnoses provide for a tough court defence. These diagnoses include various brain formation/head/cord defects (e.g. anencephaly), limb defects, dwarfism, some cardiac and renal as well as alimentary tract abnormalities and hydrops fetalis. Very often, liability of substandard care is reached quickly, as in *D* v. *L Hospital NHS Trust* (EWHC 1392 (QB), 2004) where exomphalos and cloacal maldevelopment were missed by the ultrasonographer. A missed diagnosis of fetal abnormalities carries liability per se, but often this liability is amplified by being used as grounds for a wrongful birth plea. For example, in *CW* v. *Hospital NHS Trust*, wrongful birth was claimed on the basis that an anomaly scan at 21 weeks missed the limb reduction deformity of bilateral absent ulnae [13]. The court ruled for breach of duty of care and ruled establishing the compensatory quantum at £1.8 million.

Situations such as misdiagnosed placentography may also provide serious liability charges (e.g. during amniocentesis guidance). Another source of litigation is emergency ultrasound reporting, and this should always be backed up by a more senior and experienced colleague as soon as possible in daylight hours, even if the first result appeared normal.

70.3.3.3 Birth Management

The SOC of birth management is considered to be that standard of safe and efficient practice that an ordinary and prudent obstetrician would use. The SOC required by the court is not of some super-obstetrician but of one who, given the qualifications and experience of the defendant, would practise safely and effectively, *secundum artem*. The stage of training, experience and qualifications of the defendant must be comparable to the Court's assumed ideal ordinary practitioner delivering the same intervention and in the same conditions. Thus, one cannot expect a family physician or a midwife to have the same ability as an obstetrician, or a freshly qualified obstetrician as one with 10 years of post-graduate experience.

The Intrapartum Importance of Antenatal Care

Good or bad birth management often has its roots in the antenatal care delivered to the patient: the history obtained, normal clinical and haematological parameters, confirmation of dates, maternal weight profiles and fetal growth profiles, risk category, evidence of hypertension, pre-eclampsia, diabetes etc.

In *MJ (a Minor)* v. *Dr Jonathan McLean Hayward (1) and The Royal Berkshire NHS Foundation Trust (2)*, a breach of the SOC was declared through failure to administer adequate antenatal care with the resultant antenatal hypoxic ischaemia contributing to the eventual brain damage [14]. Likewise, a history of previous mechanical problems or of a macrosomic baby, present maternal obesity, gross maternal weight gain, diabetes macrosomia or a prolonged pregnancy all render a heightened awareness and its disclosure an obligatory and basic part of the SOC.

Documentation

Labour ward documentation including partograms and CTG strips are indispensable court evidence. All entered information must be legible, dated, timed and signed. In one obstetric series, poor documentation led to 5% of cases being indefensible [15]. In a 2015 Medscape malpractice report [16], poor documentation was itself responsible for 4% of the litigation. Documented evidence is often the most important Court deciding evidence [17].

In *Baynham* v. *Royal Wolverhampton Hospitals NHS Trust* (EWHC3780GB, 2014), a cerebral palsy case, accurate and well-kept clinical records convinced the court that no medical negligence could have prevented the responsible cause of the damage, namely abruptio placentae. In conditions like pre-eclampsia, accurate and detailed documentation, fluid charts and neurological assessments are all a must. It is disconcerting to read of a 'starkly apparent' level of clinical neglect, as well as record keeping, as being prevalent in *R* v. *Inner London North Coroner* (EWCA Civ 383, 2001) where the mother of twins died from pre-eclampsia/eclampsia syndrome.

Records may be required in court, decades after birth. In *Davis* v. *City and Hackney Health Authority* (2 Med LR 366, 1991), a cerebral palsy patient born in 1963 sought court redress in 1985 with the writ being issued on 1 April 1987. Lack of availability of records such as a CTG tracing is one aspect of spoliation, defined as the intentional, reckless or negligent withholding, hiding, altering, fabricating or destroying of evidence relevant to a legal proceeding. Missing records are usually viewed negatively by the court. In *London Strategic Health Authority* v. *Whiston* (3 All ER 452, 2010), we read: 'The judge put in the scales the prejudice that the defendant would suffer by reason of the loss of the CTG.'

Praxis and Discipline

Labour ward management is essentially the obstetric equivalent of the medical intensive care unit. The same discipline, awareness, communication, ability to adapt to emergencies, sometimes multiple and concurrent and the need for precise and succinct record keeping must be continually enforced. The spirit of such an attitude was not respected in the circumstances leading to *Jill Clark (A.P.) Pursuer and Reclaimer against Greater Glasgow Health Board Defenders and Respondents* (CSIH 17, 2017): 'The midwife in charge had failed to allocate a qualified midwife to supervise the student midwife. The midwives, like the registrar, knew or ought to have known of the risks caused by the use of Syntocinon and that the labour was to be undertaken with care. They ought to have stopped or reduced the Syntocinon and sought review by a more senior midwife, or a member of the medical staff, at or around 3.05am.'

Syntocinon Stimulation and Prostaglandin 'Ripening' (familiarity breeds contempt)

The indispensable and ubiquitous use of syntocinon should be constantly judiciously tempered by an appreciation of its risks, and its careful use using infusion pumps cannot be more strongly advocated. The intrapartum CTG (I-P CTG) strip tracing renders a legal representation of the frequency of the uterine contractions – an asset (or a liability) if disaster strikes and questions are asked. Uterine activity must reveal at least a clear 60- to 90-second inter-contraction interval, and any stimulation encroaching on this is asking for problems. In *K* v. *Guy's & St Thomas' NHS Trust*, negligence was ruled when the syntocinon rate was noted to have been disastrously stepped up, instead of being immediately discontinued, in the presence of an alarming CTG tracing, leading to uterine rupture and fetal death [18].

Controversy persists regarding the use of syntocinon in the presence of a uterine scar (e.g. from a previous CS). If syntocinon is used in this circumstance, besides the maintenance of a hawkeye observation, everything must be fully documented. Rates of syntocinon exceeding 12 mu/min, are never justified in the presence of a previous scar and there are those who advocate it even in the normal patient [19]. Part of the plaintiff's plea in *Evans* v. *Birmingham and The Black Country Strategic Health Authority* (EWCA Civ 1300, 2007) concerned the use of excessive amounts of syntocinon in a case leading to cerebral palsy. In *Pauline Mckenzie Pursuer* v. *Fife Acute Hospitals NHS Trust Defenders* (CSOH 63, 2006), persistent and inappropriate syntocinon stimulation leading to acute IPH and subsequent cerebral palsy (CP) was declared by the court as constituting substandard care medical negligence: 'Accordingly, if the obstetric registrar, who was the defenders' employee, had acted with reasonable care by stopping the syntocinon infusion and arranging the prompt delivery of Kyle by 2140 hours on that date, I consider that Kyle would not have suffered the brain damage which has given rise to this action. I conclude therefore that the admitted negligence of that employee caused that damage.'

Prostaglandin use for cervical ripening also has its own potential risks, which may be falsely overlooked especially when no uterine or cervical response seems apparent. However, once prostaglandins are administered, the patient must remain admitted and regularly CTG monitored until delivery. In *Ogwang* v. *Redbridge Healthcare NHS Trust* (All ER (D) 82 (Jul) 2003), a patient with pre-eclampsia who had been administered prostaglandins for two consecutive days was discharged 10 days later, only to be re-admitted next day with an abruptio placentae, the child incurring severe cerebral palsy. The use of prostaglandins in the presence of a uterine scar retains its opponents, but if resorted to, great caution must be exercised. In the case *J* v *Birmingham Women's Hospital NHS,* uterine hyperstimulation from prostaglandin stimulation alone led to the rupture of a previous CS scar [20]. There is also no defence for the use of concurrent prostaglandin and syntocinon administration.

Intrapartum Cardiotocography (I-P CTG)

Intrapartum cardiotocography (I-P CTG) remains the only practical assessment currently available in high-risk labour monitoring. Because of its drawbacks, including its low sensitivity and high specificity, it should be considered only as a *screening* test for IPH and thus requires confirmation with fetal blood sampling (FBS) or one of the newer methods of assessment such as STAN. Medico-legally, I-P CTG monitoring tends to suffer from the *shifting sands phenomenon* as a result of both innate weaknesses such as high intra- and inter-observer error as well as constantly changing criteria and multiple classifications of abnormalities and their respective action protocols [21].

Although only 50–60% of worst-case scenario I-P CTGs can be confirmed as associated with hypoxia and acidosis [22], uterine stimulation must be stopped immediately until the underlying causation is clarified. Having said that, a severe bradycardia exceeding 3 minutes' duration necessitates intermediate and determined actions and not explanations. In *KR Pursuer against Lanarkshire Health Board Defender* (CSOH.133, U.K., 2016), it was the court's declared opinion that a persistent bradycardia of 80–90 beats per minute (bpm) should have been interpreted along National Institute for Health and Care Excellence (NICE) and Royal College of Obstetricians and Gynaecologists (RCOG) guidelines as constituting an 'acute fetal compromise'.

Ignoring I-P CTG abnormalities is indefensible. In *Popple (a child by his litigation friend, Stephen Popple)* v. *Birmingham Women's NHS Foundation Trust* (All ER, U.K., 2012), the court ruled that if the I-P CTG abnormalities had not been ignored and an episiotomy had been performed, a time period of 12 to 17 minutes would have been saved and prevented the asphyxia leading to severe dyskinetic or athetoid cerebral palsy.

Intrapartum cardiotocography interpretation must never be interpreted in isolation but in the light of all possible available detail, be it clinical, sonographic or from Doppler studies. However, this never precludes common sense when immediate delivery is clearly indicated. This should have been the case in *L* v. *West Midlands Strategic Health Authority* (EWHC 259 (QB), U.K., 2009), where the court ruled for negligence in a case of cerebral palsy and deemed that the loss of six avoidable minutes with a tight double nuchal cord was responsible for the bulk of the cerebral insult.

Ignorance of I-P CTG Interpretation –– After a good 50 years of clinical CTG monitoring, both the court and the medical community still repeatedly call for correct CTG interpretation. In *Azzam* v. *General Medical Council* (A11 ER(D) 149 (Dec), U.K., 2008), the court, backing the Medical Council's decision, declared that 'The panel's conclusion was that the appellant's assessment of the CTG scan had been inappropriate, inadequate and irresponsible, not in the best interests of the mother and below the standards which reasonably have been expected of a competent obstetrician.' Similar judgements are by no means rare, across both sides of the Atlantic. In 2007, 34% of stillbirth claims involved a clear misinterpretation of CTG traces [23]. It is morally, medically and legally untenable for a labour ward obstetrician not to be fully conversant with I-P CTG interpretation along the latest official guidelines.

Fetal Blood Sampling (FBS) – – Fetal blood sampling (FBS) retains its role of confirming or rejecting hypoxia as originally screened for by I-P CTG in high-risk cases. In spite of much surrounding controversy, FBS is superior to the assumption of intrauterine hypoxia from I-P CTG alone [24]. Furthermore, in spite of the newer and more popular methods such as STAN, both the RCOG as well as the NICE guidelines still recommend it. Furthermore here, the courts still consider FBS as the gold standard. In the 2018 Scottish case *LT Pursuer against Lothian NHS Health Board Defender* (CSOH29, U.K., 2018) we read: '. . . . In the light of the satisfactory results of the FBS at 16:58, Lord Brailsford rejected the consent case'. Again in 2018, we find in the English case *ML (a child proceeding by his Litigation Friend SL)* v. *Guy's and St Thomas' National Healthcare Foundation Trust* (EWHC 2010, U.K., 2018), the court stated: 'I understand Mr Forbes to be saying that with the history of thick meconium, and with the history of CTG abnormalities, even though the baby was fine at that moment . . . when the FBS was done.'

Intrapartum Hypoxia (IPH), Cerebral Palsy (CP) and Legal Liability

After stillbirth, the second most damaging complication from sustained, severe IPH is brain damage as often exemplified by CP. However, naturally other organ damage may occur along with CP. The most crucial point to be stressed here is that, *birth asphyxia is one preventable cause of CP, but it is a minority cause.* Much medico-legal evolution over the last 50 years has accompanied the increasing scientific recognition that preventable IPH does not cause the preponderance of cerebral palsy but only of about 14.5% of CP cases [25]. However, as an aside, this 14.5% causation cost the UK NHS in excess of £390 million between 2012 and 2016 [26]. And that, apart from the human toll of misery and suffering.

Cerebral palsy caused by IPH exhibits specific features resulting from the inevitable and preceding hypoxic ischaemic encephalopathy (HIE). Clear pH and acid-base evidence of hypoxia is accompanied by evidence of severe transient cerebral oedema clearly demonstrable on brain imagery studies. Evidence of other hypoxic organ damage may be present, and the CP itself is of a spastic quadriplegic dyskinetic form.

Over the past 50 years, court reasoning about CP has *slowly* and *generally* evolved along scientific facts showing that IPH-oriented, obstetrically liable CP is a minority cause, albeit this minority is generally preventable, due to frequently associated negligence and is the most crippling of NHS payouts. Several examples of such court-confirmed negligence have already been quoted. Furthermore, obstetric liability may not be simply limited to labour-oriented IPH. Trauma in the form of a prolonged and forceful delivery of a child's head using a Simpson's forceps instead of an indicated Kielland's forceps led to confirmation of liability in *Whiston* v. *London Strategic Health Authority* (113 BMLR 110).

However, obstetricians must prepare themselves for the legal vacuum created by the diminishing numbers of CP cases alleging damage from second-stage asphyxia and which is likely to befilled by antenatal scrutiny. For far too long have courts been distracted by sole and over-zealous scrutiny limited to second-stage labour management. Clinically, professional colleges such as the ACOG have long stressed the need to look further afield for CP causation [27]. This is likely to up the ante with a new generation of lawsuits centring on antenatal management with an emphasis on possible conditions such as hypothyroidism, infections, thrombophilia and mismanagement of obstetric complications like pre-eclampsia, multiple pregnancy and chorioamnionitis. Mismanagement of prematurity, the commonest associated factor and already the basis of much general medico-legal complaints, may itself provide liability grounds for CP [28].

There is some evidence that post-term delivery at 42 weeks may also be associated with CP [29]. In *William* v. *Blackpool Victoria Hospital NHS Trust* (EWHC 1744 (QB), U.K., 2003), although the claim failed, delivery left until 43 weeks with evidence of intrauterine growth restriction (IUGR) was put forward as a potential contributor to CP. The misdiagnosis or mismanagement of IUGR has many aspects of contention. The asymmetrical type may be claimed as a direct cause (unsuccessfully) as in *Robertson (an infant)* v. *Nottingham Health Authority* (22 BMLR 49, U.K., 1994). Similarly, untreated hypoglycaemia in the newborn was accepted as cause of the brain damage in *A H (By Her Mother and Litigation Friend M)* v. *London Strategic Health Authority known as NHS London* [30]. Although symmetrical IUGR may hint more at an innate cause of the CP such as chromosomal aberrations, it may also be caused by early intrauterine infections such as cytomegalovirus (CMV), rubella or toxoplasmosis, which may yet open another liability management facet.

The role of asymptomatic chorioamnionitis is also gaining ground in the same setting. In another failed claim, *Ludwig (by her mother and litigation friend, Ludwig)* v. *Oxford Radcliffe Hospitals NHS Trust and another* (EWHC 96 (QB), U.K., 2012), the plea centred on chorioamnionitis with group B streptococcus as a cause of the CP.

Maternal Morbidity/Mortality

Labour may result in liable maternal morbidity or mortality in both vaginal and abdominal delivery.

Obstetric Perineal Damage – – Damage to bladder/urethra/anus/rectum are all injuries which have led to litigation on morbidity claims of pain, aesthetic damage, dyspareunia, urinary and faecal urgency or incontinence or the symptoms of vesicovaginal and/or rectovaginal fistulae. Such damage should be detected at delivery, and senior obstetric management must be involved immediately with all interventions carefully noted with date and times.

Anaesthetic Problems – – Anaesthetic problems, such as severe epidural-induced maternal hypotension, may well overlap onto the obstetrician's management, dragging both anaesthetist and obstetrician into liability suits. Anaesthetic mishaps may range from failed intubation or failed epidural/spinal insertion to fatal cardiopulmonary collapse. Less harmful, but no less potentially contentious, are complications such as retained awareness during CS under general anaesthesia and inadequate pain relief in labour or during instrumental or abdominal delivery. Regional anaesthesia has its share of problems, including failure, intrathecal injections with resultant high spinal/epidural blocks, severe hypotension and nerve/cord damage.

Many problems are avoidable with due care. For example, awareness under general anaesthesia, which is a terrifying experience, may be countered both by greater anaesthetic skill, e.g. in the use of neuromuscular blocking agents and maintaining the right level of anaesthesia, and by greater attention to one's work, such as ensuring the correct state of fullness of vaporizers and cylinders and that pumps are delivering their medication and in the correct dose. Joint regular morbidity meetings attended by both labour ward obstetricians and obstetric anaesthetists may help diminish or pre-empt disasters from happening, especially on whirlwind labour ward days.

Uterine Rupture – – Reference has already been made to this catastrophic complication in conjunction with care in the use of syntocinon and prostaglandins, especially, but not solely, in the presence of a previous CS scar. Current patient autonomy demands that prior to the use of these agents, an adequate discussion with the patient is first held, and uterine rupture risks specifically disclosed in a fair and balanced way. No unnecessary panic should be induced but after the *Montgomery* case, such disclosure may prove to be wise, and ideally such discussion is held by a consultant or a senior and mature person. The disclosure should be noted in the file and the consent form for labour should specifically include reference to syntocinon/prostaglandins usage. Alternative modes of treatment (i.e. abdominal delivery) should also be discussed and recorded as discussed. Labour in such patients should be under greater vigilance than normal, and the steps taken to effect this, including discussions with all labour ward staff, should be entered in the patient's case notes. The team looking after such patients should be fully conversant with the case, and only experienced midwives should be allocated to the patient throughout all the labour.

Caesarean Section -- Many facets render this lifesaving operation a serious potential medico-legal death-trap.

Indications for CS

The indication(s) must be legally justifiable and discussed with the patient who must realize that the need lies in her own and/ or her child's interests. The only exception to this is a direct request by the patient herself for a CS. If the patient is counselled and warned about all the potential risks but is still adamant, legally the obstetrician is not in a position to refuse performing the surgery. If following the refusal of a CS by the obstetrician, the case reaches the courts, patient autonomy will definitely carry the day. All discussions must be fully documented with dates, times, witnesses' signature and signed by all concerned parties. There is a wide range of European opinion on the subject of accepting the patient's right to have an unwarranted CS. In Spain, 15% of obstetricians comply, in France 19%, in the Netherlands 22% whereas in Germany it is 75% and in the UK 79%.

Liability may be incurred both by not offering a CS where it is needed (see *Montgomery*) but also by offering it or doing it not within a reasonable time interval. In *Matthews* v. *Waltham Forest Health Authority* (Lexis Citation 2522, U.K., 1991) dealing with a case of cerebral palsy, the defendants were found liable of medical negligence for performing the required CS almost 3 hours later than when first indicated.

Valid Consent

The disclosure must include:

- A brief but clear description of the operation, its approximate duration and the pain/discomfort involved as well as its control during and after the operation.
- Any alternatives to the CS as well as their advantages, if any, and their risks and dangers.
- What may happen if the operation is not done as advised.

The patient must have the *mental capacity* to understand all this and accept the offer completely *freely* without anybody's influence. If dealing with an unaccompanied young teenager, say, below 13 years old, it is best to discuss the situation with the hospital's lawyers. Older mature teens if clearly understanding what is described to them may sign their own witnessed consents. By the ever-increasing powers of patient autonomy, the patient has every right to refuse a CS, even if maternal/fetal death is likely to follow in spite of the decision being fully against the obstetrician's principles.

Other Liabilities

All the usual potential surgery-anaesthesia complications of potential legal challenge may plague a CS. These may range from visceral damage, forgotten swabs or instruments, skin deformation, infections in the operation site, haemorrhage from any source to lingering nerve pains. The importance of good communication with the patient can never be overstressed, and by itself it may lay to rest many spectres. Furthermore, issues such as the disappointment following a failed VBAC (vaginal birth after CS) may require more delicate handling and patience. Sometimes an unjustified feeling of the patient's failure may be projected in various guises onto the obstetrician and in itself fuel unjustified litigation in or out of court.

Maternal Mortality -- In 2013–2015, maternal death rate in the UK stood at 8.76 per 100 000 maternities, with cardiac disease remaining the leading cause of indirect maternal death and thrombosis/ thromboembolism remaining the leading cause of direct maternal death. Haemorrhage has increased (non-significantly) due to a small degree of increase in abnormal placentation. Maternal suicide is the third highest cause of direct maternal deaths. All may incur liability of management if SOC is substandard. The roles of eclampsia, anaesthesia and infection should not be underplayed since they often provide preventable action (www.ukoss.org).

From 1990 to 2015, according to the UN inter-agency estimates, the global maternal mortality ratio declined by 44% from 385 deaths to 216 deaths per 100 000 live births, with the sub-Saharan Africa and South Asia regions accounting for 88% of maternal deaths worldwide [30].

For countries with substantial numbers of irregular migrants, such as Malta with its mostly sub-Saharan migrant community, perinatal morbidity and mortality demand extra vigilance. A number of cultural and socioeconomic factors may deprive such a group from benefitting from the full benefits of the recipient country's maternity services, leading to, among other things, maternal mortality [31].

70.4 Conclusion

Childbirth by its very essence is, for most people, the most beautiful and fulfilling experience surrounding femininity in the family setting. So too is the specialty of obstetrics. Awareness of current obstetric legal issues is crucial for safe and wholesome practice, but letting it take priority in management is equivalent to missing the forest for the trees. A litigious patient may sue for any reason under the sun, justifiably or otherwise. The other 99% of patients are grateful for the obstetrician's assistance in the enactment of life's greatest miracle. Do not let defensive medicine rule, for it is a cruel master. Neither go about, naively wearing a blindfold to liability. Confidently walk somewhere in between. Good practice is the best defence.

References

1. Magro M. *Five Years of Cerebral Palsy Claims – A Thematic Review of NHS Resolution Data*. London: National Health Service; 2017. https://resolution .nhs.uk/wp-content/uploads/2017/09/ Five-years-of-cerebral-palsy-claims_A-thematic-review-of-NHS-Resolution-data.pdf (Accessed 15/11/2018.)

2. Studdert DM, Mello MM, Gawande AA, et al. Claims, errors, and compensation payments in medical malpractice litigation. *N Engl J Med.* 2006;**354**:2024–33.

3. Hammond CB. The decline of the profession of medicine. *Obstet Gynaecol.* 2002;**100**(2):221–5.

4. G'Sell-Macrez F. Medical malpractice and compensation in France: Part I: the French rules of medical liability since the Patients' Rights Law of March 4, 2002. *Chicago-Kent Law Rev.* 2011;**86**(3):1093–1123.

5. Thurn P. Das patientenrechtegesetz – sicht der rechtsprechung. *MedR.* 2013;**31**:153–7.

6. Fusciani M. Rischio tecnologico e responsabilità legale in sanità. Milan: Politecnico di Milano; 20 September 2004, 2004/2.

7. Fava S. Medico-legal seminar: Medical Association of Malta – 15 October 2002. www.mam.org.mt/newsdetail.asp?i=35 2&c=1 (Accessed 12/10/2013.)

8. Economou C, Kaitelidou D, Karanikolos M, Maresso A. Greece : Health system review. *Health Syst in Transit.* 2017;**19**(5):1–166.

9. News Editor. New forensic and legal medicine findings reported from University of Coimbra – Lessons from a decade of technical-scientific opinions in obstetrical litigation. *Forensics: Health & Medicine Week.* 15 August 2014: 2711.

10. Buttigieg GG, Micallef Stafracc K. Medico-legal medicine: family practice and the latest views on disclosure of information and consent. *Int J Fam Commun Med.* 2018;**2**(2):92–5.

11. Elliman S, Spink A, Lace Mawer B. Hempsons, Havers P. Cases: failure to administer adequate antenatal care. MJ (a Minor) v Dr Jonathan McLean Hayward (1) and The Royal Berkshire NHS Foundation Trust (2). *J Patient Safety Risk Manage* 2010;**16**(1):35–8.

12. Buttigieg GG. Re-visiting Bolam and Bolitho in the light of Montgomery v Lanarkshire Health Board. *Medico-Legal J.* 2018;**86**(1):42–4.

13. Wrongful birth claim – child missing upper limbs bilaterally. CW v Hospital NHS trust. *Clin Risk.* 2011;**17**(6):234.

14. Failure to administer adequate antenatal care – MJ (a Minor) v Dr Jonathan McLean Hayward (1) and The Royal Berkshire NHS Foundation Trust (2). *Clin Risk.* 2010;**16**(1):35.

15. Ward CJ. Analysis of 500 obstetric and gynecologic malpractice claims: causes and prevention. *Am J Obstet Gynecol.* 1991;**16592**:298–304.

16. Medscape Malpractice Report. Why ob/ gyns get sued. 2015. www .medscape.com/features/slideshow/mal practice-report-2015/obgyn#page=2 (Accessed 05/02/2018.)

17. Thomas J. Medical records and issues in negligence. *Indian J Urol.* 2009;**25** 3:384–8.

18. Obstetrics: syntocinon usage, birth asphyxia, death of son – K v Guy's & St Thomas' NHS Trust. *Clin Risk.* 2002;**8**(1):37.

19. Arulkumaran S, Symonds M. Intrapartum fetal monitoring – medico-legal implications. *Obstet Gynaecol.* 1999;**1**(2):23–6.

20. Oxygen deprivation following uterine rupture at birth causing cerebral palsy J v Birmingham Women's Hospital NHS Trust. *Clin Risk.* 2008;**14**(6):246.

21. Buttigieg GG. The shifting sands of medico-legal intra-partum CTG (I-P CTG) monitoring. *Medico-Legal J.* 2016;**84**(1):42–5.

22. Hinshaw K, Ullal A. Peripartum and intra-partum assessment of the fetus.

Anaesth Intensive Care Med. 2007;**8**:331–6.

23. *Confidential Enquiry into Maternal and Child Health (CEMACH) : Perinatal Mortality 2007: United Kingdom.* London: CEMACH; 2009.

24. Steer PJ. Fetal scalp blood sampling during labour: is it a useful diagnostic test or a historical test which has no longer a place in modern clinical obstetrics? *BJOG.* 2014;**121**(13):1749–50.

25. Graham EM, Ruis KA, Hartman AL, Northington FJ, Fox HE. A systematic review of the role of intrapartum hypoxia-ischemia in the causation of neonatal encephalopathy. *Am J Obstet Gynecol.* 2008;**199**(6):587–95.

26. Magro M. Five years of cerebral palsy claims A thematic review of NHS Resolution data. September 2017 https://resolution.nhs.uk/wp-content/ uploads/2017/09/Five-years-of-cerebral-palsy-claims_A-thematic-review-of-NHS-Resolution-data.pdf (Accessed 15/11/2018.)

27. D'Alton ME, Hankins GDV, Berkowitz RL, et al. Executive summary: neonatal encephalopathy and neurologic outcome. *Obstet Gynecol.* 2014; **123**(4):896–901.

28. Thornton JG. Pre-term labour: obstetric aspects. Clinical focus – prematurity. *Clin Risk.* 1999;**5**(1):1.

29. Moster D, Wilcox AJ, Vollset SE, Markestad T, Lie RT. Cerebral palsy among term and postterm births. *JAMA.* 2010;**304** 9:976–82.

30. Nadel D, Napley K, Grace J, Partridge R. Case: Brain damage following neonatal hypoglycaemia: H (By her Mother and Litigation Friend M) v London Strategic Health Authority (known as NHS London). *Clin Risk.* 2008;**14**(5):200–1.

31. Buttigieg GG. Obstetric and medico-legal challenges posed by sudden immigrant shift in a southern Mediterranean island. *Anthropology.* 2017;**5**(3):2–7.

Research and Audit in Obstetric Practice

Paul Simpson & Martin Cameron

71.1 Research in Obstetric Practice

71.1.1 Introduction

Obstetric research is vital. It provides insights into normal physiological responses of the body, the impact of pathology on those responses and understanding about how to diagnose and treat disease.

This chapter discusses evidence-based medicine, the types of clinical study that are undertaken and how to appraise these studies. A summary of statistical terms and how clinical evidence in graded is also included to provide the additional tools needed for the assessment of the published literature. 'Scientific illiteracy is a major failing of medical education' [1]; this chapter will help you to feel more comfortable when reading the medical literature.

71.1.2 Evidence-based Medicine

A key responsibility as a doctor is to maintain an up-to date level of knowledge about your chosen specialty [2]. 'Evidence-based medicine is the conscientious, explicit and judicious use of current best evidence in making decisions about healthcare' [3]. When this evidence base is combined with the clinical expertise an individual has acquired through clinical practice, it ensures best possible clinical decisions are taken.

The volume of published medical literature means a clinician cannot read all the data available. Instead, a more selective approach is needed to ensure a focus is maintained on the most appropriate, reliable and relevant research studies to guide practice. There are five steps to this process [3]:

1. Define a clinical question.
2. Find the best evidence.
3. Appraise the evidence for validity, impact and applicability.
4. Integrate the outcome of critical appraisal with already established clinical experience, as well as patient preferences and expectations (guideline generation).
5. Review clinical practice against 'best practice' (clinical audit) as part of quality improvement and clinical governance.

Steps 3 to 5 are dealt with in further sections of this chapter. Initially, we concentrate on the process of establishing a clinical or research question and how to search the literature.

71.1.2.1 Setting a Research Question

Deciding on a research question can be for the purposes of informing your own clinical practice or as part of designing your own research study. In both circumstances, it is important to know what question you are trying to answer, which allows you to establish if the question has already been answered or needs investigating by way of a research study.

There are four components to consider: **P**opulation, **I**ntervention, **C**omparator, **O**utcome (PICO). The population should be defined in clear terms, considering factors such as age, parity, medical background and the healthcare setting in which they are being assessed. The intervention being studied is the treatment, intervention, diagnostic test or risk factor you are interested in, whereas the comparator group is an alternative population to the study population in which you hope to find a difference. The outcome is the defined consequences of the intervention you have identified.

71.1.2.2 Finding the Best Evidence

Research evidence is either primary (randomized controlled trial (RCT) or observational studies) or secondary (systematic reviews, meta-analysis or guidelines). Secondary evidence is often more helpful to answer clinical questions as pooling and analysis of data have been undertaken. When trying to answer a research question, the primary evidence is more useful. A literature search required to answer a research question may produce a systematic review, which could be published to guide other clinicians.

Literature Searching

The best resource for systematic reviews and assessment of secondary evidence is the Cochrane Library (www.cochranelibrary.com), which includes the following components for searching:

- Cochrane Database of Systematic Reviews (CDSR)
- Cochrane Central Register of Controlled Trials (CENTRAL)
- Cochrane Clinical Answers

In addition, the BMJ's Best Practice facility (https://bestpractice.bmj.com/info/) is a facility that incorporates research evidence, clinical expertise and patient preferences into specialty-specific conditions.

To access primary literature, there is a multitude of databases, with each one having some publications missing. It is helpful to conduct any literature search using two or three databases ensuring that important evidence is not excluded from your search in error. The following resources are helpful:

- MEDLINE®/PubMed® (www.ncbi.nlm.nih.gov/pubmed/) is produced by the US National Library of Medicine
- Google Scholar (https://scholar.google.co.uk)

- OVID (www.ovid.com/site/index.jsp) is provided by the Wolters Kluwer Health organization
- EMBASE (www.embase.com/login) is provided by Elsevier and has a more European emphasis with a greater focus on pharmacological content

Searching Strategy

The strategy will be influenced by the question being answered.

It is best to start with terms from your clinical question, considering all the PICO components, to create a list of free text terms including abbreviations and alternative spellings. Once this is complete, consider any controlled text terms or subject headings – known as MeSH (Medical Subject Headings) in PubMed®. These can then be combined in searches using 'and', 'or', and 'not' to create a set of results. Using 'and' will return papers containing both terms; using 'or' will return those papers with either one or both terms; 'not' should be used with caution as it will exclude papers containing a term of interest if they also include the one to be excluded. This is an iterative process which ensures the initial search net cast is very wide but then provides the facility to focus on a specific area within the literature. Although most databases track your searches for you, it is a good idea to keep a record of the steps you have taken to reach your final literature base.

71.1.2.3 Limitations of Evidence-based Medicine

The major criticisms and limitations of evidence-based medicine (EBM) were reviewed by Cohen et al in 2004. This review described the limitations in terms of five recurring themes: reliance on empiricism, narrow definition of evidence, lack of evidence of efficacy, limited usefulness for individual patients and threats to the autonomy of the doctor/patient relationship [4]. It was suggested that EBM should not be used in isolation and that the increased reliance on EBM be considered when designing studies.

This point was demonstrated by Smith and Pell's paper in the Christmas edition of the *BMJ*, where they highlight that observational data can be all that is needed to reach a safe conclusion. Their 'tongue-in-cheek' paper suggesting a double-blind, randomized, placebo-controlled, crossover trial to determine the effectiveness of parachutes during free fall was both amusing and illustrative [5].

71.1.3 Types of Research

Research begins with a question requiring an answer – the question can be prompted by observation of a phenomenon or generated by systematic reviews of the known literature. Once the question is formulated it is converted into a hypothesis to be tested. It is the testing of this hypothesis that guides the design of a research project. Consequently, formulation of the hypothesis and subsequent design is the most important step in the process – a well-designed study will predict the outcome of the results and subsequent conclusions, whereas a poorly designed study may result in incorrect conclusions or inconclusive result.

The null hypothesis (H_0) indicates that any observation has occurred by chance, while the alternative hypothesis (H_1) is the research hypothesis being tested. If the study is designed well and conducted correctly, the null hypothesis should be rejected. The results of a study rarely prove a result; rather, they provide evidence to support or refute the hypothesis. The larger the study or the more times it is repeated, the greater the weight of evidence and hence the closer one comes to proof of a hypothesis.

This concept of evidence to reject the null hypothesis is the basis of mathematical statistics, used to define how significant a result is. This is discussed in more detail later but $p < 0.05$, simply means the results of the study have a less than 5% likelihood of occurring by chance, suggesting the null hypothesis is very unlikely to be true and should be rejected. This is the accepted cut-off for the majority of studies, but it still leaves a small chance of accepting the alternative hypothesis in error (false positive or type I error – see later).

71.1.3.1 Biomedical Research

Biomedical research can be considered either basic or applied. Basic medical research tries to answer a question for the purposes of curiosity (e.g. what human placental factors trigger parturition?) and usually has no commercial value, whereas applied research tries to provide a specific solution to a problem and may have a commercial value (e.g. what biochemical changes can be used to reliably predict preterm birth?).

Basic Research

In vitro studies of biochemistry, physiology, pharmacology and genetics give insights into cellular and molecular mechanisms. This type of research can advance medical science and the understanding of pathology, which can then lead to advances in the treatment of disease.

Clinical Research

Clinical research tends to be the investigation of the safety and effectiveness of medications and treatments – first, to ensure they do no significant harm to patients, then that any side effects are tolerable and appropriate, and finally that they have a positive effect on the condition they are being suggested for.

Pre-clinical studies on human cells (in vitro) and in animal models (in vivo) provide useful information about efficacy, toxicity, pharmacokinetics and limited data on pharmacodynamics. These are a prerequisite for any new molecule that is being suggested for use in humans. Once all these data are available, they can be presented, along with a research protocol, to an ethics committee prior to commencing any in vivo study in humans.

Study Phases

Randomized controlled trials form the basis of most clinical research. They are undertaken in multiple phases:

- **Phase 0**: after pre-clinical studies, further details on pharmacodynamics are obtained by administering a subtherapeutic dose of study drug to a small cohort of volunteers (10–15 adult males), without a control group. Information on bioavailability and half-life are obtained as well as further pharmacokinetic data. Safety and efficacy cannot be determined, as the dose used is subtherapeutic.

- **Phase I**: gradually increasing doses of study drug are given to a group of 20–100 participants (usually adult male), again without a placebo control group. The main aim is establishing safety, pharmacodynamics and side effects. Phase Ia tends to be a single ascending dose and phase Ib multiple ascending doses.
- **Phase II**: administration to 100–300 participants is undertaken to establish efficacy, whilst continuing to collect safety data. There is a placebo control group to allow comparison and determine a biological effect (only 20% of studies proceed beyond this point).
- **Phase III**: a therapeutic dose is used in 1000–2000 patients to evaluate efficacy, effectiveness and safety. These are often multi-centre to aid recruitment of the numbers needed and will be placebo controlled. Two successful phase III RCTs are needed for regulatory approval, prior to marketing.
- **Phase IV**: this is post-marketing surveillance, which provides information on efficacy and side effects in the real world, whilst also giving data on more long-term use of the study drug. Even at this stage of development, safety concerns can lead to a licence being revoked and a drug being withdrawn from the market.

71.1.3.2   Qualitative vs. Quantitative Research

Quantitative research involves something that can be measured or quantified and expressed in numerical forms (e.g. percentage leading to statistical analysis and use of probability and confidence intervals to make decisions about the hypothesis being tested).

Qualitative research investigates things that cannot be expressed in numerical terms – such as opinions or behaviours. It can provide useful information about why things happen and how patients respond to certain conditions, but the conclusions can be open to the interpretation of the observer. In healthcare research, both quantitative and qualitative aspects are combined with health economics in mixed methods studies.

A paper by Porter et al highlighted the use of both types of research whilst exploring subfertility following caesarean section. Quantitative data clearly demonstrated an association, but the authors discuss how qualitative methods would be needed to explore the voluntary component of this relationship [6].

71.1.3.3   Study Design

There are two main categories of study type: observational and experimental. Data are correlated and patterns determined from usual clinical practice (e.g. descriptive studies, case series, cohort studies, case-control studies and cross-sectional studies in observational studies). An intervention takes place that is determined by the investigator and can be either controlled or non-controlled in experimental studies.

Observational Studies

Descriptive studies such as case series and questionnaires aim to describe data and characteristics about either a population or disease in a systematic and accurate manner. They are trying to determine the who, what, why, when and where of a disease: who has the disease, what disease is being studied, why the disease arose, when the disease occurs and where the disease arises ? [7]. Case series suffer from significant publication bias (for positive results) and questionnaires have problems with recall bias and participant selection, but descriptive studies are useful for rare conditions and to help inform other clinical trials. Descriptive studies cannot be used to determine a causal relationship; only analytical studies can be used for this purpose.

Analytical studies feature a comparison (or control) group, and the timing of the exposure and outcome determine the type of study. They can be used to test hypotheses and are considered to be more robust than descriptive studies.

Experimental Studies

Experimental studies, such as randomized controlled trials, are the gold standard in clinical research, as they are able to test an intervention or treatment with minimal chance for bias and incorrect conclusions.

71.1.3.4   Cohort Studies

Cohort studies are longitudinal observational studies used to investigate the causes of disease or establish links between risk factors and health outcomes. They run in logical sequence from exposure to outcome: a group of people without a disease or condition are identified, baseline measurements are taken and then they are followed over a period of time to see if disease develops [1].

The chosen cohort have a shared characteristic, experience or risk factor, which may influence the disease being studied. (e.g. do patients who smoke have a higher chance of a growth restricted baby? the cohort to be followed would be smokers). The comparison group may be the general population or another cohort of people unrelated to the study cohort who have had little or no exposure to the substance under investigation (e.g. non-smokers, in this example).

This type of study is expensive and can be conducted either prospectively or retrospectively. They are useful for calculating incidence rates, relative risks and 95% confidence interval (CI), and to study the natural history of a disease but are reliant on very specific definitions of exposure and outcome, to ensure only a single variable is being studied. However, they are unsuited to very rare conditions, as the numbers and time involved to show a result are prohibitive. The control group should be as similar as possible to the study group, but this is rarely possible – introducing additional factors that may influence the outcome (confounding factors). The long timeline involved in such studies also increases the risk of being lost to follow-up during the study, which introduces bias into the results and can lead to incorrect conclusions [8].

An excellent example of a cohort study in obstetrics is the Birthplace in England study, published in 2011 [9]. This study explored the occurrence of neonatal mortality and morbidity in different cohorts, dependent on their planned place of birth. An RCT in this situation would have been inappropriate as the primary outcome is relatively rare and randomization and blinding would have been impractical.

71.1.3.5 Case-control Studies

Case-control studies are ones in which a group of patients with the disease (the 'cases') and a group without (the 'controls') are compared on the basis of a suspected causal attribute. In the example above regarding small babies, the 'case' group would be those with small babies and the 'controls' those with normally grown babies – the smoking frequency amongst these two groups would then be determined.

In these studies, the 'control' group may not be entirely healthy and may have other, unidentified, risk factors that may influence the disease being studied. As such confounding factors are not as well controlled for. However, they are quick to deliver and as such tend to be cheaper. The results yield odds ratios (OR), which compare the proportion of individuals exposed in each group. If the incidence of the outcome in the population of interest is low (<5%) the odds ratio from a case-control study is a good estimate of relative risk [10].

When designing or evaluating such studies, consider these five areas:

- Is there an explicit criterion for the definition as a case with clear eligibility criteria?
- Do the controls come from the same population, selected independently from the exposure of interest?
- Were the data gatherers blinded to the 'case' or 'control' status of the participants (if impossible, were they blinded to the study hypothesis)?
- Did data gatherers elicit exposure from both groups using the same method?
- Have confounding factors been fully addressed in the design phase or acknowledged during analysis? [10]

71.1.3.6 Cross-sectional Studies

A cross-sectional study is one in which the disease and exposure status are measured simultaneously in a given population. They provide a snapshot of both the prevalence and disease characteristics at a particular time point. However, because they are analyzed simultaneously it is impossible to determine the order of exposure and disease occurrence and so causal relationships cannot be determined (i.e. did the exposure lead to the disease or did the disease influence the chance of finding the risk factor?) [1].

71.1.3.7 Randomized Controlled Trials (RCTs)

In order to evaluate a treatment or intervention, a study should be conducted to compare a study group and a control group. Individuals should be allocated randomly and in equal numbers to each group. This is known as a randomized controlled trial (RCT). It is better if both the participants and the study team are unaware of (or blinded to) which group a participant is in (i.e. a double-blind study). For some treatments or interventions, it is impossible to blind the participant to which group they are in. In these cases, only the study team are blinded to the intervention.

Randomized controlled trials are the gold standard as they minimize bias as well as known and unknown confounding factors. The process of randomization precludes *selection bias*; the process of blinding prevents *information bias*; and the process of protocol design eliminates *performance and detection bias*. *Attrition bias* cannot be excluded, but a well-designed protocol with clear inclusion and exclusion criteria will help to minimize it. Information on the loss of participants at each stage of a study is integral to any evaluation of attrition bias and this is why all published RCTs are required to contain a CONSORT (Consolidated Standards of Reporting Trials) diagram, which describes these data.

Despite the barriers to obstetrics research (discussed in Section 71.1.8), RCTs have been successfully carried out in obstetrics. Examples include: the Term Breech Trial [11], 'A Randomized Trial of Planned Caesarean or Vaginal Delivery for Twin Pregnancy' [12], the INFANT study looking at computer assisted cardiotocography (CTG) interpretation [13] and the TRUFFLE study exploring ductus venosus Doppler waveform compared to CTG short-term variability for the assessment of preterm, growth-restricted babies [14].

71.1.3.8 Meta-analyses and Systematic Reviews

Systematic reviews are orderly reviews of the published literature using predefined terms. An important step in the process is an evaluation of the quality of the studies identified. Those considered to be of low quality or too small to be of value are excluded from the review.

Any systematic review may also involve a meta-analysis, where the data from the collated studies are combined together for further statistical analysis. Before this can occur, an assessment of heterogeneity must be undertaken to ensure the studies are suitably similar as to warrant combining in a meta-analysis. There can be three types: clinical heterogeneity, where patient selection or clinical management is different; methodological heterogeneity, where study design or bias is difference; and statistical heterogeneity, where variation in intervention effects make comparison difficult.

An example of a systematic review and meta-analysis in obstetric practice is the Cochrane review of the use of progesterone in the prevention of preterm birth. The review considered 36 RCTs, but far fewer than this number of studies were considered to be of suitable quality to be included in the meta-analysis [15].

These types of study are considered to be the most reliable and provide strong medical evidence (see Figure 71.1). However, errors can still occur with such studies and they still do not provide proof, only strong evidence to support a particular conclusion.

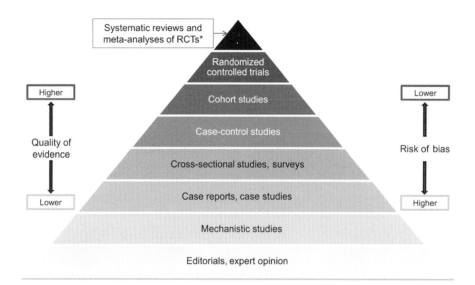

Figure 71.1 Hierarchy of Evidence
This diagram shows a model for the organization of quantitative studies – the higher up the pyramid the higher the quality of the evidence and the reduced chance of bias influencing the conclusions. (Adapted from [16])

71.1.4 Levels of Evidence

The hierarchy of evidence described in Figure 71.1 highlights how certain study designs are given a greater weighting than others. This weighting is related to the reliability of the conclusions drawn, which is influenced by the presence of confounding factors and bias. The higher up the hierarchy the lower the risk of inaccurate conclusions.

This hierarchy has been converted into 'Levels of Evidence' and shown in Table 71.1. The levels of evidence are used to define the grades of evidence, which are noted alongside recommendations in national and international guidelines.

71.1.5 Critical Appraisal

'Critical appraisal is a systematic process used to identify the strengths and weaknesses of a research article in order to assess the usefulness and validity of research findings' [18]. A review article by Young and Solomon sets out a clear 10-step guide to critical appraisal and is illustrated in Table 71.2.

The key to the process of critical appraisal is an assessment of the appropriateness of the study design and an evaluation of the methodological features of that design. The concepts of research questions and hypotheses have been outlined above and should be considered when evaluating studies. Questions about the effectiveness of a treatment or cost-effectiveness need an experimental design, whereas those with questions about incidence, prevalence, risk factors and diagnosis need observational data.

The concept of bias is very important when undertaking a critical appraisal. It is defined as a situation where the results have deviated from the truth and this can be through chance (random error) or due to the study methods (systematic bias). Random error does not influence the result in a particular direction but decreases precision and makes conclusions more difficult to draw. Systematic bias, on the other hand, does have a direction and can under- or overestimate the conclusion of a study.

The questions contained in the following sections can be used to evaluate systematic bias [18].

71.1.5.1 Systematic Reviews and Meta-analyses

- Has publication bias been considered – were studies excluded on the basis of language? What impact does the propensity to publish positive results have in this context?
- Were the studies identified and evaluated by two independent investigators?
- Was study quality assessed?
- Was heterogeneity assessed? Were the data appropriately similar to warrant meta-analysis?

71.1.5.2 Randomized Controlled Trials

- What was the process of randomization and, if the process was blinded, would participants have been able to guess their allocation?
- Were the outcomes clearly defined in the protocol and then measured objectively?
- What was the attrition rate and are all participants accounted for?

71.1.5.3 Cohort Studies

- Was the design prospective or retrospective?
- Is the cohort representative of an appropriate population?
- Have confounding factors been considered and acknowledged?
- How complete is the data set and how many were lost to follow-up?
- Was the study conducted for long enough to see a meaningful clinical effect?

71.1.5.4 Case-Control Studies

- Were the cases defined and representative of a meaningful population?
- How were controls selected and are they from the same population as cases?
- Was data collection identical in both groups?

Table 71.1 Levels of evidence

Level	Description	Recommendation grade
1a	Systematic review with homogeneity of RCTs	A: Level 1 (provided studies are consistent)
1b	Individual RCT with narrow confidence interval (CI)	
1c	All or none study	
2a	Systematic review with homogeneity of cohort studies	B: Level 2 or 3 (provided studies are consistent; extrapolations from level 1 studies)
2b	Individual cohort study; low-quality RCT (e.g. <80% follow-up)	
2c	Outcome research; ecological studies	
3a	Systematic review with homogeneity of case-control studies	
3b	Individual case-control studies	
4	Case series; poor-quality cohort or case-control studies	C: Level 4 (extrapolations from level 2 or 3)
5	Expert opinion, omitting explicit critical appraisal (includes opinion based upon physiology, bench research or first principles)	D: Level 5 (troublingly inconsistent or inconclusive studies from any level)

The Oxford Centre for Evidence-Based Medicine have defined levels of evidence based on the reliability of study undertaken. These levels of evidence can also be referred to as recommendation grades when used in guideline documents. (Reproduced from [17])

Table 71.2 Ten questions in a critical appraisal

Step	Question
1	Is the study question relevant?
2	Does the study add anything new?
3	What type of research question is being asked?
4	Was the study design appropriate for the research question?
5	Did the study methods address the most important potential sources of bias?
6	Was the study performed according to the original protocol?
7	Does the study test a stated hypothesis?
8	Were the statistical analyses performed correctly?
9	Do the data justify the conclusions?
10	Are there any conflicts of interest?

This list of 10 key questions can be used to assess the validity and relevance of a research article. (Reproduced from [18]).

▪ Were the study measures objective or subjective? Is there a risk of recall bias?

Finally, an assessment of the justification of the conclusions is required. The study may show a statistically significant result that is of no clinical value or the study may be underpowered (have too few patients) to demonstrate a statistically significant result even though there is a clear clinical difference between the groups.

Having considered all these factors, it is important to consider the significance of the research to your patient group. Does this research apply to them and should it influence your clinical practice?

71.1.6 Statistical Terms

The statistical analysis of results is the key to a study and involves the analysis, interpretation and presentation of the results data. These three steps provide the reader of the results with information about study methodology and the author's interpretation of the results in the context of the research question. The purpose of any figures, graphs and statistical tests is to provide the reader with an easy-to-understand, clear representation of the study data, which support the conclusions drawn by the author.

The mathematical explanation of statistical tests is beyond the scope of this chapter, but the following terms should facilitate interpretation and appraisal of research studies. There are three areas to consider: descriptive statistics, comparative statistics and epidemiological terms.

71.1.6.1 Descriptive Stats

Data can be described using three types of scale – interval data are called parametric data and have a normal distribution; nominal and ordinal data are 'non-parametric' [19].

▪ **Nominal**: a naming scale (data grouped according to a category, e.g. eye colour)
▪ **Ordinal**: an ordering scale (data grouped according to a category but the order relative to each other is important, e.g. five levels of satisfaction from very unhappy to very happy)
▪ **Interval**: a constant scale (the interval between data points is always the same, e.g. temperature or date)

Data sets are samples from a population and can be described in terms of the central point around which the data are scattered. The distribution of the data around the central point is important for a number of statistical tests and the normal (Gaussian) distribution is often assumed. This distribution has a characteristic symmetrical shape around a central point such that the mean, mode and median are all the same. The Shapiro–Wilk test and Kolmogorov–Smirnov test can be used to assess a data set for 'normality'.

Measurements of Central Tendency

- **Range** – spread of data in a sample (useful if a data set is skewed)
- **Mode** – the most frequently occurring value in a data set
- **Median** – the middle value in a ranked data set
- **Mean** – the average of all the terms in a data set (x or µ, for sample and population data, respectively)

Variability of Data

- **Variance** (s^2) – the average amount by which any individual measurement differs from the mean
- **Standard deviation** (s or σ, for sample and population data, respectively) – square root of variance
- **Confidence intervals** (CI) – description of the distribution of data, with 95% CI often being quoted (95% CI = mean +/− 2σ; this includes 95% of the data set with 5% lying outside in two 2.5% tails)

71.1.6.2 Comparative Statistics

Comparative statistics are a way to represent the testing of a hypothesis [19]. They are, by convention, based on the null hypothesis (H_0), which states that any variable has no effect. The null hypothesis is rejected, again by convention, if the probability of any observed outcome arising is $p<0.05$. In such a circumstance, the alternative hypothesis (H_1) would be accepted. This convention exposes the observer to two possible errors:

- **Type I error** – when H_0 is wrongly rejected, i.e. the variable has no effect but the data lead to a conclusion that there is an effect (1 in 20 trials if $p<0.05$ is used)
- **Type II error** – when H_0 is wrongly not rejected, i.e. the variable has an effect, but the data do not support that conclusion

Non-parametric Tests

- chi-square (χ^2) test, for 2 x 2 contingency tables
- Wilcoxon test, for paired data (same subject under different conditions)
- Mann–Whitney U-test, for unpaired data

Parametric Tests

- Student's *t*-test, for paired and unpaired data
- analysis of variance

T-Tests

T-tests can be undertaken on paired data (e.g. measurement of a variable under two different conditions) or unpaired data (e.g. observations on two separate groups within a population). These tests compare the mean of a sample with a predicted value (such as zero) or compare the means of two samples. The concept of comparing the means of two samples is very important for clinical trials (i.e. comparing a single variable in a control group and a treatment group).

Confidence Intervals for the Difference between Two Means

When two paired sample means are compared a confidence interval (CI) can be stated within which the difference between those means lies. If that CI contains zero, there is no significant difference between the two groups and H_0 would be accepted. However, if zero is not included, then H_1 should be accepted.

71.1.6.3 Statistical Terms

Incidence and Prevalence

The incidence (I) of a disease is the rate at which new cases occur in a population and is often expressed per 1000, 10 000, 100 000 or 1 000 000 dependent on the rate (i.e. how often a new case occurs). However, the prevalence (P) is the frequency of disease existence in any population at a given time (i.e. how much disease burden there is).

Predictive Tests

Predictive tests are assessed using the following four terms, all of which should be as high as possible:

- **Sensitivity** – the proportion of true positives identified by a test
- **Specificity** – the proportion of true negatives that are correctly identified by a test
- **Positive predictive value** – the proportion of people with a positive result who are correctly diagnosed
- **Negative predictive value** – the proportion of people with a negative result who are correctly diagnosed

Relative Risk and Odds Ratio

These terms both measure the association between an outcome variable and a predictor variable. Relative risk (RR) is the ratio of the risk of an event happening in a treatment group and the risk of an event happening in a control group (i.e. the comparison of two probabilities). Odds ratio (OR) is the ratio of the odds (number of events versus the number of non-events) of an event happening in a treatment group and the odds of an event happening in a control group (i.e. the comparison of two odds).

71.1.7 Guidelines

'Clinical guidelines are systematically produced statements to assist practitioners and patients in making decisions about specific clinical situations' [3]. The accepted methodology of such guidelines should include:

- a multidisciplinary working group,

- a well-described systematic review of the literature
- graded recommendations with links to the evidence (see Table 71.1)
- a system of quality control – an independent advisory board or peer review process

They can be found on:
- GuidelineCentral (www.guidelinecentral.com)
- OpenClinical (www.openclinical.org/guidelines.html)
- National Guideline Clearinghouse (www.ahrq.gov/gam/index.html)
- Royal College of Obstetricians & Gynaecologists (RCOG) (www.rcog.org.uk)
- National Institute for Health and Care Excellence (NICE) (www.nice.org.uk/guidance)
- Medical search engines

The most appropriate types of guidelines are those produced by international or national organizations using the above methodology. They are updated regularly (every 2–3 years) to incorporate new evidence as it is published and are the reference guides most clinicians rely on. In certain circumstances new guidelines will be commissioned in response to a significant shift in clinical practice or can result from multiple enquiries to an international or national body.

The recommendations provided in national guidelines can be considered 'best practice' but funding and practical limitations locally may mean that not all recommendations can be adhered to. This necessitates the production of regional or hospital-specific guidelines that guide local clinicians on how to deliver the best possible care with the resources available. Often the cost-effectiveness analysis found within more modern guidelines play a significant part in this local decision making.

71.1.8 Barriers to Research in Obstetric Practice

In 2015 a Scientific Impact Paper from the RCOG stated that 'obstetrics had only 1–5% of the drug pipeline of other mainstream specialties and fewer drugs in development than for some single diseases such as Crohn's disease' [20]. There can be practical and ethical barriers to conducting robust clinical research in obstetric practice but in a specialty where two patients are managed in tandem, the need for research and improved scientific understanding is never more pertinent.

There are multiple barriers, which must be considered and ameliorated in order to progress in this field. These include:

- **Two patients – mother and baby**. This makes things complex when studying interventions or drugs, which are given with the purpose of improving outcome for a single party. The unknown long-term impact and risk of teratogenicity have been highlighted by the problems of diethylstilboestrol and thalidomide exposure in utero. The balance of risks and benefits is made more complex by having to consider two patients in every clinical situation.

- **Recruitment**. This is particularly true of studies of intrapartum care, where informed consent for inclusion in a study is difficult. This is usually resolved by approaching multiple patients in the antenatal period, who may or may-not be suitable for recruitment during the intrapartum period – this is costly and time consuming.
- **Pharma company financial constraints.** Unfortunately, the cost of drug development has to be weighed against the likely profits from marketing a successful drug. As the market is relatively small and the duration of use is small the likely profit will be small – as such the payback for these companies is small, despite the fact that an intervention may be very clinically relevant. This is further compromised by the potential financial risk of litigation due to any unforeseen impact on the unborn fetus.
- **Complex obstetric conditions.** The underlying cause of obstetric conditions are often multifactorial and poorly understood, making the study population heterogeneous. This makes single interventions like a drug trial difficult to design and implement.
- **Meaningful outcomes.** When determining the measurable outcomes of an intervention looking at perinatal health, short-term measures such as perinatal morbidity have to be considered against longer-term outcomes such 3-year neurodevelopmental milestones. Any study looking at such long-term outcomes will often need to be observational in nature due to constraints such as cost and patient recruitment.
- **Novel compounds vs. repurposing.** The assessment of reproductive toxicology, pharmacokinetics and pharmacodynamics of a new compound for use in obstetrics is extremely costly. This makes repurposing a drug that already has a licensed indication a much more favourable proposition. Therefore, many drugs are routinely used 'off licence' in obstetrics despite never being formally evaluated for use in pregnancy.

71.2 Audit in Obstetric Practice

71.2.1 The Audit Cycle

'Research is concerned with discovering the right thing to do', whereas 'audit is concerned with ensuring the right thing is done' [3]. Audit and feedback are often used in healthcare organizations to improve health professionals' performance. A Cochrane review on this topic evaluated the effectiveness of this process and concluded the following:

Audit and feedback may be most effective when:
1. the health professionals are not performing well to start out with;
2. the person responsible for the audit and feedback is a supervisor or colleague;
3. they are provided more than once;
4. they are given both verbally and in writing;
5. they include clear targets and an action plan [21].

Clinical audit falls into three main types: critical incident audit, service evaluation/improvement and criterion-based audit.

71.2.2 Critical Incident Audit

An audit of maternal and perinatal mortality can be performed at a number of different levels – each adding to the depth of the audit a potential understanding of the events being audited [22]. First, this can merely take the form of simply recording the number of deaths. Second, the causes of death can be categorized into groups. Third, the potential avoidable factors or suboptimal care can be recorded against those categories to explore areas in which care could be improved.

An excellent example of this type of large-scale national audit is MBRRACE-UK, conducted by the Nuffield Department of Public Health. They use audit and confidential enquiry to evaluate and improve the care of pregnant women (www.npeu.ox.ac.uk/mbrrace-uk).

71.2.3 Service Evaluation and Quality Improvement

An audit can also be used to evaluate the structure of services, the process of care or the outcome of care. In *service evaluation*, there is guidance to suggest care is better delivered within certain structures (e.g. antenatal care of patients with complex medical needs such as diabetes or cardiac disease are better delivered within a multidisciplinary team). The delivery of this service can be evaluated or audited across a region.

Quality improvement (QI) is about making healthcare safer, effective, patient centred, timely, efficient and equitable. The aim of QI is to balance all of these aspects to strive for whole system change to achieve the following:

- better patient outcomes
- better system performance (care delivery)
- better professional development

Making large-scale changes in a single step is daunting and impractical and so smaller-scale changes are required. The Plan, Do, Study, Act (PDSA) cycle (https://improvement.nhs.uk/resources/pdsa-cycles) is a way of testing any small-scale change and evaluating its effectiveness before implementing a change. This tool allows system changes to be made in incremental steps to achieve the aims above.

71.2.4 Criterion-based Audit

A criterion-based clinical audit is the process by which a clinician evaluates their practice against the evidence base and clinical guidelines. Through a process of evaluating practice against specific criteria and then changing practice where needed, the overall quality of care offered can be improved.

The evaluation of *process measures* is the most common audit type. These audits evaluate the clinical use of an intervention that is known to alter a patient outcome (e.g. the use of antenatal magnesium sulphate preceding preterm delivery). Conversely, audits of *outcome measures* look at patient

responses to an intervention, be it improvement of symptoms or quality of life, or negative outcomes such as side effects or surgical morbidity.

The audit cycle involves five key steps:

- topic selection
- standard setting
- data collection
- implementation of change to improve care, if necessary
- subsequent data collection to evaluate the change in care

71.2.5 Topic Selection

Good planning of an audit is very important and is usually best coordinated through an audit led by a department or a specific audit department within a hospital. This ensures a multidisciplinary approach, appropriate resource allocation and feedback on the results, whilst preventing unnecessary repetition and failure to fully complete the audit cycle. This is vitally important as a clinical audit lacks purpose if it fails to improve standards where this is needed.

It is important to have a clear aim and objectives for any audit. This clarity is achieved through dialogue with stakeholders. Priority should be given to topics which have a high impact on patient care or form part of any improvement strategy within the hospital.

71.2.6 Criterion and Standard Selection

The criterion is a reference point used to measure current practice (e.g. offer of influenza vaccination in pregnancy). These must be defined so the correct data are collected as part of the audit. Once the criteria are set, a threshold of expected compliance must be set; this is known as a standard. The standard may be 100% in an ideal world but is often reduced based on known limitations within a local service or previous audit results. The process of evaluation/comparison that allows the setting of a standard is known as 'benchmarking'.

71.2.7 Data Collection

Data collection should only occur against the defined criteria to allow assessment against the set standards. Before an audit begins, it is important to define what data are needed to ensure the correct information is collected but that additional unnecessary data are not inadvertently obtained.

An audit-specific proforma (data collection tool) should be used to ensure maximum accuracy and reliability of data collection. It also allows the data to be collected in pseudo-anonymized fashion to maintain compliance with the Data Protection Act. The Act states that it is an offence to collect personally identifiable data without prior consent.

71.2.8 Data Analysis

Data analysis is arguably the most important step in the process. The data collection should be analyzed and presented to those involved in the delivery of care in the context of the defined standards. This allows the local clinicians to determine whether the care is above or below standard and facilitates a discussion about how care could be improved. If care is found to be substandard, changes should be implemented to improve care. Once improvements or changes have been introduced, a repeat round of data collection should be undertaken to see if care has been improved to the level of the predefined standard.

References

1. Grimes DA, Schulz KF. An overview of clinical research: the lay of the land. *Lancet.* 2002 Jan 5;**359**(9300):57–61.

2. General Medical Council. Good medical practice www.gmc-uk.org/ethical-guidance/ethical-guidance-for-doctors/good-medical-practice

3. Luesley DM, Baker. PN, eds. *Obstetrics & Gynaecology: An Evidence-Based Text for MRCOG*, 2nd ed. London:Hodder Education Publishers; 2010. 1–879 pp.

4. Cohen AM, Stavri PZ, Hersh WR. A categorization and analysis of the criticisms of evidence-based medicine. *Int J Med Inform.* 2004 Feb;**73**(1):35–43.

5. Smith GCS, Pell JP. Parachute use to prevent death and major trauma related to gravitational challenge: systematic review of randomised controlled trials. *BMJ.* 2003 Dec 20;**327**(7429):1459–61.

6. Porter M, Bhattacharya S, Roland Van Teilinger E. Unfulfilled expectations: How circumstances impinge on women's reproductive choices. *Soc Sci Med*, 2006;**62**(7):1757–67. doi: 10.1016/j.socscimed.2005.08.047

7. Grimes DA, Schulz KF. Descriptive studies: what they can and cannot do. *Lancet.* 2002 Jan 12;**359**(9301):145–9.

8. Grimes DA, Schulz KF. Cohort studies: marching towards outcomes. *Lancet.* 2002 Jan 26;**359**(9303):341–5.

9. Birthplace in England Collaborative Group, Brocklehurst P, Hardy P, Hollowell J, et al. Perinatal and maternal outcomes by planned place of birth for healthy women with low risk pregnancies: the Birthplace in England national prospective cohort study. *BMJ.* 2011 Nov 23;**343**(4):d7400.

10. Schulz KF, Grimes DA. Case-control studies: research in reverse. *Lancet.* 2002 Feb 2;**359**(9304):431–4.

11. Hannah ME, Hannah WJ, Hewson SA, et al. Planned caesarean section versus planned vaginal birth for breech presentation at term: a randomised multicentre trial. Term Breech Trial Collaborative Group. *Lancet.* 2000 Oct 21;**356**(9239):1375–83.

12. Barrett JFR, Hannah ME, Hutton EK, et al. A randomized trial of planned cesarean or vaginal delivery for twin pregnancy. *N Engl J Med.* 2013 Oct 3;**369**(14):1295–305.

13. Brocklehurst P, Field D, Greene K, et al. Computerised interpretation of fetal heart rate during labour (INFANT): a randomised controlled trial. *Lancet.* 2017 Apr 29;**389**(10080):1719–29.

14. Lees CC, Marlow N, van Wassenaer-Leemhuis A, et al. 2 year neurodevelopmental and intermediate perinatal outcomes in infants with very preterm fetal growth restriction (TRUFFLE): a randomised trial. *Lancet.* 2015 May 30;**385**(9983):2162–72.

15. Dodd JM, Jones L, Flenady V, Cincotta R, Crowther CA. Prenatal administration of progesterone for preventing preterm birth in women considered to be at risk of preterm birth. *Cochrane Database Syst Rev.* 2013 Jul 31;(7):CD004947.

16. Haynes RB. Of studies, syntheses, synopses, summaries, and systems: the '5S' evolution of information services for evidence-based healthcare decisions. *Evid Based Med.* 2006 Dec 1;**11**(6):162–4.

17. Howick J, Chalmers I, Glasziou P, et al. OCEBM Levels of Evidence Working Group. The Oxford Levels of Evidence 2. [Internet]. 2011 [cited 2019 Jan 22]. www.cebm.net/index.aspx?o=5653

18. Young JM, Solomon MJ. How to critically appraise an article. *Nat Clin Pract Gastroenterol Hepatol.* 2009 Jan 20;**6**(2):82–91.

19. Pipkin FB. Basic statistics. In Fiander A, Thilaganathan B, eds. *Your Essential Revision Guide MRCOG Part 1.* London:RCOG Press; 2010. 1–617 pp.

20. David A, Thornton S, Sutcliffe A, Williams P. *Developing New Pharmaceutical Treatments for Obstetric Conditions*, Scientific Impact Paper No 50. London: Royal College of Obstetricans and Gynaecologists, 2015.

21. Ivers N, Jamtvedt G, Flottorp S, et al. Audit and feedback: effects on professional practice and healthcare outcomes. *Cochrane Database Syst Rev.* 2012 Jun 13;(6):1–4.

22. Pattinson RC, Say L, Makin J, Bastos MH. Critical incident audit and feedback to improve perinatal and maternal mortality and morbidity. *Cochrane Database Syst Rev.* 2005 Oct 19;(4):CD002961.

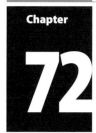

Chapter

72

Management of Malignant and Premalignant Disease of the Cervix during Pregnancy

Antonios Athanasiou, Panagiotis Cherouveim, Maria Kyrgiou & Evangelos Paraskevaidis

72.1 Introduction – Epidemiology

The rate of abnormal cytology smears during pregnancy is similar to that of non-pregnant women (around 5% in the USA). As expected, most of these abnormal smears are precancerous cervical lesions, and cervical cancer during pregnancy is a rare event. However, it remains the most common cancer diagnosed during pregnancy, with an incidence rate of 12 per 100 000 pregnancies in the USA [1].

Because pregnancy complicates the interpretation of cytology, screening should be postponed to 3 months after delivery in pregnant women whose next screening test is due during pregnancy. However, women who do not attend cervical screening regularly should be tested during pregnancy; in this non-compliant population, pregnancy might offer a unique opportunity for screening. Cytology during pregnancy might also be necessary in women with a history of abnormal cytology preceding pregnancy and requiring further follow-up, or with symptoms suspicious of cervical cancer. Staff of antenatal clinics should ensure that the cytologist is informed of the pregnant state, because pregnancy might influence the interpretation of cytological findings.

72.2 Management of Pre-cancerous Lesions during Pregnancy

In the case of abnormal cytology during pregnancy, the goal is to exclude invasion, defer any treatment for pre-cancerous lesions to the postpartum period and treat only when there is suspicion of invasion.

72.2.1 Initial Management according to Cytologic Diagnosis

According to the guidelines of the American Society for Colposcopy and Cervical Pathology (ASCCP) published in 2012 [2], the indications of colposcopy for pregnant women with abnormal cytology are similar to non-pregnant women. However, one difference is that it's acceptable to defer colposcopy until 3 months (not earlier than 6 weeks) after delivery in women with atypical squamous cells of undetermined significance (ASC-US) or low-grade squamous intraepithelial neoplasia (LSIL). Similar to non-pregnant women, colposcopy must always be performed in atypical squamous cells and cannot exclude a high-grade lesion (ASC-H), high-grade squamous intraepithelial neoplasia (HSIL), or AGC (atypical glandular cells)/AIS (adenocarcinoma in situ).

Therefore, the suggested initial approach according to ASCCP guidelines is the following:

ASC-US: Triage with human papillomavirus (HPV) testing is recommended. In case of a negative HPV test, no further follow-up is needed during pregnancy or the postpartum period. In case of a positive HPV test, colposcopy either can be deferred to 3 months after delivery or can be performed immediately, particularly as the most likely setting would be that of a first trimester pregnancy. If triage with HPV testing is not available, cytology can be repeated at 1 year.

In pregnant women, an ASC-US diagnosis may be attributed to the reactive/metaplastic reaction of cervical cells during pregnancy. According to a retrospective cohort [3], only one third of pregnant patients with ASC-US during pregnancy were found to have histologically proven cervical intraepithelial neoplasia (CIN) in biopsy during or within 6 months after pregnancy, compared to half of non-pregnant patients with biopsy within 6 months after ASC-US diagnosis (in pregnant patients, antepartum biopsy was performed only when invasion was suspected). That being said, an ASC-US diagnosis during pregnancy always warrants further investigation, as per aforementioned management strategy, and should never be overlooked and considered 'normal'. In the same study, 1 out of 45 pregnant patients with ASC-US (2.2%) were diagnosed with cervical cancer!

LSIL: Immediate colposcopy is preferred. However, deferral of colposcopy until 3 months after delivery is also acceptable.

ASC-H/HSIL: Colposcopy must always be performed in order to exclude invasive disease.

AGC/AIS: Colposcopy must always be performed. In non-pregnant patients, endocervical curettage is recommended in all women. Endometrial sampling (through endometrial biopsy or dilation and curettage (D&C)) is also recommended in non-pregnant women over 35 years old, women with risk factors for endometrial cancer or women with atypical endometrial cells in Pap smear. However, D&C and preservation of pregnancy are incompatible terms. Endometrial biopsies and endocervical curettage are also not recommended in pregnancy.

It should be emphasized that cytologists examining the smears of pregnant patients must always be informed of the pregnant state.

72.2.2 Colposcopy during Pregnancy

The various physiological changes of the cervix during pregnancy, which might persist into the puerperium as well, require an increased level of expertise during colposcopy. One of the most characteristic changes is the eversion of the endocervical columnar epithelium to the ectocervix (ectropion) because of the high oestrogen levels. An advantage of this change is that endocervical cells are easier to be sampled for cytologic examination, and an initially unsatisfactory colposcopy is expected to be satisfactory by the 20th week of gestation in most patients [4]. A disadvantage is that the exposed columnar epithelium is friable and might easily bleed or undergo inflammatory/reactive changes. In addition, the acidic pH in the vagina might result in the squamous metaplasia of the ectropion. Immature metaplasia, along with the increased vascularity of the cervix during pregnancy, might give a colposcopic impression of precancerous lesion or even cancer! Conversely, neoplastic lesions might be mistaken for the normal ectropion! Furthermore, decidualization is often observed in cervical stromata. This usually occurs in deeper cervical stromata and cannot be observed in colposcopy, but might be quite extensive and produce polyps, which are yellowish and not covered by epithelium, in contrast to the usual endocervical polyps. Decidual polyps, similar to ectropion/immature metaplasia, might be difficult to distinguish from neoplastic lesions [5].

Other pregnancy-related changes are the hyperplasia and hypersecretion of cervical glands resulting in a thick mucus plug, which 'protects' the endometrial cavity but might be difficult to remove in order to visualize the endocervix. Moreover, trophoblasts or degenerated decidual cells might shed from the endometrium and be confused with dysplastic cells by the cytologist [6]. Finally, in later stages of pregnancy, cervical effacement and cervical distortion by a low-riding fetus might cause further diagnostic problems for colposcopists [4].

According to the British guidelines published in 2016 by the National Health Service (NHS) Cervical Screening Programme (NHSCSP) [7], if the satisfactory colposcopic impression is CIN1 or less, colposcopy should be repeated at 3 months after delivery. If the satisfactory colposcopic impression is CIN2 or CIN3, colposcopy should be repeated at the end of second trimester (or just at 3 months after delivery if pregnancy is beyond that point). If the initial colposcopy in the first/second trimester is unsatisfactory, it could be repeated in 6–12 weeks or by 20th week of gestation, when most women are expected to have a satisfactory colposcopy because of the eversion of endocervical epithelium [4]. Routine punch biopsies (PBs) are not recommended when there is no suspicion of invasion. However, when invasive disease is suspected, PBs are essential. If PBs do not show invasive disease, but there remains a high suspicion of invasion, then a diagnostic excisional procedure (such as cone biopsy, wedge biopsy or loop biopsy) could be performed, but only where appropriate facilities and expertise to deal with possible haemorrhage are available.

72.2.2.1 Punch Biopsies during Pregnancy

In one study of 449 pregnant patients with colposcopically directed PBs during pregnancy [8], the concordance between colposcopy and PBs was 66%, and agreement within 1 degree

of severity was 95%. Sensitivity of colposcopy for biopsy-proven CIN2+ was 88%, specificity 87%, positive predictive value (PPV) 93%, and negative predictive value (NPV) 77%. More important, sensitivity of colposcopy for cervical cancer was 100% (two patients in this cohort had invasive disease). These data suggest that colposcopy during pregnancy might be quite reliable when performed by an experienced colposcopist (despite the confusing physiological changes of the cervix), and PBs might not be necessary. After all, the main goal during pregnancy is to exclude invasive disease and if this can be achieved through colposcopy alone, a more accurate diagnosis of the degree of the pre-cancerous lesions can be pursued after delivery. Furthermore, the ectropion that is formed during pregnancy is quite friable and vulnerable to trauma and faces the risk of bleeding [4]. These might be the reasons why NHSCSP guidelines don't suggest routine PBs during pregnancy [7]. However, some studies suggest that PBs during pregnancy are safe, such as a cohort of 128 pregnant patients, where only 1 (0.8%) patient experienced severe bleeding [9]. As a result, ASCCP guidelines recommend the routine performance of PBs when colposcopic impression is CIN2+, similar to non-pregnant population [2]. To sum up, an experienced colposcopist can probably safely omit PBs during pregnancy when they suspect no invasion, but PBs should be performed whenever invasion cannot by excluded by colposcopic impression alone, or there is any doubt.

72.2.3 Conization during Pregnancy

Conization during pregnancy should be performed only when invasive disease is suspected, because of the high number of complications. The risk of significant haemorrhage (>500 mL) during treatment increases with each trimester (<1%, 5% and 10%, respectively). The risk of intrapartum haemorrhage is increased if the patient delivers in less than 1 month after treatment when the cervix has not healed yet. Spontaneous fetal loss after conization in the first trimester and perinatal mortality are reported to be as high as 18% and 5%, respectively, although these numbers might not be very different from the overall rates of first trimester miscarriages and perinatal mortality in the general pregnant population. Finally, the risk of preterm birth is around 12%, probably caused by cervical insufficiency or chorioamnionitis occurring weeks after conization [4]. The increased risk of preterm birth is not surprising, since even non-pregnant women undergoing CIN treatment remain at increased risk of premature delivery in subsequent pregnancies [10]. Although the available data about safety of conization during pregnancy derive mainly from old studies, where patients were treated with cold-knife conization, or from studies with a small number of participants, excisional procedures during pregnancy should remain reserved only for cases with suspicion of invasion, until more robust evidence emerges.

The optimal time for conization seems to be the second trimester, between 14 and 20 weeks of gestation. A flat 'coin-shaped' or 'wedge-shaped' conization might disrupt endocervical canal to a lesser degree than a 'cone-shaped' conization and thus may limit number of complications [4]. Some authors also advocate the placement of cerclage at the time of conization in order to decrease the risk of complications. In a cohort of 13 pregnant patients treated with a 'loop-cone cerclage' technique at 13–32 weeks of gestation [11], no intraoperative or postoperative complications were observed. All patients delivered at term, except for one patient (7.7%) who delivered at 36 weeks. All infants were healthy. Unfortunately, the number of study participants was small, and more evidence is needed in order to be able to draw safe conclusions.

72.3 Prognosis – Natural History of Precancerous Lesions during Pregnancy

Conization during pregnancy should be performed only when invasion is suspected. However, even if invasion is not suspected at the time of colposcopy, the question arises whether severe pre-cancerous lesions could progress to cancer over the course of pregnancy and if conization during pregnancy should be considered to prevent progression. Fortunately, regression rates are high, and progression rates of high-grade lesions to cancer are estimated to be around 0–2% [12, 13]. In addition, of the lesions that progressed to cancer, all were limited to stage IA1. For this reason, it's safe to defer treatment of pre-cancerous lesions until the postpartum period.

Regression of CIN after the end of pregnancy is not rare. According to a study of 224 patients with an intrapartum diagnosis of CIN2/3, regression rates to less severe histology are 68–70% and to normal histology 37–39% [13]. Whether mode of delivery affects regression rates is controversial. Two studies found that the difference in regression rates between vaginal delivery (VD) and caesarean section (CS) is not statistically significant [12, 13]. On the other hand, one study found that regression rates are higher for women with VD than women with CS, but only for high-grade lesions [14]. Because of lacking robust evidence, mode of delivery should be chosen according to standard obstetric indications.

72.4 Staging of Cancer

When cancer is detected in PBs or diagnostic cone, then staging is required. Staging of cervical cancer is performed as per the International Federation of Gynecology and Obstetrics (FIGO) 2018, similar to non-pregnant women. Apart from clinical examination, the new staging system allows for any imaging techniques to be utilized for staging, depending on local resources. If available, radiologic examination for assessment of tumour dimensions, extent of local disease (parametria involvement/lymph nodes metastases), urinary tract involvement (hydronephrosis) and distant metastases (at least chest x-ray for detection of lung metastases) is recommended for all stages equal to or greater than IA2. In stage IA1, radiologic examination can be omitted.

In pregnant women, imaging with ionizing radiation should be generally avoided, especially if the fetus is within the radiation field. However, a chest x-ray (for assessment of pulmonary metastases) is very safe in pregnancy, since the fetal dose is very low (<0.01 mGy). Other ionizing radiation techniques (such as computed tomography (CT), positron emission tomography (PET)/CT, or intravenous (IV) pyelography) should be avoided. Nonetheless, even pelvic CT (with a fetal dose at around 10–50 mGy) doesn't seem to reach the estimated harm threshold dose at any pregnancy period (the lowest threshold is 60 mGy at 8–15 weeks of gestational age; higher doses during this gestational period might cause severe mental retardation). There are no safety concerns for the use of ultrasound (US) or magnetic resonance imaging (MRI) during pregnancy, but gadolinium should be withheld at any time during pregnancy, because it's associated with an increased risk of perinatal mortality and rheumatologic, inflammatory or infiltrative skin conditions in childhood/adolescence [15].

Although CT and/or MRI can detect lymph node metastases, pelvic lymph node dissection (PLND) is the gold standard. PLND should be performed for stages IA2 or greater regardless of findings on radiologic examination, but it can be omitted in stage IA1, where the risk of lymph node metastases is less than 1% [16]. However, in case of lymphovascular space invasion (LVSI), it should be considered in stage IA1 as well. Laparoscopic PLND during pregnancy is safe for both mother and child. However, increasing gestational age increases the difficulty of performing PLND, and therefore it's not recommended beyond 22–25 gestational weeks [17]. Metastasis to pelvic lymph nodes is a major prognostic factor; diagnosis of cervical cancer with positive pelvic lymph nodes before the third trimester means that definitive treatment might be required without delay (i.e. waiting until delivery at term might not be an option and that termination of pregnancy should be seriously considered) [18].

The prevalence of metastatic para-aortic lymph nodes increases with stage (5% in stage IB, 16% in stage II and 25% in stage III) and is rare in the absence of positive pelvic lymph nodes [19]. Therefore, para-aortic lymph node dissection (PALND), in addition to PLND, might not be needed when imaging doesn't suggest metastatic pelvic or para-aortic lymph nodes. If suspicious pelvic lymph nodes are encountered during PLND, then a frozen section can be performed and, if positive, PALND should be performed as well.

72.5 Management of Cancer

The first question that needs to be discussed is whether **pregnancy preservation is desirable**.

72.5.1 Pregnancy Termination

If the patient does not wish to preserve her pregnancy, then standard of care (similar to non-pregnant patients) should be provided.

If (simple or radical) hysterectomy is the treatment of choice, this can be performed with the fetus in situ, but late pregnancy might require hysterotomy and evacuation of the uterus before hysterectomy [18].

If radiation (with or without chemotherapy) is the treatment of choice, then it should be discussed whether radiation should be initiated before or after pregnancy termination. In a cohort of pregnant women with cervical cancer [20], external beam radiation therapy (EBRT) without previous termination of pregnancy resulted in fetal death within 3–4 weeks, and subsequent miscarriage in all 17 cases. However, spontaneous abortion was more delayed in the second trimester (first trimester: 7 women, mean duration between EBRT–miscarriage: 33 days, range: 27–50 days; second trimester: 10 women (9/10: <20 weeks of gestation), mean: 44 days, range: 33–66 days). Even though all miscarriages were without complications in this cohort, it should be taken into consideration that retention of a dead fetus increases the risk of disseminated intravascular coagulation (DIC), especially if miscarriage delays by more than 4 weeks after fetal demise [21]. After miscarriage occurs, brachytherapy can be added.

Conversely, evacuation of the uterus by vaginal approach before initiating radiotherapy might not be feasible or be contraindicated in advanced cancer stages, and evacuation by hysterotomy might lead to wound metastasis, enhanced radiotherapy toxicity in case of postoperative adhesions or potential delay in initiating radiotherapy in case of wound infection [18]. Therefore, a personalized decision should be made for women <20 weeks of gestation. In women >20 weeks of gestation in whom termination of pregnancy is necessary, evacuation of the uterus before radiotherapy is recommended to avoid nonlethal fetal exposure to radiation.

72.5.2 Pregnancy Preservation

If pregnancy preservation is desirable, then subsequent management depends on the cervical cancer stage and timing of diagnosis (whether cancer is diagnosed in the first/second trimester (or <22–25 weeks of gestation) or third trimester (or >22–25 weeks of gestation)).

72.5.2.1 Diagnosis in First/Second Trimester (or <22–25 weeks of gestation)

As a rule, laparoscopic PLND (+/– PALND) should be performed in all stages equal to or greater than IA2, before any decisions on further management can be made. In stage IA1, lymphadenectomy is required only in the presence of LVSI.

If lymph nodes are positive, then these patients should be advised of their poorer prognosis and the need of termination of pregnancy and immediate definitive treatment. However, if pregnancy preservation is still desirable, then neoadjuvant chemotherapy (NACT) can be administered until delivery at fetal maturity.

If lymph nodes are negative, then pregnancy preservation is a safer option, and further management depends on stage:

- Stage IA1

For micro-invasive cervical cancer, conization is advised [18]. The optimal timing for performance of conization is between 14 and 20 weeks of gestation [4]. The complications of conization during pregnancy have been already discussed (see Section 72.2.3 Conization during Pregnancy). In case of negative margins and no LVSI, this is acceptable as definitive treatment for patients who want to keep their fertility. Similar to non-pregnant women, positive margins require a repeat conization in order to exclude residual invasive disease, especially if the endocervical margin is involved. In a small cohort

of 7 non-pregnant patients with involved endocervical margins (all with CIS) after laser conization for stage IA1 and no repeat conization, no disease recurrence was observed after a median follow-up of 4 years (range 2.3–7.6 years) [22]. These results suggest that, in the case of positive margins involved with precancerous disease in pregnancy, it's safe to defer repeat conization until delivery.

- Stages IA2–IB1

In stages IA2 and IB1 (up to 2 cm according to 2018 FIGO staging), a large conization or simple trachelectomy is recommended [18]. This less radical approach is suggested by the fact that parametrial involvement rate is less than 1% in patients with early-stage cervical cancer up to stage IB1, negative LVSI and negative pelvic lymph nodes [23].

In a case series of 5 patients treated with simple trachelectomy during 12–19 weeks of gestation [24], there were no intraoperative or postoperative complications. Four out of five (80%) delivered at term and only one (20%) delivered at 28 weeks of gestation because of preterm premature rupture of membranes (PPROM). However, the latter baby was alive and healthy after 18 months of follow-up. In many case reports of trachelectomy during pregnancy, cerclage is performed at the time of the procedure. In this case series, none of the 5 patients had undergone cerclage and the authors suggested that cerclage might not be necessary, and its omission might not be associated with worse obstetric outcomes. However, the data are very limited for any safe conclusions.

In a literature review of patients treated with radical trachelectomy during pregnancy [25], the results are less favourable. Of 10 patients treated with vaginal radical trachelectomy, 2 miscarried (20%) and 5 patients had preterm birth, meaning that only 3 patients (30%) in total delivered at term. Of 11 patients treated with abdominal radical trachelectomy, 4 miscarried (36%) and 1 patient had preterm birth, meaning that only 6 patients (55%) in total delivered at term. In addition, radical trachelectomy during pregnancy is associated with a long operation time (median: 5.3 hours) and risk of significant haemorrhage (median blood loss: 1036 mL). For these reasons, radical trachelectomy should be avoided during pregnancy [18].

- Stage ≥IB2

In the case of negative PLND, NACT is the only way to preserve pregnancy [18]. As already mentioned, termination of pregnancy is advised in the case of positive PLND, but if the patient refuses to terminate her pregnancy, then NACT can be administered until fetal maturity. Therefore, if the patient is determined to keep her pregnancy and the results of PLND wouldn't change further management, then NACT can be administered without preceding PLND, which could be performed after delivery.

Conservative Management of Stage I

Conservative management of patients with stage I has been reported. In a cohort of 12 pregnant patients with intentional treatment delay until fetal maturity [26], treatment was withheld for 9–25 weeks in 8 patients with stage IA1, and for 6–15 weeks in 4 patients with stage IA2 or IB. No patients relapsed during the follow-up of 52–156 months. In a recent literature review [27], 76 pregnant patients with stage IB and a mean treatment delay of 16 weeks (minimum: 6 weeks) were identified. Only 4 (5%) died during follow-up; all these patients had either positive pelvic lymph nodes or laparoscopic PLND had not been performed. For this reason, the European Society of Gynaecological Oncology (ESGO) acknowledges treatment delay until fetal maturity as an acceptable management method for stages up to IB1 (<2 cm) with negative PLND and no observed progression during pregnancy. However, ESGO does not suggest treatment delay for stage IB2 (>2 cm) or greater [18].

72.5.2.2 Diagnosis in Third Trimester (or >22–25 weeks of gestation)

Laparoscopic PLND (+/– PALND) should be avoided during the third trimester because of the increased technical difficulty of the procedure.

- Stages IA1–IB1

Treatment delay until fetal maturity is recommended for stable disease [18]. The feasibility of delaying treatment for early-stage cervical cancer has been already discussed (see section Conservative Management of Stage I). However, in case of progression during pregnancy, then either NACT until fetal maturity or early delivery and standard of care is recommended.

Conization/trachelectomy should be avoided in the third trimester, because should the patient deliver in less than 1 month after the procedure (spontaneously or by induction) and the cervix has not yet healed, then the risk of intrapartum haemorrhage is increased [4].

- Stage ≥IB2

Treatment delay is not recommended; either NACT until fetal maturity or early delivery and immediate definitive treatment is the suggested management method [18].

72.5.2.3 Chemotherapy during Pregnancy

The role of chemotherapy in locally advanced cancer in non-pregnant women is well documented; in pregnancy, it can help control the disease and delay definitive treatment until ideally delivery occurs at term. However, chemotherapy is not without risks. General risks of chemotherapeutic regimens during the first trimester are miscarriage and congenital malformations (especially in the period of organogenesis from the second until the eighth week after fertilization). For this reason, chemotherapy should be avoided, if possible, during the first trimester. In the second/third trimester, chemotherapy is considered safer, but there is still a higher risk of preterm birth, intrauterine growth restriction and premature rupture of membranes [28].

A long-term observation (median: 22.3 months, range: 16.8–211.6 months) of 70 children born after exposure to chemotherapy in the second or third trimester (regardless of maternal cancer) concluded that chemotherapy was not associated with increased risk of neurological, cognitive, cardiac or hearing problems during childhood or adolescence, as compared to the general population [29]. However, children born prematurely had lower neurocognitive scores (IQ score increased by 11.6 points for each additional month of gestation). This study suggests that chemotherapy during second/third trimester is safe, but delivery at term should be a high priority.

A systematic review examining only pregnancies complicated with cervical cancer included 48 pregnant women treated with a platinum-based chemotherapeutic regimen at a mean gestational age of 23.9 weeks (range 17–33 weeks) [30]. Mean gestational age at delivery was 32.5 weeks (range 25–42 weeks), and mean birthweight was 2213 g (range: 1330–2990). Two thirds of babies were born healthy, while the rest were diagnosed with elevation in serum creatinine, anaemia, first degree intraventricular haemorrhage, respiratory distress syndrome, hypoglycaemia, hypotension or supraventricular tachycardia. However, all infants were healthy in the long term after a median follow-up of 12.5 months, and the authors concluded that platinum-based chemotherapy is probably safe during the second and third trimesters.

The recommended chemotherapeutic regimen for cervical cancer during pregnancy is cisplatin (75 mg/m^2 every 3 weeks) with paclitaxel (175 mg/m^2 every 3 weeks). Combination cis-platin-based chemotherapy is preferred over cisplatin alone [18]. An alternative to cisplatin with similar efficacy but less renal toxicity is carboplatin, but cisplatin remains the most studied chemotherapy drug in pregnancy [27].

The interval between the last cycle of chemotherapy and expected date of delivery should be 3 weeks in order to avoid delivery at the nadir of haematopoietic suppression. Because spontaneous preterm birth could occur at any time beyond 34 weeks of gestation, no cycles of chemotherapy should be administered after 33 weeks of gestation [28]. When a patient is diagnosed with cervical cancer after 30 weeks of gestation and there is the dilemma of early delivery without chemotherapy or term delivery with chemotherapy, ESGO suggests that initiating chemotherapy is preferable [18] (as long as it's not administered beyond 33 weeks of gestation).

72.5.2.4 Mode of Delivery

Delivery at term is preferred, as long as the disease is stable and the mother doesn't need immediate radiotherapy or radical surgery. If a bulky tumour obstructs the birth canal, then vaginal delivery VD might not be feasible at all. If the birth canal is free and VD is possible, it's controversial whether VD increases the risk of relapse. In a case-control study, VD was associated with an increased risk of recurrence compared to CS (VD vs. CS: 10/17 vs. 1/7, odds ratio (OR) 4.66, 95% confidence interval (CI) 1.05–20.8) [31], while another analysis of 44 patients concluded that there is no difference in survival [32]. However, should episiotomy be needed during VD, there is a rare but extremely dangerous possibility of recurrence at the episiotomy site. In a literature review [18], 20 cases of recurrence at the episiotomy site were identified, of which at least 7 were fatal. One of these 7 fatal cases was a patient with stage IA1 adenocarcinoma [33]. This patient had been treated with large loop excision of the transformation zone (LLETZ) during pregnancy; the invasive lesion had been 'completely' excised, but the margins were involved with pre-cancerous changes. Therefore, delivery by CS is preferable for pregnant patients diagnosed with cervical cancer [18]. Vaginal delivery might be safe only in case of stage IA1 excided during pregnancy with clear margins [5].

A 'classical' (upper segment) CS incision is recommended instead of a lower segment incision in order to avoid wound metastasis, especially if cervical cancer has spread to the corpus uterus [18]. However, the increased risk of bleeding during classical CS should be taken into consideration, which might be aggravated if chemotherapy was administered during pregnancy and the bone marrow has not yet recovered since the last dose. Chemotherapy-associated haematopoietic suppression might increase the risk of infection as well.

72.5.2.5 Definitive Treatment

Definitive treatment can be provided after delivery and should be the same as in the non-pregnant population.

72.6 Prognosis of Cancer

Similar to the general female population, most pregnancy-related cancers (>80%) are squamous, but one difference is that they are diagnosed at earlier stages (up to 83% are diagnosed at stage I) than in non-pregnant women. The detection at earlier stages might be explained by the routine Pap tests in antenatal clinics in many countries and by the fact that advanced cervical cancer might prevent conception. Prognosis per stage is comparable to that in the non-pregnant population, which means that the effect of pregnancy on the prognosis of cervical cancer is **neutral** and the diagnosis of cervical cancer during pregnancy should be considered a coincidental finding [5].

Metastasis (usually haematogenous) of cancer to the placenta or fetus is rare; a literature review in 2008 identified only 98 cases, most of them after melanoma (28 cases) [34]. Only one case of metastasis to the placenta after cervical cancer was found. Although rare, it's recommended that the placenta be examined under the microscope and, if cervical cells are detected, then the infant be followed up for signs of malignant disease.

72.7 Key Messages

- Incidence of abnormal cytology during pregnancy is similar to that of non-pregnant women. Cervical cancer is the most common pregnancy-associated cancer.
- Many physiological changes occur in the cervix during pregnancy. These changes might be confused with (pre-)cancerous lesions, and colposcopists should be aware of them.
- The risk of progression of pre-cancerous lesions to cancer during pregnancy is very low; thus, pre-cancerous lesions shouldn't be treated during pregnancy.
- If cancer is diagnosed during pregnancy, management depends on the trimester of diagnosis, staging and status of pelvic lymph nodes. Different management options include termination of pregnancy, conization, simple trachelectomy, chemotherapy, early delivery or conservative management.

- Pregnancy per se has no adverse effect on the prognosis of cervical cancer.

72.8 Key Guidelines

- Indications for colposcopy because of abnormal cytology are similar in pregnant and non-pregnant patients. Deferral of colposcopy to postpartum period is acceptable for ASC-US and LSIL.
- If the colposcopic (+/– histological) diagnosis is CIN1 or less, colposcopy should be repeated in the postpartum period. If the colposcopic (+/– histological) diagnosis is CIN2/3, colposcopy should be repeated at the end of second trimester.
- Punch biopsies can be omitted if there is no suspicion of invasion during colposcopy, but they should be performed whenever invasion is suspected or cannot be safely excluded by colposcopic impression alone. If punch biopsies are negative and suspicion of invasion remains, diagnostic conization can be performed.
- Therapeutic conization for high-grade pre-cancerous lesions should be postponed to the postpartum period.
- Diagnosis of cancer during pregnancy should be followed by staging.
- Allowed imaging techniques during pregnancy are MRI without gadolinium, ultrasound and chest x-ray for evaluation of lung metastases in stages IA2 or higher.
- Laparoscopic PLND is recommended during the first/second trimester for all stages except for IA1 without LVSI. In stages IB2 (>2 cm) or higher, it's also acceptable to postpone laparoscopic PLND until the postpartum period.
- In the case of positive PLND during first/second trimester, termination of pregnancy is recommended. If the mother doesn't consent to terminate her pregnancy, chemotherapy is required.
- Laparoscopic PLND is not recommended during the third trimester.
- If the mother doesn't wish to preserve her pregnancy or PLND is positive, definitive treatment should be provided immediately. Hysterectomy can be performed with the fetus in situ; in case of an advanced pregnancy stage, hysterotomy might be required before hysterectomy. Radiotherapy can be performed either before or after uterine evacuation; in advanced pregnancy (>20 weeks), radiotherapy should be initiated only after uterine evacuation.
- If the mother wishes to preserve her pregnancy and PLND (if performed) is negative, provisional treatment depends on the trimester of diagnosis and stage; definitive treatment similar to non-pregnant patients can be provided after delivery.
- During first/second trimester, the recommended treatment is conization for stage IA1, large conization or simple trachelectomy for stages IA2–IB1 (<2 cm), and chemotherapy for stages IB2 (>2 cm) or higher. Conservative management is also acceptable for stages IA1–IB1.
- If cancer is diagnosed during the third trimester, conservative management is recommended for stages up to IB1 (<2 cm), and chemotherapy or early delivery for stages

IB2 (>2 cm) or higher. Conization/simple trachelectomy should be avoided in the third trimester.
- Chemotherapy should be avoided during the first trimester, but it's considered safe in the second/third trimester.
- The recommended chemotherapeutic regimen during pregnancy is cisplatin with paclitaxel every 3 weeks. No cycle should be administered within 3 weeks before the expected date of delivery, or beyond 33 weeks of gestation.
- Delivery at term should be a high priority whenever the mother's health does not require immediate radiotherapy or radical surgery. Delivery by caesarean section is recommended; an upper segment uterine incision is preferable.

References

1. Yang KY. Abnormal pap smear and cervical cancer in pregnancy. *Clin Obstet Gynecol.* 2012;**55**:838–48.

2. Massad LS, Einstein MH, Huh WK, et al. 2012 updated consensus guidelines for the management of abnormal cervical cancer screening tests and cancer precursors. *J Low Genit Tract Dis.* 2013;**17**:S1–27. doi: 10.1097/LGT.0b013e318287d329

3. Broderick D, Matityahu D, Dudhbhai M, et al. Histologic and colposcopic correlates of ASCUS Pap smears in pregnancy. *J Low Genit Tract Dis.* 2002;**6**:116–19.

4. Muller CY, Smith HO. Cervical neoplasia complicating pregnancy. *Obstet Gynecol Clin North Am.* 2005;**32**:533–46. doi: 10.1016/j.ogc.2005.08.007

5. Van Calsteren K, Vergote I, Amant F. Cervical neoplasia during pregnancy: Diagnosis, management and prognosis. *Best Pract Res Clin Obstet Gynaecol.* 2005;**19**:611–30. doi: 10.1016/j.bpobgyn.2005.03.002

6. Michael CW, Esfahani FM. Pregnancy-related changes: a retrospective review of 278 cervical smears. *Diagn Cytopathol.* 1997;**17**:99–107.

7. Public Health England. *Programme and Colposcopy Management.* Guidelines for commissioners, screening providers and programme managers for NHS cervical screening. 2016.

8. Economos K, Perez Veridiano N, Delke I, et al. Abnormal cervical cytology in pregnancy: a 17-year experience. *Obstet Gynecol.* 1993;**81**:915–18.

9. Baldauf JJ, Dreyfus M, Ritter J. Benefits and risks of directed biopsy in pregnancy. *J Low Genit Tract Dis.* 1997;**1**:214–20.

10. Kyrgiou M, Koliopoulos G, Martin-Hirsch P, et al. Obstetric outcomes after conservative treatment for intraepithelial or early invasive cervical lesions: systematic review and meta-analysis. *Lancet* 2006;**367**:489–98. doi: 10.1016/S0140-6736(06)68181-6

11. Dunn TS, Ginsburg V, Wolf D. Loop-cone cerclage in pregnancy: a 5-year review. *Gynecol Oncol.* 2003;**90**:577–80. doi: 10.1016/S0090-8258(03)00395-0

12. Paraskevaidis E, Koliopoulos G, Kalantaridou S, et al. Management and evolution of cervical intraepithelial neoplasia during pregnancy and postpartum. *Eur J Obstet Gynecol Reprod Biol.* 2002;**104**:67–9.

13. Yost NP, Santoso JT, McIntire DD, et al. Postpartum regression rates of antepartum cervical intraepithelial neoplasia II and III lesions. *Obstet Gynecol.* 1999;**93**:359–62.

14. Ahdoot D, Van Nostrand KM, Nguyen NJ, et al. The effect of route of delivery on regression of abnormal cervical cytologic findings in the postpartum period. *Am J Obstet Gynecol.* 1998;**178**:1116–20.

15. American College of Obstetricians and Gynecologists. Committee Opinion No. 723: Guidelines for Diagnostic Imaging During Pregnancy and Lactation. *Obstet Gynecol.* 2017;**130**:e210–16. doi: 10.1097/AOG.0000000000002355

16. Elliott P, Coppleson M, Russell P, et al. Early invasive (FIGO stage IA) carcinoma of the cervix: a clinico-pathologic study of 476 cases. *Int J Gynecol Cancer.* 2000;**10**:42–52.

17. Favero G, Chiantera V, Oleszczuk A, et al. Invasive cervical cancer during pregnancy: laparoscopic nodal evaluation before oncologic treatment delay. *Gynecol Oncol.* 2010;**118**:123–7. doi: 10.1016/j.ygyno.2010.04.012

18. Amant F, Halaska MJ, Fumagalli M, et al. Gynecologic cancers in pregnancy: guidelines of a second international consensus meeting. *Int J Gynecol Cancer.* 2014;**24**:394–403. doi: 10.1097/IGC.0000000000000062

19. Berman ML, Keys H, Creasman W, et al. Survival and patterns of recurrence in cervical cancer metastatic to periaortic lymph nodes (a Gynecologic Oncology Group study). *Gynecol Oncol* .1984;**19**:8–16.

20. Prem KA, Makowski EL, McKelvey JL. Carcinoma of the cervix associated with pregnancy. *Am J Obstet Gynecol.* 1966;**95**:99–108. doi: 10.1016/0002-9378(66)90634-X

21. Parasnis H, Raje B, Hinduja IN. Relevance of plasma fibrinogen estimation in obstetric complications. *J Postgrad Med.* 1992;**38**:183–5.

22. Itsukaichi M, Kurata H, Matsushita M, et al. Stage Ia1 cervical squamous cell carcinoma: conservative management after laser conization with positive margins. *Gynecol Oncol.* 2003;**90**:387–9.

23. Schmeler KM, Frumovitz M, Ramirez PT. Conservative management of early stage cervical cancer: is there a role for less radical surgery? *Gynecol Oncol.* 2011;**120**:321–5. doi: 10.1016/j.ygyno.2010.12.352

24. Salvo G, Frumovitz M, Pareja R, et al. Simple trachelectomy with pelvic lymphadenectomy as a viable treatment option in pregnant patients with stage IB1 (≥2 cm) cervical cancer: bridging the gap to fetal viability. *Gynecol Oncol.* 2018;**150**:50–5. doi: 10.1016/j.ygyno.2018.05.021

25. Capilna ME, Szabo B, Becsi J, et al. Radical trachelectomy performed during pregnancy: a review of the literature. *Int J Gynecol Cancer.* 2016;**26**:758–62. doi: 10.1097/IGC.0000000000000655

26. Takushi M, Moromizato H, Sakumoto K, et al. Management of invasive carcinoma of the uterine cervix associated with pregnancy: outcome of intentional delay in treatment. *Gynecol Oncol.* 2002;**87**:185–9.

27. Morice P, Uzan C, Gouy S, et al. Gynaecological cancers in pregnancy. *Lancet.* 2012;**379**:558–69. doi: 10.1016/S0140-6736(11)60829-5

28. Peccatori FA, Azim HA, Orecchia R, et al. Cancer, pregnancy and fertility: ESMO clinical practice guidelines for diagnosis, treatment and follow-up. *Ann Oncol.* 2013;**24**:vi160–70. doi: 10.1093/annonc/mdt199

29. Amant F, Van Calsteren K, Halaska MJ, et al. Long-term cognitive and cardiac outcomes after prenatal exposure to chemotherapy in children aged 18

593

months or older: an observational study. *Lancet Oncol.* 2012;**13**:256–64. doi: 10.1016/S1470-2045(11)70363-1

30. Zagouri F, Sergentanis TN, Chrysikos D, et al. Platinum derivatives during pregnancy in cervical cancer: a systematic review and meta-analysis. *Obstet Gynecol.* 2013;**121**:337–43. doi: 10.1097/AOG.0b013e31827c5822

31. Sood AK, Sorosky JI, Mayr N, et al. Cervical cancer diagnosed shortly after

pregnancy: prognostic variables and delivery routes. *Obstet Gynecol.* 2000;**95**:832–8.

32. Van der Vange N, Weverling G, Ketting B, et al. The prognosis of cervical cancer associated with pregnancy: a matched cohort study. *Obstet Gynecol.* 1995;**85**:1022–6. doi: 10.1016/0029-7844(95)00059-Z

33. Van den Broek NR, Lopes A, Ansink A, et al. Microinvasive

adenocarcinoma of the cervix implanting in an episiotomy scar. *Gynecol Oncol.* 1995;**59**:297–9. doi: 10.1006/gyno.1995.0025

34. Pavlidis N, Pentheroudakis G. Metastatic involvement of placenta and fetus in pregnant women with cancer. *Recent Results Cancer Res Fortschritte Krebsforsch Progres Dans Rech Sur Cancer.* 2008;**178**:183–94.

Chapter

73

Breast Cancer and Pregnancy
Diagnostics, Therapy and Influence on Fertility and Further Pregnancies

Martin Weiss, Sara Y. Brucker, Diethelm Wallwiener & Eva-Maria Grischke

73.1 Introduction

The diagnosis of pregnancy-associated breast cancer is associated with serious mental strains on young patients and also leads to diagnostic and therapeutic uncertainties on the part of the treating physicians. The patients need to be thoroughly informed about diagnosis, treatment and associated risks during pregnancy, as well as breastfeeding, fertility and appropriate procedures for fertility preservation. Compared with non-pregnant women, pregnancy itself doesn't seem to significantly worsen the prognosis and outcome of breast cancer; however, breast cancer affecting young patients may be characterized by higher disease aggressiveness and higher risk of metastasis. However, with few exceptions most diagnostic and therapeutic procedures can be implemented relatively safely.

73.2 Epidemiology and Aetiology

Generally, malignant diseases of the breast in pregnancy are rare, with an incidence of breast cancer of 0.33 per 1000 individuals [1, 2]. The low coincidence of breast cancer and pregnancy is due to the typical age distribution for women with breast cancer disease. It means that only 10% of all breast cancers occur in women less than 45 years of age.

However, breast cancer is the most common carcinoma in women under the age of 35 years with an overall increasing incidence in pregnancy or 1 year postpartum between 10 and 20%. This tendency not least results from an increase in the age of women giving birth [3]. European records describe an average age of about 33 years and an average gestational age of 21 weeks when diagnosed with breast cancer [1]. Furthermore, women being diagnosed with breast cancer during pregnancy are associated with about a 50% chance in those with a positive family history, and associated with a risk of *BRCA1/BRCA2* mutations in about 30% [4, 5].

73.3 Breast Cancer Diagnostics in Pregnancy

Since breast checkups, and in particular the routine diagnostic imaging by mammography, usually do not take place in pregnancy, around 90% of all breast cancers in pregnancy are detected by the patient herself, through breast palpation. Indeed, the physiological changes of the breasts and their density significantly increase the unreliability of manual mammary exploration for the identification of a suspicious mass [6].

73.3.1 Mammography

Physiological changes in pregnancy may lead to a delay in the diagnosis of the disease. Some older studies report a delayed diagnosis of 6 months; however, more recent studies estimate the delay to be 1–2 months [7, 8]. This delay is alarming since mammography is principally a suitable imaging procedure in pregnancy when sufficient abdominal x-ray protection is guaranteed. In general, the radiation exposure for the fetus during mammography is 0.05 Gy. This level is within the current permissible dose limit that carries a risk for severe fetal impairment, which for a dose of 10 rads lies between 0.06 and 0.31 Gy at 8–15 weeks and around 0.28 Gy between 16 and 25 weeks. Thus, mammography can currently be performed at any stage of pregnancy, when ensuring appropriate safety requirements for the fetus (Table 73.1) [9, 10].

73.3.2 Ultrasound

Besides mammography, ultrasound examination of the breast is still the most suitable method, and can be performed easily and safely at any stage of pregnancy. Moreover, breast ultrasound is useful to distinguish between solid and cystic lesions of the breast, and is a very effective method to identify axillary metastases and to quickly perform percutaneous biopsies. Furthermore, it is not associated with any risk of fetal exposure to radiation [11, 12]. Thus, ultrasound examination of the breast represents the method of choice in breast cancer diagnostics. Ultrasound is also useful for assessing and following up the development of the fetus exposed to adjuvant treatments (Figure 73.1).

73.3.3 Magnetic Resonance Imaging (MRI)

In general, MRI is an ideal diagnostic procedure in young women with mammographically dense glandular breast

Table 73.1 Estimated radiation exposure doses by gestation

Time after conception (weeks)	Estimated maximum dose (Gy)	Estimated dose with adequate shielding
8	0.03	0.03
24	0.28	0.16
36	1.43	0.20

595

tissue [13, 14]. However, this procedure becomes limited during pregnancy. These limits stem from the fact that there is (1) less experience about the diagnostic information and sensitivity from the MRI images; (2) uncertainties about the safe handling of the MRI contrast agent gadolinium during pregnancy; and (3) especially during the second and third trimesters of pregnancy the required abdominal position for optimal MRI imaging is perceived as very uncomfortable. It can be useful to assess response to treatment (Figure 73.2).

73.3.4 A Practical Approach for Suspected Breast Cancer in Pregnancy

Any suspicious change in the breast that lasts longer than a month should be further clarified initially by mammography at two levels (with appropriate safety requirements and lead apron) and a supplementary ultrasound examination of both breasts and corresponding lymphatic systems. In the case of suspected malignancy, an ultrasound-guided punch biopsy is recommended for further histological evaluation. An ultrasound

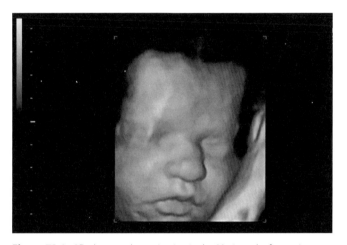

Figure 73.1 3D ultrasound examination in the 33+1 week of gestation, showing normal fetal development after neoadjuvant administration of 4 cycles of epirubicin and cyclophosphamide.

examination of the liver should follow confirmation of breast cancer and, depending on whether there is a low-risk or high-risk situation, an x-ray examination of the thorax and lungs with appropriate safety requirements and lead apron (see above). Pelvic x-ray computed tomography (CT) scan and isotope bone scans, however, are not appropriate in women during pregnancy. If there are complaints as regards the skeletal system, the spinal column should be examined by MRI without contrast agent to detect early impending transverse lesions.

73.4 Therapeutic Procedures and Investigations

As currently handled within the guidelines, the therapy of breast cancer during pregnancy should be considered, depending on the gestational age at the time of diagnosis.

As women being affected by breast cancer during pregnancy are generally young, it has to be considered that after chemotherapy women may develop infertility and a severe limitation of the quality of life, both often leading to psychological imbalances and long-term depression [15, 16]. During the first and second trimesters, therapy is mainly determined by whether or not local operability is possible.

After the 34th week of pregnancy, however, further therapy options should be considered in conjunction with the delivery of the fetus. Generally, this procedure is only influenced by inflammatory carcinoma and other highly aggressive tumours, which may necessitate different therapeutic decisions – usually in the form of immediate childbirth.

In most cases, however, the child's intrauterine maturity can be awaited before beginning a systemic therapy after delivery. Prior to the 34th week of gestation and given operability, tumour surgery will be chosen as the primary therapeutic procedure. Nevertheless, unless radiotherapy and endocrine therapy should not be performed before delivery (>35 gestational weeks), chemotherapy is an appropriate treatment regimen and can be started if required.

In the case of inoperability of breast tumours, it is crucial that neoadjuvant chemotherapy be performed promptly after the first trimester if possible, followed by tumour surgery during

(a)   (b)

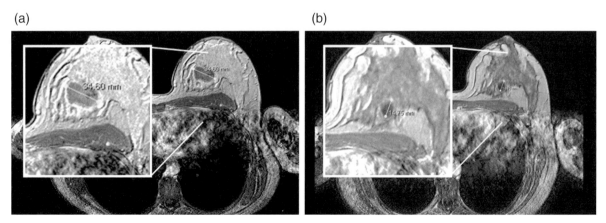

Figure 73.2 Magnetic resonance imaging (MRI) of a pregnant patient before (a; 21+2 weeks of gestation) and after (b; 33+4 weeks of gestation) administration of 4 cycles of epirubicin and cyclophosphamide.

pregnancy or immediately after delivery. Of course, all these decisions depend on the therapy response, gestational age and fetal growth. A detailed protocol is shown in Figure 73.3.

73.4.1 Surgical Interventions in Pregnancy

If primary operative therapy is a choice, ablation with axillary lymphadenectomy or breast-conserving segmental resection with axillary lymphadenectomy may be performed. However, a sentinel node biopsy is associated with some amount of radiation exposure, but it is also feasible in pregnancy, including appropriate technetium labelling. Results from cohort studies suggest that sentinel node biopsy is a safe procedure [17]. The resulting radiation exposure is a maximum of 4.3 mGy. The blue label of the

sentinel, on the other hand, is contraindicated if there is a risk for a possible anaphylactic reaction.

Moreover, isosulfan blue and methylene blue are associated with an unknown potential for fetal teratogenicity [18]. Irradiation is strictly contraindicated during pregnancy due to a high risk for fetal malformations [19, 20]. If necessary (e.g. after breast-conserving surgery), irradiation should only be performed after the end of the pregnancy.

73.4.2 Adjuvant and Neoadjuvant Systemic Therapies

Except for the first trimester, both adjuvant and neoadjuvant chemotherapy are possible in pregnancy with the appropriate

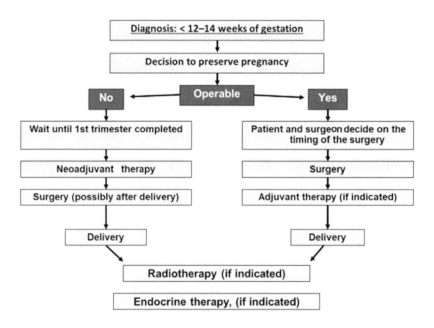

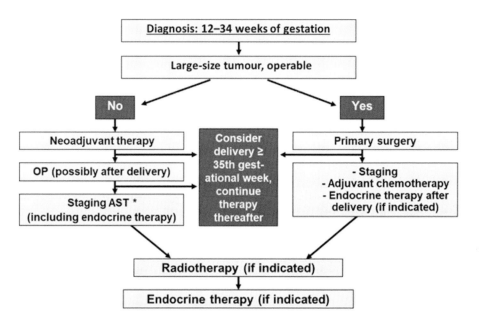

Figure 73.3 Therapeutic decisions at the time of diagnosis before 12 to 14 weeks (top diagram), and between 12 and 34 weeks of gestation (bottom diagram).
AST: aspartate aminotransferase

choice of the cytostatic agent. Substance classes that can primarily be used are *anthracyclines*, which are considered to be relatively safe; however, these substances can pass through placenta and breast milk. Regarding potential fetal cardiotoxicity, anthracyclines can be employed in the second and third trimesters [1, 9]. *Cyclophosphamide* can pass the placental barrier and can cause significant teratogenicity in the first trimester. It can be used in the second and third trimesters. Also, *5-fluorouracil* crosses the placenta. Generally, it is possible to employ 5-fluorouracil in combination with anthracyclines and cyclophosphamide; however, the available literature regarding these therapy regimens is currently insufficient. A prospective study with 57 pregnant patients treated with 5-fluorouracil 500 mg/m^2 (intravenously on days 1 and 4), doxorubicin 50 mg/m^2 (continuous infusion for 72 hours) and cyclophosphamide 500 mg/m^2 (intravenously on day 1) (FAC) have reported no significant adverse effects on mother or fetus with a mean gestational age at the time of delivery of 37 weeks [21].

The use of *methotrexate* is contraindicated, as it is known to induce abortion and otherwise may be associated with a significant risk of fetal malformation [9]. Some case reports describe the use of *taxane-containing chemotherapeutics*, without reliable evidence of significant fetal complications. Nevertheless, for the present, its use should possibly be restricted as one case of fetal malformation, possibly related to taxanes, was reported [9, 23, 24]. Table 73.2 shows an overview of the therapeutic substances.

Human studies as well as animal studies on the use of the selective oestrogen-receptor modulator *tamoxifen* revealed a significant risk for teratogenic fetal abnormalities, including craniofacial and other rare malformations [9]. Therefore, the use of tamoxifen is usually recommended after delivery.

Regarding biologics, also called targeted therapies, reports on the use of *trastuzumab* are available. This antibody crosses the placental barrier via pinocytosis. In published case reports, where trastuzumab was used, both as the adjuvant and at the metastatic stage, an amniotic fluid volume reduction was noted, thus leading to occasionally serious oligo- or anhydramnia [9, 25, 26]. A possible explanation for this could be via the inhibition of the vascular endothelial growth factor (VEGF) expression and thus influencing the regulation of the amnion permeability, followed by a corresponding decrease in the

amount of amniotic fluid volume. In addition, fetal renal perfusion appeared to be reduced. Other risks include prematurity, possibly causing neonatal lung and kidney dysfunctions [26–29]. There are two reported cases of postpartum infantile death reported among women following the use of trastuzumab in pregnancy. Thus, trastuzumab administration cannot be recommended in pregnancy (Table 73.2).

Bevacizumab as a VEGF antibody or antiangiogenesis antibody also crosses the placenta via pinocytosis. Experiments with animals showed skeletal malformations, an increased abortion rate and intrauterine growth retardation. Currently, there is no experience in humans in the context of systemic therapy during pregnancy. Thus, the data mentioned above resulted in a strict contraindication for its use in pregnancy. Besides, *lapatinib* as a tyrosine kinase inhibitor is very likely to be able to pass the placental barrier. Again, animal experiments showed an increased abortion rate, skeletal malformations and growth retardation. In a published case report, the substance was administered until the 12th week of gestation. Interestingly, within the follow-up of 18 months after delivery in the 36th gestational week, the clinical course was considered normal. However, currently, the substance should not be used during pregnancy.

73.4.3 Supportive Agents during Chemotherapy

The use of chemotherapeutics also requires effective prevention of emesis. A dose-dependent use of corticosteroids is possible, although they should not be administered in the first trimester. Among the 5-HT3 antagonists (setrons), sufficient safety data on the use of ondansetron are available, which allow its use throughout pregnancy.

The administration of growth-stimulating factors (i.e. GCSF) should be avoided since they can pass the placental barrier, possibly correlated with an increased abortion and malformation rate.

In the case of skeletal complications during metastatic breast cancer, bisphosphonates are frequently used. Published reports have described neonatal hypocalcaemia possibly due to parathyroid suppression caused by maternal hypercalcaemia but the newborns had a normal development at follow-up [9]. As a result, the authors have recommended careful monitoring of the neonatal calcium levels on the long-term basis.

Table 73.2 Cytotoxic substance use in pregnancy

Anthracyclines	Considered as relatively safe, able to pass the placenta and breast milk barrier, use in 2nd and 3rd trimesters possible, potential fetal cardiotoxicity
Cyclophosphamide	High teratogenicity in the 1st trimester, able to pass the placenta and breast milk barrier, use in 2nd and 3rd trimesters possible
5-Fluorouracil	Unclear data, able to pass placental barrier
Methotrexate	Abortion-inducing, a risk of intrauterine growth restriction (IUGR), a risk of malformations, contraindicated
Taxanes	Case reports without complications
Platine derivates	Cisplatin: risk of fetal hearing loss, a risk of IUGR, intrauterine fetal death and ventriculomegaly Carboplatin: hardly any data, no evidence for malformations

The effects of bisphosphonates on the general development and bone growth in the neonate are currently unknown.

73.4.4 Radiotherapy

Generally, radiotherapy is contraindicated during pregnancy. Routinely performed adjuvant breast or chest wall radiotherapy should be postponed until after delivery. However, if radiotherapy is considered lifesaving or to preserve essential organ functions (e.g. compression of the spinal cord), it can be considered with fetal shielding or after early elective delivery, depending on gestational age.

73.5 Pregnancy after Breast Cancer – Strategies of Fertility Preservation

Not only is the issue of late diagnosis of breast cancer diseases in pregnancy of essential importance, but also further consultation and care of patients who have not yet completed their family must be taken into consideration. They are keen to preserve their fertility after primary treatment of a breast cancer disease and wish for a child in the future. Future fertility potential depends upon the ovarian function and the recurrence of ovulation after completed chemotherapy. The following must be taken into consideration:

- The age of the patient
- The ovarian function at the time of treatment
- The choice of cytostatic drugs
- The dosage of cytostatics, which may affect fertility and ovarian function, especially in the case of alkylating agents

Temporary amenorrhoea with a median duration of 2 cycles or even permanent amenorrhoea can be expected in 21–71% of patients <40 years when employing combination chemotherapy of the cyclophosphamide, methotrexate and 5-fluorouracil (CMF) regime [30]. This rate may increase to 40–100% in older patients. Anthracycline-containing regimens have a lower rate of amenorrhoea. In the literature, several studies show a high variability depending on the individual factors mentioned [22]. Generally, it can be assumed that the functional age of the ovaries after chemotherapy is decreased by 10 years on average.

73.5.1 Medications for Ovarian Protection by Gonadotropin-releasing Hormone (GnRH) Analogues

The effectiveness of administering gonadotropin-releasing hormone (GnRH) analogues to protect the ovarian function during chemotherapy is the subject of many studies with inconsistent data. Recent work by Badawy et al and Blumenfeld and a meta-analysis by Clowse et al showed ovarian protection, while the work of Sonmezer et al and Beck-Fruchter et al summarize inconsistent data on GnRH protection of the ovaries [31–35]. In contrast, the ZORO study evaluation presented at the American Society of Clinical Oncology (ASCO) Annual Meeting 2009 showed no significant difference in the occurrence of periodic bleeding 6 months after the end of chemotherapy in both groups, with or without GnRH-a [36].

As a consequence of the inconsistent data, the application of GnRH analogues should be discussed in a differentiated way and considered against alternative methods of preserving of ovarian function.

73.5.2 Ovarian Stimulation and Oocyte Cryopreservation

Currently, ovarian stimulation followed by cryopreservation of fertilized oocytes offers an attractive option for later pregnancy. Obtaining multiple mature oocytes requires gonadotropin stimulation. For this, the time frame required is usually 14 days. The ultrasound-controlled transvaginal puncture enables the achievement of mature oocytes that are either frozen unfertilized (patients without a partner) or fertilized (patients with a partner). According to data from the FertiPROTEKT network, on average 6.1 and 5.1 pronucleosis stages could be cryopreserved within the groups of patients in the age group of 30–35 years and the age group of 36–40 years, respectively [37]. Despite ovarian stimulation, due to the use of an aromatase inhibitor, only a small increase in oestradiol occurs during gonadotropin stimulation.

73.5.3 Cryopreservation of Ovarian Tissue

Cryopreservation of ovarian tissue is another treatment option, which is not associated with an increase in oestrogen levels. With the timely planning of this procedure, the laparoscopy for the excision of ovarian tissue can be done together with the main breast cancer surgery. The ovarian tissue thus obtained is frozen by a slow freezing procedure, which is the most suitable technique for preserving the ovarian function. The aim of this procedure is to cause the complete dehydration of the cells as a first step, followed by survival rates of the frozen oocytes in the ovarian tissue of >80%. This method enables the re-transplantation of the preserved ovarian tissue in patients after having completed their cancer treatment, which subsequently leads to normal ovarian function (Figure 73.4). Principally, a pregnancy is possible thereafter and has led to many births worldwide so far [38]. Based on results from the centres in Copenhagen and Brussels, the birth rate per transplant is currently higher than 30%. The FertiPROTEKT project is a network that provides advice on the cryopreservation of ovarian tissue.

73.5.4 Special Features When Planning a Pregnancy after Breast Cancer

Generally, the desire for pregnancy after breast cancer disease and treatment is rare and amounts to about <10% of patients. Due to the fact that after completion of adjuvant therapy for breast cancer, the highest risk of cancer recurrence and metastasis is assumed (purely statistically) within the first 2 years thereafter, the planning of pregnancy is often recommended after this 2-year interval. However, there are no reliable data to support this advice.

Significant risk factors which need to be considered are:

1. Tumour stage, nodal status, grading, receptor status and other biological properties of the respective tumour must be determined.

599

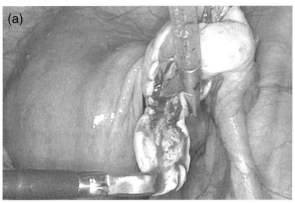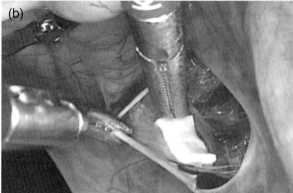

Figure 73.4 Laparoscopic procedure for ovarian cryoconservation, with laparoscopic resection of ovarian tissue (a) and re-implantation of the cryoconserved ovarian cortex into a peritoneal pocket (b).

2. Therefore, an optimal interval for the planning of pregnancy after diagnosis and treatment of breast cancer cannot be defined; however, the range should not be less than 6 months.

3. Currently, it is difficult to clarify if maternal cancer disease has a negative impact on childhood and development due to the small numbers of cases and the different forms of the treatments used.

4. One of the largest cohorts to examine this question included 84 children after an observation period of 18 years. Only a limited impact on childhood development, including a moderate increase in the tendency to develop depression, has been reported [39].

73.6 Key Messages

1. The diagnosis of breast cancer in pregnancy is not automatically associated with a prognostically unfavourable course of the disease or a worse prognosis. However, the diagnosis is often made at advanced stages.

2. According to older studies, a diagnosis with a delay of 6 months on average is possible. However, recent studies confirm a time interval of only 1–2 months to the actual diagnosis.

3. Diagnosis of breast cancer in pregnancy is challenging, especially given changes in the mass and consistency of pregnant breast tissue.

4. With few exceptions, the usual diagnostic and therapeutic procedures can be used almost without restriction.

5. For further treatment planning, the timing of the diagnosis, taking into account the respective gestational age, and the tumour stage is crucial.

6. The vital question for planning a pregnancy after breast cancer treatment includes fertility preservation measures.

73.7 Key Guidelines

- National Institute for Health and Care Excellence (NICE) guidance; www.rcog.org.uk/globalassets/documents/guidelines/gtg_12.pdf
- Arbeitsgemeinschaft Gynäkologische Onkologie (AGO); www.ago-online.de/fileadmin/downloads/leitlinien/mamma/2018-03/EN/Gesamt_PDF_Englisch/Updated_Guidelines_2018.pdf

References

1. Navrozoglou I, Vrekoussis T, Kontostolis E, et al. Breast cancer during pregnancy: a mini-review. *Eur J Surg Oncol.* 2008;**34**:837–43.

2. Azim HA Jr, Del Mastro L, Scarfone G, Peccatori FA. Treatment of breast cancer during pregnancy: regimen selection, pregnancy monitoring and more. *Breast.* 2011;**20**:1–6.

3. Csonka Y, Mosimann A. *Familien in der Schweiz – Statistischer Bericht 2017.* Neuchâtel: Swiss Federal Statistical Office (Bundesamt für Statistik); 2017.

4. Cullinane CA, Lubinski J, Neuhausen SL, et al. Effect of pregnancy as a risk factor for breast cancer in BRCA1/BRCA2 mutation carriers. *Int J Cancer.* 2005;**117**:988e91.

5. Valentini A, Lubinski J, Byrski T, et al.; Hereditary Breast Cancer Clinical Study Group. The impact of pregnancy on breast cancer survival in women who carry a BRCA1 or BRCA2 mutation. *Breast Cancer Res Treat.* 2013;**142**:177–85.

6. Framarino-Dei-Malatesta M, Piccioni MG, Brunelli R, et al. Breast cancer during pregnancy: a retrospective study on obstetrical problems and survival. *Eur J Obstet Gynecol Reprod Biol.* 2014;**173**:48–52.

7. Bonnier P, Romain S, Dilhuydy JM, et al. Influence of pregnancy on the outcome of breast cancer: a case-control study. *Int J Cancer.* 1997;**72**:720–7.

8. Shachar SS, Gallagher K, McGuire K, et al. Multidisciplinary management of breast cancer during pregnancy. *Oncologist.* 2017;**22**:324–34.

9. Ring AE, Smith IE, Ellis PA. Breast cancer and pregnancy. *Ann Oncol.* 2005;**16**:1855–60.

10. Rimawi BH, Green V, Lindsay M. Fetal implications of diagnostic radiation exposure during pregnancy: evidence-based recommendations. *Clin Obstet Gynecol.* 2016;**59**:412–18.

11. Nicklas A, Baker M. Imaging strategies in the pregnant breast cancer patient. *Semin Oncol.* 2000;**27**:623–32.

12. Amant F, Van Calsteren K, Halaska MJ, et al. Long-term cognitive and cardiac outcomes after prenatal exposure to chemotherapy in children aged 18 months or older: an observational study. *Lancet Oncol.* 2012;**13**:256–64.

13. Myers KS, Green LA, Lebron L, Morris EA. Imaging appearance and clinical impact of preoperative breast MRI in pregnancy-associated breast cancer. *AJR Am J Roentgenol.* 2017;**209**:177–83.

14. Yang WT, Dryden MJ, Gwyn K, Whitman GJ, Theriault R. Imaging of breast cancer diagnosed and treated with chemotherapy during pregnancy. *Radiology.* 2006;**239**:52–60.

15. Howard-Anderson J, Ganz PA, Bower JE, Stanton AL. Quality of life, fertility concerns, and behavioral health outcomes in younger breast cancer survivors: a systematic review. *J Natl Cancer Inst.* 2012;**104**:386e405.

16. Gerstl B, Sullivan E, Ives A, et al. Pregnancy outcomes after a breast cancer diagnosis: a systematic review and meta-analysis. *Clin Breast Cancer.* 2018;**18**:e79-e88.

17. Gropper AB, Calvillo KZ, Dominici L, et al. Sentinel lymph node biopsy in pregnant women with breast cancer. *Ann Surg Oncol.* 2014;**21**:2506–11.

18. Michieletto S, Saibene T, Evangelista L, et al. Preliminary monocentric results of biological characteristics of pregnancy associated breast cancer. *Breast.* 2014;**23**:19–25.

19. Mazonakis M, Varveris H, Damilakis J, Theoharopoulos N, Gourtsoyiannis N. Radiation dose to conceptus resulting from tangential breast irradiation. *Int J Radiat Oncol Biol Phys.* 2003;**55**:386–91.

20. Loibl S, Schmidt A, Gentilini O, et al. Breast cancer diagnosed during pregnancy: adapting recent advances in breast cancer care for pregnant patients. *JAMA Oncol.* 2015;**1**:1145–53.

21. Hahn KM, Johnson PH, Gordon N. Treatment of pregnant breast cancer patients and outcomes of children exposed to chemotherapy in utero. *Cancer.* 2006;**107**:1219–26.

22. Shalaby M, Lasheen SF, Talima S; 232P. Pregnancy associated breast cancer spotlights. *Ann Oncol.* 2017;**28**:1.

23. Gadducci A, Cosio S, Fanucchi A, et al. Chemotherapy with epirubicin and paclitaxel for breast cancer during pregnancy: case report and review of the literature. *Anticancer Res.* 2003;**23**:5225–30.

24. Mir O, Berveiller P, Goffinet F, et al. Taxanes for breast cancer during pregnancy: a systematic review. *Ann Oncol.* 2010;**21**:425–6.

25. Cheung CY. Vascular endothelial growth factor activation of intramembranous absorption: a critical pathway for amniotic fluid volume regulation. *J Soc Gynecol Invest.* 2004;**11**:63–74.

26. Bader AA, Schlembach D, Tamussimo KF, Pristauz G, Petru E. Anhydramnios associated with administration of trastuzumab and paclitaxel for metastatic breast cancer during pregnancy. *Lancet Oncol.* 2007 **8**:79–81.

27. Sekar R, Stone PR. Trastuzumab use for metastatic breast cancer in pregnancy. *Obstet Gynecol.* 2007;**110**:507–10.

28. Shrim A, Garcia-Bournissen F, Maxwell C, Farine D, Koren G. Trastuzumab treatment for breast cancer during pregnancy. *Can Fam Physician.* 2008;**54**:31–2.

29. Witzel ID, Müller V, Harps E, Janicke F, Dewit M. Trastuzumab in pregnancy associated with poor fetal outcome. *Ann Oncol.* 2008;**19**:191–2.

30. Gadducci A, Cosio S, Genazzani AR. Ovarian function and childbearing issues in breast cancer survivors. *Gynecol Endocrinol.* 2007;**23**:625–31.

31. Badawy A, Elnashar A, El-Ashry M, Shahat M. Gonadotropin-releasing hormone agonists for prevention of chemotherapy-induced ovarian damage: prospective randomized study. *Fertil Steril.* 2009;**91**:694–7.

32. Blumenfeld Z. Endocrine prevention of chemotherapy-induced ovarian failure. *Future Oncol.* 2016;**12**:1671–4.

33. Clowse ME, Behera MA, Anders CK, et al. Ovarian preservation by GnRH agonists during chemotherapy: a meta-analysis. *J Womens Health (Larchmt).* 2009 Mar;**18**(3):311–19. doi:10.1089/jwh.2008.0857. PMID: 19281314; PMCID: PMC2858300.

34. Sonmezer M, Oktay K. Fertility preservation in young women undergoing breast cancer therapy. *Oncologist.* 2006;**1**:422–34.

35. Beck-Fruchter R, Weiss A, Shalev E. GnRH agonist therapy as ovarian protectants in female patients undergoing chemotherapy: a review of the clinical data. *Hum Reprod Update.* 2008;**14**(6):553–61.

36. Gerber B, Stehle H, Ricardo F, et al. ZORO: A prospective randomized multicenter study to prevent chemotherapy-induced ovarian failure with the GnRH-agonist goserelin in young hormone-insensitive breast cancer patients receiving anthracycline containing (neo-) adjuvant chemotherapy (GBG 37). *J Clin Oncol.* 2009;**27**:526.

37. von Wolff M, Bruckner T, Strowitzki T, Germeyer A. Fertility preservation: ovarian response to freeze oocytes is not affected by different malignant diseases-an analysis of 992 stimulations. *J Assist Reprod Genet.* 2018;**35**:1713–19.

38. Van der Ven H, Liebenthron J, Beckmann M, et al.; FertiPROTEKT Network. Ninety-five orthotopic transplantations in 74 women of ovarian tissue after cytotoxic treatment in a fertility preservation network: tissue activity, pregnancy and delivery rates. *Hum Reprod.* 2016;**31**:2031–41.

39. Brown RT, Fuemmeler B, Anderson D, et al. Adjustment of children and their mothers with breast cancer. *J Pediatr Psychol.* 2007; Apr;**32**:297–308.

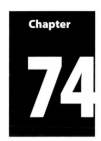

Chapter 74

Gynaecological Cancers and Pregnancy

Charlotte Maggen, Christianne A. R. Lok & Frédéric Amant

74.1 Epidemiology of Gynaecological Cancers during Pregnancy

There are few epidemiological studies on cancer in pregnancy, as national registries usually do not combine data on both cancer diagnosis and obstetrics. Nationwide linkage studies estimated the incidence of pregnancy-associated cancer, defined as a cancer diagnosis during pregnancy or within 12 months from delivery, to be 1 in 1000–2000 pregnancies [1]. The difference in estimated incidence between studies is explained by the difference in denominator used (live births, births beyond 20 weeks or pregnancies). The distribution of the various cancer types diagnosed in pregnancy is similar to that in the non-pregnant premenopausal population. Gynaecological cancers are one of the most common oncological diagnoses during pregnancy, after breast cancer, melanoma and haematological cancers [2]. Figure 74.1 represents the distribution of patients with a diagnosis during pregnancy in the registry of the international network on Cancer, Infertility and Pregnancy (www.cancerinpregnancy.org). Melanoma is probably underrepresented in this registry, as these patients are mostly diagnosed in the early stage and often not referred to centres that participate in the registration study.

74.2 General Aspects

Diagnosing cancer without delay is as important in pregnant women as it is in non-pregnant women. Preferably, the same imaging modalities as advised in the regular guidelines are used in order to avoid a suboptimal diagnostic process.

Physical examination is important but can be challenged by the physiological changes of pregnancy, certainly if the breast or abdomen is to be examined.

The plasma concentration of tumour markers can be influenced by pregnancy [3]. In the first trimester, the cancer antigen 125 (CA125) is commonly elevated (up to 35% of the normal value), whereas the squamous cell carcinoma antigen (SCC) is more often elevated in the third trimester. However, very high concentrations are not expected in pregnancy and can be indicative of disease. Human epididymis secretory protein 4 (HE4), inhibin B, anti-Müllerian hormone (AMH) and lactate dehydrogenate (LDH) remain stable during pregnancy. Tumour markers of ovarian germ cell tumours (hCG, alpha-fetoprotein) cannot be reliably assessed during pregnancy. Biomarker assessment is often reliable again after 2 to 10 weeks after delivery.

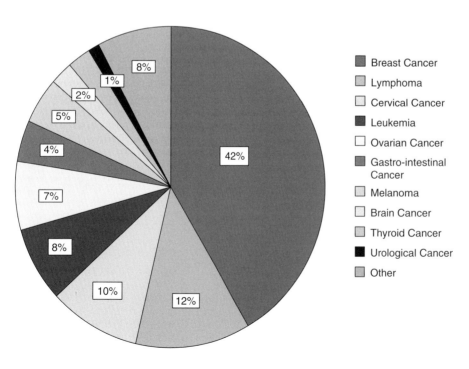

Figure 74.1 Distribution of cancer types during pregnancy, INCIP database, update August 2019 (n=2049)

- Breast Cancer
- Lymphoma
- Cervical Cancer
- Leukemia
- Ovarian Cancer
- Gastro-intestinal Cancer
- Melanoma
- Brain Cancer
- Thyroid Cancer
- Urological Cancer
- Other

Radiation-free imaging (ultrasound and magnetic resonance imaging (MRI)) is preferred in the staging of cancer during pregnancy; however, optimal imaging is essential to decide on further management in treatment and follow-up of the patient. Gynaecological ultrasound should be performed by an expert sonographer, as pregnancy might complicate interpretation. For example, decidualization of endometrioma due to gestational hormonal changes can hamper correct differentiation from ovarian cancer. The simple rules, consisting of five features typical of benign tumours (unilocular, solid components <7, acoustic shadow, smooth multilocular tumour <100, no blood flow) and five features typical of malignant tumours (irregular solid tumour, ascites, ≥4 papillary structures, irregular multilocular-solid tumour ≥100 mm, very strong blood flow), were defined to guide physicians in further management of ovarian masses [4]. Radiographic imaging in pregnancy is possible and sometimes necessary, but only those examinations that will influence management should be performed. Cumulative fetal radiation exposure should be estimated and may not exceed 100 mGy, preferably 50 mGy [5]. MRI without contrast is validated during all trimesters of pregnancy (see Figure 74.2) [6, 7]. Diffusion-weighted MRI of the whole body is validated for the staging during pregnancy and is for many cancer types the preferred method to avoid computed tomography (CT) scanning, which exposes the fetus to significantly more radiation [6]. Table 74.1 summarizes the estimated fetal absorbed doses from common radiologic procedures [5, 8].

Contrast products should to be used with caution in imaging. Fetal gadolinium exposure is associated with rheumatologic, inflammatory or infiltrative skin conditions, stillbirth and neonatal death [7]. Iodinated contrast may cause neonatal thyroid dysfunction. If it is used during pregnancy, the thyroid function of the neonate has to be controlled after birth.

Nuclear imaging such as PET-CT and bone scans are possible but preferably avoided if it does not change the treatment plan. Sentinel node biopsies are feasible and safe in breast cancer, but rarely investigated in gynaecological cancer [9].

The use of radiographic and nuclear imaging should be carefully considered and adaptations for the pregnant patient (i.e. shielding or dosages) should comply with the ALARA principle (as low as reasonably achievable). It is recommended to discuss imaging with a physicist and to estimate fetal dose as accurately as possible using a phantom model in order to counsel parents on the potential toxicity.

74.3 General Aspects of Surgery during Pregnancy

A surgical intervention can often be performed safely during pregnancy, However, physiological changes in pregnancy necessitate a different anaesthetic approach compared to non-pregnant patients. The maternal haemodynamic condition should remain as stable as possible, as this may directly influence fetal well-being. A stable oxygenation and stable blood pressure are mandatory to maintain an optimal fetal condition. In pregnancy, there is an increase in oxygen demand and functional residual lung capacity is reduced, resulting in a faster desaturation when apnoea occurs. Maternal hypotension as a result of deep anaesthesia, hypovolaemia and vena cava compression may cause uterine hypoperfusion. Therefore, left lateral tilt position with 15 or 30 degrees from 20 weeks of gestational age onwards is advised. From a viable duration of pregnancy (usually 24 weeks of gestation, depending on local hospital policies and patient's perspective), intraoperative fetal monitoring is an option whenever possible. Tocolytics should be considered during the second half of pregnancy if uterine manipulation during surgery is inevitable [10, 11].

A laparoscopic intervention during pregnancy can be performed until 26–28 weeks of gestational age, depending on the surgeon's expertise and the target organ. However, the gravid uterus challenges surgery and might be an obstacle for optimal pelvic and para-aortic lymphadenectomy in gynaecological cancer. An open introduction with a Hasson trocar is the preferred method. The umbilical port should be located at least 3–4 cm above the uterine fundus, even if this location is supra-umbilical. Carbon dioxide (CO_2) insufflation of 10–15 mm Hg can be safely used, and the estimated maximal duration of the intervention should be 90 minutes.

Postoperative analgesia is important, as pain may provoke preterm uterine contractions. Paracetamol and opiates can be used safely. Nonsteroidal anti-inflammatory drugs are contraindicated in pregnancy, especially in the third trimester because of the risk of preterm closure of the ductus arteriosus.

In the postoperative or hospitalization setting, prevention of thromboembolism with low molecular weight heparin is indicated because of the prothrombogenic condition of cancer, pregnancy and relative immobilization [12].

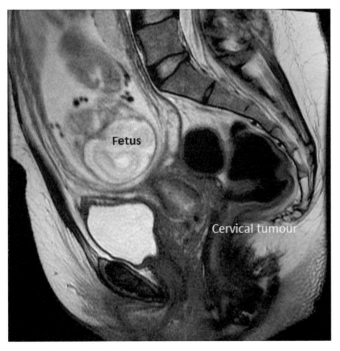

Figure 74.2 MRI pelvis, cervical tumour at 22 weeks of gestational age

Table 74.1 Estimated fetal radiation exposure according to radiographic examinations

Procedure	Fetal dose (mGy)	Procedure	Fetal dose (mGy)
Chest x-ray	0.0001–0.43	CT lumbar spine	2–8.6
Abdominal x-ray	1.4–4.2	CT pulmonary embolism	0.2–0.7
Pelvic x-ray	0.16–22	CT chest	0.02–0.2
Intravenous pyelography	0.7–55.0	CT abdomen	4.0–60.0
Lumbosacral spine x-ray	0.2–40.0	CT pelvis	6.7–114
Mammography	<0.1	CT head	<0.1
Hips and femur x-ray	0.73–14.0	Tc bone scan	4.0–5.0
CT liver	2.0–4.4	^{18}F PET/CT whole body scintigraphy	10–50

X-ray: rontgen radiation; CT: computed tomography; PET: positron emission tomography; Tc: technetium. Reference: Dauer et al 2012 [5], ACOG 2017 [8]

74.4 General Aspects of Chemotherapy during Pregnancy

According to current knowledge, based on animal studies and clinical experience, oncological treatment can often be initiated during pregnancy. The key principle is that the same treatment should be offered to pregnant patients as is offered to non-pregnant patients. However, from a fetal perspective, some treatments are not advised or are even contraindicated during pregnancy. If a pregnant patient presents with a very aggressive or metastatic disease early in pregnancy, it makes sense to question whether the pregnancy can be continued. Preferably, decision making should be performed in a specialized centre by a multidisciplinary team, taking the patient's perspective into account.

Chemotherapy is contraindicated in the first trimester because it can potentially disturb organogenesis (which occurs between 2 and 8 weeks after conception) and is associated with miscarriage, fetal death and congenital malformations. Starting from the second trimester of pregnancy, the administration of several cytotoxic drugs seems to be safe.

74.4.1 Transplacental Passage of Chemotherapy and Pharmacokinetics

The transplacental passage of cytotoxic agents, including paclitaxel, carboplatin, doxorubicin and epirubicin, are investigated in mouse and baboon models and the fetal plasma concentrations were (considerably) lower than maternal plasma concentrations (Table 74.2) [13, 14]. Cyclophosphamide passes the placenta up to 20%. Platinum-based chemotherapy (carboplatin, cisplatin) has a high potential to cross the placenta (up to 60%). In contrast, the placental transfer of taxanes is very low (±2%). However, baboon studies revealed an accumulation of taxanes of up to 14% of the maternal plasma concentration in fetal tissues, likely explained by the immature hepatic metabolism of neonates [14].

Currently, the administered dose during pregnancy is calculated from the actual body weight on the day of treatment, as no studies to date justify a change in dosage. However, van Hasselt et al have shown that physiological changes in pregnancy lead to a decrease in peak plasma concentrations and active medication in plasma (area under the curve, AUC), as well as an elevated distribution volume and elimination [15]. This finding may suggest that a standard treatment dose of cytotoxic agents that is based on the actual body weight may be suboptimal. But so far the prognosis of patients treated for cancer during pregnancy does not seem to differ from that of non-pregnant patients [16]. More studies on follow-up data and pharmacokinetics are indicated.

74.4.2 Maternal and Fetal Consequences of Chemotherapy

Maternal risks are similar to those for non-pregnant patients, including myelosuppression, in particular neutropenia and sepsis. Our clinical experience suggests that pregnant patients endure chemotherapy the same as or better than (less nausea) non-pregnant patients; however, studies on toxicity in pregnancy are needed to confirm this.

The administration of chemotherapy during the second or third trimester is associated with low birthweight and prematurity [2]. Both taxanes and platinum derivatives during the second or third trimester of pregnancy increase the risk of low birthweight (odds ratio (OR) 2.07, 95% confidence interval (CI) 1.11–3.86; OR 3.12, 95% CI 1.45–6.70, respectively) [2].

A systematic review in 2012 that addressed the effect of taxanes during the second or third trimester of pregnancy in ovarian cancer patients did not find a negative effect on fetal organ development, although there was limited information on the long-term outcome of the offspring [17].

Ototoxicity is a known complication of platinum-based chemotherapy and cisplatin carries the greatest risk. Few cases of hearing loss after prenatal exposure to cisplatin have been reported, and this effect seems to be dose dependent [18, 19]. Amant et al assessed auditory functioning in 21 children between 6 and 18 years of age who had been exposed to platinum-based

Table 74.2 Pre-clinical data of placental transfer for most common cytotoxic drugs in gynaecological cancers during pregnancy

Drug class	Drug	Transplacental passage (animal models)
Platinum compounds	Carboplatin, (cisplatin)	± 60%
Alkylating agents	Cyclophosphamide	± 20%
Antitumour antibiotics	Epirubicin	<10%
	Doxorubicin	<10% (active metabolite)
Taxanes	Paclitaxel, docetaxel	<2%, Up to 14% accumulation in fetal tissue
Vinca alkaloids	Vinblastine	± 20%

Reference: Calsteren et al [14], van Hasselt et al [15]

treatment in utero [20]. While 18 children showed no abnormalities, 3 children had hearing loss. In reported cases, infection, the use of aminoglycosides and neurodevelopmental problems in these children were confounding factors. This risk should be carefully weighed, and follow-up of hearing after birth is recommended. Where possible, the second generation compound carboplatin should be the preferred option during pregnancy, as it is less nephrotoxic and ototoxic than cisplatin.

74.5 Obstetric Management

Decisions about the best management in pregnancy should be based on the balance of maternal and fetal risks. Maternal risks mostly depend on the consequences on prognosis if adequate oncological treatment is postponed.

The most important fetal risk is prematurity. Iatrogenic preterm delivery is not uncommon, as delivery will often be planned to start oncological treatment soon thereafter. However, prematurity is associated with neonatal mortality and morbidity [21]. Therefore, the tendency to avoid iatrogenic preterm delivery and to start treatment during pregnancy needs to be balanced against the neonatal risks such as fetal growth restriction and fetal loss (including stillbirth). Ideally, delivery after 37 weeks of gestation should be aimed for. Delivery within 2–3 weeks following the last administration of cytotoxic drugs (depending on the regimen used) should be avoided to reduce the risk of myelosuppression and systemic infection and to allow fetal drug excretion via the placenta. A vaginal delivery is preferable, unless there is an obstetric or oncological contraindication. If indicated, a caesarean section can be performed simultaneously with surgical treatment. Although placental metastases are rare, sending the placenta for histological examination should be considered [22].

74.6 Cervical Cancer

74.6.1 Background

Cervical cancer (CC) is the most common gynaecological cancer diagnosed during pregnancy, with an estimated incidence between 1 and 12/10 000 pregnancies [23]. However, its incidence is geographically and socioculturally defined, depending on national screening programmes for CC. Approximately 30% of patients with CC are diagnosed during their reproductive years, whereas 3% of CC are diagnosed during pregnancy.

74.6.2 Diagnosis

In pregnant patients, CC is most frequently diagnosed at early International Federation of Gynecology and Obstetrics (FIGO) stages and in the first half of pregnancy, due to a low threshold for referral for medical assistance and subsequent gynaecological examination when a pregnant patient presents with vaginal bleeding. Mean age at diagnosis is 35 years, with a mean gestational age at diagnosis of 19.5 weeks [18]. Staging should follow the standard steps as closely as possible. As stated, CA125 can be elevated in pregnancy, whereas SCC is more often elevated in the third trimester [3]. Examination under general anaesthesia can be considered during all stages of pregnancy. Gynaecological ultrasound and MRI are preferred methods of imaging, as radiation of more than 100 mGy during pregnancy is associated with miscarriage, fetal malformations and cancers in the offspring (see Table 74.1: 100 mGy is equivalent to a pelvic CT) [5].

Pregnancy is not an absolute contraindication of a clinically justified ^{18}F-FDG PET scan; however, radiation exposure is considerable and safer alternatives are available [24].

74.6.3 Treatment Options

When CC is diagnosed during pregnancy, the management will depend upon gestational age at diagnosis, histological subtype, stage of disease, size of the lesion, lymph node involvement and patient's desire about both her actual pregnancy and future fertility. This implies either to initiate treatment during pregnancy, wait for fetal maturity before definitive treatment or terminate pregnancy.

74.6.3.1 Surgery

Tumour size and lymph node involvement are the most important prognostic factors in patients diagnosed with CC. Under 22 weeks of gestation, pelvic lymphadenectomy is safe and reproducible and has good oncological and obstetric outcome.

This procedure can be performed laparoscopically in experienced centres in order to reduce treatment-related morbidity. Several authors report the safety and efficacy of this technique and absence of intraoperative complications when performed by experienced surgeons.

Pelvic sentinel node biopsy is contraindicated using patent blue (risk of anaphylactic reaction) or technetium (radiation dose too high). Indocyanine green appears to be an alternative, but more evidence is needed.

If lymph node metastases are present, management is challenging and depends on the nodal involvement (micro metastasis, micro with extracapsular growth). The prognostic importance of node positivity should be taken into consideration while counselling further management during pregnancy (termination versus chemotherapy). Patients without lymph node metastasis can safely continue pregnancy, and in these patients initiation of neo-adjuvant chemotherapy can be considered. As increasing number of studies in non-pregnant women demonstrates that in small tumours without lymph nodes metastases, the risk of parametrial involvement is negligible and there is a growing support for simple trachelectomy/conization only. Radical trachelectomy during pregnancy is possible; however, it is discouraged because of the high incidence of patient-related and fetal complications [10, 11].

When CC is diagnosed after approximately 22 weeks of gestation, pelvic lymph node dissection is difficult to perform; therefore, decision making cannot rely on the nodal status. In small tumours (less than 2 cm), delay of treatment until fetal maturity can be considered under strict monitoring of tumour size, with an adequate surgical staging following delivery. Alternatively, chemotherapy can be initiated during pregnancy in order to prevent tumour progression. For larger tumours, chemotherapy is the only way to preserve pregnancy and reach fetal maturity [10, 11].

74.6.3.2 Neo-adjuvant Chemotherapy (NACT)

When delivery needs to be delayed until the fetus reaches maturity or in locally advanced tumours, neo-adjuvant chemotherapy (NACT) helps in controlling the disease and prevents tumour progression until delivery. Although no randomized trials have been published, the available case series suggest that NACT is a viable option in the management of CC during pregnancy. Most patients respond to treatment, allowing prolongation of pregnancy until fetal maturity is reached, but strict monitoring is essential. If the tumour grows under chemotherapy, pregnancy should be terminated or premature delivery by caesarean section should be performed. Platinum-based chemotherapy in combination with paclitaxel is the recommended regimen for CC. Where possible, cisplatin should be replaced by carboplatin with a more favourable toxicity profile.

74.6.3.3 Radiation Therapy

In advanced CC stages, chemoradiation is indicated and this is not compatible with pregnancy at any gestational age. Therefore, pregnancy preservation is difficult or impossible and could lead to worse maternal outcome. External beam radiation therapy will result in spontaneous abortion in the first trimester or to fetal loss within 4 weeks after treatment in the second trimester. In the second trimester, termination of pregnancy by hysterotomy before the initiation of radiation therapy is supported to avoid obstetric complications as haemorrhage and infection. Also from a psychological point of view, this approach seems more favourable; however, management should always be balanced individually [11].

74.6.4 Obstetric Management

Vaginal delivery is only possible if the cervix is microscopically clear of tumour (after a conization with clear margins for FIGO IA1-2 CC). In the presence of tumour, caesarean section is the preferred route of delivery to prevent recurrence in a perineal lesion (i.e. episiotomy or perineal rupture) or other location [10, 11]. During caesarean section, a wall wound protective system or a corporeal incision is recommended to prevent possible abdominal spilling. Simultaneous oncological surgery as radical hysterectomy and rarely trachelectomy can be performed. As preterm delivery is associated with increased neonatal morbidity, a term delivery (after 37 weeks of gestation) is recommended where possible [21].

74.6.5 Maternal Outcome

Pregnancy does not seem to have a negative effect on the prognosis of CC [23]. In a large Norwegian population-based linkage study maternal prognosis of CC does not seem to be influenced by pregnancy or lactation [25]. A recent cohort study revealed a similar survival of cervical cancer of 132 pregnant and 256 non-pregnant patients, matched for age and FIGO (2009) stage, with a median follow-up of 84 months [26]. However, caution is warranted, as Xia et al noted decreased survival in pregnant patients who delayed definitive treatment for CC (this cohort had a high proportion of tumours >4 cm) [27].

74.7 Borderline Ovarian Cancer

74.7.1 Background

Ovarian masses are detected in 0.2–2% of all pregnant women. This occurs mostly in the first trimester because of the routine obstetric ultrasound [28]. The majority of the masses (up to 90%) are benign tumours, such as dermoid cysts, serous and mucinous adenomas and persistent corpus luteum and endometrioid cysts. The vast majority of ovarian masses will resolve spontaneously. The malignancy rate of persistent ovarian masses in pregnancy is 1–6%. The most frequent are germ cell tumours, borderline ovarian tumours (between 21 and 35%) and invasive epithelial ovarian cancers [23].

74.7.2 Diagnosis

Most patients with borderline tumours are asymptomatic. Abdominal discomfort or pain and an increased abdominal circumference can occur. They have a risk of torsion and rupture.

Most borderline ovarian tumours are detected in the first trimester of pregnancy, usually in FIGO stage 1. Around 20% are diagnosed in FIGO stages II and III [29]. Histopathology shows atypical proliferation of stromal cells. The serous subtype is most frequently diagnosed (53–65%). It develops bilaterally in 20–30% of patients. Transvaginal ultrasound may reveal typical sonographic features (Figure 74.3) [4]. Borderline ovarian tumours are characterized by a cystic and partly solid type of lesion with papillations and septa. In general, serous and endocervical-type mucinous subtypes have a higher rate of unilocular-solid lesions, more papillar formations, a higher vascuularization, a lower percentage of multilocular lesions and fewer locules compared to the intestinal type of mucinous borderline ovarian tumours. This type typically is an unilocular large, multicystic tumour with smooth capsule, hyperechoic-connecting multiple locules and no clear solid tissue or papillary projections. (Diffusion-weighted) MRI may be a good alternative in the case of diagnostic doubts and to exclude intra-abdominal metastases or implants [6, 7]. Pelvic CT is not recommended since it exposes the fetus to a radiation dose of at least 20–40 mGy. As mentioned earlier, the level of CA125 should be interpreted with caution, as it may be increased in pregnancy [3].

74.7.3 Treatment Options

Borderline tumours can be treated by adnexectomy, and according to local protocol further staging by peritoneal washings, biopsies, omentectomy or appendectomy can be performed. Conservative treatment (cystectomy) can be considered in selected patients. The early second trimester is generally considered optimal for surgical interventions because of the minimal miscarriage risk and the acceptable accessibility of the peritoneal cavity. The surgery should be performed by a team trained in oncological interventions in pregnant patients, and mass rupture must be avoided. If access to the peritoneal cavity is poor because of advanced gestational age, definitive surgical staging can be postponed until 3–6 weeks after vaginal delivery or be performed immediately after caesarean section. Surgical intervention can be performed by laparotomy or laparoscopy, based on gestational age, size of ovarian mass and surgeon's expertise.

74.7.4 Obstetric Management

The measures for surgery during pregnancy as described earlier should be followed. After surgery, routine prenatal care is sufficient. Preterm delivery is seldom necessary. Term vaginal delivery is likely to be achieved. Caesarean section should only be performed for obstetric indications. However, the caesarean section can be combined with oncological surgery if necessary.

74.7.5 Maternal Outcome

Maternal prognosis is excellent. Pregnancy does not influence outcome. Even with expectant management, adverse outcome is very unlikely. The most challenging is not to miss an invasive ovarian cancer.

74.8 Invasive Ovarian Cancer

74.8.1 Background

Ovarian cancer is the second most common gynaecological cancer diagnosed during pregnancy, with an estimated incidence of 1 in 12 000–47 000 pregnancies [28]. As stated, 1–6% of persistent ovarian masses are estimated to be malignant. Improved diagnostic procedures and more interaction between specialized health services during pregnancy contribute to early detection [30].

74.8.2 Diagnosis

The presence of an ovarian mass is usually an incidental finding on standard prenatal ultrasound. Therefore, ovarian cancer is often diagnosed in the first or second trimester of pregnancy

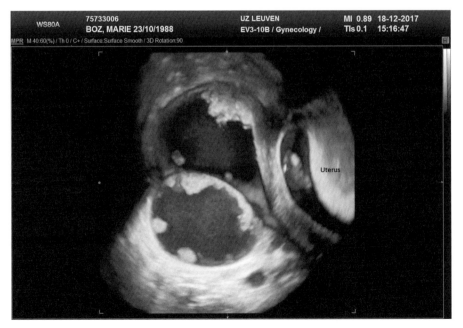

Figure 74.3 Mucinous borderline ovarian tumour, diagnosed in the first trimester of pregnancy by vaginal ultrasound (left side: mobile 10 cm multilocular-solid mass with irregular papillar formations with flow, color score 3; and right side: intrauterine pregnancy)

and at an early stage. Epithelial malignant and borderline tumours are the most frequent histological types, while germ cell tumours are less common. Expert gynaecological ultrasound is the preferred imaging technique to evaluate ovarian masses during pregnancy. Sonographic features suggesting malignancy are the same as they are in non-pregnant patients [4]. MRI can be used to help determine the nature of the ovarian mass and to exclude metastases.

74.8.3 Treatment Options

74.8.3.1 Surgery

Clinical early-stage ovarian cancer can be staged with laparoscopic or open surgery. The extent of staging depends on gestational age, local protocol and the histological type of ovarian cancer. A frozen section can be performed to guide surgical management, and a definitive histology conveyed [10, 11]. Complete debulking surgery in pregnant patients is almost impossible and neo-adjuvant chemotherapy should be initiated if the pregnancy is continued. Advanced stage epithelial ovarian cancer is rarely reported in the literature. Termination of pregnancy should be discussed in pregnancies with lower gestational age. Obviously, in these cases individualization and extensive counselling of the patient and her partner are indispensable.

For non-epithelial ovarian cancer, surgical treatment with pregnancy preservation is often feasible, as almost 90% of reported cases are diagnosed in early-stage disease [23]. Peritoneal staging is generally sufficient and lymph node dissection is not recommended.

When a bilateral adnexectomy is aimed for, this should be ideally performed after 14–16 weeks of gestation, as from then onwards the placenta is capable of sufficient supply to maintain pregnancy [10, 11].

74.8.3.2 Chemotherapy for Epithelial Ovarian Cancer

Chemotherapy can be indicated after surgical staging for epithelial ovarian cancer. In advanced stages, neo-adjuvant chemotherapy can be the only option to preserve pregnancy. Paclitaxel and carboplatin are the standard agents for epithelial ovarian cancer and are also recommended during pregnancy [10, 11].

The use of targeted therapy such as poly(ADP-ribose) polymerase (PARP) inhibitors or bevacizumab is discouraged because of the limited experience with these agents during pregnancy. Using these drugs may be associated with fetal anomalies as specific molecular changes in cancer development are targeted, which may also be mechanisms in fetal development. Bevacizumab inhibits angiogenesis and directly interferes with fetal development. More preclinical studies are needed to support their safety. Also, intraperitoneal chemotherapy is contraindicated during pregnancy.

74.8.3.3 Chemotherapy for Non-epithelial Ovarian Cancer

Non-epithelial ovarian cancers (germ cell tumours, sex cord stromal tumours) are primarily treated by surgical resection (Figure 74.4). Following the general recommendations, advanced stages require adjuvant chemotherapy. Standard treatment, as in the non-pregnant population, is an etoposide-platinum combination

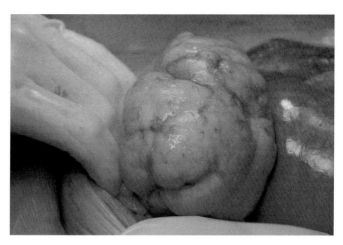

Figure 74.4 Ovarian dysgerminoma, surgery performed at 14 weeks of pregnancy. A black and white version of this figure will appear in some formats. For the colour version, please refer to the plate section.

(BEP or EP). Etoposide and platinum derivatives are possible when initiated after the first trimester of pregnancy. There are some reports of adverse neonatal events when bleomycin was used in the second or third trimester of pregnancy, such as ventriculomegaly with cerebral atrophy, plagiocephaly, syndactyly and pectus excavatum [31]. However, because of the aggressivity of some non-epithelial ovarian cancers, the use of the (B)EP regimen is encouraged with or without bleomycin in pregnant patients, as overall survival is superior to other regimens [11]. Cisplatin in this regimen is used in lower dosages (20 mg/m^2) compared to the case reports where neonatal ototoxicity was described [21]. However, the long-term effects of the use of BEP during pregnancy are still unknown. Carboplatinum-paclitaxel might be an alternative. For pregnant patients with relapsed germ cell tumours, the combination of cisplatin (75 mg/m^2) and weekly paclitaxel (80 mg/m^2) is recommended after the first trimester [32].

74.8.4 Obstetric Management

Prematurity, fetal growth restriction and fetal loss (including stillbirth) are the most frequent reported events [28, 33]. Adequate timing of surgery and chemotherapy regimens, serial fetal scans with umbilical and middle cerebral Doppler flow and a cautious planning of (preferably) term delivery are important strategies to achieve good obstetric outcome.

74.8.5 Maternal Outcome

A Norwegian registry-based study reported on oncological outcome of pregnancy-associated cancer [25]. Cause-specific death was increased in lactating women with ovarian cancer (2.23; 95% CI 1.05–4.73; P=0.036), but not in pregnant patients. Undifferentiated histology and advanced stage were associated with poor 2-year survival in 105 pregnant patients with epithelial ovarian cancer with survival rates of 30% (stage III) and 25% (stage IV), respectively. To date there is no evidence that pregnancy may affect the survival outcomes of patients with epithelial ovarian cancer.

74.9 Endometrial Cancer

Endometrial cancer diagnosed in association with pregnancy is extremely rare, as it is mainly a disease in perimenopausal or postmenopausal women.

The diagnosis is usually made following curettage for persistent bleeding after miscarriage or postpartum. One case series describes 35 patients with pregnancy-associated endometrial cancer [34]. Most patients (n=31) presented with FIGO stage I. Twenty patients were diagnosed after curettage for a spontaneous abortion at delivery or postpartum.

74.10 Vulvar and Vaginal Cancer

74.10.1 Background

The gestational incidence of other malignancies of the female genital organs, including vulvar and vaginal cancers, is estimated at 0.1 to 0.5 in 100 000 pregnancies [35, 36]. Lower genital tract malignancy during pregnancy is very rare due to the fact that it is rarely diagnosed before the age of 40–45 years. A systematic review reported on 36 patients with vulvar cancer during pregnancy diagnosed between 1955 and 2014 [37]. Vaginal cancer is even rarer, with, to our knowledge, only 12 case reports in the literature [38].

74.10.2 Diagnosis

The diagnosis of lower genital tract malignancies during pregnancy is often delayed, because symptoms can mimic physiological gestational changes (i.e. vaginal discharge) and the reluctance of performing invasive procedure during pregnancy (i.e. biopsy). Therefore, any suspicious lesion presented in all trimesters of pregnancy should be biopsied to obtain histological diagnosis. Most lesions are likely human papillomavirus (HPV) related and further screening for systemic immunosuppressive risk factors such as HIV or smoking and cervical intra-epithelial neoplasia (CIN) is recommended. MRI can be helpful in large tumours to determine local growth and relation with surrounding structures.

Vulvar cancer is mostly diagnosed in the second trimester of pregnancy by a symptomatic vulvar lesion or swelling [37]. Vulvar cancers in pregnancy mostly have squamous histology (47.2%) and are stage I disease (60.0%) [37].

In available case reports of vaginal cancer, all patients presented with stage I or II disease (50% and 50%, respectively). Most patients were diagnosed at the third trimester of pregnancy (42%) [38].

74.10.3 Treatment Options

During pregnancy, the standard surgical care should be provided, depending on tumour size, tumour stage and gestational age at diagnosis [38]. As lower genital tract malignancies are rarely diagnosed during pregnancy, management should always be individually discussed within a multidisciplinary team.

For vulvar cancer, radical local excision or radical vulvectomy with unilateral or bilateral lymph node dissection or sentinel node procedure is performed in patients with clinical negative lymph nodes. Because of the increased vascularity of tissues in the third trimester, haemostasis might be challenging, and the surgery is recommended before 36 weeks of gestation. Radical surgical margins are essential to avoid postoperative radiation therapy or a second procedure. Patients with lymph node metastasis require additional treatment. When nodal involvement is evident after inguinofemoral lymphadenectomy, pregnancy should be terminated or delivery planned, depending on the gestational age followed by postpartum irradiation. Delay of radiotherapy by 6 to 8 weeks is within the safety limits [10, 11].

When inguinal lymph node involvement is suggested by preoperative examinations, the prognosis is less favourable and lymph node dissection and adjuvant inguinal radiotherapy to prevent groin recurrence become vital. Termination of the pregnancy in the first and second trimesters is indicated, as immediate treatment is primordial [10, 11]. Neo-adjuvant chemotherapy remains experimental.

For early-stage superficial vaginal cancer, surgical resection with clear margins is primordial. For tumours invading the upper part of the vagina surgical treatment might be very extensive, including hysterectomy, colpectomy and pelvic lymphadenectomy and should be performed after pregnancy termination.

74.10.4 Obstetric Management

In the third trimester, a caesarean delivery is performed to prevent vulvar wound dehiscence. In case of smaller wounds without reconstructive surgery that have already healed well, vaginal delivery is an option. Standard treatment follows delivery.

74.10.5 Maternal Outcome

If standard therapy can be offered, the maternal prognosis is likely to be similar to that of non-pregnant patients, although the literature is very scarce [38]. In the review of Matsuo et al [37], delay in diagnosis was associated with a prognosis of vulvar cancer. A delay in diagnosis of more than 8 weeks versus ≤8 weeks had a disease-free survival of 5 years of respectively 0% and 69%, leading to a hazard ratio (HR) of 7.86 (95% CI 2.03–30.6, p=0.001).

References

1. Smith LH, Danielsen B, Allen ME, Cress R. Cancer associated with obstetric delivery: results of linkage with the California cancer registry. *Am J Obstet Gynecol.* 2003 Oct;**189**(4):1128–35.

2. de Haan J, Verheecke M, Van Calsteren K, et al. Oncological management and obstetric and neonatal outcomes for women diagnosed with cancer during pregnancy: a 20-year international cohort study of 1170

patients. *Lancet Oncol.* 2018;**19** (3):337–46.

3. Han SN, Lotgerink A, Gziri MM, et al. Physiologic variations of serum tumor markers in gynecological malignancies during pregnancy: a systematic review. *BMC Med.* 2012 Aug 8;**10**:86.

4. Timmerman D, Van Calster B, Testa A, et al. Predicting the risk of malignancy in adnexal masses based on the Simple Rules from the International Ovarian Tumor Analysis group. *Am J Obstet Gynecol.* 2016 Apr;**214**(4):424–37.

5. Dauer LT, Thornton RH, Miller DL, et al. Radiation management for interventions using fluoroscopic or computed tomographic guidance during pregnancy: a joint guideline of the Society of Interventional Radiology and the Cardiovascular and Interventional Radiological Society of Europe with Endorsement by the Canadian Interventional Radiology Association. *J Vasc Interv Radiol.* 2012 Jan;**23**(1):19–32.

6. Han SN, Amant F, Michielsen K et al. Feasibility of whole-body diffusion-weighted MRI for detection of primary tumour, nodal and distant metastases in women with cancer during pregnancy: a pilot study. *Eur Radiol.* 2018 May;**28**(5):1862–74.

7. Ray JG, Vermeulen MJ, Bharatha A, Montanera WJ, Park AL. Association between MRI exposure during pregnancy and fetal and childhood outcomes. *JAMA.* 2016 Sep 6;**316** (9):952–61.

8. Committee on Obstetric Practice. *Guidelines for Diagnostic Imaging during Pregnancy and Lactation*, ACOG Committee Opinion No 723. October 2017.

9. Han SN, Amant F, Cardonick EH, et al. Axillary staging for breast cancer during pregnancy: feasibility and safety of sentinel lymph node biopsy. *Breast Cancer Res Treat.* 2018;**168**(2):551–7.

10. Amant F, Halaska MJ, Fumagalli M, et al. Gynecologic cancers in pregnancy: guidelines of a second international consensus meeting. *Int J Gynecol Cancer.* 2014 Mar;**24** (3):394–403.

11. Amant F, Berveiller P, Boere I, et al. Gynecologic cancers in pregnancy: guidelines based on a third international consensus meeting. *Ann Oncol.* 2019;**30**(10):1601–12.

12. *Thrombosis and Embolism during Pregnancy and the Puerperium,* *Reducing the Risk*, Green-top Guideline No 37a. London: Royal College of Obstetricians and Gynaecologists, 13 April 2015.

13. Berveiller P, Marty O, Vialard F, Mir O. Use of anticancer agents in gynecological oncology during pregnancy: a systematic review of maternal pharmacokinetics and transplacental transfer. *Expert Opin Drug Metab Toxicol.* 2016 May;**12** (5):523–31.

14. Calsteren KV, Verbesselt R, Devlieger R, et al. Transplacental transfer of paclitaxel, docetaxel, carboplatin, and trastuzumab in a baboon model. *Int J Gynecol Cancer.* 2010 Dec;**20**(9):1456–64.

15. van Hasselt JG, van Calsteren K, Heyns L, et al. Optimizing anticancer drug treatment in pregnant cancer patients: pharmacokinetic analysis of gestation-induced changes for doxorubicin, epirubicin, docetaxel and paclitaxel. *Ann Oncol.* 2014 Oct;**25** (10):2059–65.

16. Amant F, von Minckwitz G, Han SN, et al. Prognosis of women with primary breast cancer diagnosed during pregnancy: results from an international collaborative study. *J Clin Oncol.* 2013 Jul 10;**31**(20):2532–9.

17. Zagouri F, Sergentanis TN, Chrysikos D, Filipits M, Bartsch R. Taxanes for ovarian cancer during pregnancy: a systematic review. *Oncology.* 2012;**83**(4):234–8.

18. Zagouri F, Sergentanis TN, Chrysikos D, Bartsch R. Platinum derivatives during pregnancy in cervical cancer: a systematic review and meta-analysis. *Obstet Gynecol.* 2013 Feb;**121**(2 Pt 1):337–43.

19. Geijteman EC, Wensveen CW, Duvekot JJ, van Zuylen L. A child with severe hearing loss associated with maternal cisplatin treatment during pregnancy. *Obstet Gynecol.* 2014 Aug;**124**(2Pt 2 Suppl 1):454–6.

20. Amant F, Van Calsteren K, Halaska MJ, et al. Long-term cognitive and cardiac outcomes after prenatal exposure to chemotherapy in children aged 18 months or older: an observational study. *Lancet Oncol.* 2012 Mar;**13** (3):256–64.

21. Amant F, Vandenbroucke T, Verheecke M, et al. Pediatric outcome after maternal cancer diagnosed during pregnancy. *N Engl J Med.* 2015 Nov 5;**373**(19):1824–34.

22. Pentheroudakis G, Pavlidis N. Cancer and pregnancy: poena magna, not anymore. *Eur J Cancer.* 2006 Jan;**42** (2):126–40.

23. Morice P, Uzan C, Gouy S, Verschraegen C, Haie-Meder C. Gynaecological cancers in pregnancy. *Lancet.* 2012 Feb 11;**379** (9815):558–69.

24. Zanotti-Fregonara P, Chastan M, Edet-Sanson A, et al. New fetal dose estimates from 18F-FDG administered during pregnancy: standardization of dose calculations and estimations with voxel-based anthropomorphic phantoms. *J Nucl Med.* 2016 Nov;**57** (11):1760–3.

25. Stensheim H, Moller B, van Dijk T, Fossa SD. Cause-specific survival for women diagnosed with cancer during pregnancy or lactation: a registry-based cohort study. *J Clin Oncol.* 2009 Jan 1;**27**(1):45–51.

26. Halaska MJ, Uzan C, Han SN, et al. Characteristics of patients with cervical cancer during pregnancy: a multicenter matched cohort study. An initiative from the International Network on Cancer, Infertility and Pregnancy. *Int J Gynecol Cancer.* 2019 Mar 20;ijgc-2018-000103.

27. Xia T, Gao Y, Wu B, Yang Y. Clinical analysis of twenty cases of cervical cancer associated with pregnancy. *J Cancer Res Clin Oncol.* 2015 Sep;**141** (9):1633–7.

28. Fruscio R, de Haan J, Van Calsteren K, et al. Ovarian cancer in pregnancy. *Best Pract Res Clin Obstet Gynaecol.* 2017 May;**41**:108–17.

29. Gui T, Cao D, Shen K, et al. Management and outcome of ovarian malignancy complicating pregnancy: an analysis of 41 cases and review of the literature. *Clin Transl Oncol.* 2013 Jul;**15**(7):548–54.

30. Nazer A, Czuzoj-Shulman N, Oddy L, Abenhaim HA. Incidence of maternal and neonatal outcomes in pregnancies complicated by ovarian masses. *Arch Gynecol Obstet.* 2015 Nov;**292** (5):1069–74.

31. Cardonick E, Usmani A, Ghaffar S. Perinatal outcomes of a pregnancy complicated by cancer, including neonatal follow-up after in utero exposure to chemotherapy: results of an international registry. *Am J Clin Oncol.* 2010 Jun;**33**(3):221–8.

32. Peccatori FA, Azim HA Jr, Orecchia R, et al. Cancer, pregnancy and fertility:

ESMO Clinical Practice Guidelines for diagnosis, treatment and follow-up. *Ann Oncol.* 2013 Oct;**24**(Suppl 6): vi160–70.

33. Blake EA, Kodama M, Yunokawa M, et al. Feto-maternal outcomes of pregnancy complicated by epithelial ovarian cancer: a systematic review of literature. *Eur J Obstet Gynecol Reprod Biol.* 2015 Mar;**186**:97–105.

34. Hannuna KY, Putignani L, Silvestri E, et al. Incidental endometrial adenocarcinoma in early pregnancy: a case report and review of the literature. *Int J Gynecol Cancer.* 2009 Dec;**19**(9):1580–4.

35. Lee YY, Roberts CL, Dobbins T, et al. Incidence and outcomes of pregnancy-associated cancer in Australia, 1994–2008: a population-based linkage study. *BJOG.* 2012 Dec;**119** (13):1572–82.

36. Parazzini F, Franchi M, Tavani A, Negri E, Peccatori FA. Frequency of pregnancy related cancer: a population based linkage study in Lombardy, Italy. *Int J Gynecol Cancer.* 2017 Mar;**27** (3):613–19.

37. Matsuo K, Whitman SA, Blake EA, et al. Feto-maternal outcome of pregnancy complicated by vulvar cancer: a systematic review of literature. *Eur J Obstet Gynecol Reprod Biol.* 2014 Aug;**179**:216–23.

38. Soo-Hoo S, Luesley D. Vulval and vaginal cancer in pregnancy. *Best Pract Res Clin Obstet Gynaecol.* 2016 May;**33**:73–8.

Chapter 75

Non-Gynaecological Cancers and Pregnancy

Chiara Benedetto, Emilie Marion Canuto & Francesca Salvagno

75.1 Introduction

The management of cancer during pregnancy is a clinical dilemma since it involves two persons, the mother and the fetus. The complex medical, ethical, psychological and religious issues in pregnant women diagnosed with cancer are best addressed by a dedicated multidisciplinary team composed of obstetricians, oncologists, radiation oncologists, radiologists, surgeons, paediatricians, psychologists, pharmacologists, anaesthetists and clinical nurses.

Obstetricians and oncologists will need to provide optimal treatment of the mother and optimal protection of the fetus [1].

Available guidelines for healthcare practitioners attending cancer patients during pregnancy are based mainly on expert opinion, as most scientific articles are retrospective case series and reviews based on these.

Recent data show that pregnant women can and should be treated just as effectively as non-pregnant women. Nonetheless, a survey of European and non-European physicians potentially involved in the care of pregnant cancer patients showed that, contrary to the available evidence, most preferred terminating the pregnancy, postponing the treatment or anticipating delivery [2].

Indeed, curing the mother remains the main priority and treatment should be the same as that for non-pregnant patients, as we know that, with some adaptations, in most cases, cancer treatment is possible during pregnancy without jeopardizing fetal safety [3].

75.2 Epidemiology

The estimated incidence of cancer during pregnancy is 1 in 1000 pregnancies, but this number is growing with the increase in maternal age at first childbirth [4]. The most frequent among non-gynaecological cancers diagnosed during pregnancy are haematological cancers (lymphoma and leukaemia) and malignant melanoma, followed by thyroid, gastrointestinal and brain tumours (see Figure 74.1, p. 602).

75.3 Clinical Features and Investigations: General Considerations

Since cancer-related symptoms and signs may be confused with normal gestational symptoms (nausea, fatigue, anaemia, pain, hyperpigmentation), it is important that clinicians pay attention to persisting/worsening complaints because ignoring a sign can delay the diagnosis of malignancy [5] (Table 75.1).

Table 75.1 Common symptoms of malignancy overlapping with symptoms of pregnancy

Nausea and vomiting

Appetite changes

Constipation / haemorrhoids/ rectal bleeding

Abdominal discomfort / pain

Anaemia

Hyperpigmentation / changes in nevi

Fatigue

Staging should be as comprehensive as outside pregnancy. A prestaging multidisciplinary discussion should be conducted to avoid unnecessary radiographic examinations.

Ultrasound and magnetic resonance imaging (MRI) (without gadolinium) are the preferred staging instruments during pregnancy. MRI should be deferred until after the first trimester due to the risk of heating effects causing biological damage to the fetus. The 2007 American College of Radiology (ACR) guidelines admit the use of MRI also in the first trimester if the benefits outweigh the potential risks to the fetus.

If radiographic examinations are necessary, total fetal radiation exposure should be kept as low as reasonably achievable (ALARA). Below the limit of 100 mGy, no deterministic effect (e.g. mortality, malformations, microcephaly or mental retardation of the fetus) are expected (Table 75.2), and less than 1% of stochastic effects are seen (e.g. cancer and hereditary mutations).

For medico-legal reasons, a fetal ultrasound to screen for fetal anomaly should be performed before cancer staging procedures during pregnancy [6]. Non-abdominal x-ray with proper abdominal shielding implies fetal radiation exposure of <0.1 mGy. Abdominal x-ray involves higher fetal exposure and is not indicated for cancer diagnosis and staging.

As for computed tomography (CT), except for pelvic CT, all ionizing diagnostic techniques remain far below the threshold of 100 mGy. A CT is particularly useful in case of doubt after MRI or when MRI is contraindicated (e.g. pacemaker). Data on iodinated contrast agents are insufficient to consider them safe.

Positron emission tomography (PET) can be proposed during the second and third trimesters; accumulation of the

Table 75.2 Fetal radiation exposure for different diagnostic tests in different body regions

Body region	mGy
X-ray chest	0.0001–0.43
X-ray abdomen	1.4–4.2
X-ray pelvis	0.16–22
CT head	<0.005
CT chest	0–02–0.2
CT pulmonary embolism	0.2–0.7
CT abdomen	4–60
CT pelvis	6.7–114
PET	1.1–2.43

tracer should be prevented by using a bladder catheter and providing hydration [5].

Finally, the pathologist should always be informed that the patient is pregnant since gestational hyperproliferative changes may influence tissue characteristics and interpretation of the findings.

75.4 Clinical Management: General Considerations

Decisions in the treatment of cancer in pregnancy should be made by an interdisciplinary team, individualized to the patient, and made together with her after carefully weighing the risks and benefits of treatment.

75.5 Chemotherapy

The potential fetal risks associated with chemotherapy during pregnancy depend on the gestational period at exposure.

During the first 10 days post-conception (fertilization/implantation), cells are omnipotent and can develop in the three different embryological layers. Toxic exposure at this stage will result in an 'all-or-nothing' phenomenon.

During organogenesis (between 10 days and 8 weeks after conception) the risk of congenital malformations is highest. The risk of major malformations due to chemotherapy exposure during the first trimester varies from 10 to 20%, while it does not differ from that of the general population when chemotherapy is administered during the second or third trimester (3–5%) [6–7].

Cytotoxic treatment during the second and third trimesters is not expected to cause major malformations; however, cases of growth restriction, prematurity, intrauterine and

neonatal death and haematopoietic suppression have been reported. Short-term outcome studies report an increased risk of preterm delivery (frequently iatrogenic), intrauterine growth restriction, haematopoietic suppression and stillbirth. The International Network on Cancer, Infertility and Pregnancy (INCIP) published the results of an ongoing 20-year cohort study of cancer and obstetric management and outcomes in 1170 patients: multivariate analysis revealed an increased risk of small for gestational age (SGA) at birth after antenatal chemotherapy exposure, especially after exposure to platinum derivates or taxanes (odds ratio (OR) 3.12, 95% confidence interval (CI) 1.45–6.70 and OR 2.07, 95% CI 1.11–3.86, respectively). SGA is a known risk factor for neonatal morbidity, stillbirth and neonatal mortality [8, 9]. Recent data suggest that chemotherapy exposure during pregnancy increases oxidative DNA damage and that this could alter placental cellular growth and increase the incidence of fetal growth restriction [10].

The long-term outcomes (neurodevelopmental delay, sterility, carcinogenesis) remain to be determined, as large data on long-term follow-up are lacking [8].

The decision to administer chemotherapy should follow the same guidelines as those for non-pregnant patients, taking into account gestational age, tumour stage and characteristics (e.g. indolent or aggressive) and the overall treatment plan (timing of surgery, need for radiotherapy, etc.).

Generally speaking, chemotherapy is considered safe starting from 14 up to 35 weeks of gestation to allow the recovery of bone marrow and to minimize fetal and maternal risk of sepsis and haemorrhage during delivery. Deferring delivery for 2 to 3 weeks after chemotherapy can allow the excretion of fetal drug through the placenta, especially in preterm babies in which the ability to metabolize or excrete drugs is limited due to immaturity of the liver and kidneys [7].

The side effects of chemotherapy (nausea, vomiting, myelosuppression) can be detrimental for both mother and fetus and therefore should be minimized. Dehydration needs to be prevented. Antiemetics considered safe during pregnancy are metoclopramide and 5HT3 antagonists (e.g. ondansetron). As for glucocorticosteroids, methylprednisolone and hydrocortisone are usually chosen because they do not cross the placenta. Limited existing data suggest that granulocyte-colony stimulating factor (G-CSF) does not cause significant sequelae, and so can be used if clinically necessary, even if it can cross the human placenta during the second and third trimesters [11].

Targeted drugs are aimed at specific molecular changes in tumour development, which may also be physiological in fetal development, thus leading to fetal abnormalities. The majority of targeted drugs are contraindicated during pregnancy (i.e. trastuzumab, imatinib), while others, despite the scarce safety data, may be used with caution during pregnancy (i.e. rituximab) [11].

75.6 Surgery

Surgery can be safely performed during pregnancy. The surgical technique is similar to that used in non-pregnant cancer patients, except for colorectal cancer surgery, as carrying out surgery after 20 weeks of gestation will be very difficult due to the enlarged uterus.

Surgical and anaesthetic management require some modifications due to the anatomic and physiological changes during pregnancy. Objectives include optimal surgical outcome as well as maternal and fetal safety [3].

75.7 Radiotherapy

Fetal exposure to ionizing radiation is associated with an increased risk of biological effects on the fetus. The risk of deterministic effects is certain when the fetal dose is above 100 mGy, uncertain between 50 and 100 mGy and weak when below 50 mGy; there is no dose limit for stochastic effects. The decision to carry out radiotherapy during pregnancy should be discussed with an expert radiotherapist, who will estimate the dose delivered to the fetus [3].

75.8 Obstetric and Perinatal Management

Pregnancy in patients diagnosed with cancer is considered high risk and should be managed at a referral centre. Fetal well-being must be regularly monitored during pregnancy. The timing of delivery will depend on tumour type, planned cancer treatment, maternal conditions, fetal growth and, ultimately, the woman's choice. Term delivery (>37 weeks) should be the target, except for late cancer diagnosis during the third trimester when delivery at 35 weeks and prompt start of chemotherapy during the immediate postpartum period can be planned. Late prematurity is associated with neonatal and long-term morbidity, while prematurity and low birthweight seem to be factors contributing to delays in cognitive and emotional development.

The mode of delivery should be determined based on obstetric indications. Generally, vaginal delivery is preferable to caesarean section because of the lower risk of infection and quicker recovery. Exceptions include cancer metastasis to the long bones or pelvis (risk of fracture during labour and delivery) and central nervous system metastases (risk of increased intracranial pressure) [6]. The placenta should always be examined for metastatic disease, as metastasis in the placenta can be found in 30% of cases of melanoma and 15% of cases of haematological malignancies [1].

Chemotherapy can be restarted immediately after vaginal delivery and 1 week after uncomplicated caesarean section. Breastfeeding is not recommended if chemotherapy is continued into the postpartum period or was administered in the last weeks before delivery.

75.9 Maternal Prognosis

Theoretically, the physiological changes in pregnancy (e.g. relative immunosuppression, hypervascularization and increased hormonal exposure in particular) may negatively influence maternal prognosis. Another possible negative prognostic factor

is a late diagnosis, resulting in a higher stage of cancer at diagnosis. However, two recent studies (each involving 500 pregnant women with cancer) reported a prognosis similar to that in non-pregnant women [12].

75.10 Haematological Cancer

After breast cancer, haematological cancer is the second most frequent cancer diagnosed during pregnancy, with Hodgkin lymphoma (HL) and non-Hodgkin lymphoma (NHL) accounting for roughly 14% and leukaemia for up to 7% of cancers diagnosed during pregnancy [13].

75.10.1 Hodgkin Lymphoma

Epidemiology: Hodgkin lymphoma (HL) is the most common haematological malignancy diagnosed during pregnancy (approximately 1 per 1000 pregnancies); about 3% of HL is diagnosed during pregnancy [14]. This may be due to its occurrence during a woman's reproductive age, as no data support an association between HL and pregnancy.

Pathology: The typical finding at microscopic examination of tissue biopsy is the Reed–Sternberg cell, which is classically large (15–45 μ), with abundant basophilic cytoplasm, a binucleate or bilobed nucleus and a thick, irregular nuclear membrane.

Clinical Features: Typical symptoms include painless swelling of lymph nodes, persistent fatigue, fever, night sweats, unexplained weight loss and severe itching.

Investigations: Diagnostic procedures include physical examination, blood tests, imaging studies (x-ray, CT), lymph node biopsy and bone marrow biopsy.

Clinical Management (Figure 75.1): The gold standard therapy for HL is a combination of Adriamycin, bleomycin, vinblastine and dacarbazine (ABVD), which is considered safe after the first trimester, as no significant fetal complications have been described. To date, no safety data exist for other chemotherapeutic combinations such as BEACOPP (bleomycin, etoposide, Adriamycin, cyclophosphamide, oncovin, procarbazine, prednisone), and their use is not recommended during pregnancy [15].

Few patients present with early stage IA/IB or IIA non-mediastinal disease; for these patients, watchful waiting can be considered and treatment may be postponed until after delivery, especially if diagnosis is made during the third trimester. If diagnosis is made during the first trimester, chemotherapy may be started during the second trimester. For patients diagnosed with advanced HL during the first trimester, pregnancy termination should be considered. Two possible reasons for keeping patients for their treatment in the second trimester are the administration of single-agent vinblastine or steroid administration [14–16]. Prognosis does not seem to be inferior to that in non-pregnant patients: the estimated 5-year survival rate is about 90% for stages I–II HL, 80% for stage III and about 65% for stage IV [1].

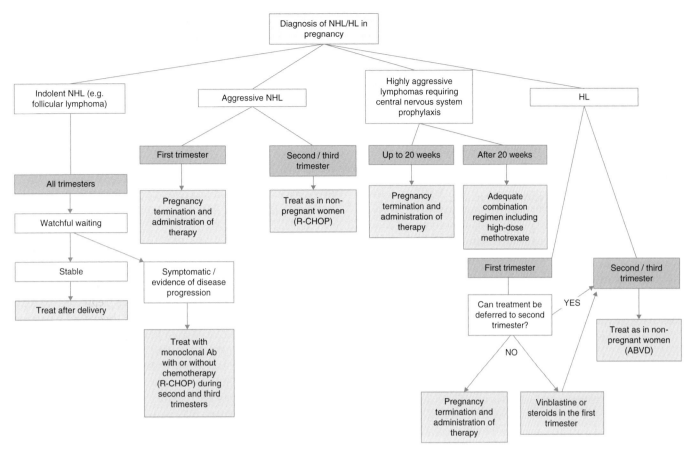

Figure 75.1 Therapeutic approaches in women diagnosed with Non-Hodgkin Lymphoma (NHL) or Hodgkin Lymphoma (HL) during pregnancy. Adapted from Lishner M et al 2016 [13].
Ab: antibodies; R-CHOP: rituximab, Cytoxan, hydroxyrubicin, oncovin, prednisone; ABVD: Adriamycin, bleomycin, vinblastine, dacarbazine

75.10.2 Non-Hodgkin Lymphoma

Epidemiology: Non-Hodgkin lymphoma (NHL) occurs in 1–5 per 100 000 pregnancies [17].

Pathology: The most common subtype is diffuse, large B-cell lymphoma, followed by follicular lymphoma and T-cell lymphoma. Furthermore, lymphomas can be divided into indolent lymphomas, which grow and spread slowly (e.g. follicular lymphoma), and aggressive lymphomas, which grow and spread quickly (e.g. diffuse large B-cell lymphoma).

Clinical Features: NHL can cause many different signs and symptoms depending on the type of lymphoma and where it is located in the body. Sometimes it may not cause any symptoms until it has grown quite large. Common signs and symptoms include enlarged lymph nodes, weight loss, anorexia, fatigue, swollen abdomen, chest pain or pressure, shortness of breath or cough, severe or frequent infections and easy bleeding.

Investigations: The key to the diagnosis of NHL is lymph node biopsy, with immunophenotypic, cytogenetic and molecular analysis. Essential workup includes a complete physical examination, blood tests, CT scan, echocardiogram and bone marrow biopsy. Optional procedures, depending on the type of lymphoma, include endoscopic ultrasound, head CT and lumbar puncture.

Clinical Management (Figure 75.1): Evaluation and management of NHL during pregnancy are particularly complex because the disease is pathologically and clinically heterogeneous. Staging may be delayed due to overlapping symptoms of pregnancy and lymphoma, especially in very aggressive lymphomas. Furthermore, extra-nodal involvement, especially in the reproductive organs (e.g. breast, ovary, cervix) is more frequent in pregnant women. This may be due to either hormone-dependent growth or hyperproliferative state. The decision to administer therapy during pregnancy depends on such factors as type of NHL (indolent or aggressive), gestational age and patient's wishes.

For patients diagnosed with indolent lymphoma, treatment may be postponed until after delivery or deferred to the second trimester. For patients with aggressive NHL, immediate treatment is mandatory; for patients diagnosed with NHL during the first trimester, pregnancy termination should be contemplated; for patients diagnosed during the second and third trimesters, an R-CHOP regimen (rituximab, Cytoxan, hydroxyrubicin, oncovin, prednisone) may be considered safe, as there are no data on increased fetal morbidity. Rituximab, a chimeric antibody targeting CD20, crosses the placenta, and this passage increases with gestational age; however, data from a retrospective analysis showed that its administration during the second and third trimesters seems to be relatively

615

safe, despite the increased risk of transient cell depletion without related infection, albeit not clinically significant [15]. In highly aggressive lymphomas, central nervous system (CNS) prophylaxis may be required to prevent spread of the lymphoma in the CNS; the most commonly used drug is high-dose methotrexate, for which fetal teratogenicity (aminopterin syndrome: cranial dysostosis, delayed ossification, hypertelorism, wide nasal bridge, ear abnormalities) and myelosuppression have been reported, especially when administered before 20 weeks of pregnancy [13]. Therefore, antimetabolite therapy for NHL during pregnancy is challenging.

A population-based study reported that NHL was associated with a higher statistically significant risk of pre-eclampsia, preterm birth, postpartum blood transfusions, infectious morbidity, venous thromboembolism, intrauterine fetal death and coagulation abnormalities [16]. The overall 5-year relative survival rate for NHL is 71% but varies widely depending on NHL type, patient age, NHL stage, patient's performance status and blood tests. The survival rates of pregnant patients with NHL are similar to those of non-pregnant controls matched for tumour grade [17].

75.10.3 Chronic Myeloid Leukaemia

Chronic myeloid leukaemia (CML) is a myeloproliferative disorder characterized by increased proliferation of the granulocytic cell line without the loss of their capacity to differentiate.

Epidemiology: CML occurs in approximately 1 in 100 000 pregnancies.

Clinical Features; Typical signs and symptoms of CML can be interpreted as normal pregnancy signs and symptoms (e.g. leukocytosis, abdominal bloating, weight loss, night sweats, bone pain, enlarged spleen).

Investigations: The workup for CML entails complete blood cell count with differential, peripheral blood smear and bone marrow analysis. Diagnosis is suggested by blood test anomalies (leukocytosis with mildly increased basophils and eosinophils, anaemia, thrombocytopenia; the peripheral blood smear will demonstrate leukoerythroblastosis with circulating immature cells from the bone marrow) and is confirmed by the presence of t (9;22) cytogenetic abnormality and/or the fusion oncogene *BCR-ABL1*. Complementary imaging studies include ultrasound, CT and MRI.

Clinical Management: A variety of medications have been used for treating CML, including myelosuppressive agents and interferon alpha. The 5-year survival rate has doubled from 31% in the early 1990s to 67% for patients diagnosed from 2005 to 2014 thanks to earlier diagnosis, improved therapy with targeted drugs, bone marrow transplantation and better supportive care. Prognosis has dramatically improved after the introduction of tyrosine kinase inhibitors (TKIs): 90% of patients are now expected to have long-lasting response with one of the five available TKIs, among which the most commonly used is imatinib. Currently, bone marrow transplantation is reserved for patients who do not achieve molecular remission or show resistance to imatinib and failure of second generation TKIs.

Unfortunately, TKIs are contraindicated during pregnancy, as they inhibit important kinases for embryonic implantations, gonadal development and fetal maturation. Data for imatinib administration during pregnancy show a higher incidence of skeletal malformations and renal and gastrointestinal abnormalities. Other therapeutic approaches, including leukapheresis and IFN-alpha, have been proposed when white blood cell count (WBC) is >100 x 10^9 and/or platelet count is >500 x 10^9. When the platelet count is >1000 x 10^9, the addition of aspirin or low molecular weight heparin (LMWH) should be considered to reduce the risk of thrombosis. In lymphoblast crisis during early pregnancy, the recommended management is similar to that for acute leukaemia. [13, 18].

75.10.4 Acute Leukaemia

Acute myeloid leukaemia (AML) is a malignant disease of the bone marrow in which haematopoietic precursors are arrested at an early stage of development. Most AML subtypes are distinguished from other related blood disorders by the presence of more than 20% of lymphoblasts in the bone marrow. Acute lymphoblastic leukaemia (ALL) is a malignant (clonal) disease of the bone marrow in which early lymphoid precursors proliferate and replace the normal haematopoietic cells of the marrow; more than 20% of lymphoblasts are typically found in the bone marrow.

Epidemiology: AML is reported in 1 per 75 000 to 1 per 100 000 pregnancies. AML accounts for two thirds and ALL for one third of cases. Prompt treatment is mandatory because deferral of treatment may compromise maternal outcome without improving fetal outcome: without treatment, maternal death can occur within weeks or months.

Clinical Features: Some patients present with acute symptoms that develop over a few days to 1–2 weeks; the presenting signs and symptoms result from bone marrow failure, organ infiltration with leukaemic cells or both. Symptoms of bone marrow failure are related to anaemia, neutropenia and thrombocytopenia: fatigue, dyspnoea on exertion, dizziness, history of upper respiratory infection symptoms that have not improved despite empiric treatment with oral antibiotics and ecchymoses. Symptoms of organ infiltration with leukaemic cells include pain in the left upper quadrant of the abdomen and early satiety or skin rash due to infiltration of the skin with leukaemic cells. Patients with a high leukaemic cell burden may present with bone pain caused by increased bone marrow pressure. Patients with markedly elevated WBC counts (>100 000 cells/µL) can present with symptoms of leukostasis (i.e. respiratory distress and altered mental status), a medical emergency that calls for immediate intervention. Poor prognostic factors are leukocytosis, thrombosis and disseminated intravascular coagulation (DIC), which are aggravated by the gestational thrombogenic milieu.

Investigations: Essential investigations include complete blood count and blood film examination, vitamin B12, folate and ferritin measurements, coagulation screen, renal and liver function tests and bone marrow biopsy. Immunophenotyping by flow cytometry of bone marrow or peripheral blood samples can be useful to distinguish AML from ALL and further classify the AML subtype. Findings from cytogenetic analysis of the bone marrow constitute one of the most important prognostic factors. Patients with t(8;21), t(15;17) or inversion 16 have the best prognosis, with 10-year overall survival rates of approximately 65%. Patients with normal cytogenetic findings have an intermediate prognosis and a long-term survival rate of approximately 35%. Patients with poor-risk cytogenetic findings (especially –7, –5 or monosomal karyotype) have a poor prognosis, with a long-term survival rate of less than 10%. In patients with signs or symptoms suggesting CNS involvement, CT or MRI should be performed. Lumbar puncture is indicated in these patients if no CNS mass or lesion is detected on CT or MRI.

Clinical Management (Figure 75.2): In AML diagnosed during the first trimester, the mother should be informed of the higher risk of spontaneous miscarriage in women with AML and of the risk of fetal malformation due to chemotherapy in the first trimester; this is why elective pregnancy termination followed by conventional induction therapy (anthracycline plus cytarabine) is recommended.

Patients diagnosed later (second and third trimesters) must be carefully counselled, as they can receive conventional induction therapy (anthracycline plus cytarabine), although this seems to be associated with increased risk of fetal growth restriction and even fetal loss. In detail, cytarabine is an antimetabolite, which can cause intrauterine growth restriction (IUGR) in approximately 13% of fetuses, intrauterine fetal death in 6% and cytopenia in 5%. The effect of anthracycline on the fetal heart seems to be low and is usually reversible, though data on long-term cardiotoxicity are scarce. Serial prenatal sonographic assessment of fetal cardiac function may have a role in monitoring anthracycline cardiotoxicity or cardiac failure. A neonatologist should discuss with the patient the mortality and morbidity rates specific to the stage of pregnancy. Between 24 and 28 weeks, delivery will not usually be advised, as fetal risks related to prematurity are high. Treatment should not be deferred in an effort to balance the risks of fetal exposure to chemotherapy against the risks of prematurity. For patients diagnosed during the third trimester, delivery before initiating chemotherapy may be considered reasonable after a course of corticosteroids. If delivery is planned before 32 weeks, magnesium sulphate

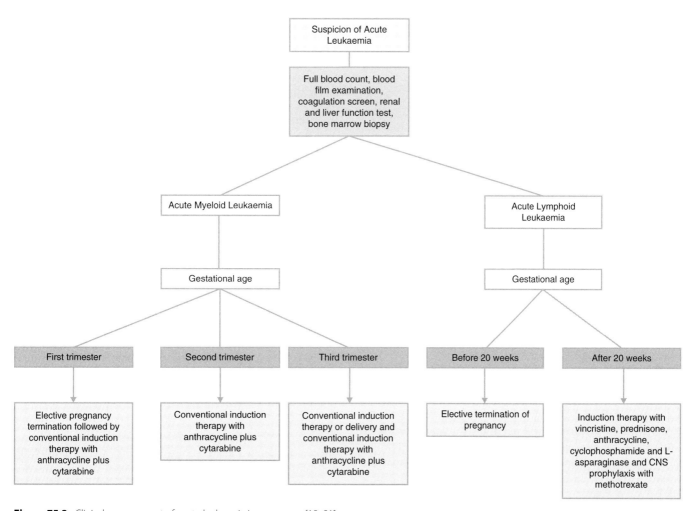

Figure 75.2 Clinical management of acute leukaemia in pregnancy [18–21]
CNS: Central nervous system

617

within 24 hours before delivery should be considered for fetal neuroprotection. Vaginal planned delivery is generally preferred, and involvement of the anaesthesia team is recommended. Similarly, in the presence of severe neutropenia (<1 x 10^9/L) or thrombocytopenia (<80 x 10^9/L), epidural analgesia is not recommended, and alternatives need to be considered. Women with AML receiving chemotherapy are at an increased risk of sepsis. Because its signs and symptoms may be less typical than in the non-pregnant population, if there is evidence of sepsis the patient should be managed by a senior team of haematologists, obstetricians and anaesthetists. Women with AML are also at increased risk of postpartum haemorrhage; therefore, in addition to active management of the third stage of delivery, consideration should be given to prophylactic oxytocin infusion over the first 4 hours following delivery [19]. Regarding the fetus, leukaemia transfer to the fetus seems remarkably low. Leukapheresis is well tolerated in pregnancy and is useful in the presence of severe leukocytosis- and leukostasis-related signs and symptoms.

Acute promyelocytic leukaemia (APL) accounts for approximately 5% of AML; it is more likely to occur than other AML subtypes to present during pregnancy. APL is often accompanied by DIC. Standard treatment includes anthracycline combined with all-trans retinoic acid (ATRA), which induces differentiation of leukaemic cells but is highly teratogenic during the first trimester. Termination of pregnancy is recommended before initiating therapy, whereas it can be administered during the second and third trimesters. Arsenic trioxide is emerging as standard care in combination with ATRA and anthracycline. However, the European LeukemiaNet for APL recommends not using it during pregnancy as it seems to be associated with an increased risk of malformation, growth retardation and fetal death [20].

Acute lymphoblastic leukaemia raises additional therapeutic issues. Unlike patients with acute AML, some have meningeal disease at the time of initial diagnosis. As a result, CNS prophylaxis with intrathecal chemotherapy is essential. Standard induction therapy typically includes a five-drug regimen (vincristine, prednisone, an anthracycline, cyclophosphamide, and L-asparaginase) given over the course of 4–6 weeks. Maintenance therapy consists of prednisone, vincristine, and methotrexate (MTX). MTX, cyclophosphamide and L-asparaginase are fetotoxic. The use of MTX is prohibited before week 20 of gestation, while L-asparaginase may increase the already high risk for thromboembolic events. TKIs, which are essential for treating Philadelphia chromosome-positive ALL, are teratogenic. For these reasons, patients diagnosed with ALL before week 20 of gestation should undergo termination of pregnancy and begin conventional treatment. After week 20, conventional chemotherapy can be administered during pregnancy and TKIs during the postpartum period. However, in the general population, poor outcome has been reported in a retrospective analysis: complete remission was obtained in 65–85% of patients, with a 5-year survival of 38% [21].

75.11 Malignant Melanoma

Epidemiology: The estimated incidence of malignant melanoma during pregnancy is between 0.14 and 2.8 cases per 1000 births and accounts for 4 to 8% of malignancies diagnosed during pregnancy. According to the registry of the German Dermatological Society, 1% of female melanoma patients were pregnant [22]. The incidence of stage I and II melanoma in young adults is 95%, with a 5-year survival of 93%. In pregnant women, late diagnosis is probably due to the tendency to view changes in nevi size and pigmentation as physiological during pregnancy; this means that about 50% of patients are found to be stage III or IV, where 5-year survival falls to 63 and 20%, respectively [6].

Clinical Features: The morphological changes in nevi during pregnancy must be considered a pathological sign, just as in the non-pregnant population. The signs and symptoms of melanoma are similar to those seen in the non-pregnant population. The anatomical location of the primary tumour does not differ between pregnant and non-pregnant women. The ABCDs for differentiating early melanomas from benign nevi are:

- A – Asymmetry (melanoma lesion more likely to be asymmetrical)
- B – Border irregularity (melanoma more likely to have irregular borders)
- C – Colour (melanoma more likely to be very dark black or blue and to vary more in colour than a benign mole would, which more often is uniform in colour and light tan or brown)
- D – Diameter (<6 mm is usually benign)

Investigations: Excisional biopsy is the recommended procedure for any suspicious lesion. Clinical staging includes assessment of the local tumour site and adjacent skin, regional lymph node areas and distant organs that are frequently the site of metastatic disease. Intensive radiological investigation is not required for patients with early disease, while imaging studies (chest CT, brain MRI) are required for patients with suspicion of metastasis.

Clinical Management: Surgical removal of the melanoma with adequate margins (1 or 2 cm depending on Breslow thickness) remains the standard primary therapy for early melanoma. Elective lymph node dissection is not recommended. Sentinel node biopsy using technetium-99 is recommended especially for patients with stage IB or higher. For most patients, this procedure can be done under local anaesthesia. It has been calculated that the fetal radiation exposure is <5 mGy when using technetium-99. Therefore, when maternal outcome is expected to benefit from sentinel node biopsy, it should not be avoided for fear of fetal radiation exposure [5].

Adjuvant therapy is used for metastatic or unresectable melanoma. Multiple options for adjuvant treatment of node-positive melanoma have become available. A critical question for guiding the choice of regimen is whether the tumour contains a *BRAF* V600 mutation. In patients with no *BRAF* mutation, current National Comprehensive Cancer Network (NCCN) guidelines recommend single-agent immunotherapy with pembrolizumab or nivolumab. For patients with a *BRAF* mutation, the NCCN recommends targeted combination therapy with vemurafenib. Unfortunately, these therapies are not recommended during pregnancy [23]. Promising results have been obtained with these therapies; nonetheless, the decision whether or not to induce preterm birth should be discussed by a team of melanoma experts, obstetricians, neonatologists and oncologists to weigh the impact of therapy on maternal prognosis and the risks of premature birth.

75.12 Thyroid Cancer

EPIDEMIOLOGY: Thyroid cancer accounts for 3 to 6% of cancers diagnosed in pregnancy, with approximately 14 cases per 100 000 [7].

Pathogenesis and Pathology: No endocrine association has been found between maternal hormonal changes and thyroid cancer. Tumour types are similar to those in non-pregnant patients. Most pregnant patients present with well-differentiated, localized disease (follicular or papillary carcinoma) and very good prognosis: the 10-year survival rate for differentiated thyroid cancer in pregnant women is more than 99%. Poorly or undifferentiated carcinoma (anaplastic) thyroid cancer carries a poor prognosis, with a median survival of less than 5 months even with treatment [24]. The impact of pregnancy on thyroid cancer is still controversial: several studies reported pregnancy as a negative prognostic factor, whereas large population studies did not confirm this relationship. Prognosis depends on histological type and stage of disease and patient age [25].

CLINICAL FEATURES: Signs and symptoms of thyroid carcinoma are painless, palpable, solitary thyroid nodule, abnormal thyroid function tests and cervical lymphadenopathy.

INVESTIGATIONS: The International Society of Endocrinology guidelines recommend a diagnostic and therapeutic approach via team care (endocrinologist, surgeon, obstetrician-gynaecologist, anaesthesiologist, psychologist), taking into account tumour stage and aggressiveness, the patient's clinical conditions and expectations [24]. Diagnostic procedures include high-resolution ultrasound in combination with fine needle aspiration cytology (FNAC), which has high sensitivity and specificity (97–98%). Ultrasound criteria for FNAC include a hypo-echogenic irregular nodule margins, absent peripheral halo of nodule, increased intranodular vascularization, presence of laterocervical adenopathies, presence of microcalcifications, nodules taller than wider and presence of microcalcifications. Cytology can fall into six categories based on the Bethesda System: nondiagnostic, benign, atypia of undetermined significance (AUS) or follicular lesion of undetermined significance (FLUS), follicular neoplasm (FN) or suspicious for follicular neoplasm (SFN), suspicious for malignancy, and malignant [24] (Figure 75.3).

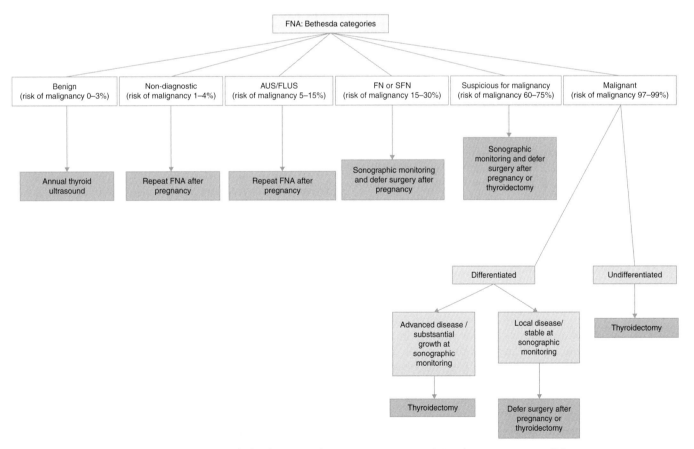

Figure 75.3 Thyroid cancer: Bethesda categories, risk of malignancy and management recommendations for pregnant women [24]
FNA: fine needle aspiration; AUS: atypia of undetermined significance; FLUS: follicular lesion of undetermined significance; FN: follicular neoplasm; SFN: suspicious for follicular neoplasm

Computed tomograpy or MRI may be considered in selected patients to better characterize tumour invasion and bulky, inferiorly located or posteriorly located lymph nodes. A PET CT is not generally indicated but it may be reserved for patients with high risk of distant metastases, where management and maternal outcome depend on it.

CLINICAL MANAGEMENT: Surgery remains the treatment of choice for well-differentiated thyroid cancer [26]. Standard treatment for non-pregnant patients is total thyroidectomy or lobectomy in selected cases, sometimes followed by radioactive iodine administration to ablate the normal remnant thyroid or as an adjuvant therapy to eliminate suspected micro-metastases.

Due to its relatively indolent course but potential impact on long-term survival, therapy during pregnancy can be tailored to gestational age. The Endocrine Society recommends surgery after delivery in patients with pregnancy-related differentiated thyroid cancer and no evidence of advanced disease or rapid progression, as deferring surgery does not affect outcome and surgery performed during pregnancy is associated with greater risk of complications (hypoparathyroidism and hypothyroidism to the fetus), longer hospital stays and higher costs. Thyroidectomy is suggested during pregnancy in differentiated tumours with evidence of advanced disease or with substantial growth at sonographic monitoring or for undifferentiated tumours. Surgery may be deferred until after delivery in patients diagnosed during the third trimester.

Radioiodine therapy is contraindicated during pregnancy, as it can cross the placenta and cause fetal hypothyroidism, cognitive disorders and mental retardation. In patients requiring radioiodine therapy after delivery, breastfeeding should be stopped at least 6 weeks before ablative therapy. The endocrinological management of thyroid cancer during pregnancy is of utmost importance. A patient with thyroid cancer during pregnancy needs levothyroxine (LT4) treatment for various different indications: as suppressive treatment for those who decide to postpone surgery until the second trimester or after delivery in order to keep thyroid-stimulating hormone (TSH) levels below 0.1–1 mU/L; as replacement therapy after thyroidectomy because maternal hypothyroidism has serious consequences for fetal development; and as suppressive therapy for patients with residual disease [27].

75.13 Colorectal Cancer

Epidemiology: Colorectal cancer (CRC) in pregnancy is rare, with an incidence of 0.8 in 100 000 pregnancies.

Clinical Features: The presenting symptoms of CRC are frequently attributed to pregnancy (abdominal pain, rectal bleeding, constipation, nausea and vomiting), which is why presentation of advanced disease during pregnancy occurs in approximately 59% of cases.

Investigations: Abdominal CT is the standard staging method for non-pregnant patients but is contraindicated during pregnancy. Because abdominal ultrasound has a moderate sensitivity (50–76%), MRI is preferred since it does not expose the fetus to ionizing radiation and has an accuracy similar to CT. Thoracic CT has the highest sensitivity for pulmonary metastases, exposing the fetus to low doses of radiation. Serum carcinoembryonic antigen (CEA) levels can be used to monitor the response to therapy as its levels are not modified by pregnancy.

Clinical Management: If possible, surgery should be performed before 20 weeks of gestation when complete resection is still feasible, and the miscarriage rate is similar to that in the general pregnant population (14%). After 20 weeks, radical surgery is challenging and almost impossible because of the enlarged uterus, so postpartum surgery is preferred. If delivery is made vaginally, surgery can be performed several weeks later; if a caesarean section is planned, colon cancer can be resected at the same time, while rectal cancer is more challenging. Some 17% of patients present with bowel perforation or obstruction requiring emergency laparotomy [28]. Colorectal cancer chemotherapy is usually based on 5-fluorouracil and oxaliplatin, which are considered relatively safe during pregnancy even if a higher incidence of SGA is reported (OR 3.12, 95% CI 1.45–6.70) [10]. Angiogenesis inhibitors should be considered contraindicated in pregnancy because of the lack of studies in humans, negative outcomes in animals, theoretical fetal exposure and their high-risk angiogenesis target [29]. Radiotherapy is generally indicated preoperatively for locally advanced rectal cancer; however, it is contraindicated during pregnancy.

Despite a higher incidence of advanced disease, the data report a similar stage-by-stage survival rate between pregnant and non-pregnant patients. Regarding fetal outcome, the literature reports a higher incidence of SGA and a higher rate of iatrogenic preterm delivery, as radiotherapy or surgery needs to be started postpartum.

75.14 Brain Cancer

Epidemiology: Primary intracranial tumours are the fifth leading cause of cancer-related death in women aged 20 to 39 years.

Clinical Features: Common clinical features are focal neurological symptoms or disorders, epileptic seizures and nonfocal symptoms (headache, nausea, vomiting).

Pathology: The most frequent histotypes are malignant glioma (anaplastic, astrocytoma, glioblastoma), low-grade astrocytoma and medulloblastoma.

Investigations: The diagnosis is based on MRI or CT findings.

Clinical Management: Treatment for malignant tumours and growing benign intracranial tumours is neurosurgical resection. Timing of surgery during pregnancy remains debated: if possible, surgery should be deferred until after the first trimester to lower miscarriage risk, while surgery in the second and the third trimesters is considered safe. The importance of not deferring surgery to after pregnancy is that complete surgical resection is a favourable prognostic factor, whereas deferrals can cause neurological deterioration and expose the patient to the risk of incomplete resection. Adjuvant chemotherapy and/or radiotherapy improves the outcome of aggressive brain tumours like glioblastoma. Brain radiotherapy exposes the fetus to 0.02–0.1 Gy; these radiotherapy schedules can therefore be considered safe. Proper shielding should always be used to reduce the fetal dose, and treatment should be discussed with an expert radiotherapist to estimate the fetal dose and counsel the parents on the potential risks of radiation-induced toxicity. The mode of delivery should be discussed in a multidisciplinary team: if there is risk of increased intracranial pressure during the second stage of labour, an elective caesarean section can be planned, whereas if the patient is stable, a vaginal term delivery is preferred whenever possible [30].

75.15 Key Messages

- Non-gynaecological cancers in pregnancy are estimated at 1 in 1000 pregnancies.
- Multidisciplinary management in a referral centre is pivotal.
- Staging should be as comprehensive as outside pregnancy, but an examination should be performed only if it changes the clinical plan.
- Pregnant women with cancer can and should be treated just as effectively as non-pregnant women, while keeping in mind that surgery is usually feasible during all trimesters, chemotherapy is considered safe between 14 and 35 weeks of gestation and radiotherapy is generally contraindicated.
- Term delivery should always be aimed for, as prematurity and low birthweight seem to be contributing factors to later cognitive and emotional development of the baby. The mode of delivery should be planned according to obstetric conditions.
- Prognosis does not seem to be inferior to that of non-pregnant women.

References

1. Mitrou S, Zarkavelis G, Fotopoulos G, Petrakis D, Pavlidis N. A mini review on pregnant mothers with cancer: a paradoxical coexistence. *J Adv Res.* 2016 Jul;7 (4):559–63.

2. Han SN, Kesic VI, Van Calsteren K, Petkovic S, Amant F; ESGO 'Cancer in Pregnancy' Task Force. Cancer in pregnancy: a survey of current clinical practice.*Eur J Obstet Gynecol Reprod Biol.* 2013 Mar;**167**(1):18–23.

3. Amant F, Han SN, Gziri MM, et al. Management of cancer in pregnancy. *Best Pract Res Clin Obstet Gynaecol.* 2015 Jul;29(5):741–53.

4. De Geus KF, Maggen C, de Haan J, Amant F. Implementation of cancer treatment during pregnancy in daily practice: the important role of perinatologists. *Oncotarget.* 2018 Aug 7; 9(61):31795–6.

5. De Haan J, Vandecaveye V, Han SN, Van de Vijver KK, Amant F. Difficulties with diagnosis of malignancies in pregnancy. *Best Pract Res Clin Obstet Gynaecol.* 2016 May; 33:19–32.

6. Van Calsteren K, Amant F. Cancer during pregnancy. *Acta Obstet Gynecol Scand.* 2014 May;93(5):443–6.

7. Ngu SF, Ngan HY. Chemotherapy in pregnancy. *Best Pract Res Clin Obstet Gynaecol.* 2016 May;33:86–101.

8. De Haan J, Verheecke M, Van Calsteren K, et al.; International Network on Cancer and Infertility Pregnancy (INCIP). Oncological management and obstetric and neonatal outcomes for women diagnosed with cancer during pregnancy: a 20-year international cohort study of 1170 patients.

Lancet Oncol. 2018 Mar;**19**(3): 337–46.

9. Peccatori FA, Fumagalli M. Long and winding road of cancer and pregnancy: a need for action. *J Clin Oncol.* 2017 May 10;35(14):1499–1500.

10. Verheecke M, Cortès Calabuig A, Finalet Ferreiro J, et al. Genetic and microscopic assessment of the human chemotherapy-exposed placenta reveals possible pathways contributive to fetal growth restriction. *Placenta.* 2018 Apr;**64**:61–70.

11. Boere I, Lok C, Vandenbroucke T, Amant F. Cancer in pregnancy: safety and efficacy of systemic therapies. *Curr Opin Oncol.* 2017 Sep;29(5):328–34.

12. Stensheim H, Moller B, Van Dijk T, Fossa SD. Cause specific survival for women diagnosed with cancer during pregnancy or lactation: a registry-based cohort study. *J Clin Oncol* 2009;27:45–51.

13. Lishner M, Avivi I, Apperley JF, et al. Hematologic malignancies in pregnancy: management guidelines from an international consensus meeting. *J Clin Oncol.* 2016 Feb 10; **34**(5):501–8.

14. Moshe Y, Bentur OS, Lishner M, Avivi I. The management of Hodgkin lymphomas in pregnancies. *Eur J Haematol.* 2017 Nov;99(5):385–91.

15. Zagouri F, Dimitrakakis C, Marinopoulos S, Tsigginou A, Dimopoulos MA. Cancer in pregnancy: disentangling treatment modalities. *ESMO Open.* 2016 May 4;**1** (3):e000016.

16. Paydas S. Management of hemopoietic neoplasias during pregnancy. *Crit Rev Oncol Hematol.* 2016 Aug;**104**:52–64.

17. Pereg D, Koren G, Lishner M. The treatment of Hodgkin's and non-Hodgkin's lymphoma in pregnancy. *Hematologica.* 2007;**92**:1230–7.

18. Berman E. Pregnancy in patients with chronic myeloid leukemia. *J Natl Compr Canc Netw.* 2018 May; 16(5S):660–2.

19. Ali S, Jones GL, Culligan DJ, et al. British Committee for Standards in Haematology Guidelines for the diagnosis and management of acute myeloid leukaemia in pregnancy. *Br J Haematol.* 2015 Aug;170(4):487–95.

20. Verma V, Giri S, Manandhar S, Pathak R, Bhatt VR. Acute promyelocytic leukemia during pregnancy: a systematic analysis of outcome. *Leuk Lymphoma.* 2016; **57**(3):616–22.

21. Vlijm-Kievit A, Jorna NGE, Moll E, et al. Acute lymphoblastic leukemia during the third trimester of pregnancy. *Leuk Lymphoma.* 2018 May;**59**(5):1274–6.

22. De Haan J, Lok CA, de Groot CJ, et al.; International Network on Cancer, Infertility and Pregnancy (INCIP). Melanoma during pregnancy: a report of 60 pregnancies complicated by melanoma. *Melanoma Res.* 2017 Jun; **27**(3):218–23.

23. De Haan J, van Thienen JV, Casaer M, et al. Severe adverse reaction to vemurafenib in a pregnant woman with metastatic melanoma. *Case Rep Oncol.* 2018 Feb 15;**11**(1):119–24.

24. Yu SS, Bischoff LA. Thyroid cancer in pregnancy. *Semin Reprod Med.* 2016 Nov;**34**(6):351–5.

25. Boucek J, de Haan J, Halaska MJ, et al.; International Network on Cancer, Infertility, and Pregnancy. Maternal

and obstetrical outcome in 35 cases of well-differentiated thyroid carcinoma during pregnancy. *Laryngoscope.* 2018 Jun;**128** (6):1493–1500.

26. Modesti C, Aceto P, Masini L, et al. Approach to thyroid carcinoma in pregnancy. *Updates Surg.* 2017 Jun; **69**(2):261–5.

27. Khaled H, Al Lahloubi N, Rashad N. A review on thyroid cancer during pregnancy: Multitasking is required. *J Adv Res.* 2016 Jul; **7**(4):565–70.

28. Kocián P, De Haan J, Cardonick EH, et al.; Writing Committee of the International Network on Cancer, Infertility and Pregnancy (INCIP). Management and outcome of colorectal cancer during pregnancy: report of 41 cases. *Acta Chir Belg.* 2018 Jul;**16**:1–10.

29. Rogers JE, Dasari A, Eng C. The treatment of colorectal cancer during pregnancy: cytotoxic chemotherapy and targeted therapy challenges. *Oncologist.* 2016 May;**21**(5):563–70.

30. Verheecke M, Halaska MJ, Lok CA, et al.; ESGO Task Force 'Cancer in Pregnancy'. Primary brain tumours, meningiomas and brain metastases in pregnancy: report on 27 cases and review of literature. *Eur J Cancer.* 2014 May;**50**(8): 1462–71.

Chapter 76

Simulation for Obstetric Emergencies

Cécile Monod & Irene Hösli

76.1 Background

Appropriate management of obstetric emergencies requires the immediate coordinated action of multidisciplinary and multiprofessional teams, composed of midwifes, obstetricians, anaesthetists and neonatologists. As most of these emergencies do not happen very frequently and are unforeseeable, adequate regular training of skills and communication is essential. Most often, the situation is charged with emotions; suddenly, not only the mother but also the fetus or the newborn might be involved, and communication within the team and to the patient becomes impaired.

76.2 Maternal and Perinatal Mortality

Over the past two decades, the UK Confidential Enquiries into Maternal and Neonatal Deaths analyzed maternal and perinatal deaths in order to improve the standard of care for mothers and neonates. Nowadays, two thirds of maternal deaths in the UK are caused by indirect medical and mental health problems in pregnancy and one third from direct complications of pregnancy such as bleeding [1]. The Confidential Enquiries into Maternal Deaths in the UK 2011 [2] identified substandard care in 70% of direct and 55% of indirect maternal deaths. The 2017 MBRRACE-UK Perinatal Confidential Enquiry into term, singleton, intrapartum stillbirth and intrapartum-related neonatal death identified 80% with elements of substandard care [3]. In the last two MBRRACE-UK reports on maternal death, about one quarter of maternal deaths were attributed to sepsis [1, 2]. Particularly for sepsis, substandard care was identified in 75% of cases.

76.3 Recommendations for Obstetric Team Training

For the past 20 years, ongoing simulation team training for obstetric emergencies has been recommended for all obstetric units in the UK (Confidential Enquiry into Stillbirths and Deaths in Infancy (CESDI) 4th annual report 1997) [4]. As human factors were identified as major contributors to preventable maternal deaths, specific team training for human factors has been newly recommended too [1].

Several professional societies have set up working groups to facilitate simulation courses in obstetrics and gynaecology, including the European Union of Medical Specialists (UEMS) section [5], the American College of Obstetricians and Gynecologists (ACOG) Simulations Working Group [6], the Canadian society [7] and the Royal College of Obstetricians and Gynaecologists (RCOG) [8].

Table 76.1 lists possible simulation training topics, which are illustrated in Figures 76.1 to 76.4.

76.4 Simulation for Obstetric Emergencies: Available Evidence

Available evidence strongly supports the use of simulation training for obstetric emergencies to improve perinatal outcomes, but not all training exhibited the same efficacy.

76.4.1 Impact on Self-confidence and Self-perceived Competencies

A one-day simulation training for obstetric emergencies can improve self-confidence and self-perceived competencies of both obstetricians and midwives, as shown in these two series [9, 10].

Table 76.1 Simulation training in obstetrics: examples of possible emergency scenarios, skills training and routine procedures

Simulation training in obstetrics
Emergencies and skills training
Eclampsia
Shoulder dystocia
Vaginal operative delivery
Twin delivery
Breech delivery
Umbilical cord prolapse
Caesarean section in the second stage of labour
Emergency caesarean section
Postpartum haemorrhage
Maternal life support
Maternal sepsis
Routine procedures
Spontaneous vaginal delivery, episiotomy, third and fourth degree perineal tears repair, caesarean section, amniocentesis, cordocentesis

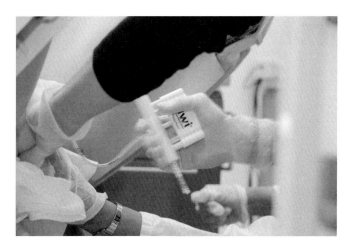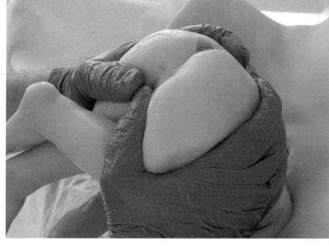

Figure 76.1 Simulation training for vaginal operative and breech delivery

76.4.2 Impact on Outcomes in a Simulation Setting: Lessons from the SaFE Study

The Simulation and Fire-drill Evaluation (SaFE) study is a large randomized study requested by the Department of Health in the UK to evaluate different methods of simulation for obstetric emergencies. The SaFE study used three simulated emergency scenarios: shoulder dystocia, eclampsia and postpartum haemorrhage. The study showed an overall improvement of clinical obstetric emergency knowledge in a multiple-choice questionnaire after the multiprofessional simulation training. There was no difference in evolution of knowledge if the training was performed in a local hospital or a simulation centre and no additional benefit of a specific teamwork training [11]. The study also demonstrated an improvement in team performance in a simulation setting. The proportion of teams who managed to deliver the baby in a simulated shoulder dystocia improved from 49% pre-training to 85% post-training [12]. Training on high-fidelity birth simulators showed an advantage compared with low-fidelity mannequins in managing shoulder dystocia [13]. The management of a simulated eclampsia was improved after the training: increase in completion and rapidity to perform basic tasks, increase in proportion of teams who administer a loading dose of magnesium (61% pre-training to 92% post-training) and rapidity to perform the task [14]. Additionally, perception of care (communication, safety, respect) by a patient-actor improved after the training. The perception of communication and safety by a patient-actor during a simulation for postpartum haemorrhage was significantly improved after training in a local hospital where a patient-actor was used compared with training with a computerized full-body simulator in a simulation centre [15].

76.4.3 Impact on Clinical Outcomes

In 2006, Draycott et al demonstrated improved perinatal outcomes after introduction of a one-day multiprofessional simulation training in the Southmead Hospital, Bristol, UK. The training programme was compulsory for all midwives, obstetricians and anaesthetists. The course consisted of cardiotocography (CTG) training and six simulation training stations for shoulder dystocia, postpartum haemorrhage, eclampsia, twins, breech and adult resuscitation and neonatal resuscitation. In comparison to the pre-training period (1998–1999), rates of 5 minutes of Apgar <7 (86.6–44.6 per 10 000 births) and rates of hypoxic ischaemic encephalopathy (27.3–13.6 per 10 000 births) decreased significantly in the post-training period [16]. This simulation training programme evolved to become the PROMPT training programme (PRactical Obstetric Multi-Professional Training) [17]. This programme has been successfully implemented in different settings with similar results in Kansas, USA, or in Victoria, Australia [18, 19]. Introduction of the PROMPT programme in the Mpilo Central Hospital, Zimbabwe, led to a 34% reduction in maternal mortality [20]. In contrast, other studies did not show any improvement of Apgar <7 [21] or a composite outcome of obstetrics complications [22].

76.4.3.1 Shoulder Dystocia

Annual simulation training for shoulder dystocia in Southmead Hospital, Bristol, UK, showed sustainable improvement of perinatal outcomes [12, 23, 24]. Brachial plexus injury at birth was reduced from 7.4% in the pre-training period to 2.3% in the early (2–5 years) post-training period and to 1.3% in the late training period after 12 years [24]. Additionally, permanent brachial plexus injury (injury still present at 12 months or injury requiring operative intervention) decreased from 1.9% pre-training to 0.8% in the early post-training period and to 0% in the late post-training period. Implementation of the PROMPT programme in other settings led to similar changes in rate of brachial plexus injury [18]. On the contrary, some other training programmes didn't demonstrate improvement in clinical outcomes [25]. A study by MacKenzie et al even observed an increase in the rate of brachial plexus injury after shoulder dystocia between 1991 and 2005 [26]. This increase was seen despite the introduction of training and increased use of the McRoberts manoeuvre over time.

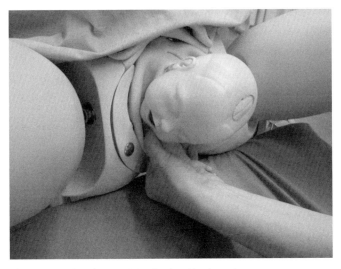

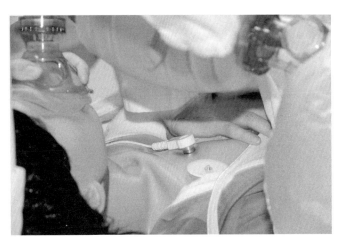

Figure 76.3 Simulation training for maternal life support

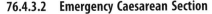

Figure 76.2 Simulation training for shoulder dystocia

76.4.3.2 Emergency Caesarean Section

Two studies observed a shorter diagnosis/decision-to-delivery interval for emergency caesarean section after introducing a simulation drill for cord prolapse and emergency caesarean section. Siassakos et al observed a significant reduction in diagnosis-to-delivery interval from 25 to 14.5 minutes in a retrospective cohort study [27]. Fuhrmann et al also noticed an increase in emergency caesarean sections performed within a 30 minutes decision-to-delivery interval in a 'before-after' study introducing a multiprofessional multidisciplinary training [28].

76.4.4 Cost-effectiveness of Simulation Training Programmes for Obstetric Emergencies

Adverse events in maternity care are not always preventable but are often identified as avoidable. Litigation costs for adverse events in maternity care is rising worldwide [29]. After introducing a simulation programme for obstetric emergencies, some hospitals or countries observed a substantial reduction of litigation costs for unsafe care. In Bristol, UK, there was a reduction of 91% of litigation costs and there are similar reports in the USA and Australia [29, 30]. Implementing simulation training for obstetric teams is not cheap, but it can be cost-effective [31]. In the Netherlands, van de Ven et al also concluded that such training can be cost-effective [32].

76.5 Communication and Teamwork

Human factors play an essential role in avoidable adverse events in maternity care. The MBRRACE-UK 2014 reports recognized problems in communication and teamwork as a cause for preventable maternal adverse events [1]. Particularly, problematic communication and teamwork led junior doctors to seek senior support from experienced obstetricians and anaesthetists too late and teams failed to recognize and communicate the severity of the woman's condition to all members of the obstetric team. Therefore, specific teamwork training was newly recommended [1, 2, 33]. However, thus far training communication and teamwork issues in isolation did not show improvement in clinical outcomes in obstetric simulation studies [22, 34]. Nevertheless, Siassakos et al identified some key elements of non-technical skills in analyzing a series of simulation training for eclampsia [33, 35]. The teams who administered essential medication (magnesium sulphate) earlier were the ones who recognized and verbalized the problem earlier, used structured communication techniques (SBAR, close-loop) and had fewer exits out of the delivery room as a reflection of better teamwork [36]. Furthermore, an adult resuscitation simulation study showed that teams receiving a brief leadership instruction had more hands-on time in heart massage than those who received technical resuscitation training [37]. Nowadays, it seems that an integrated team and clinical training in multiprofessional multidisciplinary teams offers the best opportunity to improve teamwork and communication issues [33]: 'Who works together should train together.'

76.6 Which Elements Make an Effective Simulation Training Programme for Obstetric Emergencies?

Current evidence suggests some key features for implementing effective simulation training programmes for obstetric emergencies. Bergh et al concluded in a review of 23 studies that multiprofessional training performed locally was the best way to organize obstetric team training [38]. A proposed explanation is that using local, practice-based training tools, such as clinical checklists and tool boxes, and training in communities of practice, may represent more essential elements of effective training than transfer of new knowledge [39]. Key elements of teamwork should be best incorporated in the clinical simulation training scenario. A patient-actor should be preferred to a computerized mannequin simulator as it appears to improve perception of care. Which birth simulator is best has yet to be determined. The RCOG guidelines recommend the use of high-fidelity birth

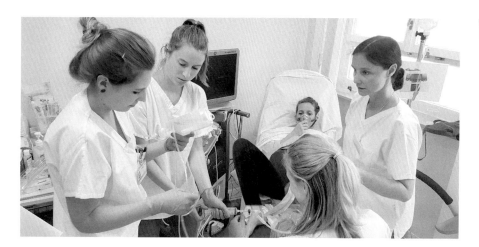

Figure 76.4 Simulation training for postpartum haemorrhage: teamwork

simulators for team training in their most current guidelines [30].

Debriefing and feedback after simulation were demonstrated to enhance the learning effect of the simulation session [40] and also represent a key point in implementing effective training programmes.

Exploring the underlying mechanisms that make a training session effective was proposed by different authors as a further area of research, thus moving from the question 'Does the training work?' to 'How does the training work?' and 'Why does the training work?' [38].

References

1. Knight M, Kenyon S, Brocklehurst P, et al. eds. *Saving Lives, Improving Mothers' Care: Lessons Learned to Inform Future Maternity Care from the UK and Ireland Confidential Enquiries into Maternal Deaths and Morbidity 2009–2012.* Oxford: National Perinatal Epidemiology Unit, University of Oxford; 2014.

2. Cantwell R, Clutton-Brock T, Cooper G, et al. Saving mothers' lives: reviewing maternal deaths to make motherhood safer: 2006–2008. The Eighth Report of the Confidential Enquiries into Maternal Deaths in the United Kingdom. *BJOG.* 2011;**118**(Suppl 1): 1–203.

3. Draper ES, Kurinczuk JJ, Kenyon S. eds. *MBRRACE-UK Perinatal Confidential Enquiry: Term, Singleton, Intrapartum Stillbirth and Intrapartum-Related Neonatal Death.* Leicester: Department of Health Sciences, University of Leicester; 2017.

4. *Confidential Enquiry into Stillbirths and Deaths in Infancy: 4th Annual Report, 1 January–31 December 1995.* London: Maternal and Child Health Research Consortium; 1997.

5. European Training Requirements in Obstetrics and Gynaecology, UEMS Section Obstetrics and Gynaecology / European Board and College of Obstetrics and Gynaecology, Standing Committee on Training and Assessment, Version 2018.

6. ACOG Simulations Working Group, www.acog.org/About-ACOG/ACOG-Departments/Simulations-Consortium?IsMobileSet=false.

7. Craig C, Posner GD. Developing a Canadian curriculum for simulation-based education in obstetrics and gynaecology: a Delphi study. *J Obstet Gynaecol Can.* 2017;**39** (9):757–63.

8. Royal College of Obstetricians and Gynaecologists. Run emergency obstetric skills and drills training, www.rcog.org.uk/en/careers-training/workplace-workforce-issues/improving-workplace-behaviours-dealing-with-undermining/undermining-toolkit/departmental-and-team-interventions/run-emergency-obstetric-skills-and-drills-training/.

9. Monod C, Voekt CA, Gisin M, Gisin S, Hoesli IM. Optimization of competency in obstetrical emergencies: a role for simulation training. *Arch Gynecol Obstet.* 2014;**289**(4):733–8.

10. Reynolds A, Ayres-de-Campos D, Lobo M. Self-perceived impact of simulation-based training on the management of real-life obstetrical emergencies. *Eur J Obstet Gynecol Reprod Biol.* 2011;**159**(1):72–6.

11. Crofts JF, Ellis D, Draycott TJ, et al. Change in knowledge of midwives and obstetricians following obstetric emergency training: a randomised controlled trial of local hospital, simulation centre and teamwork training. *BJOG.* 2007;**114** (12):1534–41.

12. Crofts JF, Bartlett C, Ellis D, et al. Management of shoulder dystocia: skill retention 6 and 12 months after training. *Obstet Gynecol.* 2007;**110** (5):1069–74.

13. Crofts JF, Bartlett C, Ellis D, et al. Training for shoulder dystocia: a trial of simulation using low-fidelity and high-fidelity mannequins. *Obstet Gynecol.* 2006;**108**(6): 1477–85.

14. Ellis D, Crofts JF, Hunt LP, et al. Hospital, simulation center, and teamwork training for eclampsia management: a randomized controlled trial. *Obstet Gynecol.* 2008;**111** (3):723–31.

15. Crofts JF, Bartlett C, Ellis D, et al. Patient-actor perception of care: a comparison of obstetric emergency training using manikins and patient-actors. *Qual Saf Health Care.* 2008; **17**(1):20.

16. Draycott T, Sibanda T, Owen L, et al. Does training in obstetric emergencies improve neonatal outcome? *BJOG.* 2006;**113**(2):177–82.

17. PROMPT: PRactical Obstetric Multi-Professional Training. www.promptmaternity.org/

18. Weiner CP, Collins L, Bentley S, Dong Y, Satterwhite CL. Multi-professional training for obstetric emergencies in a U.S. hospital over a 7-year interval: an observational study. *J Perinatol.* 2016;**36**(1):19–24.

19. Shoushtarian M, Barnett M, McMahon F, Ferris J. Impact of introducing practical obstetric multi-professional training (PROMPT) into maternity units in Victoria, Australia. *BJOG.* 2014;**121**(13):1710–18.

20. Crofts JF, Mukuli T, Murove BT, et al. Onsite training of doctors, midwives and nurses in obstetric emergencies, Zimbabwe. *Bull World Health Organ.* 2015;**93**(5):347–51.

21. Millde Luthander C, Källen K, Nyström ME, et al. Results from the National Perinatal Patient Safety Program in Sweden: the challenge of evaluation. *Acta Obstet Gynecol Scand.* 2016;**95**(5):596–603.

22. Fransen AF, van de Ven J, Schuit E, et al. Simulation-based team training for multi-professional obstetric care teams to improve patient outcome: a multicentre, cluster randomised controlled trial. *BJOG.* 2017;**124**(4):641–50.

23. Draycott TJ, Crofts JF, Ash JP, et al. Improving neonatal outcome through practical shoulder dystocia training. *Obstet Gynecol.* 2008;**112**(1):14–20.

24. Crofts JF, Lenguerrand E, Bentham GL, et al. Prevention of brachial plexus injury-12 years of shoulder dystocia training: an interrupted time-series study. *BJOG.* 2016;**123**(1):111–18.

25. Walsh JM, Kandamany N, Ni Shuibhne N, et al. Neonatal brachial plexus injury: comparison of incidence and antecedents between 2 decades. *Am J Obstet Gynecol.* 2011;**204**(4):324.e1–.e6.

26. MacKenzie IZ, Shah M, Lean K, et al. Management of shoulder dystocia: trends in incidence and maternal and neonatal morbidity. *Obstet Gynecol.* 2007;**110**(5):1059–68.

27. Siassakos D, Hasafa Z, Sibanda T, et al. Retrospective cohort study of diagnosis-delivery interval with umbilical cord prolapse: the effect of team training. *BJOG.* 2009;**116**(8):1089–96.

28. Fuhrmann L, Pedersen TH, Atke A, Møller AM, Østergaard D. Multidisciplinary team training reduces the decision-to-delivery interval for emergency caesarean section. *Acta Anaesthesiol Scand.* 2015;**59**(10):1287–95.

29. Draycott T, Sagar R, Hogg S. The role of insurers in maternity safety. *Best Pract Res Clin Obstet Gynaecol.* 2015;**29**(8):1126–31.

30. Draycott TJ, Collins KJ, Crofts JF, et al. Myths and realities of training in obstetric emergencies. *Best Pract Res Clin Obstet Gynaecol.* 2015;**29**(8):1067–76.

31. Yau CWH, Pizzo E, Morris S, et al. The cost of local, multi-professional obstetric emergencies training. *Acta Obstet Gynecol Scand.* 2016;**95**(10):1111–19.

32. van de Ven J, van Baaren GJ, Fransen AF, et al. Cost-effectiveness of simulation-based team training in obstetric emergencies (TOSTI study).

Eur J Obstet Gynecol Reprod Biol. 2017 Sep;**216**:130–7.

33. Siassakos D, Fox R, Bristowe K, et al. What makes maternity teams effective and safe? Lessons from a series of research on teamwork, leadership and team training. *Acta Obstet Gynecol Scand.* 2013;**92**(11):1239–43.

34. Nielsen PE, Goldman MB, Mann S, et al. Effects of teamwork training on adverse outcomes and process of care in labor and delivery: a randomized controlled trial. *Obstet Gynecol.* 2007;**109**(1):48–55.

35. Siassakos D, Fox R, Crofts JF, et al. The management of a simulated emergency: better teamwork, better performance. *Resuscitation.* 2011;**82**(2):203–6.

36. Siassakos D, Bristowe K, Draycott TJ, et al. Clinical efficiency in a simulated emergency and relationship to team behaviours: a multisite cross-sectional study. *BJOG.* 2011;**118**(5):596–607.

37. Hunziker S, Bühlmann C, Tschan F, et al. Brief leadership instructions improve cardiopulmonary resuscitation in a high-fidelity simulation: a randomized controlled trial. *Crit Care Med.* 2010;**38**(4):1086–91.

38. Bergh A-M, Baloyi S, Pattinson RC. What is the impact of multi-professional emergency obstetric and neonatal care training? *Best Pract Res Clin Obstet Gynaecol.* 2015;**29**(8):1028–43.

39. Draycott T. Not all training for obstetric emergencies is equal, or effective. *BJOG.* 2017;**124**(4):651.

40. Hattie J. *Visible Learning.* Abingdon and New York: Routledge; 2009.

Index